Kinesiology

The Mechanics and Pathomechanics of Human Movement

Second Edition

Carol A. Oatis, PT, PhD

Professor
Department of Physical Therapy
Arcadia University
Glenside, Pennsylvania

With contributors

Acquisitions Editor: Emily J. Lupash
Managing Editor: Andrea M. Klingler
Marketing Manager: Missi Carmen
Production Editor: Sally Anne Glover
Designer: Doug Smock
Typesetter: International Typesetting and Composition

Second Edition
Copyright © 2009, 2004 Lippincott Williams & Wilkins, a Wolters Kluwer business.

351 West Camden Street   530 Walnut Street
Baltimore, MD 21201   Philadelphia, PA 19106

Printed in India.

9 8 7 6 5 4 3 2 1

Library of Congress Cataloging-in-Publication Data

Oatis, Carol A.
    Kinesiology : the mechanics and pathomechanics of human movement /
Carol A. Oatis, with contributors.—2nd ed.
        p. ; cm.
    Includes bibliographical references and index.
    ISBN-13: 978-0-7817-7422-2
    ISBN-10: 0-7817-7422-5
    1. Kinesiology.   2. Human mechanics.   3. Movement disorders.
I. Title.
    [DNLM: 1. Biomechanics.   2. Kinesiology, Applied.
3. Movement—physiology.   4. Movement Disorders.   WE 103 O11k 2009]
    QP303.O38 2009
    612.7'6—dc22

                                2007037068

DISCLAIMER

This book is dedicated to the memories of two people who have graced my life and whose friendships have sustained me:

Marian Magee, PT, MS, a scholar–clinician whose respect for patient, student, and colleague can serve as a model for all practitioners. She demonstrated the value of interprofessional practice and mutual respect in her everyday interactions. She generously shared her wisdom, humor, and friendship with me.

Steven S. Goldberg, JD, PhD, educator, author, negotiator, and colleague. He demanded much of his students and of himself. He was a generous colleague and friend who listened carefully, offered wise and thoughtful advice, and never failed to make me laugh.

FEATURES OF THE SECOND EDITION

- **Clinical Relevance** boxes allow us to emphasize the applicability of the information contained in this textbook. These were one of the most popular aspects of the first edition and are intended to once again help focus information and enhance understanding. We have added new Clinical Relevance boxes throughout the text to provide additional examples of how a clinician can use the information in this text to understand a dysfunction or choose an intervention strategy.

- **Muscle Action** tables introduce the discussion of muscle actions for each muscle. Actions of each muscle are now introduced in table format and include the conclusions drawn from the evidence regarding each action. The evidence is discussed in detail after the table. This format allows the reader to identify at a glance which reported actions are supported by evidence, which are refuted, and which remain controversial.

- **Examining the Forces** boxes and **Muscle Attachment** boxes explain and highlight more advanced mathematical concepts and provide muscle innervation and attachment information, respectively. The Muscle Attachment boxes now also include brief descriptions of palpation strategies.

- **New and updated artwork,** including illustrations and photographs, have been created and revised specifically for this text.

- **Updated references** continue to lend current, evidence-based support to chapter content and direct the student to further research resources

ANCILLARIES

- **Approximately 150 video clips** provide dynamic illustrations of concepts discussed in the textbook and demonstrate movement disorders that can occur as a result of impairments. The clips also include demonstrations of palpations of bony landmarks for each anatomical region. A **video icon** is used throughout the text to identify concepts with related video material. These added elements will help the reader integrate the relationships among structure, force, movement, and function and provide examples for students and teachers to analyze and discuss.

- **Laboratory Manuals** for both students and instructors continue to offer activities for students to enhance learning and applications. The instructors' laboratory manual includes solutions and brief discussions of most activities. The student manual for Chapter 1 now has 10 additional problems for students to test their analytical skills. The solutions are provided in the Instructors' Manual.

- The **Instructors' Guide** is a chapter-by-chapter outline to assist instructors with preparing class lectures. This ancillary has been updated to include the materials added to the revised chapters.

Contributors

PAUL F. BEATTIE, PHD, PT, OCS
Clinical Associate Professor
Program in Physical Therapy
Department of Exercise Science
School of Public Health
University of South Carolina
Columbia, SC

EMILY L. CHRISTIAN, PHD, PT
Restore Management Co, LLC
Pelham, AL

JULIE E. DONACHY, PHD, PT
Restore Management Co, LLC
Pelham, AL

Z. ANNETTE IGLARSH, PT, PHD, MBA
Chair and Professor
Department of Physical Therapy
University of the Sciences in Philadelphia
Philadelphia, PA

ANDREW R. KARDUNA, PHD
Assistant Professor
Department of Exercise and Movement Science
University of Oregon
Eugene, OR

MARGERY A. LOCKARD, PT, PHD
Clinical Associate Professor
Pathway to Health Professions Program
Drexel University
Philadelphia, PA

JOSEPH M. MANSOUR, PHD
Professor
Department of Mechanical and Aerospace Engineering
Case Western Reserve University
Cleveland, OH

THOMAS P. MAYHEW, PT, PHD
Associate Professor and Chair
Department of Physical Therapy
School of Allied Health Professions
Virginia Commonwealth University
Richmond, VA

STUART M. McGILL, PHD
Professor
Department of Spine Biomechanics
University of Waterloo
Waterloo, Canada

SUSAN R. MERCER, PHD, BPHTY (HON), FNZCP
Senior Lecturer
Department of Anatomy & Developmental Biology
The University of Queensland
Brisbane, Australia

PETER E. PIDCOE, PT, DPT, PHD
Associate Professor
Department of Physical Therapy
School of Allied Health Professions
Virginia Commonwealth University
Richmond, VA

NEAL PRATT, PHD, PT
Emeritus Professor of Rehabilitation Sciences
Drexel University
Philadelphia, PA

L. D. TIMMIE TOPOLESKI, PHD
Professor
Department of Mechanical Engineering
University of Maryland, Baltimore County
Baltimore, MD

Reviewers

ROSCOE C. BOWEN, PHD
Associate Professor
Campbellsville University
Campbellsville, KY

BETH KIPPING DESCHENES, PT, MS, OCS
Clinical Assistant Professor
Department of Physical Therapy
UT Southwestern Medical Center at Dallas
Dallas, TX

JEFF LYNN, PHD
Assistant Professor
Slippery Rock University
Slippery Rock, PA

CORRIE A. MANCINELLI, PT, PHD
Associate Professor
West Virginia University School of Medicine
Morgantown, WV

ROBIN MARCUS, PT, PHD, OCS
Assistant Professor
University of Utah
Salt Lake City, UT

LEE N MARINKO, PT, OCS, FAAOMPT
Clinical Assistant Professor
Boston University
Sargent College of Health and Rehabilitative Sciences
Boston, MA

PATRICIA ANN McGINN, PHD, ATC, CSCS, LAT
Assistant Professor of Athletic Training
Nova Southeastern University
Ft. Lauderdale, FL

MARCIA MILLER SPOTO, PT, DC, OCS
Associate Professor
Nazareth College of Rochester
Rochester, NY

KEITH SPENNEWYN, MS
Department Head
Globe University
Minneapolis, MN

Foreword

This new edition of *Kinesiology: The Mechanics and Pathomechanics of Human Movement* is a very timely arrival! Hardly a day goes by without a newspaper or magazine article extolling the values of exercise as a regular and enduring part of daily activity. Exercise can only become a sustained part of daily activity if it does not cause injury, but any exercise regimen creates the potential for injury to the musculoskeletal system. A challenge of exercise is finding the right balance between activity that enhances tissue health versus that which injures tissues. Optimizing the precision of movement is the key to achieving this balance. A clear understanding of the precision of movement and its contributing factors requires a thorough knowledge of kinesiology. In the field of physical therapy, the focus is on movement and movement-related dysfunctions or impairments; thus kinesiology is the science that provides physical therapy's major foundation.

Since the first kinesiological texts were published, the depth of material has grown immensely. Although knowledge in the fields of kinesiology, pathokinesiology, and kinesiopathology has increased substantially since the first kinesiological texts were published, the changes that may come from this new knowledge are not always reflected in clinical practice. All physical therapy students study kinesiology during their education, but the information is often not retained for application in the clinic, nor is it expanded by additional study. The emphasis on functional performance, prompted in part by reimbursement criteria, has detracted from improving the depth of knowledge of impairments underlying the compromises in performance. Similarly, focus on treatment techniques applied to conditions without attention to the underlying movement dysfunction or the techniques' effects compromises patient care and the status of the profession. *Kinesiology: The Mechanics and Pathomechanics of Human Movement* is a wonderful example of both the breadth and depth of the expansion of kinesiological knowledge and the clinical application of that knowledge. How fortunate for rehabilitation specialists that the information they need is readily available in this text.

A strong emphasis is currently being placed on evidence-based practice. It may be a long time before even a small percentage of our treatment procedures have met level 3 evidence, and all evidence is only the best available at a given time. In the fields of physical therapy, occupational therapy, and athletic training, evidence for the best treatments and the methods used when addressing a person's movement will change, just as it has for the physicians' treatments of metabolic, cardiopulmonary, or neurological conditions. The improvement in the diagnosis and treatment of any body system is based on increased understanding of mechanisms and pathophysiology. We therefore have to continue to pursue an understanding of the mechanisms related to any body system that therapists, trainers, and exercise instructors address during their care, especially the systems involved in movement and its dysfunctions or impairments.

Kinesiology: The Mechanics and Pathomechanics of Human Movement is truly unique in its thoroughly researched approach and provides convincing evidence to debunk old and inaccurate theories. This scientific approach to the clinical application of biomechanics means the information contained in this text is of particular importance to anyone involved in a rehabilitation specialty.

I have had many opportunities to interact with therapists and trainers around the world, and I am struck by how few have a thorough understanding of basic kinesiology, such as an understanding of scapulohumeral rhythm, lumbar range of motion, and the determinants of gait. Coupled with this is a deficiency in the ability to observe movement and recognize subtle deviations and variations in normal patterns. I attribute this to an emphasis on both passive techniques and the lack of a strong basic knowledge about exercise program development.

Kinesiology: The Mechanics and Pathomechanics of Human Movement is an invaluable resource for people seeking to correct this deficiency. Physical therapists must clearly demonstrate themselves to be movement experts and diagnosticians of movement dysfunctions. This book is the key to acquiring the knowledge that will enable students and practitioners to achieve the required level of expertise. The essentials of kinesiology are all present in this text. The basics of tissue biomechanics are well explained by experts in the field. The specifics of muscle action and the biomechanical basis of those actions, kinetics, and kinematics for each region of the body are analyzed and well described. This text is suited for readers who are interested in acquiring either an introductory and basic knowledge as well as those who want to increase their understanding of the more detailed and biomechanically focused knowledge of kinesiology. In selecting the authors for each chapter, Dr. Oatis has chosen well; each expert has provided an excellent and relevant presentation of normal and abnormal kinesiology. This text is a must-have textbook for every student and reference for every practitioner of physical therapy, as well any other rehabilitation specialist or individual desiring knowledge of the biomechanical aspects of the human movement system.

Shirley Sahrmann, PT, PhD, FAPTA
Professor of Physical Therapy
Departments of Physical Therapy, Neurology,
Cell Biology, and Physiology
Washington University School of Medicine—St. Louis
St. Louis, Missouri

Preface from the First Edition

A clinician in rehabilitation treats patients with many and varied disorders, and usually goals of intervention include improving the individual's ability to move [1]. Physical therapists prevent, identify, assess, and correct or alleviate movement dysfunction [3]. Similarly, occupational therapists work to restore or optimize "purposeful actions." Optimizing movement and purposeful actions and treating movement disorders require a firm foundation in **kinesiology,** the scientific study of movement of the human body or its parts.

To evaluate and treat movement disorders effectively, the clinician must address two central questions: What is required to perform the movement, and what effects does the movement produce on the individual? This textbook will help the reader develop knowledge and enhance skills that permit him or her to answer these questions.

Two general factors govern the movement of a structure: the composition of the structure and the forces applied to it. A central principle in kinesiology is that the form or shape of a biological structure is directly influenced by its function. In fact, the relationship among movement, structure, and force is multidirectional. It is a complex interdependent relationship in which structure influences a body's movement, its movement affects the forces applied to the structure, and the forces, in turn, influence the structure (*see Figure*). For example, the unique *structure* of the tibiofemoral joint produces complex three-dimensional *motion* of the knee, leading to intricate loading patterns (*forces*) on the tibia and femur that may contribute to *structural changes* and osteoarthritis later in life. Similarly, the type of movement or function and its intensity influence the forces sustained by a region, which in turn alter the structure. For instance, as muscles hypertrophy with exercise and activity, they stimulate bone growth at their attachment sites; physically active individuals tend to have more robust skeletons than inactive people.

Function is interdependent among structure, force, and movement, so that structure affects both the forces on a structure and the motion of that structure. Similarly, forces on a structure influence its structure and movement. Finally, movement affects both the structure and the forces sustained by the structure.

An abnormal structure produces abnormal movement as well as abnormal forces on a structure, contributing to further alterations in structure. Excessive anteversion of the hip, for example, leads to torsional deformities at the knee, which may contribute to abnormal loading patterns at the hip as well as at the knee or foot, ultimately leading to pain and dysfunction. The clinician needs to understand these interrelationships to design and direct the interventions used to restore or optimize human movement.

An understanding of the relationship among structure, force, and movement requires a detailed image of the structure of a region as well as a grasp of the basic laws of motion and the basic material properties of the tissues comprising the musculoskeletal system. The purposes of this textbook are to:

- Provide a detailed analysis of the structures of the musculoskeletal system within individual functional regions.
- Discuss how the structures affect function within each region.
- Analyze the forces sustained at the region during function.

This textbook will help the clinician recognize the relationships between form and function, and abnormal structure and dysfunction. This foundation should lead to improved evaluation and intervention approaches to movement dysfunction.

This book uses terminology that is standard within health care to describe elements of disablement based on a classification of function developed by the World Health Organization (WHO) and others. In this classification scheme, a disease process, or **pathology,** alters a tissue, which then changes a structure's function, producing an **impairment.** The impairment may cause an individual to have difficulty executing a task or activity, producing an **activity limitation** or **dysfunction.** When the dysfunction alters the individual's ability to participate in life functions, the individual has **participation restriction** or a **disability** [2,4].

Although improving activity and participation are usually the primary objectives in rehabilitation, the WHO model of disease provides a vision of how clinicians can improve function not only by intervening directly at the level of the dysfunction, but also by addressing the underlying impairments. By understanding the detailed structure and precise movement of an anatomical region, the clinician has tools to identify impairments and their influence on function and devise interventions

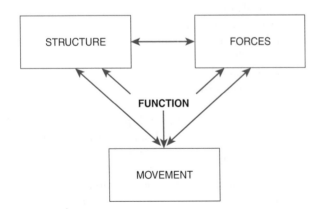

that focus on the mechanism producing the dysfunction. This textbook allows the reader to examine normal structure and function and then consider the impairments that result from alterations in structure at anatomical regions, thus providing insight into the dysfunctions that may follow. For example, by understanding the normal glenohumeral rhythm of the shoulder the clinician can appreciate the consequences of an unstable scapula during arm trunk elevation and develop strategies to improve function.

The needs of individual readers vary, and I have designed this book to allow readers to use it in ways that best meet their needs. Part I of this textbook introduces the reader to the principles of biomechanics and material properties and then examines the material properties of the major component tissues of the musculoskeletal system: bone, muscle, cartilage, and dense connective tissue. These chapters lay out the biomechanical foundation for examining human movement. Parts II through IV explore movement by anatomical region, investigating the detailed structure of the bones, joints, and muscles in that region and examining how their structures influence its movement. The ability of the region to sustain the forces generated during movements and function also is explored in Parts II through IV. Finally, Part V considers more global, or whole-body, movements, specifically posture and locomotion.

Detailed discussions of forces at joints are presented in separate chapters so that readers may access that information as they need it. Although many readers will be interested in delving into the mathematical analyses used to determine forces on joint structures, others will find little need for such detail. The actual calculations are set apart in boxes that accompany the chapters. Conclusions based on the calculations are contained within the chapters' text so that readers can read the chapter and glean the essential information and return to the specific analyses as desired.

Conclusions regarding structure, function, and dysfunction in this text are based on the best available evidence, and each chapter is extensively referenced using both current and classic resources. I believe that the clinician is best equipped to evaluate current practice and to debunk long-held beliefs by having access to the classic resources that have established a concept and to the most current evidence that confirms or refutes standard impressions. Throughout this book, common clinical beliefs that are unsupported—or actually refuted—by strong evidence are explicitly identified so that the clinician hones the skill of healthy skepticism and develops the practice of demanding the evidence to support a concept. The book also notes where the evidence is meager or inconclusive or the conclusion is the opinion of the author. A strong, evidence-based background in kinesiology also helps develop clinician scholars who can contribute to our understanding of movement and movement dysfunction through the systematic, thoughtful observation and reporting of clinical phenomena. Despite the comment made long ago by a fellow graduate student that there was "nothing left to learn in gross anatomy," there is much to be learned yet in functional anatomy and kinesiology.

Today one can discover the errors of yesterday,
And tomorrow obtain a new light on what seemed
*   certain today.*

—*Prayer of Maimonides*

References

1. Guide to Physical Therapy Practice, 2nd ed. Phys Ther 2001; 81: 6–746.
2. Nagi SZ: An epidemiology of disability among adults in the United States. Milbank Mem Fund Q Health Soc 1976; 54: 439–467.
3. Sahrmann SA: Moving precisely? Or taking the path of least resistance? Twenty-ninth Mary McMillan Lecture. Phys Ther 1998; 78: 1208–1218.
4. www3.who.int/icf/icftemplate.cfm?myurlintroduction.html%20&mytitle=Introduction

Preface to the Second Edition

The purposes of *Kinesiology: The Mechanics and Pathomechanics of Human Movement* were articulated in the Preface to the first edition and are unchanged in this new edition. They are to:

- Provide a detailed analysis of the structures of the musculoskeletal system within individual functional regions
- Discuss how the structures affect function within each region
- Analyze the forces sustained at the region during function

If the purposes of this textbook remain the same what is the point of a second edition? Is there a compelling reason to undertake a second edition? As I considered these questions, I recalled the conclusion of the Preface to the first edition, the Prayer of Maimonides. That prayer provides the impetus for a second edition:

> *Today one can discover the errors of yesterday,*
> *And tomorrow obtain a new light on what seemed certain*
> *today.*

> —*Prayer of Maimonides*

A new edition provides the opportunity to correct "the errors of yesterday" and offer suggestions on where to look for "new light" tomorrow. The primary goal of this second edition of *Kinesiology: The Mechanics and Pathomechanics of Human Movement* is to ensure that it reflects the most current understanding of kinesiology and biomechanics science. Chapter contributors reviewed the literature and updated chapters wherever necessary. We have also explicitly identified new knowledge and emerging areas of study or controversy. These additions will aid the reader in the quest for principles that underlie and drive best practice in the fields of rehabilitation and exercise.

The second purpose of the revision has been to build on the strong clinical links available from the first edition. We provide additional examples of the interrelationships among structure, force, and movement and their effects on function (as described in the Preface from the First Edition). A strong and clear understanding of the interdependency of these factors allows practitioners to recognize abnormal movement and systematically search for and identify the underlying pathomechanics. By recognizing underlying mechanisms, practitioners will be able to intervene at the level of the mechanism to normalize or remediate dysfunction. One means to demonstrate these relationships and enhance the applicability of the information contained in this textbook is through the use of the Clinical Relevance boxes. We have added more of these boxes

throughout the text to provide more direct examples of how structure, function, and forces affect movement, demonstrating ways a clinician can use the information in this text to understand a dysfunction or choose an intervention strategy.

Updating the content to reflect new information and current research and practice also has helped us build on those clinical links. Although little has changed in the biomechanical principles outlined in Chapter 1, Dr. Karduna has clarified certain aspects of analysis. He has also provided additional "practice problems" for students to access on the associated website. Drs. Topoleski and Mansour have reorganized their chapters on basic material properties (Chapters 2) and on the properties of bone and cartilage (Chapters 3 and 5) and added clinical examples to help readers see the connections between engineering principles and the clinical issues important to practitioners. Dr. Lockard has included emerging evidence regarding tissue response to activity gleaned from new research technologies (Chapter 6). Drs. Pidcoe and McGill reorganized their chapters to help the readers utilize the information and understand the evidence (Chapters 27, 33, and 34). Dr. McGill also updated evidence and addressed some contemporary issues. Drs. Beattie and Christian reviewed the literature to ensure that their chapters reflected an understanding based on the most current scientific evidence (Chapters 32, 35, and 36).

The final purpose of producing a second edition was to provide dynamic illustrations of the principles and concepts presented in this text. We all know that a "picture is worth a thousand words," but kinesiology is the study of movement, and video provides benefits not found in still images. Recognizing that movement is the central theme of kinesiology and biomechanics, we have produced a DVD with approximately 150 video clips to provide action videos of concepts discussed in the textbook and demonstrate movement disorders that can occur as the result of impairments. These will help the reader integrate the relationships among structure, force, movement, and function and provide examples for students and teachers to analyze and discuss.

In the second edition we have also slightly modified the format of the chapters that address muscles of specific regions. The format change will help the reader quickly recognize the strength of the evidence supporting the identified muscle actions. Actions of each muscle are now presented in table format, which includes the conclusions drawn from the evidence regarding each action.

These changes have been made because I firmly believe that people with musculoskeletal disorders or those who want to optimize their already normal function require the wisdom and guidance of individuals who have a clear, evidence-based understanding of musculoskeletal structure and function, a firm grasp of biomechanical principles, and the ability to observe and document movement. This second edition is meant to help further advance the ability of exercise and rehabilitation specialists to serve this role.

— *Carol A. Oatis*

Acknowledgments

Completion of this second edition required the work and commitment of several individuals. Revising chapters is often less "fun" than writing the original piece. I want to thank the contributing authors for undertaking the project willingly and enthusiastically. Their efforts to identify changes in knowledge or perspective help ensure that this textbook remains at the forefront of kinesiologic science. I am also grateful to the contributors to the functional region chapters who also reviewed and revised their chapters as necessary.

An extensive team at Lippincott Williams & Wilkins has provided invaluable developmental, managerial, and technical support throughout the project. Peter Sabatini, Acquisitions Editor, helped me articulate my goals for the project and provided me the freedom and support to undertake new approaches. Andrea Klingler, Managing Editor, has been patient, persistent, and enthusiastic—frequently at the same time! She has held me to deadlines while simultaneously acknowledging the exciting challenges we were facing. She also brought together an exceptional team of talented individuals to produce the accompanying DVD. This team included Freddie Patane, Art Director (video); Ben Kitchens, Director of Photography (video); and his wonderful crew: Andrew Wheeler, Gaffer, David Mattson, Grip, and Kevin Gallagher, Grip. These people made the production of the DVD not only exciting and successful but wonderfully fun. They provided extraordinary artistic insight and technical skill, but always remained focused on the learning objectives for each clip, wanting to ensure that each clip met the needs of the student and teacher. Brett McNaughton, the Art Director of Photography/Illustration, coordinated the models for video and photography and coordinated the photography shoot. His wisdom and experience helped make the whole process of producing videos and photography smooth and successful. I also want to thank all of the people who were filmed or photographed, including students and people with disabilities, who willingly participated so others could learn.

I am indebted to three people who provided clinical insight, technical and organizational assistance, and moral support during the production of the DVD. Amy Miller, DPT, assisted with setting up the EMGs and monitored those activities. Her understanding of EMG and kinesiology was invaluable for the production of these clips. Additionally her enthusiasm for the entire project was a constant support. Marianne Adler, PT, worked with me to write the scripts for the video clips. Her understanding of the subject matter and her logical thinking yielded clear, concise scripts to describe the action and articulate the principles to be learned. Michele Stake, MS, DPT, coordinated the overall video and photography program, from finding and scheduling patients to helping to direct each shoot and ensuring that the video or photograph told the story we intended. Without these women's commitment to the project and their friendship, I could not have completed the job.

I had the wonderful good fortune of working again with Kim Battista, the talented artist who created the artwork in the original textbook. She contributed new art with the same skill and artistry as in the first edition. Similarly, Gene Smith, the photographer for the first edition, returned to work with me again and has provided new photographs that, like the ones in the first text, "tell the story." These two artists together have created images that bring kinesiology and biomechanics alive. Jennifer Clements, Art Director, oversaw the entire art program and coordinated the production of new and revised art. She was wonderfully patient and receptive to the little "tweaks" we requested to optimize the art program.

I am grateful to Jon McCaffrey, DPT, who provided essential help in tracking down references as well as proofreading and offering helpful editorial suggestions, and to Luis Lopez, SPT, who played a pivotal role in final manuscript production. Again I wish to thank the Department of Physical Therapy and Arcadia University for their support during this process. I am particularly grateful for the support provided by Margaret M. Fenerty, Esq., who listened to my fears, tolerated my stress, and encouraged my efforts.

Finally, I wish to thank all the students and colleagues who have used the first edition and provided insightful feedback and valuable suggestions that have informed this new edition. They helped identify errors, offered new ideas, and graciously told me what worked. I look forward to hearing new ideas and suggestions for this second edition.

Contents

xiv   CONTENTS

Biomechanical Principles

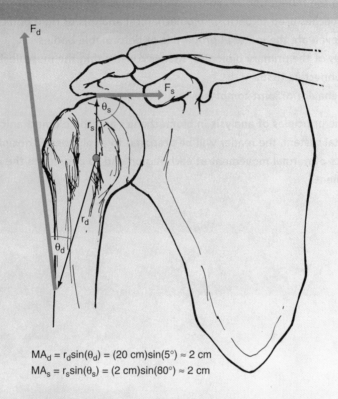

$$MA_d = r_d\sin(\theta_d) = (20\ cm)\sin(5°) \approx 2\ cm$$
$$MA_s = r_s\sin(\theta_s) = (2\ cm)\sin(80°) \approx 2\ cm$$

PART I

This part introduces the reader to the basic principles used throughout this book to understand the structure and function of the musculoskeletal system. Biomechanics is the study of biological systems by the application of the laws of physics. The purposes of this part are to review the principles and tools of mechanical analysis and to describe the mechanical behavior of the tissues and structural units that compose the musculoskeletal system. The specific aims of this part are to

- Review the principles that form the foundation of biomechanical analysis of rigid bodies
- Review the mathematical approaches used to perform biomechanical analysis of rigid bodies
- Examine the concepts used to evaluate the material properties of deformable bodies
- Describe the material properties of the primary biological tissues constituting the musculoskeletal system: bone, muscle, cartilage, and dense connective tissue
- Review the components and behavior of joint complexes

By having an understanding of the principles of analysis in biomechanics and the biomechanical properties of the primary tissues of the musculoskeletal system, the reader will be prepared to apply these principles to each region of the body to understand the mechanics of normal movement at each region and to appreciate the effects of impairments on the pathomechanics of movement.

Introduction to Biomechanical Analysis

ANDREW R. KARDUNA, PH.D.

CHAPTER CONTENTS

Although the human body is an incredibly complex biological system composed of trillions of cells, it is subject to the same fundamental laws of mechanics that govern simple metal or plastic structures. The study of the response of biological systems to mechanical forces is referred to as **biomechanics.** Although it wasn't recognized as a formal discipline until the 20th century, biomechanics has been studied by the likes of Leonardo da Vinci, Galileo Galilei, and Aristotle. The application of biomechanics to the musculoskeletal system has led to a better understanding of both joint function and dysfunction, resulting in design improvements in devices such as joint arthroplasty systems and orthotic devices. Additionally, basic musculoskeletal biomechanics concepts are important for clinicians such as orthopaedic surgeons and physical and occupational therapists.

Biomechanics is often referred to as the link between structure and function. While a therapist typically evaluates a patient from a kinesiologic perspective, it is often not practical or necessary to perform a complete biomechanical analysis. However, a comprehensive knowledge of both biomechanics and anatomy is needed to understand how the musculoskeletal system functions. Biomechanics can also be useful in a critical evaluation of current or newly proposed patient evaluations and treatments. Finally, a fundamental understanding of biomechanics is necessary to understand some of the terminology associated with kinesiology (e.g., torque, moment, moment arms).

The purposes of this chapter are to

- Review some of the basic mathematical principles used in biomechanics
- Describe forces and moments
- Discuss principles of static analysis
- Present the basic concepts in kinematics and kinetics

The analysis is restricted to the study of rigid bodies. Deformable bodies are discussed in Chapters 2–6. The material in this chapter is an important reference for the force analysis chapters throughout the text.

MATHEMATICAL OVERVIEW

This section is intended as a review of some of the basic mathematical concepts used in biomechanics. Although it can be skipped if the reader is familiar with this material, it would be helpful to at least review this section.

Units of Measurement

The importance of including units with measurements cannot be emphasized enough. Measurements must be accompanied by a unit for them to have any physical meaning. Sometimes, there are situations when certain units are assumed. If a clinician asks for a patient's height and the reply is "5-6," it can reasonably be assumed that the patient is 5 feet, 6 inches tall. However, that interpretation would be inaccurate if the patient was in Europe, where the metric system is used. There are also situations where the lack of a unit makes a number completely useless. If a patient was told to perform a series of exercises for two, the patient would have no idea if that meant two days, weeks, months, or even years.

The units used in biomechanics can be divided into two categories. First, there are the four **fundamental units** of length, mass, time, and temperature, which are defined on the basis of universally accepted standards. Every other unit is considered a **derived unit** and can be defined in terms of these fundamental units. For example, velocity is equal to length divided by time and force is equal to mass multiplied by length divided by time squared. A list of the units needed for biomechanics is found in *Table 1.1*.

Trigonometry

Since angles are so important in the analysis of the musculoskeletal system, trigonometry is a very useful biomechanics tool. The accepted unit for measuring angles in the clinic is the degree. There are 360° in a circle. If only a portion of a circle is considered, then the angle formed is some fraction of 360°. For example, a quarter of a circle subtends an angle of 90°. Although in general, the unit degree is adopted for this text, angles also can be described in terms of radians. Since there are 2π radians in a circle, there are 57.3° per radian. When using a calculator, it is important to determine if it is set

TABLE 1.1: Units Used in Biomechanics

Quantity	Metric	British	Conversion
Length	meter (m)	foot (ft)	1 ft = 0.3048 m
Mass	kilogram (kg)	slug	1 slug = 14.59 kg
Time	second (s)	second (s)	1 s = 1 s
Temperature	Celsius (°C)	Fahrenheit (°F)	°F = (9/5) × °C + 32°
Force	newton (N = kg × m/s²)	pound (lb = slug × ft/s²)	1 lb = 4.448 N
Pressure	pascal (Pa = N/m²)	pounds per square inch (psi = lb/in²)	1 psi = 6895 Pa
Energy	joule (J = N × m)	foot pounds (ft-lb)	1 ft-lb = 1.356 J
Power	watt (W = J/s)	horsepower (hp)	1 hp = 7457 W

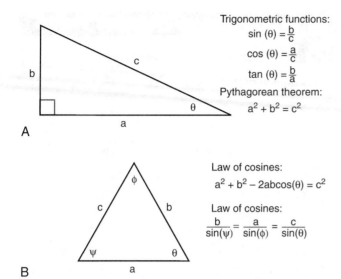

Trigonometric functions:
$$\sin(\theta) = \frac{b}{c}$$
$$\cos(\theta) = \frac{a}{c}$$
$$\tan(\theta) = \frac{b}{a}$$
Pythagorean theorem:
$$a^2 + b^2 = c^2$$

Law of cosines:
$$a^2 + b^2 - 2ab\cos(\theta) = c^2$$

Law of cosines:
$$\frac{b}{\sin(\psi)} = \frac{a}{\sin(\phi)} = \frac{c}{\sin(\theta)}$$

Figure 1.1: Basic trigonometric relationships. These are some of the basic trigonometric relationships that are useful for biomechanics. **A.** A right triangle. **B.** A general triangle.

to use degrees or radians. Additionally, some computer programs, such as Microsoft Excel, use radians to perform trigonometric calculations.

Trigonometric functions are very useful in biomechanics for resolving forces into their components by relating angles to distances in a right triangle (a triangle containing a 90° angle). The most basic of these relationships (**sine, cosine,** and **tangent**) are illustrated in *Figure 1.1A*. A simple mnemonic to help remember these equations is **sohcahtoa**—**s**ine is the **o**pposite side divided by the **h**ypotenuse, **c**osine is the **a**djacent side divided by the **h**ypotenuse, and **t**angent is the **o**pposite side divided by the **a**djacent side. Although most calculators can be used to evaluate these functions, some important values worth remembering are

$$\sin(0°) = 0, \sin(90°) = 1 \qquad \text{(Equation 1.1)}$$
$$\cos(0°) = 1, \cos(90°) = 0 \qquad \text{(Equation 1.2)}$$
$$\tan(45°) = 1 \qquad \text{(Equation 1.3)}$$

Additionally, the Pythagorean theorem states that for a right triangle, the sum of the squares of the sides forming the right angle equals the square of the hypotenuse (Fig. 1.1A). Although less commonly used, there are also equations that relate angles and side lengths for triangles that do not contain a right angle (Fig. 1.1B).

Vector Analysis

Biomechanical parameters can be represented as either **scalar** or **vector** quantities. A scalar is simply represented by its magnitude. Mass, time, and length are examples of scalar quantities. A vector is generally described as having both **magnitude** and **orientation.** Additionally, a complete description of a vector also includes its **direction** (or **sense**) and **point of application.** Forces and moments are examples of vector quantities. Consider the situation of a 160-lb man

sitting in a chair for 10 seconds. The force that his weight is exerting on the chair is represented by a vector with magnitude (160 lb), orientation (vertical), direction (downward), and point of application (the chair seat). However, the time spent in the chair is a scalar quantity and can be represented by its magnitude (10 seconds).

To avoid confusion, throughout this text, bolded notation is used to distinguish vectors (**A**) from scalars (B). Alternative notations for vectors found in the literature (and in classrooms, where it is difficult to bold letters) include putting a line under the letter (A), a line over the letter Ā, or an arrow over the letter $\vec{A}$. The **magnitude** of a given vector (**A**) is represented by the same letter, but not bolded (A).

By far, the most common use of vectors in biomechanics is to represent forces, such as muscle, joint reaction and resistance forces. These vectors can be represented graphically with the use of a line with an arrow at one end (*Fig. 1.2A*). The length of the line represents its magnitude, the angular position of the line represents its orientation, the location of the arrowhead represents its direction, and the location of the line in space represents its point of application. Alternatively, this same vector can be represented mathematically with the use of either **polar coordinates** or **component resolution.** Polar coordinates represent the magnitude and orientation of the vector directly. In polar coordinates, the same vector would be 5 N at 37° from horizontal (Fig. 1.2B). With components, the vector is resolved into its relative contributions from both axes. In this example, vector **A** is resolved into its components: $A_X = 4$ N and $A_Y = 3$ N (Fig. 1.2C). It is often useful to break down vectors into components that are aligned with anatomical directions. For instance, the x and y axes may correspond to superior and anterior directions, respectively.

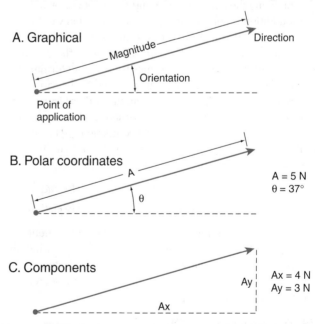

Figure 1.2: Vectors. **A.** In general, a vector has a magnitude, orientation, point of application, and direction. Sometimes the point of application is not specifically indicated in the figure. **B.** A polar coordinate representation. **C.** A component representation.

Although graphical representations of vectors are useful for visualization purposes, analytical representations are more convenient when adding and multiplying vectors.

Note that the directional information (up and to the right) of the vector is also embedded in this information. A vector with the same magnitude and orientation as the vector represented in Figure 1.2C, but with the opposite direction (down and to the left) is represented by $A_X = -4$ N and $A_Y = -3$ N, or 5 N at 217°. The description of the point-of-application information is discussed later in this chapter.

VECTOR ADDITION

When studying musculoskeletal biomechanics, it is common to have more than one force to consider. Therefore, it is important to understand how to work with more than one vector. When adding or subtracting two vectors, there are some important properties to consider. Vector addition is commutative:

$$\mathbf{A} + \mathbf{B} = \mathbf{B} + \mathbf{A} \qquad \text{(Equation 1.4)}$$
$$\mathbf{A} - \mathbf{B} = \mathbf{A} + (-\mathbf{B}) \qquad \text{(Equation 1.5)}$$

Vector addition is associative:

$$\mathbf{A} + (\mathbf{B} + \mathbf{C}) = (\mathbf{A} + \mathbf{B}) + \mathbf{C} \qquad \text{(Equation 1.6)}$$

Unlike scalars, which can just be added together, both the magnitude and orientation of a vector must be taken into account. The detailed procedure for adding two vectors ($\mathbf{A} + \mathbf{B} = \mathbf{C}$) is shown in *Box 1.1* for the graphical, polar coordinate, and component representation of vectors. The graphical representation uses the "tip to tail" method. The first step is to draw the first vector, **A.** Then the second vector, **B,** is drawn so that its tail sits on the tip of the first vector. The vector representing the sum of these two vectors (**C**) is obtained by connecting the tail of vector **A** and the tip of vector **B.** Since vector addition is commutative, the same solution would have been obtained if vector **B** were the first vector. When using polar coordinates, the vectors are drawn as in the graphical method, and then the law of cosines is used to determine the magnitude of **C** and the law of sines is used to determine the direction of **C** (see Fig 1.1 for definitions of these laws).

For the component resolution method, each vector is broken down into its respective x and y components. The components represent the magnitude of the vector in that direction. The x and y components are summed:

$$C_X = A_X + B_X \qquad \text{(Equation 1.7)}$$
$$C_Y = A_Y + B_Y \qquad \text{(Equation 1.8)}$$

The vector **C** can either be left in terms of its components, C_X and C_Y, or be converted into a magnitude, C, using the Pythagorean theorem, and orientation, θ, using trigonometry. This method is the most efficient of the three presented and is used throughout the text.

VECTOR MULTIPLICATION

Multiplication of a vector by a scalar is relatively straightforward. Essentially, each component of the vector is individually multiplied by the scalar, resulting in another vector. For

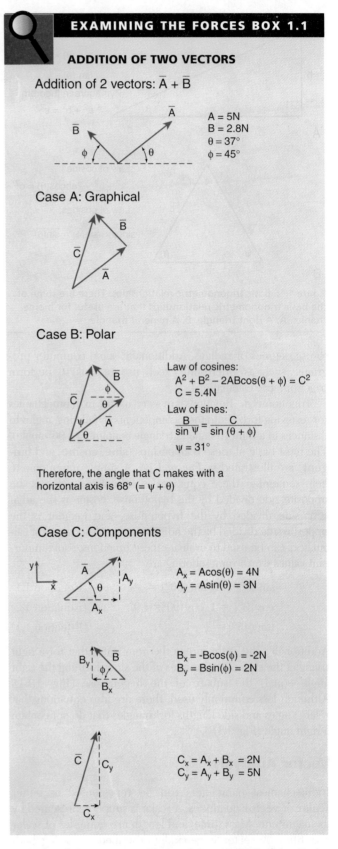

EXAMINING THE FORCES BOX 1.1

ADDITION OF TWO VECTORS

Addition of 2 vectors: $\bar{A} + \bar{B}$

A = 5N
B = 2.8N
θ = 37°
ϕ = 45°

Case A: Graphical

Case B: Polar

Law of cosines:
$A^2 + B^2 - 2AB\cos(\theta + \phi) = C^2$
C = 5.4N

Law of sines:
$$\frac{B}{\sin \psi} = \frac{C}{\sin (\theta + \phi)}$$
ψ = 31°

Therefore, the angle that C makes with a horizontal axis is 68° (= ψ + θ)

Case C: Components

$A_x = A\cos(\theta) = 4N$
$A_y = A\sin(\theta) = 3N$

$B_x = -B\cos(\phi) = -2N$
$B_y = B\sin(\phi) = 2N$

$C_x = A_x + B_x = 2N$
$C_y = A_y + B_y = 5N$

example, if the vector in Figure 1.2 is multiplied by 5, the result is $A_X = 5 \times 4$ N = 20 N and $A_y = 5 \times 3$ N = 15 N. Another form of vector multiplication is the **cross product,** in which two vectors are multiplied together, resulting in

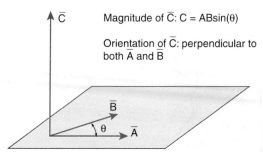

Magnitude of $\bar{C}$: C = ABsin(θ)

Orientation of $\bar{C}$: perpendicular to both $\bar{A}$ and $\bar{B}$

Figure 1.3: Vector cross product. **C** is shown as the cross product of **A** and **B**. Note that **A** and **B** could be any two vectors in the indicated plane and C would still have the same orientation.

another vector ($\mathbf{C} = \mathbf{A} \times \mathbf{B}$). The orientation of **C** is such that it is mutually perpendicular to **A** and **B.** The magnitude of **C** is calculated as C = A × B × sin (θ), where θ represents the angle between A and B, and × denotes scalar multiplication. These relationships are illustrated in *Figure 1.3*. The cross product is used for calculating joint torques later in this chapter.

Coordinate Systems

A three-dimensional analysis is necessary for a complete representation of human motion. Such analyses require a coordinate system, which is typically composed of anatomically aligned axes: medial/lateral (ML), anterior/posterior (AP), and superior/inferior (SI). It is often convenient to consider only a two-dimensional, or planar, analysis, in which only two of the three axes are considered. In the human body, there are three perpendicular anatomical planes, which are referred to as the **cardinal planes.** The **sagittal plane** is formed by the SI and AP axes, the **frontal (or coronal) plane** is formed by the SI and ML axes, and the **transverse plane** is formed by the AP and ML axes (*Fig. 1.4*).

The motion of any bone can be referenced with respect to either a **local** or **global** coordinate system. For example, the motion of the tibia can be described by how it moves with respect to the femur (local coordinate system) or how it moves with respect to the room (global coordinate system). Local coordinate systems are useful for understanding joint function and assessing range of motion, while global coordinate systems are useful when functional activities are considered.

Most of this text focuses on two-dimensional analyses, for several reasons. First, it is difficult to display three-dimensional information on the two-dimensional pages of a book. Additionally, the mathematical analysis for a three-dimensional problem is very complex. Perhaps the most important reason is that the fundamental biomechanical principles in a two-dimensional analysis are the same as those in a three-dimensional analysis. It is therefore possible to use a simplified two-dimensional representation of a three-dimensional problem to help explain a concept with minimal mathematical complexity (or at least less complexity).

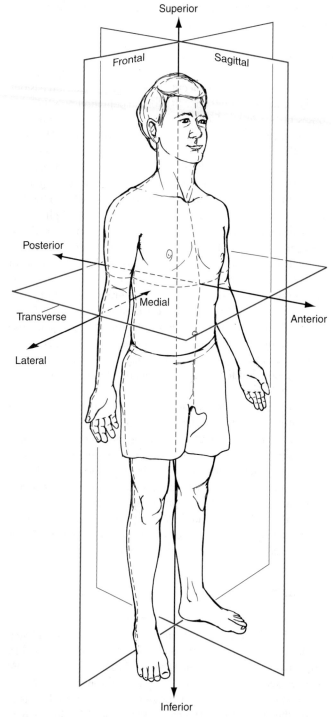

Figure 1.4: Cardinal planes. The cardinal planes, sagittal, frontal, and transverse, are useful reference frames in a three-dimensional representation of the body. In two-dimensional analyses, the sagittal plane is the common reference frame.

FORCES AND MOMENTS

The musculoskeletal system is responsible for generating forces that move the human body in space as well as prevent unwanted motion. Understanding the mechanics and pathomechanics of human motion requires an ability to study the forces and moments applied to, and generated by, the body or a particular body segment.

Forces

The reader may have a conceptual idea about what a force is but find it difficult to come up with a formal definition. For the purposes of this text, a **force** is defined as a "push or pull" that results from physical contact between two objects. The only exception to this rule that is considered in this text is the force due to gravity, in which there is no direct physical contact between two objects. Some of the more common force generators with respect to the musculoskeletal system include muscles/tendons, ligaments, friction, ground reaction, and weight.

A distinction must be made between the **mass** and the **weight** of a body. The mass of an object is defined as the amount of matter composing that object. The weight of an object is the force acting on that object due to gravity and is the product of its mass and the acceleration due to gravity ($g = 9.8$ m/s^2). So while an object's mass is the same on Earth as it is on the moon, its weight on the moon is less, since the acceleration due to gravity is lower on the moon. This distinction is important in biomechanics, not to help plan a trip to the moon, but for ensuring that a unit of mass is not treated as a unit of force.

As mentioned previously, force is a vector quantity with magnitude, orientation, direction, and a point of application. *Figure 1.5* depicts several forces acting on the leg in the frontal plane during stance. The forces from the abductor and adductor muscles act through their tendinous insertions, while the hip joint reaction force acts through its respective joint center of rotation. In general, the point of application of a force (e.g., tendon insertion) is located with respect to a fixed point on a body, usually the joint center of rotation. This information is used to calculate the **moment** due to that force.

Moments

In kinesiology, a moment (**M**) is typically caused by a force (**F**) acting at a distance (**r**) from the center of rotation of a segment. A moment tends to cause a rotation and is defined by the cross product function: **M = r × F.** Therefore, a moment is represented by a vector that passes through the point of interest (e.g., the center of rotation) and is perpendicular to both the force and distance vectors (*Fig. 1.6*). For a two-dimensional analysis, both the force and distance vectors are in the plane of the paper, so the moment vector is always directed perpendicular to the page, with a line of action through the point of interest. Since it has only this one orientation and line of action, a moment is often treated as a scalar quantity in a two-dimensional analysis, with only magnitude and direction. **Torque** is another term that is synonymous with a scalar moment. From the definition of a cross product, the magnitude of a moment (or torque) is calculated as M = r × F × sin (θ). Its direction is referred to as the direction in which it would tend to cause an object to rotate (*Fig. 1.7A*).

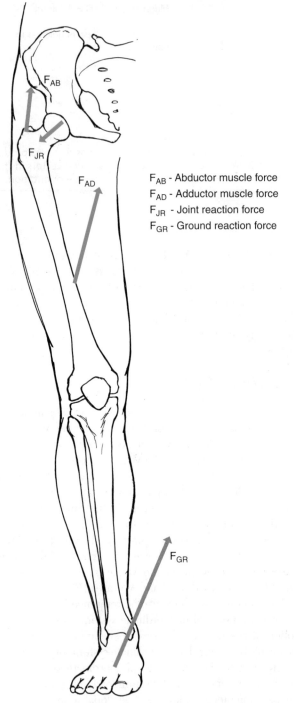

F_{AB} - Abductor muscle force
F_{AD} - Adductor muscle force
F_{JR} - Joint reaction force
F_{GR} - Ground reaction force

Figure 1.5: Vectors in anatomy. Example of how vectors can be combined with anatomical detail to represent the action of forces. Some of the forces acting on the leg are shown here.

Although there are several different distances that can be used to connect a vector and a point, **the same moment is calculated no matter which distance is selected** (Fig. 1.7B). The distance that is perpendicular to the force vector is referred to as the **moment arm** (MA) of that force (r_2 in Fig. 1.7B). Since the sine of 90° is equal to 1, the use of a moment arm simplifies the calculation of moment to

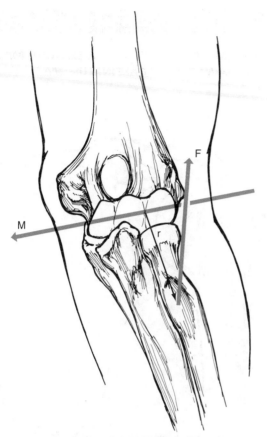

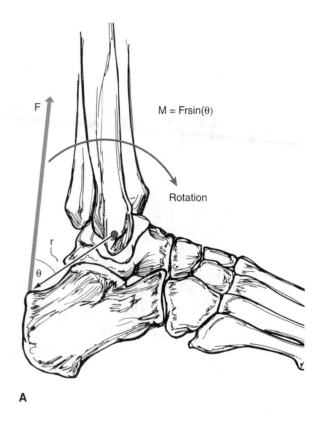

A

Figure 1.6: Three-dimensional moment analysis. The moment acting on the elbow from the force of the biceps is shown as a vector aligned with the axis of rotation. *F,* force vector; r, distance from force vector to joint COR; *M,* moment vector.

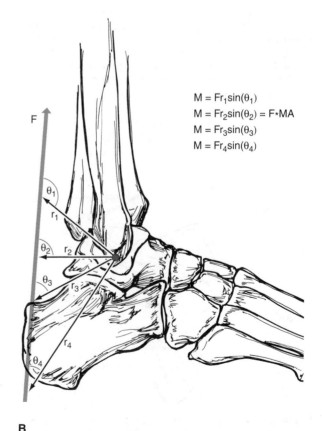

B

Figure 1.7: *Continued*

$M = MA \times F$. The moment arm can also be calculated from any distance as $MA = r \times \sin(\theta)$. Additionally, although there are four separate angles between the force and distance vectors, all four angles result in the same moment calculation (Fig. 1.7C).

The examples in Figures 1.6 and 1.7 have both force and moment components. However, consider the situation in *Figure 1.8A.* Although the two applied forces create a moment, they have the same magnitude and orientation but opposite directions. Therefore, their vector sum is zero. This is an example of a **force couple.** A pure force couple results in rotational motion only, since there are no unbalanced forces. In the musculoskeletal system, all of these conditions are seldom met, so pure force couples are rare. In general, muscles are responsible for producing both forces and moments, thus resulting in both translational and rotational motion. However, there are examples in the human body in which two or more muscles work in concert to produce a moment, such as the upper trapezius and serratus anterior (Fig. 1.8B). Although these muscles do not have identical magnitudes or orientations, this situation is frequently referred to as a force couple.

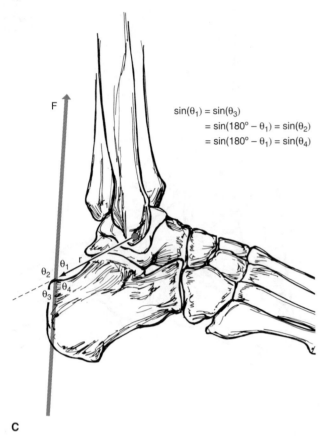

$$\sin(\theta_1) = \sin(\theta_3)$$
$$= \sin(180° - \theta_1) = \sin(\theta_2)$$
$$= \sin(180° - \theta_1) = \sin(\theta_4)$$

C

Figure 1.7: Two-dimensional moment analysis. **A.** Plantar flexion moment created by force at the Achilles tendon. **B.** Note that no matter which distance vector is chosen, the value for the moment is the same. **C.** Also, no matter which angle is chosen, the value for the sine of the angle is the same, so the moment is the same.

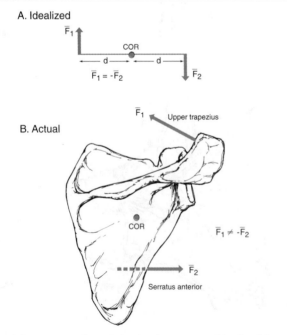

Figure 1.8: Force couples. Distinction between an idealized force couple **(A)** and a more realistic one **(B).** Even though the scapular example given is not a true force couple, it is typically referred to as one. *COR,* center of rotation.

EXAMINING THE FORCES BOX 1.2

MOMENT ARMS OF THE DELTOID (MA_d) AND THE SUPRASPINATUS (MA_s)

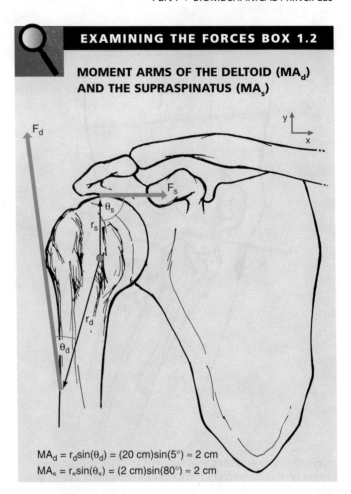

$$MA_d = r_d\sin(\theta_d) = (20\ cm)\sin(5°) \approx 2\ cm$$
$$MA_s = r_s\sin(\theta_s) = (2\ cm)\sin(80°) \approx 2\ cm$$

Muscle Forces

As mentioned previously, there are three important parameters to consider with respect to the force of a muscle: orientation, magnitude, and point of application. With some care, it is possible to measure orientation and line of action from cadavers or imaging techniques such as magnetic resonance imaging (MRI) and computed tomography (CT) [1,3]. This information is helpful in determining the function and efficiency of a muscle in producing a moment. As an example, two muscles that span the glenohumeral joint, the supraspinatus and middle deltoid, are shown in *Box 1.2.* From the information provided for muscle orientation and point of application in this position, the moment arm of the deltoid is approximately equal to that of the supraspinatus, even though the deltoid insertion on the humerus is much farther away from the center of rotation than the supraspinatus insertion.

Clinical Relevance

MUSCLE FORCES: *In addition to generating moments that are responsible for **angular motion** (rotation), muscles also produce forces that can cause **linear motion** (translation).*

(continued)

(Continued)

This force can be either a stabilizing or a destabilizing force. For example, since the supraspinatus orientation shown in Box 1.2 is primarily directed medially, it tends to pull the humeral head into the glenoid fossa. This compressive force helps stabilize the glenohumeral joint. However, since the deltoid orientation is directed superiorly, it tends to produce a destabilizing force that may result in superior translation of the humeral head.

These analyses are useful, since they can be performed even if the magnitude of a muscle's force is unknown. However, to understand a muscle's function completely, its force magnitude must be known. Although forces can be measured with invasive force transducers [13], instrumented arthroplasty systems [6], or simulations in cadaver models [9], there are currently no noninvasive experimental methods that can be used to measure the in vivo force of intact muscles. Consequently, basic concepts borrowed from freshman physics can be used to predict muscle forces. Although they often involve many simplifying assumptions, such methods can be very useful in understanding joint mechanics and are presented in the next section.

STATICS

Statics is the study of the forces acting on a body at rest or moving with a constant velocity. Although the human body is almost always accelerating, a static analysis offers a simple method of addressing musculoskeletal problems. This analysis may either solve the problem or provide a basis for a more sophisticated dynamic analysis.

Newton's Laws

Since the musculoskeletal system is simply a series of objects in contact with each other, some of the basic physics principles developed by Sir Isaac Newton (1642-1727) are useful. Newton's laws are as follows:

First law: An object remains at rest (or continues moving at a constant velocity) unless acted upon by an unbalanced external force.

Second law: If there is an unbalanced force acting on an object, it produces an acceleration in the direction of the force, directly proportional to the force (f = ma).

Third law: For every action (force) there is a reaction (opposing force) of equal magnitude but in the opposite direction.

From Newton's first law, it is clear that if a body is at rest, there can be no unbalanced external forces acting on it. In this situation, termed **static equilibrium,** all of the external forces acting on a body must add (in a vector sense) to zero. An extension of this law to objects larger than a particle is that

the sum of the external moments acting on that body must also be equal to zero for the body to be at rest. Therefore, for a three-dimensional analysis, there are a total of six equations that must be satisfied for static equilibrium:

$$\Sigma F_X = 0 \quad \Sigma F_Y = 0 \quad \Sigma F_Z = 0$$
$$\Sigma M_X = 0 \quad \Sigma M_Y = 0 \quad \Sigma M_Z = 0 \qquad \text{(Equation 1.9)}$$

For a two-dimensional analysis (in the x–y plane), there are only two in-plane force components and one perpendicular moment (torque) component:

$$\Sigma F_X = 0 \quad \Sigma F_Y = 0 \quad \Sigma M_Z = 0 \qquad \text{(Equation 1.10)}$$

Under many conditions, it is reasonable to assume that all body parts are in a state of static equilibrium and these three equations can be used to calculate some of the forces acting on the musculoskeletal system. When a body is not in static equilibrium, Newton's second law states that any unbalanced forces and moments are proportional to the acceleration of the body. That situation is considered later in this chapter.

Solving Problems

A general approach used to solve for forces during static equilibrium is as follows:

Step 1 Isolate the body of interest.
Step 2 Sketch this body and all external forces (referred to as a **free body diagram**).
Step 3 Sum the forces and moments equal to zero.
Step 4 Solve for the unknown forces.

As a simple example, consider the two 1-kg balls hanging from strings shown in *Box 1.3*. What is the force acting on the top string? Although this is a very simple problem that can be solved by inspection, a formal analysis is presented. Step 1 is to sketch the entire system and then place a dotted box

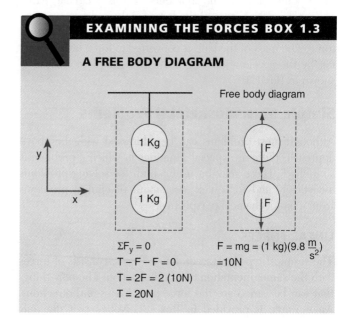

EXAMINING THE FORCES BOX 1.3

A FREE BODY DIAGRAM

Free body diagram

$\Sigma F_y = 0$

$T - F - F = 0$

$T = 2F = 2 \ (10N)$

$T = 20N$

$F = mg = (1 \ kg)(9.8 \ \frac{m}{s^2})$

$= 10N$

around the body of interest. Consider a box that encompasses both balls and part of the string above the top one, as shown in Box 1.3.

Proceeding to step 2, a free body diagram is sketched. As indicated by Newton's first law, only external forces are considered for these analyses. For this example, everything inside the dotted box is considered part of the body of interest. External forces are caused by the contact of two objects, one inside the box and one outside the box. In this example, there are three external forces: tension in the top string and the weight of each of the balls.

Why is the tension on the top string considered an external force, but not the force on the bottom string? The reason is that the tension on the top string is an **external force** (part of the string is in the box and part is outside the box), and the force on the bottom string is an internal force (the entire string is located inside the box). This is a very important distinction because it allows for isolation of the forces on specific muscles or joints in the musculoskeletal system.

Why is the weight of each ball considered an external force? Although gravity is not caused by contact between two objects, it is caused by the interaction of two objects and is treated in the same manner as a contact force. One of the objects is inside the box (the ball) and the other is outside the box (the Earth). In general, as long as an object is located within the box, the force of gravity acting on it should be considered an external force.

Why is the weight of the string not considered an external force? To find an exact answer to the problem, it should be considered. However, since its weight is far less than that of the balls, it is considered negligible. In biomechanical analyses, assumptions are often made to ignore certain forces, such as the weight of someone's watch during lifting.

Once all the forces are in place, step 3 is to sum all the forces and moments equal to zero. There are no forces in the x direction, and since all of the forces pass through the same point, there are no moments to consider. That leaves only one equation: sum of the forces in the y direction equal to zero. The fourth and final step is to solve for the unknown force. The mass of the balls is converted to force by multiplying by the acceleration of gravity. The complete analysis is shown in Box 1.3.

Simple Musculoskeletal Problems

Although most problems can be addressed with the above approach, there are special situations in which a problem is simplified. These may be useful both for solving problems analytically and for quick assessment of clinical problems from a biomechanical perspective.

LINEAR FORCES

The simplest type of system, linear forces, consists of forces with the same orientation and line of action. The only things that can be varied are the force magnitudes and directions. An example is provided in Box 1.3. Notice that the only

equation needed is summing the forces along the y axis equal to zero. When dealing with linear forces, it is best to align either the x or y axis with the orientation of the forces.

PARALLEL FORCES

A slightly more complicated system is one in which all the forces have the same orientation but not the same line of action. In other words, the force vectors all run parallel to each other. In this situation, there are still only forces along one axis, but there are moments to consider as well.

LEVERS

A **lever** is an example of a parallel force system that is very common in the musculoskeletal system. Although not all levers contain parallel forces, that specific case is focused on here. A basic understanding of this concept allows for a rudimentary analysis of a biomechanical problem with very little mathematics.

A lever consists of a rigid body with two externally applied forces and a point of rotation. In general, for a musculoskeletal joint, one of the forces is produced by a muscle, one force is provided by contact with the environment (or by gravity), and the point of rotation is the center of rotation of the joint. The two forces can either be on the same side or different sides of the **center of rotation (COR).**

If the forces are on different sides of the COR, the system is considered a **first class lever.** If the forces are on the same side of the COR and the external force is closer to the COR than the muscle force, it is a **second class lever.** If the forces are on the same side of the COR and the muscle force is closer to the COR than the external force, it is a **third class lever.** There are several cases of first class levers; however, most joints in the human body behave as third class levers. Second class levers are almost never observed within the body. Examples of all three levers are given in Figure 1.9.

If moments are summed about the COR for any lever, the resistive force is equal to the muscle force times the ratio of the muscle and resistive moment arms:

$$F_R = F_M \times (MA_M/MA_R) \qquad \text{(Equation 1.11)}$$

The ratio of the muscle and resistive moment arms (MA_M/MA_R) is referred to as the **mechanical advantage** of the lever. Based on this equation and the definition of levers, the mechanical advantage is greater than one for a second class lever, less than one for a third class lever, and has no restriction for a first class lever. A consequence of this is that since most joints behave as third class levers, muscle forces are greater than the force of the resistive load they are opposing. Although this may appear to represent an inefficient design, muscles sacrifice their mechanical advantage to produce large motions and high-velocity motions. This equation is also valid in cases where the two forces are not parallel, as long as their moment arms are known. The effects of a muscle's moment arm on joint motion is discussed in Chapter 4.

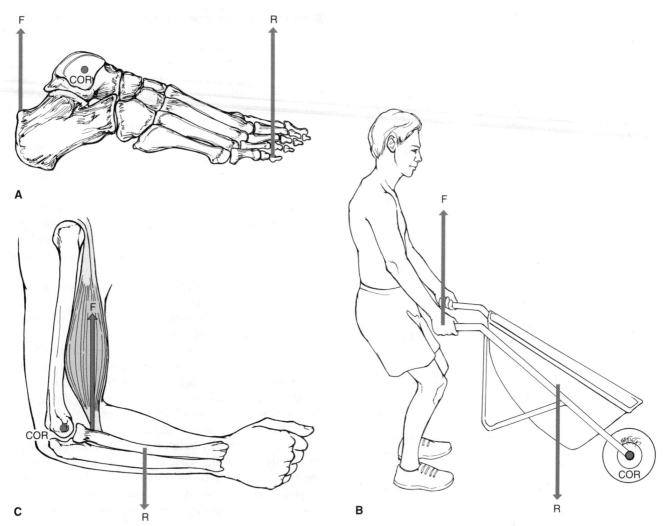

Figure 1.9: Classification of lever systems. Examples of the three different classes of levers, where F is the exerted force, R is the reaction force, and COR is the center of rotation. Most musculoskeletal joints behave as third class levers. **A.** First class lever. **B.** Second class lever. **C.** Third class lever.

Center of Gravity and Stability

Another example of a parallel force system is the use of the **center of gravity** to determine stability. The center of gravity of an object is the point at which all of the weight of that body can be thought to be concentrated, and it depends on a body's shape and mass distribution. The center of gravity of the human body in the anatomical position is approximately at the level of the second sacral vertebra [8]. This location changes as the shape of the body is altered. When a person bends forward, his or her center of gravity shifts anteriorly and inferiorly. The location of the center of gravity is also affected by body mass distribution changes. For example, if a person were to develop more leg muscle mass, the center of mass would shift inferiorly.

The location of a person's center of gravity is important in athletics and other fast motions because it simplifies the use of Newton's second law. More important from a clinical point of view is the effect of the center of gravity on stability. For motions in which the acceleration is negligible, it can be shown with Newton's first law that the center of gravity must be contained within a person's base of support to maintain stability.

Consider the situation of a person concerned about falling forward. Assume for the moment that there is a ground reaction force at his toes and heel. When he is standing upright, his center of gravity is posterior to his toes, so there is a counterclockwise moment at his toes (*Fig. 1.10A*). This is a stable position, since the moment can be balanced by the ground reaction force at his heel. If he bends forward at his hips to touch the ground and leans too far forward, his center of gravity moves anterior to his toes and the weight of his upper body produces a clockwise moment at his toes (Fig. 1.10B). Since there is no further anterior support, this moment is unbalanced and the man will fall forward. However, if in addition to hip flexion he plantarflexes at his ankles while keeping his knee straight, he is in a stable position with his center of gravity posterior to his toes (Fig. 1.10C).

Advanced Musculoskeletal Problems

One of the most common uses of static equilibrium applied to the musculoskeletal system is to solve for unknown muscle forces. This is a very useful tool because as mentioned above, there are currently no noninvasive experimental methods that can be used to measure in vivo muscle forces. There are typically 3 types of forces to consider in a musculoskeletal problem: *(a)* the joint reaction force between the two articular surfaces, *(b)* muscle forces and *(c)* forces due to the body's interaction with the outside world. So how many unknown parameters are associated with these forces? To answer this, the location of all of the forces with their points of application must be identified. For the joint reaction force nothing else is known, so there are two unknown parameters: magnitude and orientation. The orientation of a muscle force can be measured, so there is one unknown parameter, magnitude. Finally, any force interaction with the outside world can theoretically be measured, possibly with a handheld dynamometer, force plate, or by knowing the weight of the segment, so there are no unknown parameters (*Table 1.2*) [5,8].

Consequently, there are two unknown parameters for the joint reaction force and one unknown parameter for each muscle. However, there are only three equations available from a two-dimensional analysis of Newton's first law. Therefore, if there is more than one muscle force to consider, there are more unknown parameters than available equations. This situation is referred to as **statically indeterminate,** and there are an infinite number of possible solutions. To avoid this problem, only one muscle force can be considered. Although this is an oversimplification of most musculoskeletal situations, solutions based on a single muscle can provide a general perspective of

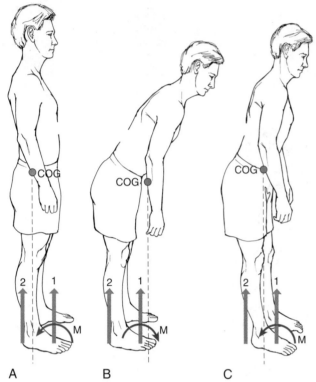

Figure 1.10: Center of gravity. For the man in the figure to maintain his balance, his center of gravity must be maintained within his base of support. This is not a problem in normal standing **(A).** When he bends over at the waist, however, his center of gravity may shift anterior to the base of support, creating an unstable situation **(B).** The man needs to plantarflex at the ankles to maintain his balance **(C).**

TABLE 1.2: Body Segment Parameters [12]

	Mass (% of Total Body Weight)	Location of the Center of Mass (% of Limb Segment Length from Proximal End)	Radius of Gyration (% of Limb Segment Length from Proximal End)
Head and neck	8.1	100.0[a]	11.6
Trunk	49.7	50.0	NA
Upper extremity	5.0	53.0	64.5
Arm	2.8	43.6	54.2
Forearm and hand	2.2	68.2	82.7
Forearm	1.6	43.0	52.6
Hand	0.6	50.6	58.7
Lower extremity	16.1	44.7	56.0
Thigh	10.0	43.3	54.0
Leg and foot	6.1	60.6	73.5
Leg	4.7	43.3	52.8
Foot	1.5	50.0	69.0

[a]Measured from C7-T1 to ear.
NA, not available.

the requirements of a task. Options for solving the statically indeterminate problem are briefly discussed later.

FORCE ANALYSIS WITH A SINGLE MUSCLE

There are additional assumptions that are typically made to solve for a single muscle force:

- Two-dimensional analysis
- No deformation of any tissues
- No friction in the system
- The single muscle force that has been selected can be concentrated in a single line of action
- No acceleration

The glenohumeral joint shown in *Box 1.4* is used as an example to help demonstrate the general strategy for approaching these problems. Since only one muscle force can be considered, the supraspinatus is chosen for analysis. The same general approach introduced earlier in this chapter for addressing a system in static equilibrium is used.

Step one is to isolate the body of interest, which for this problem is the humerus. In step two, a free body diagram is drawn, with all of the external forces clearly labeled: the weight of the arm (F_G), the supraspinatus force (F_S), and the glenohumeral joint reaction force (F_J) in Box 1.4. Note that external objects like the scapula are often included in the free body diagram to make the diagram complete. However, the scapula is external to the analysis and is only included for convenience (which is why it is drawn in gray). It is important to keep track of which objects are internal and which ones are external to the isolated body.

The next step is to sum the forces and moments to zero to solve for the unknown values. Since the joint reaction force acts through the COR, a good strategy is to start by summing the moments to zero at that point. This effectively eliminates the joint reaction force from this equation because its moment arm is equal to zero. The forces along the x and y axes are summed to zero to find those components of the joint reaction force. The fourth and final step is to solve for the unknown parameters in these three equations. The details of these calculations are given in Box 1.4. In this example, the magnitude of the joint reaction force is 180 N directed laterally and 24 N directed superiorly. Those components represent the force of the scapula acting on the humerus. Newton's third law can then be used to find the force of the humerus acting on the scapula: 180 N medial and 24 N inferior, with a total magnitude of 182 N.

Note that the muscle force is much larger than the weight of the arm. This is expected, considering the small moment arm of the muscle compared with the moment arm of the force due to gravity. While this puts muscles at a mechanical disadvantage for force production, it enables them to amplify their motion. For example, a 1-cm contraction of the supraspinatus results in a 7.5-cm motion at the hand. This is discussed in more detail in Chapter 4.

The problem can be solved again by considering the middle deltoid instead of the supraspinatus. For those conditions,

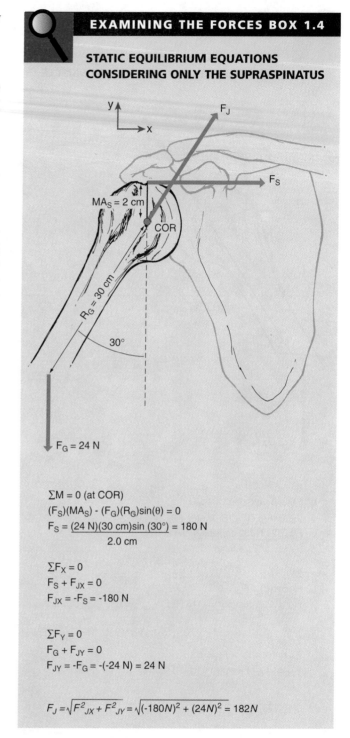

EXAMINING THE FORCES BOX 1.4

STATIC EQUILIBRIUM EQUATIONS CONSIDERING ONLY THE SUPRASPINATUS

$MA_S = 2$ cm

COR

$R_G = 30$ cm

30°

$F_G = 24$ N

$\Sigma M = 0$ (at COR)

$(F_S)(MA_S) - (F_G)(R_G)\sin(\theta) = 0$

$F_S = \dfrac{(24 \text{ N})(30 \text{ cm})\sin(30°)}{2.0 \text{ cm}} = 180$ N

$\Sigma F_X = 0$

$F_S + F_{JX} = 0$

$F_{JX} = -F_S = -180$ N

$\Sigma F_Y = 0$

$F_G + F_{JY} = 0$

$F_{JY} = -F_G = -(-24 \text{ N}) = 24$ N

$F_J = \sqrt{F^2_{JX} + F^2_{JY}} = \sqrt{(-180N)^2 + (24 N)^2} = 182N$

Box 1.5 shows that the deltoid muscle force is 200 N and the force of the humerus acting on the scapula is 115 N directed medially and 140 N directed superiorly, with a total magnitude of 181 N. Notice that although the force required of each muscle and the total magnitude of the joint reaction force is similar for both cases, the deltoid generates a much higher superior force and the supraspinatus generates a much higher medial force.

Although the magnitude of the muscle and joint reaction forces in this example is similar, this might not be the case

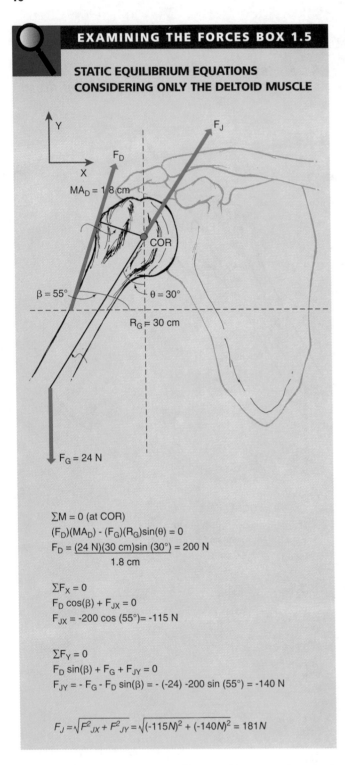

EXAMINING THE FORCES BOX 1.5

STATIC EQUILIBRIUM EQUATIONS CONSIDERING ONLY THE DELTOID MUSCLE

$\sum M = 0$ (at COR)

$(F_D)(MA_D) - (F_G)(R_G)\sin(\theta) = 0$

$F_D = \dfrac{(24\ N)(30\ cm)\sin(30°)}{1.8\ cm} = 200\ N$

$\sum F_X = 0$

$F_D \cos(\beta) + F_{JX} = 0$

$F_{JX} = -200 \cos(55°) = -115\ N$

$\sum F_Y = 0$

$F_D \sin(\beta) + F_G + F_{JY} = 0$

$F_{JY} = -F_G - F_D \sin(\beta) = -(-24) - 200 \sin(55°) = -140\ N$

$F_J = \sqrt{F_{JX}^2 + F_{JY}^2} = \sqrt{(-115N)^2 + (-140N)^2} = 181N$

Clinical Relevance

SUPRASPINATUS AND DELTOID MUSCLE FORCES:
A clinical application of these results is that under normal conditions the supraspinatus serves to maintain joint stability with its medially directed force. However, if its integrity is compromised, as occurs with rotator cuff disease, and the deltoid plays a larger role, then there is a lower medial stabilizing force and a higher superior force that may cause impingement of the rotator cuff in the subacromial region.

The analysis presented above serves as a model for analyzing muscle and joint reaction forces in subsequent chapters. Although some aspects of the problem will clearly vary from joint to joint, the basic underlying method is the same.

FORCE ANALYSIS WITH MULTIPLE MUSCLES

Although most problems addressed in this text focus on solving for muscle forces when only one muscle is taken into consideration, it would be advantageous to solve problems in which there is more than one muscle active. However such systems are statically indeterminate. Additional information is needed regarding the relative contribution of each muscle to develop an appropriate solution.

One method for analyzing indeterminate systems is the **optimization method.** Since an indeterminate system allows an infinite number of solutions, the optimization approach helps select the "best" solution. An optimization model minimizes some cost function to produce a single solution. This function may be the total force in all of the muscles or possibly the total stress (force/area) in all of the muscles. While it might make sense that the central nervous system attempts to minimize the work it has to do to perform a function, competing demands of a joint must also be met. For example, in the glenohumeral example above, it might be most efficient from a force production standpoint to assume that the deltoid acts alone. However, from a stability standpoint, the contribution of the rotator cuff is essential.

Another method for analyzing indeterminate systems is the **reductionist model** in which a set of rules is applied for the relative distribution of muscle forces based on electromyographic (EMG) signals. One approach involves developing these rules on the basis of the investigator's subjective knowledge of EMG activity, anatomy, and physiological constraints [4]. Another approach is to have subjects perform isometric contractions at different force levels while measuring EMG signals and to develop an empirical relationship between EMG and force level [2,7]. Perhaps the most common approach is based on the assumption that muscle force is proportional to its cross-sectional area and EMG level. This method has been attempted for many joints, such as the shoulder [10], knee, and hip. One of the key assumptions in all these approaches is that there is a known relationship between EMG levels and force production.

for other problems. Consequently, an alternative approach is to simply document the joint **internal moment** (generated by the joint muscles and ligaments) that is necessary to balance the joint **external moment** (generated by the external forces, gravity in this example). Therefore, in both cases (supraspinatus and deltoid), the external moment is equal to a 360 N cm (from $F_G \cdot R_G \cdot \sin[\theta]$) adduction moment. Consequently, the internal moment is a 360 N cm abduction moment.

KINEMATICS

Until now, the focus has been on studying the static forces acting on the musculoskeletal system. The next section deals with **kinematics,** which is defined as the study of motion without regard to the forces that cause that motion. As with the static force analysis, this section is restricted to two-dimensional, or planar, motion.

Rotational and Translational Motion

Pure linear, or **translatory, motion** of an entire object occurs when all points on that object move the same distance (*Fig. 1.11A*). However, with the possible exception of passive manipulation of joints, pure translatory motion does not often occur at musculoskeletal articulations. Instead, **rotational motion** is more common, in which there is one point on a bone that remains stationary (the COR), and all other points trace arcs of a circle around this point (Fig. 1.11*B*). For three-dimensional motion, the **COR** would be replaced by an **axis of rotation,** and there could also be translation along this axis.

Consider the general motion of a bone moving from an initial to a final position. The rotational component of this motion can be measured by tracking the change in orientation of a line on the bone. Although there are an infinite number of lines to choose from, it turns out that no matter which line is selected, the amount of rotation is always the same. Similarly, the translational component of this motion can be measured by tracking the change in position of a point on the bone. In this case, however, the amount of translatory motion is *not* the same for all points. In fact, the displacement of a point increases linearly as its distance from the COR increases (Fig. 1.11*B*). Therefore, from a practical standpoint, if there is any rotation of a bone, a description of joint translation or displacement must refer to a specific point on the bone.

Consider the superior/inferior translation motion of the humerus in *Figure 1.12A*, which is rotated 90°. Point 1 represents the geometric center of the humeral head and does not translate from position 1 to 2. However, point 2 on the articular surface of the humeral head translates inferiorly. The motion in Figure 1.12*B* is similar, except now point 1 translates

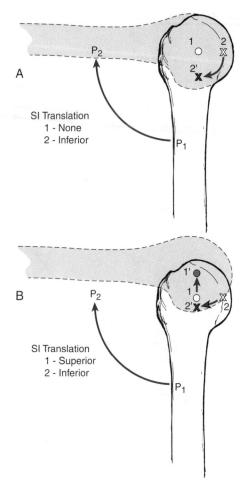

Figure 1.12: Translations and rotations within a joint. For both of these examples, it is fairly straightforward to describe the rotational motion of the humerus—it rotates 90°. However, translational motion is more complicated, and it is important to refer to a specific point. Consider the superior/inferior (SI) translation of two points: point 1 is located at the center of the humeral head and point 2 sits closer to the articular surface. **A.** The center of the rotation of the motion is at point 1, so there is no translation at point 1, but point 2 moves inferiorly. **B.** Point 1 moves superiorly, and point 2 moves inferiorly.

superiorly, while point 2 still translates inferiorly. This example demonstrates how important the point of reference is when describing joint translations.

Displacement, Velocity, and Acceleration

Both linear and angular displacements are measures of distance. **Position** is defined as the location of a point or object in space. **Displacement** is defined as the distance traveled between two locations. For example, consider the knee joint during gait. If its angular position is 10° of flexion at heel strike and 70° of flexion at toe off, the angular displacement from heel strike to toe off is 60° of flexion.

Change in linear and angular position (displacement) over time is defined as linear and angular **velocity,** respectively.

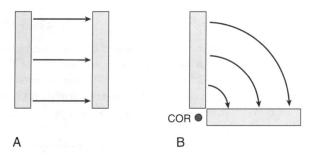

Figure 1.11: Translations and rotations. In biomechanics, motion is typically described in terms of translations and rotations. **A.** In translatory motion, all points on the object move the same distance. **B.** In rotational motion, all points on the object revolve around the center of rotation (*COR*), which is fixed in space.

TABLE 1.3: Kinematic Relationships

	Position	Velocity		Acceleration	
		Instantaneous	Average	Instantaneous	Average
Linear	P	$v = \dfrac{dp}{dt}$	$v = \dfrac{P_2 - P_1}{t_2 - t_1}$	$a = \dfrac{dv}{dt}$	$a = \dfrac{v_2 - v_1}{t_2 - t_1}$
Angular	0	$\omega = \dfrac{d\theta}{dt}$	$\omega = \dfrac{\theta_2 - \theta_1}{t_2 - t_1}$	$\alpha = \dfrac{d\omega}{dt}$	$\alpha = \dfrac{\omega_2 - \omega_1}{t_2 - t_1}$

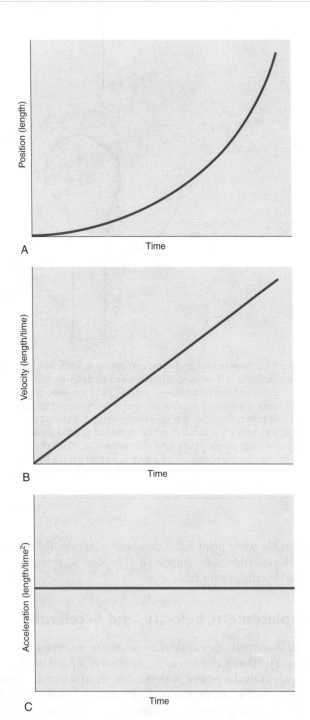

A

B

C

Figure 1.13: Acceleration, velocity, and displacement. Schematic representation of the motion of an object traveling at constant acceleration. The velocity increases linearly with time, while the position increases nonlinearly.

Finding the instantaneous velocity at any given point in time, requires the use of calculus. *Instantaneous velocity* is defined as the differential of position with respect to time. Average velocity may be calculated by simply considering two separate locations of an object and taking the change in its position and dividing by the change in time (*Table 1.3*). As the time interval becomes smaller and approaches zero, the average velocity approaches the instantaneous velocity.

Similarly, changes in linear and angular velocity over time are defined as linear and angular **acceleration.** *Instantaneous acceleration* is defined as the differential of velocity with respect to time. Average acceleration may be calculated by simply considering two separate locations of an object and taking the change in its velocity and dividing by the change in time (Table 1.3). An example of the effect of constant acceleration on velocity and position is shown in *Figure 1.13*.

KINETICS

Until now, forces and motion have been discussed as separate topics. **Kinetics** is the study of motion under the action of forces. This is a very complex topic that is only introduced here to give the reader some working definitions. The only chapter in this text that deals with these terms in any detail is Chapter 48 on gait analysis.

Inertial Forces

Kinematics and kinetics are bound by Newton's second law, which states that the external force (f) on an object is proportional to the product of that object's mass (m) and linear acceleration (a):

$$f = ma \qquad \text{(Equation 1.12)}$$

For conditions of static equilibrium, there are no external forces because there is no acceleration, and the sum of the external forces can be set equal to zero. However, when an object is accelerating, the so-called **inertial forces** (due to acceleration) must be considered, and the sum of the forces is no longer equal to zero.

Consider a simple example of a linear force system in which someone is trying to pick up a 20-kg box. If this is performed very slowly so that the acceleration is negligible, static equilibrium conditions can be applied (sum of forces equal zero), and the force required is 200 N (*Box 1.6*). However, if this same box is lifted with an acceleration of 5 m/s^2, then the

EXAMINING THE FORCES BOX 1.6

STATIC AND DYNAMIC EQUILIBRIUM

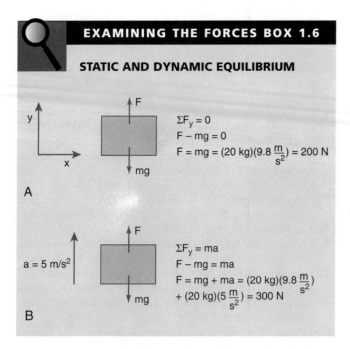

A

$\Sigma F_y = 0$
$F - mg = 0$
$F = mg = (20\ kg)(9.8\ \frac{m}{s^2}) = 200\ N$

B

$a = 5\ m/s^2$

$\Sigma F_y = ma$
$F - mg = ma$
$F = mg + ma = (20\ kg)(9.8\ \frac{m}{s^2})$
$+ (20\ kg)(5\ \frac{m}{s^2}) = 300\ N$

EXAMINING THE FORCES BOX 1.7

CALCULATING THE RADIUS OF GYRATION AND MOMENT OF INERTIA OF THE LOWER EXTREMITY ABOUT THE HIP JOINT

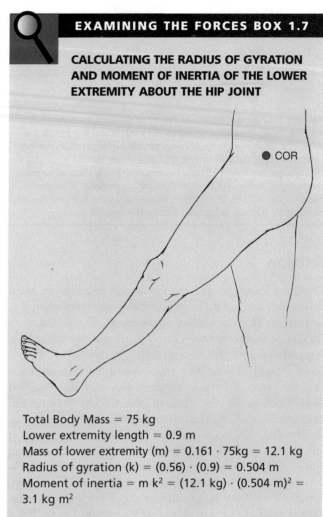

● COR

Total Body Mass = 75 kg
Lower extremity length = 0.9 m
Mass of lower extremity (m) = 0.161 · 75kg = 12.1 kg
Radius of gyration (k) = (0.56) · (0.9) = 0.504 m
Moment of inertia = m k² = (12.1 kg) · (0.504 m)² = 3.1 kg m²

sum of the forces is *not* equal to zero, and the force required is 300 N (*Box 1.6*).

There is an analogous relationship for rotational motion, in which the external moment (M) on an object is proportional to that object's **moment of inertia** (I) and angular acceleration (α):

$$M = I\alpha \qquad \text{(Equation 1.13)}$$

Just as mass is a measure of a resistance to linear acceleration, moment of inertia is a measure of resistance to angular acceleration. It is affected both by the magnitude of all the point masses that make up a body and the distance that each mass is from the center of rotation (r) as follows:

$$I = \Sigma mr^2 \qquad \text{(Equation 1.14)}$$

So the further away the mass of an point mass is from the center of rotation, the larger its contribution to the moment of inertia. For example, when a figure skater is spinning and tucks in her arms, she is moving more of her mass closer to the center of rotation, thus reducing her moment of inertia. The consequence of this action is that her angular velocity increases.

Although equation 1.14 can theoretically be used to calculate the moment of inertia of a segment, a more practical approach is to treat the segment as one object with a single mass (m) and radius of gyration (k):

$$I = mk^2 \qquad \text{(Equation 1.15)}$$

The radius of gyration of an object represents the distance at which all the mass of the object would be concentrated in order to have the same moment of inertia as the object itself. The radius of gyration for various human body segments is given in Table 1.2. An example of how to calculate a segment's moment of inertia about its proximal end is presented in *Box 1.7*.

Work, Energy, and Power

Another combination of kinematics and kinetics comes in the form of **work,** which is defined as the force required to move an object a certain distance (work = force × distance). The standard unit of work in the metric system is a joule (J; newton × meter). For example, if the 20-kg box in Box 1.6 is lifted 1 m under static equilibrium conditions, the work done is equal to 200 joules (200 N × 1 m). By analogy with the analysis in Box 1.6, under dynamic conditions, the work done is equal to 300 J (300 N × 1 m).

Power is defined as the rate that work is being done (power = work/time). The standard unit of power is a watt (W; watt = newton × meter/second). Continuing with the above example, if the box were lifted over a period of 2 seconds, the average power would be 100 W under static conditions and 150 W under dynamic conditions. In practical terms, the static lift is generating the same amount of power needed to light a 100 W light bulb for 2 seconds.

The *energy* of a system refers to its capacity to perform work. Energy has the same unit as work (J) and can be divided into potential and kinetic energy. While **potential energy** refers to stored energy, **kinetic energy** is the energy of motion.

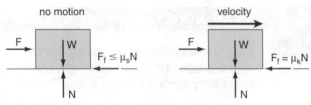

Figure 1.14: Friction. **A.** Under static conditions (no motion), the magnitude of the frictional force (F_f) exerted on the box is the same as the applied force (F) and cannot be larger than the coefficient of static friction (μ_s) multiplied by the normal force (N). If the applied force exceeds the maximum static frictional force, the box will move and shift to dynamic conditions. **B.** Under dynamic conditions, the friction force is equal to the coefficient of dynamic friction (μ_k) multiplied by the normal force.

Friction

Frictional forces can prevent the motion of an object when it is at rest and resist the movement of an object when it is in motion. This discussion focuses specifically on Coulomb friction, or friction between two dry surfaces [11]. Consider a box with a weight (W) resting on the ground (*Fig. 1.14*). If a force (F) applied along the *x* axis is equal to the frictional force (F_f), the box is in static equilibrium. However, if the applied force is greater than the frictional force, the box accelerates to the right because of an unbalanced external force.

The frictional force matches the applied force until it reaches a critical value, $F = \mu_s N$, where N is the reaction force of the floor pushing up on the box and μ_s is the coefficient of *static* friction. In this example, N is equal to the magnitude of the force due to the weight of the box. Once this critical value is reached, there is still a frictional force, but it is now defined by: $F = \mu_k N$, where μ_k is the coefficient of *dynamic* friction.

The values for the coefficient of friction depend on several parameters, such as the composition and roughness of the two surfaces in contact. In general, the dynamic coefficient of friction is lower than the static coefficient of friction. As a consequence, it would take less force the keep the box in Figure 1.14 moving than it would take to start it moving.

SUMMARY

This chapter starts with a review of some important mathematical principles associated with kinesiology and proceeds to cover statics, kinematics, and kinetics from a biomechanics perspective. This information is used throughout the text for analysis of such activities as lifting, crutch use, and single-limb stance. The reader may find it useful to refer to this chapter when these problems are addressed.

References

1. An KN, Takahashi K, Harrigan TP, Chao EY: Determination of muscle orientations and moment arms. J Biomech Eng 1984; 106: 280–282.

2. Arwert HJ, de Groot J, Van Woensel WWLM, Rozing PM: Electromyography of shoulder muscles in relation to force direction. J Shoulder Elbow Surg 1997; 6: 360–370.
3. Chao EY, Lynch JD, Vanderploeg MJ: Simulation and animation of musculoskeletal joint system. J Biomech Eng 1993; 115: 562–568.
4. Dempster WT: Space requirements of the seated operator. In: Human Mechanics; Four Monographs Abridged AMRL-TDR-63-123. Krogman WM, Johnston FE, eds. Wright-Patterson Air Force Base, OH: Behavioral Sciences Laboratory, 6570th Aerospace Medical Research Laboratories, Aerospace Medical Division, Air Force Systems Command, 1963; 215–340.
5. Fuller JJ, Winters JM: Assessment of 3-D joint contact load preditions during postural/stretching exercises in aged females. Ann Biomed Eng 1993; 21: 277–288.
6. Krebs DE, Robbins CE, Lavine L, Mann RW: Hip biomechanics during gait. J Orthop Sports Phys Ther 1998; 28: 51–59.
7. Laursne B, Jensen BR, Németh G, Sjøgaard G: A model predicting individual shoulder muscle forces based on relationship between electromyographic and 3D external forces in static position. J Biomech 1998; 31: 731–739.
8. LeVeau BF: Williams and Lissner's Biomechanics of Human Motion, 3rd ed. Philadelphia: WB Saunders, 1992.
9. McMahon PJ, Debski RE, Thompson WO, et al.: Shoulder muscle forces and tendon excursions during glenohumeral abduction in the scapular plane. J Shoulder Elbow Surg 1995; 4: 199–208.
10. Poppen NK, Walker PS: Forces at the glenohumeral joint in abduction. Clin Orthop 1978; 135: 165–170.
11. Stevens KK: Statics and Strength of Materials. Englewood Cliffs, NJ: Prentice-Hall, 1987.
12. Winter DA: Biomechanics and Motor Control of Human Movement, 3rd ed. Hoboken, NJ: John Wiley & Sons, 2005.
13. Xu WS, Butler DL, Stouffer DC, et al.: Theoretical analysis of an implantable force transducer for tendon and ligament structures. J Biomech Eng 1992; 114: 170–177.

Musculoskeletal Biomechanics Textbooks

Bell F: Principles of Mechanics and Biomechanics. Cheltenham, UK: Stanley Thornes Ltd, 1998.

Enoka R: Neuromechanics of Human Movement, 3rd ed. Champaign, IL: Human Kinetics, 2002.

Hall S: Basic Biomechanics, 5th ed. Boston: WCB/McGraw-Hill, 2006.

Hamill J, Knutzen K. Biomechanical Basis of Human Movement, 2nd ed. Philadelphia: Lippincott Williams & Wilkins, 2003.

Low J, Reed A: Basic Biomechanics Explained. Oxford, UK: Butterworth-Heinemann 1996.

Lucas G, Cooke F, Friis, E: A Primer of Biomechanics. New York: Springer, 1999.

McGinnis P: Biomechanics of Sports and Exercise. Champaign, IL: Human Kinetics, 2005.

Nigg B, Herzog W: Biomechanics of the Musculo-skeletal System, 3rd ed. New York: John Wiley and Sons, 2007.

Nordin M, Frankel V: Basic Biomechanics of the Musculoskeletal System, 3rd ed. Philadelphia: Lippincott Williams & Wilkins, 2001.

Özkaya N, Nordin M: Fundamentals of Biomechanics: Equilibrium, Motion and Deformation, 2nd ed. New York: Springer, 1999.

Mechanical Properties of Materials

L.D. TIMMIE TOPOLESKI, PH.D.

CHAPTER CONTENTS

There are over 1,000 types of properties (reactions to external stimuli) that describe a material's behavior. Since all human tissue is composed of one material or another, the same material properties that describe materials like steel, concrete, and rubber can be applied to the behavior of human tissue. Readers may have an intuitive sense that different tissues behave differently; for example, skin and muscle seem to stretch or deform more easily than bone. It is also easier to cut skin or muscle than to cut bone. Defining and measuring properties of different materials quantifies the differences between materials (how much easier is it to cut muscle than bone?), and predicts how a material will behave under a known environment (how much force is required to break a bone during, say, a skiing accident?).

The purposes of this chapter are to

- Familiarize readers with basic definitions of mechanics and materials terms
- Describe some of the most useful and general properties of materials
- Provide an appreciation of the clinical relevance of mechanical properties of biological tissues

BASIC MATERIAL PROPERTIES

Most people, regardless of their background, can name some material properties. An initial thought might be **weight.** Weight, however, is defined by the acceleration of a mass in Earth's gravity. So **mass** may be a better candidate for a material property. But then someone may ask, which has more mass, a kilogram of gold or a kilogram of paper? Well, a kilogram is a kilogram, so the mass of a kilogram of gold is the same as the mass of a kilogram of paper. But it certainly takes less gold than paper to make up a kilogram. So, the mass of an object depends on how much of the material there is. Properties that depend on the amount of a material are called **extensive properties. Volume** and **internal energy** are other examples of extensive properties.

It is easier to compare the behavior of materials without worrying about whether they are of the same mass or volume. So properties are often *normalized* by dividing by the mass or volume. For example, the mass/unit volume is the **density** of a material. The density of gold is the same for an ounce, a kilogram, or a stone of gold (a stone is an old British unit of weight, equal to 14 pounds). Density is an example of an **intensive** property, a property that does not depend on the amount of a material. Many of the useful material properties in biomechanics are intensive properties.

One of the most important properties of a material is the material's **strength.** People are especially likely to wonder about the strength of a material when crossing over a bridge, for example. Perhaps every person who has ever lived has wondered at some point "is this object strong enough?" meaning, will the object in use break during the intended use? Some materials seem to break readily and at inconvenient times. For example, many people will remember when the tines from the plastic fork broke at the picnic, when the tire blew out on the highway, or when shoelaces snapped while being tied. Engineers have devoted much time and effort to ensure that materials do not break, especially when people's lives depend on the integrity of materials (e.g., materials used in a bridge).

Many factors other than strength influence how and when a material will break. A simple experiment with a paper clip should convince the reader that material failure may occur under conditions that are not initially obvious (*Box 2.1*).

Before considering the details of how strength is measured, consider whether strength is an intensive or an extensive property. Can a thin strand of steel wire hold the same

EXAMINING THE FORCES BOX 2.1

THE PAPER CLIP EXPERIMENT

Most readers have experienced a remarkable phenomenon. "Uncoil" a common paper clip, and grab both ends, say with a pair of pliers. You are unlikely to break the paper clip, even if you pull with all of your strength; yet if you bend the paper clip back and forth, you will eventually break a piece of steel with your bare hands! How is this possible? The answer is that whether a material breaks depends on the conditions applied to the material; pulling the two ends of a paper clip creates different conditions from bending the paper clip back and forth. The first relates to the tensile strength of the metal, and the second to a form of fatigue strength; both are discussed in detail soon.

EXAMINING THE FORCES BOX 2.2

EXPERIMENT TO TEST THE BREAKING POINT OF WIRES OF DIFFERENT THICKNESS

Perform a simple experiment to answer the question. For this experiment, we need wires of different diameters made from the same material. Most hardware stores have some kind of wire, for example copper or lead, available in different diameters. Lead solder is a good material to use, since it usually breaks under moderate loads. Hang the wires from a convenient ledge, and place the same weight (or mass) on each of the wires. Next, add more weight to each wire, keeping the weight on each wire equal. Which wire breaks first? The thinnest, of course, and you probably predicted it. The experiment demonstrates a very important fact: *strength,* defined as the maximum weight a wire can hold before breaking, is an extensive property.

weight as a thick beam? No, because strength is an extensive property. Another simple experiment demonstrates that the thickness of a wire, for example, influences when that wire breaks (*Box 2.2*).

STRESS AND STRAIN

The results of the experiment in Box 2.2 present a problem. It would be much more convenient if a material, whether it is a type of steel or polymer, artificial or biological, had a single value for strength; that is, if strength were an intensive property. To arrive at a definition of strength that is an intensive property, some additional background is necessary, specifically the definition and understanding of two concepts, **stress** and **strain.** Long before the words were used to describe how students feel before final exams, stress and strain were used as measures of a material's behavior. Most importantly, stress and strain have distinct meanings; they are not synonyms and cannot be used interchangeably. **Stress** is defined by units of force/area, the same units used for pressure (e.g., pounds per square inch, newtons per square meter). Stress is a measure that is independent of the amount of a material. This simple concept is incredibly useful. A 10-lb weight hanging on a wire with a cross-sectional area of 0.1 in^2 produces a stress inside the wire of 10 lb/0.1 in^2 (force/area), or 100 psi (pounds per square inch; 1 psi is equal to about 6,900 N/m^2) (*Fig. 2.1*). A thinner wire, for example one with a cross-sectional area of 0.05 in^2, requires less applied force to sustain the same 100-psi stress. The full calculation of stress in the thinner wire is presented in *Box 2.3*. Note that stress is a measure of load (or energy) that is in an object. Stress is similar to an internal pressure in a solid material or a normalized load (or weight)

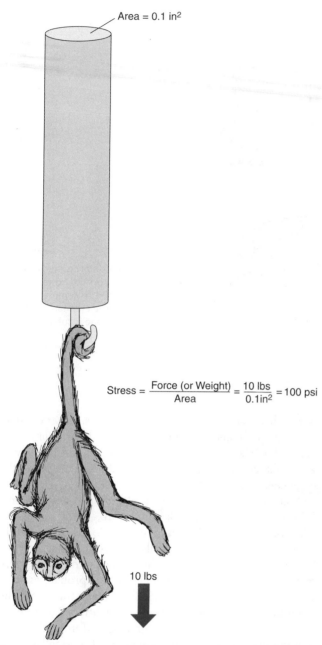

Area = 0.1 in²

$$\text{Stress} = \frac{\text{Force (or Weight)}}{\text{Area}} = \frac{10\text{ lbs}}{0.1\text{in}^2} = 100\text{ psi}$$

10 lbs

Figure 2.1: Stress in a simple bar is defined as the load (in this case the weight of the monkey) divided by the cross-sectional area of the bar (with units of psi, pounds per square inch).

on a material. While it is not a material property, stress has the *sense* of being intensive, because it does not depend on the amount of material.

Stress has a complementary measure, called **strain.** Just as stress is like a force normalized by the cross-section (or amount of material) of a wire, strain is like a normalized stretch or displacement of a material (*Box 2.4*).

To define stress or strain more formally, imagine a cylinder of any material under an applied load (or force). The length and the diameter of the cylinder have been measured. The cross-sectional area is easily calculated from the diameter. The direction in which the cylinder is loaded is important;

EXAMINING THE FORCES BOX 2.3

CALCULATION OF STRESS IN A WIRE

How much weight must be added to a wire with a cross-section of 0.05 in² to produce a stress of 100 psi?

Set up an equation:

$$\frac{100\text{ lb}}{\text{in}^2} = \frac{X}{0.05\text{ in}^2}$$

where X is the necessary weight, in pounds. As noted in Chapter 1, it is always important to keep track of units when performing any mechanics calculations. Readers who do not think units are important should not have any trouble giving the author a $20 bill, and accepting 20 cents in return! After all, 20 is 20, if the units are disregarded. Solving the equation, X is equal to 5 lb. Therefore, to achieve 100 psi of stress in a 0.1-in² wire, use 10 lb of weight, but in a 0.05-in² wire use only 5 lb of weight.

pushing along the axis of the cylinder is called *compression*, or in other words, the cylinder is under a compressive load (Fig. 2.2A). Pulling the cylinder is called *tension*, or the cylinder is under a tensile load (Fig. 2.2B).

Knowing the force applied to the cylinder, the stress in the cylinder is calculated as

$$\sigma = \frac{F}{A} \qquad \text{(Equation 2.1)}$$

where σ is a generally accepted symbol for stress, F is the applied load, and A is the cross-sectional area. For any force

EXAMINING THE FORCES BOX 2.4

EXPERIMENT TO ASSESS THE STRAIN IN RUBBER BANDS OF DIFFERENT LENGTHS

Take rubber bands of the same material and thickness but of different lengths, and place on the same convenient ledge as in Box 2.2. Hang the same size weight from each. Which stretches the farthest? The longest rubber band. Think of it this way: suppose that the rubber bands, pulled by the weight in the experiment, stretch by 25%. A 1-in rubber band stretches to 1.25 in, adding 0.25 in, but the 10-in rubber band stretches to 12.5 in, adding 2.5 in. The absolute stretch, or gain in length, depends on the original length of the material. But, you say, the original premise was that each rubber band stretched 25% of its original length, so on a percentage basis, the relative stretch is the same.

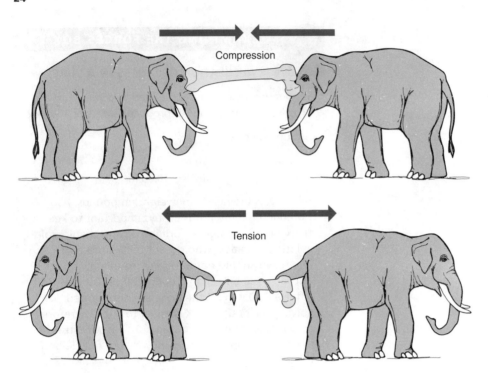

Figure 2.2: A. Compression. As the elephants push on the bone, the bone is subjected to compression. **B.** Tension. As the elephants pull on the bone, the bone is subjected to tension.

F, if the stress is calculated on the basis of the original cross-sectional area (call it A_0), then the stress is called the **engineering stress.** Why is this important? It turns out that when a material is in tension, the diameter decreases (this is easy to see in a rubber cylinder), and if the material is in compression, the diameter increases (the cylinder bulges). The more you pull (or push), the more the diameter decreases (or increases). For many metals and other materials, it is difficult to detect the squeeze or bulge, and a difference of a few square micrometers in area doesn't change the value of stress much. Thus, it may not be necessary to measure the cylinder's diameter for every force. For other materials, such as rubber, the bulge can be a significant percentage of change, and so it is important to know the exact cross-sectional area (called the **instantaneous area**). Using the instantaneous or actual area in the stress calculation (equation 2.1) gives the **true stress.**

Strain also comes in "engineering" and "true" definitions. The **engineering strain** (e) is defined as the change in length of a specimen divided by the original length:

$$e = \frac{\Delta L}{L_0} = \frac{L - L_0}{L_0} \qquad \text{(Equation 2.2)}$$

where L is the length at the time of measurement, L_0 is the original length, and ΔL is then the calculated change in length. The **true strain** (ε) is defined by

$$\varepsilon = \ln \frac{L}{L_0} \qquad \text{(Equation 2.3)}$$

Notice that strain appears to be dimensionless. However, strain is usually presented in terms of inches/inch, or millimeters/millimeter. The units cancel each other out, but they give a sense of scale and often impart information on the size of the specimens tested.

Many materials (e.g., the structural metals) strain only a little before they break. Therefore, their useful life takes place at *small strains*. The definitions of strains (in equations 2.2 and 2.3) are really approximations, and they hold only for small strains. The definition of *small strain* may vary from person to person, but it is probably safe to say that anything less than 1% is a small strain, and the definitions above are applicable. Equation 2.3 for *true strain* is determined by integrating differential length increments over the entire specimen. For small strains, less than 1%, engineering strain is a reasonable approximation to true strain. Certain simplifying assumptions are used in calculating strain for small strains. Between 1 and 10%, the definitions may be useful, depending on the material system and the accuracy of the information that is needed. If the strains are larger than 10%, as they may be for some soft tissues, then those assumptions are no longer valid. More complex treatments are needed to define "large" or "finite strains." In biomechanics, the definitions for finite strains are important, because many tissues undergo finite strains; however, a discussion of finite strain is beyond the scope of this book. With stress, it doesn't matter so much. Both stress and strain have precise mathematical definitions and actually have several different definitions, which are based largely on the point of view the definer takes. The in-depth treatments of stress and strain appear in courses in continuum mechanics and finite deformations.

There is one additional topic to be discussed related to small strains. Tension is defined by forces that tend to pull something apart. That is like pulling hands apart before clapping. Compression is the force applied when the hands come together for the clap. To continue the hand/stress analogy, consider a person rubbing his or her hands together, for example, when the hands are cold. The back-and-forth motion can occur in materials, and it is known as **shear strain** (usually designated by the Greek γ). Shear strain has a counterpart, **shear stress** (designated by the Greek τ) (*Fig. 2.3*). The shear stress, τ is defined as the shear force, F_s, divided by the area over which it acts, A:

$$\tau = \frac{F_s}{A} \qquad \text{(Equation 2.4)}$$

Shear stresses are very important, because many failure theories for ductile materials (defined below) show that failure occurs when the **maximum shear stress** is reached. If an experimenter pulled apart a cylinder of copper, a ductile material, it would fracture at a 45° angle to the direction of the applied forces. Why? Because that is the direction of the maximum shear stress.

The concepts of stress and strain are not necessarily easy to grasp. Many readers may feel comfortable with the description of stress as an "internal pressure." Strain may best be thought of as a percentage change in length. Once stress and strain are no longer a mystery, however, defining most of the mechanical properties is relatively straightforward.

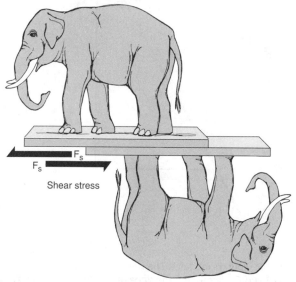

Figure 2.3: Shear. As the elephants slide relative to each other, the boards they are standing on are subjected to shear.

THE TENSION TEST

The Basics (Young's Modulus, Poisson's Ratio)

The definitions of stress and strain are the first steps toward understanding and defining some of the most useful properties of a material, such as the nebulous concept of strength discussed earlier. It is easier to make sense of some of the most important material properties in the context of a simple tensile test on a cylindrical specimen of material. Everything that applies to the simple tension test also applies to a simple compression test; however, the values of the properties in tension and compression may not be simple negatives of each other!

Imagine that the director of new materials development at a huge, multinational biotechnology corporation has just received samples of a new material developed by one of the engineers. The engineer believes that the new material is an excellent bone replacement candidate. The new material would be most useful if it had properties similar to those of natural bone. The first task that the materials engineers must tackle is determining the properties of the new material and comparing them to the properties of bone (assume that appropriately sized cylinders are available to perform the test).

To test the properties of the new material, the test specimens are carefully placed in the grips of a tension-testing machine, and the test begins (with the stress and strain both initially zero). More and more tensile force is gradually applied to the specimen. Most tension-testing machines provide force and displacement data, rather than stress and strain. However, this is no problem; stress and strain are easily calculated from equations 2.1 through 2.3, since the specimen diameter and length are known. A **stress–strain diagram** (or graph) is a plot of the stress for each strain. At first, the engineer may tend to be a little cautious, perhaps because there is only a limited supply of the sample material. So the test is programmed to produce only 20–30 lb of force. After calculating the stress and strain for the initial test, a stress–strain diagram is generated, which may look something like *Figure 2.4*.

Notice that in the figure, when the specimen is unloaded, the stress–strain curve goes back down the same line that it went up and stops right where it started. That means the strain is zero at the end of the test, just as at the beginning. When a material returns back to its original shape after it is loaded and unloaded, the deformations, or strains, that occurred during loading are said to be **elastic.** This is a different definition than most people are used to. For example, the term *elastic* may produce images of elastic bands in clothing; elastic is sometimes taken to mean "stretchy." In the language of mechanics of materials, *elastic* has a precise definition. Elastic means that the material returns to its original shape after loading. What happens if the material does not return to its original shape? The experiment must continue for the answer to be revealed.

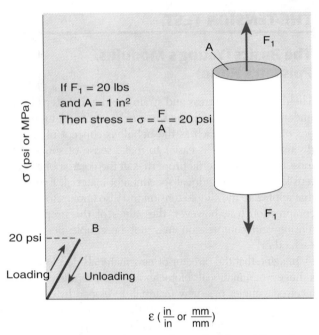

Figure 2.4: Stress–strain diagram. The applied force (F_1) on the test specimen is the independent variable. The displacement is measured after the force is applied, and thus displacement is the dependent variable. Traditionally, however, stress–strain diagrams are created with the stress acting as the dependent (or "y") variable, and the strain as the independent (or "x") variable. A cylindrical test specimen (cross-sectional area = 1 in²) is loaded with an applied force of 20 lb, and thus the uniform stress in the specimen is 20 psi. The stress–strain diagram is linear from zero stress to the maximum stress at 20 psi (point B).

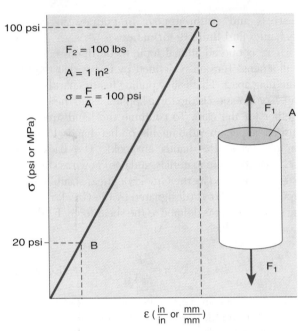

Figure 2.5: Stress–strain diagram for larger forces. The test specimen is loaded with a force (F_2) of 100 lb. The corresponding engineering stress is 100 psi. The stress–strain diagram shows that the stress–strain relationship remains linear from point B (20 psi) to point C (100 psi). Note that the corresponding strains at point B (0.0005 $\frac{in}{in}$) and point C (0.0025 $\frac{in}{in}$) are also recorded.

Because the specimen appears to have suffered no damage, the engineers become a little braver and increase the load on the specimen, perhaps to about 100 lb. The new, extended plot on the stress–strain diagram still looks like a straight line (*Fig. 2.5*). Indeed, many materials exhibit this **linear** behavior (e.g., steel, concrete, glass). It is extremely important, however, to know that most soft tissue (e.g., muscle, skin, ligament, tendon, cartilage) does not show this linear behavior; the materials exhibit **nonlinear** behavior. Nonlinear materials are more difficult to understand and require a fundamental knowledge of how linear materials behave.

The slope of the straight line in a stress–strain diagram is one of the most important and fundamental properties of any material; the slope is called the **Young's modulus, or modulus of elasticity** (engineers often use the letter E to represent the Young's modulus) (*Fig. 2.6*). The Young's modulus is similar to a spring constant, except it relates to stress and strain, not force and displacement. The Young's modulus indicates either (*a*) how much a material stretches or strains when it is subjected to a certain stress or (*b*) how much stress builds up in a material when it is stretched or strained by a certain amount. The Young's modulus also is sometimes called the material's **stiffness**. A material with a high Young's modulus undergoes less strain under a given load than a material with a lower Young's modulus (*Fig. 2.7*), and hence it is a stiffer material. The Young's modulus is an intensive property, since

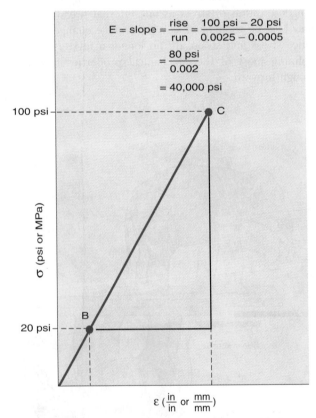

Figure 2.6: Young's modulus. The stress–strain relationship between points B and C is linear, and the slope of the line is the Young's modulus, or modulus of elasticity. In the case of the test specimen, the calculations show that the Young's modulus, E, is 40,000 psi.

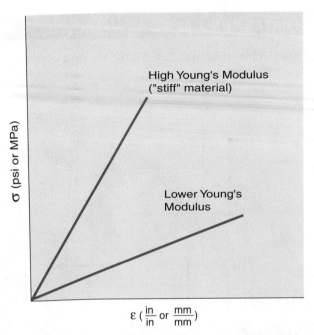

Figure 2.7: Young's moduli for two different materials. On this stress–strain diagram are illustrated two different materials, one with a slope greater than the other. The material with the greater slope (or Young's modulus) is "stiff" relative to the material with the lower slope (or Young's modulus).

it is based on stress and strain and does not depend on the size of the specimen.

The engineers have carefully observed the specimen during the testing and notice that the diameter of the specimen decreases as the specimen is pulled! Just as strain is measured in the direction that the specimen is pulled (along the axis of the cylinder), strain can also be measured in the direction across the cylinder. The true strain in the direction perpendicular to the loading direction can also be calculated as

$$\varepsilon = 2 \ln \left(\frac{D_0}{D} \right) \qquad \text{(Equation 2.5)}$$

where D_0 is the original diameter and D is the current diameter. The ratio of the axial strain to the lateral strain is called **Poisson's ratio** and denoted by the Greek letter nu, v:

$$v = \frac{-\text{lateral strain}}{\text{axial strain}} \qquad \text{(Equation 2.6)}$$

The negative sign appears because while the material is stretched in the axial direction (a positive strain), the material is shrinking in the lateral direction (a negative strain). The negative sign ensures that the resultant Poisson's ratio will always be positive.

The Young's modulus and the Poisson's ratio allow a basic comparison of material behavior of the new material and human bone. If the values are the same, the engineers can be confident that the new material behaves somewhat like human bone. There are several different ways to measure the Young's modulus and Poisson's ratio; the tension test is only one potential and simple way. Young's modulus and Poisson's ratio are

material properties because their values are the same regardless of the type of test or the specimen geometry. They are also intensive properties, since they are the same regardless of the amount of the material. There may be only a subtle distinction between a material property and an intensive property. A material property must be the same regardless of the way the material is tested; it is conceivable that there could be two different test methods that use the same amount of material. Of course, there may be no difference at all. Therefore, if the cylinders have different diameters but are of the same material and the Young's modulus is determined for each type of specimen, the value should be the same each time!

The Young's modulus and the Poisson's ratio also allow calculation of stresses and strains in directions other than that of the load, through the relationship between stress and strain called **Hooke's law** (Box 2.5).

Load to Failure

Once the Young's modulus of the new material is known with some confidence, the next testing objective is to discover when the specimen breaks. As the specimen is loaded more and more, one of two things commonly happens. In the first case, the stress and strain continue to increase in a straight line, and then suddenly . . . WHAM! the specimen breaks. This is quite an exciting event when it happens, because (although it is not calculated here) lots of elastic energy has been stored in the material, and the remaining fragments spring rapidly back to their original shape. The largest stress that the material withstands before it breaks is called the **ultimate tensile stress,** or **ultimate tensile strength,** or just the **ultimate strength.** The ultimate strength is an intensive definition of strength based on the maximum stress a material can withstand (Fig. 2.8).

The second possible material response to the increasing stress is that as the test progresses, the stress–strain line deviates from the nice straight line it had been following since the beginning of the test. Usually, the slope of the line decreases (Fig. 2.9). If the test is reversed after the "bend" in the stress–strain plot becomes evident, the specimen does not unload along the same line it described when the load was increasing. The plot exhibits hysteresis (Fig. 2.10). When the stress reaches zero, the strain does not return to zero, as it did in the elastic deformation case. The permanent deformation is known as **inelastic,** or **plastic, deformation.** A material deforms plastically when it does not return to its original shape when the load is removed. It is quite easy to demonstrate plastic deformation (e.g., by bending a paperclip).

When a material begins to deform plastically, the material has **yielded.** The point on the stress–strain graph where the bend and plastic deformation begin is called the **yield point,** or **elastic limit.** The stress at which the material begins to deform plastically is called the **yield strength.** It is important to reiterate that once a material has exceeded its yield strength, it is permanently deformed, and it will *not* recover to its original shape. This introduces an interesting twist to the concept of "failure." It is easy to say that a broken piece of

HOOKE'S LAW

The general form of Hooke's law is three equations, one for each direction (x, y, z):

$$\varepsilon_x = \frac{1}{E}(\sigma_x - \nu(\sigma_y + \sigma_z))$$

$$\varepsilon_y = \frac{1}{E}(\sigma_y - \nu(\sigma_x + \sigma_z))$$

$$\varepsilon_z = \frac{1}{E}(\sigma_z - \nu(\sigma_x + \sigma_y))$$

where ε_x, ε_y, and ε_z are the strains in the x, y, and z directions; σ_x, σ_y, and σ_z are the stresses in the x, y, and z directions; and E is the Young's modulus. There are analogous relationships between shear stress (τ) and shear strain (γ), also part of Hooke's law:

$$\gamma_{xy} = \frac{\tau_{xy}}{G}$$

$$\gamma_{yz} = \frac{\tau_{yz}}{G}$$

$$\gamma_{xz} = \frac{\tau_{xz}}{G}$$

where γ_{ij} is the shear strain on an i-facing surface in the j direction, τ_{ij} is the shear stress on an i-facing surface in the j direction (figure), and G is called the *shear modulus* (analogous to the Young's modulus). The shear modulus, Young's modulus, and Poisson's ratio are related by

$$G = \frac{E}{2(1 + \nu)}$$

where G is the shear modulus, E is the Young's modulus, and ν is Poisson's ratio.

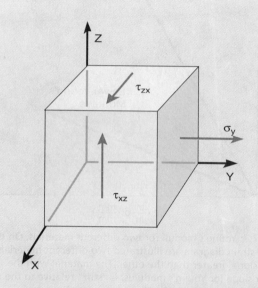

Shear stresses. Shear stresses are designated by two subscripts (e.g., τ_{xy}), where the first subscript indicates the face on which the shear stress is acting, and the second subscript indicates the direction in which it is acting. Officially, in mechanics, the normal stresses also have two subscripts. The equations use a frequently adopted shorthand: the normal stress in the y direction, which is designated σ_y, is more correctly written as σ_{yy}, which indicates that the stress is acting on an "y" face in a y direction.

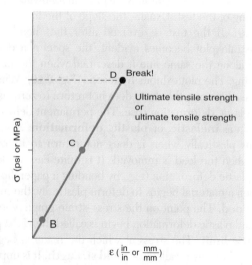

Figure 2.8: Brittle failure. One scenario for the failure of the test specimen illustrated in Figures 2.4 and 2.5. is that with a continued increase in load on the specimen, the specimen breaks at point D. Note that the stress–strain relationship remains linear. Point D represents the ultimate tensile strength of the material.

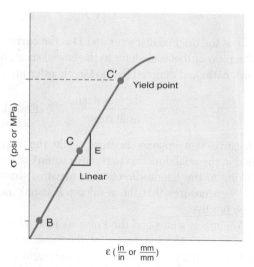

Figure 2.9: Yield. Another scenario for failure of the test specimens illustrated in Figures 2.4 and 2.5 is that the material's behavior is linear until point C'. At point C', the yield point, the stress–strain relationship is no longer linear, although the material does not break.

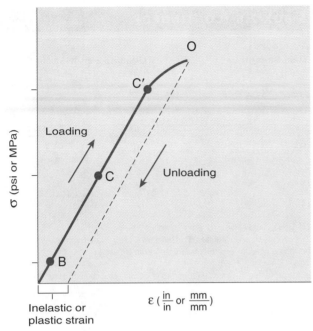

Figure 2.10: Permanent deformation. After the stress in the specimen has passed point C′, say to point O, the load is removed from the specimen. When there is no load on the specimen, there is still a measurable strain; the specimen has not returned to its original shape and is permanently deformed. The onset of inelastic or plastic strain at point C′ identifies C′ as the yield point (or yield stress) of the material.

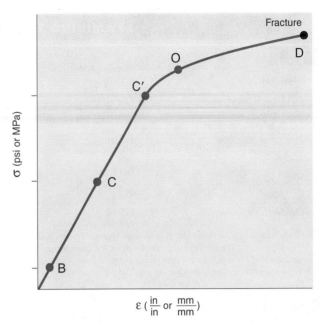

Figure 2.11: Ductile failure. After the specimen yields, with a continued increase in the applied load, the specimen eventually fractures (point D). Because the specimen yields before fracture, this is an example of a ductile fracture. For this ductile material, point D represents the ultimate tensile strength.

metal has "failed" when it has exceeded its ultimate tensile strength and is in two pieces. However, a material need not be in two pieces to fail. Engineers speak of a failure when the part or material no longer functions as it was designed. So, for example, if a bridge were made of a material that yielded a little every time a person walks over it, say an inch or two, eventually that bridge may yield all the way into the water! The bridge is no longer functioning as designed (i.e., to keep feet dry as people walk over the water), and therefore the bridge fails because of excessive yielding. If sharks are in the water, then the point is even clearer.

When the tensile test is continued, and the specimen is pulled beyond its yield point, eventually the specimen will break. The breaking point, again, is sometimes called the

ultimate strength, even though the material has yielded before reaching its breaking point (*Fig. 2.11*). *Box 2.6* provides comparisons of some material properties, including ultimate strength of several materials.

Figures 2.8 and 2.11 illustrate two ways that a material can behave before it breaks. The first is that the deformation before fracture is all elastic (Fig. 2.8). If there is no plastic deformation before the material breaks, then that material's behavior is **brittle.** Notice that only the material's *behavior* is described as brittle; the *material* itself is not brittle. Some will not worry about the distinction, but it is important. If the material deforms plastically before it breaks, that is, it yields first (Fig. 2.11), then the material's behavior is **ductile.** Everyday materials with brittle behavior include glass, concrete, and ceramic coffee mugs. If a material's behavior is not brittle, then it is ductile; the only question is one of degree. One interesting point is that for almost all materials, temperature plays a big role in

---

EXAMINING THE FORCES BOX 2.6

PROPERTIES OF DIFFERENT MATERIALS

A given material property varies over a considerable range. This should be no surprise, however. The reader has likely handled many different materials, even in the past week. We notice, for instance, that items made from plastics (e.g., a CD jewel case or plastic drinking cup) are light and somewhat flexible, while items made from metal (e.g., a hammer) are heavier and tend to be less flexible. The table lists some

common materials and their Young's moduli and yield strengths. Students should make use of the given data to perform a valuable exercise: On a single sheet of graph paper (or using a computer program) plot the stress-strain behavior of the materials in the table up to their yield strengths. Note the differences in yield strengths. The graphic representation may help to build an appreciation for the differences in material behaviors.

(Continued)

EXAMINING THE FORCES BOX 2.6 (CONTINUED)

Material	Young's Modulus (GPa)	Yield Strength (MPa)	Ultimate Tensile Strength (MPa)
2014-T4 Al alloy[a]	73	324	469
Cortical bone[b]	17–20 (compressive)	182	195
304 L stainless steel[a]	193	206	517
Ti6Al4V[a]	114	965	1103
Gold[c]	75	207	220
Tungsten[a]	407	(1,516)[e]	1,516
PMMA (bone cement)[d]	2.0	(40)[e]	40

[a]From Budinski KG, Budinski MK: Engineering Materials, Properties and Selection, 6th ed. Upper Saddle River, NJ: Prentice Hall, 1999.
[b]From Cowin SC: The mechanical properties of cortical bone tissue. In: Bone Mechanics. Cowin SC, ed. Boca Raton, FL: CRC Press, 1989. Note that the measured
  properties of bone vary widely, depending on age of bone, method of testing, etc., and the numbers given are "reasonable" example values.
[c]From Properties of Some Metals and Alloys, 3rd ed, a publication of the International Nickel Company, 1968.
[d]Values are approximate and are based on the summary of different experimental measures presented in Lewis G: Properties of acrylic bone cement: state of the
  art review. J Biomed Mater Res Appl Biomater 1997; 38: 155–182.
[e]Brittle (no yield before fracture).

whether the behavior is brittle or ductile. Many readers have witnessed the demonstration in which a bouncy ball is placed into liquid nitrogen, after which it no longer bounces. Instead it shatters when it is dropped! Materials undergo a **ductile–brittle transition** at a specific temperature. Thus, a material that shows ductile behavior in the laboratory may be brittle in outer space. A material that appears to be brittle in the laboratory may be ductile at body temperature.

MATERIAL FRACTURE

Fracture Toughness

An in-depth discussion on the fracture of materials is beyond the scope of this book, but this section introduces some of the more important concepts. For several reasons, it is difficult to quantify the fracture properties of a material from the tension-test data. In the middle of the 20th century, around the 1940s–1950s, people noticed, for example, that large ships split apart while sitting in the harbor, even though they were not loaded past their yield point. Seeing a big ship split in the harbor probably made quite an impression, and people who questioned why this occurred created a branch of mechanics called **fracture mechanics.** From fracture mechanics came the concept of **fracture toughness.** Fracture toughness is analogous to the ultimate tensile strength of a material but really is a measure of how fracture resistant a material is *if a small crack or flaw already exists*. Fracture toughness can be determined by experiments similar to the tensile test, which are discussed only briefly here. It is interesting that the units of ultimate tensile stress or yield stress are the same as those for stress, for example, pounds per square inch (psi) or mega-pascals (MPa; where one pascal = one newton/meter²). The units for fracture toughness are in psi (inches)$^{1/2}$ or MPa (m)$^{1/2}$. The square root of length appears because the fracture toughness depends on the length of the crack in the material.

It turns out that the longer the starting crack, the less force is necessary to break the material.

Another way to quantify the fracture strength of a material is by using the impact test. The most common is called the **Charpy impact test** (*Fig. 2.12*). In the Charpy test, a heavy pendulum is released with the specimen in its path. The pendulum swings through, and presumably breaks, the specimen. The difference in the starting height and the final height of the pendulum represents an energy loss. That energy loss is the energy that is needed to break the specimen. The fracture strength from a Charpy test is given in energy units, such

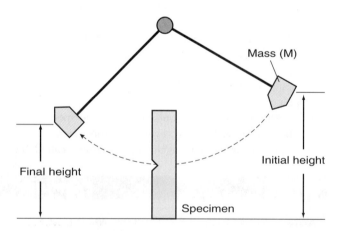

Potential energy = mgh

Energy loss from fracture
= mg (initial height − final height)

Figure 2.12: The Charpy impact test. In the Charpy impact test, a mass on a pendulum is raised to some initial height (and thus has an initial potential energy, mass × acceleration due to gravity × height). The pendulum is released and swings through an arc that brings it into contact with the test specimen, causing it to fracture. The final height of the specimen (and thus the final potential energy) can be measured. The difference in potential energy is equal to the energy absorbed by the specimen as it fractures.

as newton-meters or joules. A Charpy impact test, for example, can provide useful information on whether a bone breaks under a certain impact.

Fatigue

Another common word found in the engineering failure dictionary is "fatigue." A person who is tired is said to be "fatigued." Fatigue fracture is a type of material fracture that potentially can be very dangerous, because it can sneak up unexpectedly. Consider the example of a paper clip discussed earlier. Although the paper clip cannot be pulled apart, it eventually breaks after repeated bending. This is a form of fatigue. **Fatigue fracture** occurs when a material is loaded and unloaded, loaded and unloaded, repeatedly, and the maximum loads are below the ultimate tensile strength or yield strength. When a paper clip is bent a lot, it stays bent, and thus it has yielded. Fatigue can occur at loads above or below yield. Fatigue failure is harder to quantify than any of the behaviors discussed so far. It is difficult to identify an intensive material property for fatigue failure. One property that may be of interest is called the **fatigue, or endurance, limit.** For a given test setup, the endurance limit is defined as the stress below which the material will never fail in fatigue. For example, a paper clip can withstand countless small back and forth bends. If the bending is increased, however, the paper clip breaks. Somewhere between "a lot" and "a little" is the endurance limit. Life is complicated more, because some materials appear to have no endurance limit, and some materials appear to have an endurance limit under certain conditions. The fatigue behavior of a material, including the endurance limit, depends on many variables such as temperature, which determines whether the material's behavior is brittle or ductile.

Another factor that controls the failure of a material that is loaded so that the maximum stress is lower than the yield or fracture stress is the initial (or nominal) maximum stress. The **nominal maximum stress** is the maximum stress at the start of a fatigue test, before any damage occurs to a specimen. In general, the higher the nominal stress, the sooner the material fails. An S–N curve (S, nominal maximum stress; N, number of loading cycles to failure; bending the paperclip in the previous example once, back and forth, is considered one cycle) is one graphic tool that researchers use to understand how the initial load affects the life of a material in fatigue (*Fig. 2.13*).

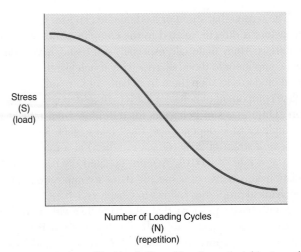

Figure 2.13: Fatigue life. The fatigue life of a material is strongly influenced by the loads (and thus the stresses) applied to the material. The higher the stress, the shorter the fatigue life, or the fewer cycles needed for failure.

LOADING RATE

Many materials behave differently if they are loaded at different rates. **Stress rates** may be given in psi/second or megapascals/second. **Strain rates** may be given as either a pure frequency, per second, or in units such as inch/inch/second or millimeter/millimeter/second. In general, the faster a material is loaded, the more brittle it behaves. Anyone who has played with modeling clay, Silly Putty® or even bread dough has experienced this. When the clay is pulled apart rapidly, it seems to snap apart. When it is pulled apart slowly, it sags, and extends for quite a while before breaking. Another illustration is putting a hand in water. When the palm of the hand is slapped rapidly on the water, it stings as if hitting concrete. Put a hand in slowly, and the water moves readily out of the way. Most structural materials, like steel and concrete, behave the same way regardless of the strain rate. Polymers and many soft (biological) tissues, on the other hand, are sensitive to strain rate. In this case, *sensitive* means that the materials behave differently under different loading conditions. It is especially important to realize this in the context of injuries, for example, bone fracture or ligament injuries. Chapters 3 and 6 discuss this issue for bone and ligaments, respectively.

Clinical Relevance

STRESS FRACTURES: *Biological tissues exhibit fatigue failure. Repeated loadings that generate stresses less than the ultimate tensile stress may lead to fatigue failures; when this occurs in bone, the injury is referred to as a stress fracture. The term **stress fracture** is really a misnomer, since the reader has, by now, learned that all fractures are caused by stress, in the language of engineering mechanics. Thus, the clinical stress fracture may be better termed* subcritical fatigue damage.

Clinical Relevance

LOADING RATES: *Fast or slow strain rates can lead to different types of injury. For example, some ligaments fail under very high loading rates, while the bone where the ligament attaches fails at lower loading rates. Low loading rates appear to produce avulsion fractures at the bone–ligament interface, while high loading rates produce failures in the central portions of ligaments. The type of tissue damaged or the kind of injury sustained is useful in explaining the mechanism of injury. Biomechanics experts are often called as "expert witnesses" in trials to establish the mechanism of injury in personal injury cases.*

The reason that strain or loading rate can lead to different behaviors is directly related to the complex structure of the materials. Many materials, especially soft tissue, have a fluid-like component to their behavior, very much like the dampers used on doors to keep them from banging into walls. The fluidlike component of behavior leads to time-dependent behaviors. Differences in behaviors for different strain rates is an example of time dependence, for it takes much less time to achieve a strain of 20% (or 0.2 mm/mm) at a rate of 0.05/s than at a rate of 0.001/s. A more detailed discussion of the relationships between a specific tissue's composition and its mechanical properties follows in Chapters 3–6.

Fluids have a property that all are familiar with, informally known as "gooeyness," formally known as **viscosity.** Fluids with a high viscosity (e.g., honey) flow slowly. Fluids with a lower viscosity (e.g., water) flow quickly. Ice at the bottom of a glacier, under the tremendous weight of all the ice on top, acts like an extremely viscous fluid, perhaps moving only a few inches per year. Therefore, solids that have time-dependent mechanical behaviors, because of a fluidlike component, are **viscoelastic.** The simplest models of viscoelastic behaviors in materials contain a single elastic element, such as a spring, and a viscous element, represented by a dashpot (the damper on the door), either in series (lined up one after another, the "Maxwell model") or in parallel (lined up next to each other, the "Kelvin-Voigt model") (*Fig. 2.14*). The

viscoelastic nature of materials leads to two important and related behaviors, **creep** and **stress relaxation.**

Creep is the continued deformation of a material over time as the material is subjected to a constant load. The simplest illustration of creep is a cylindrical material loaded with a fixed weight applied in the axial direction for a long time. Initially, the weight creates a stress in the material, and the material deforms according to the elastic strain. Because the material in this case is viscoelastic, the material continues to deform and stretch over time, usually very slowly. In creep experiments, a fixed load is maintained on the specimen, and the strain is measured as a function of time. The slow, steady closing of a door with a damper is an example of creep. The door (and possibly the door spring) applies a constant force on the damper. The damper slowly deforms and allows the door to close.

The complementary experiment to the creep experiment is the stress relaxation test. *Stress relaxation* is the reduction of stress within a material over time as the material is subjected to a constant deformation. For the stress relaxation test, instead of applying a fixed load to the specimen, a fixed displacement, or strain, is maintained, and the resisting force (from which stress is calculated) is measured as a function of time. Stress generally decreases with time and hence the label "relaxation." Both creep and stress relaxation are important behaviors in biological soft tissue.

A. The Maxwell Model

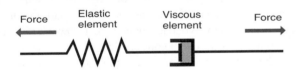

B. The Kelvin-Voigt Model

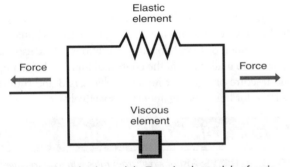

Figure 2.14: Viscoelastic models. Two simple models of a viscoelastic material behavior. **A.** In the Maxwell model the viscous element, or dashpot, is in series with the spring. The displacement of the dashpot does not recover like that of the spring does. When the load is removed, the spring returns to its original position, but the dashpot does not, and thus there is permanent or plastic deformation of the model. **B.** In the Kelvin-Voigt model, the spring and dashpot are in parallel. When the load is removed, the spring recovers, and pulls the dashpot back with it; there is no plastic deformation. In each case, the deformation of the dashpot depends on the loading rate.

BENDING AND TORSION

Bending

Many bones act as structural beams in the body. Thus, they are subjected to various forces, like beams, and may be analyzed as beams. Beams that are used in bridges or buildings that are oriented vertically often are subjected to compressive loads. The beams that are oriented horizontally, however, are often loaded at or near the midspan and are subjected to **bending.** Most readers have, for example, broken a stick by bending it.

EXAMINING THE FORCES BOX 2.7

THE BEAM BENDING EQUATION

For a beam of single material (concrete, steel, or bone, for example), the stresses generated by pure bending of a beam may be calculated from

$$\sigma = \frac{My}{I}$$

where σ is the stress calculated at position y, M is the applied bending moment, and I is the moment inertia (a function of the beam's cross-sectional area).

What is most amazing about the formula for stress in a beam subjected to bending is that *material properties are absent!* (*Box 2.7*) This means that for a beam of concrete, steel, or bone, if the cross section has the same geometry and the applied loads are the same, the stresses are exactly the same. Thus, the difference in behavior of beams is largely controlled by the Young's modulus (to determine how much the beam will deform) and by the failure strength of the material. Another interesting result of beam analysis is that there is an axis along which there is no stress, called the **neutral axis.** Stresses on one side of the neutral axis are compressive and on the opposite side, tensile. For beams with symmetric cross-sectional geometries, the neutral axis is through the center of the beam. *Box 2.8* calculates the stresses in a beam subjected to bending and uses the calculation to determine the stress in the ulna when lifting a 5-lb load.

Torsion

This section considers torsion of a cylinder. The treatment of torsion for cross sections that are not cylindrical is beyond the scope of this text. Torsion of cylinders, however, is directly applicable to the torsion in long bones, where the cross section can be approximated as a cylinder. In torsion, a torque, or twisting, is applied to the beam instead of a bending moment (*Box 2.9*). Torsion generates shear stresses in a beam, and the equation to calculate the shear stress is directly analogous to the bending equation.

EXAMINING THE FORCES BOX 2.8

WILL THE ULNA BREAK WHEN "BENT" BY LIFTING A LOAD?

To determine whether a beam fails under a bending moment, consider only the maximum value of y, the distance from the neutral axis (Fig. A). For a beam with a rectangular cross section, the maximum value is $h/2$ or one half the beam's height. For a beam with a circular cross section, the maximum value is r, the radius of the beam. Using the formulas shown in the figure, the maximum stress in a beam with a rectangular cross section is $6M/(b \times h^2)$, and in a beam with a circular cross section is $4M/(\pi \times r^3)$.

Results calculated elsewhere in this textbook (Chapter 13) can be used to estimate the stresses in one of the forearm bones (e.g., in the midshaft of the ulna). Assume that the ulna can be modeled as a beam with a circular cross section (albeit hollow) (Fig. B), with an outer radius of r_o and an inner radius of r_i. Chapter 13 (Box 13.2), reports an *internal moment* of 13.4 Nm; that is, the moment that exists within the bone material to resist external forces (lifting a 5-lb load) and keep the bone in equilibrium, is 13.4 Nm. Box 2.7 demonstrates calculation of the stresses in a beam under a bending moment. For a beam with a circular cross section, like the model of the ulna, the neutral axis is the geometric center of the beam. Therefore, the maximum stress occurs at $y = r_o$, the distance farthest from the neutral axis. The bending moment, M, is 13.4 Nm. The only information that is missing is the moment of inertia of the ulna, I_{ulna}. To calculate I for a hollow circle, first calculate I for the bone as if it were a solid cylinder, and then subtract I for the inner hollow circle. Thus,

$$I_{outer\ circle} = \frac{\pi (r_o)^4}{4}$$

$$I_{inner\ circle} = \frac{\pi (r_i)^4}{4}$$

$$I_{ulna} = I_{outer\ circle} - I_{inner\ circle} = \frac{\pi (r_o)^4}{4} - \frac{\pi (r_i)^4}{4}$$

$$= \frac{\pi}{4}[(r_o)^4 - (r_i)^4]$$

Now it is easy to calculate I_{ulna} for any values of r_o and r_i. For the sake of this example, assume that the outer radius is 25 mm (0.025 m), and the inner radius is 20 mm (0.020 m). Hence, $I_{ulna} = 180 \times 10^{-9}$ m^4. Apply the equation in Box 2.7 to find

$$\sigma = \frac{13.4\ Nm \times (0.025\ m)}{180 \times 10^{-9} m^4}$$

$$= 185 \times 10^6\ N/m^2,\ or\ 1.85\ Mpa.$$

Recall that in a beam subjected to bending, one side of the beam is in compression and the other is in tension. Comparison of the calculated stress value with the strength values listed in the table in Box 2.6 clearly shows that the stress in the ulna is well below the yield or ultimate tensile stress of bone. This is, of course, a good thing and what is expected, since people rarely break their ulnas when lifting a 5-lb bag of sugar!

(Continued)

EXAMINING THE FORCES BOX 2.8 (CONTINUED)

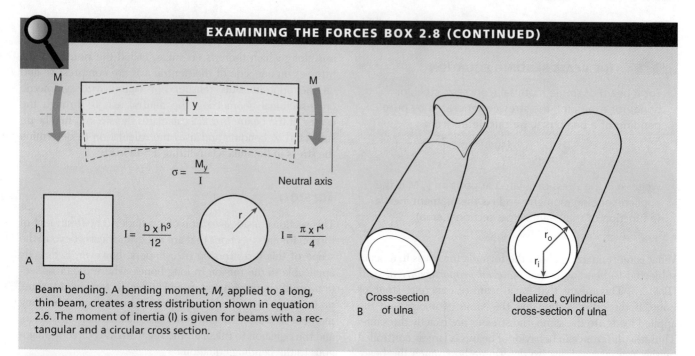

$$\sigma = \frac{My}{I}$$

$$I = \frac{b \times h^3}{12}$$

$$I = \frac{\pi \times r^4}{4}$$

Beam bending. A bending moment, *M,* applied to a long, thin beam, creates a stress distribution shown in equation 2.6. The moment of inertia (I) is given for beams with a rectangular and a circular cross section.

A   Cross-section of ulna
B

Idealized, cylindrical cross-section of ulna

EXAMINING THE FORCES BOX 2.9

SHEAR STRESSES IN A BEAM SUBJECTED TO TORSION

The shear stress in a beam that is subjected to torsion or "twisting" is calculated from:

$$\tau = \frac{Tr}{J}$$

where the shear stress, τ, is calculated at radius *r, T* is the applied torque, or twist, and J is the polar moment of inertia.

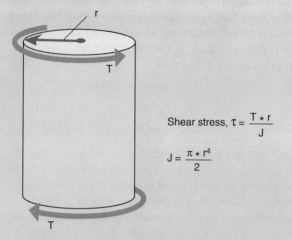

Shear stress, $\tau = \frac{T \star r}{J}$

$$J = \frac{\pi \star r^4}{2}$$

A torque T twisting a cylinder creates a shear stress distribution shown in the equation. The polar moment of inerta (J) is for the cylindrical cross-section.

Clinical Relevance

BENDING VERSUS TORSION FRACTURES: *Many bone fractures occur because of either excessive bending or torsion on the bone. For example, a torsional fracture may occur during a skiing accident if a ski is caught, say, on a tree, and the bindings do not release. The momentum of the skier causes the body to spin, thus applying torsion to the bone. Depending on the speed at which the torsion is applied, this may result in a complex "spiral" fracture or an even more serious shattering of the bone. If a bone breaks under bending loads, however, the fracture is likely to be a simpler, linear-type fracture. Another common skiing injury, a boot-top fracture, occurs with a bending load as the skier tumbles forward over a relatively motionless ski and the tibia "bends" over the stationary boot.*

SUMMARY

This chapter discusses the basic definitions of intensive (e.g., density) and extensive (e.g., volume) material properties. Using an example of a simple tension test, some of the most important material properties are defined in the language of mechanics of materials: tensile or compressive modulus (modulus of elasticity, or Young's modulus), Poisson's ratio, ultimate tensile strength, yield point and yield strength, endurance limit, and fracture toughness. The simple tension test also allows the introduction of the concepts of load and deformation, stress and strain, materials testing, and brittle versus ductile behavior. Additional concepts that are important to understanding the behavior of biological materials include fatigue failure, beam bending, torsion, and loading rate (viscoelasticity). The properties specific to biological materials such as bone, tendons, and ligaments are discussed in detail in the appropriate chapters.

Additional Reading

Beer FP, Johnston ER: Mechanics of Materials, 2nd ed. New York: McGraw-Hill, 1992.

Gere JM, Timoshenko SP: Mechanics of Materials, 4th ed. Boston: PWS Publishing, 1997.

Panjabi MM, White AA III. Biomechanics in the Musculoskeletal System. New York: Churchill Livingstone, 2001.

Popov EP: Mechanics of Materials, 2nd ed. Englewood Cliffs, NJ: Prentice Hall, 1976.

Ruoff AL: Materials Science. Englewood Cliffs, NJ: Prentice Hall, 1973.

CHAPTER 3

Biomechanics of Bone

L.D. TIMMIE TOPOLESKI, PH.D.

All living organisms have a strategy for supporting and protecting their bodies' parts. Marine invertebrates like the jellyfish rely on the balance of the internal and external water pressure for support. A jellyfish out of water is really pretty much a blob of jelly (as readers who are beach walkers have witnessed). Insects, lobsters, and other small skittering creatures may make use of an external or exoskeleton (a hard outer layer composed of chitin in many cases) to give support and keep their insides in. Biomechanically, an exoskeleton does not work for larger animals; the animals and their organs get too heavy. Larger land-dwelling animals are equipped with the familiar endoskeleton (or internal skeleton) for support. The skeleton in the human body provides support for the body, acts as a rigid system of levers that transfer forces from muscles, and provides protection for vital organs (e.g., the skull for the brain and the ribcage for the heart and thoracic organs). There are also some curious little bones in the ears of some animals (including humans) that are needed to transmit sound to enable hearing.

Chapter 2 introduced the reader to the language and principles needed to understand the general mechanical behavior of materials. This chapter discusses the structural and support aspects of bone, providing information on the mechanical properties of bone as a specific material. The purposes of this chapter are to

- Briefly review basic bone biology and terminology
- Describe mechanical properties of human bone
- Discuss the clinical relevance of understanding bone properties

Research on the mechanical properties of bone continues. The review provided in this chapter is meant to offer the reader only an introductory understanding of bone's mechanical properties. The mechanical properties of bone are not nearly as well understood as those of the engineering materials mentioned in Chapter 2; bone is more complex than steel, for example. Many of the references cited are perhaps "old" in the context of the relatively young field of biomedical engineering. In the case of bone, however, old does not mean "invalid." Much of the original work from the 1970s and 1980s is still valuable to students, clinicians, and researchers in biomechanics. The more recent work on the mechanical properties of bone involves details of bone behavior that are beyond the scope of this book, for example numerical models of the micromechanics of bone remodeling, or investigating the complex interactions within a network of trabeculae [e.g., 7,10,12,17,19]. Indeed, it would require a substantial monograph to justly review all of the work on bone properties. Readers who are interested in a specific aspect of bone behavior are encouraged to consult the primary literature.

BRIEF REVIEW OF BONE BIOLOGY, STRUCTURE, AND CHEMICAL COMPOSITION

The mechanical properties of bone are determined primarily by the structural components of bone. Bone contains two principal structural components: **collagen** and **hydroxyapatite** (HA). Collagen is an organic material that is found in all of the body's connective tissue (see Chapters 5 and 6). Organic components of bone make up approximately 40% of the bone's dry weight, and collagen is responsible for about 90% of bone's organic content. The collagen in bone is primarily **type I** collagen (bone = b + *one*, or I). Other types of collagen are found in other connective tissues; for example, types II, IX, and X are known as *cartilage-specific collagens* because they seem to be found only in cartilage [6]. An excellent research project for the reader is to determine the number of different types of collagen and where they are all located.

The inorganic, or mineral, components make up approximately 60% of the bone's dry weight. The primary mineral component is HA, which is a calcium phosphate–based mineral: $Ca_{10}(PO_4)_6(OH)_2$. The HA crystals are found primarily between the collagen fibers. HA is related to, but distinct from, the Ca minerals found in marine corals (they are calcium carbonates). Pure HA is a ceramic and can be found in crystal form as a mineral (e.g., apatite). Because HA is a ceramic, bone can be expected to have ceramic-like properties. For example, ceramics are generally brittle, tolerating little deformation before fracture. Ceramics and bone are also relatively strong in compression but weak in tension.

The structure of human bone changes with age. The bone in children is different from the bone in adults. Immature bone is composed of **woven bone.** In woven bone, the cartilage fibers are more or less randomly distributed (as they are in skin). The random distribution of fibers gives some strength in all directions (i.e., no preferred direction), but woven bone is not as strong as mature bone. Woven bone of children is also more flexible than adult bone, presumably to provide resilience for all the falls and tumbles of childhood.

As bone matures, cells in the bone, called *osteoclasts*, essentially dig tunnels in the bone. Other cells, called *osteoblasts*, line the tunnels with type I collagen. The collagen is then mineralized with HA. The mineralization may be controlled by cells called *osteocytes*, which are "older" osteoblasts that have been trapped in the collagen matrix. The osteocytes play a role in controlling the extracellular calcium and phosphorus. The result of all the osteoclast, osteoblast, and osteocyte activity is a series of tubes, called haversian canals, which are lined with layers of bone (**lamellae**) and are oriented in the primary load-bearing direction of the bone (e.g., along the long axis of a femur). The haversian canals, also known as *osteons*, represent the structural units of bone. The hollow osteons are also passageways for blood vessels and nerves in the bone. Other passageways, which tend to be perpendicular to the haversian canals, called *Volkmann's canals*, allow the blood vessels to connect across the bone and form a network throughout the bone (*Fig. 3.1*) [3,8,13].

The first set of osteons to develop in mature bone are called the *primary osteons*. Throughout life, however, the osteoclasts/blasts/cytes remain active, and new haversian canals are constantly formed. The new osteons are formed on top of the old and are called *secondary osteons*. Haversian canals are formed by secondary osteons.

Once the woven bone has been replaced by the system of osteons, the bone is considered mature. There are two primary types of mature human bone: **cortical bone** and **cancellous bone.** Cortical bone (also known as *compact bone*) is hard, dense bone. Cancellous bone (also known as *spongy* or *trabecular bone*) is not as dense as cortical bone

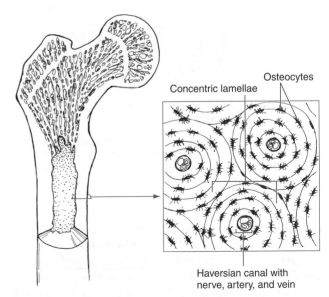

Figure 3.1: Schematic drawing showing the microstructural organization of bone.

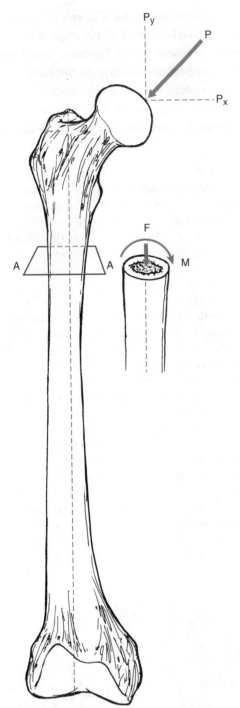

Figure 3.2: Schematic drawing of a femur, a "long bone" of the body. The force (*P*) applied to the femur through the joint is offset from the center line of the bone's long axis. The offset creates bending moments (*M*) in the bone.

bone is determined only by static loading" [13]. Today, it is clear that dynamic loading of bone plays an important, if not pivotal, role in the bone' s structure. Thus, Nigg and Grimston suggest restating Wolff's Law as "Physical laws are a major factor influencing bone modeling and remodeling. [13]" A less formal, though perhaps more elegant and to the point, statement of Wolff's law is "Form follows function."

Most readers are familiar with the general shape of a long bone, such as a human femur or tibia (*Fig. 3.2*). Where two bones connect and rub against each other, the bone is coated with articular cartilage, which allows very low friction articulation at the **joints** (where two bones come together). Note that not all joints are mobile; for example, the bones of the skull are not supposed to move relative to each other. In children, the bone grows from the ends out, in the **metaphysis** and **epiphysis.** The regions where bone actually grows are called *growth plates*. If a child's growth plate is damaged, the bone may stop growing altogether and will not reach a normal length.

The previous description of bone structure and biology gives only the briefest introduction to allow readers to become familiar with some of the language and architecture of bone. Readers are urged to investigate one or more of the references at the end of this chapter to learn more of the details of bone.

MECHANICAL PROPERTIES OF BONE

The mechanical properties of bone vary with both the type of bone (e.g., cancellous vs. cortical) and with the location of the bone (e.g., rib vs. femur). Because of the wide variety of properties, there is no "standard value" for the strength or elastic modulus of bone, for example. The analysis and examination of bone mechanics thus requires that the student or investigator research the unique properties of the specific bones that are in question. Knowing only a few of the fundamental properties of bone, however, it is possible to predict general behavior, since the focus here is the structural function of bone.

In a general sense, the important properties of a particular bone may be deduced by carefully considering the bone's function(s). For example, the femur carries all of the body's weight during each step a person makes while walking. The weight comes largely from above, so the bone must be both stiff (high Young's modulus) and strong in compression in the direction of the long axis. The bone must be stiff so that for each step, the bone does not compress like a spring. Bone would be an ineffective structural material if, for each step taken, the legs shortened by an inch or two. Bone would also be ineffective if, when loaded more severely than it is loaded in standard walking (e.g., in running or jumping), the bone fractured or was crushed in compression. Examination of the femur's functional demands reveals that the bone must be strong in compression. However, if most of the apparent load is compressive, must bone also resist tension? Ultimately, how strong does bone need to be?

Biomechanical studies of joint forces show that the force on the femur varies with activity. For example, simply standing on

and is filled with spaces. The bone between the spaces can be thought of as small beams that are called *trabeculae*. Cortical bone is found, for example, in the midshaft of the femur, and cancellous bone is found in the interior of the femoral head. In the late 19th century, Wolff observed that bone, especially cancellous bone, is oriented to resist the primary forces to which bone is subjected. Wolff suggested that "the shape of

one leg can result in a force on the femur of 1.8–2.7 times body weight. Leg lifting in bed can result in a force of 1.5 times body weight, and walking at a fairly good pace can exert a force of up to 6.9 times body weight [1]! But, an individual weighs only one body weight, so where does this "extra" weight come from? Chapter 1 explains the analytical approach to determining the forces in the muscles applied to the joints during activity. That chapter reveals that muscles with their small moment arms must generate large forces to balance the large moments produced by external loads such as body weight. Figure 3.2 demonstrates that the femoral head is offset medially from the centerline of the femoral shaft. The offset implies that mechanical moments are applied to the bone (by muscles) to balance the body. Dynamic activities like walking and running demand even larger muscle moments because the body is accelerating. Chapter 48 discusses the forces generated during normal locomotion. The additional moments from the muscles result in increased joint forces. So, a bone is required not only to support the body weight, but also to sustain loads that are potentially several times the body weight during normal activity.

The preceding discussion reveals that the femur must withstand large compression loads. The femur also helps illustrate why bone must withstand tensile loads. Because the load on the femoral head is off center, (eccentric), the offset creates a bending moment in the bone. In Chapter 2, the equation in Box 2.7 shows that an applied bending moment creates both compression and tension in a beam or bone. Thus, according to mechanical principles, the stresses in the bone are determined by the superposition (addition) of the compressive and bending loads. On the medial side of the femur, for example, the compressive axial load and compressive bending loads add, so that stresses are predominantly compressive. On the lateral side, in contrast, the compressive axial loads and the tensile bending loads are opposite, and tensile stresses may occur. Under particularly intense loading conditions (e.g., a skiing accident), the tensile forces on a bone may be substantial and indeed can lead to fracture. Depending on the type of accident, torsional forces that are generated can also lead to severe fractures. Thus, bone must be able to withstand both compressive and tensile loads (as well as torsion).

Clinical Relevance

FRACTURES RESULTING FROM DIFFERENT KINDS OF LOADING: *Bones are subjected to different forms of loading and fail under different conditions. Long bones such as the tibia and femur sustain large compressive loads at the joint but commonly fail as the result of torsional forces, such as those applied to the tibia in a spiral fracture described in Chapter 2. Vertebral fractures, on the other hand, are more commonly the result of compressive forces on the vertebral body. Tensile forces produce avulsion fractures when ligaments or tendons are pulled away from their bony attachments.*

Material Properties versus Geometry

The mechanical response of materials used in building skyscrapers and bridges depends on their geometry. For example, the shape of a beam's cross section controls how much the beam deflects under a load. Beams with a circular cross section behave differently than I-beams of the same height, for example. The structural geometry of bone contributes to its mechanical response, and thus different bones have different shapes [11]. The long bones of the legs, for example, have cross sections that are roughly hollow cylinders. The cylindrical cross section allows a tibia, for example, to support bending forces approximately equally in any direction. An I-beam, on the other hand, is good at supporting bending loads when it is upright, but when it is sideways (like an "H"-beam), it does not support bending loads as well. Note the orientation of the steel beams the next time you pass under an overpass on the highway.

Anisotropy

Bone is an **anisotropic material;** it has different properties in different directions. The Young's modulus in the axial direction of the femur, for example, differs from the Young's modulus in the transverse direction (lateral to medial). Many common structural materials, like steel, are usually treated as **isotropic materials,** and a single value of Young's modulus or of yield stress is sufficient to analyze the deformation or failure characteristics respectively. Bone, however, like some other special anisotropic materials (e.g., wood), has a structure that gives rise to differences in the mechanical properties acting at right angles. Although the properties of bone are different in the longitudinal and transverse directions, it may not make any difference which transverse direction is chosen, the properties are nearly the same in all directions within the transverse plane (*Fig. 3.3*). Such a material is called

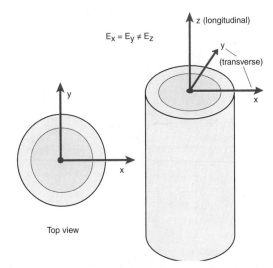

Figure 3.3: Bone can be considered a transversely isotropic material, which means that the properties, such as modulus of elasticity and ultimate strength, are the same in the *x* and *y* directions (and it makes no difference where those directions are assigned), but differ in the *z* direction.

EXAMINING THE FORCES BOX 3.1

AN EXPERIMENT TO DEMONSTRATE ANISOTROPIC BEHAVIOR

The concept of anisotropy, and more specifically, orthotropy, can be illustrated by a simple experiment. For this experiment, find six sheets of $8\frac{1}{2} \times 11$-in paper and some tape. Roll each piece of paper into a tube $8\frac{1}{2}$ in tall, and tape it so it stays rolled. Tape all six tubes together into a pyramid structure (*Fig. 3.4*). With the taped tubes standing on end, you can place your textbook or another book on top, and the tubes easily carry the weight. Next lay the tubes on their side, and place the book on top. The tubes collapse and are crushed by the weight of the book. The stiffness and the strength are different in the different directions, greater in the direction parallel to the length of the rolls than in the direction perpendicular to their lengths. Although the Young's modulus, or the strength of the paper itself, is a constant, when the paper has a distinct structure, similar to that of cortical bone, properties in directions that are at right angles to each other are different.

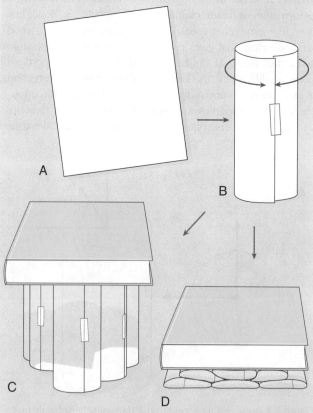

Figure 3.4: Demonstration of anisotropy. The strength of a bundle of tubes (B) is different if they are loaded from the top (C) or from the side (D).

transversely orthotropic (*Box 3.1*). A good first approximation for bone is that it is transversely orthotropic.

Stress and *strain* are defined in Chapter 2 as force per area and the ratio of the change in shape to the material's original shape, respectively. They are related by Hooke's law (Box 2.5). The relationship between stress and strain is called a **constitutive equation.** The constitutive equations for anisotropic or orthotropic materials are far more complex than equation 2.6. Two material property constants are required to relate stress and strain for an isotropic material: its stiffness, or Young's modulus, E, and a measure of the amount of bulging the material undergoes in compression, known as Poisson's ratio, v. For an anisotropic material, 21 material property constants are required to relate stress and strain! A general orthotropic material is a bit simpler, requiring 9 constants. For a transversely orthotropic material such as bone, only 5 constants are needed. *Only* is a relative term, of course. The constants can be evaluated only by careful experimentation; given the geometry of bone, however, such experiments can be quite difficult. Consequently, a complete description of bone's response to loading (i.e., the precise definition of the relationship between stress and strain in bone) is a complex analysis, beyond the scope of this text.

Elastic Constants of Bone

Since bone may be considered to be either orthotropic or transversely isotropic, we must define more than the two constants (the Young's modulus and Poisson's ratio) indicated in Box 2.5. In an elementary sense, a Young's modulus is required for each of the three primary directions: along the long axis, in the radial direction, and in the circumferential direction. For an excellent and more detailed summary of the work on mechanical properties of bone, see Cowin's book [5]. The Young's modulus along the long axis of either human or bovine cortical bone ranges from 17 to 27 GPa, and in the circumferential or radial directions, ranges from about 7 to 20 GPa. The transverse stiffnesses, therefore, are roughly half that of the longitudinal stiffness. To place these stiffnesses in a context familiar to the reader, the Young's modulus (*a*) of steel is approximately 200 GPa; (*b*) of the titanium alloy used in artificial joints (Ti6Al4V), approximately 115 GPa; (*c*) of aluminum, approximately 70 GPa; and (*d*) of acrylic, approximately 2 GPa. The elastic constants that correspond to the Poisson's ratio are more difficult to interpret and are not reported here.

The elastic constants of cancellous bone present an interesting challenge. The overall, or bulk, properties of a piece of cancellous bone depend on the structure, arrangement, and density of the component trabeculae. An individual trabecula, or beam of bone, may actually have properties close to those of cortical bone. When many small beams of bone are linked together, however, in a network like cancellous bone, the apparent properties change. Experimental studies suggest relationships, for example, between the compressive modulus and apparent (or measured) density of the material. Hayes gives a relationship for the compressive Young's modulus of cancellous bone (E) as

$$E = 2,915 \, \rho^3 \qquad \text{(Equation 3.1)}$$

where ρ is the apparent density [8]. Research on the elastic constants of both cortical and cancellous bone continues.

Strength

The ultimate strength of bone is also not represented by a single value. The reported values vary depending on the test method used and type of bone tested. The tensile strength of

cortical bone in the longitudinal direction varies from approximately 100 to 150 MPa or higher. The compressive strength in the longitudinal direction is greater than the tensile strength and varies from approximately 130 to 230 MPa or higher [5]. For comparison, the ultimate strength for a standard structural steel is approximately 400 MPa, for Ti6Al4V it is 900 MPa, and for bone cement it is approximately 25–40 MPa.

Fracture Toughness

Chapter 2 explains that fracture toughness is a measure of a material's ability to resist crack growth if a crack has already initiated. The reported values of fracture toughness vary (depending on the study, location of bone, methods, etc.) from about 3.3 to 6.4 MPa-m$^{1/2}$ [14,15,18]. The range of fracture toughnesses shows about a factor of 2 difference between the minimum and maximum reported values. It is difficult, therefore, to assign a single value of fracture toughness to bone, and the fracture toughness has not been measured for many bone locations. The relative magnitude (3–6 MPa-m$^{1/2}$) of bone's fracture toughness compared with that of other materials provides a useful perspective. The fracture toughness of bone is comparable, for example, to that of PMMA (like Plexiglas)® with a fracture toughness of about 1.5 MPa-m$^{1/2}$, or a ceramic like alumina (Al$_2$O$_3$, the basic mineral of ruby and sapphire) with a fracture toughness of 2.7–4.8 MPa-m$^{1/2}$. The fracture toughness of bone is low compared with that of aluminum alloys (20–30 MPa-m$^{1/2}$), steel (70–140 MPa-m$^{1/2}$), or titanium alloys (70–110 MPa-m$^{1/2}$). Cortical bone has a relatively low fracture toughness because it is brittle and does not easily absorb strain energy by deforming plastically. Thus, bone's fracture toughness is consistent with that of nonbiological ceramics.

Strain Rate

Not only are the material properties of bone different in different directions, but also the properties depend on the strain rate, or how fast the bone is loaded; that is, bone is viscoelastic. In general, both the modulus of elasticity and the strength of bone increase with loading rate. For example, models based on experimental results predict that the longitudinal elastic modulus of bone can vary by as much as 15% because of the differences in strain rates encountered in everyday activity [5]. The dependence of materials properties on strain rate may be one of the body's protective mechanisms; bone is able to withstand greater stresses during traumatic, rapid loading when needed. Recall that bone has two primary constituent materials: collagen and HA crystals. Collagen imparts the viscoelastic component to bone behavior (see Chapter 2). Bone's viscoelastic behavior is an example in which the behavior of bone differs from standard structural ceramics.

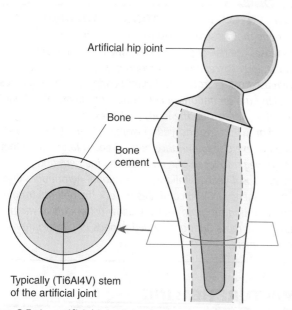

Artificial hip joint

Bone

Bone cement

Typically (Ti6Al4V) stem of the artificial joint

Figure 3.5: An artificial joint introduces several different materials into a bone. The system can no longer be modeled as a beam of homogeneous bone. The effects of the joint replacement stem and bone cement (if used) must be accounted for.

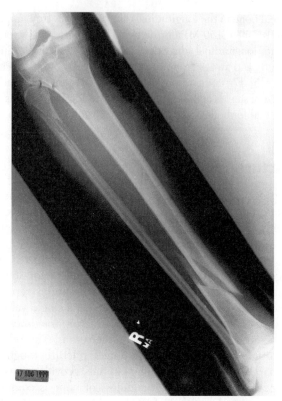

Figure 3.6: Torsional Fracture. The radiograph illustrates the typical spiral oblique fractures of the tibia and fibula resulting from a torsional injury such as a skiing accident.

Clinical Relevance

EFFECTS OF LOADING RATE IN BONE: *Skiers know that a fall comes quickly and suddenly. Most skiers are able to get up and continue to ski down the mountain after even seemingly horrendous falls. Part of the explanation is the viscoelastic property of bone, which allows bones to withstand larger loads when those loads are applied at a rapid rate. However, there are limits to such protection, and when the loads exceed the strength of the bone, the bone fractures. Many skiers sustain tibial fractures when they fall. Before the advent of modern binding release mechanisms, skiers catching their skis could subject their leg bones to rapid torsional loading (Fig. 3.6).*

Understanding how bone responds to different loading rates helps to explain the kind of fracture an individual sustains. Fractures resulting from extremely high velocity projectiles such as bullets are characterized by bony fragments from the shattered bone. Fractures from slower-velocity loading events such as falls typically consist of only two or three fragments.

CHANGES IN MECHANICAL PROPERTIES WITH AGE AND ACTIVITY

Both bone geometry and the fundamental material properties of bone appear to change with age, although the subject has not been studied in depth. In a study of bones between 35

and 92 years old, several of the mechanical properties tested decreased with age [21]. For example, the Young's modulus, predicted by a least squares linear curve fit to the experimental data, decreased by about 2.3% for every 10 years after age 35, beginning with a value of 15.2 GPa (which is reasonably consistent with values summarized by Cowin [5]). The resistance of bone to fracture, as measured by the fracture toughness, decreased with age at a rate of about 4% per 10 years (from 6.4 MPa-m$^{1/2}$), and the bending strength decreased by about 3.7% per 10 years (from 170 MPa) [21]. The decreases in properties may be the result of changes in the bone's mineral content or perhaps changes in the bone's structure. Additional studies are needed to fully understand how the mechanical properties of bone change with age.

Activity translates into increased loading on the bone. When bone is loaded or stressed, it tends to build up; bone becomes denser with use. When activity decreases and the loads on the bone decrease, the bone loses mass through remodeling [2]. One of the concerns with extended voyages in the low-gravity environment of space (e.g., human flights to Mars or long-term stays on a permanent space station) is that bone is not loaded as it is on Earth, and the bone mass decreases [4,9]. Investigators sometimes induce **osteoporosis,** or an osteoporotic state, by restricting bone loading or mimicking low gravity in experimental animal models [e.g., 16,20]. Osteoporosis is a disease or condition that is more common in older people. It is the loss of bone density caused by the failure of osteoblasts to lay down new bone in the holes created by osteoclasts. Osteoporosis is thought to be mediated by hormones, for example, in the case of postmenopausal women.

Clinical Relevance

PREVENTING AND TREATING OSTEOPOROSIS: *Loss of bone mass (osteoporosis) through inactivity or disease increases the risk of fractures. Postmenopausal women are particularly susceptible to osteoporosis and thus are at increased risk of fractures. Weight-bearing exercises such as walking are an important component of maintaining bone health by increasing the loads on bones and stimulating bone growth. Girls and young women should be encouraged to exercise to enhance bone strength long before they might begin to lose bone mass during the peri- and postmenopausal years. Similarly, the National Aeronautics and Space Agency (NASA) continues to seek the optimal training and nutrition program that will allow astronauts to maintain bone mass during extended periods in a microgravity environment.*

FRACTURE HEALING

When a bone breaks, the body initiates a cascade of events to repair the injury. The first step is similar to an inflammatory response: the bone bleeds at the fracture and possibly the surrounding tissues, and a blood clot forms. The cells that repair the fracture gather at the fracture site. In about 2 weeks, a **callus** begins to form. A callus is the precursor to the calcified bone. When the callus calcifies, it becomes woven bone, much like the immature bone in children. The woven bone undergoes remodeling; that is, the osteoclasts tunnel holes, and the osteoblasts lay down collagen to fill them in and create the haversian systems of mature or lamellar bone. The remodeling process continues long after the bone has healed. Eventually, the bone reforms itself into its natural shape (e.g., a hollow cylinder for a tibia or femur), and the intermedullary space is filled again with bone marrow. The woven bone of the callus is not as strong as the mature bone, but is more flexible and is more isotropic than lamellar bone. This appears to be the body's mechanism to allow the bone to heal and to reduce the potential for damaging the new bone. Almost all of the data on the strength of the callus during bone healing comes from animal models, and it is difficult to determine material property values for healing bone in humans. We do know, qualitatively, that the strength of the callus increases as the bone mineral density increases, that is only logical; however, the elastic constants and tensile/compressive strengths are not known.

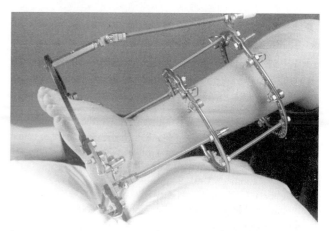

Figure 3.7: An Ilizarov fixator. The Ilizarov construct is applied externally to stabilize fractures and lengthen limbs. (Photo courtesy of James J. McCarthy, MD, Shriners Hospitals for Children, Philadelphia, PA)

SUMMARY

Bone serves as mechanical support, as a system of levers to transmit forces, and as protection for vital organs in the human body. Mechanically, bone is an anisotropic material; it has different mechanical properties in different directions. Bone is a composite material, consisting primarily of collagen and HA mineral. In many respects, because of the HA, bone behaves like a ceramic material: it is stronger in compression than in tension, and it exhibits brittle fracture. The collagen imparts some viscoelastic behavior, as well as increased tensile strength. Several of the referenced texts (especially 5 and 8) give an excellent overview of the properties of bone. The reader is strongly urged to consult the primary publications that report on the mechanical properties, however, when a specific property of a specific bone is needed for analysis.

Clinical Relevance

A LIMB-LENGTHENING PROCEDURE: *A fascinating example of an "artificial" use of the bone healing process is in limb-lengthening. Limb-lengthening was pioneered by a Russian physician named Gavril Ilizarov. Today, the Ilizarov procedure is used to lengthen unnaturally short bones caused by either a congenital condition or growth plate damage, to correct bone deformities, and to help heal difficult fractures. The Ilizarov procedure makes use of an external mechanical construct that is fixed to the bone by percutaneous pins and wires (Fig. 3.7). In the case of a lengthening, the surgeon first attaches the frame and then breaks the bone. The bone is gradually pulled apart over the course of several days; in most instances, the patient makes adjustments on the external fixator to separate the ends of the broken bone. In what can only be called a wonder of nature, new bone begins to grow in the gap as the bone is distracted. The new bone, called a **callus,** is like the woven bone that forms during "standard" fracture healing. The method pioneered by Ilizarov uses the patient's own weight to help bone healing. Over the course of treatment, the bone gradually bears more of the patient's weight. The weight bearing stimulates blood flow in the new bone and thereby stimulates bone formation. As the patient progresses, the bone hardens until it can fully support the patient's weight. The frame is then removed.*

References

1. An K-N, Chao EYS, Kaufman KR: Analysis of muscle and joint loads. In: Basic Orthopaedic Biomechanics. Mow VC, Hayes WC, eds. New York: Raven Press, 1991; 1–50.
2. Bikle DD, Halloran BP: The response of bone to unloading. J Bone Miner Metab 1999; 17: 233–244.
3. Brinker MR: Basic sciences, section 1, Bone. In: Review of Orthopaedics, 3rd ed. Miller MD, ed. Philadelphia: WB Saunders, 2000; 1–22.
4. Buckey JC Jr: Preparing for Mars: the physiologic and medical challenges. Eur J Med Res 1999; 4: 353–356.
5. Cowin SC: The mechanical properties of cortical bone tissue. In: Bone Mechanics. Cowin SC, ed. Boca Raton: CRC Press, 1989; 97–128.
6. Eyre DR, Wu JJ, Niyibizi C, Chun L: The cartilage collagens—analysis of their cross-linking interactions and matrix organizations. In: Methods in Cartilage Research. Maroudas A, Kuettner K, eds. San Diego: Academic Press, 1990; 28–32.
7. Fenech CM, Keaveny TM: A cellular solid criterion for predicting the axial-shear failure properties of bovine trabecular bone. J Biomech Eng 1999; 121: 414–422.

8. Hayes WC: Biomechanics of cortical and trabecular bone: implications for assessment of fracture risk. In: Basic Orthopaedic Biomechanics. Mow VC, Hayes WC, eds. New York: Raven Press, 1991; 93–142.

9. Holick MF: Perspective on the impact of weightlessness on calcium and bone metabolism. Bone 1998; 22(5 Suppl): 105S–111S.

10. Kabel J, van Rietbergen B, Odgaard A, Huiskes R: Constitutive relationships of fabric, density, and elastic properties in cancellous bone architecture. Bone 1999; 25: 481–486.

11. Martin RB: Determinants of the mechanical properties of bones. J Biomech 1991; 24(Suppl 1): 79–88.

12. Niebur GL, Yuen JC, Hsia AC, Keaveny TM: Convergence behavior of high-resolution finite element models of trabecular bone. J Biomech Eng 1999; 121: 629–635.

13. Nigg BM, Grimston SK: Bone. In: Biomechanics of the Musculo-Skeletal System. Nigg BM, Herzog W, eds. Chichester: John Wiley & Sons, 1994; 47–78.

14. Norman TL, Nivargikar SV, Burr DB: Resistance to crack growth in human cortical bone is greater in shear than in tension. J Biomech 1996; 29: 1023–1031.

15. Norman TL, Vashishth D, Burr DB: Fracture toughness of human bone under tension. J Biomech 1995; 28: 309–320.

16. Thomas T, Vico L, Skerry TM, et al.: Architectural modifications and cellular response during disuse-related bone loss in calcaneus of the sheep. J Appl Physiol 1996; 80: 198–202.

17. Van Rietbergen B, Muller R, Ulrich D, et al.: Tissue stresses and strain in trabeculae of a canine proximal femur can be quantified from computer reconstructions. J Biomech 1999; 32: 443–451.

18. Wang X, Agrawal CM: Fracture toughness of bone using a compact sandwich specimen: effects of sampling sites and crack orientations. J Biomed Mater Res (Appl Biomater) 1996; 33: 13–21.

19. Weiner S, Traub W, Wagner HD: Lamellar bone: structure-function relations. J Struct Biol 1999; 30; 126: 241–255.

20. Wimalawansa SM, Wimalawansa SJ: Simulated weightlessness-induced attenuation of testosterone production may be responsible for bone loss. Endocrine 1999; 10: 253–260.

21. Zioupos P, Currey JD: Changes in the stiffness, strength, and toughness of human cortical bone with age. Bone 1998; 22: 57–66.

Biomechanics of Skeletal Muscle

CHAPTER CONTENTS

Skeletal muscle is a fascinating biological tissue able to transform chemical energy to mechanical energy. The focus of this chapter is on the mechanical behavior of skeletal muscle as it contributes to function and dysfunction of the musculoskeletal system. Although a basic understanding of the energy transformation from chemical to mechanical energy is essential to a full understanding of the behavior of muscle, it is beyond the scope of this book. The reader is urged to consult other sources for a discussion of the chemical and physiological interactions that produce and affect a muscle contraction [41,52,86].

Skeletal muscle has three basic performance parameters that describe its function:

- Movement production
- Force production
- Endurance

The production of movement and force is the mechanical outcome of skeletal muscle contraction. The factors that influence these parameters are the focus of this chapter. A brief description of the morphology of muscles and the physiological processes that produce contraction needed to understand these mechanical parameters are also presented here. Specifically the purposes of this chapter are to

- Review briefly the structure of muscle and the mechanism of skeletal muscle contraction
- Examine the factors that influence a muscle's ability to produce a motion
- Examine the factors that influence a muscle's ability to produce force
- Consider how muscle architecture is specialized to optimize a muscle's ability to produce force or joint motion
- Demonstrate how an understanding of these factors can be used clinically to optimize a person's performance
- Discuss the adaptations that muscle undergoes with prolonged changes in length and activity

STRUCTURE OF SKELETAL MUSCLE

The functional unit that produces motion at a joint consists of two discrete units, the muscle belly and the tendon that binds the muscle belly to the bone. The structure of the muscle belly itself is presented in the current chapter. The structure and mechanical properties of the tendon, composed of connective tissue, are presented in Chapter 6. The muscle belly consists of the muscle cells, or fibers, that produce the contraction and the connective tissue encasing the muscle fibers. Each is discussed below.

Structure of an Individual Muscle Fiber

A skeletal muscle fiber is a long cylindrical, multinucleated cell that is filled with smaller units of filaments (*Fig. 4.1*). These

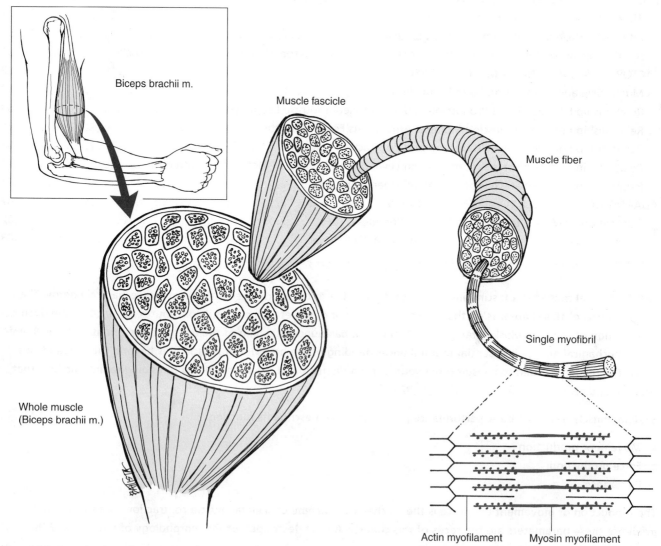

Figure 4.1: Organization of muscle. A progressively magnified view of a whole muscle demonstrates the organization of the filaments composing the muscle.

filamentous structures are roughly aligned parallel to the muscle fiber itself. The largest of the filaments is the myofibril, composed of subunits called *sarcomeres* that are arranged end to end the length of the myofibril. Each sarcomere also contains filaments, known as *myofilaments*. There are two types of myofilaments within each sarcomere. The thicker myofilaments are composed of myosin protein molecules, and the thinner myofilaments are composed of molecules of the protein actin. Sliding of the actin myofilament on the myosin chain is the basic mechanism of muscle contraction.

THE SLIDING FILAMENT THEORY OF MUSCLE CONTRACTION

The sarcomere, containing the contractile proteins actin and myosin, is the basic functional unit of muscle. Contraction of a whole muscle is actually the sum of singular contraction events occurring within the individual sarcomeres. Therefore, it is necessary to understand the organization of the sarcomere. The thinner actin chains are more abundant than the myosin myofilaments in a sarcomere. The actin myofilaments are anchored at both ends of the sarcomere at the Z-line and project into the interior of the sarcomere where they surround a thicker myosin myofilament (*Fig. 4.2*). This arrangement of myosin myofilaments surrounded by actin myofilaments is repeated throughout the sarcomere, filling its interior and giving the muscle fiber its characteristic striations. The amount of these contractile proteins within the cells is strongly related to a muscle's contractile force [6,7,27].

Contraction results from the formation of cross-bridges between the myosin and actin myofilaments, causing the actin

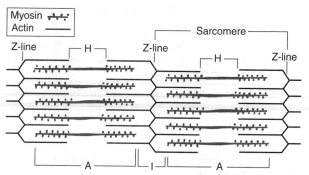

Figure 4.2: Organization of actin and myosin within a muscle fiber. The arrangement of the actin and myosin chains in two adjacent sarcomeres within a fiber produces the characteristic striations of skeletal muscle.

chains to "slide" on the myosin chain (*Fig. 4.3*). The tension of the contraction depends upon the number of cross-bridges formed between the actin and myosin myofilaments. The number of cross-bridges formed depends not only on the abundance of the actin and myosin molecules, but also on the frequency of the stimulus to form cross-bridges.

Contraction is initiated by an electrical stimulus from the associated motor neuron causing depolarization of the muscle fiber. When the fiber is depolarized, calcium is released into the cell and binds with the regulating protein troponin. The combination of calcium with troponin acts as a trigger, causing actin to bind with myosin, beginning the contraction. Cessation of the nerve's stimulus causes a reduction in calcium levels within the muscle fiber, inhibiting the cross-bridges between actin and myosin. The muscle relaxes [86]. If

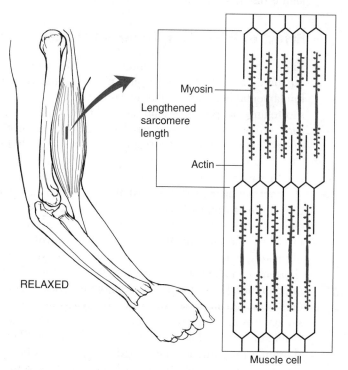

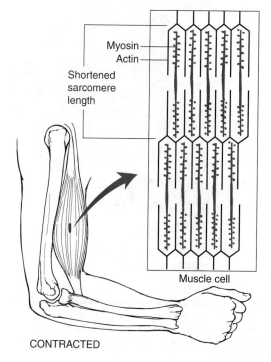

Figure 4.3: The sliding filament model. Contraction of skeletal muscle results from the sliding of the actin chains on the myosin chains.

stimulation of the muscle fiber occurs at a sufficiently high frequency, new cross-bridges are formed before prior interactions are completely severed, causing a fusion of succeeding contractions. Ultimately a sustained, or tetanic, contraction is produced. Modulation of the frequency and magnitude of the initial stimulus has an effect on the force of contraction of a whole muscle and is discussed later in this chapter.

The Connective Tissue System within the Muscle Belly

The muscle belly consists of the muscle cells, or fibers, and the connective tissue that binds the cells together (*Fig. 4.4*). The outermost layer of connective tissue that surrounds the entire muscle belly is known as the *epimysium*. The muscle belly is divided into smaller bundles or fascicles by additional connective tissue known as *perimysium*. Finally individual fibers within these larger sheaths are surrounded by more connective tissue, the endomysium. Thus the entire muscle belly is invested in a large network of connective tissue that then is bound to the connective tissue tendons at either end of the muscle. The amount of connective tissue within a muscle and the size of the connecting tendons vary widely from muscle to

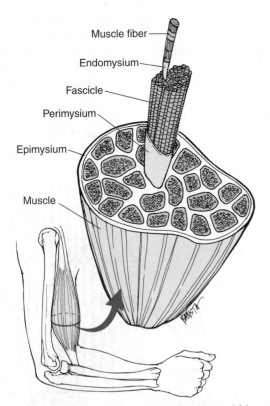

Figure 4.4: Organization of the connective tissue within muscle. The whole muscle belly is invested in an organized system of connective tissue. It consists of the epimysium surrounding the whole belly, the perimysium encasing smaller bundles of muscle fibers, and the endomysium that covers individual muscle fibers.

muscle. The amount of connective tissue found within an individual muscle influences the mechanical properties of that muscle and helps explain the varied mechanical responses of individual muscles. The contribution of the connective tissue to a muscle's behavior is discussed later in this chapter.

FACTORS THAT INFLUENCE A MUSCLE'S ABILITY TO PRODUCE A MOTION

An essential function of muscle is to produce joint movement. The passive range of motion (ROM) available at a joint depends on the shape of the articular surfaces as well as on the surrounding soft tissues. However the joint's active ROM depends on a muscle's ability to pull the limb through a joint's available ROM. Under normal conditions, active ROM is approximately equal to a joint's passive ROM. However there is a wide variation in the amount of passive motion available at joints throughout the body. The knee joint is capable of flexing through an arc of approximately 140°, but the metacarpophalangeal (MCP) joint of the thumb usually is capable of no more than about 90° of flexion. Joints that exhibit large ROMs require muscles capable of moving the joint through the entire range. However such muscles are unnecessary at joints with smaller excursions. Thus muscles exhibit structural specializations that influence the magnitude of the excursion that is produced by a contraction. These specializations are

- The length of the fibers composing the muscle
- The length of the muscle's moment arm.

How each of these characteristics affects active motion of a joint is discussed below.

Effect of Fiber Length on Joint Excursion

Fiber length has a significant influence on the magnitude of the joint motion that results from a muscle contraction. The fundamental behavior of muscle is shortening, and it is this shortening that produces joint motion. The myofilaments in each sarcomere are 1 to 2 μm long; the myosin myofilaments are longer than the actin myofilaments [125,149]. Thus sarcomeres in humans are a few micrometers in length, varying from approximately 1.25 to 4.5 μm with muscle contraction and stretch [90–92,143]. Each sarcomere can shorten to approximately the length of its myosin molecules. Because the sarcomeres are arranged in series in a myofibril, the amount of shortening that a myofibril and, ultimately, a muscle fiber can produce is the sum of the shortening in all of the sarcomeres. Thus the total shortening of a muscle fiber depends upon the number of sarcomeres arranged in series within each myofibril. The more sarcomeres in a fiber, the longer the fiber is and the more it is able to shorten (*Fig. 4.5*). The amount a muscle fiber can shorten is proportional to its length [15,89,155]. A fiber can shorten roughly 50 to 60% of its length [44,155], although

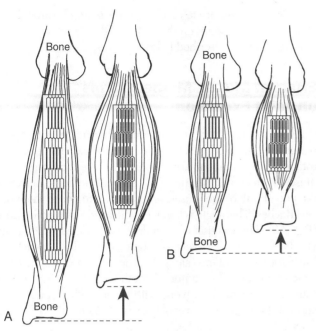

Figure 4.5: The relationship between fiber length and shortening capacity of the whole muscle. A muscle with more sarcomeres in series **(A)** can shorten more than a fiber with fewer sarcomeres in series **(B)**.

there is some evidence that fibers exhibit varied shortening capabilities [15].

The absolute amount of shortening a fiber undergoes is a function of its fiber length. Similarly, the amount a whole muscle can shorten is dictated by the length of its constituent fibers. An individual whole muscle is composed mostly of fibers of similar lengths [15]. However there is a wide variation in fiber lengths found in the human body, ranging from a few centimeters to approximately half a meter [86,146]. The length of the fibers within a muscle is a function of the architecture of that muscle rather than of the muscle's total length. The following describes how fiber length and muscle architecture are related.

ARCHITECTURE OF SKELETAL MUSCLE

Although all skeletal muscle is composed of muscle fibers, the arrangement of those fibers can vary significantly among muscles. This fiber arrangement has marked effects on a muscle's ability to produce movement and to generate force. Fiber arrangements have different names but fall into two major categories, **parallel** and **pennate** [42] (*Fig. 4.6*). In general, the fibers within a parallel fiber muscle are approximately parallel to the length of the whole muscle. These muscles can be classified as either **fusiform** or **strap** muscles. Fusiform muscles have tendons at both ends of the muscle so that the muscle fibers taper to insert into the tendons. Strap

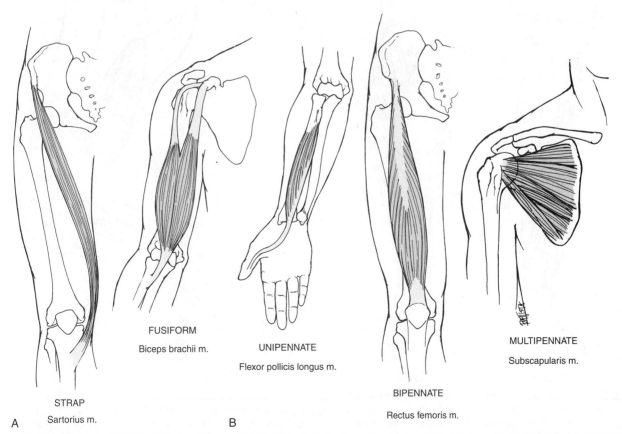

Figure 4.6: Muscle architecture. **A.** Muscles with parallel fibers include fusiform (biceps brachii) and strap (sartorius) muscles. **B.** Pennate muscles include unipennate (flexor pollicis longus), bipennate (rectus femoris), and multipennate (subscapularis).

muscles have less prominent tendons, and therefore their fibers taper less at both ends of the whole muscle. Parallel fiber muscles are composed of relatively long fibers, although these fibers still are shorter than the whole muscle. Even the sartorius muscle, a classic strap muscle, contains fibers that are only about 90% of its total length.

In contrast, a pennate muscle has one or more tendons that extend most of the length of the whole muscle. Fibers run obliquely to insert into these tendons. Pennate muscles fall into subcategories according to the number of tendons penetrating the muscle. There are **unipennate, bipennate,** and **multipennate** muscles. A comparison of two muscles of similar total length, one with parallel fibers and the other with a pennate arrangement, helps to illustrate the effect of fiber arrangement on fiber length (*Fig. 4.7*). The muscle with parallel fibers has longer fibers than those found in the pennate muscle. Because the amount of shortening that a muscle can undergo depends on the length of its fibers, the muscle with parallel fibers is able to shorten more than the pennate muscle. If fiber length alone affected joint excursion, the muscle with parallel fibers would produce a larger joint excursion than the muscle composed of pennate fibers

[90]. However, a muscle's ability to move a limb through an excursion also depends on the length of the muscle's moment arm. Its effect is described below.

Effect of Muscle Moment Arms on Joint Excursion

Chapter 1 defines the moment arm of a muscle as the perpendicular distance between the muscle and the point of rotation. This moment arm depends on the location of the muscle's attachment on the bone and on the angle between the line of pull of the muscle and the limb to which the muscle attaches. This angle is known as the **angle of application** (*Fig. 4.8*). The location of an individual muscle's attachment on the bone is relatively constant across the population. Therefore, the distance along the bone between the muscle's attachment and the center of rotation of the joint can be estimated roughly by anyone with a knowledge of anatomy and can be measured precisely as well [57,81,95,151]. This

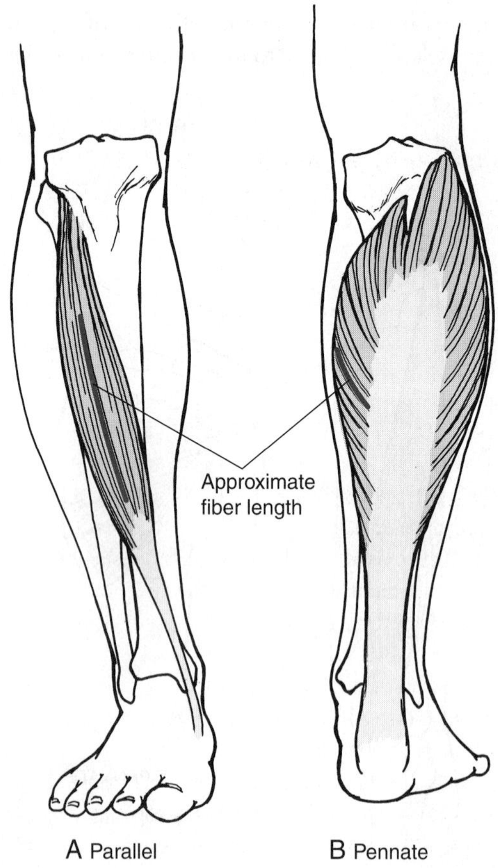

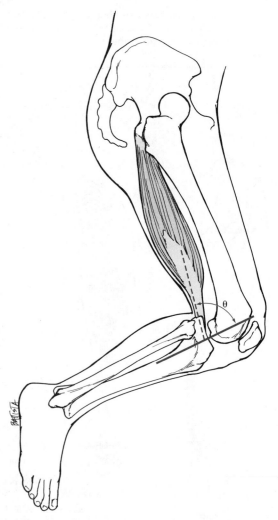

Figure 4.7: The relationship between muscle architecture and muscle fiber length. The fibers in a muscle with parallel fibers are typically longer than the fibers in a muscle of similar overall size but with pennate fibers.

A Parallel   B Pennate

Figure 4.8: Angle of application. A muscle's angle of application is the angle formed between the line of pull of the muscle and the bone to which the muscle attaches.

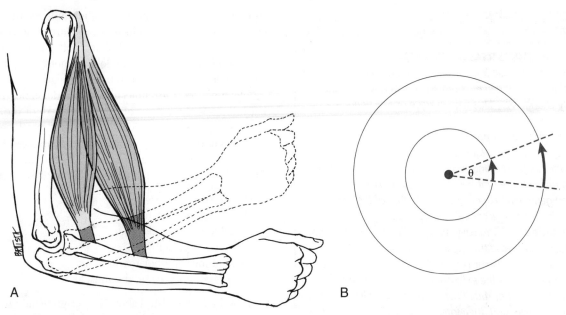

Figure 4.9: The relationship between a muscle's moment arm and excursion. The length of a muscle's moment arm affects the excursion that results from a contraction. **A.** Movement through an angle, θ, requires more shortening in a muscle with a long moment arm than in a muscle with a short moment arm. **B.** The arc subtended by an angle, θ, is larger in a large circle than in a small circle.

distance is related to the true moment arm by the sine of the angle of application, θ, which can also be estimated or measured directly.

A muscle's moment arm has a significant effect on the joint excursion produced by a contraction of the muscle. A muscle with a short moment arm produces a larger angular excursion than another muscle with a similar shortening capacity but with a longer moment arm. Principles of basic geometry help explain the relationship between muscle moment arms and angular excursion. Given two circles of different sizes, an angle, θ, defines an arc on each circle (*Fig. 4.9*). However, the arc of the larger circle is larger than the arc of the smaller circle. Thus the distance traveled on the larger circle to move through the angle θ is greater than that on the smaller circle. Similarly, a muscle with a long moment arm must shorten more to produce the same angular displacement as a muscle with a short moment arm [76,77].

Joint Excursion as a Function of Both Fiber Length and the Anatomical Moment Arm of a Muscle

The preceding discussion reveals that both a muscle's fiber length and its moment arm have direct effects on the amount of excursion a muscle contraction produces. These effects can be summarized by the following:

- Because muscle fibers possess a similar relative shortening capability, longer fibers produce more absolute shortening than shorter fibers.

- Because muscles with parallel fibers generally have longer fibers than pennate muscles, whole muscles composed of parallel fibers have a larger shortening capacity than whole muscles of similar length composed of pennate fibers.
- Muscles with shorter anatomical moment arms are capable of producing greater angular excursions of a joint than muscles of similar fiber length with larger anatomical moment arms.

It is interesting to see how these characteristics are combined in individual muscles. Muscles combine these seemingly opposing attributes in various ways, resulting in diverse functional capacities. It appears that some muscles, like the gluteus maximus, possess both long fibers and relatively short moment arms. Such muscles are capable of producing relatively large joint excursions [62]. Others, like the brachioradialis muscle at the elbow, combine relatively long muscle fibers with large moment arms [89]. The long fibers enhance the muscle's ability to produce a large excursion. However, the large moment arm decreases the muscle's ability to produce a large excursion. This apparent contradiction is explained in part by the recognition that the factors that influence production of movement, muscle architecture and anatomical moment arm, also influence force production capabilities in a muscle. Muscles must find ways to balance the competing demands of force production and joint excursion. The ratio of a muscle's fiber length to its moment arm is a useful descriptor of a muscle's ability to produce an excursion and its torque-generating capability [99]. This ratio helps surgeons determine appropriate donor muscles to replace dysfunctional ones.

Clinical Relevance

CONSIDERATIONS REGARDING TENDON TRANSFERS: *Muscle fiber arrangement and muscle moment arms are inherent characteristics of a muscle and normally change very little with exercise or functional use. However, surgeons commonly transfer a muscle or muscles to replace the function of paralyzed muscles [15,16]. Successful restoration of function requires that the surgeon not only replace the nonfunctioning muscle with a functional muscle but also must ensure that the replacement muscle has an excursion-generating capacity similar to that of the original muscle. This may be accomplished by choosing a structurally similar muscle or by surgically manipulating the moment arm to increase or decrease the excursion capability [155].*

For example, the flexor carpi radialis muscle at the wrist is a good substitute for the extensor digitorum muscle of the fingers in the event of radial nerve palsy. The wrist flexor has long muscle fibers and, therefore, the capacity to extend the fingers through their full ROM. In contrast, the flexor carpi ulnaris, another muscle of the wrist, has very short fibers and lacks the capacity to move the fingers through their full excursion. Thus the functional outcome depends on the surgeon's understanding of muscle mechanics, including those factors that influence the production of motion.

FACTORS THAT INFLUENCE A MUSCLE'S STRENGTH

Strength is the most familiar characteristic of muscle performance. However, the term *strength* has many different interpretations. Understanding the factors affecting strength requires a clear understanding of how the term is used. The basic activity of muscle is to shorten, thus producing a tensile force. As noted in Chapter 1, a force also produces a moment, or a tendency to rotate, when the force is exerted at some distance from the point of rotation. The ability to generate a tensile force and the ability to create a moment are both used to describe a muscle's strength. Assessment of muscle strength in vivo is typically performed by determining the muscle's ability to produce a moment. Such assessments include determination of the amount of manual resistance an individual can sustain without joint rotation, the amount of weight a subject can lift, or the direct measurement of moments using a device such as an isokinetic dynamometer. In contrast, in vitro studies often assess muscle strength by measuring a muscle's ability to generate a tensile force. Of course the muscle's tensile force of contraction and its resulting moment are related by the following:

$$M = r \times F \qquad \text{(Equation 4.1)}$$

where M is the moment generated by the muscle's tensile force (F) applied at a distance (r, the muscle's moment arm) from the point of rotation (the joint axis). Therefore, muscle strength as assessed typically in the clinic by the measurement of the moment produced by a contraction is a function of an array of factors that influence both the tensile force of contraction, F, and the muscle's moment arm, r [54]. To obtain valid assessments of muscle strength and to optimize muscle function, the clinician must understand the factors that influence the output of the muscle. All of the following factors ultimately influence the moment produced by the muscle's contraction. Some affect the contractile force, and others influence the muscle's ability to generate a moment. The primary factors influencing the muscle's strength are

- Muscle size
- Muscle moment arm
- Stretch of the muscle
- Contraction velocity
- Level of muscle fiber recruitment
- Fiber types composing the muscle

Each of the factors listed above has a significant effect on the muscle's moment production. An understanding of each factor and its role in moment production allows the clinician to use these factors to optimize a person performance and to understand the alteration in muscle performance with pathology. The effects of size, moment arm, and stretch are most apparent in isometric contractions, which are contractions that produce no discernable joint motion. Consequently, the experiments demonstrating these effects usually employ isometric contractions. However, the reader must recognize that the effects are manifested in all types of contraction. Each factor is discussed below.

Muscle Size and Its Effect on Force Production

As noted earlier in this chapter, the force of contraction is a function of the number of cross-links made between the actin and myosin chains [1,39]. The more cross-links formed, the stronger the force of contraction. Therefore, the force of contraction depends upon the amount of actin and myosin available and thus on the number of fibers a muscle contains. In other words, the force of contraction is related to a muscle's size [67,126]. In fact, muscle size is the most important single factor determining the tensile force generated by a muscle's contraction [44,60]. Estimates of the maximal contractile force per unit of muscle range from approximately 20 to 135 N/cm^2 [15,22, 120,155]. These data reveal a wide disparity in the estimates of the maximum tensile force that muscle can produce. Additional research is needed to determine if all skeletal muscle has the same potential maximum and what that maximum really is.

Although the estimates presented above vary widely, they do demonstrate that the maximum tensile force produced by an individual muscle is a function of its area. However, the overall size of a muscle may be a poor indication of the number of fibers contained in that muscle. The relationship between muscle size and force of contraction is complicated by the muscle's architecture. The **anatomical cross-sectional area** of the muscle is the cross-sectional area at the muscle's widest point and perpendicular to the length of the whole muscle. In a parallel fiber muscle this cross-sectional area cuts across most of the fibers of the muscle (*Fig. 4.10*). However, in a pennate muscle the anatomical cross-sectional area cuts across only a portion of the fibers composing the muscle. Thus the anatomical cross-sectional area underestimates the number of fibers contained in a pennate muscle and hence its force production capabilities.

The standard measure used to approximate the number of fibers of a whole muscle is its **physiological cross-sectional area (PCSA).** The PCSA is the area of a slice that passes through all of the fibers of a muscle [15]. In a parallel fiber

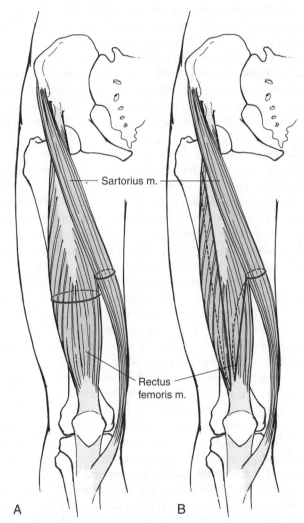

Figure 4.10: The relationship between muscle architecture and muscle size. **A.** The anatomical cross-sectional area of a muscle is the area of a slice through the widest part of the muscle perpendicular to the muscle's length. It is similar in a parallel fiber muscle and a pennate muscle of similar overall size. **B.** The physiological cross-sectional area of a muscle is the area of a slice that cuts across all of the fibers of the muscle. It is quite different for a parallel fiber muscle and a pennate muscle.

muscle the PCSA is approximately equal to the anatomical cross-sectional area. However, in a pennate muscle the PCSA is considerably larger than its anatomical cross-sectional area. The PCSAs of two muscles of similar overall size demonstrate the influence of muscle architecture on force production. Although their anatomical cross-sectional areas are very similar, the pennate muscle has a much larger PCSA. Thus if all other factors are equal, the pennate muscle is capable of generating more contraction force than the muscle with parallel fibers [64,90,114].

The angle at which the fibers insert into the tendon also influences the total force that is applied to the limb by a pennate muscle. This angle is known as the *angle of pennation*. The tensile force generated by the whole muscle is the vector sum of the force components that are applied parallel to the muscle's tendon (*Fig. 4.11*). Therefore, as the angle of pennation increases, the tensile component of the contraction force decreases. However, the larger the pennation angle is, the larger the PCSA is [2]. In most muscles the pennation angle is 30° or less, and thus pennation typically increases the tensile force produced by contraction [86,146]. Resistance training increases the fibers' angle of pennation (and the muscle's PCSA). This increase appears to result from increases, or hypertrophy, in the cross-sectional area of individual muscle fibers [2,13].

Muscle architecture demonstrates how muscles exhibit specializations that enhance one performance characteristic or another. Long fibers in a muscle promote the excursion-producing capacity of the muscle. However, spatial constraints of the human body prevent a muscle with long fibers from having a very large cross-sectional area and hence a large force-production capacity. On the other hand, muscles with a large PCSA can be fit into small areas by arranging the fibers in a pennate pattern. However, the short fibers limit the excursion capacity of the muscle. Thus fiber arrangement suggests that pennate muscles are specialized for force production but have limited ability to produce a large excursion. Conversely, a muscle with parallel fibers has an improved ability to produce an excursion but produces a smaller contractile force than a pennate muscle of the same overall size. Thus the intrinsic structural characteristics of a muscle help define the performance of the muscle by affecting both the force of contraction and the amount of the resulting joint excursion. These intrinsic factors respond to an increase or decrease in activity over time [27,64,119,145]. However, instantaneous changes in the muscle also result in large but temporary responses in a muscle's performance. These changes include stretching the muscle and altering its moment arm. These effects are described below.

Relationship between Force Production and Instantaneous Muscle Length (Stretch)

Since the strength of muscle contraction is a function of the number of cross-links made between the actin and myosin chains within the sarcomeres, alterations in the proximity of

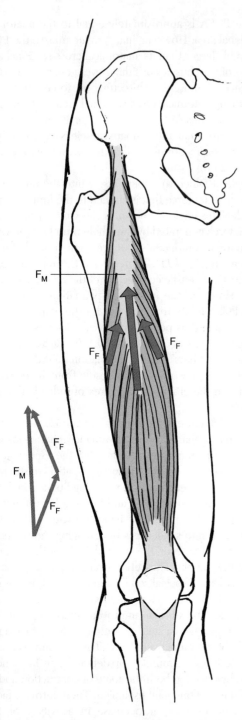

Figure 4.11: The pull of a pennate muscle. The overall tensile force (F_M) of a muscle is the vector sum of the force of contraction of the pennate fibers (F_F).

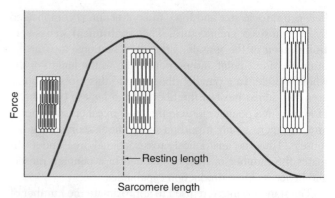

Figure 4.12: The length–tension curve of a sarcomere. The length–tension curve of a sarcomere demonstrates how the length of the sarcomere influences its force production.

the actin and myosin chains also influence a muscle's force of contraction. The maximum number of cross-links between the actin and myosin myofilaments and hence the maximum contractile force in the sarcomere occurs when the full length of the actin strands at each end of the sarcomere are in contact with the myosin molecule [34,50,125] (*Fig. 4.12*). This length is operationally defined as the **resting length** of the muscle. The sarcomere can shorten slightly from this point, maintaining the maximum cross-linking. However, increased shortening causes the actin strands from each end of the sarcomere to interfere with each other. This reduces the number of available sites for cross-bridge formation, and the force of contraction decreases. Similarly, when the sarcomere is stretched from its resting length, contact between the actin and myosin myofilaments decreases, and thus the number of cross-links that can be made again diminishes. Consequently, the force of contraction decreases.

Investigation of the effects of stretch on the whole muscle reveals that the muscle's response to stretch is affected both by the behavior of the sarcomere described above and by the elastic properties of the noncontractile components of the muscle, including the epimysium, perimysium, endomysium, and tendons [43,45,53,121]. The classic studies of the length–tension relationships in muscle were performed by Blix in the late 19th century but have been repeated and expanded by others in the ensuing 100 years [43,45, 88,90,121]. These studies, performed on whole muscle, consistently demonstrate that as a muscle is stretched in the absence of a contraction, there is some length at which the muscle begins to resist the stretch (*Fig. 4.13*). As the stretch of the muscle increases, the muscle exerts a larger pull against the stretch. This pull is attributed to the elastic recoil of the passive structures within the muscle, such as the investing connective tissue. These components are known as the **parallel elastic components.** The tendons at either end of the muscle also provide a force against the stretch. These are described as the **series elastic components.**

The combined effects of muscle contraction and stretch of the elastic components are represented mechanically by a contractile element in series and in parallel with the elastic components (*Fig. 4.14*). The response of both the contractile and elastic components together is examined by measuring the resistance to increasing stretch while simultaneously stimulating the muscle to induce a contraction. Such experiments reveal that when the muscle is very short, allowing no passive recoil force, stimulation produces a small contractile force. As the stretch increases and stimulations continue, the tension in

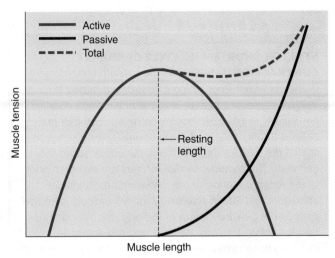

Figure 4.13: The length–tension curve of a whole muscle. The length–tension curve of a whole muscle demonstrates how muscle length affects the force production of the whole muscle. The contractile, or active, component; the passive component primarily due to the connective tissue; and the total muscle tension all are affected by the stretch of the muscle.

the muscle increases. In the middle region of stretch, the muscle's force plateaus or even decreases, even with stimulation. This plateau occurs at approximately the resting length of the muscle. With additional stretch, the tension in the whole muscle begins to increase again and continues to increase with further stretch. By subtracting the results of the passive test from the results of the combined test, the contribution of the active, or contractile, component to muscle

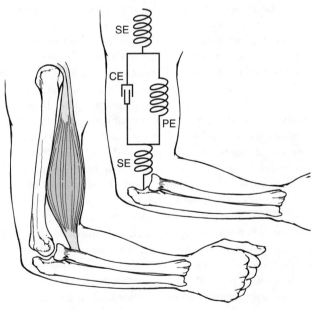

Figure 4.14: A mechanical model of the contractile and elastic components of a muscle. A muscle's contractile (actin and myosin) and elastic (connective tissue) components are often modeled mechanically as a combination of a contractile element (CE) with springs that represent the elastic elements that are both in series (SE) and in parallel (PE) with the contractile component.

tension is determined. The active contribution to muscle tension in the whole muscle is similar to the length–tension relationship seen in the individual sarcomeres. These results demonstrate that while the contractile contribution to muscle tension peaks in the midregion of stretch, the passive components of the muscle make an increasing contribution to force after the midrange of stretch. Thus the overall tension of the muscle is greatest when the muscle is stretched maximally.

It is important to recognize that the experiments described above are performed on disarticulated muscles. Consequently, the extremes of shortening and lengthening tested are nonphysiological. An intact human muscle functions somewhere in the central portion of the length–tension curve, although the precise shape of the length–tension curve varies across muscles [45,152]. The response to stretch depends on the architecture of the individual muscle as well as the ratio of contractile tissue to connective tissue in the muscle [45]. In addition, the exact amount of stretch and shortening sustained by a muscle depends on the individual muscle and the joint. Muscles that cross two or more joints undergo more shortening and lengthening than muscles that span only one joint. The force output of such multijointed muscles is influenced significantly by the length–tension relationship [56,123].

Clinical Relevance

THE LENGTH–TENSION RELATIONSHIP OF MUSCLES IN VIVO: *Weakness is a common impairment in individuals participating in rehabilitation. Sometimes individuals are too weak to be able to move the limb much at all. By positioning the patient's limb so that the contracting muscles are functioning in the stretched position, the clinician enhances the muscle's ability to generate tension. For example, hyperextension of the shoulder increases elbow flexion strength by stretching the biceps brachii. Conversely, placing muscles in a very shortened position decreases their ability to generate force. Muscles of the wrist and fingers provide a vivid example of how the effectiveness of muscles changes when they are lengthened or shortened (Fig. 4.15). It is difficult to make a forceful fist when the wrist is flexed because the finger flexor muscles are so short they produce insufficient force. This phenomenon is known as **active insufficiency.** Inspection of the wrist position when the fist is clenched normally reveals that the wrist is extended, thereby stretching the muscles, increasing their contractile force, and avoiding active insufficiency.*

The classic length–tension relationship described so far has been studied by altering the length of a muscle passively and then assessing the strength of contraction at the new length. More recent studies have investigated the effects of

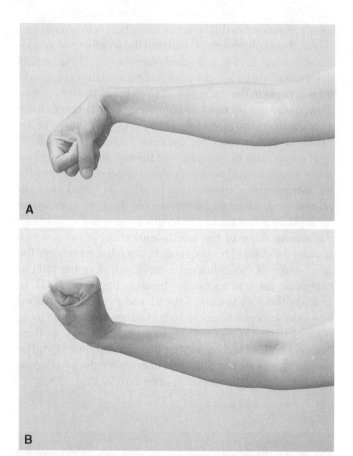

Figure 4.15: The effects of muscle length on performance. A. When the wrist is in flexion it is difficult to flex the fingers fully because the finger flexors are so shortened. B. When the wrist is in extension, the fingers readily flex to make a fist since the finger flexors are lengthened.

Clinical Relevance

STRETCH-SHORTENING CYCLE OF MUSCLE CONTRACTION IN SPORTS: *The strength enhancement that comes from lengthening a contracting muscle prior to using it to produce motion is visible in countless activities, particularly in sports. For example the wind-up that precedes a throw or the backswing of a golf swing serves to stretch the muscles that will throw the ball or swing the golf club. The shoulder medial rotators are stretched prior to the forward motion of the throw, and the shoulder abductors and lateral rotators of the left arm are stretched prior to the forward motion of the golf swing for a right-handed golfer. Similarly the start of a running sprint event is characterized by a brief stretch of the plantar flexors, knee extensors and hip extensors before these same muscles shorten to push the runner down the track. The stretch of all of these muscles occurs as they are contracting and consequently amplifies even more the strength gains resulting from the stretch itself. (See the jumping activity in Chapter 4 laboratory.)*

length changes on isometric strength while the muscle is actively contracting. These studies consistently demonstrate that the traditional length-tension relationships are amplified if the length changes occur during contraction. Specifically, if a contracting muscle is lengthened and then held at its lengthened position, the force generated at the lengthened position is greater than the strength measured at that same position with no preceding length change [55,128]. Similarly, shortening a muscle as it contracts produces more strength reduction than placing the relaxed muscle at the shortened position and then measuring its strength [124,128]. Many vigorous functional activities occur utilizing muscle contractions that consist of a lengthening then shortening contraction cycle [102]. Such a pattern of muscle activity appears to utilize the length–tension relationship to optimize a muscle's ability to generate force.

A muscle's length, and therefore its force of contraction, changes as the joint position changes. However, the length of the muscle is only one factor that changes as the joint position changes. The moment arm of the muscle also varies with joint position. The influence of a muscle's moment arm on muscle performance is described below.

Relationship between a Muscle's Moment Arm and Its Force Production

As noted earlier, a muscle's ability to rotate a joint depends upon the muscle's force of contraction and on its moment arm, the perpendicular distance from the muscle force to the point of rotation [125]. The previous discussion reveals that muscle size and the stretch of the muscle have a significant impact on the force of contraction. However, the muscle's moment arm is critical in determining the moment generated by the muscle contraction. The larger the moment arm, the larger the moment created by the muscle contraction. The relationship between a muscle's moment arm and its angle of application is described earlier in the current chapter. The moment arm is determined by the sine of the angle of application and the distance between the muscle's attachment and the joint's axis of rotation (*Fig. 4.16*). The muscle's moment arm is maximum when the muscle's angle of application is 90°, since the sine of 90° equals 1. A muscle with a large moment arm produces a larger moment than a muscle with a shorter moment arm if both muscles generate equal contractile forces (*Fig. 4.17*). The moment arms of some muscles such as the hamstrings change several centimeters through the full ROM of the joint, while others such as the flexor digitorum profundus demonstrate very little change (*Fig. 4.18*) [57,70,71,81, 113,135,151]. Therefore, a muscle's ability to produce a moment varies with the joint position.

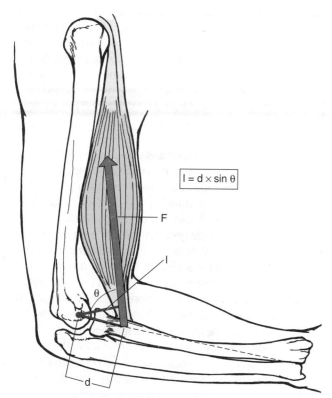

Figure 4.16: Moment arm of a muscle. A muscle's moment arm (l) is easily calculated using the muscle's angle of application (θ) and the distance (d) from the muscle attachment to the axis of rotation.

$$l = d \times \sin \theta$$

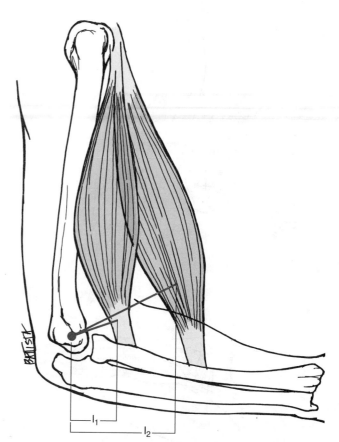

Figure 4.17: The effect of moment arm of a muscle on the muscle's performance. A muscle with a short moment arm (l_1) generates a smaller moment than a muscle with a longer moment arm (l_2) that generates the same contraction force.

INTERACTION BETWEEN A MUSCLE'S MOMENT ARM AND ITS LENGTH WITH CHANGING JOINT POSITIONS

It is easy to observe the positions that shorten or lengthen a muscle. For example, elbow flexion lengthens the elbow extensor muscles and shortens the elbow flexors. Although somewhat less obvious, a knowledge of anatomy allows the clinician to estimate the effects of joint position on a muscle's angle of application and thus on its moment arm. The angle of application of the biceps brachii is almost zero with the elbow extended and increases to over 90° with the elbow flexed maximally. In this case, the muscle's moment arm is at a minimum when the muscle's length is at a maximum. In contrast, the angle of application is greatest when the length is shortest. The optimal angle of application, 90°, occurs when the elbow is flexed to approximately 100° of elbow flexion [4,113]. Thus the muscle's ability to generate a large contractile force as a result of stretch is maximum in the very position in which the muscle's ability to produce a moment is smallest by virtue of its moment arm. Consequently, the biceps produces peak moments in the midrange of elbow flexion where neither the muscle's length nor angle of application is optimal. The relative contribution of moment arm

and muscle length to a muscle's ability to produce a moment varies among the muscles of the body and depends on the individual characteristics of each muscle and joint [62,82, 87,100,112,148].

In a series of elegant experiments Lieber and colleagues assessed the combined effects of muscle size, moment arm, and length on the ability of the primary wrist muscles, the flexor carpi ulnaris, flexor carpi radialis, extensor carpi ulnaris, and extensor carpi radialis longus and extensor carpi radialis brevis to produce a joint torque in the directions of wrist flexion, extension, and radial and ulnar deviation [88,94,95]. These investigations reveal that the influence of moment arms and muscle lengths differs markedly among these muscles of the wrist. The output from the wrist extensor muscles correlates well with the muscles' moment arms, suggesting that their output depends largely on their moment arms and is less influenced by muscle length. In contrast, the output of the wrist flexors is nearly maximum over a large portion of the wrist range, suggesting that both moment arm and muscle length have significant impact on the muscles' performance.

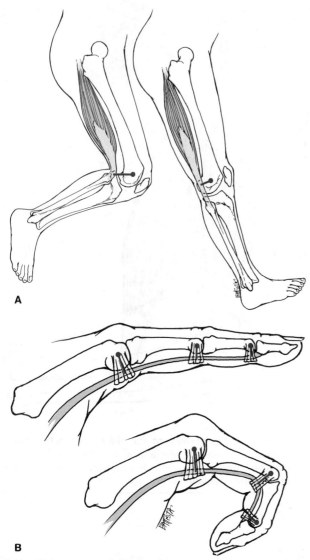

A

B

Figure 4.18: Changes in muscle moment arms. **A.** The hamstrings' moment arm at the knee is small with the knee extended and much larger with the knee flexed. **B.** The moment arm of a tendon of the flexor digitorum profundus at the finger changes little with the fingers extended or flexed.

Clinical Relevance

JOINT POSITION'S INFLUENCE ON MUSCLE
STRENGTH: *Joint position is likely to have a dramatic effect on the output from a muscle contraction, since joint position affects both the stretch and the moment arm of a muscle. The exact influence is revealed through careful testing and varies across muscles and joints. Similarly, only careful investigation provides an explanation for the precise nature of the relationship between joint position and muscle force. However, a valid clinical assessment of strength requires that the joint position at which strength is assessed*

be maintained for each subsequent test. The clinician must consider the effects of joint position on muscle output when measuring strength and also when designing intervention strategies to improve muscle function. Unless the effects of muscle moment arm and muscle length are held constant, changes in strength resulting from intervention cannot be distinguished from changes resulting from the mechanical change in the muscle.

The following scenario provides a helpful demonstration. In the initial visit to a patient treated at home, the clinician measures hip flexion strength while the patient is sitting in a wheelchair. Weakness is identified, and exercises are provided. On the next visit, 2 days later, the clinician finds the patient in bed and so measures hip flexion strength in bed with the hip extended. Hip flexion strength is greater at this measurement than in the previous measurement. The astute therapist recognizes that the apparent increase in strength may be attributable to the change in position, since muscle hypertrophy as a result of exercise is unlikely after only 2 days. Research demonstrates that the hip flexors are strongest with the hip close to extension where the muscles are in a lengthened position (Chapter 39). It is noteworthy to recognize that in this position the angle of application is relatively small as well, suggesting that muscle length is a larger influence on hip flexion strength than is angle of application.

Relationship between Force Production and Contraction Velocity

The chapter to this point has examined the influence of muscle factors on force production only in isometric contractions, contractions with no visible change in muscle length. However in nonisometric contractions, the direction and speed of contraction influence the muscle's output. Speed of movement and its direction are described together by the vector quantity velocity. This section examines the effects of contraction velocity on muscle output. Both the direction and the magnitude of the velocity are important influences and are discussed individually below.

EFFECTS OF THE MAGNITUDE OF THE CONTRACTION VELOCITY ON FORCE PRODUCTION IN MUSCLE

Contractile velocity of a muscle is determined usually by the macroscopic change in length per unit time. Thus an **isometric contraction** has zero contraction velocity. It is important to recognize that on the microscopic level there is a change in length of the muscle even in an isometric contraction. In contrast, a **concentric contraction,** also known as a **shortening contraction,** is defined as a contraction in which there is visible shortening of the muscle [37]. Thus a concentric contraction has a positive contraction velocity.

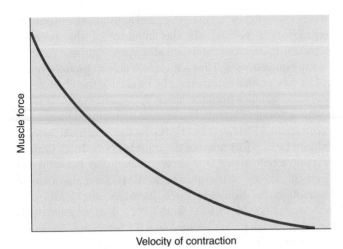

Figure 4.19: The relationship between contractile force and the velocity of contraction in isometric and concentric contractions. A plot of contractile force and the velocity of contraction from isometric (F_i) to concentric contractions shows that the strength of the contraction decreases with increasing contractile velocity.

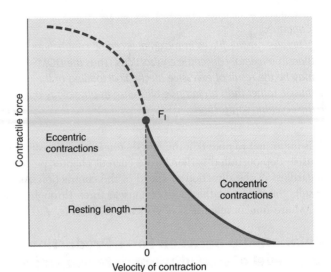

Figure 4.20: The relationship between contractile force and the velocity of contraction in isometric, concentric, and eccentric contractions. A plot of contractile force and the velocity of contraction from eccentric to concentric contractions shows that an eccentric contraction is stronger than either isometric (F_i) or concentric contractions.

The relationship between contractile force and speed of contraction in isometric and shortening contractions has been studied for most of the 20th century and is well understood [36,38,68,75,122,141,147]. A plot of a muscle's force of contraction over contractile velocity for isometric and concentric contractions reveals that contractile force is maximum when contraction velocity is zero (isometric contraction) and decreases as contraction velocity increases (*Fig. 4.19*). Thus an isometric contraction produces more force than a concentric contraction of similar magnitude. Similarly, a rapid shortening contraction produces less force than a slow shortening contraction.

Clinical Relevance

EXAMINING MUSCLE STRENGTH IN THE CLINIC: *Both isometric and concentric contractions are used in the clinic to assess strength. For example, one form of the standardized manual muscle testing procedures examines the force of an isometric contraction at the end of range, while another form measures the force of a concentric contraction through the full ROM to grade a muscle's force [59]. Similarly, clinicians use isokinetic dynamometers to measure both isometric and concentric strength. Each of these tests is valid, and there is a correlation among maximum force at various contraction velocities [74,118]. However, it is important for clinicians to recognize that the absolute force produced depends on the testing mode. If all other factors of muscle performance are constant, the isometric contractions produce greater forces than the concentric forces. Judgments regarding the adequacy of an individual's strength must consider the effects of contraction velocity.*

EFFECTS OF THE DIRECTION OF CONTRACTION ON FORCE PRODUCTION IN MUSCLE

As noted earlier, both the magnitude and direction of the contraction influence a muscle's performance. A contraction that occurs as a muscle visibly lengthens is called an **eccentric contraction.** Eccentric contractile strength is less well understood than isometric and concentric strength, at least in part because it is difficult to study lengthening contractions over a large spectrum of speeds in intact muscles. Despite this limitation, many studies have been completed and provide important information regarding the comparative contractile force of eccentric contractions. A plot of muscle tension over the whole spectrum of contraction velocities reveals that eccentric contractions produce more force than either isometric or concentric contractions [28,36,46,58,61,78,80,117,127,132,140,154] (*Fig. 4.20*). Maximum eccentric strength is estimated to be between 1.5 and 2.0 times maximum concentric strength [127,144]. The plot of muscle force as a function of contraction velocity also reveals that the effect of the magnitude of contraction velocity on force production plateaus in an eccentric contraction [28,36,91].

Clinical Relevance

POST-EXERCISE MUSCLE SORENESS: *Studies indicate that delayed-onset muscle soreness (DOMS) typically is associated with exercise using resisted eccentric exercise [11,40]. Although this phenomenon has not been thoroughly explained, one possible explanation is that a muscle*

(continued)

(Continued)

generates greater forces in maximal eccentric contractions than in maximal concentric contractions. Thus the DOMS may be the result of excessive mechanical loading of the muscle rather than an intrinsic difference in physiology of the eccentric contraction.

It is important to note that the length–tension relationship in muscle demonstrated earlier in the current chapter persists regardless of the direction or speed of the contraction. As a result, the shape of the plots of muscle force through the ROM are similar, regardless of velocity [75,79] (*Fig. 4.21*).

Relationship between Force Production and Level of Recruitment of Motor Units within the Muscle

Earlier in the current chapter it is reported that the strength of the cross-links between actin and myosin is influenced by the frequency of stimulation by the motor nerve. Examination of the function of a whole muscle reveals a similar relationship. A whole muscle is composed of smaller units called *motor units*. A **motor unit** consists of the individual muscle fibers innervated by a single motor nerve cell, or motoneuron. The force of contraction of a whole muscle is modulated by the frequency of stimulation by the motor nerve and by the number of motor units active. A single stimulus of low intensity from the motor nerve produces depolarization of the muscle and a **twitch** contraction of one or more motor units. As the frequency of the stimulus increases, the twitch is repeated. As in the single fiber, if the stimulus is repeated before the muscle

relaxes, the twitches begin to fuse, and a sustained, or **tetanic,** contraction is elicited. As the intensity of the stimulus increases, more motor units are stimulated, and the force of contraction increases. Thus a muscle is able to produce maximal or submaximal contractions by modifying the characteristics of the stimulus from the nerve.

The amount of activity of a muscle is measured by its electromyogram (EMG). The EMG is the electrical activity induced by depolarization of the muscle fibers. In an isometric contraction, there is a strong relationship between the electrical activity of the muscle, its EMG, and the force of contraction. As isometric force increases, the EMG also increases [24,30,31,78,130,136,137,142]. This relationship is logical, since the force of contraction is a function of the number of cross-links formed between the actin and myosin chains and thus a function of the number of muscle fibers contracting. The EMG reflects the number of active fibers as well as their firing frequency [8,10,12,26,134]. However, the relationship of the muscle's EMG and its force of contraction is more complicated when the muscle is free to change length and the joint is free to move.

This chapter demonstrates that the size and stretch of the muscle, the muscle's moment arm, and the velocity of contraction all contribute to the force produced by contraction. The EMG merely serves to indicate the electrical activity in a muscle. Thus a larger muscle produces a larger EMG pattern during a maximal contraction than a smaller muscle performing a maximal contraction, since there are more motor units firing in the larger muscle. However, within the same muscle, a maximal eccentric contraction elicits an EMG pattern similar to that produced during a maximal concentric contraction, even though the force of contraction is greater in the eccentric contraction [78,127]. In the case of maximal contractions, the muscle recruits approximately the same number of motor units regardless of the output. The magnitude of the force output from concentric and eccentric contractions varies primarily because of the mechanical effects of contraction velocity.

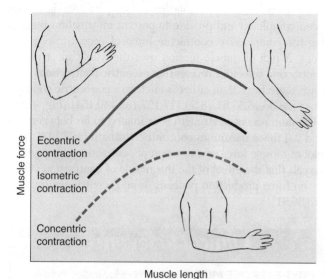

Figure 4.21: Comparison of eccentric, isometric, and concentric muscle strengths with changing muscle length. A comparison of eccentric, isometric, and concentric muscle strengths through an ROM reveals that the force of an eccentric contraction is greater than the force of an isometric contraction, which is greater than the force of a concentric contraction, regardless of the length of the muscle.

Clinical Relevance

ASSESSMENT OF PEAK STRENGTH: *The basic premise of strength assessment is that the test subject is producing a maximal contraction; that is, the subject is maximally recruiting available motor units. The validity and reliability of muscle testing depends upon the tester's ability to motivate the individual to produce a maximal contraction. A classic study of the reliability of manual muscle testing reveals that an important factor explaining the lack of reliability is that some testers failed to elicit a maximal contraction, erroneously grading a submaximal contraction [65]. Encouraging a subject to produce a maximal effort requires both psychological and mechanical skills that are developed with knowledge and practice but are essential to valid and reliable measures of strength.*

Maximal contractions are assumed to activate all of the motor units of the muscle. In young healthy adults this appears to be the case; that is they can typically activate 98–100% of the available motor units [103]. In contrast individuals who have pain or who are chronically inactive may be unable to fully activate the muscle, even though they are attempting to perform a maximal voluntary contraction (MVC) and appear to have an intact neuromuscular system [63,106,138]. These individuals exhibit **activation failure** in which, despite their best efforts and in the presence of intact muscles and nerves, they are unable to recruit all of the available motor units of the muscle. It is important that the clinician be able to determine if muscle weakness is the result of morphological changes in the muscles or nerves or activation failure.

Clinical Relevance

ACTIVATION FAILURE IN INDIVIDUALS WITH OSTEOARTHRITIS: *Individuals with either hip or knee osteoarthritis exhibit activation failure in the involved joints [63,138]. This failure is also described as **arthrogenic inhibition**, suggesting, that joint pain inhibits full muscle activation. Yet similar activation failure is found in individuals 1 year following total knee replacements when pain is no longer a complaint. Traditional exercises appear to have little effect on the activation failure, but more dynamic functional exercises have produced improved recruitment in patients with knee osteoarthritis [63]. Neuromuscular electrical stimulation also reduces activation failure. Identifying activation failure as a cause of muscle weakness may alter the intervention strategies used to improve strength.*

In a submaximal contraction, the muscle recruits enough motor units to produce the necessary muscle force. A muscle that is lengthened or positioned with a large moment arm is said to be at a **mechanical advantage.** It can produce the same moment with less recruitment and consequently a smaller EMG than when the muscle is at a mechanical disadvantage, positioned at a shortened length, or with a small moment arm [66,109]. When a muscle is at a mechanical advantage or when it is stronger, it needs fewer motor units to generate a moment; when the muscle is at a mechanical disadvantage or is weaker, it must recruit more motor units to generate the same moment [9,30,108].

This literature review demonstrates that EMG reflects the relative activity of a muscle rather than providing a direct measure of the force of that muscle's contraction. The literature is filled with studies of the EMG activity of muscles during function. These studies are used to explain the role of muscles during activity. Reference to such articles is made frequently throughout this textbook. However, caution is needed when interpreting these studies, since EMG reflects only the relative activity of a muscle. Muscle size and mechanical advantage affect the recorded electrical activity. There are also several technical factors that influence the magnitude of EMG produced during muscle contraction. These include the type and size of the recording electrodes and the signal-processing procedures. These issues are beyond the scope of this book, but they serve as a warning to the clinician that interpretation of EMG and comparisons across studies must proceed with caution. To improve the generalizability of EMG data, analysis of the electrical activity of a muscle typically involves some form of **normalization** of the data. A common normalizing procedure is to compare the activity of a muscle to the EMG produced by a maximal voluntary contraction (MVC). The basic premise in this approach is that an MVC requires maximal recruitment of a muscle's motor units, which then produces a maximum electrical signal. This maximal activity is used as the basis for comparing the muscle's level of activity in other activities. Processing of the electrical signal also affects the interpretation of the signal [8]. A discussion of the issues involved in the analysis of EMG data is beyond the scope of this book. However, the reader is urged to use EMG data cautiously when analyzing the roles of individual muscles.

Relationship between Force Production and Fiber Type

The last characteristic of muscle influencing the force of contraction to be discussed in this chapter is the type of fibers composing an individual muscle. Different types of muscle fibers possess different contractile properties. Therefore, their distribution within a muscle influences the contractile performance of a whole muscle. However, because human muscles are composed of a mix of fiber types, fiber type has less influence on the force-producing capacity of a muscle than do the factors discussed to this point.

There are a variety of ways to categorize voluntary muscle fibers based on such characteristics as their metabolic processes, their histochemical composition, and their phenotype. Although each method examines different properties, each identifies groups ranging from fatigue-resistant fibers with slow contractile properties to rapidly fatiguing cells with faster contractile velocities [153]. A common cataloging system based on metabolic properties classifies most human muscle fibers as type I, type IIa, or type IIb fibers. Characteristics of these three fiber types are listed in *Table 4.1*. For the purposes of the current discussion, a closer examination of the mechanical properties of these fibers is indicated. In general, the contractile force of a type IIb fiber is greater than that of a type I fiber [14]. Thus muscles composed of more type IIb fibers are likely to generate larger contractile forces than a comparable muscle consisting of mostly type I fibers [110]. Type I fibers are innervated by small-diameter axons of the motor nerve. They are recruited first in a muscle contraction. Type IIb fibers are innervated by large axons and are recruited only after type I and type IIa fibers. Type IIb fibers are recruited as the resistance increases [105,107].

TABLE 4.1: Basic Performance Characteristics of Types I, IIa, and IIb Muscle Fibers

	I	IIa	IIb
Contraction velocity	Slow	Moderately fast	Fast
Contractile force	Low	Variable	High
Fatigability	Fatigue resistant	Somewhat fatigue resistant	Rapidly fatiguing

The velocity of contraction also differs among fiber types [3,14]. Consequently, the force–velocity relationship also varies among the fiber types. Data from human muscles suggest that type IIb fibers exert larger forces at higher velocities, while type I fibers have slower maximal contractile velocities as well as lower peak forces [14]. Thus muscles with a preponderance of type II fibers have a higher rate of force production and a higher contractile force than muscles with more type I fibers [1].

Postural muscles typically are composed largely of type I fibers, while muscles whose functions demand large bursts of force consist of more type II fibers [1,133]. However, as already noted, human muscles contain a mixture of fiber types [32,33,104,107]. Therefore, the contractile properties of whole muscles reflect the combined effects of the fibers types. Consequently, the other factors influencing force production such as muscle size and mechanical advantage appear to have a larger influence on contractile force [25]. However, muscle fibers demonstrate different responses to changes in activity and thus play a significant role in muscle adaptation. The adaptability of muscle is discussed briefly below.

ADAPTATION OF MUSCLE TO ALTERED FUNCTION

Muscle is perhaps the most mutable of biological tissues. A discussion of the mechanical properties of muscle cannot be complete without a brief discussion of the changes in these mechanical properties resulting from changes in the demands placed on muscle. The following provides a brief discussion of the changes in muscle that occur in response to sustained changes in

- Muscle length
- Activity level

Understanding the effects of sustained changes in muscle length or activity level is complicated by the recognition that these factors are often combined in investigations. Studies assessing the effects of length changes often use immobilization to apply the length change. Consequently, the muscles respond to both the altered length and decreased activity. As a result, a complete understanding of the influence of these factors on muscle function continues to elude investigators. The following briefly reviews the current state of knowledge of muscles' adaptation to altered function.

Adaptation of Muscle to Prolonged Length Changes

The relationship between stretch of a muscle and its force of contraction is presented in detail elsewhere in this chapter. This relationship is a function of both the contractile and noncontractile components of muscle. However, it also is important to ponder the effect of prolonged length change on the length–tension relationship. Since muscles are organized in groups of opposing muscles, when one muscle is held on stretch, another muscle is held in a shortened position. Therefore, it is important to consider a muscle's response to both prolonged lengthening and prolonged shortening. The vast majority of studies examining alterations in muscle resulting from prolonged length changes use immobilization procedures to provide the length change. Therefore, the reader must exert caution when attempting to generalize these results to other cases such as postural abnormalities that do not involve immobilization.

CHANGES IN MUSCLE WITH PROLONGED LENGTHENING

In general, prolonged stretch of a muscle induces protein synthesis and the production of additional sarcomeres [48,49,139, 150,153]. The muscle hypertrophies, and as a result, peak contractile force is increased with prolonged stretch. The addition of sarcomeres in series increases the overall length of the muscle fibers. This remodeling appears important in allowing the muscle to maintain its length–tension relationship. There also is evidence of changes in the metabolic characteristics of muscle cells subjected to prolonged stretch. Some muscles exhibit changes in mRNA consistent with a transition from type II to type I fibers [153].

Although hypertrophy is the typical muscle response to prolonged stretch, studies report more varied responses among individual muscles. Changes in muscle mass, peak strength, and even gene expression with prolonged stretch vary across muscles and appear to depend upon the muscle's fiber type composition and its function [86,96].

CHANGES IN MUSCLE HELD IN A SHORTENED POSITION FOR A PROLONGED PERIOD

Investigation into the effects of prolonged shortening also demonstrates a complex response. Prolonged shortening produced by immobilization appears to accelerate atrophy, and muscles demonstrate a loss of sarcomeres [48,139,153]. Some muscles immobilized in a shortened position also show evidence of a transition toward type II fibers. Yet a study examining the effects of shortening without immobilization reports an increase in sarcomeres [77]. Results of this study suggest that tendon excursion may be a stronger factor than the shortening itself in determining the muscle's remodeling. In addition, like prolonged stretch, prolonged shortening yields different responses in different muscles [86].

Clearly, complete understanding of the factors inducing muscle adaptation requires further investigation. The studies reported here demonstrate that the adaptability of muscle to prolonged length changes is complex and depends on many factors besides the specific change in length. Yet these studies do consistently demonstrate changes that seem directed, at least in part, at maintaining a safe and functional length–tension relationship in each muscle [86,125,139].

Clinical Relevance

PROLONGED LENGTH CHANGES IN MUSCLE AS THE RESULT OF POSTURAL ABNORMALITIES: *Postural abnormalities reportedly produce prolonged lengthening of some muscles and prolonged shortening of other muscles [69]. This has led to the belief that abnormal posture produces changes in muscle strength. Studies have attempted to identify such changes in strength and changes in the length-tension relationships of muscles that appear to be affected by postural abnormalities [23,116]. However, these studies fail to demonstrate a clear change in strength attributable to length changes. Yet clinicians continue to treat abnormal postural alignment with strengthening and stretching exercises. Although current studies neither prove nor disprove the existence of clinically measurable changes in muscle as the result of prolonged length changes, they emphasize the need for clinicians to use caution in assuming relationships between postural alignment and muscular strength.*

Adaptations of Muscle to Sustained Changes in Activity Level

Muscle's basic response to changes in activity level is well known: increased activity results in hypertrophy and increased force production, and decreased activity leads to atrophy and decreased force production. Of course the exact response is far more complicated than this. The response depends on the nature of the activity change and on the nature of the muscle whose activity is altered.

Resistance exercise leads to muscle hypertrophy and increased strength in both men and women of virtually all ages [18,72,83,119,145]. Strengthening exercises in humans produce an increase in the cross-sectional area (CSA) of both type I and type II fibers, although there is evidence that there is a greater increase in the CSA of type II fibers

[25,27,61,97,101,115]. In addition, animal studies reveal that protein synthesis is consistent with a transition from type IIb fibers to type I fibers [6,86].

In contrast, decreased activity produces a decrease in CSA and loss of strength [47,85,115]. One study reports a 13% decrease in some lower extremity strength in 10 healthy subjects who underwent only 10 days of non-weight-bearing activity [9]! Disuse atrophy is apparent in both type I and type II fibers. In addition, there is evidence supporting a transition from type I fibers to type II fibers [5,6,96].

Although the preceding discussion demonstrates general patterns of muscle response to changes in activity level, the response is actually quite muscle dependent [85,86]. One study reports a 26% loss in plantarflexion strength with no significant loss in dorsiflexion strength in healthy individuals following 5 weeks of bed rest [85]. Animal studies show similar differences among muscle groups [19,86]. Other mechanical factors such as stretch also affect a muscle's response to reduced activity [96].

Clinical Relevance

DISUSE ATROPHY IN PATIENTS: *Patients who have spent prolonged periods in bed are likely to demonstrate significant loss of strength resulting directly from the inactivity and unrelated to other simultaneous impairments or comorbidities. However, the effects of inactivity may be manifested differently in the various muscle groups of the body. The clinician must be aware of the likely loss of strength and also must consider the possible loss of muscular endurance that may result from a transition from type I to type II muscle fibers. In addition, the clinician also must screen carefully for these changes to identify those muscle groups that are most affected by disuse.*

Astronauts and cosmonauts experience a unique case of disuse atrophy resulting from their time spent in a microgravity environment. As with bed rest, microgravity induces atrophy of both Type I and Type II with evidence of a transition toward more Type II fibers [29]. Motor unit recruitment also appears altered. The resulting muscle weakness and decreased muscular endurance present significant challenges for protracted space travel and particularly for re-entry to earth's gravitational field.

Clinical Relevance

EXERCISING IN SPACE: *The International Space Lab is designed to allow prolonged stays in space and may serve as an intermediate stop for travelers to farther locations*

(continued)

(Continued)

such as Mars. However, unless these space travelers can exercise sufficiently to prevent the loss of muscle function that currently accompanies space travel, travel to outer space will remain limited to a select few individuals who can tolerate these changes. Exercise and rehabilitation experts who devise exercise equipment and regimens for microgravity use will find a very interested audience at the National Aeronautics and Space Agency (NASA) and other international space agencies.

AGING AS ANOTHER MODEL OF ALTERED ACTIVITY

Loss of strength is a well-established finding in aging adults [17,83,93,98,119,131]. This loss of strength is attributed to a decreased percentage of, and greater atrophy in, type II fibers [73,84,129]. As in the other adaptations of muscle described above, changes in muscle with age vary across muscles [20]. Some muscle groups appear to be more susceptible to age-related change; others seem impervious to such changes. Again these data reveal that the clinician must assess strength in the aging individual. However, the clinician must also take care to identify those muscle groups that are weakened and those that are relatively unaffected, to target the intervention specifically for optimal results.

Clinical Relevance

DECREASED STRENGTH WITH AGING: *Decreased functional ability is a frequent finding with aging. Although many factors contribute to diminished function with age, investigations demonstrate a relationship between diminished functional ability and decreased strength [21,23,51]. Similarly, increasing strength in elders improves functional ability [35,111]. One of the challenges in rehabilitation is to identify successful strategies to prevent or reduce strength loss and preserve functional ability in the aging population.*

SUMMARY

This chapter reviews the basic mechanisms of muscle shortening and discusses in detail the individual factors that influence a muscle's ability to produce motion and to generate force. The primary factors influencing a muscle's ability to produce joint motion are the length of the muscle fibers within the muscle and the length of the muscle's moment arm. Muscle strength, including its tensile force of contraction and its resulting moment, is a function of muscle size, muscle moment arm length, stretch of the muscle, contraction velocity, fiber types within the muscle, and amount of muscle fiber recruitment. Each factor is described and examples are provided to demonstrate how an understanding of the factor can be used in the clinic to explain or optimize performance. The

discussion also demonstrates that often as one factor is enhancing a performance characteristic another factor may be detracting from that performance. The final output of a muscle is the result of all of the factors influencing performance. Thus to understand the basis for a patient's performance, the clinician must be able to recognize how the individual factors influencing muscle performance change as joint position and motion change.

References

1. Aagaard P, Andersen JL: Correlation between contractile strength and myosin heavy chain isoform composition in human skeletal muscle. Med Sci Sports Exerc 1998; 30: 1217–1222.
2. Aagaard P, Andersen JL, Dyhre-Poulsen P, et al.: A mechanism for increased contractile strength of human pennate muscle in response to strength training: changes in muscle architecture. J Physiol 2001; 534: 613–623.
3. Adam C, Eckstein F, Milz S, Putz R: The distribution of cartilage thickness within the joints of the lower limb of elderly individuals. J Anat 1998; 193: 203–214.
4. An KN, Kaufman KR, Chao EYS: Physiological considerations of muscle force through the elbow joint. J Biomech 1989; 22: 1249–1256.
5. Andersen JL, Gruschy-Knudsen T, Sabdri C, et al.: Bed rest increases the amount of mismatched fibers in human skeletal muscle. J Appl Physiol 1999; 86: 455–460.
6. Baldwin KM: Effects of altered loading states on muscle plasticity: what have we learned from rodents? Med Sci Sports Exerc 1996; 28: S101–S106.
7. Baldwin KM, Valdez V, Herrick RE, et al.: Biochemical properties of overloaded fast-twitch skeletal muscle. J Appl Physiol 1982; 52: 467–472.
8. Basmajian JV, DeLuca CJ: Muscles Alive. Their Function Revealed by Electromyography. Baltimore: Williams & Wilkins, 1985.
9. Berg HE, Tesch PA: Changes in muscle function in response to 10 days of lower limb unloading in humans. Acta Physiol Scand 1996; 157: 63–70.
10. Bergstrom RM: The relation between the number of impulses and the integrated electrical activity in electromyogram. Acta Physiol Scand 1959; 45: 97–101.
11. Berry CB, Moritani T, Tolson H: Electrical activity and soreness in muscles after exercise. Am J Phys Med Rehabil 1990; 69: 60–66.
12. Bigland B, Lippold OCJ: The relation between force, velocity and integrated electrical activity in human muscles. J Physiol 1954; 123: 214–224.
13. Blazevich AJ, Gill ND, Deans N, Zhou S: Lack of human muscle architectural adaptation after short-term strength training. Muscle Nerve 2007; 35: 78–86.
14. Bottinelli R, Pellegrino MA, Canepari M, et al.: Specific contributions of various muscle fibre types to human muscle performance: an in vitro study. J Electromyogr Kinesiol 1999; 9: 87–95.
15. Brand PW, Beach RB, Thompson DE: Relative tension and potential excursion of muscles in the forearm and hand. J Hand Surg [Am]. 1999; 6: 209–219.
16. Brand PW, Hollister A: Clinical Mechanics of the Hand. St. Louis, MO: Mosby-Year Book, 1993.

17. Brown DA, Miller WC: Normative data for strength and flexibility of women throughout life. Eur J Appl Physiol 1998; 78: 77–82.

18. Brown M: Exercising and elderly person. Phys Ther Pract 1992; 1: 34–42.

19. Brown M, Hasser EM: Weight-bearing effects on skeletal muscle during and after simulated bed rest. Arch Phys Med Rehabil 1995; 76: 541–546.

20. Brown M, Hasser EM: Complexity of age-related change in skeletal muscle. J Gerontol 1996; 51A: B117–B123.

21. Brown M, Sinacore D, Host H: The relationship of strength to function in the older adult. J Gerontol 1995; 50A: 55–59.

22. Buchanan TS: Evidence that maximum muscle stress is not a constant: differences in specific tension in elbow flexors and extensors. Med Eng Phys 1995; 17: 529–536.

23. Buchner DM, Beresford SAA, Larson EB, et al.: Effects of physical activity on health status in older adults II: intervention studies. Annu Rev Public Health 1992; 13: 469–488.

24. Clancy EA, Hogan N: Relating agonist-antagonist electromyograms to joint torque during isometric, quasi-isotonic, nonfatiguing contractions. IEEE Trans Biomed Eng 1997; 44: 1024–1028.

25. Clarkson PM, Kroll W, Melchionda AM: Isokinetic strength, endurance, and fiber type composition in elite American paddlers. Eur J Appl Physiol 1982; 48: 67–76.

26. Coburn JW, Housh TJ, Malek MH, et al.: Mechanomyographic and electromyographic responses to eccentric muscle contractions. Muscle Nerve 2006; 33: 664–671.

27. Cress NM, Conley KE, Balding SL, et al.: Functional training: muscle structure, function and performance in older women. J Orthop Sports Phys Ther 1996; 24: 4–10.

28. Cress NM, Peters KS, Chandler JM: Eccentric and concentric force-velocity relationships of the quadriceps femoris muscle. J Orthop Sports Phys Ther 1992; 16: 82–86.

29. di Prampero PE, Narici MV: Muscles in microgravity: from fibres to human motion. J Biomech 2003; 36: 403–412.

30. Dolan P, Adams MA: The relationship between EMG activity and extensor moment generation in the erector spinae muscles during bending and lifting activities. J Biomech 1993; 26: 513–522.

31. Dolan P, Kingman I, DeLooze MP, et al: An EMG technique for measuring spinal loading during asymmetric lifting. Clin Biomech 2001; 16 Suppl: S17–S24.

32. Edgerton VR, Smith JL, Simpson DR: Muscle fibre type populations of human leg muscles. Histochem J 1975; 7: 259–266.

33. Elder GCB, Bradbury K, Roberts R: Variability of fiber type distributions within human muscles. J Appl Physiol 1982; 53: 1473–1480.

34. Elftman H: Biomechanics of muscle, with particular application to studies of gait. J Bone Joint Surg [AM] 1966; 48: 363–377.

35. Evans WJ: Exercise training guidelines for the elderly. Med Sci Sports Exerc 1999; 31: 12–17.

36. Evetovich TK, Housh TJ, Johnson GO, et al.: Gender comparisons of the mechanomyographic responses to maximal concentric and eccentric isokinetic muscle actions. Med Sci Sports Exerc 1998; 30: 1697–1702.

37. Faulkner JA: Terminology for contractions of muscles during shortening, while isometric, and during lengthening. J Appl Physiol 2003; 95: 455–459.

38. Fenn WO, Marsh BS: Muscular force at different speed of shortening. Proc R Soc B [Lond] 1998; 277–297.

39. Fitts RH, McDonald KS, Schluter JM: The determinants of skeletal muscle force and power: their adaptability with changes in activity pattern. J Biomech 1991; 24: 111–122.

40. Fitzgerald GK, Rothstein JM, Mayhew TP, Lamb RL: Exercise-induced muscle soreness after concentric and eccentric isokinetic contractions. Phys Ther 1991; 71: 505–513.

41. Foss ML, Keteyian SJ: Fox's physiological basis of exercise and sport. Boston: WCB/McGraw-Hill, 1998.

42. Fukunaga T, Kawakami Y, Kuno S, et al.: Muscle architecture and function in humans. J Biomech 1997; 30: 457–463.

43. Gandevia SC, McKenzie DK: Activation of human muscles at short muscle lengths during maximal static efforts. J Physiol [Lond] 1988; 407: 599–613.

44. Gans C: Fiber architecture and muscle function. Exerc Sports Sci Rev 1982; 10: 160–207.

45. Gareis H, Solomonow M, Baratta R, et al.: The isometric length-force models of nine different skeletal muscles. J Biomech 1992; 25: 903–916.

46. Ghena DR, Kurth AL, Thomas M, Mayhew J: Torque characteristics of the quadriceps and hamstring muscles during concentric and eccentric loading. J Orthop Sports Phys Ther 1991; 14: 149–154.

47. Gogia PP, Schneider VS, LeBlanc AD, et al.: Bed rest effect on extremity muscle torque in healthy men. Arch Phys Med Rehabil 1988; 69: 1030–1032.

48. Goldspink G: The influence of immobilization and stretch in protein turnover of rat skeletal muscle. J Physiol 1977; 264: 267–282.

49. Goldspink G: Changes in muscle mass and phenotype and the expression of autocrine and systemic growth factors by muscle in response to stretch and overload. J Anat 1999; 194: 323–334.

50. Gordon AM, Huxley AF, Julian FJ: The variation in isometric tension with sarcomere length in vertebrate muscle fibres. J Physiol 1966; 184: 170–192.

51. Graafmans WC, Ooms ME, Hofstee HMA, et al.: Falls in the elderly: a prospective study of the risk factors and risk profiles. Am J Epidemiol 1996; 143: 1129–1136.

52. Harms-Ringdahl K: Muscle strength. Edinburgh: Churchill Livingstone, 1993.

53. Hawkins D, Bey M: Muscle and tendon force-length properties and their interactions in vivo. J Biomech 1997; 30: 63–70.

54. Hawkins DA, Hull ML: A computer simulation of muscle-tendon mechanics. Comput Biol Med 1991; 21: 369–382.

55. Herzog W, Leonard TR: The role of passive structures in force enhancement of skeletal muscles following active stretch. J Biomech 2005; 38: 409–415.

56. Herzog W, Leonard TR, Renaud JM, et al.: Force-length properties and functional demands of cat gastrocnemius, soleus, and plantaris muscles. J Biomech 1992; 25: 1329–1335.

57. Herzog W, Read LJ: Lines of action and moment arms of the major force-carrying structures crossing the human knee joint. J Anat 1993; 182: 213–230.

58. Higbie EJ, Cureton KJ, Warren GLI, Prior BM: Effects of concentric and eccentric training on muscle strength, cross-sectional area, and neural activation. J Appl Physiol 1996; 81: 2173–2181.

59. Hislop HJ, Montgomery J: Daniel's and Worthingham's Muscle Testing: Techniques of Manual Examination. Philadelphia: WB Saunders, 1995.

60. Holzbaur KR, Delp SL, Gold GE, Murray WM: Moment-generating capacity of upper limb muscles in healthy adults. J Biomech 2007; 40(4): 742–749.

61. Hortobagyi T, Hill JP, Houmard JA, et al.: Adaptive responses to muscle lengthening and shortening in humans. J Appl Physiol 1996; 80: 765–772.

62. Hoy MG, Zajac FE: A musculoskeletal model of the human lower extremity: the effect of muscle, tendon, and moment arm on the moment-angle relationship of musculotendon actuators at the hip, knee, and ankle. J Biomech 1990; 23: 157–169.

63. Hurley MV, Newham DJ: The influence of arthrogenous muscle inhibition on quadriceps rehabilitation of patients with early, unilateral osteoarthritic knees. Br J Rheumatol 1993; 32: 127–131.

64. Ichinose Y: Relationship between muscle fiber pennation and force generation capability in Olympic athletes. Int J Sports Med 1998; 19: 541–546.

65. Iddings DM, Smith LK, Spencer WA: Muscle testing: Part 2. Reliability in clinical use. Phys Ther Rev 1960; 41: 249–256.

66. Inman VT, Ralston HJ, Saunders JBDM, et al.: Relation of human electromyogram to muscular tension. Electroenceph Clin Neurophysiol 1952; 4: 187–194.

67. Kanehisa H, Ikegawa S, Fukunaga T: Force-velocity relationships and fatigability of strength and endurance-trained subjects. Int J Sports Med. 1997; 18: 106–112.

68. Katz B: The relation between force and speed in muscular contraction. J Physiol 1939; 96: 45–64.

69. Kendall FP, McCreary EK, Provance PG: Muscle Testing and Function. Baltimore: Williams & Wilkins, 1993.

70. Ketchum LD, Thompson D, Pocock G, Wallingford D: A clinical study of forces generated by the intrinsic muscles of the index finger and the extrinsic flexor and extensor muscles of the hand. J Hand Surg [Am]. 1978; 3: 571–578.

71. Klein P, Mattys S, Rooze M: Moment arm length variations of selected muscles acting on talocrural and subtalar joints during movement: an in vitro study. J Biomech 1996; 29: 21–30.

72. Klinge K, Magnusson SP, Simonsen EB, et al.: The effect of strength and flexibility training on skeletal muscle electromyographic activity, stiffness, and viscoelastic stress relaxation response. Am J Sports Med. 1997; 25: 710–716.

73. Klitgaard H, Mantoni M, Schiaffino S, et al.: Function, morphology and protein expression of ageing skeletal muscle: a cross-sectional study of elderly men with different training backgrounds. Acta Physiol Scand. 1990; 140: 41–54.

74. Knapik JJ: Isokinetic, isometric and isotonic strength relationships. Arch Phys Med Rehabil 1983; 64: 77–80.

75. Knapik JJ, Wright JE, Mawdsley RH, Braun J: Isometric, isotonic, and isokinetic torque variations in four muscle groups through a range of joint motion. Phys Ther 1983; 63: 938–947.

76. Koh TJ, Herzog W: Increasing the moment arm of the tibialis anterior induces structural and functional adaptation: implications for tendon transfer. J Biomech 1998; 31: 593–599.

77. Koh TJ, Herzog W: Excursion is important in regulating sarcomere number in the growing rabbit tibialis anterior. J Physiol [Lond] 1998; 508: 267–280.

78. Komi PV: Relationship between muscle tension, EMG, and velocity of contraction under concentric and eccentric work. In: New Developments in Electromyography and Clinical Neurophysiology. Desmedt JE, ed. Basel: Karger, 1973; 596–606.

79. Komi PV: Measurement of the force-velocity relationship in human muscle under concentric and eccentric contractions. Biomechanics III 1979; 224–229.

80. Krylow AM, Sandercock TG: Dynamic force responses of muscle involving eccentric contraction. J Biomech 1997; 30: 27–33.

81. Kuechle DK, Newman SR, Itoi E, et al.: Shoulder muscle moment arms during horizontal flexion and elevation. J Shoulder Elbow Surg 1997; 6: 429–439.

82. Kulig K, Andrews JG, Hay JG: Human strength curves. Exerc Sports Sci Rev 1984; 12: 417–466.

83. Laforest S, St-Peirre DMM, Cyr J, Gayton D: Effects of age and regular exercise on muscle strength and endurance. Eur J Appl Physiol 1990; 60: 104–111.

84. Larsson L, Grimby G, Karlsson J: Muscle strength and speed of movement in relation to age and muscle morphology. J Appl Physiol 1979; 46: 451–456.

85. LeBlanc A, Gogia P, Schneider VS, et al.: Calf muscle area and strength changes after 5 weeks of horizontal bed rest. Am J Sports Med 1988; 16: 624–629.

86. Lieber RL: Skeletal Muscle Structure and Function: Implications for Rehabilitation and Sports Medicine. Baltimore: Williams & Wilkins, 1992.

87. Lieber RL, Boakes JL: Sarcomere length and joint kinematics during torque production in frog hindlimb. Am J Phys 1988; 254: C759–C768.

88. Lieber RL, Friden J: Musculoskeletal balance of the human wrist elucidated using intraoperative laser diffraction. J Electromyogr Kinesiol 1998; 8: 93–100.

89. Lieber RL, Jacobson MD, Fazeli BM, et al.: Architecture of selected muscles of the arm and forearm: anatomy and implications for tendon transfer. J Hand Surg [Am]. 1992; 17: 787–798.

90. Lieber RL, Ljung B, Friden J: Intraoperative sarcomere length measurements reveal differential design of human wrist extensor muscles. J Exp Biol 1997; 200: 19–25.

91. Lieber RL, Ljung B, Friden J: Sarcomere length in wrist extensor muscles, changes may provide insights into the etiology of chronic lateral epicondylitis. Acta Orthop Scand 1997; 68: 249–254.

92. Lieber RL, Loren GJ, Friden J: In vivo measurement of human wrist extensor muscle sarcomere length changes. J Neurophysiol. 1994; 71: 874–881.

93. Lindle RS, Metter EJ, Lynch NA, et al.: Age and gender comparisons of muscle strength in 654 women and men aged 20–93 yr. J Appl Physiol 1997; 83: 1581–1587.

94. Loren GJ, Lieber RL: Tendon biomechanical properties enhance human wrist muscle specialization. J Biomech 1995; 28: 791–799.

95. Loren GJ, Shoemaker SD, Burkholder TJ, et al.: Human wrist motors: biomechanical design and application to tendon transfers. J Biomech 1996; 29: 331–342.

96. Loughna PT: Disuse and passive stretch cause rapid alterations in expression of developmental and adult contractile protein genes in skeletal muscle. Development 1990; 109: 217–223.

97. MacDougall JD, Elder GCB, Sale DG, et al.: Effects of strength training and immobilization on human muscle fibers. J Appl Physiol 1980; 43: 25–34.

98. Maclennan WJ, Hall MPR, Timithy JI, Robinson M: Is weakness in old age due to muscle wasting? Age Ageing 1980; 9: 188–192.

99. Maganaris CN, Baltzopoulos V, Tsaopoulos D: Muscle fibre length-to-moment arm ratios in the human lower limb determined in vivo. J Biomech 2006; 39: 1663–1668.

100. Marshall RN, Mazur SM, Taylor NAS: Three-dimensional surfaces for human muscle kinetics. Eur J Appl Physiol 1990; 61: 263–270.

101. McCall GE, Byrnes WC, Dickinson A, et al.: Muscle fiber hypertrophy, hyperplasia, and capillary density in college men after resistance training. J Appl Physiol 1996; 81: 2004–2012.

102. Mero A, Kuitunen S, Harland M, et al.: Effects of muscle-tendon length on joint moment and power during sprint starts. J Sports Sci 2006; 24: 165–173.

103. Miller M, Holmback AM, Downham D, Lexell J: Voluntary activation and central activation failure in the knee extensors in young women and men. Scand J Med Sci Sports 2006; 16: 274–281.

104. Miller AEJ, MacDougall JD, Tarnopolsky MA, Sale DG: Gender differences in strength and muscle fiber characteristics. Eur J Appl Physiol. 1993; 66: 254–262.

105. Milner-Brown HS, Stein RB, Yemm R: The orderly recruitment of human motor units during voluntary isometric contractions. J Physiol 1973; 230: 359–370.

106. Mizner RL, Petterson SC, Stevens JE, et al.: Early quadriceps strength loss after total knee arthroplasty: the contributions of muscle atrophy and failure of voluntary muscle activation. J Bone Joint Surg Am 2005; 87: 1047–1053.

107. Mizuno M, Secher NH, Quistorff B: 31P-NMR spectroscopy, rsEMG, and histochemical fiber types of human wrist flexor muscles. J Appl Physiol. 1994; 76: 531–538.

108. Moritani T: 1998 ISEK Congress Keynote Lecture: The use of electromyography in applied physiology. International Society of Electrophysiology and Kinesiology. J Electromyogr Kinesiol. 1998; 8: 363–381.

109. Moritani T, DeVries HA: Reexamination of the relationship between the surface integrated electromyogram (IEMG) and force of isometric contraction. Am J Phys Med. 1978; 57: 263–277.

110. Moss CL: Comparison of the histochemical and contractile properties of human gastrocnemius muscle. J Orthop Sports Phys Ther 1991; 13: 322–327.

111. Mulrow CD, Gerety MB, Kanten D, et al.: A randomized trial of physical rehabilitation for very frail nursing home residents. JAMA 1994; 271: 519–524.

112. Murphy AJ, Wilson GJ, Pryor JF, Newton RU: Isometric assessment of muscular function: the effect of joint angle. J Appl Biomech 1995; 11: 205–214.

113. Murray WM, Delp SL, Buchanan TS: Variation of muscle moment arms with elbow and forearm position. J Biomech 1995; 28: 513–525.

114. Narici M: Human skeletal muscle architecture studied in vivo by non-invasive imaging techniques: functional significance and applications. J Electromyogr Kinesiol 1999; 9: 97–103.

115. Narici MV, Roi GS, Landoni L, et al.: Changes in force, cross-sectional area and neural activation during strength training and detraining of the human quadriceps. Eur J Appl Physiol. 1989; 59: 310–319.

116. Neumann DA, Soderberg GL, Cook TM: Comparison of maximal isometric hip abductor muscle torques between hip sides. Phys Ther 1988; 68: 496–502.

117. Olson VL, Smidt GL, Johnston RC: The maximum torque generated by the eccentric, isometric, and concentric contractions of the hip abductor muscles. Phys Ther 1972; 52: 149–158.

118. Osternig LR, Bates BT, James SL: Isokinetic and isometric torque force relationships. Arch Phys Med Rehabil 1977; 58: 254–257.

119. Payne VG, Morrow JR Jr, Johnson L, Dalton SN: Resistance training in children and youth: a meta-analysis. Res Q Exerc Sport 1997; 68: 80–88.

120. Powell PL, Roy RR, Kanim P, et al.: Predictability of skeletal muscle tension from architectural determinations in guinea pig hindlimbs. J Appl Physiol 1984; 57: 1715–1721.

121. Ralston HJ, Inman VT, Strait LA, Shaffrath MD: Mechanics of human isolated voluntary muscle. Am J Phys 1947; 151: 612–620.

122. Ralston HJ, Polissar MJ, Inman VT, et al.: Dynamic features of human isolated voluntary muscle in isometric and free contractions. J Appl Physiol 1949; 1: 526–533.

123. Raschke U, Chaffin DB: Support for a linear length-tension relation of the torso extensor muscles: an investigation of the length and velocity EMG-force relationships. J Biomech 1996; 29: 1597–1604.

124. Rassier DE, Herzog W: Effects of shortening on stretch-induced force enhancement in single skeletal muscle fibers. J Biomech 2004; 37: 1305–1312.

125. Rassier DE, MacIntosh BR, Herzog W: Length dependence of active force production in skeletal muscle. J Appl Physiol. 1999; 86: 1445–1457.

126. Raty HP, Kujala U, Videman T, et al.: Associations of isometric and isoinertial trunk muscle strength measurements and lumbar paraspinal muscle cross-sectional areas. J Spinal Disord 1999; 12: 266–270.

127. Rogers KL, Berger RA: Motor-unit involvement and tension during maximum voluntary concentric, eccentric and isometric contractions of elbow flexors. Med Sci Sports 1974; 6: 253–254.

128. Rousanoglou EN, Oskouei AE, Herzog W: Force depression following muscle shortening in sub-maximal voluntary contractions of human adductor pollicis. J Biomech 2007; 40: 1–8.

129. Scelsi R, Marchetti C, Poggi P: Histochemical and ultrastructural aspects of muscle vastus lateralis in sedentary old people (age 65–89). Acta Neuropathol 1980; 51: 99–105.

130. Seroussi RE, Pope MH: The relationship between trunk muscle electromyography and lifting moments in the sagittal and frontal planes. J Biomech 1987; 20: 135–146.

131. Shephard RJ, Sidney KH: Exercise and aging. Exerc Sports Sci Rev 1978; 6: 1–57.

132. Shklar A, Dvir Z: Isokinetic strength relationships in shoulder muscles. Clin Biomech 1995; 10: 369–373.

133. Sirca A, Kostevc V: The fibre type composition of thoracic and lumbar paravertebral muscles in man. J Anat 1985; 141: 131–137.

134. Solomonow M, Baratta R, Shoji H, D'Ambrosia R: The EMG-force relationships of skeletal muscle; dependence on contraction rate, and motor units control strategy. Electromyogr Clin Neurophysiol 1990; 30: 141–152.

135. Spoor C, Van Leeuwen J, Meskers C, et al.: Estimation of instantaneous moment arms of lower-leg muscles. J Biomech 1990; 23: 1247–1259.

136. Stokes IAF: Relationships of EMG to effort in the trunk under isometric conditions: force-increasing and decreasing effects and temporal delays. Clin Biomech 2005; 20: 9–15.

137. Stokes IAF, Moffroid M, Rush S, Haugh LD: EMG to torque relationship in rectus abdominis muscle: results with repeated testing. Spine 1989; 14: 857–861.

138. Suetta C, Aagaard P, Rosted A, et al.: Training-induced changes in muscle CSA, muscle strength, EMG, and rate of force development in elderly subjects after long-term unilateral disuse. J Appl Physiol 2004; 97: 1954–1961.

139. Tabary JC, Tabary C, Tardieu C, et al.: Physiological and structural changes in the cat's soleus muscle due to immobilization at different lengths by plaster casts. J Physiol 1972; 224: 231–244.

140. Tesch PA, Dudley GA, Duvoisin MR, et al.: Force and EMG signal patterns during repeated bouts of concentric or eccentric muscle actions. Acta Physiol Scand. 1990; 138: 263–271.

141. Thorstensson A, Grimby G, Karlsson J: Force-velocity relations and fiber composition in human knee extensor muscles. J Appl Physiol 1976; 40: 12–16.

142. Vogt R, Nix WA, Pfeifer B: Relationship between electrical and mechanical properties of motor units. J Neurol Neurosurg Psychiatry 1990; 53: 331–334.

143. Walker SM, Schrodt GR: I segment lengths and thin filament periods in skeletal muscle fibers of the rhesus monkey and human. Anat Rec 1974; 178: 63–81.

144. Webber S, Kriellaars D: Neuromuscular factors contributing to in vivo eccentric moment generation. J Appl Physiol. 1997; 83: 40–45.

145. Welle S, Totterman S, Thornton C: Effect of age on muscle hypertrophy induced by resistance training. J Gerontol A Biol Sci Med Sci 1996; 51: M270–M275

146. Wickiewicz TL, Roy RR, Powell PL, Edgerton VR: Muscle architecture of the human lower limb. Clin Orthop 1983; 179: 275–283.

147. Wilkie DR: The relation between force and velocity in human muscle. J Physiol 1950; 110: 249–286.

148. Williams M, Stutzman L: Strength variation through the range of joint motion. Phys Ther Rev 1959; 39: 145–152.

149. Williams P, Bannister L, Berry M, et al.: Gray's Anatomy, The Anatomical Basis of Medicine and Surgery, Br. ed. London: Churchill Livingstone, 1995.

150. Williams P, Kyberd P, Simpson H, et al.: The morphological basis of increased stiffness of rabbit tibialis anterior muscles during surgical limb-lengthening. J Anat 1998; 193: 131–138.

151. Wilson DL, Zhu Q, Duerk JL, et al.: Estimation of tendon moment arms from three-dimensional magnetic resonance images. Ann Biomed Eng 1999; 27: 247–256.

152. Winters J, Stark L, Seif-Naraghi A: An analysis of the sources of musculoskeletal system impedance. J Biomech 1988; 21: 12: 1011–1025.

153. Yang H, Alnaqeeb M, Simpson H, Goldspink G: Changes in muscle fibre type, muscle mass and IGF-I gene expression in rabbit skeletal muscle subjected to stretch. J Anat 1997; 190: 613–622.

154. Yeadon MR, King MA, Wilson C: Modelling the maximum voluntary joint torque/angular velocity relationship in human movement. J Biomech 2006; 39: 476–482.

155. Zajac FE: How musculotendon architecture and joint geometry affect the capacity of muscles to move and exert force on objects: a review with application to arm and forearm tendon transfer design. J Hand Surg [Am]. 1992; 17: 799–804.

Biomechanics of Cartilage

JOSEPH M. MANSOUR, PH.D.

The materials classed as cartilage exist in various forms and perform a range of functions in the body. Depending on its composition, cartilage is classified as articular cartilage (also known as hyaline), fibrocartilage, or elastic cartilage. Elastic cartilage helps to maintain the shape of structures such as the ear and the trachea. In joints, cartilage functions as either a binder or a bearing surface between bones. The annulus fibrosus of the intervertebral disc is an example of a fibrocartilaginous joint with limited movement (an amphiarthrosis). In the freely moveable synovial joints (diarthroses) articular cartilage is the bearing surface that permits smooth motion between adjoining bony segments. Hip, knee, and elbow are examples of synovial joints. This chapter is concerned with the mechanical behavior and function of the articular cartilage found in freely movable synovial (diarthroidal) joints.

In a typical synovial joint, the ends of opposing bones are covered with a thin layer of articular cartilage (*Fig. 5.1*). On the medial femoral condyle of the knee, for example, the cartilage averages 0.41 mm in rabbit and 2.21 mm in humans [2]. Normal articular cartilage is white, and its surface is smooth and glistening. Cartilage is aneural, and in normal mature animals, it does not have a blood supply. The entire joint is enclosed in a fibrous tissue capsule, the inner surface of which is lined with the synovial membrane that secretes a fluid known as *synovial fluid*. A relatively small amount of fluid is present in a normal joint: less than 1 mL, which is less than one fifth of a teaspoon. Synovial fluid is clear to yellowish and is stringy. Overall, synovial fluid resembles egg white, and it is this resemblance that gives these joints their name, *synovia*, meaning "with egg."

Cartilage clearly performs a mechanical function. It provides a bearing surface with low friction and wear, and because of its compliance, it helps to distribute the loads between opposing bones in a synovial joint. If cartilage were a stiff material like bone, the contact stresses at a joint would be much higher, since the area of contact would be much smaller. These mechanical functions alone would probably not be sufficient to justify an in-depth study of cartilage biomechanics. However, the apparent link between osteoarthritis and mechanical factors in a joint adds a strong impetus for studying the mechanical behavior of articular cartilage.

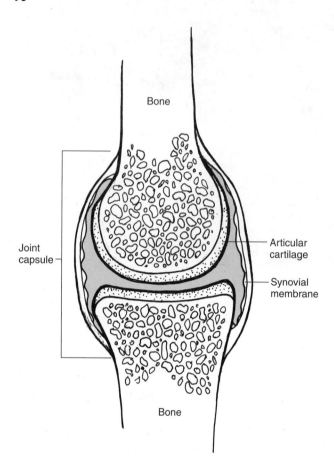

Figure 5.1: Schematic representation of a synovial joint. Articular cartilage forms the bearing surface on the ends of opposing bones. The space between the capsule and bones is exaggerated in the figure for clarity.

The specific goals of this chapter are to

- Describe the structure and composition of cartilage in relation to its mechanical behavior
- Examine the material properties of cartilage, what they mean physically, and how they can be determined
- Describe modes of mechanical failure of cartilage
- Describe the current state of understanding of joint lubrication
- Describe the etiology of osteoarthritis in terms of mechanical factors

Before proceeding through this chapter, the reader should be familiar with the basic concepts and terminology introduced in Chapters 1 and 2.

COMPOSITION AND STRUCTURE OF ARTICULAR CARTILAGE

Articular cartilage is a living material composed of a relatively small number of cells known as *chondrocytes* surrounded by a multicomponent matrix. Mechanically, articular cartilage is a composite of materials with widely differing properties. Approximately 70 to 85% of the weight of the whole tissue is water. The remainder of the tissue is composed primarily of proteoglycans, collagen, and a relatively small amount of lipids. Proteoglycans consist of a protein core to which glycosaminoglycans (chondroitin sulfate and keratan sulfate) are attached to form a bottlebrush-like structure. These proteoglycans can bind or aggregate to a backbone of hyaluronic acid to form a macromolecule with a weight up to 200 million daltons [76] (*Fig. 5.2*). Approximately 30% of the dry weight of articular cartilage is composed of proteoglycans. Proteoglycan concentration and water content vary through the depth of the tissue. Near the articular surface, proteoglycan concentration is relatively low, and the water content is the highest in the tissue. In the deeper regions of the cartilage, near subchondral bone, the proteoglycan concentration is greatest, and the water content is the lowest [67,74]. Collagen is a fibrous protein that makes up 60 to 70% of the dry weight of the tissue. Type II is the predominant collagen in articular cartilage, although other types are present in smaller amounts [25]. Collagen architecture varies through the depth of the tissue.

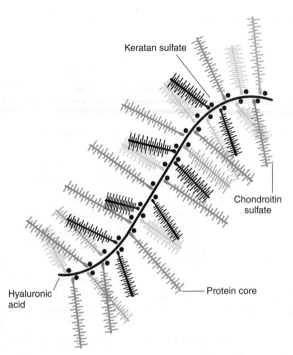

Figure 5.2: A proteoglycan aggregate showing a collection of proteoglycans bound to a hyaluronic acid backbone. Proteoglycans are the bottlebrush-like structures consisting of a protein core with side chains of chondroitin sulfate and keratan sulfate. Negatively charged sites on the chondroitin and keratan sulfate chains cause this aggregate to spread out and occupy a large domain when placed in an aqueous solution.

The structure of articular cartilage is often described in terms of four zones between the articular surface and the sub-chondral bone: the surface or superficial tangential zone, the intermediate or middle zone, the deep or radiate zone, and the calcified zone (*Fig. 5.3*). The calcified cartilage is the boundary between the cartilage and the underlying subchondral bone. The interface between the deep zone and calcified cartilage is known as the *tidemark*. Optical microscopy (e.g., polarized light), scanning electron microscopy, and transmission electron microscopy have been used to reveal the structure of articular cartilage [10,11,36,37,53,76,111]. While each of these methods suggests somewhat similar collagen orientation for the superficial and deep zones, the orientation of fibers in the middle zone remains controversial.

Using scanning electron microscopy to investigate the structure of cartilage in planes parallel and perpendicular to split lines, Jeffery and coworkers [37] have given some new insights into the collagen structure (Fig. 5.3). **Split lines** are formed by puncturing the cartilage surface at multiple sites with a circular awl. The resulting holes are elliptical, not circular, and the long axes of the ellipses are aligned in what is called the *split line direction*. In the plane parallel to a split line, the collagen is organized in broad layers or leaves, while in the plane orthogonal to the split lines the structure has a ridged pattern that is interpreted as the edges of the leaves (Fig. 5.3). In the calcified and deep zones, collagen fibers are oriented radially and are arranged in tightly packed bundles. The bundles are linked by numerous fibrils. From the upper deep zone into the middle

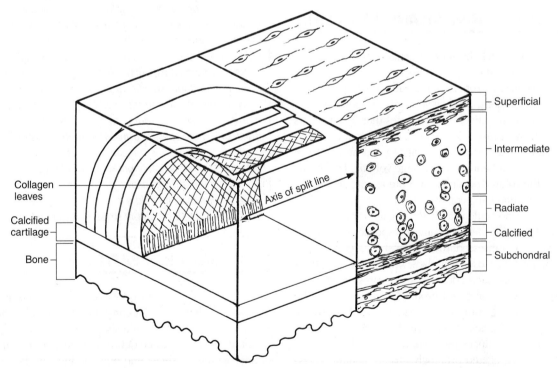

Figure 5.3: Cross sections cut through the thickness of articular cartilage on two mutually orthogonal planes. These planes are oriented parallel and perpendicular to split lines on the cartilage surface. The background shows the four zones of the cartilage: superficial, intermediate, radiate, and calcified. The foreground shows the organization of collagen fibers into "leaves" with varying structure and organization through the thickness of the cartilage. The leaves of collagen are connected by small fibers not shown in the figure.

zone, the radial orientation becomes less distinct, and collagen fibrils form a network that surrounds the chondrocytes. In the superficial zone, the fibers are finer than in the deeper zones, and the collagen structure is organized into several layers. An amorphous layer that does not appear to contain any fibers is found on the articular surface.

Scanning electron microscopy is also used to investigate the structure of osteoarthritic cartilage [16,53]. These investigations demonstrate two primary structural changes associated with degeneration: rolling of delaminated sheets into fronds, and formation and propagation of large cracks. In delaminated regions of tissue below the superficial layer, and in large fissures, cracks appear to propagate by separation or peeling of parallel collagen fibrils, rather than fracture of fibrils [53]. This observation suggests a mechanism that binds fibrils into a parallel structure [9,53].

Clinical Relevance

STRUCTURE: *On a structural level, osteoarthritis is characterized by surface fibrillation, fissures, and eventual removal of cartilage from underlying bone. Scanning electron microscopy provides a detailed picture of specific structural changes that occur in osteoarthritis. Recognizing that peeling of collagen fibrils in delaminated and fissured regions may involve failure of a component that "glues" fibrils together, could lead to new procedures for treating osteoarthritis.*

MECHANICAL BEHAVIOR AND MODELING

The mechanical behavior of articular cartilage is determined by the interaction of its predominant components: collagen, proteoglycans, and interstitial fluid. In an aqueous environment, proteoglycans are polyanionic; that is, the molecule has negatively charged sites that arise from its sulfate and carboxyl groups. In solution, the mutual repulsion of these negative charges causes an aggregated proteoglycan molecule to spread out and occupy a large volume. In the cartilage matrix, the volume occupied by proteoglycan aggregates is limited by the entangling collagen framework. The swelling of the aggregated molecule against the collagen framework is an essential element in the mechanical response of cartilage. When cartilage is compressed, the negatively charged sites on aggrecan are pushed closer together, which increases their mutual repulsive force and adds to the compressive stiffness of the cartilage. Nonaggregated proteoglycans would not be as effective in resisting compressive loads, since they are not as easily trapped in the collagen matrix. Damage to the collagen framework also reduces the compressive stiffness of the tissue, since the aggregated proteoglycans are contained less efficiently.

The mechanical response of cartilage is also strongly tied to the flow of fluid through the tissue. When deformed, fluid flows through the cartilage and across the articular surface [56]. If a pressure difference is applied across a section

of cartilage, fluid also flows through the tissue [66]. These observations suggest that cartilage behaves like a sponge, albeit one that does not allow fluid to flow through it easily.

Recognizing that fluid flow and deformation are interdependent has led to the modeling of cartilage as a mixture of fluid and solid components [74–76]. This is referred to as the *biphasic model of cartilage*. In this modeling, all of the solid-like components of the cartilage, proteoglycans, collagen, cells, and lipids are lumped together to constitute the solid phase of the mixture. The interstitial fluid that is free to move through the matrix constitutes the fluid phase. Typically, the solid phase is modeled as an incompressible elastic material, and the fluid phase is modeled as incompressible and inviscid, that is, it has no viscosity [75]. Under impact loads, cartilage behaves as a single-phase, incompressible, elastic solid; there simply isn't time for the fluid to flow relative to the solid matrix under rapidly applied loads. For some applications, a viscoelastic model is used to describe the behavior of cartilage in creep, stress relaxation, or shear. Although the mathematics of modeling cartilage is outside the scope of this chapter, some examples illustrate the fundamental fluid–solid interaction in cartilage.

Clinical Relevance

BIPHASIC MODEL OF CARTILAGE: *Mathematical simulations, using the biphasic model for cartilage, show that when a compressive load is applied to a joint, pressure in the interstitial fluid, not stress in the solid matrix, supports a significant portion of the load [2]. If the load is maintained over hundreds of seconds, fluid pressure decreases, and stress in the solid matrix increases. The biphasic model shows that fluid pressure shields the solid matrix from the higher level of stress that it would experience if cartilage were a simple elastic material without significant interaction of its fluid and solid components. In osteoarthritic cartilage that is more permeable than normal, stress shielding by fluid pressurization is diminished, and more stress is transferred to the solid matrix.*

Biphasic behavior is sometimes described using an analogy of a balloon that is tightly packaged within a cardboard box. Pressure in the balloon allows the box to support more compressive load than it could if it were empty. If the pressure in the balloon is reduced, more stress is transferred to the box.

MATERIAL PROPERTIES

Modeling cartilage as an isotropic biphasic material requires two independent material constants for the solid matrix, and one for fluid flow. As with a simple elastic material, multiple material constants can be determined for the solid matrix (the elastic, aggregate, shear, and bulk moduli, and Poisson's ratio) but only two of these are independent. The constant associated with fluid flow is called the permeability. Typically, these constants are determined from confined or unconfined compression. Shear tests are also used to determine the intrinsic material properties of the solid matrix.

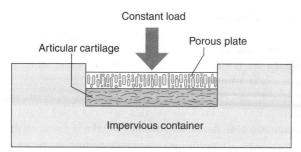

Constant load

Articular cartilage

Porous plate

Impervious container

Figure 5.4: Schematic drawing of an apparatus used to perform a confined compression test of cartilage. A slice of cartilage is placed in an impervious, fluid-filled well. The tissue is loaded through a porous plate. In the configuration shown, the load is constant throughout the test, which can last for several thousand seconds. Since the well is impervious, flow through the cartilage will only be in the vertical direction and out of the cartilage.

A confined compression test is one of the commonly used methods for determining material properties of cartilage (*Fig. 5.4*). A disc of cartilage is cut from the joint and placed in an impervious well. Confined compression is used in either a "creep" mode or a "relaxation" mode. In the creep mode, a constant load is applied to the cartilage through a porous plate, and the displacement of the tissue is measured as a function of time. In relaxation mode, a constant displacement is applied to the tissue, and the force needed to maintain the displacement is measured.

In creep mode, the cartilage deforms under a constant load, but the deformation is not instantaneous, as it would be in a single-phase elastic material such as a spring. The displacement of the cartilage is a function of time, since the fluid cannot

escape from the matrix instantaneously (*Fig. 5.5*). Initially, the displacement is rapid. This corresponds to a relatively large flow of fluid out of the cartilage. As the rate of displacement slows and the displacement approaches a constant value, the flow of fluid likewise slows. At equilibrium, the displacement is constant and fluid flow has stopped. In general, it takes several thousand seconds to reach the equilibrium displacement.

By fitting the mathematical biphasic model to the measured displacement, two material properties of the cartilage are determined: the aggregate modulus and permeability. The aggregate modulus is a measure of the stiffness of the tissue at equilibrium when all fluid flow has ceased. The higher the aggregate modulus, the less the tissue deforms under a given load. The aggregate modulus of cartilage is typically in the range of 0.5 to 0.9 MPa [3]. There is no analogous material constant for solid materials, but using the aggregate modulus and representative values of Poisson's ratio (described below), the Young's modulus of cartilage is in the range of 0.45 to 0.80 MPa. For comparison, the Young's modulus of steel is 200 GPa and for many woods is about 10 GPa parallel to the grain. These numbers show that cartilage has a much lower stiffness (modulus) than most engineering materials.

In addition to the aggregate modulus, the permeability of the cartilage is also determined from a confined compression test. The permeability indicates the resistance to fluid flow through the cartilage matrix. Permeability was first introduced in the study of flow through soils. The average fluid velocity through a porous sample (v_{ave}) is proportional to the pressure gradient (∇p) (*Fig. 5.6*). The constant of proportionality (k) is called the *permeability*. This relationship is expressed by Darcy's law, as shown in *Box 5.1*.

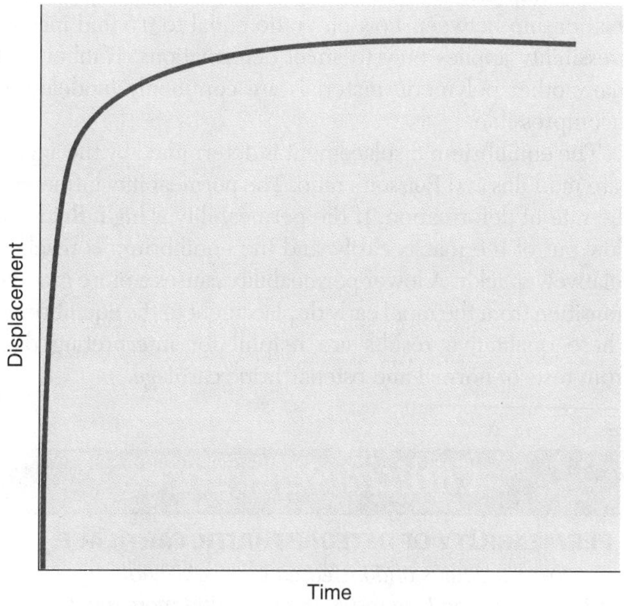

Displacement

Time

Figure 5.5: Typical displacement of cartilage tested in a confined compression creep test. A constant load is applied to the cartilage, and the displacement is measured over time. Initially, the deformation is rapid, as relatively large amounts of fluid are exuded from the cartilage. As the displacement reaches a constant value, the flow slows to zero. Two material properties are determined from this test.

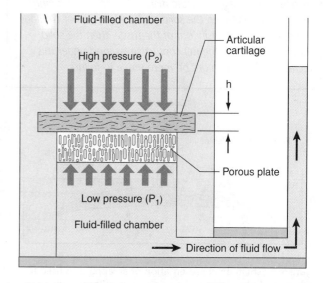

Fluid-filled chamber

Articular cartilage

High pressure (P_2)

h

Porous plate

Low pressure (P_1)

Fluid-filled chamber

Direction of fluid flow

Figure 5.6: Schematic representation of a device used to measure the permeability of cartilage. A slice of cartilage is supported on a porous plate in a fluid-filled chamber. High pressure applied to one side of the cartilage drives fluid flow. The average fluid velocity through the cartilage is proportional to the pressure gradient, and the constant of proportionality is called the *permeability*.

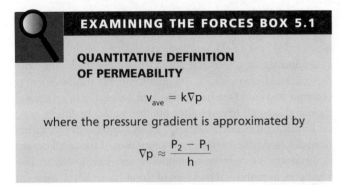

In SI units, the permeability of cartilage is typically in the range of 10^{-15} to 10^{-16} m^4/Ns. If a pressure difference of 210,000 Pa (about the same pressure as in an automobile tire) is applied across a slice of cartilage 1 mm thick, the average fluid velocity will be only $1 \cdot 10^{-8}$ m/s, which is about 100 million times slower than normal walking speed.

Permeability is not constant through the tissue. The permeability of articular cartilage is highest near the joint surface (making fluid flow relatively easy) and lowest in the deep zone (making fluid flow relatively difficult) [65–67]. Permeability also varies with deformation of the tissue. As cartilage is compressed, its permeability decreases [49,63]. Therefore, as a joint is loaded, most of the fluid that crosses the articular surface comes from the cartilage closest to the joint surface. Under increasing load, fluid flow will decrease because of the decrease in permeability that accompanies compression.

Clinical Relevance

VARIABLE PERMEABILITY: *Deformation-dependent permeability may be a valuable mechanism for maintaining load sharing between the solid and fluid phases of cartilage. If the fluid flowed easily out of the tissue, then the solid matrix would bear the full contact stress, and under this increased stress, it might be more prone to failure.*

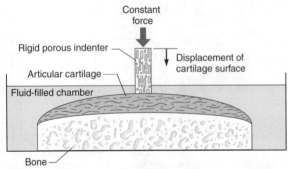

Figure 5.7: Schematic representation of an apparatus used to perform an indentation test on articular cartilage. Unlike the confined compression and most permeability tests, the cartilage remains attached to its underlying bone, which provides a more natural environment for testing. A constant load is applied to a small area of the cartilage through a porous indenter. The displacement of the cartilage is similar to that shown in Figure 5.6. Three material properties are determined from this test.

An indentation test provides an attractive alternative to confined compression [29,31,42,60,73,106] (*Fig. 5.7*). Using an indentation test, cartilage is tested in situ. Since discs of cartilage are not removed from underlying bone, as must be done when using confined compression, indentation may be used to test cartilage from small joints. In addition, three independent material properties are obtained from one indentation test, but only two are obtained from confined compression. Typically, an indentation test is performed under a constant load. The diameter of the indenter varies depending on the curvature of the joint surface, but generally is no smaller than 0.8 mm. Under a constant load, the displacement of the indenter resembles that for confined compression and requires several thousand seconds to reach equilibrium. By fitting the biphasic model of the test to the measured indentation, the aggregate modulus, Poisson's ratio, and permeability are determined. Poisson's ratio is typically less than 0.4 and often approaches zero. This finding is a significant departure from earlier studies, which assumed that cartilage was incompressible and, therefore, had a Poisson's ratio of 0.5. This assumption was based on cartilage being mostly water, and water may often be modeled as an incompressible material. However, when cartilage is loaded, fluid flows out of the solid matrix, which reduces the volume of the whole cartilage. Recognizing that cartilage is a mixture of a solid and fluid leads to the whole tissue behaving as a compressible material, although its components are incompressible.

The interpretation of Poisson's ratio used here is somewhat different from the commonly used definition, the ratio of transverse to axial strain. However, a material that has a Poisson's ratio of 0.5, as commonly defined, will deform as if it is incompressible; that is, its volume will not change. The relationship between Poisson's ratio equal to 0.5 and incompressibility applies only to small deformations. Rubber and many other polymeric materials are commonly modeled as incompressible.

The equilibrium displacement is determined by the aggregate modulus and Poisson's ratio. The permeability influences the rate of deformation. If the permeability is high, fluid can flow out of the matrix easily, and the equilibrium is reached relatively quickly. A lower permeability causes a more gradual transition from the rapid early displacement to the equilibrium. These qualitative results are helpful for interpreting data from tests of normal and osteoarthritic cartilage.

Clinical Relevance

PERMEABILITY OF OSTEOARTHRITIC CARTILAGE: *The lower modulus and increased permeability of osteoarthritic cartilage result in greater and more-rapid deformation of the tissue than normal. These changes may influence the synthetic activity of the chondrocytes, which are known to respond to their mechanical environment. [13,114,123].*

Pure shear provides a means for evaluating the intrinsic properties of the solid matrix. Small torsional displacements of cylindrical samples (which produce pure shear), result in no volume change of the cartilage to drive fluid flow. Furthermore, the interstitial fluid is water. It has low viscosity and does not make an appreciable contribution to resisting shear. Therefore, the resistance to shear is due to the solid matrix. Tests of cartilage in shear show that the matrix behaves as a viscoelastic solid [27–29]. Mathematical models of cartilage deformation also suggest that the matrix may behave as a viscoelastic solid [59,103].

RELATIONSHIP BETWEEN MECHANICAL PROPERTIES AND COMPOSITION

In addition to the qualitative descriptions given above, quantitative correlations between the mechanical properties of cartilage and glycosaminoglycan content, collagen content, and water content have been established. The compressive stiffness of cartilage increases as a function of the total glycosaminoglycan content [45] (*Fig. 5.8*). In contrast, there is no correlation of compressive stiffness with collagen content. In these cases, compressive stiffness is measured in creep, 2 seconds after a load is applied to the tissue. Permeability and compressive stiffness, as measured by the aggregate modulus, are both highly correlated with water content. As the water content increases, cartilage becomes less stiff and more permeable [1] (*Fig. 5.9*). Note that the inverse of permeability is plotted in Figure 5.9B. This is done for convenience, since the permeability becomes very large as the water content increases.

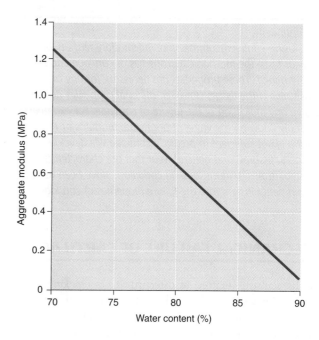

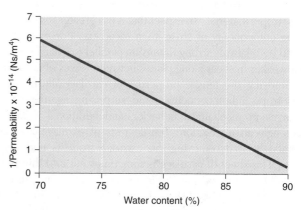

Figure 5.9: A. Correlation of the aggregate modulus with water content of articular cartilage. A regression line obtained from tests of a large number of samples is plotted. As the water content increases, the aggregate modulus decreases. **B.** Correlation of the inverse of permeability with water content. A regression line obtained from tests of a large number of samples is plotted. As the water content increases, the permeability increases.

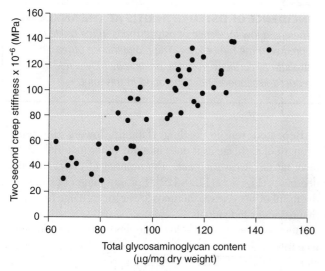

Figure 5.8: Correlation of compressive stiffness with the total glycosaminoglycan concentration. As the total glycosaminoglycan concentration decreases, the compressive stiffness also decreases.

Clinical Relevance

MATERIAL PROPERTIES OF CARTILAGE: The relationships between material properties and water content help to explain early cartilage changes in animal models of osteoarthritis. Proteoglycan content and equilibrium stiffness decrease and the rate of deformation and water content increases in these models [50,71]. Decreasing proteoglycan content allows more space in the tissue for fluid. An increase in water content correlates with an increase in permeability. Increasing permeability allows fluid to flow out of the tissue more easily, resulting in a more rapid rate of deformation.

(continued)

> *(Continued)*
>
> *Using confined compression, indentation, tension, and shear tests, the mechanical properties of cartilage can be determined. These properties are necessary for any analysis of stress in the tissue. However, material properties do not give any indication of the failure of cartilage. For example, simply knowing the value of aggregate modulus or Poisson's ratio is not sufficient to predict if cartilage will develop the cracks, fissures, and general wear that are characteristic of osteoarthritis. Various loading conditions have been used to gain better insight into the failure properties of cartilage.*

MECHANICAL FAILURE OF CARTILAGE

A characteristic feature of osteoarthritis is cracking, fibrillation, and wear of cartilage. This appears to be a mechanically driven process, and it motivates numerous investigations aimed at identifying the stresses and deformations responsible for the failure of articular cartilage. Since cartilage is an anisotropic material, we expect that it has greater resistance to some components of stress than to others. For example, it could be relatively strong in tension parallel to collagen fibers, but weaker in shear along planes between leaves of collagen.

Studying the tensile properties of cartilage illustrates its anisotropy, inhomogeneity, some surprising age-dependent changes in mechanical behavior, and additional collagen–proteoglycan interaction. Tensile tests of cartilage are performed by first removing the cartilage from its underlying bone. This sheet of cartilage is sometimes cut into thin slices (200–500 μm thick) parallel to the articular surface, using a microtome. Dumbbell-shaped specimens are cut from each slice with a custom-made cookie cutter.

A particularly thorough study of the tensile properties of cartilage shows that samples oriented parallel to split lines have a higher tensile strength and stiffness than those perpendicular to the split lines. In skeletally mature animals (closed physis), tensile strength and stiffness decrease from the surface to the deep zone. In contrast, tensile strength and stiffness increase with depth from the articular surface in skeletally immature (open physis) animals [96].

The relative influence of the collagen network and proteoglycans on the tensile behavior of cartilage depends on the rate of loading [100]. When pulled at a slow rate, the collagen network alone is responsible for the tensile strength and stiffness of cartilage. At high rates of loading, interaction of the collagen and proteoglycans is responsible for the tensile behavior; proteoglycans restrain the rotation of the collagen fibers when the tissue is loaded rapidly.

Tensile failure of cartilage has been of particular interest, since it was generally believed that vertical cracks in cartilage were initiated by relatively high tensile stresses on the articular surface. More-recent computational models of joint contact show that the tensile stress on the surface is lower than originally thought, although tensile stress still exists within the

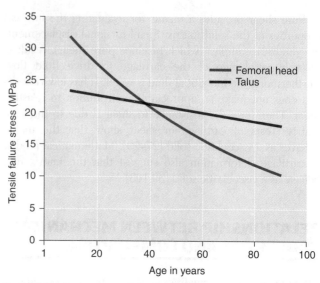

Figure 5.10: Comparison of the tensile failure stress of cartilage from the hip and talus. There is a statistically significant drop in the failure stress, as a function of age, for cartilage from the hip, but not for cartilage from the talus. Interestingly, there is a relatively high occurrence of osteoarthritis in the hip compared with that in the ankle (talus).

cartilage [20–22]. It now appears that failure by shear stress may dominate. Studies of the tensile failure of cartilage are primarily concerned with variations in properties among joints, the effects of repeated load, and age.

Kempson and coworkers report a decrease in tensile failure stress with age for cartilage from hip and knee [40,41,43, 44]. However, they find no appreciable age-dependent decrease in tensile failure stress for cartilage from the talus (*Fig. 5.10*).

Clinical Relevance

INCIDENCE OF OSTEOARTHRITIS AT THE ANKLE:
There is a low incidence of osteoarthritis in the ankle compared with the hip or knee. The maintenance of tensile strength of cartilage from the ankle may play a role in the reduced likelihood of degeneration in this joint.

Repeated tensile loading (fatigue) lowers the tensile strength of cartilage as it does in many other materials. As the peak tensile stress increases, the number of cycles to failure decreases (*Fig. 5.11*) [120–122]. For any value of peak stress, the number of cycles to failure is lower for cartilage from older than younger individuals.

Repeated compressive loads applied to the cartilage surface in situ also cause a decrease in tensile strength, if a sufficient number of load cycles are applied [68]. Following 64,800 cycles of compressive loading, there is no change in the tensile strength of cartilage, but after 97,200 cycles, tensile strength is reduced significantly. Surface damage is not found in any sample. This shows that damage may be induced

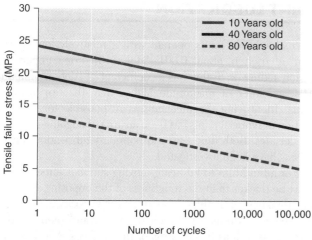

Figure 5.11: The effects of repeated tensile loading on the tensile strength of cartilage. As the tensile loading stress increases, fewer cycles of loading are needed to cause failure. Age is also an important factor. Cartilage from older individuals fails at a lower stress than that from younger people. Regression lines fit to multiple tests are plotted.

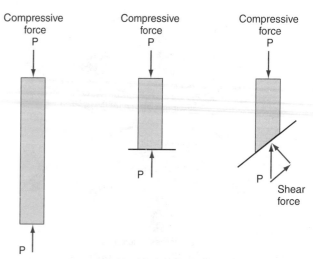

Figure 5.12: Illustration of shear stress in a simple loading condition. **A.** A free body diagram of a bar loaded in compression. **B.** A free body diagram of the same bar cut perpendicular to the load at an arbitrary location. On the cut surface, the resultant force must be *P* to maintain equilibrium. **C.** The same bar cut at an arbitrary angle. Again, to be in equilibrium the resultant force parallel to the bar must be equal to *P*. This force can always be decomposed into components parallel and perpendicular to the cut. The component parallel to the cut is a shear force that gives rise to a shear stress on the inclined surface.

within the tissue before any signs of surface fibrillation are apparent.

How do the number of cycles used in this test relate to human activity? Running a 26-mile marathon with a 6-foot step length corresponds to 11,440 cycles of load on each leg. Bicycling for 4 hours with a cadence of 90 revolutions per minute corresponds to 21,600 cycles per leg.

Some caution must be exercised when evaluating the effects of repeated loading on cartilage. In many cases failure occurs under large strain applied to samples removed from underlying bone. The strain to failure may be greater than that experienced in vivo. In addition, the properties of most biological materials change with the applied strain; the collagen network becomes aligned with the direction of the tensile strain, and the material becomes strongly anisotropic. Lastly, repeated loading of dead tissue does not include any biological response, and therefore may not give a complete picture of the effects of loading.

Rather than assume that tensile stress is responsible for fibrillation of the articular surface, the feasibility of several criteria is considered in a combined experimental and computational approach to cartilage failure [4–6]. Dropping three different-sized spherical indenters (2, 4, and 8 mm) onto the articular surface produces three different states of stress and, in some instances, a crack through the surface. Based on the stresses in the cartilage in each test and the presence or absence of a crack, a regression is used to determine the condition that is most likely to cause a crack to develop. The maximum shear stress in the cartilage is the most likely predictor of crack formation based on the location of the crack with respect to the calculated stresses.

Since cartilage is loaded in compression, the idea of failure by shear stress may seem unrealistic. Shear stresses do exist in cartilage, although the orientation of these stresses is not always obvious. To illustrate this, imagine a loading situation that is simpler than a joint, namely a straight bar loaded in compression (*Fig. 5.12*). If the bar is cut by a plane perpendicular to its length, then the resultant force on the cross section must also be compressive and equal to the applied force to maintain equilibrium. Now imagine the bar is cut at a 45° angle to its length (the exact angle is not important). The resultant force must still be equal to the applied force. Resolving the resultant force into components parallel and perpendicular to the cut surface gives rise to a shear force and a normal force. The shear stress (force per unit area) comes from the shear force acting over the inclined cut area of the bar. The same concept applies in any loading situation, including the cartilage in a synovial joint. However, in a synovial joint the stresses are multiaxial, not uniaxial as in the bar.

Radin and coworkers also show that cartilage failure could be induced by shear stress [86]. However, they are particularly interested in failure at the cartilage–bone interface, not the articular surface. Motivation for this investigation comes from postmortem studies that show cracks at the cartilage–bone interface and the recognition that under rapid loading, cartilage behaves as an incompressible elastic material, that is, its Poisson's ratio is 0.5. The relatively compliant, but incompressible cartilage experiences large lateral displacement (due to its high Poisson's ratio) when loaded in compression, but this expansion is constrained by the stiff underlying bone (*Fig. 5.13*). Under these conditions, high shear stress develops at the cartilage–bone boundary.

Most studies of cartilage failure are based directly on the values of ultimate stress or strain. An alternative is to use

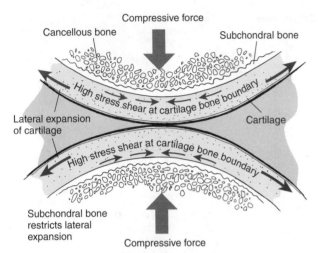

Figure 5.13: Under impulsive compressive loads, the cartilage experiences a relatively large lateral displacement due to its high Poisson's ratio. This expansion is restrained by the much stiffer subchondral bone, causing a high shear stress at the cartilage bone interface.

parameters that more directly represent the propagation of a crack in a loaded material sample. The feasibility of using two methods to determine fracture parameters of cartilage is evaluated extensively by Chin-Purcell and Lewis (*Fig. 5.14*) [14]. The so-called J integral is a measure of the fracture energy dissipated per unit of crack extension. As used, the J integral also assumes that a crack propagates in the material, as opposed to deformation or flow of the material, which results in a more ductile failure. Since cracks may not propagate in soft biological materials, a tear test is also evaluated. The tear test yields a fracture parameter similar to the J integral. As with tensile-stress-based ideas of failure, it is necessary to apply large strains to cause failure of the samples: these strains may be far greater than those found in any in vivo loading conditions. To date, the application of these fracture parameters is limited to the normal canine patella.

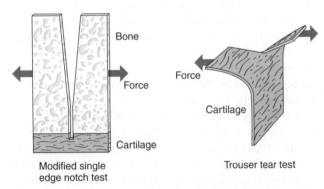

Figure 5.14: Sample shape and load application for the modified single-edge notch and trouser tear tests. Each test yields a specific measure of fracture, the energy required to propagate a crack in the material.

JOINT LUBRICATION

Normal synovial joints operate with a relatively low coefficient of friction, about 0.001 [54,69,113]. For comparison, Teflon sliding on Teflon has a coefficient of friction of about 0.04, an order of magnitude higher than that for synovial joints. Identifying the mechanisms responsible for the low friction in synovial joints has been an area of ongoing research for decades. Both fluid film and boundary lubrication mechanisms have been investigated.

For a fluid film to lubricate moving surfaces effectively, it must be thicker than the roughness of the opposing surfaces. The thickness of the film depends on the viscosity of the fluid, the shape of the gap between the parts, and their relative velocity, as well as the stiffness of the surfaces. A low coefficient of friction can also be achieved without a fluid film through a mechanism known as boundary lubrication. In this case, molecules adhered to the surfaces are sheared rather than forming a fluid film.

It now appears that a combination of fluid film lubrication and boundary lubrication are responsible for the low friction in synovial joints [55,90,92].

Numerous mechanisms for developing a lubricating fluid film on the articular surface have been postulated [19,38,62,69,116,118,119]. If cartilage is modeled as a rigid material, it is not possible to generate a fluid film of sufficient thickness to separate the cartilage surface roughness. However, models that include deformation of the cartilage and its surface roughness have shown that a sufficiently thick film can be developed [38]. This is known as microelastohydrodynamic lubrication. Deformation also causes fluid flow across the cartilage surface, which modifies the film thickness, although there is some question as to the practical importance of this component of flow [32,33,38].

Boundary lubrication of the articular surface appears to be linked to a glycoprotein fraction in synovial fluid known as lubricin [17,24,26,30,69,85,90,93,94,98,101,108–110]. Recent evidence suggests that lubricin may be a carrier for lubricating molecules known as surface active phospholipids that may provide the boundary lubricating property of synovial joints [101]. Surface active phospholipids are believed to be boundary lubricants not just in synovial joints, but in other parts of the body such as the pleural space.

MODELS OF OSTEOARTHRITIS

Animal models are used to provide a controlled environment for studying the progression of osteoarthritis. Although osteoarthritis may be induced by numerous means, models based on disruption of the mechanical environment of the joint, either by surgical alteration of periarticular structures or by abnormal joint load, are commonly used [34,35, 72,83,89,91,104].

Surgical resection of one or combinations of the anterior cruciate ligament, the medial collateral ligament, and a partial medial meniscectomy produce osteoarthritis of the knee. These models are thought to produce an unstable joint, but kinematic studies show varying degrees of deviation from normal joint kinematics.

Small differences in kinematics between control and operated knees (anterior cruciate ligament release and partial medial meniscectomy) are reported in rabbit [64]. At 4 weeks after surgery, there is a statistically significant change in the maximum anterior displacement of the knee, but anterior displacement is not significantly different from normal at 8 or 12 weeks after surgery. The most notable kinematic changes are in external rotation at 8 weeks and adduction at 4, 8, and 12 weeks after surgery. In dog, which has a more extended knee, greater anterior-posterior drawer is found after anterior (cranial) cruciate ligament release [48,115]. The relatively small changes in kinematics in unstable joints (particularly in rabbit) suggests that altered forces and possibly sensory input may be more important than joint displacements in the development of osteoarthritis [39].

Repetitive impulse loading also produces osteoarthritis in animal joints [87,89,91]. An advantage of this model is that it is more controlled than surgical models; the force applied to the limb is known and can be altered. This model has demonstrated the effect of loading rate on the development of osteoarthritis. Impulsively applied loads were found to produce osteoarthritis, while higher loads applied at a lower rate do not. The importance of impulsive loading to the development of osteoarthritis also appears in humans; persons with knee pain, but no history to suggest its origin, load their legs more rapidly at heel strike than persons without knee pain.

Although biochemical, metabolic, and mechanical assays have been used to evaluate the properties of cartilage from animal models of osteoarthritis, this chapter concentrates on the mechanical properties of cartilage. Following resection of the anterior cruciate ligament in dog, tensile stiffness, aggregate modulus, and shear modulus are lower than those in cartilage from unoperated control joints [102]. Permeability increases significantly 12 weeks after surgery. There is a significant increase in water content of samples from the medial tibial plateau and the lateral condyle and femoral groove.

In summary, various mechanical alterations of a joint lead to the development of osteoarthritis. The kinematic instability induced by surgical alterations may be small, suggesting that altered forces are primarily responsible for the developing osteoarthritis. Models based solely on abnormal joint loading support the view that alterations in force can lead to osteoarthritis. Following resection of the anterior cruciate ligament, cartilage is less stiff in both compression and shear, and fluid flows more easily through the tissue in joints with osteoarthritis. This implies greater displacement of osteoarthritic cartilage than normal (decreased stiffness) and a greater rate of deformation (increased permeability).

Clinical Relevance

OSTEOARTHRITIS: *Osteoarthritis is a leading cause of disability in developed countries [15]. In the United States, it is second to cardiovascular disease as the most common cause of disability [82]. Despite the widespread occurrence of osteoarthritis, it is difficult to study in human populations. Early physical symptoms such as fibrillation and cracking of the articular surface cannot be detected by an individual since cartilage is aneural. Insults to the cartilage may take years to progress to the point at which symptoms are detected by the surrounding joint structures and underlying bone. Although numerous epidemiological studies of osteoarthritis have been performed, they have been described as "disappointing" since they have not led to an explanation of the mechanisms underlying the development of osteoarthritis [82]. However, what seems to be clear is that the development of osteoarthritis depends on a combination of factors, including age, sex, heredity, joint mechanics and cartilage biology, and biochemistry [18,61,70].*

Although it is not an inescapable consequence of aging, osteoarthritis is more prevalent in the elderly [77,81]. In the United States, approximately 80% of people over the age of 65 and essentially everyone over the age of 80 has osteoarthritis, although it is uncommon before the age of 40. After 55 years of age, osteoarthritis is more common in women than men. Typically the distal interphalangeal, first carpometacarpal, and knee joints are the first joints affected [77]. However, specific links between aging and osteoarthritis are not known.

Excessive mechanical loading may also predispose joints to osteoarthritis. Workers in physically strenuous occupations (coal miners) have a higher incidence of osteoarthritis than those in less strenuous lines of work (office workers) [82]. Interestingly, evidence of osteoarthritis of the shoulder and elbow is found in relatively young individuals in ancient populations dependent on hunting [82]. However, strenuous work may not be the only risk factor for osteoarthritis, since people who use pneumatic drills or physical education teachers do not have an increased risk of osteoarthritis [82].

Radin argues that it is not the magnitude of the load, but rather the loading rate that is the determining factor in the development of osteoarthritis. Osteoarthritis develops only when impulsive loads are applied; that is, the load reaches its maximum value over a relatively short time. This is demonstrated in animal models using externally applied loads, and in sheep walking on soft and hard surfaces [84,88,89,91,104]. The role of impulsive rather than more slowly applied loads is also supported by tests in humans. Individuals with knee pain who are diagnosed as "prearthrotic" have a higher loading rate at heel strike than normal subjects [86]. These studies suggest that particular activities alone do not necessarily predispose an individual to osteoarthritis. Rather, the way in

(continued)

(Continued
which the activity is performed may be the factor that deter-
mines if osteoarthritis will develop.

Obesity is also correlated with an increasing risk of devel-
oping osteoarthritis, particularly in the tibio-femoral,
patellofemoral, and carpometacarpal joints [15]. Although
increased weight would be expected to increase the load on
joints of the lower extremity, and possibly predispose an indi-
vidual to osteoarthritis, obesity has no direct mechanical
effect on the carpometacarpal joint.

EXERCISE AND CARTILAGE HEALTH

Participation in certain sports also appears to increase the risk of developing osteoarthritis. Based on a review of existing literature, Saxon et al. [99] concluded that activities that involve torsional loading, fast acceleration and deceleration, repetitive high impact, and high levels of participation appear to increase the risk of developing osteoarthritis. Track and field events, racket sports, and soccer are among the sports that are linked to a higher risk of osteoarthritis. Swimming and cycling are not linked with an increased risk of developing osteoarthritis at the hip, although cycling may be related to osteoarthritis of the patella.

Injuries to the anterior cruciate ligament, collateral ligament, or meniscus are implicated in the development of osteoarthritis in the knee [51]. Loss of the anterior cruciate ligament may impair sensory function and protective mechanisms at the knee. Disruption of internal joint structures may alter joint alignment and the areas of cartilage that are loaded. If ligament damage results in a loss of joint stability, then joint loads may be increased by active muscle contraction trying to stabilize the joint. Partial or total meniscectomy can also be expected to increase the stress on the joint since the joint force is concentrated over a smaller area [117].

Despite an increased risk of developing osteoarthritis from excessive or abnormal joint loading, some level of loading or exercise appears to be beneficial for joint heath. In an in vivo study with 37 healthy human volunteers, Tiderius et al. [112] show that glycosaminoglycan content in medial and lateral femoral condyle cartilage is lower in sedentary subjects than those who exercise regularly. After an exercise regimen there is also an increase in glycosaminoglycan content in the knee of patents at risk for developing osteoarthritis [95]. These latter two studies use an MRI imaging technology known as dGEMRIC [7, 8] to quantitatively measure glycosaminoglycan content in vivo. They show a biochemical adaptation to exercise, although there appears to be no adaptation of cartilage morphology to exercise as determined by tissue mass [23]. Since exercise can enhance production of matrix molecules, it may seem reasonable to expect that it can have a positive effect on joint health.

Clinical Relevance

EXERCISE THERAPY: *Smidt et al. [105] review the literature on the effectiveness of exercise therapy for patients with disorders of the musculoskeletal, nervous, respiratory, and cardiovascular systems. They conclude that among musculoskeletal disorders, exercise therapy is effective in patients with osteoarthritis of the knee, and subacute and chronic low back pain. They also find indications that exercise therapy is effective for patients with osteoarthritis of the hip and ankylosing spondylitis. However, existing evidence is not sufficient to support or refute the effectiveness of exercise therapy for neck and shoulder pain or repetitive strain injury, and they conclude that exercise therapy is not effective for patients with acute low back pain. Exercise in people with osteoarthritis is shown to have positive effects on several outcome measures such as pain, strength, self-reported disability, observed disability in walking, and self-selected walking and stepping speed [46,80]. Although mild to moderate exercise is often recommended, the optimal therapeutic exercise protocol for people with osteoarthritis is not known [46,58,80].*

Although exercise that is actively controlled by a person with osteoarthritis has multiple positive effects, passive joint motion may be superior for healing of articular cartilage defects. Using surgically created defects in an animal model, Salter et al. [97] show a significantly higher healing rate in joints subjected to continuous passive motion (44% of defects healed) than those subjected to intermittent active motion (5% of defects healed) or immobilization (3% of defects healed).

It should not be surprising that active or passive joint motion can have positive effects on articular cartilage. As established earlier in this chapter, cartilage is a fluid-saturated deformable porous material. Active or passive joint motion results in cartilage deformation, and hydrostatic pressure and movement of interstitial fluid in the cartilage matrix. A large body of research, not reviewed in this chapter, shows that cartilage matrix production is sensitive to applied hydrostatic pressure or deformation. Varying pressure or deformation applied within defined amplitude and frequency ranges can enhance or inhibit matrix production [12,47,52,78,79, 114,123]. The effects of active and passive exercise on the health of articular cartilage are consistent with accepted models and carefully controlled experimental results.

SUMMARY

In summary, articular cartilage provides an efficient load-bearing surface for synovial joints that is capable of functioning for the lifetime of an individual. The mechanical behavior of this tissue depends on the interaction of its fluid and solid components. Numerous factors can impair the function of cartilage and lead to osteoarthritis and a painful and nonfunctional joint. Mechanical factors are strongly implicated in the development of osteoarthritis, although exact mechanisms are still not known. Exercise has both beneficial and detrimental effects on cartilage. It produces positive biochemical changes and reduces pain and increases function in people with arthritis. Conversely, sports injuries are significant contributors to osteoarthritis.

References

1. Armstrong CG, Mow VC: Variations in the intrinsic mechanical properties of human articular cartilage with age, degeneration, and water content. J Bone Joint Surg [Am] 1982; 64: 88–94.

2. Ateshian, G.A., W.M. Lai, W.B. Zhu, and V.C. Mow, *An asymptotic solution for the contact of two biphasic cartilage layers.* J Biomech, 1994. 27(11): p. 1347–60.

3. Athanasiou KA, Rosenwasser MP, Buckwalter JA, et al.: Interspecies comparisons of in situ intrinsic mechanical properties of distal femoral cartilage. J Orthop Res 1991; 9: 330–340.

4. Atkinson TS, Haut RC, Altiero NJ: A poroelastic model that predicts some phenomenological responses of ligaments and tendons. J Biomech Eng 1997; 119: 400–405.

5. Atkinson TS, Haut RC, Altiero NJ: Impact-induced fissuring of articular cartilage: an investigation of failure criteria. J Biomech Eng 1998; 120: 181–187.

6. Atkinson TS, Haut RC, Altiero NJ: An investigation of biphasic failure criteria for impact-induced fissuring of articular cartilage. J Biomech Eng 1998; 120: 536–537.

7. Bashir, A.; Gray, M. L.; Boutin, R. D.; and Burstein, D.: Glycosaminoglycan in articular cartilage: in vivo assessment with delayed Gd(DTPA)(2-)-enhanced MR imaging. *Radiology*, 205(2): 551–8, 1997.

8. Bashir, A.; Gray, M. L.; Hartke, J.; and Burstein, D.: Nondestructive imaging of human cartilage glycosaminoglycan concentration by MRI. *Magn Reson Med*, 41(5): 857–65, 1999.

9. Broom, N. D.: An enzymatically induced structural transformation in articular cartilage. Its significance with respect to matrix breakdown. *Arthritis Rheum*, 31(2): 210–8, 1988.

10. Broom ND: Further insights into the structural principles governing the function of articular cartilage. J Anat 1984; 139 (Pt 2): 275–294.

11. Broom ND, Myers DD: Fibrous waveforms or crimp in surface and subsurface layers of hyaline cartilage maintained in its wet functional condition. Connect Tissue Res 1980; 7: 165–175.

12. Buschmann, M. D.; Gluzband, Y. A.; Grodzinsky, A. J.; and Hunziker, E. B.: Mechanical compression modulates matrix biosynthesis in chondrocyte/agarose culture. *J Cell Sci*, 108 (Pt 4): 1497–508., 1995.

13. Buschmann MD, Kim YJ, Wong M, et al.: Stimulation of aggrecan synthesis in cartilage explants by cyclic loading is localized to regions of high interstitial fluid flow. Arch Biochem Biophys 1999; 366: 1–7.

14. Chin-Purcell MV, Lewis JL: Fracture of articular cartilage. J Biomech Eng 1996; 118: 545–556.

15. Cicuttini FM, Baker JR, Spector TD: The association of obesity with osteoarthritis of the hand and knee in women: a twin study. J Rheumatol 1996; 23: 1221–1226.

16. Clark, J. M., and Simonian, P. T.: Scanning electron microscopy of "fibrillated" and "malacic" human articular cartilage: technical considerations. *Microsc Res Tech*, 37(4): 299–313, 1997.

17. Davis, W. H., Jr.; Lee, S. L.; and Sokoloff, L.: Boundary lubricating ability of synovial fluid in degenerative joint disease. *Arthritis Rheum*, 21(7): 754–6, 1978.

18. Dijkgraaf LC, de Bont LG, Boering G, Liem RS: The structure, biochemistry, and metabolism of osteoarthritic cartilage: a review of the literature. J Oral Maxillofac Surg 1995; 53: 1182–1192.

19. Dowson D: Lubrication and wear of joints. Physiotherapy 1973; 59: 104–106.

20. Eberhardt AW, Keer LM, Lewis JL, Vithoontien V: An analytical model of joint contact. J Biomech Eng 1990; 112: 407–413.

21. Eberhardt AW, Lewis JL, Keer LM: Contact of layered elastic spheres as a model of joint contact: effect of tangential load and friction. J Biomech Eng 1991; 113: 107–108.

22. Eberhardt AW, Lewis JL, Keer LM: Normal contact of elastic spheres with two elastic layers as a model of joint articulation. J Biomech Eng 1991; 113: 410–417.

23. Eckstein, F.; Hudelmaier, M.; and Putz, R.: The effects of exercise on human articular cartilage. *J Anat*, 208(4): 491–512, 2006.

24. Elsaid, K. A.; Jay, G. D.; Warman, M. L.; Rhee, D. K.; and Chichester, C. O.: Association of articular cartilage degradation and loss of boundary-lubricating ability of synovial fluid following injury and inflammatory arthritis. *Arthritis Rheum*, 52(6): 1746–55, 2005.

25. Eyre DR: The collagens of articular cartilage. Semin Arthritis Rheum 1991; 21(Suppl 2): 2–11.

26. Foy JR, Williams PF 3rd, Powell GL, et al.: Effect of phospholipidic boundary lubrication in rigid and compliant hemiarthroplasty models. Proc Inst Mech Eng [H] 1999; 213: 5–18.

27. Hayes W: Some viscoelastic properties of human articular cartilage. Acta Orthop Belg 1972; 38(Suppl 1): 23–31.

28. Hayes WC, Bodine AJ: Flow-independent viscoelastic properties of articular cartilage matrix. J Biomech 1978; 11: 407–419.

29. Hayes WC, Mockros LF: Viscoelastic properties of human articular cartilage. J Appl Physiol 1971; 31: 562–568.

30. Hills, B. A., and Monds, M. K.: Enzymatic identification of the load-bearing boundary lubricant in the joint. *Br J Rheumatol*, 37(2): 137–42, 1998.

31. Hirsch C: The pathogenesis of chondromalacia of the patella. Acta Chir Scand 1944; 83(Suppl): 1–106.

32. Hou JS, Holmes MH, Lai WM, Mow VC: Boundary conditions at the cartilage-synovial fluid interface for joint lubrication and theoretical verifications. J Biomech Eng 1989; 111: 78–87.

33. Hou JS, Mow VC, Lai WM, Holmes MH: An analysis of the squeeze-film lubrication mechanism for articular cartilage. J Biomech 1992; 25: 247–259.

34. Hulth A: Experimental osteoarthritis: a survey. Acta Orthop Scand 1982; 53: 1–6.

35. Hulth A, Lindberg L, Telhag H: Experimental osteoarthritis in rabbits. Preliminary report. Acta Orthop Scand 1970; 41: 522–530.

36. Hwang WS, Li B, Jin LH, et al.: Collagen fibril structure of normal, aging, and osteoarthritic cartilage. J Pathol 1992; 167: 425–433.

37. Jeffery AK, Blunn GW, Archer CW, Bentley G: Three-dimensional collagen architecture in bovine articular cartilage. J Bone Joint Surg [Br] 1991; 73: 795–801.

38. Jin ZM, Dowson D, Fisher J: Effect of porosity of articular cartilage on the lubrication of a normal human hip joint. Proc Inst Mech Eng Part H J Eng Med 1992; 206: 117–124.

39. Johansson H, Sjolander P, Sojka P: A sensory role for the cruciate ligaments. Clin Orthop 1991; 268: 161–178.

40. Kempson GE: Age-related changes in the tensile properties of human articular cartilage: a comparative study between the femoral head of the hip joint and the talus of the ankle joint. Biochim Biophys Acta 1991; 1075: 223–230.

41. Kempson GE: Relationship between the tensile properties of articular cartilage from the human knee and age. Ann Rheum Dis 1982; 41: 508–511.

42. Kempson GE, Freeman MA, Swanson SA: The determination of a creep modulus for articular cartilage from indentation tests of the human femoral head. J Biomech 1971; 4: 239–250.

43. Kempson GE, Freeman MA, Swanson SA: Tensile properties of articular cartilage. Nature 1968; 220: 1127–1128.

44. Kempson GE, Muir H, Pollard C, Tuke M: The tensile properties of the cartilage of human femoral condyles related to the content of collagen and glycosaminoglycans. Biochim Biophys Acta 1973; 297: 456–472.

45. Kempson GE, Muir H, Swanson SAV, Freeman MAR: Correlations between stiffness and the chemical constituents of cartilage on the human femoral head. Biochim Biophys Acta 1970; 215: 70–77.

46. Kettunen, J. A., and Kujala, U. M.: Exercise therapy for people with rheumatoid arthritis and osteoarthritis. *Scand J Med Sci Sports,* 14(3): 138–42, 2004.

47. Kim, Y. J.; Bonassar, L. J.; and Grodzinsky, A. J.: The role of cartilage streaming potential, fluid flow and pressure in the stimulation of chondrocyte biosynthesis during dynamic compression. *J Biomech,* 28(9): 1055–66., 1995.

48. Korvick DL, Pijanowski GJ, Schaeffer DJ: Three-dimensional kinematics of the intact and cranial cruciate ligament-deficient stifle of dogs [published erratum appears in J Biomech 1994; 27: 1295]. J Biomech 1994; 27: 77–87.

49. Lai WM, Mow VC: Drag-induced compression of articular cartilage during a permeation experiment. Biorheology 1980; 17: 111–123.

50. Lane JM, Chisena E, Black J: Experimental knee instability: early mechanical property changes in articular cartilage in a rabbit model. Clin Orthop 1979; 140: 262–265.

51. Lane NE, Buckwalter JA: Exercise: a cause of osteoarthritis? Rheum Dis Clin North Am 1993; 19: 617–633.

52. Lee, D. A., and Bader, D. L.: Compressive strains at physiological frequencies influence the metabolism of chondrocytes seeded in agarose. *J Orthop Res,* 15(2): 181–8, 1997.

53. Lewis, J. L., and Johnson, S. L.: Collagen architecture and failure processes in bovine patellar cartilage. *J Anat,* 199(Pt 4): 483–92, 2001.

54. Linn FC: Lubrication of animal joints. I. The arthrotripsometer. J Bone Joint Surg [Am] 1967; 49: 1079–1098.

55. Linn FC, Radin EL: Lubrication of animal joints. 3. The effect of certain chemical alterations of the cartilage and lubricant. Arthritis Rheum 1968; 11: 674–682.

56. Linn FC, Sokoloff L: Movement and composition of interstitial fluid of cartilage. Arth Rheum 1965; 8: 481–494.

57. Lipshitz H, Etheredge Rd, Glimcher MJ: In vitro wear of articular cartilage. J Bone Joint Surg [Am] 1975; 57: 527–534.

58. Lucas, B.: Treatment options for patients with osteoarthritis of the knee. *Br J Nurs,* 14(18): 976–81, 2005.

59. Mak AF: The apparent viscoelastic behavior of articular cartilage—the contributions from the intrinsic matrix viscoelasticity and interstitial fluid flows. Trans. ASME J Biomech Eng 1986; 108: 108–130.

60. Mak AF, Lai WM, Mow VC: Biphasic indentation of articular cartilage—I. Theoretical analysis. J Biomech 1987; 20: 703–714.

61. Malemud CJ: Changes in proteoglycans in osteoarthritis: biochemistry, ultrastructure and biosynthetic processing. J Rheumatol Suppl 1991; 27: 60–62.

62. Mansour JM, Mow VC: Natural lubrication of synovial joints' normal and degenerate. Trans Asme Ser F 1977; 99: 163–173.

63. Mansour JM, Mow VC: The permeability of articular cartilage under compressive strain and at high pressures. J Bone Joint Surg [Am] 1976; 58: 509–516.

64. Mansour JM, Wentorf FA, Degoede KM: In vivo kinematics of the rabbit knee in unstable models of osteoarthritis. Ann Biomed Eng 1998; 26: 353–360.

65. Maroudas A: Physicochemical properties of cartilage in the light of ion exchange theory. Biophys J 1968; 8: 575–595.

66. Maroudas A, Bullough P: Permeability of articular cartilage. Nature 1968; 219: 1260–1261.

67. Maroudas A, Bullough P, Swanson SA, Freeman MA: The permeability of articular cartilage. J Bone Joint Surg [Br] 1968; 50: 166–177.

68. McCormack T, Mansour JM: Reduction in tensile strength of cartilage precedes surface damage under repeated compressive loading in vitro. J Biomech 1998; 31: 55–61.

69. McCutchen C: Mechanism of animal joints. Nature 1959; 184: 1284–1285.

70. McDevitt CA, Miller RR: Biochemistry, cell biology, and immunology of osteoarthritis. Curr Opin Rheumatol 1989; 1: 303–314.

71. McDevitt CA, Muir H: Biochemical changes in the cartilage of the knee in experimental and natural osteoarthritis in the dog. J Bone Joint Surg [Br] 1976; 58: 94–101.

72. Moskowitz RW, Davis W, Sammarco J, et al.: Experimentally induced degenerative joint lesions following partial meniscectomy in the rabbit. Arthritis Rheum 1973; 16: 397–405.

73. Mow VC, Gibbs MC, Lai WM, et al.: Biphasic indentation of articular cartilage—II. A numerical algorithm and an experimental study. J Biomech 1989; 22: 853–861.

74. Mow VC, Holmes MH, Lai WM: Fluid transport and mechanical properties of articular cartilage: a review. J Biomech 1984; 17: 377–394.

75. Mow VC, Kuei SC, Lai WM, Armstrong CG: Biphasic creep and stress relaxation of articular cartilage in compression? Theory and experiments. J Biomech Eng 1980; 102: 73–84.

76. Mow VC, Lai WM: Recent developments in synovial joint biomechanics. SIAM Rev 1980; 22: 275–317.

77. Oddis CV: New perspectives on osteoarthritis. Am J Med 1996; 100: 10S–15S.

78. Parkkinen, J. J.; Lammi, M. J.; Inkinen, R.; Jortikka, M.; Tammi, M.; Virtanen, I.; and Helminen, H. J.: Influence of short-term hydrostatic pressure on organization of stress fibers in cultured chondrocytes. *J Orthop Res,* 13(4): 495–502, 1995.

79. Parkkinen, J. J.; Lammi, M. J.; Pelttari, A.; Helminen, H. J.; Tammi, M.; and Virtanen, I.: Altered Golgi apparatus in hydrostatically loaded articular cartilage chondrocytes. *Ann Rheum Dis,* 52(3): 192–8, 1993.

80. Petrella, R. J.: Is exercise effective treatment for osteoarthritis of the knee? *Br J Sports Med,* 34(5): 326–31, 2000.

81. Peyron JG: Osteoarthritis. The epidemiologic viewpoint. Clin Orthop 1986; 213: 13–19.

82. Peyron JG: Clinical features of osteoarthritis, diffuse idiopathic skeletal hyperostosis, and hypermobility syndromes. Curr Opin Rheumatol 1991; 3: 653–661.

83. Pond MJ, Nuki G: Experimentally-induced osteoarthritis in the dog. Ann Rheum Dis 1973; 32: 387–388.

84. Radin EL: The effects of repetitive loading on cartilage. Advice to athletes to protect their joints. Acta Orthop Belg 1983; 49: 225–232.

85. Radin, E. L.: Synovial fluid as a lubricant. *Arthritis Rheum,* 11(5): 693–5, 1968.

86. Radin EL, Burr DB, Caterson B, et al.: Mechanical determinants of osteoarthritis. Semin Arthritis Rheum 1991; 21 (3 Suppl 2): 12–21.

87. Radin EL, Ehrlich MG, Chernack R, et al.: Effect of repetitive impulsive loading on the knee joints of rabbits. Clin Orthop 1978; 131: 288–293.

88. Radin EL, Orr RB, Kelman JL, et al.: Effect of prolonged walking on concrete on the knees of sheep. J Biomech 1982; 15: 487–492.

89. Radin EL, Parker HG, Pugh JW, et al.: Response of joints to impact loading—III Relationship between trabecular microfractures and cartilage degeneration. J. Biomech 1973; 6: 51–57.

90. Radin EL, Paul IL: A consolidated concept of joint lubrication. J Bone Joint Surg 1972; 54-A: 607–616.

91. Radin EL, Paul IL: Response of joints to impact loading. I. In vitro wear. Arthritis Rheum 1971; 14: 356–362.

92. Radin EL, Paul IL, Pollock D: Animal joint behavior under excessive loading. Nature 1970; 226: 554–555.

93. Radin, E. L.; Swann, D. A.; and Weisser, P. A.: Separation of a hyaluronate-free lubricating fraction from synovial fluid. *Nature,* 228(5269): 377–8, 1970.

94. Roberts, B. J.; Unsworth, A.; and Mian, N.: Modes of lubrication in human hip joints. *Ann Rheum Dis,* 41(3): 217–24, 1982.

95. Roos, E. M., and Dahlberg, L.: Positive effects of moderate exercise on glycosaminoglycan content in knee cartilage: a four-month, randomized, controlled trial in patients at risk of osteoarthritis. *Arthritis Rheum,* 52(11): 3507–14, 2005.

96. Roth V, Mow VC: The intrinsic tensile behavior of the matrix of bovine articular cartilage and its variation with age. J Bone Joint Surg [Am] 1980; 62: 1102–1117.

97. Salter, R. B.; Simmonds, D. F.; Malcolm, B. W.; Rumble, E. J.; MacMichael, D.; and Clements, N. D.: The biological effect of continuous passive motion on the healing of full-thickness defects in articular cartilage. An experimental investigation in the rabbit. *J Bone Joint Surg Am,* 62(8): 1232–51, 1980.

98. Sarma, A. V.; Powell, G. L.; and LaBerge, M.: Phospholipid composition of articular cartilage boundary lubricant. *J Orthop Res,* 19(4): 671–6, 2001.

99. Saxon, L.; Finch, C.; and Bass, S.: Sports participation, sports injuries and osteoarthritis: implications for prevention. *Sports Med,* 28(2): 123–35, 1999.

100. Schmidt MB, Mow VC, Chun LE, Eyre DR: Effects of proteoglycan extraction on the tensile behavior of articular cartilage. J Orthop Res 1990; 8: 353–363.

101. Schwarz IM, Hills BA: Surface-active phospholipid as the lubricating component of lubricin. Br J Rheumatol 1998; 37: 21–26.

102. Setton, L. A.; Mow, V. C.; and Howell, D. S.: Mechanical behavior of articular cartilage in shear is altered by transection of the anterior cruciate ligament. *J Orthop Res,* 13(4): 473–82, 1995.

103. Setton LA, Zhu W, Mow VC: The biphasic poroviscoelastic behavior of articular cartilage: role of the surface zone in governing the compressive behavior [see comments]. J Biomech 1993; 26: 581–592.

104. Simon SR, Radin EL, Paul IL: The response of joints to impact loading—II In vivo behavior of subchondral bone. J Biomech 1972; 5: 267.

105. Smidt, N. et al.: Effectiveness of exercise therapy: a best-evidence summary of systematic reviews. *Aust J Physiother,* 51(2): 71–85, 2005.

106. Sokoloff L: Elasticity of aging cartilage. Fed Proc 1966; 25: 1089–1095.

107. Suh J-K, DiSilvestro MR: Biphasic poroviscoelastic behavior of hydrated biological soft tissues. Trans ASME J Appl Mech 1999; 66: 538–535.

108. Swann, D. A.; Bloch, K. J.; Swindell, D.; and Shore, E.: The lubricating activity of human synovial fluids. *Arthritis Rheum,* 27(5): 552–6, 1984.

109. Swann DA, Hendren RB, Radin EL, et al.: The lubricating activity of synovial fluid glycoproteins. Arthritis Rheum 1981; 24: 22–30.

110. Swann, D. A., and Radin, E. L.: The molecular basis of articular lubrication. I. Purification and properties of a lubricating fraction from bovine synovial fluid. *J Biol Chem,* 247(24): 8069–73, 1972.

111. Teshima R, Otsuka T, Takasu N, et al.: Structure of the most superficial layer of articular cartilage. J Bone Joint Surg [Br] 1995; 77: 460–464.

112. Tiderius, C. J.; Svensson, J.; Leander, P.; Ola, T.; and Dahlberg, L.: dGEMRIC (delayed gadolinium-enhanced MRI of cartilage) indicates adaptive capacity of human knee cartilage. *Magn Reson Med,* 51(2): 286–90, 2004.

113. Unsworth A, Dowson D, Wright V: The frictional behaviour of human synovial joints. I. Natural joints. Trans Asme Ser F 1975; 97: 369–376.

114. Urban JP: The chondrocyte: a cell under pressure. Br J Rheumatol 1994; 33: 901–908.

115. Vilensky JA, O'Connor BL, Brandt KD, et al.: Serial kinematic analysis of the unstable knee after transection of the anterior cruciate ligament: temporal and angular changes in a canine model of osteoarthritis. J Orthop Res 1994; 12: 229–237.

116. Walker PS, Dowson D, Longfield MD, Wright V: Lubrication of human joints. Ann Rheum Dis 1969; 28: 194.

117. Walker PS, Erkman MJ: The role of the menisci in force transmission across the knee. Clin Orthop 1975; 109: 184–192.

118. Walker PS, Sikorski J, Dowson D, et al.: Features of the synovial fluid film in human joint lubrication. Nature 1970; 225: 956–957.

119. Walker PS, Unsworth A, Dowson D, et al.: Mode of aggregation of hyaluronic acid protein complex on the surface of articular cartilage. Ann Rheum Dis 1970; 29: 591–602.

120. Weightman B: In vitro fatigue testing of articular cartilage. Ann Rheum Dis 1975; 34(Suppl): 108–110.

121. Weightman B: Tensile fatigue of human articular cartilage. J Biomech 1976; 9: 193–200.

122. Weightman B, Chappell DJ, Jenkins EA: A second study of tensile fatigue properties of human articular cartilage. Ann Rheum Dis 1978; 37: 58–63.

123. Wong M, Wuethrich P, Buschmann MD, et al.: Chondrocyte biosynthesis correlates with local tissue strain in statically compressed adult articular cartilage. J Orthop Res 1997; 15: 189–196.

Biomechanics of Tendons and Ligaments

MARGERY A. LOCKARD, P.T., PH.D.

Tendons and ligaments are dense connective tissue structures that connect muscle to bone and bone to bone, respectively. Both are located in and around the joints of the body, and as a result, they are both subjected to large distractive or tensile loads. These are the structures that are largely responsible for providing joint stability during movement and function. Tendons and ligaments are biologically active structures, and as a result, injuries, aging, and abnormal conditions such as joint immobilization produce alterations in their composition and structure. These changes in structure affect the mechanical properties of tendons and ligaments as well as the functioning of the joints with which they are associated. It is important for clinicians who are treating patients with tendon and ligament injuries to understand these structural and mechanical changes so that the treatments selected will stimulate positive tissue adaptations and improve joint and overall function.

The specific goals of this chapter are to

- Describe the components and organization of dense regular connective tissues, particularly tendons and ligaments
- Discuss the mechanical behavior of tendons and ligaments in response to tensile loads
- Describe physical factors affecting the mechanical properties of tendons and ligaments
- Describe biological factors affecting the mechanical properties of tendons and ligaments
- Discuss the response of tendons and ligaments to immobilization and remobilization

- Describe the mechanical properties of tendons and ligaments during healing
- Describe the effects of stress enhancement on the mechanical properties of tendons and ligaments

Prior to reading this chapter, the reader should understand the mechanical properties of viscoelastic tissues that are described in Chapter 2.

STRUCTURE OF CONNECTIVE TISSUE

Tendons and ligaments are composed of connective tissue. Connective tissues provide and maintain form in the body, functioning mechanically to connect and bind cells and organs together, thus giving support to the body. Connective tissues are typically classified into three major groups: connective tissue proper, supporting connective tissues, and specialized connective tissues. Supporting connective tissues include bone and cartilage. The histological and mechanical properties of these tissues are described in Chapters 3 and 5. Specialized connective tissues include adipose tissue and hematopoietic tissue. Connective tissue proper is described as loose or dense. Loose, or areolar, connective tissue is the "packing material" that is found within and between muscle sheaths, supporting epithelial tissue, and encircling neurovascular bundles. Loose connective tissue is very delicate and not very resistant to stress or strain. Dense connective tissue is less flexible and more resistant to stress. The dermis of skin is classified as dense, irregular connective tissue since the fiber bundles are disorganized and lack specific orientation. Tendons and ligaments are classified as dense, regular connective tissue. Fiber bundles in tendons and ligaments are densely packed and are oriented parallel to one another as well as to frequently applied forces. This arrangement makes them particularly well adapted to resisting traction or tensile forces.

Composition of Tendons and Ligaments

Like all dense connective tissues, tendons and ligaments are composed of two major compartments, cells and extracellular matrix. The primary cell type in tendons and ligaments is the fibrocyte, also called the *fibroblast*, when it is actively manufacturing proteins. Cells, however, make up only about 20% of the total tissue volume. Fibroblasts manufacture and secrete the components of the extracellular matrix that makes up the remaining 80%. The extracellular matrix is composed of fibers (collagen and elastin) and the ground substance. The ground substance is the gelatinous material that fills the spaces between cells and fibers. It is composed of non-collagenous structural glycoproteins (fibronectin), proteoglycans (decorin, biglycan), and water (*Fig. 6.1*).

EXTRACELLULAR MATRIX: FIBERS

The fibrous component of tendons and ligaments is composed primarily of collagen, giving tendons and ligaments their white appearance. Collagen, which has strength similar to that of steel, is manufactured in the rough endoplasmic

reticulum of fibroblasts. It is composed of amino acids that are assembled into long polypeptide chains in which every third residue is glycine. Three polypeptide chains become attached together to form a triple helix called *procollagen*. Procollagen, an organic crystal, is secreted from the fibroblast into the extracellular matrix, end components are cleaved, and the slightly shorter molecule is now called *tropocollagen*. Tropocollagen molecules in the extracellular space polymerize into collagen microfibrils, which in turn aggregate into subfibrils, fibrils, and finally fibers [64] (*Fig. 6.2*). Tropocollagen molecules are initially attracted to each other by weak hydrogen, hydrophobic, hydrophilic, and covalent bonds. Once aggregation into microfibrils has occurred, changes in the intra- and intermolecular attachments progress from less, to more, stable bonding. As the collagen matures, there is an increase in both the density and the stability of bonding, which results in increased tissue strength and stiffness [6]. This is a brief overview of how collagen is manufactured in connective tissues. A more detailed description can be found in a histology textbook.

The amino acid sequence of the polypeptide chains that constitute the tropocollagen molecules is not always the same.

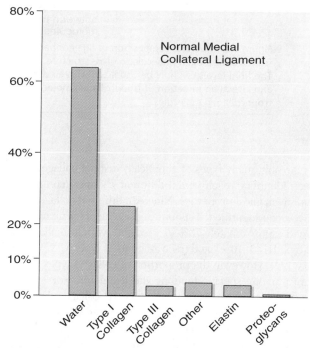

Figure 6.1: Biochemical composition of normal rabbit medial collateral ligament. This graph demonstrates the proportion of components in ligament (based on analysis of rabbit ligament).

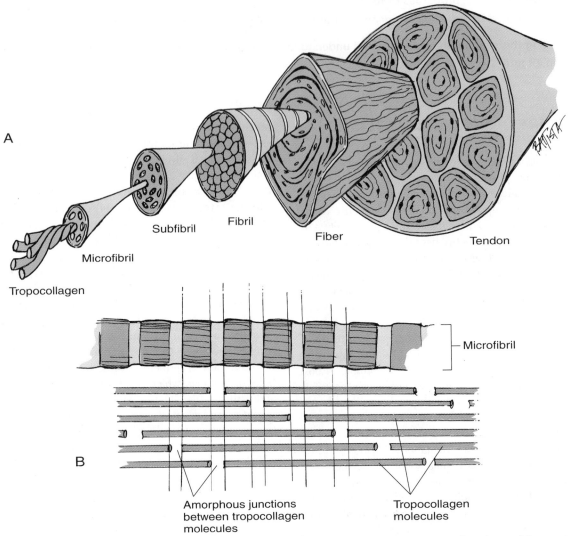

Figure 6.2: Structural composition of ligament and tendon. **A.** The hierarchical organization of tendon and ligament from tropocollagen molecule to gross structure. Fibers and their crimp pattern can be seen with optical microscopy. The fibril levels can only be visualized with electron microscopy. **B.** The formation of microfibrils from end-to-end and lateral aggregation of tropocollagen molecules. Microfailures occur at the amorphous junctions at the ends of tropocollagen molecules.

As a result, many types of genetically distinct collagens have been identified, each with a different chemical composition and mechanical properties. Nineteen different collagen types have been identified. Tendons and ligaments primarily have type I (approximately 70%, dry weight), with a small amount of type III (3–10%), and trace amounts of types V, X, VII, and XIV [92]. However, the proportion of collagen types present varies among specific tendons and ligaments. For example, tendons typically have very little type III collagen; ligaments have a greater proportion. The cruciate ligaments of the knee have a greater proportion of type III collagen than medial collateral ligaments. Granulation tissue has a very high proportion of type III collagen. Variations in collagen type composition may contribute to variations in the mechanical behavior of different ligaments and tendons.

Clinical Relevance

GENETIC DISORDERS AFFECTING COLLAGEN: *Ehlers-Danlos syndrome (EDS) is a genetically inherited connective tissue disorder resulting from defective collagen types I, II, III, or V. There are several types of EDS, each with a unique clinical presentation. However, in all types, various genetic abnormalities cause defective collagen that is unable to form fibrils properly. As a result, connective tissues with this defective collagen are very weak. Some patients suffer from joint hypermobility, subluxations, and dislocations. Other symptoms due to the defective connective tissues include mitral valve prolapse, gastrointestinal tract problems, tendency to bruise easily, and slow-healing skin wounds.*

(continued)

(Continued)

Another genetic disorder that results from defects of a gene that codes for collagen type I is osteogenesis imperfecta. Mutations result in failure to form the collagen triple helix correctly, which interferes with subsequent fibril formation. The result is brittle bones, manifested clinically in varying degrees of severity and producing multiple low-load fractures.

Elastin fibers constitute a much smaller proportion of the fibrous composition of tendons and ligaments. Tendons have very little elastin. The proportion of elastin to collagen fibers varies among ligaments. However, in most ligaments of the joints, as in tendons, collagen is present in a much higher proportion than elastin. The ligamentum flavum, an interlaminar ligament in the spine, however, has more elastin than collagen [66].

EXTRACELLULAR MATRIX: GROUND SUBSTANCE

The ground substance, or nonfibrous part of the extracellular matrix, is composed of structural glycoproteins, proteoglycans, and water. Structural glycoproteins contain a large protein fraction and a small carbohydrate component. These glycoproteins, such as fibronectin, thrombospondin, tenascin-C, and undulin, play an important role in the adhesion of cells to fibers and other extracellular matrix components [43].

Although proteoglycans constitute less than 1% of a tendon's or ligament's total dry weight, they play a key role in ligament and tendon functioning (Fig. 6.1). Proteoglycans are large, complex macromolecules with a protein core to which one or more glycosaminoglycans (GAGs) are covalently attached. GAGs are linear molecules of repeating disaccharide units, which are bound to the protein core at one end and radiate from it to form a "bottlebrush" configuration (see Fig. 5.2). The concentration of GAGs is considerably smaller in tendon and ligament than in cartilage. However, due to their high charge density and charge-to-charge repulsion force, proteoglycan molecules are stiffly extended and thus contribute to tendons' and ligaments' ability to resist compression and tensile forces [43]. The polar nature of these molecules also attracts and holds water within the connective tissues. This hydrophilic characteristic helps to maintain tendon and ligament extensibility in response to tensile forces. For example, wet tendon is able to elongate easily in response to a distraction force, while dry tendon loses compliance [100]. The hydrophilic property of proteoglycans also enables rapid diffusion of water-soluble molecules and migration of cells within the extracellular matrix of the tendon or ligament [43].

Proteoglycans also help to regulate and maintain the structural organization of the tissue by providing support and spacing for the cellular and fibrous connective tissue components. Attachments between GAGs and collagen fibers occur in connective tissue, which contributes to the aggregation of collagen into fiber bundles and to tissue strength. The crimp pattern (wavy appearance of collagen fibers in dense regular connective tissue) has been attributed to the attachments of GAGs to collagen [9]. Examples of GAGs include chondroitin sulfate, dermatan sulfate, and hyaluronic acid, although dermatan sulfate is usually most common in tendons and ligaments. Examples of proteoglycans common in tendons and ligaments include decorin and biglycan.

MECHANICAL PROPERTIES

The mechanical properties of tendons and ligaments are measured by subjecting tissue preparations to uniaxial tensile loads to failure. Tissue preparations typically consist of bone–ligament–bone complexes or tendon. Data collected from these tests are used to create load–deformation curves by plotting the externally applied load against the corresponding amount of elongation of the tissue. These load–deformation curves represent the structural properties of the tissue tested (*Fig. 6.3*). As described in Chapter 2, load–deformation curves can be converted to stress–strain curves that mathematically describe the mechanical properties of the tendon or ligament tested. These mechanical properties depend on the composition of the tissue, the orientation of the collagen fibers, and the interaction between collagen and the components of the ground substance. This method of determining ligament and tendon mechanical properties, however, requires extraction of whole tissues. Thus, studies that employ these methods use tissues from a variety of animal models or human tissue removed during surgery (e.g., degenerated ligaments removed for insertion of total knee replacement prosthetic components).

More recently tendon strain has been measured in vivo in humans using real-time ultrasound scanning methods. These emerging methods allow researchers to study the effects of various factors, such as aging and exercise, on tendon mechanical properties directly in humans during movement [57].

Determination of Stress and Strain

Tensile **strain** is defined as the elongation per unit length of a material in response to a tensile load. It is represented by the formula strain = $(l - l_o)/l_o$, where l_o is the length before the tensile load is applied, and l is the length after the load has been applied. Thus, strain has no units and is usually expressed as a percentage. Length can be measured directly in extracted tissues by placing markers on the soft tissue in the region to be studied. It can also be measured by using devices such as linearly variable differential transformers (LVDT), which are instruments that measure voltage change during elongation and convert this change to a corresponding change in length. This method can be used to collect data in vivo during joint movement, but requires invasive methods to attach the device directly to the tissue

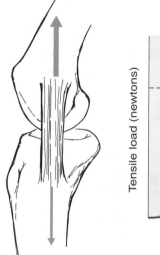

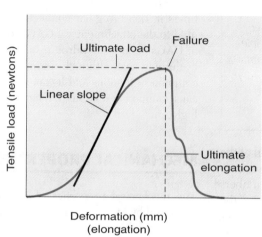

Figure 6.3: A typical load–deformation curve for a bone–ligament–bone complex. When tensile forces (loads) are applied to a bone–ligament–bone complex, a load–deformation curve can be drawn to represent its structural properties.

[13,92]. Noninvasive in vivo ultrasound methods are also used to measure tendon elongation, strain, and tissue stiffness during joint movement, but require the subject to be stationary [30].

Tensile **stress** is defined as the externally applied tensile load per cross-sectional area of the tendon or ligament tested. It is represented by the formula stress = F/A, where F is the amount of the externally applied distraction force and A is the cross-sectional area of the material tested. It is usually expressed as newtons per square millimeter. Although this is a simple relationship, accurate determination of the cross-sectional area of the structure can be difficult. Various methods to determine area are used, ranging from low-tech calipers to measure the width and thickness of the specimen to sophisticated noncontact laser methods [92]. This method requires tissue explants from animal models or human tissues discarded at surgery.

The forces or stresses within tendon and ligaments are also measured in vivo during movement using devices that are placed in or around the midsubstance of the tissue of interest. Examples of these instruments include buckle transducers, fiberoptic sensors, and other implantable force probes [30].

Stress–Strain Curve for Tendons and Ligaments

A stress–strain curve typical for a tendon or ligament is drawn in *Figure 6.4*. Five major regions can be identified on the stress–strain curve of a tendon or ligament. These regions are called the **toe region,** the **linear** or **elastic region,** the progressive failure or **plastic region,** the region of **major failure,** and **complete failure** [84].

The first region is the toe region. In this region there is very little increase in stress as the tissue elongates. Strain is also very low (1.2–1.5%). The stresses that produce strains in the toe region have been equated to those applied by an evaluator

during clinical ligament stress tests. In tendons, toe region stress is sufficient to straighten collagen's crimp pattern and is equivalent to the force produced by a maximum tetanic contraction of the corresponding muscle (*Fig. 6.5*).

In the linear, or elastic, region of the curve, elongation in response to the applied load continues to increase. Stiffness or resistance to elongation also increases, but the relationship between stress and strain remains consistently linear. Micro- and macro-examination of the strain response of tendons to tensile loading shows that loads that exceed those that produce crimp straightening result in tissue elongation by means

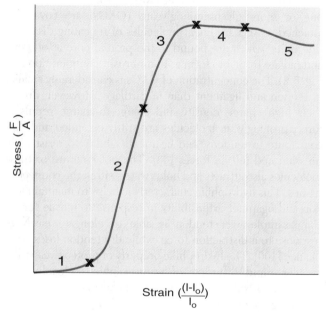

Figure 6.4: Stress–strain curve for tendon or ligament. Five regions are labeled: *1*, toe region; *2*, linear, or elastic, region; *3*, progressive failure, or plastic, region; *4*, major failure region; and *5*, complete rupture region or failure.

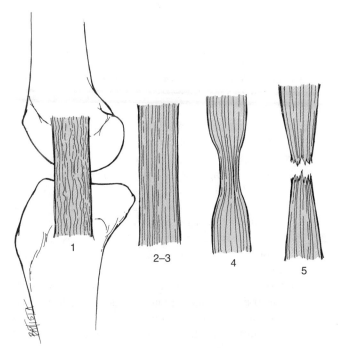

Figure 6.5: Changes in the internal structure of the collagenous tissue of tendons and ligaments in response to tensile loads. The drawing demonstrates the changes that occur in collagenous tissue during stretching. *1,* Toe region, in which the stretch straightens the wavy pattern of the collagen. Regions *2* and *3* are the elastic and plastic regions, in which the crimp is eliminated, and tissue elongation occurs because of stretching of the straightened collagen fibers. Region *4* is the site of major failure where the ligament is still intact, but there is visible narrowing, or necking, of the structure. Region *5* is characterized by complete failure.

TABLE 6.1: Peak Strain in Human Anterior Cruciate Ligaments during Selected Rehabilitation Activities (n = 8–18)

Activity	Peak Strain (%)
Isometric quads contraction @15°	4.4
Squatting with sport cord	4.0
Active flexion/extension of knee with 45 N weight boot	3.8
Lachman test (150 N anterior shear load)	3.7
Squatting	3.6
Active flexion/extension (no weight)	2.8
Stationary bike	1.7

display considerably greater peak and yield stress and elastic modulus as compared with the posterior portion of the tendons [36]. Regional variation of the strain within tendons may also be affected by joint position. Researchers who examined tensile strain in patellar tendons with the knee in various positions report uniform strains throughout the tendon with the knee in full extension. However, when the knee is flexed, the tensile strain increases on the anterior side of the tendon and decreases on the posterior side [3]. A better understanding of these regional variations in the biomechanical properties and stresses and strains within tendons and ligaments may contribute to our comprehension of tendinopathy and other microtrauma injuries.

The slope of the elastic, or linear, portion of the stress–strain curve is called **Young's modulus of elasticity** and is represented numerically as stress divided by strain (see Fig. 2.6). It represents the resistance of the tissue to elongation. When the slope of the curve is steep and the modulus is high, the material exhibits a high degree of stiffness, or resistance to elongation. When the slope of the curve is gradual and the modulus is low, the tissue is more compliant and easily deformed when subjected to a tensile force (see Fig. 2.7).

The third region of the curve is the region of progressive microfailures, also called the **plastic range.** The point at which the elastic region transitions to the plastic region is called the **yield point.** Plastic region tensile forces disrupt enough collagen fibers and bonds to produce a slow unraveling of the collagen fibers and a decrease in the slope of the stress–strain curve [78]. Thus, when the deforming force is removed, the structure is not able to return completely to its prestretched dimension. The tissue remains permanently deformed, even though, to the naked eye, it appears normal and intact. Stresses in this range could occur during an injury that causes a ligamentous sprain. A ligament sprained to this extent may remain overstretched or lax, causing joint instability and future reinjury.

When the plastic range is exceeded, the slope of the curve flattens dramatically. This is the region of major failure. Although the tendon or ligament is still intact, there is visible narrowing, or necking, of the structure (Fig. 6.5). Elongation

of collagen fibers sliding with respect to one another [78]. When the tensile force is removed, the tendon or ligament returns to its prestressed length and shape. However, depending on the duration of this elastic range deformation, additional time may be required for full recovery to the original prestressed length. The persistence of elongation demonstrates the hysteresis property of viscoelastic material. The stress and strain that occur in tendons and ligaments because of normal physiological motions fall in this elastic, or linear, region of the curve and strain is estimated to be up to 6%. Physiological strains in the anterior cruciate and medial collateral ligaments at the knee are in the range of 4–5% (*Table 6.1*) [12,13]. A current view is that during normal movements, tendon elongation does not exceed 4% [43,84].

Physiological strains vary among different tendons and ligaments and among different regions within the same tendon. For example, optical methods examining the strain behavior in normal anterior tibialis tendons reveal that the strain measured in the region close to the muscle was five times greater than that measured in either the mid-tendon or the region of the tendon close to the bone [9]. Tendon fascicles from patellar tendons of young men also demonstrate regional variation in strain. Fascicles from the anterior portion of these tendons

of the material may occur without additional force. This stage is followed by complete failure. The stress and strain at the failure point are called the **ultimate stress** and the **ultimate strain**, respectively. During physiological loading, a tendon is subjected to tensile strains of up to 6% [78]. When an acute stress causes an elongation of 8% or more, the tendon or ligament will probably rupture, depending on the specific structure and the method of loading [43]. These are properties of the tendon or ligament tissue, thus they can only be determined if failure is through the substance of the ligament or tendon tissue itself. However, ultimate failure in a tendon or ligament can occur in three different ways. Failure can occur by rupture in which there is tearing through the substance of the tissue, by failure through the enthesis (tendon or ligament insertional site), or by pulling away a portion of the bony attachment of the ligament or tendon. Failure at the bony site is called an **avulsion fracture**.

Modes of Failure

The nature of failure varies among different tendons and ligaments and may be influenced by several factors including age or skeletal maturity, structural differences among different ligaments and tendons, and the speed or rate at which the elongation force is applied. Failure modes in ligaments, in particular, depend on age or skeletal maturity. For example, collateral ligaments at the knee fail by tibial avulsion in animals with open epiphyses, whereas in animals with closed epiphyses, failure is by ligamentous disruption [98]. Structural differences within the ligament or tendon and differences in the nature of their attachment to bone also influence the method of failure. For example, in animal studies, the collateral ligaments at the knee typically fail by midsubstance rupture, while anterior cruciate ligaments (ACLs) fail by tibial avulsion. Patellar tendons fail by avulsion from the inferior pole of the patella [24]. However, clinical observations show that knee ligament injuries in humans typically result in ligament failures by midsubstance rupture. Thus, there may be species differences as well as differences among different tendons and ligaments within a subject.

Effects of Physical Conditions on Mechanical Properties

The biomechanical properties of tendons and ligaments and their behavior in response to tensile loads are affected by physical conditions. Two conditions that have been studied extensively include the speed, or rate, of application of the stretching force and the temperature of the structures at the time of stretching.

EFFECTS OF RATE OF FORCE APPLICATION

The effect of the rate of stretch, or strain rate, on the biomechanical properties of tendons and ligaments has been investigated and debated for many years. Studies using human

tendons and ligaments demonstrate that the speed of stretch has an effect on their stress–strain curves [68,86]. It had been suggested that the rate of strain that occurred during injury had an effect on the nature of the resulting ligament injury. For example, as the rate of force application increases, stiffness and ultimate load also increase, and failure is more likely to occur by rupture. Conversely, at slow speeds, failure occurs predominantly by avulsion [22,68]. However, data from more-recent studies suggest that the effects of strain rate are overestimated [92]. Ligaments tested at low, medium, and high rates of elongation show similar biomechanical responses. Small differences are observed in the modulus of elasticity between the slow and medium strain rates, but the modulus at the fast extension rate is only 30% higher [24]. Consistent with this finding, tendons also show moderate increases in elastic modulas and ultimate tensile strength as strain rate increases [62]. Failure modes (avulsion versus substance rupture) in ligaments are independent of strain rate but depend on age and skeletal maturity. In animals with open epiphyses, all failures occur by avulsion, regardless of strain rate, whereas in animals with closed epiphyses, failures occur by ligament disruption [70].

EFFECTS OF TEMPERATURE

Temperature has an important effect on the molecular and mechanical properties of collagen. When an unrestrained tendon or ligament is heated to 59–60°C, it undergoes irreversible shrinkage [65]. This critical temperature, called the *melting temperature*, is presumed to cause breaking of chemical bonds that maintain the structure and organization of collagen fibers.

Clinical Relevance

USING HEAT TO STABILIZE THE SHOULDER: *In the young, active population, a common cause of shoulder pain is joint instability due to capsular injury. Once shoulder instability is present, the incidence of reinjury is high. As a result, surgical intervention may be required to restore the joint stability necessary for return to an active lifestyle. Open surgical procedures to retense lax ligaments require a lengthy healing and rehabilitation time. As a result, another procedure, thermal capsulorraphy, has been developed in which thermal energy is used to shrink the lax capsule and ligaments, thus restoring joint stability. Thermal energy, produced by lasers or radiofrequency (RF) electrothermal probes, denatures the collagen and disrupts the covalent molecular bonds, producing a condensed collagen coil that results in decreased tissue length. The amount of tissue shrinkage is variable and increases with increasing applied thermal energy, tissue temperature, and the duration of application [55].*

Arthroscopically applied thermal energy at a temperature between 55 and 65°C is commonly used to produce the

(continued)

(Continued)

tissue shrinkage and associated histological changes [38]. Biomechanical analysis has demonstrated that gleno-humeral thermal capsulorraphy results in decreased humeral head translation on the glenoid and reestablishment of intraarticular pressure within the shoulder joint [71,83]. Although the joint appears to be stabilized by the heat-tightened ligaments, studies have shown that heat-treated ligaments have an increase in ultimate and yield strain and a decrease in tissue stiffness [71,80]. The failure load of shrunken ligaments is also reduced as a result of the thermal treatment. Patients who have received this treatment and their therapists must protect the treated joints from excessive tensile loads during the postoperative period to allow for healing and restoration of strength in the shrunken tissue. Researchers tested heat shrunken ligaments to failure at 3-week intervals for 9 weeks after thermal treatment. They found that the highest failure load occurred in the third week after treatment; that is, the treated ligaments were the strongest at 3 weeks after treatment. However, at 9 weeks after thermal treatment, those heat shrunken ligaments that had also been immobilized were significantly weaker than they were at 3 weeks after treatment and were also weaker than those in which motion was permitted [25]. Total immobilization seems to have a negative effect on the healing ligament. However, the ideal timing for remobilization is still controversial. Joint instability in other regions that is also treated with thermal shrinking procedures include chronic lateral ankle instability and the medial patellar retinaculum for recurrent patellar instability [21,41].

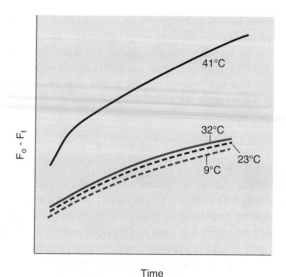

Figure 6.6: The effect of temperature on the stress relaxation curves. Stress relaxation curves for rat tail tendon at a given strain for several temperatures above and below thermal transition. F_o, original force; F_t, force at the end of the period of sustained strain. Note that as stress relaxation increases, the difference between F_o and F_t increases. (Data from Rigby BJ, Hirai N, Spikes JD: The mechanical behavior of rat tail tendon. J Gen Physiol 1959; 43: 265–283.)

A less severe temperature increase to 37–40°C is termed *thermal transition*. When collagen in tendons and ligaments is heated to temperatures in the thermal transition range, the viscoelastic properties of the structure are affected, including stress relaxation, rate of creep, and rupture strain and load [84]. When tendons are held under tension during load–deformation studies, stress relaxation is independent of temperature until 37°C is reached. Above this temperature, stress relaxation increases as temperature increases (*Fig. 6.6*) [76]. Recovery from stress relaxation is also temperature dependent. For example, when tendons heated to 37°C and subjected to strains between 1 and 4% are allowed to cool, they return to their original stress. However, in tendons heated to 40°C, the change is irreversible [75].

Heating tendons to thermal transition temperatures also increases the rate of creep. That is, it takes less time to reach a given strain in response to application of a stretching load when tendons are heated [91] (*Fig. 6.7*). Heated tendons demonstrate increased rates of creep in response to both cyclic stretching and constant loading. Both loading conditions produce similar increases in creep in response to the heating [51].

The rupture load and strain of tendons are also affected by heating. For example, tendons heated to 40°C demonstrate a

rupture strain of only 3–4%, compared with 8–14% for tendons at temperatures lower than 37°C. These results support the conclusion that heating to 40°C can produce structural damage to collagen [75]. Additionally, tendons that are heated and then cooled while the tensile load is maintained rupture at lower strains than those in which loading was not maintained during cooling. This suggests that cooling in an elongated position inhibits reestablishment of structural bonds, thus structurally weakening the tendon [91]. These conclusions are drawn from in vitro studies conducted on rat tail and

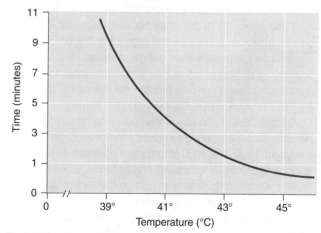

Figure 6.7: Effect of temperature on tendon elongation time. The graph demonstrates the effect of temperatures above thermal transition on the time required to achieve a 2.6% strain (elongation) in rat tail tendon. (Data from Warren CG, Lehman JF, Koblanski JN: Elongation of rat tail tendon: effect of load and temperature. Arch Phys Med Rehabil 1971; 52: 465–484.)

canine tendon. A more recent in vivo study examined the effect of immersing the legs of young men in water at 5°C or 42°C for 30 minutes. No changes in the strain behavior of their Achilles tendons were found. These results provide evidence that the general application of superficial heat or cooling agents may not affect the mechanical properties of tendons [48].

Clinical Relevance

CLINICAL RELEVANCE: USING HEAT TO INCREASE RANGE OF MOTION: *Clinicians are often confronted with patients who have restricted joint range of motion that interferes with functional activities. Joint restriction can be produced by dense connective tissues within muscles and in joint capsules as well as in tendons and ligaments. Treatment to increase joint range of motion is often focused on increasing the length of dense connective tissues that have shortened as a result of immobilization or healing. Treatments involve the application of stretching forces. Among the methods that can be used to produce stretching are brief, intense methods, such as joint mobilization or manual osteokinematic stretching, as well as low-load, prolonged stretching techniques using splints, casts, or other devices. Increased connective tissue extensibility is helpful in the administration of any of these stretching techniques. The studies described above have shown that heating dense connective tissue to about 40°C affects the bonding between tropocollagen molecules, resulting in increased ductility. The increased rate of creep and stress relaxation that occurs in heated dense connective tissue should facilitate the effectiveness of stretching techniques. Preheating or heating applied simultaneously with stretch allows clinicians to produce elongation in shortened connective tissues with less force, thus reducing the risk of injuring healing, or other adjacent, tissues. However, heating also results in reduced rupture load and strain. When 2% strain has been exceeded, collagen begins to yield. Since heated connective tissues fail at significantly lower loads than unheated tissues, clinicians applying stretching forces to heated connective tissues during treatment must carefully monitor the amount of stretching force applied to avoid unwanted tissue tearing.*

Another clinical consideration is how to achieve the temperature increase required to produce the desired effect in the target tissue. The 40°C temperature necessary to produce increased tissue extensibility refers to the temperature of the collagen, not the temperature on the surface of the body. Since most methods of heating used in the clinic require transmission of thermal energy through skin and perhaps overlying muscle and fat before the target tissue can be reached, clinicians must be knowledgeable about the depth of penetration of the heating method selected. Heating modalities with superficial depths of penetration, such as moist hot packs, may not achieve the necessary

temperature elevation in dense connective tissue structures such as tendons and ligaments that are located beneath overlying muscles. As a result, insufficient heating will compromise treatment effectiveness.

Biological Effects on Mechanical Properties

The biomechanical properties of tendons and ligaments are affected by several biological factors. Biological factors discussed in this chapter include skeletal maturity, aging, sex, and hormones.

EFFECTS OF MATURATION AND AGING

Skeletal maturation and aging have significant effects on the biomechanical properties of ligaments and tendons. In general, tensile strength, load to failure, and elastic modulus all improve rapidly during maturation until skeletal maturity (closing of the epiphyses) is achieved. Stress relaxation and creep in response to both static and cyclic loads are also greater in very young animals and improve with maturation. Maximal tissue strength is achieved around the time of skeletal maturity. It declines gradually during adulthood and into senescence [96,97]. Thus ligaments and tendons from very young and old animals withstand lower maximal tensile loads than those from young and middle-aged adults [96] (*Fig. 6.8*). In addition to affecting the

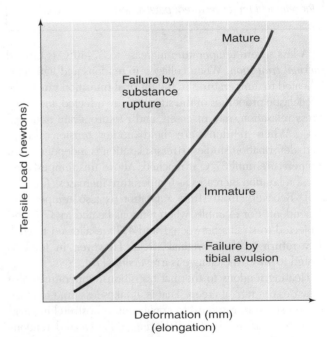

Figure 6.8: Mechanical properties of the bone–ligament–bone complexes of skeletally mature and immature rabbits. A load–deformation curve demonstrates the mechanical properties of the bone–ligament–bone complexes of skeletally mature and immature rabbits. Skeletally immature rabbits have open epiphyses; mature rabbits have closed epiphyses.

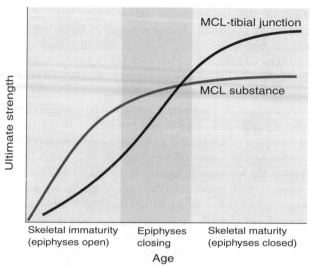

Figure 6.9: Comparison of the strength of the insertional site and the ligament substance during skeletal maturation in rabbit medial collateral ligaments. The graph demonstrates the differences in ultimate strength between insertion site and the ligament substance of rabbit medial collateral ligaments as the animals mature. In skeletally immature animals, failure is most often by ligament tibial avulsion because its ultimate strength is less than that of the ligament substance. In skeletally mature animals, failure occurs by ligament substance rupture, which is now weaker than the insertion site. (Adapted from Woo SL-Y, Ohland KJ, Weiss JA: Aging and sex-related changes in the biomechanical properties of the rabbit medial collateral ligament. Mech Ageing Dev 1990; 56: 129–142.)

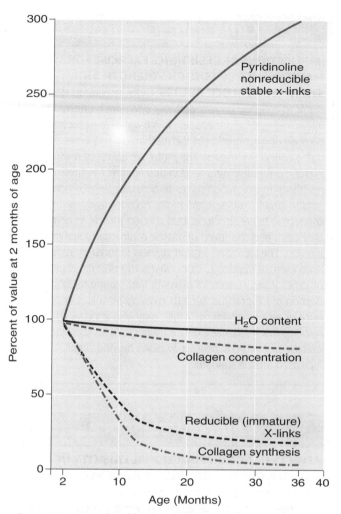

Figure 6.10: Age-related biochemical changes in anterior cruciate and medial collateral ligaments of rabbits. Two-month-old rabbits are skeletally immature (open epiphyses), while 12- and 36-month-old rabbits have closed epiphyses; 36-month-old rabbits are considered aged or elderly. (Data from Amiel D, Kuiper SD, Wallace D, et al: Age-related properties of medial collateral ligament and anterior cruciate ligament: a morphologic and collagen maturation study in the rabbit. J Gerontol 1991; 46: B159–B165.)

mechanical properties of ligaments, maturation also changes the mode of failure caused by tensile loading. In young animals with open epiphyses, the mechanism of failure that occurs most often is avulsion fracture of bone. In mature animals with closed epiphyses, ligament failure is more likely to occur by midsubstance rupture [96] (*Fig. 6.9*).

Biochemical and histological alterations also occur during maturation and aging and may explain some of the mechanical changes associated with aging. During maturation, collagen fibril size increases, and collagen concentration and synthesis are greater than in adults [43]. Prior to skeletal maturity there is a greater number of immature, reducible collagen cross-links, which corresponds to collagen synthesis. Adults have a higher proportion of the more stable pyridinoline cross-links [6] (*Fig. 6.10*). The mechanical superiority of adult ligaments may be related to the shift in the predominant type of collagen cross-linking and increased fibril size. Aged tendons and ligaments have reduced collagen concentration and an increased number of small-diameter collagen fibrils [82]. In addition, collagen type V, a known regulator of collagen fibril diameter, is found in aged tendons and ligaments, but not in those of young animals [27]. Other in vitro analyses of aged tendons show that aging is also associated with a reduction in the collagen fibril crimp angle, an increase in elastin content, and a reduction in extracellular water and proteoglycan content. The net effect of these changes is a reduction of tendon stiffness in aged tendons [59].

Although most of these findings were taken from investigations using animal models, studies on human tissues also demonstrate the mechanical inferiority of older tendons and ligaments. For example, the stiffness, ultimate load, and elastic modulus of ACL specimens from young adults (age 22–35 years) are about three times higher than those from older people [69,95]. Anterior and posterior spinal ligaments taken from humans at the time of surgery show a strong inverse relationship between age and tensile strength [42,60]. Elderly human patellar tendons also show more compliance and loss of stiffness [73]. However, recent studies in both animals and humans show that the reduction in tendon and ligament stiffness that occurs with aging can be minimized, if not reversed, in response to low or moderately intense resistance exercise [18,49,74].

Clinical Relevance

IMPLICATIONS OF RESISTANCE EXERCISE FOR MAINTENANCE OF TENDON STRENGTH AND STIFFNESS IN OLDER ADULTS: *Older individuals who desire to continue athletic activities often are hampered by musculoskeletal strain injuries, which are at least partially because of deterioration in the mechanical properties of aging connective tissues. The protective effects of resistance exercise on maintaining tendon and ligament stiffness and resistance to elongation forces may reduce the likelihood of tendon strain injuries. Additionally, because tendons are the connective tissue structures that connect muscle to bone, they can affect the speed of muscle contraction force transmission. The increased tendon stiffness induced by resistance exercise training is associated with faster development of joint torque. Functional activities that require rapid production of joint torque, such as recovery from loss of balance as well as athletic activities, may also improve as a result of this resistance exercise training. Thus, resistance exercise training has benefits to elders beyond simply increased muscle strength.*

Clinical Relevance

AFFECTS OF AGE ON FUNCTIONAL CAPACITY OF LIGAMENTS AND TENDONS: *Ligaments and tendons help to maintain joint stability. As tendons and ligaments age, they are less able to withstand tensile loads. As a result they may be less effective in stabilizing a joint in response to repetitive or high forces that occur during functional activities. Joint instability may result in abnormal joint mechanics during movement. This alteration in joint mechanics may place excessive stress on joint structures and lead to degenerative joint disease.*

EFFECT OF HORMONES

Hormones can affect the mechanical properties of dense connective tissues also. The adrenocorticotropic hormone of the pituitary and cortisone of the adrenal cortex both lower the GAG content of the extracellular matrix of connective tissues. Excessive levels of cortisol also reduce the synthesis of type I collagen. Both of these effects reduce connective tissue strength. Another hormone, relaxin, which is produced during pregnancy, softens and increases the extensibility of pelvic ligaments. The female sex hormone estrogen may also play a role in determining the tensile properties of ligaments. Observations that more female than male athletes experience ACL injuries led some clinicians and researchers to hypothesize a role for estrogen in determining ligament strength [8]. Functional estrogen and progesterone receptors have been

found in the ligaments of rabbits and humans [77]. Additionally, in vitro incubation of rabbit ACLs with estrogen produces alterations in cell behavior, including downregulation (reduced transcription) of type I collagen synthesis [54]. The mechanical behavior of ligaments is also affected by alterations in hormone concentration. For example, increasing the concentration of circulating estrogen is associated with reduced tensile properties in ACLs of rabbits [81]. This finding prompted others to attempt to find a relationship between menstrual cycle phase and incidence of ACL injury [35]. A recent study, however, shows that there are no significant differences in ACL ligament laxity in any of the three menstrual phases, either before or after exercise [58]. Further, a well-designed and controlled investigation examines the influence of estrogen and estrogen receptors on knee ligament mechanical properties in an animal model. These authors report that estrogen treatment has no significant effect on the viscoelastic or tensile properties of the MCL or ACL. Thus, it does not seem likely that estrogen plays a significant role in explaining the high incidence of ACL injuries in women [90].

RESPONSE OF TENDONS AND LIGAMENTS TO IMMOBILIZATION

Decreased joint mobility has significant effects on both bone and soft tissues. Wolff's law describes the effect of mechanical stresses on bone remodeling. This law is often restated as the specific adaptation to imposed demand (SAID) principle, which is used to explain remodeling in response to alterations in external loading in soft tissues such as tendons and ligaments [17]. Joint immobilization by casting or pinning is often used to study the effects of stress reduction on tendons and ligaments. This immobilization model enables examination of the responses of normal soft tissues as well as soft tissues that have been injured and are healing. The importance of understanding the effects of immobilization on healing connective tissue is obvious, since many tendon and ligament injuries are treated with periods of rest and immobilization. Clinicians need to decide when to begin and how much movement is desirable to facilitate joint motion without producing negative effects on the healing tissue. However, noninjured connective tissues may also be immobilized. For example, bed rest or pain following surgical procedures may result in joint immobility. Neuromuscular conditions such as stroke or spinal cord injury may also cause muscle paralysis, weakness, or pain resulting in loss of joint motion. Understanding the effects of immobilization on healing as well as normal joint structures is important to provide effective and safe rehabilitation treatments.

Immobilization and Remobilization of Normal Connective Tissue

Joint immobilization, which reduces the tensile forces normally applied to tendons and ligaments during joint movement, alters the biomechanical properties of the joint structures. These alterations include reduction of the load at failure, reduced stiffness and elastic modulus, and increased elongation at failure load [44] (*Fig. 6.11*). In addition, on load-to-failure testing, the frequency of failure by avulsion at the insertional site, rather than by midsubstance tear, is increased significantly in immobilized ligaments. This is related to increased subperiosteal osteoclastic activity, which results in subperiosteal bone resorption.

Biochemical and histological changes also occur in immobilized tendons and ligaments, which may help to explain the biomechanical changes. Both collagen synthesis and degradation increase, resulting in increased collagen turnover. This increase in collagen turnover is time dependent. For example, when immobilization is limited to 9 weeks, collagen turnover increases, but the total collagen mass does not change [7]. However, when immobilization is continued to 12 weeks, the increased collagen turnover results in reduced collagen mass or atrophy [4]. Ligaments subjected to extended periods of joint immobilization also demonstrate disorganization of collagen fiber orientation and alteration in collagen fiber size [15,28,44]. These changes may contribute to the reduced failure load and reduced stiffness observed in immobilized tissue. Collagen cross-linking is also affected by immobilization. Chemical analysis of immobilized dense connective tissue shows an overall increase in the quantity of collagen cross-links. However, the greatest increase is found in the proportion of cross-links associated with newly synthesized collagen, indicating the presence of increased amounts of immature collagen [2]. Water content and total GAGs decrease during immobilization [1]. These losses may be associated with the development of connective tissue contractures in immobilized dense connective tissue structures [5].

Joint position during an immobilization period affects the nature of the biomechanical changes that occur in both tendons and ligaments. For example, immobilization of ligaments with some tension results in less deterioration of their tensile properties than does immobilization without tension [61]. Collagen fiber disorganization occurs in tendons maintained in a stress-reduced position in immobilized joints. However, recasting the joint in a position in which the tendon is elongated can reverse the fiber disorganization [28]. Thus, in both ligaments and tendons, maintaining tensile load in the tissue during joint immobilization provides some protection from reduction of their biomechanical properties.

Stress-shielding experiments without joint immobilization also demonstrate the protective role of tension in maintaining tissue strength [37]. In these studies, patellar tendons were either totally (100%) or partially (70%) shielded from tensile load while animals were permitted full use of knee joint range of motion and weight bearing. After 2 weeks of stress shielding, bone–tendon–bone complexes were tested to failure. Although all stress-shielded tendons show reduced failure load, those that maintained some tensile stress were much less affected [37] (*Fig. 6.12*).

Fortunately, the deleterious histological, biochemical, and mechanical changes associated with joint immobilization are reversible. Reestablishment of normal stresses to the tissues restores normal structure and function. However, full recovery of the biomechanical characteristics of the complex may take longer than the time required to produce the undesirable change. Restoration of mechanical properties also appears to vary among specific structures and among animals of different species. For example, in a study of the ACLs of primates, 5 months of remobilization (following 2 months of

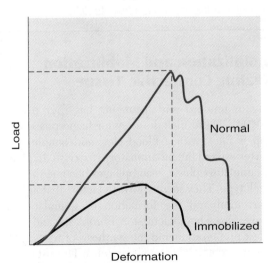

Figure 6.11: Typical load–deformation curves from normal and immobilized ligaments. The graph demonstrates typical load-deformation curves for bone–ligament–bone complexes from normal and normal immobilized joints.

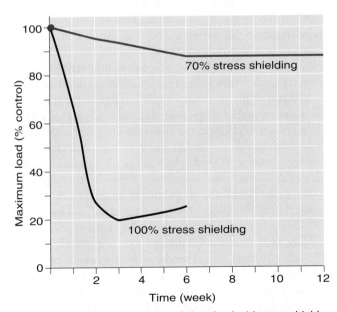

Figure 6.12: Changes in maximum failure load with stress shielding. The graph demonstrates the difference in maximum failure load of rabbit patellar tendons in response to complete (100%) or partial (70%) stress shielding. (Data from Hayashi K: Biomechanical studies of the remodeling of knee joint tendons and ligaments. J Biomech 1996; 29: 707–716.)

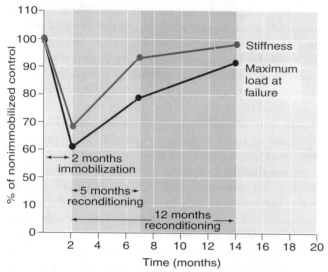

Figure 6.13: Effect of immobilization and reconditioning on mechanical properties of ligaments. This graph demonstrates the effect of 2 months of knee joint immobilization on the mechanical properties of the anterior cruciate ligament in primates. Recovery after 5 and 12 months of remobilization is only partial. (Data from Noyes FR: Functional properties of knee ligaments and alterations induced by immobilization: a correlative biomechanical and histological study in primates. Clin Orthop 1977; 123: 210–242.)

immobilization) are required to recover about 80% of the maximum load at failure. After 12 months of recovery, ligament strength is still only about 90% of preimmobilization values [67] (*Fig. 6.13*). With rabbit medial collateral ligament complexes, 12 weeks of immobilization requires 9 to 12 weeks of remobilization to restore most of the biomechanical properties of the ligaments [93]. Insertional sites, however, are more resistant to recovery and require 3–4 months of increased activity to reverse the detrimental effects of immobilization. In general, prolonged recovery time is required for recovery from relatively brief periods of stress deprivation.

Because of the methods required to determine mechanical tissue properties in the past, the findings reported on the effects of immobilization and stress shielding discussed above come from studies that used a variety of animal models, from rats to primates. Recent advances in ultrasound scanning have enabled the in vivo assessment of the effects of disuse on some of the mechanical properties of intact human tendon. Using this methodology short-term (20 days) and long-term (90 days) bed-rest studies show that tendon stiffness is reduced by approximately 30% and 40%, respectively [47,72]. The adaptive responses of tendon to loss of normal mechanical loading are also studied by measuring tendon stiffness and elastic modulus in tendons from paralyzed muscles in patients with spinal cord injuries (SCI) of longstanding duration (1.5 to 24 years) [56]. Investigators report that tendon stiffness and elastic modulus were lower by 77% in the subjects with SCI as compared with healthy age-matched controls. Although tendon length was maintained in the paralyzed muscles, cross-sectional area (CSA) was reduced by 17%.

This reduction in tendon CSA that occurs with paralyzed muscles differs from nonparalyzed immobilized muscles, in which CSA is maintained. These findings concerning the mechanical properties of tendons from paralyzed muscles have safety implications for clinicians using electrical stimulation protocols with patients with SCI.

Clinical Relevance

TREATMENT DURING AND FOLLOWING IMMOBILIZATION: *Clinicians must consider these biomechanical changes when treating patients with joints that are immobilized for any reason. Application of safe tensile loads to affected ligaments and tendons during immobilization may minimize the amount of connective tissue atrophy and loss of mechanical integrity that might otherwise occur. This can be accomplished by very simple methods, such as having patients perform isometric contractions of immobilized muscles to load the immobilized tendons or by moving joints that are not being used functionally through their range of motion.*

Clinicians must also exercise caution when applying forces during exercise to remobilize joint structures that have been immobilized for extended periods. Immobilized connective tissues may have developed contractures during the immobilization period. As a result, clinicians often select therapeutic techniques to stretch or elongate the shortened tissues. These techniques involve application of a tensile load in an attempt to lengthen the restricted joint structures. In addition to being shortened, these tissues and their bony insertion sites may be weaker and more susceptible to disruption in response to tensile loads. Thus, to avoid inadvertent injury, when treating shortened connective tissue post-immobilization, it may be prudent to select techniques that apply low-load, prolonged stretch rather than brief, but intense or high-load stretch.

Immobilization and Mobilization in Healing Connective Tissue

Healing in tendons and ligaments has four overlapping phases [94]. These include a hemorrhagic phase in which the gap is filled with a blood clot, and lymphocytes and leukocytes expand the inflammatory response. In phase two, the inflammatory phase, macrophages become the predominant cell type. They secrete growth factors that induce neovascularization and the formation of granulation tissue. They are also chemotactic for fibroblasts and stimulate fibroblast proliferation and the synthesis of types I, III, and V collagen and noncollagenous proteins. The last cell type to become prominent is the fibroblast. This event signals the beginning of the third, or proliferative, phase of healing. During this stage, fibroblasts produce collagen and other matrix proteins. This usually occurs within 1 week of injury.

The last stage, remodeling and maturation, is marked by a gradual decrease in the cellularity of the healed tissue. The matrix becomes more dense and longitudinally oriented. Collagen turnover, water content, the ratio between types I and III collagens, and the ratio among the various collagen cross-links begin to approach normal levels.

During the last stage of healing, various biochemical and mechanical signals are critical in facilitating the remodeling process. Tension or physiological loading is an important signal necessary to trigger the changes required for the healed ligament to recover normal tensile strength and other biomechanical properties. Certain growth factors also influence healing and facilitate the restoration of strength. The healed tissue continues to mature for many months but may never attain normal morphological characteristics or mechanical properties. The degree of recovery of normal composition, organization, and tensile strength varies among structures within an individual as well as among species. For example, in the knee, ACLs do not heal after disruption, while collateral ligaments do. Additionally, tendons and ligaments heal much more slowly than a wound in the skin. Variation in healing time among tissues occurs for a variety of reasons, including the amount of blood supply to the tissue and the method by which the tissue receives nutrition and has metabolites removed.

Biomechanical testing of healing tendons and ligaments shows that like normal ligaments that have been immobilized, healing dense connective tissues have poorer stress–strain characteristics, including lower failure loads and reduced stiffness (lower elastic modulus). Healing tendons and ligaments demonstrate smaller-diameter collagen fibers, a greater proportion of type III collagen, and a higher proportion of reducible cross-links, indicating immature collagen. The effect of joint immobilization versus free joint movement on tendon and ligament healing has been studied to determine the most beneficial method of treatment. For many years, the clinical management of healing tendons and ligaments included protection from tensile loads by casting or splinting for long periods. Current practice focuses on early mobilization during healing, since prolonged protection of tendon and ligament wounds from stress is detrimental to restoration of normal strength and stress–strain characteristics. Movement within physiological limits introduced immediately after repair results in stronger unions than delayed mobilization or prolonged immobilization [29,33,34]. Additionally, compared with the outcome of delayed activity, early motion to healing connective tissue results in faster healing and reduced scar tissue adhesions [23].

As the proportion of the population classified as elderly increases and more older adults choose surgical treatments of musculoskeletal injuries rather than reduction of activity level, clinicians require specific knowledge about the effects of aging on healing in tendons and ligaments to make sound clinical decisions about patient care. Many studies describe the detrimental effects of aging in healing dermal wounds;

however, little is known about tendon and ligament healing in older adults. Interestingly, at least one animal study using healthy elderly rabbits has demonstrated that the biomechanical properties of healing tendons in old animals (age 4.8 years) are equally as good as those for young (age 1 year) rabbits. It appears that age does not negatively influence the biomechanical properties of healing patellar tendon repairs [26]. In fact, the tensile strength of the healing scar tissue in tendon wounds of the older rabbits was just as strong as the scar tissue in the tendons of the young rabbits. However, more study is required to determine interactions among the processes of tendon and ligament healing, comorbid factors often present in elders that are known to affect healing (e.g., diabetes mellitus, poor nutrition, and smoking) and exercise on the biomechanical properties of healing tendons and ligaments in elders.

Clinical Relevance

EARLY MOBILIZATION OF TENDON REPAIRS: *The most commonly used treatment approaches for postoperative management of primary tendon repairs in the hand use early passive mobilization. During the inflammatory and early fibroblastic stages of healing (the first 3 weeks after surgical repair), the repaired tendon is protected from active motion. However, with the joints of the hand and wrist positioned so that the repaired tendon is protected from excessive tension or elongating stresses that might rupture or attenuate the repair site, each joint of the finger is moved passively through its full range of motion. Healing tendons subjected to this type of passive motion during the first 3 weeks of healing are two to three times as strong as immobilized tendons [40]. In fact, repaired tendons that are immobilized for 3 weeks are no stronger than immediately after suture [32].*

Growth factors also affect the outcome of healing in tendons and ligaments. Endogenous growth factors and growth factor receptors increase during the first 2 weeks after ligament injury [50,53]. This observation led researchers to add selected growth factors to healing ligaments. When exogenous growth factors, such as platelet-derived growth factor-BB and transforming growth factor 1, are applied individually to healing ligaments, tensile strength and stiffness increase significantly [39,46]. This effect is greatest when the growth factors are applied within 24 hours of injury [10]. Although growth-factor-treated healing ligaments are stronger than untreated healing ligaments, their tensile strength still does not approach that of uninjured ligaments [10]. Continuing study of the effects of growth factors to facilitate and enhance tendon and ligament healing is needed as clinical applications emerge.

Clinical Relevance

TREATMENT OF TENDON AND LIGAMENT TEARS:
Not all tendons and ligaments heal in the same manner. The healing capability of collateral and cruciate ligaments at the knee and extrasynovial versus intrasynovial grafts for tendon injuries have been compared [99]. Isolated injuries of the medial collateral ligament heal reliably without surgical intervention. Conversely, there is little chance that the cruciate ligaments will heal after disruption. As a result, when a cruciate ligament tear results in functional joint instability, ligament reconstruction with a connective tissue graft is usually performed.

Reviews from the clinical literature on anterior cruciate reconstructions report approximately a 30% incidence of postoperative laxity [19,52]. There is concern that excessive loading during rehabilitation may contribute to elongation of ligament grafts [13,63]. As a result, it is important for clinicians to understand the creep properties of ligament grafts over time and the effect of joint immobilization and mobilization on these properties. Autografts for medial collateral ligaments in rabbits are more susceptible to creep than normal medial collateral ligament controls. Additionally, immobilization of the autografts during healing results in increased vulnerability of the grafts to creep. Progressive elongation of the grafts could occur over time because of their inability to recover from the imposed creep strain, compared with normal ligaments [16]. As a result, most postoperative protocols for rehabilitation following ACL reconstruction include early mobilization rather than extended periods of immobilization. Moreover, to prevent excessive creep from accumulating over time, it is important for clinicians to understand the effect of postoperative exercises on ligament and graft strain. Exercises that may be effective in increasing muscle strength may apply excessive strain to the ligament graft and thus potentially contribute to recurrence of ligament instability due to graft creep (Table 6.1) [12].

RESPONSE OF TENDONS AND LIGAMENTS TO STRESS ENHANCEMENT

Since immobilization and reduction of stress in tendons and ligaments has a deleterious effect on the their biomechanical properties, researchers have become interested in the effect of exercise and stress enhancement on dense connective tissues. Studies to determine if exercise affects normal tendons and ligaments identified some positive effects on the strength of ligaments and tendons and their insertion sites [20,85, 87,88]. For example, following an endurance exercise regimen, trained animals have ligaments with smaller-diameter collagen fiber bundles, higher collagen content, increased tensile strength, and maximum load at failure. Animals that performed nonendurance exercise did not exhibit these

adaptations [89]. However, the results of a more recent study show that a lifelong endurance exercise training program (420–557 weeks of training) had little or no effect on the biomechanical properties of medial collateral ligaments from normal adult animals [98]. Thus, it appears that exercise may only protect against the weakening effect of inactivity and not strengthen normal tendons and ligaments. A drawback of all of these studies is that the amount of load actually applied to the tendons and ligaments by the exercise is not known. Studies previously discussed in this chapter (see Effects of Maturation and Aging) show that low and moderately intense resisted exercise can minimize or reverse the loss of tendon stiffness that occurs with aging [49,73]. Aerobic endurance exercise, however, does not have the same protective effect on aging tendons, even though an in vitro study in which cyclic tensile strain was applied to tendon explants showed collagen synthesis up-regulation and retention of the newly synthesized collagen after the tensile loading had ceased [45,79]. These findings are very interesting, but additional study is required to help develop clinical applications.

In addition to altering the tensile load to tendons and ligaments by exercise, stress enhancement in tendons and ligaments is studied in animals by partial removal of tissue from the structure [37]. For example, by cutting away both edges of the rabbit patellar tendon, the cross-sectional area of the remaining tendon is reduced, and the remaining tendon is subjected to higher stress when the animal performs normal activity (force remains the same, but cross-sectional area decreases). Biomechanical tests performed on tendons from animals that experienced stress enhancement by this method show that when stress is elevated 33% above the normal stress, there is no significant difference between the tensile

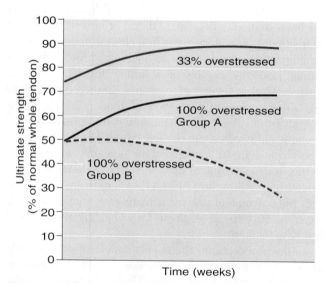

Figure 6.14: Effect of stress enhancement on tensile strength. This graph demonstrates the effect of stress enhancement on the ultimate tensile strength of rabbit patellar tendons. (Data from Hayashi K: Biomechanical studies of the remodeling of knee joint tendons and ligaments. J Biomech 1996; 29: 707–716.)

strength of experimental (tendons reduced in cross-sectional area) and control (normal) tendons. Interestingly, the cross-sectional area of these stress-enhanced tendons increases back to normal over 6 to 12 weeks. However, when stress is elevated 100%, although all tendons gradually increase in cross-sectional area, not all tendons respond in the same way to biomechanical testing. One group of stress-enhanced tendons (group A) show no change in the stress–strain behavior, no histological differences, and only a small change in tensile strength. However, another group of stress-enhanced tendons (group B) show reduced tensile strength and stiffness as well as histological changes including an increased number of fibroblasts and breakage of collagen bundles [37] (*Fig. 6.14*). These results indicate that knee joint tendons and ligaments seem to have the ability to adapt to overstressing within a certain range, (less than 100% overstress). However, they cannot adapt if stress exceeds this limit [37].

Clinical Relevance

PATELLAR TENDON GRAFTS: *The middle third of the patellar tendon is commonly used as an autogenous graft in ACL reconstruction surgery. The remaining tendon is subjected to tensile loads caused by quadriceps muscle contraction and weight bearing. Patients do not typically experience difficulty with quadriceps function as a result of the reduction of the patellar tendon; however, occasionally a patient develops patellar tendinitis. This may be related to overstress to a susceptible tendon.*

SUMMARY

Tendons and ligaments provide passive and dynamic stability to joints. They are collagenous structures with a molecular and gross structure designed to resist tensile loads. Changes in physical and biological conditions alter the biochemical composition, histological structure and organization, and biomechanical properties of the tissue. These changes can occur by physical means, such as breaking of intermolecular bonds, or by biological means. Alteration by biological means is called *remodeling*. During remodeling, various factors affect the fibroblasts within the tissue, causing a cellular response that alters the components of the extracellular matrix and the way in which it responds to loading. Factors that cause deterioration of the biomechanical properties of tendons and ligaments include immobilization, aging, healing, and stress shielding. The application of physiological loads during immobilization and healing reduces the amount of deterioration of the biomechanical properties. Normal ligaments can withstand increased stress loading within a range (about 133% of normal), after which the biomechanical properties of the overstressed ligaments deteriorate. Maintenance of

normal biomechanical functioning of tendons and ligaments is important to ensure normal joint kinematics and tolerance to loading during functional activities.

References

1. Akeson WH, Amiel D, LaViolette D: The connective tissue response to immobility: a study of the chondroitin-4 and 6-sulfate and dermatan-sulfate changes in periarticular connective tissue of control and immobilized knees of dogs. Clin Orthop 1967; 51: 183.
2. Akeson WH, Amiel D, Mechanic GL, et al.: Collagen cross-linking alterations in joint contractures: changes in the reducible cross-links in periarticular connective tissue collagen after nine weeks of immobilization. Connect Tissue Res 1977; 5: 15.
3. Almekinders LC, Vellema JH, Weinhold PS: strain patterns in the patellar tendon and the implications for patellar tendinopathy. Knee Surg Sports Traumatol Arthroscop 2002; 10:.2–5.
4. Amiel D, Akeson WH, Harwood FL, Frank CB: Stress deprivation effect on metabolic turnover of the medial collateral ligament collagen: a comparison between nine- and 12-week immobilization. Clin Orthop 1983; 172: 265–270.
5. Amiel D, Frey C, Woo SL-Y: Value of hyaluronic acid in the prevention of contracture formation. Clin Orthop 1985; 196: 306–311.
6. Amiel D, Kuiper SD, Wallace D, et al.: Age-related properties of medial collateral ligament and anterior cruciate ligament: a morphologic and collagen maturation study in the rabbit. J Gerontol 1991; 46: B159–B165.
7. Amiel D, Woo SL-Y, Harwood FL, Akeson WH: The effect of immobilization on collagen turnover in connective tissue: a biochemical-biomechanical correlation. Acta Orthop Scand 1982; 53: 325–332.
8. Arendt E, Dick R: Knee injury patterns among men and women in collegiate basketball and soccer: NCAA data and review of literature. Am J Sports Med 1995; 23: 694–701.
9. Arruda EM, Calve S, Dennis RG et al.: Regional variation of tibialis anterior tension mechanics is lost following denervation. J Appl Physiol 2001; 90:164–171.
10. Batten ML, Hansen JC, Dahners LE: Influence of dosage and timing of application of platelet-derived growth factor on early healing of the rat medial collateral ligament. J Orthop Res 1996; 14: 736–741.
11. Betsch EF, Baer E: Structure and mechanical properties of rat tail tendon. Biorheology 1980; 17: 83–94.
12. Beynnon BD, Fleming BC: Anterior cruciate ligament strain in vivo: a review of previous work. J Biomech 1998; 31: 519–525.
13. Beynnon BD, Fleming BC, Johnson RJ, et al.: Anterior cruciate ligament strain behavior during rehabilitation exercises in vivo. Am J Sports Med 1995; 23: 24–34.
14. Beynnon BD, Johnson RJ, Fleming BC, et al.: The strain behavior of the anterior cruciate ligament during squatting and active flexion-extension: a comparison of open and a closed kinetic chain exercise. Am J Sports Med 1997; 25: 223–229.
15. Binkley JM, Peat M: The effects of immobilization on the ultrastructure and mechanical properties of the medial collateral ligament of rats. Clin Orthop 1986; 203: 301–308.
16. Boorman RS, Shrive NG, Frank CB: Immobilization increases the vulnerability of rabbit medial collateral ligament autografts to creep. J Orthop Res 1998; 16: 682–689.

17. Brody LT: Mobility impairment. In: Therapeutic Exercise: Moving toward Function. Hall CM, Brody LT, eds. Philadelphia: Lippincott Williams & Wilkins, 1999; 88.

18. Buchanan CI, Marach RL: Effects of long-term exercise on the biomechanical properties of Achilles tendon of guinea fowl. J Appl Physiol 2001; 90:164–171.

19. Byum EB, Barrack RL, Alexander AH: Open versus closed chain kinetic exercises after anterior cruciate ligament reconstruction: a prospective randomized study. Am J Sports Med 1995; 23: 401–406.

20. Cabaud HE, Chatty A, Gildengorin V, Feltman RJ: Exercise effects on the strength of the rat anterior cruciate ligament. Am J Sports Med 1980; 8: 79–886.

21. Coons DA, Barber FA: Thermal medial retinaculum shrinkage and lateral release for the treatment of recurrent patellar instability. Arthroscopy: J Arthroscop Rel Surg 2006; 22: 166–171.

22. Crowninshield RD, Pope MH: The strength and failure characteristics of rat medial collateral ligaments. J Trauma 1976; 16: 99–105.

23. Cummings GS, Tillman LJ: Remodeling of dense connective tissue in normal adult tissues. In: Dynamics of Human Biologic Tissues. Currier DP, Nelson RM, eds. Philadelphia: FA Davis, 1992; 60.

24. Danto MI, Woo SL-Y: The mechanical properties of skeletally mature rabbit anterior cruciate ligament and patellar tendon over a range of strain rates. J Orthop Res 1993; 11: 58–67.

25. Demirham M, Uysal M, Kilioylu O, et al.: tensile strength of ligaments after thermal shrinkage depending on time and immobilization: in vivo study in the rabbit. J Shoulder Elbow Surg 2005; 12: 193–200.

26. Dressler MR, Butler DL, Boivin GP: Age-related changes in the biomechanics of healing patellar tendon. J Biomech 2006; 39: 2205–2213.

27. Dressler MR, Butler DL, Wenstrup R, et al.: A potential mechanism for age-related declines in patellar tendon biomechanics. J Orthop Res 2006; 20: 1315–1322.

28. Enwemeka CS: Connective tissue plasticity: ultrastructural, biomechanical and morphometric effects of physical factors on intact and regenerating tendons. J Orthop Sports Phys Ther 1991; 12: 198–212.

29. Frank C, Woo SL-Y, Amiel D: Medial collateral ligament healing: a multidisciplinary assessment in rabbits. Am J Sports Med 1983; 11: 379–389.

30. Flemming BC, Beynnon BD: In vivo measurement of ligament/tendon strains and forces: a review. Annals Biomed Eng 2004; 32: 318–328.

31. Fung YC: Biomechanics: Mechanical Properties of Living Tissues. New York: Springer-Verlag, 1981.

32. Gelberman RH: Effects of early intermittent passive mobilization on healing canine flexor tendons. J Hand Surg 1982; 7: 170–175.

33. Gelberman RH, Vande Berg JS, Lundborg GN: Flexor tendon healing and restoration of the gliding surface: an ultrastructural study in dogs. J Bone Joint Surg 1983; 65A: 70–80.

34. Gomez MA, Woo SL-Y, Amiel D, et al.: The effects of increased tension on healing medial collateral ligaments. Am J Sports Med 1991; 19: 347–354.

35. Griffin LY, Agel J, Albohm MJ, et al.: Noncontact anterior cruciate ligament injuries: risk factors and prevention strategies. J Am Acad Orthop Surg 2000; 8: 141–150.

36. Haraldsson BT, Aagaard P, Krogsgaard M et al.: Region-specific mechanical properties of the human patellar tendon. J Appl Physiol 2005; 98: 1006–1012.

37. Hayashi K: Biomechanical studies of the remodeling of knee joint tendons and ligaments. J Biomech 1996; 29: 707–716.

38. Hayashi K, Thabit G, Massa KL: The effect of thermal heating on the length and histological properties of the glenohumeral joint capsule. Am J Sports Med 1997; 25: 107–112.

39. Hildebrand KA, Woo SL-Y, Smith DW: The effects of platelet-derived growth factor-BB on healing of the rabbit medial collateral ligament: an in vivo study. Am J Sports Med 1998; 26: 549–554.

40. Hitchcock T: The effect of immediate constrained digital motion on strength of flexor tendon repairs in chickens. J Hand Surg 1987; 12A: 590–595.

41. Hyer CF, VanCourt R: Arthroscopic repair of lateral ankle instability by using the thermal-assisted capsular shift procedure: a review of four cases. J Foot Ankle Surg 2004; 43: 104–109.

42. Iida T, Abumi K, Kotani Y et al.: Effects of aging and spinal degeneration on mechanical properties of lumbar supraspinous and interspinous ligaments. Spine J 2002; 2: 95–100.

43. Kannus P: Structure of the tendon connective tissue. Scand J Med Sci Sports 2000; 10: 312–320.

44. Kannus P, Jozsa L, Renstrom P, Jarvinen M: The effects of training, immobilization and remobilization on musculoskeletal tissue. I. Training and immobilization. Scand J Med Sci Sports 1992; 2: 100–118.

45. Karamanidis K, Arampatzis A: Mechanical and morphological properties of human quadriceps femoris and triceps surae muscle-tendon unit in relation to aging and running. J Biomech 2006; 39: 406–417.

46. Kobayashi D, Kurosaka M, Yoshiya S, Mizuno K: Effect of basic fibroblast growth factor on the healing of defects in the canine anterior cruciate ligament. Knee Surg Sports Traumatol Arthrosc 1997; 5: 189–194.

47. Kubo K, Akima H, Ushiyama J, et al.: Effects of 20 days of bedrest on the viscoelastic properties of tendon structures in lower limb muscles. Br J Sports Med 2004; 38: 324–330.

48. Kubo K, Kanehisa H, Fukunaga T: Effects of cold and hot water immersion on the mechanical properties of human muscle and tendon in vivo. Clin Biomech 2005; 20: 291–300.

49. Kubo K, Kanehisa M, Miyatani M, et al.: Effect of low load resistance training on the tendon properties of middle aged and elderly women. Acta Physiol Scand 2003; 178: 25–32.

50. Lee J, Chamberlin TA, Schreck PJ, Amiel D: In situ localization of growth factors during the early healing of knee ligaments: Trans Orthop Res Soc 1995; 20: 158.

51. Lehman JF, Masock AJ, Warren CG: Effect of therapeutic temperatures on tendon extensibility. Arch Phys Med Rehabil 1970; 50: 481–487.

52. Lerat JL, Moyen BJ, Mandrino A, et al.: A prospective study of the outcome of anterior laxity of the knee after anterior cruciate ligament reconstruction with procedures using two different patellar tendon grafting methods. Rev Chir Orthop 1997; 83: 217–228.

53. Letson AK, Dahners LE: The effect of combinations of growth factors on ligament healing. Clin Orthop 1994; 308: 207–212.

54. Liu SH, al-Shaikh RA, Panossian V, et al.: Estrogen affects the cellular metabolism of the anterior cruciate ligament: a potential explanation for female athletic injury. Am J Sports Med 1997; 25: 704–709.

55. Lopez MJ, Hayaski K, Vanderby R, el al.: Effects of monopolar radiofrequency energy on ovine joint capsular mechanical properties. Clin Orthop Rel Res 2000; 374:286–297.

56. Maganaris CN, Reeves ND, Rittwegner J, et. al.: Adaptive response of human tendon to paralysis. Muscle Nerve 2006; 33:85–92.

57. Maganaris CN: Tensile properties of in vivo human tendinous tissue. J Biomech 2002; 35:1019–1027.

58. Moore MJ, Crisco DC, Fadale JJ, et al.: Knee laxity does not vary with menstrual cycle, before or after exercise. Am J Sports Med 2004; 32:1150–1157.

59. Narici MV, Maganaris CN, Reeves ND: Myotendinous alterations and effects of resistive loading in old age. Scand J Med Sci Sports 2005; 12:392–401.

60. Neuman P, Ekstrom LA, Keller B, et al.: Aging, vertebral density, and disc degeneration alter the tensile stress-strain characteristics of human anterior longitudinal ligament. J Orthop Res 1994; 12: 103–112.

61. Newton PO, Woo SL-Y, MacKenna DA, Akeson WH: Immobilization of the knee joint alters the mechanical and ultrastructural properties of the rabbit anterior cruciate ligament. J Orthop Res 1995; 13: 191–200.

62. Ng BH, Chou SM, Lim BH, et al.: Strain rate effect on failure properties of tendons. Proc Inst Mech Eng 2004; 218:203–206.

63. Ng GY, Oakes BW, Deacon OW, et al.: Biomechanics of patellar tendon autograft for reconstruction of the anterior cruciate ligament in the goat: three-year study. J Orthop Res 1995; 13: 602–608.

64. Nimni ME: Collagen: structure, function, and metabolism in normal and fibrotic tissues. Semin Arthritis Rheum 1983; 13: 1–83.

65. Nordschow CD: Aspects of aging in human collagen: an exploratory thermoelastic study. Exp Molec Pathol 1966; 5: 350–373.

66. Norkin CC, Levangie PK: Joint Structure and Function: A Comprehensive Analysis, 2nd ed. Philadelphia: FA Davis, 1992; 75–76.

67. Noyes FR: Functional properties of knee ligaments and alterations induced by immobilization: a correlative biomechanical and histological study in primates. Clin Orthop 1977; 123: 210–242.

68. Noyes FR, DeLucas JL, Torvik PJ: Biomechanics of anterior cruciate ligament failure: an analysis of strain-rate sensitivity and mechanisms of failure in primates. J Bone Joint Surg 1974; 56A: 236–241.

69. Noyes FR, Grood ES: The strength of the anterior cruciate ligament in humans and rhesus monkeys. J Bone Joint Surg 1976; 58A: 1074–1082.

70. Peterson RH, Gomez MA, Woo SL-Y: The effects of strain rate on the biomechanical properties of the medial collateral ligament: a study of immature and mature rabbits. Trans Orthop Res Soc 1987; 12: 127.

71. Pullin J, Collier M, Johnson L: Holmium:YAG laser-assisted capsular shift in a canine model: intraarticular pressure and histological observations. J Shoulder Elbow Surg 1997; 6: 272–285.

72. Reeves ND, Maganaris CN, Ferretti G et al.: Influence of 90-day simulated microgravity on human tendon mechanical properties and the effect of resistive countermeasures. J Appl Physiol 2005; 98:2278–2286.

73. Reeves ND, Maganaris CN, Narici MV: Effect of strength training on human patellar tendon mechanical properties of older individuals. J Physiol (Lond) 2003; 548:971–981.

74. Reeves ND, Narici MV, Maganaris CN: Strength training alters the visoelastic properties of tendons in elderly humans. Muscle Nerve 2003; 28: 74-81.

75. Rigby BJ: The effect of mechanical extension upon the thermal stability of collagen. Biochim Biophys Acta 1964; 79: 634–636.

76. Rigby BJ, Hirai N, Spikes JD: The mechanical behavior of rat tail tendon. J Gen Physiol 1959; 43: 265–283.

77. Sciore P, Frank CB, Hart DA: Identification of sex hormone receptors in human and rabbit ligaments of the knee by reverse transcription-polymerase chain reaction: evidence that receptors are present in tissue from both male and female subjects. J Orthop Res 1998; 16: 604–610.

78. Screen HR, Lee DA, Bader DL, et al.: An investigation into the effects of the hierarchical structure of tendon fascicles on micromechanical properties. Proc Inst Mech Eng (H) 2004; 218: 109–119.

79. Screen HR, Shelton JC, Bader DL, et al.: Cyclic tensile strain upregulates collagen synthesis in isolated tendon fascicles. Biochem Biophys Res Comm 2005; 21: 424–429.

80. Selecky MT, Vangsness T, Lias WL: The effects of laser induced collagen shortening on the biomechanical properties of the inferior glenohumeral ligament complex. Am J Sports Med 1999; 27: 168–172.

81. Slauterbeck J, Clevenger C, Lundberg W, Burchfield DM: Estrogen level alters the failure load of the rabbit anterior cruciate ligament. J Orthop Res 1999; 17: 405–408.

82. Strocchi R, DePasquale V, Facchini A, et al.: Age-related changes in human anterior cruciate ligament collagen fibrils. Ital J Anat Embryol 1996; 101: 213–220.

83. Tibone JE, McMahon PJ, Shrader TA. Glenohumeral joint translation after arthroscopic nonablative thermal capsuloplasty with a laser. Am J Sports Med 1998; 26: 495–598.

84. Tillman LJ, Cummings GS: Biologic mechanisms of connective tissue mutability. In: Dynamics of Human Biologic Tissues. Currier DP, Nelson RM, eds. Philadelphia: FA Davis, 1992; 17–22.

85. Tipton CM, Vailas AC, Matthes RD: Experimental studies on the influences of physical activity on ligaments, tendons and joints: a brief review. Acta Med Scand Suppl 1986; 711: 157–168.

86. Van Brocklin JD, Ellis DG: A study of the mechanical behavior of toe extensor tendons under applied stress. Arch Phys Med Rehabil 1965; 46: 369–370.

87. Viidik A: Elasticity and tensile strength of the anterior cruciate ligament in rabbits and influenced by training. Acta Physiol Scand 1968; 74: 372–380.

88. Viidik A: Interdependence between structure and function in collagenous tissue. In: Biology of Collagen. Viidik A, Vuust J, eds. London: Academic Press, 1980; 257–280.

89. Wang CW, Weiss JA, Albright JP, et al.: The effects of long term exercise on the structural and mechanical properties of the canine medial collateral ligament. In: 1989 Biomechanics Symposium. Torzilli PA, Friedman MH, eds. New York: ASME, 1989; 69–72.

90. Warden SJ, Saxon LK, Castillo AB, et al.: knee ligament mechanical properties are not influenced by estrogen or its receptors. Am J Physiol Endocrimol Metab 2006; 290: E1034–E1040.

91. Warren CG, Lehman JF, Koblanski JN: Elongation of rat tail tendon: effect of load and temperature. Arch Phys Med Rehabil 1971; 52: 465–484.

92. Woo SL-Y, Debski RE, Withrow JD, Janaushek MA: Biomechanics of knee ligaments. Am J Sports Med 1999; 27: 533–542.

93. Woo SL-Y, Gomez MA, Sites TJ, et al.: The biomechanical and morphological changes in the medial collateral ligament of the rabbit after immobilization and remobilization. J Bone Joint Surg 1987; 69A: 1200–1211.

94. Woo SL-Y, Hildebrand K, Watanabe N, et al.: Tissue engineering of ligament and tendon healing. Clin Orthop 1999; 367S: S312–S323.

98. Woo SL-Y, Hollis JM, Adams DJ, et al.: Tensile properties of the human femur-anterior cruciate ligament-tibia complex: the effects of specimen age and orientation. Am J Sports Med 1991; 19: 217–225.

96. Woo SL-Y, Ohland KJ, Weiss JA: Aging and sex-related changes in the biomechanical properties of the rabbit medial collateral ligament. Mech Ageing Dev 1990; 56: 129–142.

97. Woo SL-Y, Orlando CA, Gomez MA, Frank CB: Tensile properties of the medial collateral ligament as a function of age. J Orthop Res 1986; 4: 133–141.

98. Woo SL-Y, Peterson RH, Ohland KJ, et al.: The effects of strain rate on the properties of the medial collateral ligament in skeletally immature and mature rabbits: a biomechanical and histological study. J Orthop Res 1990; 8: 712–721.

99. Woo SL-Y, Suh JK, Parson IM, et al.: Biological intervention in ligament healing effect of growth factors. Sports Med Arthrosc Rev 1998; 6: 74–82.

100. Yannas IV, Huang C: Fracture of tendon collagen. J Polymer Sci 1972; 10: 577–584.

Biomechanics of Joints

MARGERY A. LOCKARD, P.T., PH.D.
CAROL A. OATIS, P.T., PH.D.

Joints, the sites of motion between articulating bones, are joined to one another by various connective tissue structures that must maintain the integrity of the junction while allowing motion between the bones. Thus, the architectural challenge of joints is to create a balance between mobility and stability. The amount of mobility or stability varies widely throughout the joints of the body. For example, the primary function of the joints within the skull is to provide stability between articulating bones. Other joints, such as the glenohumeral joint of the shoulder, allow remarkable mobility between the adjacent bones and exhibit much less stability. Most movable joints must demonstrate a combination of stability and mobility, producing stable motion capable of supporting functional use of the body part in which the joint is located. Thus, the structure of joints must be able to support a wide range of functions from extreme stability, permitting almost no movement at all, to maximum mobility.

The body exhibits a wide variety of joint designs and structures. Despite the variations in structure from joint to joint, the connective tissues discussed in the preceding chapters—bone, cartilage, and dense, fibrous connective tissues—are used in each joint design. Thus, the reader is encouraged to review the biomechanical properties of each connective tissue type to understand how each joint component contributes to the overall function of the joint.

The specific goals of this chapter are to

- Describe the design and general structure of human joints
- Discuss the factors that influence the stability and mobility of the joint
- Classify joints anatomically and biomechanically
- Define the terminology used to describe joint motion biomechanically
- Discuss the production and control of joint motion

CLASSIFICATION AND STRUCTURE OF HUMAN JOINTS

The broadest level of classification divides joints into two groups on the basis of the amount of motion available at the joint. **Diarthroses** permit free bone movement, while **synarthroses** permit very limited or no movement at all. Synarthroses are subclassified as **synostoses, synchondroses,** and **syndesmoses.**

In a **synostosis,** bone is connected to bone by bone. No movement takes place. In elderly persons, the sutures of the skull are synostoses. In synchondroses and syndesmoses, bone is connected to bone by cartilage or fibrous connective tissue, respectively. The connective tissue connection between adjacent bones is solid, allowing only a slight-to-moderate amount of motion. A **synchondrosis** contains either hyaline cartilage or fibrocartilage. The attachments of the ribs to the sternum are synchondroses formed by hyaline cartilage. They furnish a great deal of stability, which is necessary for the rib cage to protect the vital organs within the chest. However, they also permit the mobility needed to allow the chest wall to expand and relax during ventilation.

The symphysis pubis is a synchondrosis composed of fibrocartilage. This joint transmits forces between the weight-bearing lower extremities and the pelvis. It must withstand high loads and thus must be very stable, permitting little movement. However, during pregnancy, hormones soften the fibrocartilage in the symphysis to permit movement necessary for the baby to pass through the birth canal. Typically, cartilaginous joints allow more motion than fibrous joints.

In a **syndesmosis,** or fibrous joint, adjacent bones are connected by a fibrous connective tissue membrane that allows some movement but is primarily designed for stability. The distal tibiofibular articulation is a syndesmosis in which the shafts of the tibia and fibula are connected and stabilized by the syndesmotic membrane. Additionally, early in life the sutures of the skull are connected in synarthroses by fibrous membranes. Although inherently stable, these fibrous connections allow some movement to occur. This is necessary to allow molding of the infant's head during passage through the birth canal and to allow for growth.

Diarthroses

Diarthroses, or **synovial joints,** are joints that are free to move because there is a space between the ends of the bones that meet in the joint. The ends of long bones are usually united in this type of articulation. The ends of the adjacent long bones are connected by a fibrous joint capsule that encloses a sealed cavity called the **articular cavity** (see Fig. 5.1). A **synovial membrane** lines the capsule and produces **synovial fluid** that is contained within the cavity. The ends of the bones within the articular cavity are covered with a smooth layer of **articular cartilage,** which is usually hyaline cartilage. Articular cartilage has no perichondrium. The smooth articular surfaces, coupled with the lubricating

properties of the synovial fluid, facilitate low-friction movement within these joints.

In addition to the common components of diarthroses or synovial joints, some may contain additional structures that protect the joint and guide movement. For example, synovial joints may contain fibrocartilaginous menisci, or discs, or fat pads to increase the protection of the bony surfaces from compressive loads. Fibrocartilage labra and menisci deepen concave joint surfaces, thus improving joint congruency and stability. Joints are protected from tensile loads, or forces that tend to pull the surfaces apart, by both ligaments and tendons as well as by the contraction of muscles whose tendons cross the joint.

JOINT CAPSULE AND SYNOVIAL MEMBRANE

Joint capsules have an external **fibrous layer** and an inner **synovial layer.** The fibrous layer, composed of dense fibrous connective tissue, attaches to the periosteum, which in turn attaches to the subjacent bone via Sharpey's fibers, fibers which originate in the periosteum and perforate into the underlying bone [4,23].

Although the fibrous layer of the joint capsule has a meager blood supply, it is richly innervated. Capsules typically receive innervation from articular nerves that are branches of adjacent peripheral nerves and from branches of nerves that supply muscles controlling the joint. Several nerves usually supply joint capsules, and their distributions tend to overlap. Joint receptors, located in capsules, tendons, and ligaments, transmit information about the status of the joint to the central nervous system. This afferent information is used by the central nervous system to coordinate muscle activity around the joint to maintain appropriate balance between joint mobility and stability [12]. Joint capsules contain various types of joint receptors, which, along with receptors located in skin, other connective tissues, and muscle, contribute to static joint position sense, sense of movement, direction of movement, change in movement, and regulation of muscle tone [25,29].

Clinical Relevance

JOINT SPRAIN: *When joint capsules and ligaments are injured, as in a sprain, clinicians have observed continued reduced functional performance, even after all impairments such as swelling, pain, restricted range of motion, and decreased strength have been corrected. Further examination often reveals reduced proprioception (position sense) at the injured joint, even after healing of the original injury appears to be complete. Patients may continue to complain that the joint "feels unstable," even when results of tests for structural stability are normal. These deficits may be due to reduced or abnormal sensory input from the joint receptors that may also be injured during a sprain. As a result, clinicians may need to include balance and coordination activities on unstable surfaces, such as a rocker board, to improve the patient's functional abilities [6,7].*

Additional ligaments in areas that are subjected to great strain may also reinforce the fibrous outer layer of the joint capsule. Some of these reinforcing ligaments may be separate or discrete from the capsule itself. Others may be thickenings of the capsule substance and cannot be separated from the capsule. For example, at the knee, the lateral collateral ligament is a discrete structure separate from, and outside of, the joint capsule, which resists varus forces, or forces that adduct the tibia on the femur. The medial collateral ligament, however, is a thickening of the medial aspect of the knee joint capsule and cannot be separated from the capsule. It restrains valgus forces, or forces that abduct the tibia on the femur.

The tendons of muscles that cross a joint may insert into bone outside the joint capsule, such as the semitendinosus tendon on the medial aspect of the knee. In this case the tendon helps to reinforce the capsule and protect it from tensile stresses. Tendons, however, may also attach to bone within the joint capsule. In this case, the tendon must pierce the joint capsule, such as the attachment of the long head of the biceps brachii at the shoulder.

The inner layer of the joint capsule, lining the joint cavity, is the **synovial layer.** This layer is more cellular than the fibrous layer. Cells on its surface synthesize hyaluronic acid and proteins that are secreted into the synovial fluid. These components of synovial fluid are essential for reducing friction and providing joint lubrication. The structure of the synovial membrane is variable. In some joints, it simply lines the fibrous capsule. Other joints have folds that project quite far into the joint cavity. Folds of the synovial membrane may be transient formations, depending on the position of the joint, or they may be permanent villi that extend into the joint cavity. Loose or dense connective tissue and adipose tissue lie below the surface cells of the synovium. Although the synovium is poorly innervated compared with the fibrous capsule, it contains numerous blood and lymphatic vessels.

Clinical Relevance

RHEUMATOID ARTHRITIS: *Rheumatoid arthritis (RA) is a disease characterized by chronic inflammatory changes in the synovial membranes of joints. As a result of chronic inflammation, the synovium becomes congested and edematous, infiltrated by leukocytes and inflammatory cells, and further thickened by the proliferation of synovial cells and hypertrophy of the synovial villi. Chronic synovitis resulting in synovial hypertrophy can contribute to stretching of the fibrous capsule of a joint, resulting in joint instability and, ultimately, the joint deformities characteristic of RA.*

Synovial fluid, produced by the synovial membrane, is contained within the joint capsule. Normal synovial fluid is a clear, pale yellow, viscous fluid. Its composition is similar to that of blood plasma, with the addition of hyaluronate and other proteins that aid joint lubrication. Synovial fluid also plays an important role in supplying nutrition to, and removing metabolic wastes from articular cartilage and intraarticular fibrocartilage. This occurs by diffusion and imbibition between the synovial fluid and the cartilage. Intermittent compression and distraction of the joint surfaces that occur during weight bearing and active movement of the joints facilitate diffusion of nutrients and are required to maintain healthy joint function [17,18].

Clinical Relevance

EARLY REMOBILIZATION FOLLOWING JOINT INJURY: *An understanding of the mechanics and pathomechanics of joint structure and tissues supports the current practice of early mobilization following fractures and sprains. Ankle sprains are frequently treated with splints that limit motions that stress the injured ligaments, but allow other ankle motions in order to promote normal joint lubrication during the healing period. Early mobilization minimizes the deleterious effects of immobilization and facilitates return to normal function more quickly [24]. Safe early joint motion during the healing process requires clinicians to apply their knowledge of tissue and joint mechanics.*

JOINT MOTION

Classification of Motion

As described in Chapter 1, the two basic types of motion are rotation and translation. **Rotation** is motion about an axis, causing points on the rotating body to travel different distances depending upon their distance from the point of rotation (see Fig. 1.11). **Translation** produces a linear movement in which all points in the body travel the same distance regardless of their location in the body. Most cartilaginous and fibrous joints allow translation, or linear movement. Synovial joints, on the other hand, allow both rotation and translation.

PLANES AND AXES OF MOTION

Rotation about an axis produces motion in a plane that is perpendicular to that axis. Thus flexion of most joints occurs about a medial–lateral axis and takes place in the sagittal plane (*Fig. 7.1*). Similarly, abduction of most joints occurs in the frontal plane about an anterior–posterior axis. Rotation of most joints occurs in the transverse plane about a longitudinal axis.

DEGREES OF FREEDOM

Another way of describing the kind of motion available at a joint is to describe its **degrees of freedom** (DOF). A movement can be described completely by describing it with

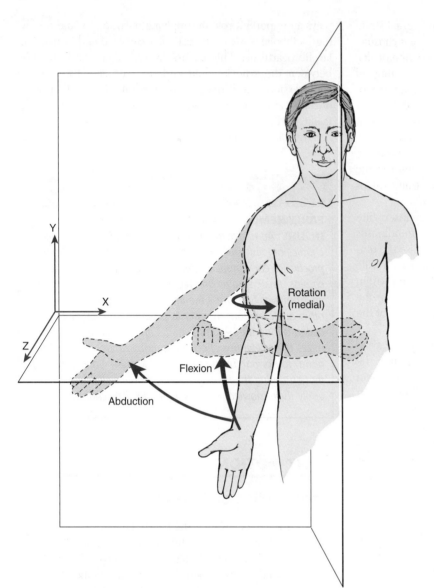

Figure 7.1: Axes of motion. Axes of motion are perpendicular to the plane in which the segment rotates. The flexion extension axis *(X)* is medial–lateral and perpendicular to the sagittal plane, the plane of flexion and extension. The abduction–adduction axis *(Z)* is anterior–posterior and perpendicular to the frontal plane, the plane of abduction and adduction. The rotation axis *(Y)* is usually a long axis through the length of the bone and perpendicular to the transverse plane, the plane of medial and lateral rotation.

respect to a coordinate system. Movement in a two-dimensional space can be described as some combination of translation along the x and y axes and a rotation about the z axis (*Fig. 7.2*). Thus movement in two-dimensional space is said to have three DOF. In contrast, a body in three-dimensional space can translate along all three axes, x, y, and z and also can rotate about the three axes. Thus a body moving in three-dimensional space can have up to six DOF [5].

COMBINING TRANSLATION AND ROTATION IN A SYNOVIAL JOINT

Although most of the movements that occur at synovial joints are rotations, they also allow translation. This translation is often subtle but essential to the normal motion of the joint. To understand the combinations of motions that occur in most synovial joints, it is necessary to understand how an object that typically rotates may undergo simultaneous

translation. An object that demonstrates pure rotation with no translation has a fixed axis, and the resulting movement is described as **spin** (*Fig. 7.3*). An automobile tire that lacks traction on ice spins with its axle fixed in space. As the tire spins, all points on the tire eventually come in contact with a single point on the pavement. In contrast, normal progression of a car on the road results when the tires **roll** on the surface of the road. Rolling motion causes each point on the tire surface to contact a unique location on the road. Finally, pure translation of the articulating surfaces is often referred to as **glide,** analogous to a car in a skid, when a single point on the tire glides over several points on the road [19].

Many synovial joints exhibit a combination of rotation and translation during normal motion. When knee flexion is viewed from the tibia, the femur rolls posteriorly (*Fig. 7.4*). During knee extension, the femur rolls anteriorly. Early two-dimensional research suggested that during knee flexion, the

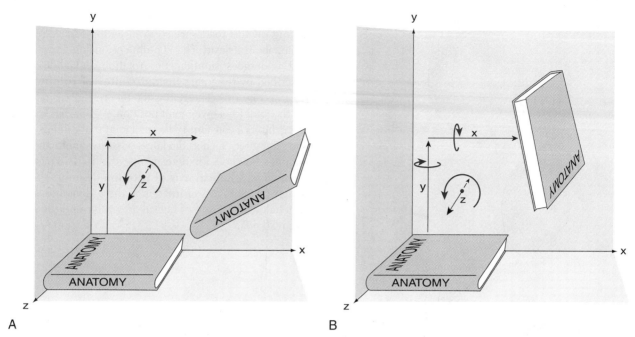

Figure 7.2: Degrees of freedom (DOF). **A.** An object moving in two-dimensional space has up to three DOF, translation along the *x* and *y* axes and rotation in the plane of the two axes about the *z* axis. **B.** An object moving in three-dimensional space has up to six DOF, translation about the *x, y,* and *z* axes, and rotation about the three axes.

femur also translated anteriorly, giving rise to the so-called **concave–convex rule,** which suggested that the direction of the intraarticular glide accompanying rotation could be predicted by the shape of the moving articular surface. This rule was used by clinicians to help determine the particular joint glide that was needed to restore a specific limited joint movement. More recent three-dimensional studies, however, show that during knee flexion slight femoral translation may occur in both anterior and posterior directions within the same flexion movement (Fig 7.4). Other biomechanical analyses demonstrate that many other synovial joints with convex and concave articular surfaces also do not behave according to the concave–convex rule. For example, studies of the glenohumeral joint demonstrate that there is slight superior glide of the humeral head as it rolls superiorly during shoulder flexion and abduction [10,26]. The humeral head also glides posteriorly during lateral rotation and anteriorly during medial rotation [10,20,26]. These studies show that the convex humeral head rolls and glides in the same direction during shoulder motion, contradicting the concave–convex rule.

The metacarpal joints, also composed of concave and convex surfaces, have fixed axes of motion during flexion and extension, with no appreciable glide [9,30]. Motion at these joints is essentially pure rotation. Thus, it appears that the concave–convex rule is neither correct nor clinically useful. However, current understanding of joint motion continues to indicate a need to restore joint glides as well as rotations when attempting to improve joint mobility.

Synovial joints move by combining rotation and translation or by pure rotation. The rotational movement of one

bone on another is described as the **osteokinematics** of the joint. The gliding motions of the joint surfaces that may accompany the joint rotations are described as the **arthrokinematics** of the joint [19,28]. These joint glides are usually much smaller, more-subtle movements than the accompanying rotations and are known as **component** or **accessory motions** of a joint. Although small, component motions are essential to the normal mechanics of the joint. Inadequate glide may inhibit the restoration of normal motion, while excessive glide may contribute to damage of the soft tissues surrounding a joint.

Clinical Relevance

JOINT MOBILIZATION: *Joint mobilization is a manual therapy technique used to restore the joint glides necessary for normal joint range of motion (ROM). The specific mobilizations used at a joint usually are based on the normal arthrokinematics of that joint. For example, to increase knee flexion and extension ROM, a clinician may work to restore normal anterior and posterior glides of the tibia on the femur while also stretching the surrounding soft tissues into flexion and extension.*

INSTANT CENTER OF ROTATION

Joints that exhibit pure rotation move about a fixed axis. Joints that rotate while simultaneously gliding, are rotating

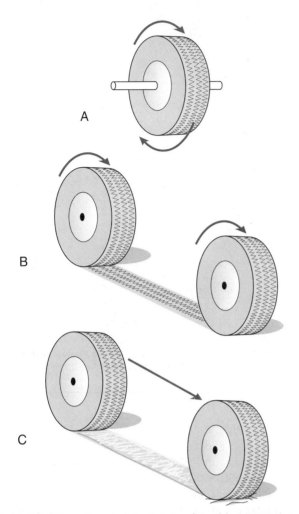

Figure 7.3: Spin, roll, and glide. **A.** Spin of an object is rotation about a fixed axis so that all of the points on the spinning object contact a single point on the stationary surface. **B.** Roll of an object is rotation about a moving axis so that all of the points on the spinning object contact unique points on the stationary surface. **C.** Glide of an object is translation without any rotation, a single point on the gliding object contacting several points on the stationary surface.

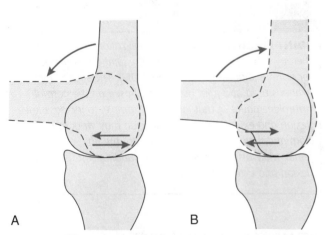

Figure 7.4: Roll and glide of the knee. In flexion (**A**) the femur rolls posteriorly. In extension (**B**) the femur rolls anteriorly. In both, the femur may glide both anteriorly and posteriorly.

about an axis that moves in space, just as the car that skids is gliding on the road surface even as the tire continues to rotate about its axle. The two-dimensional motion of a joint that undergoes simultaneous rotation and glide is often described by the joint's **instant center of rotation** (ICR) [21,27] (*Fig. 7.5*). The ICR is the theoretical axis of rotation for the joint for a given joint position. A joint that has a fixed axis exhibits a constant ICR, but a joint that exhibits rotation and joint glide, such as the knee, possesses multiple ICRs. A common method for determining the ICR is pictured in *Figure 7.6*. A **helical axis of rotation** describes the movement of a joint's axis of rotation in three-dimensional space. A detailed discussion of helical axes is beyond the scope of this textbook.

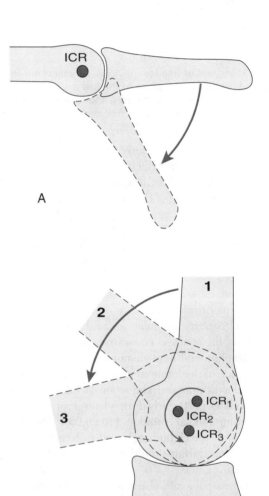

Figure 7.5: Instant center of rotation (ICR). The ICR is the theoretical axis of rotation at a specific joint position. It is constant in pure rotation (**A**) but is variable in motions that combine rotation and glide (**B**).

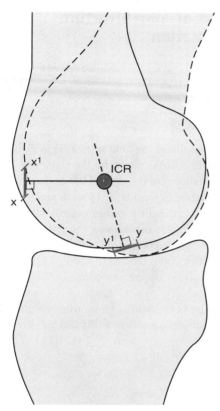

Figure 7.6: Method to determine the instant center of rotation. A common method to determine the ICR is to locate two points on the moving segment and draw a line connecting two locations of each point. The intersection of lines drawn perpendicular to the first lines identifies the ICR. By repeating this procedure at several consecutive joint positions, the ICR is identified through the range of motion.

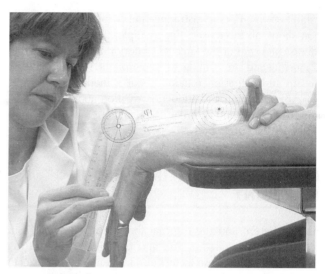

Figure 7.7: A single-axis goniometer to measure joint motion. The single-axis goniometer measures the angular position of a joint.

Clinical Relevance

GONIOMETRY: *Assessment of ROM is a common clinical approach to identify joint impairment. A single-axis goniometer allows determination of the angular position of one limb segment with respect to another when the device is aligned appropriately at the joint (Fig. 7.7). An understanding of a joint's motion helps the clinician align the goniometer correctly to obtain an accurate measure of the joint's ROM.*

Classification of Synovial Joints

Most joints in the body are freely moving diarthrodial, or synovial joints. While sharing several structural characteristics, they also demonstrate considerable variation in structure that produces a broad spectrum of functional capabilities. Synovial joints are classified anatomically by their surface shapes and kinds of motion or biomechanically by the number of axes of motion they possess [23,28] (*Table 7.1*). For example, a hinge joint is also called a *uniaxial joint* because motion occurs about a single axis. The superior radioulnar joint and the distal interphalangeal joints of the fingers are classified as uniaxial joints, although they can also be classified separately as pivot and hinge joints, respectively. From a rehabilitation standpoint, the mechanical classification based on axes of motion is helpful because it identifies the kind of motion that is normally available at a given joint.

Classification of synovial joints by the number of axes of rotation implies that these joints allow only rotational movement. However, many synovial joints demonstrate both translation and rotation during normal movement [28]. A uniaxial joint that allows pure rotation has a single DOF. Most synovial joints possess at least three DOF. Joints such as the knee

TABLE 7.1: Classification of Synovial Joints

Anatomical Classification	Mechanical Classification	Example
Hinge (ginglymus)	Uniaxial	Distal interphalangeal joint
Pivot (trochoid)	Uniaxial	Superior radioulnar joint
Condyloid	Biaxial	Metacarpophalangeal joint of the fingers
Ellipsoid	Biaxial	Wrist (radiocarpal) joint
Saddle	Triaxial	Carpometacarpal joint of the thumb
Ball-and-socket	Triaxial	Glenohumeral joint
Gliding (plane or sliding)	No rotation is available	Midtarsal joint of the foot

exhibit six DOF, demonstrating translation along, and rotation about, all three axes. For example, the following movements can occur at the knee: (1) anterior and posterior glide, (2) medial and lateral glide, (3) superior and inferior glide, (4) flexion and extension rotation about a medial-lateral (ML) axis, (5) abduction and adduction rotation about an AP axis, and (6) internal and external rotation about a vertical (longitudinal) axis.

FACTORS INFLUENCING MOTION AT A JOINT

Joint structure and the external forces applied to the joint together determine the type and quantity of motion that occurs at a joint. These factors also influence the nature and amount of internal forces required of the joint's muscles and ligaments to control the joint effectively (*Fig. 7.8*). The interaction between a joint and its adjacent joints and the external environment also affects the joint's motion.

The Effect of Joint Structure on Joint Motion

The structure of a joint is described by its articular surfaces and ligamentous supporting structures. Each has a significant effect on the motion available at a joint.

JOINT SURFACES

Both the amount and the kind of motion available at a joint are dictated to a large extent by the shapes of its articular surfaces. The shapes of the ends of bones that meet at a joint are quite variable. For example, in some joints, the shapes of the adjacent surfaces fit together congruently like adjacent puzzle pieces, while in other joints, the surfaces that meet are quite dissimilar, or **incongruent** (*Fig. 7.9*). Joints with more-congruent articulations tend to restrain motion and are more stable, while those having less-congruent surfaces typically allow more mobility.

The amount of curvature of the surfaces of the articulating surfaces also affects a joint's mobility and stability. The **radius**

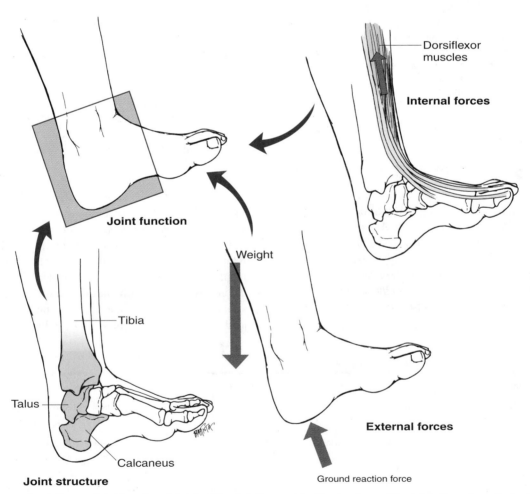

Figure 7.8: Factors that influence joint function. Joint function is influenced by the structure of the joint, the externally applied forces such as limb weight and external loads, and the internal forces applied by the muscles and ligaments of the joint.

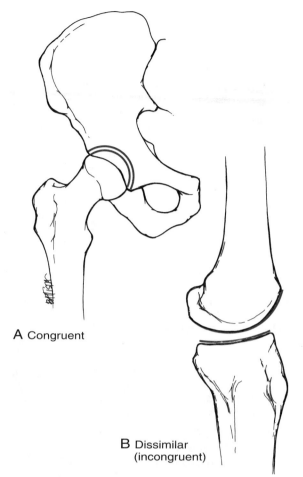

A Congruent

B Dissimilar
(incongruent)

Figure 7.9: Congruent and incongruent joint surfaces. **A.** Some joint surfaces consist of similarly shaped surfaces such as the hip joint and are described as congruent. **B.** Others consist of dissimilar surfaces (incongruent) such as the knee.

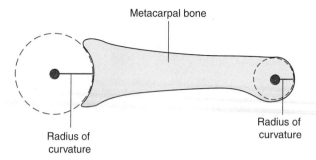

Metacarpal bone

Radius of
curvature

Radius of
curvature

Figure 7.10: Radius of curvature. The radius of curvature describes the amount of curvature of a joint surface. It is the length of the radius of a circle of the same curvature.

of curvature describes the curvature of an articular surface. The radius of curvature of an articular surface equals the radius of a circle that possesses the same curved surface as the articular surface (*Fig. 7.10*). The more curved the surface, the smaller the radius of curvature. Articulating surfaces that possess similar radii of curvatures are **congruent.** The amount of curvature of the articulating surfaces and their congruence affect the combination of translation and rotation that occurs at the joint.

Clinical Relevance

THE KNEE JOINT: *The knee includes four articulating surfaces between the femur and the tibia, each with a different radius of curvature. These differences help produce the combination of rotation and translation that accompanies knee flexion and extension. Clinicians need a clear understanding of these complex motions to restore normal joint motion.*

Joints with relatively flat surfaces allow translation, while the more-curved surfaces allow rotation. Curved surfaces vary in their shapes, defining still further the kinds of motions that occur at the joint. For example, the pulley-shaped, or trochlear, surfaces found at the articulation between the ulna and the humerus or between the middle and distal phalanges of the fingers constrain the available motion to rotation about a single axis, much like a train rolling along a track. Other articular surfaces exhibit shapes that appear to be parts of spheres, with surfaces that are either concave in two directions (typically anterior–posterior and medial–lateral) or convex in two directions. These surfaces are called **biconcave** and **biconvex,** respectively. Articulations between biconvex and biconcave surfaces allow freer motion, with rotations about two or three axes, compared with the trochlear surfaces. An example of a joint with these types of articular surfaces is the radiocarpal joint. In this articulation, the carpus is the biconvex surface, which articulates with the biconcave distal end of the radius.

Even joints composed of convex on concave surfaces with similar curvatures exhibit a wide spectrum of motions. Both the glenohumeral and hip joints consist of convex bony surfaces fitting onto concave surfaces with articular surfaces that are relatively congruent. Yet these two joints allow very different amounts of mobility. The glenoid fossa covers less than half of the articular surface of the humeral head [13,15], but approximately three quarters of the femoral head is covered by the acetabulum at the hip [11,14]. As a result the glenohumeral joint is more mobile than the hip, and the hip is more stable than the glenohumeral joint. These two joints demonstrate how the shapes of the articular surfaces influence both the mobility and stability of a joint.

LIGAMENTOUS SUPPORT

The ligamentous support of a joint also influences its mobility and stability. Ligaments exhibit unique designs to provide stabilization without limiting too much motion. Many synovial joint capsules have folds that unfold as the capsule is stretched to allow more joint movement. For example, the inferior portion of the glenohumeral joint capsule lies in folds when the shoulder is in the neutral position (next to the body), but unfolds during shoulder flexion and abduction. This allows considerable mobility, although the consequence is that the inferior joint capsule adds little to the stability of the glenohumeral joint.

Clinical Relevance

GLENOHUMERAL JOINT STABILITY: *Inferior subluxations of the glenohumeral joint appear most frequently in individuals with severe muscle weakness and are observed with the shoulder in neutral. Muscles contribute important stabilizing forces because the folded inferior glenohumeral joint capsule is unable to stabilize the joint.*

Another common design characteristic in ligaments is seen in collateral ligaments that are found on the medial and lateral sides of most hinge and biaxial joints. Collateral ligaments provide stability, preventing or limiting side-to-side movement. Many collateral ligaments radiate from a small, rather localized proximal attachment to a broader, more extensive distal attachment (*Fig. 7.11*). This arrangement allows some part of the ligament to remain taut throughout the ROM of the joint, providing a side-to-side stabilizing force in any joint position. The medial collateral ligaments of the elbow and knee are large triangular ligaments that maintain some stabilizing ability regardless of where in flexion or extension the joints lie [3,8,16,22].

External Forces on a Joint

Chapter 1 describes the interaction between forces applied to a joint from the environment and the internal forces produced by the muscles and ligaments of a joint. The weight of the limb and the forces of additional loads, such as the manual resistance applied by a therapist or the resistance from a weight-training machine, all apply moments or torques to the joint, producing rotation at the joint. These are counteracted by the moments, or torques produced by the muscles and ligaments (*Fig. 7.12*). If the external forces and moments balance the internal forces and moments, static equilibrium exists, and the joint remains at rest or in uniform motion. Identification and characterization of the external forces applied to a joint during activity helps clinicians determine which muscles and ligaments are needed to move or stabilize the joint.

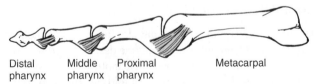

Figure 7.11: Typical collateral ligaments. Typical collateral ligaments attach to a small location proximal to the joint and radiate distally to a broader attachment across the joint.

Distal
pharynx

Middle
pharynx

Proximal
pharynx

Metacarpal

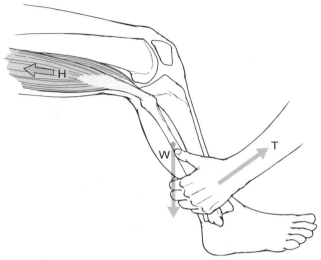

Figure 7.12: The external and internal moments on a joint. A joint is controlled by the externally applied loads including the weight (*W*) of the limb and any additional force such as the manual resistance (*T*) from a therapist and by the internally applied loads (*H*) of the muscles and ligaments.

Clinical Relevance

MUSCLES USED TO DESCEND AND ASCEND STAIRS: *An individual who is descending a step gradually moves from hip and knee extension to hip and knee flexion as the opposite foot is lowered onto the step below (Fig. 7.13). Does the individual need hip and knee flexor or extensor muscles to lower the body onto the step? To answer this question, the clinician must recognize that the weight of the head, arms, trunk, and opposite lower extremity produces a flexion moment on the weight-bearing hip and knee joints (Fig. 7.14). Consequently, the individual must use hip and knee extensor muscles to lower the body and control the hip and knee flexion produced by body weight. When climbing the stair, the individual also uses the hip and knee extensor muscles to lift the body onto the next step. In this case, the hip and knee joints are extending, but the body weight continues to produce a flexion moment at each joint. The hip and knee extensor muscles must produce torques that exceed the flexion torque produced by body weight. In both ascending and descending a step, the extensor muscles of the weight-bearing leg are used. The difference is in the type of contraction produced by the extensor muscles in each case. When descending the step, the extensor muscles contract eccentrically. While ascending stairs, the extensor muscles contract concentrically. In both cases, identification of the external loads and their effect on joint movement allows the practitioner to determine what muscles must contract and the kind of contraction needed.*

Many joints in the body sustain very large joint reaction forces during normal daily activities. The surface area over

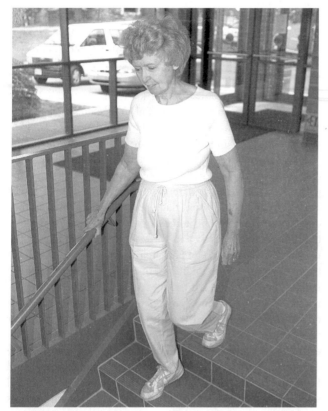

Figure 7.13: Stair descent. As an individual descends a step, the weight-bearing hip and knee move from a position of extension to a position of flexion.

which the joint reaction force is applied determines the stress (force/area) that a joint sustains during the activity. Changes in joint surface or alignment can alter the stresses applied to a joint. Joint reaction forces and the resulting stresses appear to play a role in the production of joint pain and degeneration [1,2]. The joint reaction forces that occur during exercise and functional activities are influenced by various factors, including joint position and the method of application of external loads. Clinicians must design exercises and functional activities that minimize joint reaction forces, to protect the joint surfaces.

Clinical Relevance

JOINT PROTECTION TECHNIQUES: *Joint protection techniques are methods of performing common daily activities in a way that minimizes joint reaction forces. These techniques are important for patients with arthritis or other conditions in which joints are at risk for degeneration. For example, joint reaction forces in the carpometacarpal (basal) joint of the thumb are extremely high during lateral pinch, commonly used to turn a key in the ignition of a car or to open a jar lid. To reduce the joint reaction forces during these activities, devices can be used so that two hands can be substituted for the lateral pinch of one hand.*

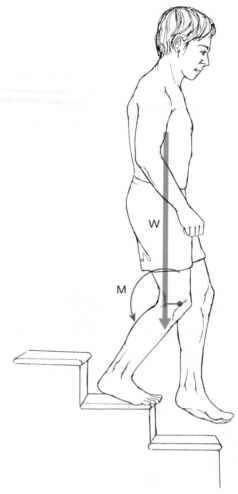

Figure 7.14: Joint moments on the knee during stair descent. In stair descent the weight (*W*) of the head, arms, trunk, and opposite lower extremity produce a flexion moment on the weight-bearing knee. The quadriceps muscle must apply an extension moment to control the descent onto the lower step.

Interactions between Joints and the External Environment

The human body consists of well over 150 joints. Movement of one joint may affect several nearby joints. This is particularly true when the moving limb is fixed to a relatively immovable object. For example, when one is standing upright with the arm at the side of the body and the hand free, elbow flexion can occur without movement in adjacent joints. In contrast, when an individual performs a push-up, elbow flexion requires simultaneous wrist and shoulder movements. In the first case, when the elbow moves in isolation, it is functioning as part of an **open chain.** Other terms used to describe the same condition include *open kinetic chain* and *open kinematic chain.* When the elbow flexes during performance of a push-up, it is functioning as part of a **closed chain** (*closed kinetic chain,* or *closed kinematic chain*). This is described as a closed chain condition since the moving joints of the upper extremity lie between the relatively immovable loads of the body and the floor. Movement at any of the joints in the closed chain will influence movement at adjacent joints. The lower extremity also functions under both open- and closed-chain conditions. For example, when kicking a ball, the end of the kicking leg is not fixed, and joint movement in the hip, knee, and ankle are independent of one another. However, in the stance leg with the foot fixed on the unmoving floor, movement at one joint influences movement at adjacent joints. For example, flexion of the stance knee requires ankle dorsiflexion and hip flexion. Joints of the upper and lower extremities can function under both open- and closed-chain conditions, and both are required during functional activities.

Clinical Relevance

LOCOMOTION: *Normal human locomotion is divided into a weight-bearing and a non-weight-bearing phase for each lower extremity. During the non-weight-bearing (swing) phase of gait, the lower extremity functions in an open chain, and the motions of the hip, knee, and foot are mechanically independent of one another. However, during the weight-bearing (stance) phase of gait, the limb functions in a closed chain. Abnormal movements at a joint, perhaps due to pain, may cause abnormal compensatory movements in adjacent joints. These abnormal compensatory movements may place excessive stress on the soft tissue limiters of the compensating joints. As a result, abnormal movements or positions at one joint in the lower extremity may cause pain or other symptoms in an adjacent but compensating joint. Accurate diagnosis of painful conditions at a weight-bearing joint requires a thorough assessment of the function of all the surrounding joints, and successful intervention at one joint often includes interventions at adjacent joints. An example is an individual with excessive pronation at the subtalar joint of the foot during running. This individual may develop knee pain due to compensatory movements at the knee. Treatment directed only at the knee will not be effective until the abnormal subtalar joint movement is addressed.*

SUMMARY

Articulating bones are attached to one another at joints. Joints are composed of a variety of connective tissue structures arranged to provide a combination of mobility and stability. The structure of some joints favors stability, while other joints favor mobility. Synarthroses permit very little movement and are designed for extreme stability. Types of synarthroses include synostoses, synchondroses, and syndesmoses. Diarthroses, or synovial joints, are moveable joints. Diarthroses are

subclassified either anatomically according to the shapes of the articular surfaces or biomechanically according to the number of axes about which movement occurs. Movement within synovial joints includes rotation and gliding or translation. Although these movements may occur in isolation, more typically they occur together during joint movement. Rotations describe the osteokinematics of joint movement, while glides, or accessory movements, describe the arthrokinematics of joint movement. The amount and nature of the movement that occurs at a synovial joint is influenced by the shapes of the articular surfaces, the connective tissue structures present at the joint (e.g., ligaments and menisci), and the external forces applied to the joint. Forces that are applied to joints and produce movement include forces from contraction of muscles that cross the joint as well as forces from body weight or the weight of other limb segments. Joint movement can occur in open- or closed-chain conditions. In open-chain conditions, the ends of the extremity (arm or leg) are free; thus the joints within the extremity can move independently of one another. In closed-chain conditions, the ends of the extremity are fixed or relatively immovable, thus, movement at one joint within the extremity will affect movement at the other joints in the extremity. A thorough understanding of joint structure and function is essential to appreciate the mechanics of normal joints and the pathomechanics of abnormal joint movements associated with painful conditions.

References

1. Ateshian GA, Ark JW, Rosenwasser MP, et al.: Contact areas in the thumb carpometacarpal joint. J Orthop Res 1995; 13: 450–458.
2. Ateshian GA, Rosenwasser MP, Mow VC: Curvature characteristics and congruence of the thumb carpometacarpal joint: differences between female and male joints. J Biomech 1992; 25: 591–607.
3. Brantigan OC, Voshell AF: The mechanics of the ligaments and menisci of the knee joint. J Bone Joint Surg 1941; 23: 44–65.
4. Cooper RR, Misra S: Tendon and ligament insertion: a light and electron microscopic study. J Bone Joint Surg 1970; 52: A1–A21.
5. Dvir Z: Clinical Biomechanics. Philadelphia: Churchill Livingstone, 2000.
6. Fitzgerald GK, Axe MJ, Snyder-Mackler L: Efficacy of perturbation training in nonoperative anterior cruciate ligament rehabilitation programs for physically active individuals. Phys Ther 2000; 80: 128–140.
7. Freeman MAR: Treatment of ruptures of the lateral ligament of the ankle. J Bone Joint Surg 1965; 47B: 661–668.
8. Fuss FK: The ulnar collateral ligament of the human elbow joint. Anatomy, function and biomechanics. J Anat 1991; 175: 203–212.
9. Hagert CG: Anatomical aspects on the design of metacarpophalangeal implants. Reconstr Surg Traumatol 1981; 18: 92–110.
10. Harryman DT II, Sidles JA, Harris SL, Matsen FA III: The role of the rotator interval capsule in passive motion and stability of the shoulder. J Bone Joint Surg [AM] 1992; 74: 53–66.
11. Harty M.: Symposium on surface replacement arthroplasty of the hip: anatomic considerations. 1982; 13, 667–679.

12. Hertling D, Kessler R: Management of Common Musculoskeletal Disorders: Physical Therapy Principles and Methods. Philadelphia: JB Lippincott, 1996.

13. Jobe CM, Iannotti JP: Limits imposed on glenohumeral motion by joint geometry. J Shoulder Elbow Surg 1995; 4: 281–285.

14. Johnston RC: Mechanical considerations of the hip joint. Arch Surg 1973; 107: 411–417.

15. Kent BE: Functional anatomy of the shoulder complex: a review. Phys Ther 1971; 51: 867–888.

16. Lloyd DG, Buchanan TS: A model of load sharing between muscles and soft tissues at the human knee during static tasks. J Biomech Eng 1996; 118: 367–376.

17. Mankin HJ: The reaction of articular cartilage to injury and osteoarthritis. N Engl J Med 1974; 291: 1285–1292.

18. Mankin HJ: The reaction of articular cartilage to injury and osteoarthritis. N Engl J Med 1974; 291: 1335–1340.

19. Neumann DA: Joint deformity and dysfunction: a basic review of underlying mechanisms. Arthritis Care Res 1999; 12: 139–151.

20. Novotny JE, Beynnon BD, Nichols CE: Modeling the stability of the human glenohumeral joint during external rotation. J Biomech 2000; 33: 345–354.

21. Panjabi MM, Goel VK, Walters SD, et al.: Errors in the center and angle of rotation of a joint; an experimental study. J Biomech Eng 1982; 104: 232–237.

22. Regan WD, Korinek SL, Morrey BF, An KN: Biomechanical study of ligaments around the elbow joint. Clin Orthop 1991; 271: 170–179.

23. Romanes GJE: Cunningham's Textbook of Anatomy. Oxford: Oxford University Press, 1981.

24. Salter RB: Textbook of Disorders and Injuries of the Musculoskeletal System, 3rd ed. Baltimore: Williams & Wilkins, 1999.

25. Skoglund S: Anatomic and physiologic studies of knee joint innervation in the cat. Acta Physiol Scand 1956; 124: 1–100.

26. Soslowsky LJ, Flatow EL, Bigliani L, et al.: Quantitation of in situ contact areas at the glenohumeral joint: a biomechanical study. J Orthop Res 1992; 10: 524–534.

27. Volz RG: Basic biomechanics: lever arm, instant center of motion, moment force, joint reactive force. Orthop Rev 1986; 15: 101–108.

28. Williams P, Bannister L, Berry M, et al.: Gray's Anatomy, The Anatomical Basis of Medicine and Surgery, Br. ed. London: Churchill Livingstone, 1995.

29. Wyke B: The neurology of joints. Ann R Coll Surg Engl 1967; 41: 25–50.

30. Youm Y: Instantaneous center of rotation by least square method. J Bioeng 1978; 2: 129–137.

Kinesiology of the Upper Extremity

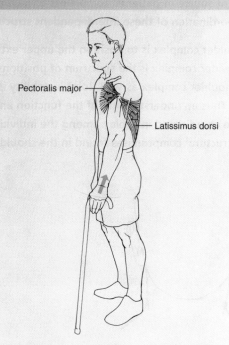

Pectoralis major

Latissimus dorsi

The shoulder complex is the functional unit that results in movement of the arm with respect to the trunk. This unit consists of the clavicle, scapula, and humerus; the articulations linking them; and the muscles that move them. These structures are so functionally interrelated to one another that studying their individual functions is almost impossible. However, a careful study of the structures that compose the shoulder unit reveals an elegantly simple system of bones, joints, and muscles that together allow the shoulder an almost infinite number of movements (Figure). An important source of patients' complaints of pain and dysfunction at the shoulder complex is an interruption of the normal coordination of these interdependent structures.

The primary function of the shoulder complex is to position the upper extremity in space to allow the hand to perform its tasks. The wonder of the shoulder complex is the spectrum of positions that it can achieve; yet this very mobility is the source of great risk to the shoulder complex as well. Joint instability is another important source of patients' complaints of shoulder dysfunction. Thus an understanding of the function and dysfunction of the shoulder complex requires an understanding of the coordinated interplay among the individual components of the shoulder complex as well as an appreciation of the structural compromises found in the shoulder that allow tremendous mobility yet provide sufficient stability.

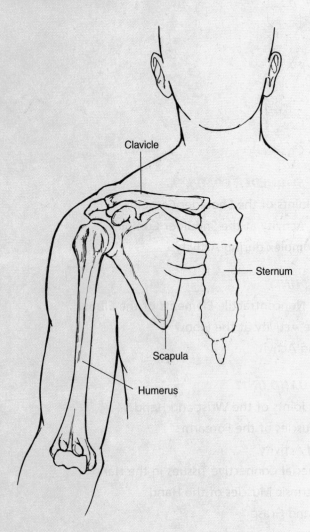

Clavicle

Sternum

Scapula

Humerus

The shoulder complex. The shoulder complex consists of the humerus, clavicle, and scapula and includes the sternoclavicular, acromioclavicular, glenohumeral, and scapulothoracic joints.

This three-chapter unit on the shoulder complex describes the structure of the shoulder complex and its implications for function and dysfunction. The purposes of this unit are to

- Provide the clinician with an understanding of the morphology of the individual components of the complex
- Identify the functional relationships among the individual components
- Discuss how the structures of the shoulder complex contribute to mobility and stability
- Provide insight into the stresses that the shoulder complex sustains during daily activity

The unit is divided into three chapters. The first chapter presents the bony structures making up the shoulder complex and the articulations that join them. The second chapter presents the muscles of the shoulders and their contributions to function and dysfunction. The third chapter investigates the loads to which the shoulder complex and its individual components are subjected during daily activity.

Structure and Function of the Bones and Joints of the Shoulder Complex

CHAPTER CONTENTS

T his chapter describes the structure of the bones and joints of the shoulder complex as it relates to the function of the shoulder. The specific purposes of this chapter are to

- Describe the structures of the individual bones that constitute the shoulder complex
- Describe the articulations joining the bony elements
- Discuss the factors contributing to stability and instability at each joint
- Discuss the relative contributions of each articulation to the overall motion of the shoulder complex
- Review the literature's description of normal range of motion (ROM) of the shoulder
- Discuss the implications of abnormal motion at an individual articulation to the overall motion of the shoulder complex

STRUCTURE OF THE BONES OF THE SHOULDER COMPLEX

The shoulder complex consists of three individual bones: the clavicle, the scapula, and the humerus. Each of these bones is discussed in detail below. However, the complex itself is connected to the axioskeleton via the sternum and rests on the thorax, whose shape exerts some influence on the function of the entire complex. Therefore, a brief discussion of the sternum and the shape of the thorax as it relates to the shoulder complex is also presented.

Clavicle

The clavicle functions like a strut to hold the shoulder complex and, indeed, the entire upper extremity suspended on the axioskeleton [84]. Other functions attributed to the clavicle are to provide a site for muscle attachment, to protect underlying nerves and blood vessels, to contribute to increased ROM of the shoulder, and to help transmit muscle force to the scapula [52,69]. This section describes the details of the clavicle that contribute to its ability to perform each of these functions. How these characteristics contribute to the functions of the clavicle and how they are implicated in injuries to the clavicle are discussed in later sections of this chapter.

The clavicle lies with its long axis close to the transverse plane. It is a crank-shaped bone when viewed from above, with its medial two thirds convex anteriorly, approximately conforming to the anterior thorax, and its lateral one third convex posteriorly (*Fig. 8.1*). The functional significance of this unusual shape becomes apparent in the discussion of overall shoulder motion.

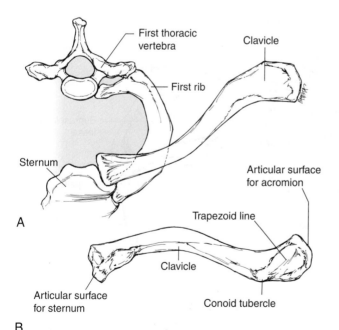

Figure 8.1: Clavicle. **A.** View of the superior surface. **B.** View of the inferior surface.

The superior surface of the clavicle is smooth and readily palpated under the skin. Anteriorly, the surface is roughened by the attachments of the pectoralis major medially and the deltoid laterally. The posterior surface is roughened on the lateral one third by the attachment of the upper trapezius. Inferiorly, the surface is roughened medially by attachments of the costoclavicular ligament and the subclavius muscle and laterally by the coracoclavicular ligament. The latter produces two prominent markings on the inferior surface of the lateral aspect of the clavicle, the conoid tubercle and, lateral to it, the trapezoid line.

The medial and lateral ends of the clavicle provide articular surfaces for the sternum and acromion, respectively. The medial aspect of the clavicle expands to form the head of the clavicle. The medial surface of this expansion articulates with the sternum and intervening articular disc, or meniscus, as well as with the first costal cartilage. The articular surface of the clavicular head is concave in the anterior posterior direction and slightly convex in the superior inferior direction [93,101]. Unlike most synovial joints, the articular surface of the mature clavicle is covered by thick fibrocartilage. The lateral one third of the clavicle is flattened with respect to the other two thirds and ends in a broad flat expansion that articulates with the acromion at the acromioclavicular joint. The actual articular surface is a small facet typically facing inferiorly and laterally. It too is covered by fibrocartilage rather than hyaline cartilage. The medial and lateral aspects of the clavicle are easily palpated.

Scapula

The scapula is a flat bone whose primary function is to provide a site for muscle attachment for the shoulder. A total of 15 major muscles acting at the shoulder attach to the scapula [58,101]. In quadrupedal animals, the scapula is long and thin and rests on the lateral aspect of the thorax. In primates, there is a gradual mediolateral expansion of the bone along with a gradual migration from a position lateral on the thorax to a more posterior location (*Fig. 8.2*). The mediolateral expansion is largely the result of an increased infraspinous fossa and costal surface that provide attachment for three of the four rotator cuff muscles as well as several other muscles of the shoulder [40,83]. These changes in structure and location of the scapula reflect the gradual change in the function of the upper extremity from its weight-bearing function to one of reaching and grasping. These alterations in function require a change in the role of muscles that now must position and support a scapula and glenohumeral joint that are no longer primarily weight bearing and instead are free to move through a much larger excursion.

The scapula has two surfaces, its costal, or anterior, surface and the dorsal, or posterior surface (*Fig. 8.3*). The costal surface is generally smooth and provides proximal attachment for the subscapularis muscle. Along the medial border of the anterior surface, a smooth narrow surface gives rise to the serratus anterior muscle.

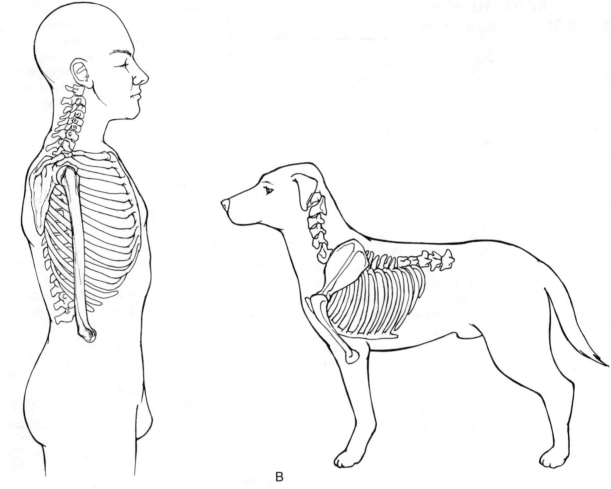

Figure 8.2: Location of the scapula. **A.** In humans the scapula is located more posteriorly. **B.** The scapula is located on the lateral aspect of the thorax in quadrupedal animals.

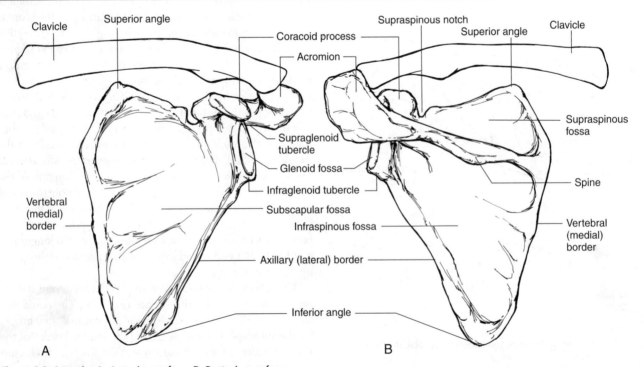

Figure 8.3: Scapula. **A.** Anterior surface. **B.** Posterior surface.

The dorsal surface of the scapula is divided into two regions by the spine of the scapula, a small superior space called the supraspinous fossa and a large inferior space known as the infraspinous fossa. The spine is a large dorsally protruding ridge of bone that runs from the medial border of the scapula laterally and superiorly across the width of the scapula. The spine ends in a large, flat surface that projects laterally, anteriorly, and somewhat superiorly. This process is known as the acromion process. The acromion provides a roof over the head of the humerus. The acromion has an articular facet for the clavicle on the anterior aspect of its medial surface. Like the clavicular surface with which it articulates, this articular surface is covered by fibrocartilage rather than hyaline cartilage. This facet faces medially and somewhat superiorly. The acromion is generally described as flat. However Bigliani et al. describe various shapes of the acromion including flat, rounded, and hooked processes [4]. These authors suggest that the hooked variety of acromion process may contribute to shoulder impingement syndromes. Additional factors contributing to impingement syndromes are discussed throughout this chapter.

The scapula has three borders: the medial or vertebral border, the lateral or axillary border, and the superior border. The medial border is easily palpated along its length from inferior to superior. The medial border bends anteriorly from the root of the spine to the superior angle, thus conforming to the contours of the underlying thorax. It joins the superior border at the superior angle of the scapula that can be palpated only in individuals with small, or atrophied, muscles covering the superior angle, particularly the trapezius and levator scapulae.

Projecting from the anterior surface of the superior border of the scapula is the coracoid process, a fingerlike projection protruding superiorly then anteriorly and laterally from the scapula. It is located approximately two thirds of the width of the scapula from its medial border. The coracoid process is readily palpated inferior to the lateral one third of the clavicle on the anterior aspect of the trunk. Just medial to the base of the coracoid process on the superior border is the supraspinous notch through which travels the suprascapular nerve.

The medial border of the scapula joins the lateral border at the inferior angle, an important and easily identified landmark. The lateral border of the scapula is palpable along its inferior portion until it is covered by the teres major, teres minor, and latissimus dorsi muscles. The lateral border continues superiorly and joins the superior border at the anterior angle or head and neck of the scapula. The head gives rise to the glenoid fossa that provides the scapula's articular surface for the glenohumeral joint. The fossa is somewhat narrow superiorly and widens inferiorly resulting in a "pear-shaped" appearance. The depth of the fossa is increased by the surrounding fibrocartilaginous labrum. Superior and inferior to the fossa are the supraglenoid and infraglenoid tubercles, respectively.

The orientation of the glenoid fossa itself is somewhat controversial. Its orientation is described as

- Lateral [2]
- Superior [2]
- Inferior [80]
- Anterior [2,84]
- Retroverted [85]

Only the lateral orientation of the glenoid fossa appears uncontested. Although the differences in the literature may reflect real differences in measurement or in the populations studied, at least some of the variation is due to differences in reference frames used by the various investigators to describe the scapula's position. The reference frames used include one imbedded in the scapula itself and one imbedded in the whole body. The scapula-fixed reference frame allows comparison of the position of one bony landmark of the scapula to another landmark on the scapula. The latter body-fixed reference frame allows comparison of the position of a scapular landmark to other regions of the body.

To understand the controversies regarding the orientation of the glenoid fossa, it is useful to first consider the orientation of the scapula as a whole. Using a body-fixed reference frame, the normal resting position of the scapula can be described in relationship to the sagittal, frontal, and transverse planes. In a transverse plane view, the scapula is rotated inwardly about a vertical axis. The **plane of the scapula** is oriented approximately 30–45° from the frontal plane (*Fig. 8.4*) [46,86]. This position directs the glenoid anteriorly with respect to the body. However, a scapula-fixed reference frame reveals that the glenoid fossa is retroverted, or rotated posteriorly, with respect to the neck of the scapula [14,85].

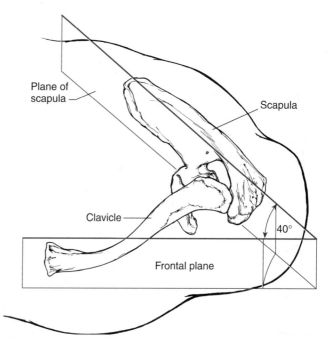

Figure 8.4: Plane of the scapula. A transverse view of the scapula reveals that the plane of the scapula forms an angle of approximately 40° with the frontal plane.

Thus the glenoid fossa is directed anteriorly (with respect to the body) and at the same time is retroverted (with respect to the scapula).

Rotation of the scapula in the frontal plane about a body-fixed anterior–posterior (AP) axis is also described (*Fig. 8.5*). This frontal plane rotation of the scapula is described by either the upward or downward orientation of the glenoid fossa or by the medial or lateral location of the scapula's inferior angle [2,25,80]. A rotation about this AP axis that tips the glenoid fossa inferiorly, moving the inferior angle of the scapula medially (i.e., closer to the vertebral column), is described as **downward** or **medial rotation** of the scapula. A rotation that tilts the glenoid fossa upward, moving the inferior angle laterally away from the vertebral column, is **upward** or **lateral rotation.** Two investigations report that the glenoid fossa is upwardly inclined in quiet standing [2,61]. Two other studies report a downward inclination of approximately 5° [25,80]. The posture of the studies' subjects may help to explain these reported differences. Perhaps subjects who demonstrate an upward inclination are instructed to pull their shoulders back into an "erect" posture while those who have a downward inclination of the glenoid fossa have slightly drooping

shoulders (*Fig. 8.6*). A final determination of the normal orientation of the scapulae in the frontal plane requires an accepted definition of normal postural alignment of the shoulder. That definition unfortunately is presently

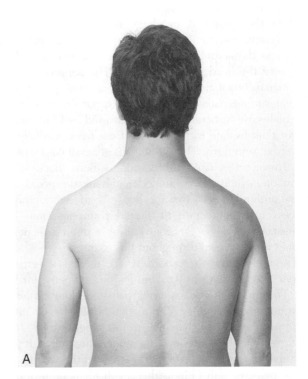

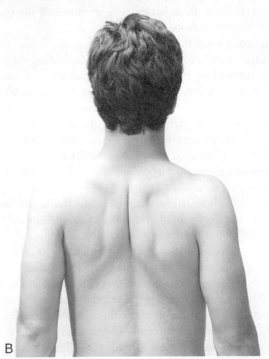

Figure 8.6: Postural changes of the scapula. **A.** This individual is standing with drooping, or rounded, shoulders, and the scapulae are rotated so that the glenoid fossa tilts downward. **B.** This individual stands with the shoulders pulled back and the scapulae tilted upward.

Figure 8.5: Scapular rotation. Rotation of the scapula about an anterior–posterior (AP) axis causes the glenoid fossa to face upward (2) or downward (3).

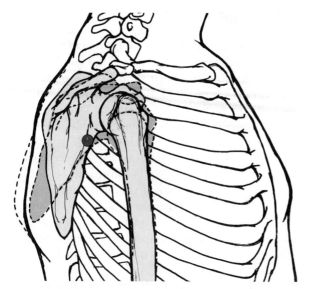

Figure 8.7: Scapular rotation. Rotation of the scapula about a ML axis tilts the scapula anteriorly and posteriorly.

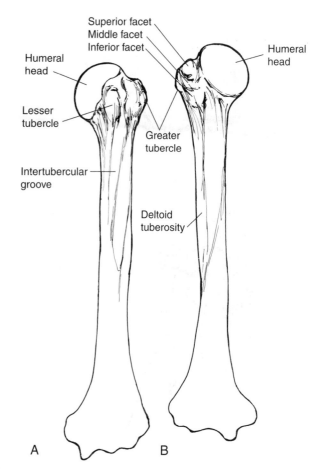

Figure 8.8: Proximal humerus. **A.** Anterior view. **B.** Posterior view.

lacking. Therefore, the controversy regarding the orientation of the scapula and its glenoid fossa in the frontal plane continues.

Viewed sagittally, the scapula tilts forward from the frontal plane approximately 10° about a medial lateral axis (*Fig. 8.7*) [17]. This forward tilting is partly the result of the scapula's position on the superior thorax, which tapers toward its apex. Additional forward tilt of the scapula causes the inferior angle of the scapula to protrude from the thorax.

Clinical Relevance

SCAPULAR POSITION IN SHOULDER DYSFUNCTION:
Abnormal scapular positions have been implicated in several forms of shoulder dysfunction. Abnormal orientation of the glenoid fossa has been associated with instability of the glenohumeral joint [2,85,91]. In addition, excessive anterior tilting is found in individuals with shoulder impingement syndromes during active shoulder abduction [61]. Careful evaluation of scapular position is an essential component of a thorough examination of patients with shoulder dysfunction.

Proximal Humerus

The humerus is a long bone composed of a head, neck, and body, or shaft. The body ends distally in the capitulum and trochlea. This chapter presents only those portions of the humerus that are relevant to a discussion of the mechanics and pathomechanics of the shoulder complex. The rest of the

humerus is discussed in Chapter 11 with the elbow. The articular surface of the head of the humerus is most often described as approximately half of an almost perfect sphere (*Fig. 8.8*) [39,89,99,101]. The humeral head projects medially, superiorly, and posteriorly with respect to the plane formed by the medial and lateral condyles (*Fig. 8.9*) [40]. The humeral head ends in the anatomical neck marking the end of the articular surface.

On the lateral aspect of the proximal humerus is the greater tubercle, a large bony prominence that is easily palpated on the lateral aspect of the shoulder complex. The greater tubercle is marked by three distinct facets on its superior and posterior surfaces. These facets give rise from superior to posterior to the supraspinatus, infraspinatus, and teres minor muscles, respectively. On the anterior aspect of the proximal humerus is a smaller but still prominent bony projection, the lesser tubercle. It too has a facet that provides attachment for the remaining rotator cuff muscle, the subscapularis. Separating the tubercles is the intertubercular, or bicipital, groove containing the tendon of the long head of the biceps brachii. The greater and lesser tubercles continue onto the body of the humerus as the medial and lateral lips of the groove. The surgical neck is a slight narrowing of the shaft of the humerus just distal to the tubercles.

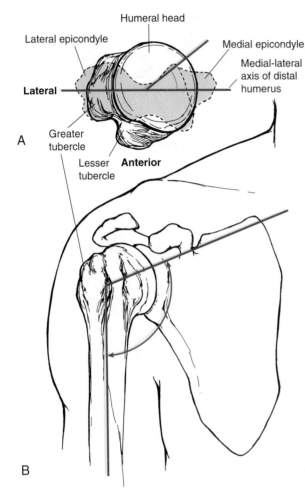

Figure 8.9: Orientation of the head of the humerus. **A.** In the transverse plane, the humeral head is rotated posteriorly with respect to the condyles of the distal humerus. **B.** In the frontal plane, the head of the humerus is angled medially and superiorly with respect to the shaft of the humerus.

Clinical Relevance

THE DEPTH OF THE BICIPITAL GROOVE: *The depth of the bicipital groove varies. A shallow groove appears to be a contributing factor in dislocations of the biceps tendon [56,58].*

Approximately midway distally on the body of the humerus is the deltoid tuberosity on the anterolateral surface. It provides the distal attachment for the deltoid muscle. The spiral groove is another important landmark on the body of the humerus. It is found on the proximal half of the humerus, spiraling from proximal to distal and medial to lateral on the posterior surface. The radial nerve travels in the spiral groove along with the profunda brachii vessels. The radial nerve is particularly susceptible to injury as it lies in the spiral groove.

Sternum and Thorax

Although the sternum and thorax are not part of the shoulder complex, both are intimately related to the shoulder; therefore, a brief description of their structure as it relates to the shoulder complex is required. Both the sternum and thorax are covered in greater detail in Chapter 29. The superior portion of the sternum, the manubrium, provides an articular surface for the proximal end of each clavicle (*Fig. 8.10*). The articular surface is a shallow depression called the clavicular notch covered with fibrocartilage like the clavicular head with which it articulates. Each notch provides considerably less articular surface than the clavicular head that articulates with it. The two clavicular notches are separated by the sternal or jugular notch on the superior aspect of the manubrium. This notch is very prominent and is a useful landmark for identifying the sternoclavicular joints. Another reliable and useful landmark is the angle formed by the junction of the manubrium with the body of the sternum, known as the sternal angle, or angle of Louis. This is also the site of the attachment of the second costal cartilage to the manubrium and body of the sternum.

The bony thorax forms the substrate on which the two scapulae slide. Consequently, the shape of the thorax serves as a constraint to the movements of the scapulae [97]. Each scapula rides on the superior portion of the thorax, positioned in the upright posture approximately from the first through the eighth ribs and from the vertebral bodies of about T2 to T7 or T8. The medial aspect of the spine of the scapula is

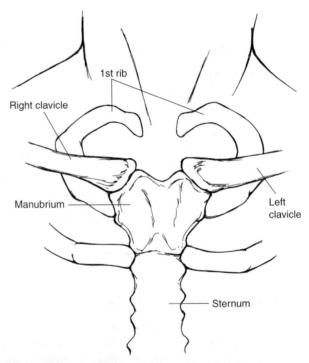

Figure 8.10: The sternum's articular surface. The sternum provides a shallow articular surface for the head of the clavicle.

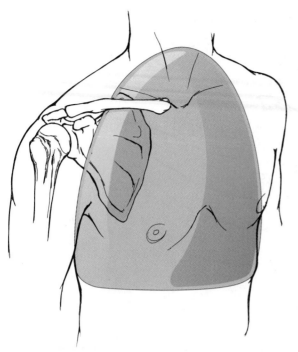

Figure 8.11: Shape of the thorax. The elliptical shape of the thorax influences the motion of the scapula.

typically described as in line with the spinous process of T2. The inferior angle is usually reported to be in line with the spinous process of T7. It is important to recognize, however, that postural alignment of the shoulder and vertebral column can alter these relationships significantly.

The dorsal surface of the thorax in the region of the scapulae is characterized by its convex shape, known as a thoracic kyphosis. The superior ribs are smaller than the inferior ones, so the overall shape of the thorax can be described as ellipsoid (*Fig. 8.11*) [99]. Thus as the scapula glides superiorly on the thorax it also tilts anteriorly. An awareness of the shape of the thorax on which the scapula glides helps to explain the resting position of the scapula and the motions of the scapula caused by contractions of certain muscles such as the rhomboids and pectoralis minor [17,49].

In conclusion, as stated at the beginning of this chapter, the shoulder complex is an intricate arrangement of three specific bones, each of which is unique. These three bones are also functionally and structurally related to parts of the axioskeleton (i.e., to the sternum and the thorax). A clear image of each bone and its position relative to the others is essential to a complete and accurate physical examination. The palpable bony landmarks relevant to the shoulder complex are listed below:

- Sternal notch
- Sternal angle
- Second rib
- Head of the clavicle
- Sternoclavicular joint

- Superior surface of the clavicle
- Anterior surface of the clavicle
- Acromion
- Acromioclavicular joint
- Coracoid process
- Vertebral border of the scapula
- Spine of the scapula
- Inferior angle of the scapula
- Axillary border of the scapula
- Greater tubercle of the humerus
- Lesser tubercle of the humerus
- Intertubercular groove of the humerus

The following section describes the structure and mechanics of the joints of the shoulder complex formed by these bony components.

STRUCTURE OF THE JOINTS AND SUPPORTING STRUCTURES OF THE SHOULDER COMPLEX

The shoulder complex is composed of four joints:

- Sternoclavicular
- Acromioclavicular
- Scapulothoracic
- Glenohumeral

All but the scapulothoracic joint are synovial joints. The scapulothoracic joint falls outside any traditional category of joint because the moving components, the scapula and the thorax, are not directly attached or articulated to one another and because muscles rather than cartilage or fibrous material separate the moving components. However, it is the site of systematic and repeated motion between bones and thus justifiably can be designated a joint. This section presents the structure and mechanics of each of the four joints of the shoulder complex.

Sternoclavicular Joint

The sternoclavicular joint is described by some as a ball-and-socket joint [84] and by others as a saddle joint [93,101]. Since both types of joints are triaxial, there is little functional significance to the distinction. The sternoclavicular joint actually includes the clavicle, sternum, and superior aspect of the first costal cartilage (*Fig. 8.12*). It is enclosed by a synovial capsule that attaches to the sternum and clavicle just beyond the articular surfaces. The capsule is relatively weak inferiorly but is reinforced anteriorly, posteriorly, and superiorly by accessory ligaments that are thickenings of the capsule itself. The anterior and posterior ligaments are known as the anterior and posterior sternoclavicular ligaments. These ligaments serve to limit anterior and posterior glide of the sternoclavicular joint. They also provide some limits to the joint's normal transverse plane movement, known as *protraction* and *retraction*.

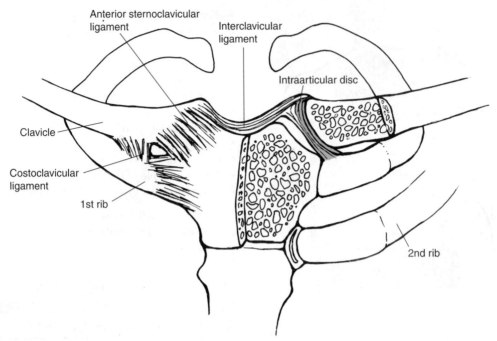

Figure 8.12: The sternoclavicular joint. The supporting structures of the sternoclavicular joint include the capsule, the intraarticular disc, the anterior and posterior sternoclavicular ligaments, the interclavicular ligament, and the costoclavicular ligament.

The superior thickening of the joint capsule comes from the interclavicular ligament, a thick fibrous band extending from one sternoclavicular joint to the other and covering the floor of the sternal notch. This ligament helps prevent superior and lateral displacements of the clavicle on the sternum. The capsule with its ligamentous thickenings is described as the strongest limiter of excessive motion at the sternoclavicular joint [3].

The capsule and ligaments described so far are the primary limiters of anterior, posterior, and lateral movements. However, other structures provide additional limits to medial translation and elevation of the clavicle. As noted in the descriptions of the bones, the articular surface of the clavicle is considerably larger than the respective surface on the sternum. Consequently, the superior aspect of the clavicular head projects superiorly over the sternum and is easily palpated. This disparity between the articular surfaces results in an inherent joint instability that allows the clavicle to slide medially over the sternum. Such migration can be precipitated by a medially directed force on the clavicle, such as those that arise from a blow to, or a fall on, the shoulder (*Fig. 8.13*). An intraarticular disc interposed between the clavicle and sternum increases the articular surface on which the clavicle moves and also serves to block any medial movement of the clavicle. The disc is attached inferiorly to the superior aspect of the first costal cartilage and superiorly to the superior border of the clavicle's articular surface dividing the joint into two separate synovial cavities. The specific attachments of the disc help it prevent medial migration of the clavicle over the sternum. A blow to the lateral aspect of the shoulder applies a medial force on the clavicle, tending to push it medially on the sternum. The clavicle is anchored to the underlying first costal cartilage by the intraarticular disc resisting any medial movement of the clavicle. However a cadaver study suggests that the disc can be torn easily from its attachment on the costal cartilage [3]. Therefore, the magnitude of its role as a

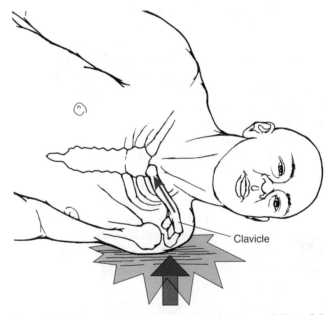

Figure 8.13: Forces that tend to move the clavicle medially. A fall on the lateral aspect of the shoulder produces a force on the clavicle, tending to push it medially.

stabilizer of the sternoclavicular joint, particularly in limiting medial translation of the clavicle on the sternum, remains unclear. The disc may also serve as a shock absorber between the clavicle and sternum [50].

Another important stabilizing structure of the sternoclavicular joint is the costoclavicular ligament, an extracapsular ligament lying lateral to the joint itself. It runs from the lateral aspect of the first costal cartilage superiorly to the inferior aspect of the medial clavicle. Its anterior fibers run superiorly and laterally, while the posterior fibers run superiorly and medially. Consequently, this ligament provides significant limits to medial, lateral, anterior, and posterior movements of the clavicle as well as to elevation.

A review of the supporting structures of the sternoclavicular joint reveals that despite an inherently unstable joint surface, these supporting structures together limit medial, lateral, posterior, anterior, and superior displacements of the clavicle on the sternum. Inferior movement of the clavicle is limited by the interclavicular ligament and by the costal cartilage itself. Thus it is clear that the sternoclavicular joint is so reinforced that it is quite a stable joint [72,96].

Clinical Relevance

FRACTURE OF THE CLAVICLE: *The sternoclavicular joint is so well stabilized that fractures of the clavicle are considerably more common than dislocations of the sternoclavicular joint. In fact the clavicle is the bone most commonly fractured in humans [32]. Trauma to the sternoclavicular joint and clavicle most commonly occurs from forces applied to the upper extremity. Although clavicular fractures are commonly believed to occur from falls on an outstretched hand, a review of 122 cases of clavicular fractures reports that 94% of the clavicular fracture cases (115 patients) occurred by a direct blow to the shoulder [92]. Falls on the shoulder are a common culprit. As an individual falls from a bicycle, for example, turning slightly to protect the face and head, the shoulder takes the brunt of the fall. The ground exerts a force on the lateral and superior aspect of the acromion and clavicle. This force pushes the clavicle medially and inferiorly [96]. However, the sternoclavicular joint is firmly supported against such movements, so the ground reaction force tends to deform the clavicle. The first costal cartilage inferior to the clavicle is a barrier to deformation of the clavicle, and as a result, the clavicle is likely to fracture (Fig. 8.14). Usually the fracture occurs in the middle or lateral one third of the clavicle, the former more frequently than the latter [32]. The exact mechanism of fracture is unclear. Some suggest that it is a fracture resulting from bending, while others suggest it is a direct compression fracture [32,92]. Regardless of the mechanism, it is clear that fractures of the clavicle are more common than sternoclavicular joint dislocations, partially because of the firm stabilization provided by the disc and ligaments of the sternoclavicular joint [15,96].*

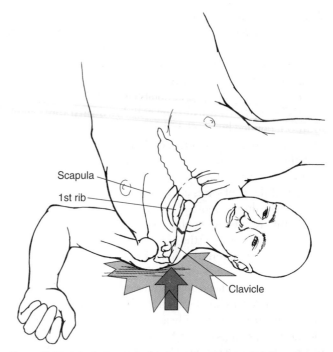

Figure 8.14: A typical way to fracture the clavicle. A fall on the top of the shoulder produces a downward force on the clavicle, pushing it down onto the first rib. The first rib prevents depression of the medial aspect of the clavicle, but the force of the fall continues to depress the lateral portion of the clavicle, resulting in a fracture in the middle third of the clavicle.

Whether regarded as a saddle or ball-and-socket joint, motion at the sternoclavicular joint occurs about three axes, an anterior–posterior (AP), a vertical superior–inferior (SI), and a longitudinal (ML) axis through the length of the clavicle (*Fig 8.15*). Although these axes are described as slightly

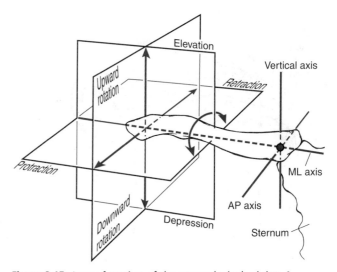

Figure 8.15: Axes of motion of the sternoclavicular joint. **A.** Elevation and depression of the sternoclavicular joint occur about an anterior–posterior axis. **B.** Protraction and retraction of the sternoclavicular joint occur about a vertical axis. **C.** Upward and downward rotation of the sternoclavicular joint occur about a medial–lateral axis.

oblique to the cardinal planes of the body [93], the motions of the clavicle take place very close to these planes. Movement about the AP axis yields **elevation** and **depression,** which occur approximately in the frontal plane. Movements about the SI axis are known as **protraction** and **retraction** and occur in the transverse plane. Rotations around the longitudinal axis are **upward (posterior)** and **downward (anterior) rotation,** defined by whether the anterior surface of the clavicle turns up (upward rotation) or down (downward rotation).

Although movement at the sternoclavicular joint is rotational, the prominence of the clavicular head and the location of the joint's axes allow easy palpation of the head of the clavicle during most of these motions. This palpation frequently results in confusion for the novice clinician. Note that retraction of the clavicle causes the head of the clavicle to move anteriorly on the sternum as the body of the clavicle rotates posteriorly (*Fig. 8.16*). Similarly in protraction the clavicular head rolls posteriorly as the body moves anteriorly. Likewise in elevation the body of the clavicle and the acromion rise, but the head of the clavicle descends on the sternum; depression of the sternoclavicular joint is the reverse. These movements of the proximal and distal clavicular surfaces in opposite directions are consistent with rotations of the sternoclavicular joint and are the result of the location of the axes within the clavicle itself. The exact location of the axes about which the movements of the sternoclavicular joint occur are debated, but probably the axes lie somewhat lateral to the head of the clavicle [3,82]. This location explains the movement of the lateral and medial ends of the clavicle in apparently opposite directions. With the axes of motion located between the two ends of the clavicle, pure rotation results in opposite movements of the two ends, just as the two ends of a seesaw move in opposite directions during pure rotation about the pivot point.

Few studies are available that investigate the available ROM of the sternoclavicular joint. The total excursion of elevation and depression is reportedly 50 to 60°, with depression being less than 10° of the total [69,93]. Elevation is limited by the costoclavicular ligament, and depression by the superior portion of the capsule and the interclavicular ligament [3,93]. Some suggest that contact between the clavicle and the first rib also limits depression of the sternoclavicular joint [82]. Facets found in some cadaver specimens between the clavicle and first costal cartilage provide strong evidence for contact between these structures in at least some individuals [3,82].

Protraction and retraction appear to be more equal in excursion, with a reported total excursion ranging from 30 to 60° [82,93]. Protraction is limited by the posterior sternoclavicular ligament limiting the backward movement of the clavicular head and by the costoclavicular ligament limiting the forward movement of the body of the clavicle. Retraction is limited similarly by the anterior sternoclavicular ligament and by the costoclavicular ligament. The interclavicular ligament assists in limiting both motions [3].

Upward and downward rotations appear to be more limited than the other motions, with estimates of upward rotation ROM that vary from 25 to 55° [3,40,82]. Although there are no known studies of downward rotation ROM, it appears to be much less than upward rotation, probably less than 10°. Regardless of the exact amount of excursion available at the sternoclavicular joint, it is well understood that motion at the sternoclavicular joint is intimately related to motions of the other joints of the shoulder complex. How these motions are related is discussed after each joint is presented.

Acromioclavicular Joint

The acromioclavicular joint is generally regarded as a gliding joint with flat articular surfaces, although the surfaces are sometimes described as reciprocally concave and convex [93,101] (*Fig. 8.17*). Both articular surfaces are covered by fibrocartilage rather than hyaline cartilage. The joint is supported by a capsule that is reinforced superiorly and inferiorly by acromioclavicular ligaments (*Fig. 8.18*). Although the capsule is frequently described as weak, the acromioclavicular ligaments may provide the primary support to the joint in instances of small displacements and low loads [26,55]. In addition, the acromioclavicular ligaments appear to provide important limitations to posterior glide of the acromioclavicular joint regardless of the magnitude of displacement or load [26]. The inferior acromioclavicular ligament also may provide substantial resistance to excessive anterior displacement of the clavicle on the scapula [55]. The joint also possesses an intraarticular meniscus that is usually less than a whole disc and provides no known additional support.

The other major support to the acromioclavicular ligament is the extracapsular coracoclavicular ligament that runs from the base of the coracoid process to the inferior surface of the

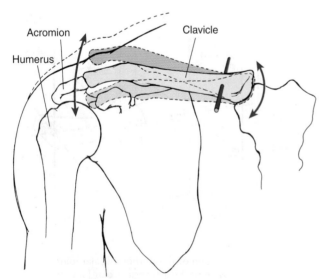

Figure 8.16: Movement of the head of the clavicle. Rotation of the sternoclavicular joint about an axis causes the head of the clavicle to move in a direction opposite the motion of the rest of the clavicle just as the two ends of a seesaw move in opposite directions about a central pivot point.

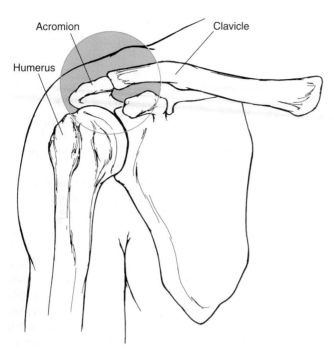

Figure 8.17: The articular surfaces of the acromioclavicular joint are relatively flattened and beveled with respect to one another.

acromioclavicular, coracoacromial, and superior glenohumeral ligaments [13].

It is curious that a ligament that does not even cross the joint directly can be so important in providing stability. An understanding of the precise orientation of the ligament helps explain its role in stabilizing the joint. The ligament is composed of two parts, the conoid ligament that runs vertically from the coracoid process to the conoid tubercle on the clavicle and the trapezoid ligament that runs vertically and laterally to the trapezoid line. The vertically aligned portion, the conoid ligament, reportedly limits excessive superior glides at the acromioclavicular joint. The acromioclavicular ligaments purportedly limit smaller superior displacements [26,55].

The more obliquely aligned trapezoid ligament protects against the shearing forces that can drive the acromion inferiorly and medially under the clavicle. Such forces can arise from a fall on the shoulder or a blow to the shoulder. The shape of the articular surfaces of the acromioclavicular joint causes it to be particularly prone to such displacements. As stated earlier, the articular facet of the clavicle faces laterally and inferiorly, while that of the acromion faces medially and superiorly. These surfaces give the acromioclavicular joint a beveled appearance that allows medial displacement of the acromion underneath the clavicle. Medial displacement of the acromion results in simultaneous displacement of the coracoid process, since it is part of the same scapula. Examination of the trapezoid ligament shows that it is aligned to block the medial translation of the coracoid process, thus helping to keep the clavicle with the scapula and preventing dislocation (*Fig. 8.19*) [82]. Dislocation of the acromioclavicular

clavicle. This ligament provides critical support to the acromioclavicular joint, particularly against large excursions and medial displacements [26,55]. It is regarded by many as the primary suspensory ligament of the shoulder complex. Mechanical tests reveal that it is substantially stiffer than the

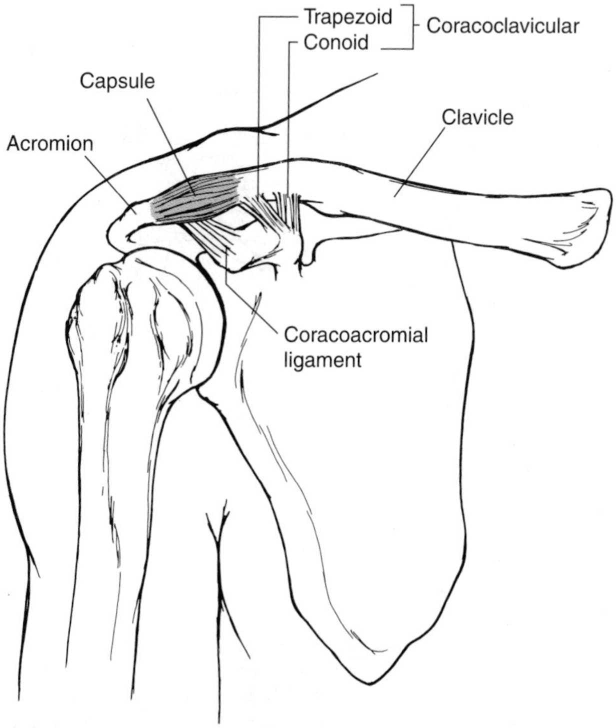

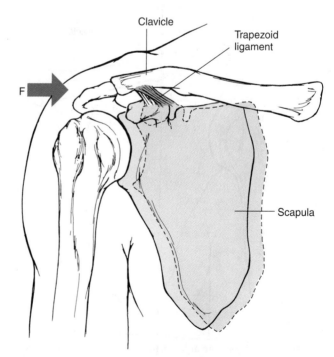

Figure 8.18: Acromioclavicular joint. The acromioclavicular joint is supported by the capsule, acromioclavicular ligaments, and the coracoclavicular ligament.

Figure 8.19: Trapezoid ligament. The trapezoid ligament helps prevent medial displacement of the acromion under the clavicle during a medial blow to the shoulder.

joint can be accompanied by disruption of the coracoclavicular ligament and by fractures of the coracoid process.

The coracoacromial ligament is another unusual ligament associated with the acromioclavicular joint. It is unusual because it crosses no joint. Instead it forms a roof over the glenohumeral joint by attaching from one landmark to another landmark on the scapula (*Fig. 8.20*). This ligament provides protection for the underlying bursa and supraspinatus tendon. It also provides a limit to the superior gliding of the humerus in a very unstable glenohumeral joint [58]. The coracoacromial ligament also is implicated as a factor in impingement of the structures underlying it and is thicker in some shoulders with rotator cuff tears. The question remains whether the thickening is a response to contact with the unstable humerus resulting from the disrupted rotator cuff or whether the thickening is itself a predisposing factor for rotator cuff tears [88]. Additional research is needed to clarify the relationship between the morphology of the coracoacromial ligament and the integrity of the rotator cuff muscles.

Few studies report objective measurements of the excursions of the acromioclavicular joint. Sahara et al. report total translations of approximately 4 mm in the anterior and posterior directions and approximately 2 mm in inferior/superior directions during shoulder movement [87].

Although gliding joints allow only translational movements, many authors describe rotational movement about specific axes of motion at the acromioclavicular joint [17,82,101]. The axes commonly described are vertical, AP, and medial/lateral (ML) (*Fig. 8.21*). The vertical axis allows motion of the scapula that brings the scapula closer to, or farther from, the clavicle in the transverse plane. Motion about the AP axis results in enlarging or shrinking the angle formed by the clavicle and spine of the scapula in the frontal plane. Motion about the ML axis tips the superior border of the scapula toward the clavicle or away from it. Direct measurements of angular excursions vary and range from less than 10° to 20° about individual axes [40,82]. Using a screw axis (a single axis that describes the total rotation and translation), Sahara et al. report a total of 35° of rotation with full shoulder abduction [87]. These studies suggest that the acromioclavicular joint allows significant motion between the scapula and clavicle.

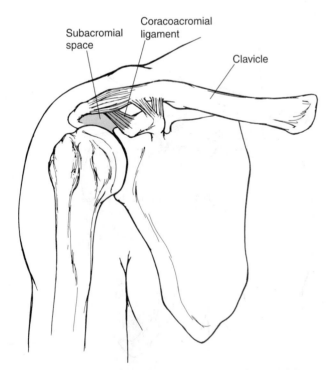

Figure 8.20: Coracoacromial ligament. The coracoacromial ligament forms a roof over the humeral head and helps create the subacromial space.

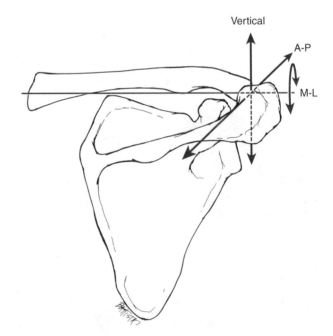

Figure 8.21: Axes of motion of the acromioclavicular joint. Motion about a vertical axis of the acromioclavicular joint moves the scapula in the transverse plane. Motion about an anterior–posterior *(AP)* axis turns the glenoid fossa upward and downward. Motion about a medial–lateral *(ML)* axis tilts the scapula anteriorly and posteriorly.

Viewed in the context of the shoulder complex, the acromioclavicular joint is responsible for maintaining articulation of the clavicle with the scapula, even as these two bones move in separate patterns. Whether this results in systematic rotational motions or in a gliding reorientation of the bones is not critical to the clinician, since in either case the motions cannot be readily measured. What is essential is the recognition that although the clavicle and scapula move together, their contributions to whole shoulder motion require that they also move somewhat independently of one another. This independent movement requires motion at the acromioclavicular joint.

Clinical Relevance

OSTEOARTHRITIS OF THE ACROMIOCLAVICULAR JOINT: *The acromioclavicular joint is a common site of osteoarthritis particularly in individuals who have a history of heavy labor or athletic activities. The normal mobility of the joint helps explain why pain and lost mobility in it from arthritic changes can produce significant loss of shoulder mobility and function.*

Scapulothoracic Joint

The scapulothoracic joint, as stated earlier, is an atypical joint that lacks all of the traditional characteristics of a joint except one, motion. The primary role of this joint is to amplify the motion of the glenohumeral joint, thus increasing the range and diversity of movements between the arm and trunk. In addition, the scapulothoracic joint with its surrounding musculature is described as an important shock absorber protecting the shoulder, particularly during falls on an outstretched arm [50].

Primary motions of the scapulothoracic joint include two translations and three rotations (*Fig. 8.22*). Those motions are

- Elevation and depression
- Abduction and adduction
- Downward (medial) and upward (lateral) rotations
- Internal and external rotations
- Scapular tilt

Elevation is defined as the movement of the entire scapula superiorly on the thorax. **Depression** is the opposite. **Abduction** is defined as the entire medial border of the scapula moving away from the vertebrae, and **adduction** as movement toward the vertebrae. Abduction and adduction of the scapulothoracic joint are occasionally referred to as protraction and retraction. However, protraction also is used by some to refer to the combination of abduction and upward rotation of the scapula. Others use the term protraction to refer to a rounded shoulder posture that may include abduction and downward rotation of the scapula. Therefore to avoid confusion, this text describes scapular movements discretely as elevation and depression, abduction and adduction, and upward and downward rotation. *Protraction* and *retraction*

refer solely to the motions of the sternoclavicular joint in the transverse plane.

Downward (medial) rotation of the scapula is defined as a rotation about an AP axis resulting in downward turn of the glenoid fossa as the inferior angle moves toward the vertebrae. **Upward (lateral) rotation** is the opposite. The location of the axis of downward and upward rotation is controversial but appears to be slightly inferior to the scapular spine, approximately equidistant from the vertebral and axillary borders [97]. It is likely that the exact location of the axis varies with ROM of the shoulder.

Internal and external rotations of the scapula occur about a vertical axis. Internal rotation turns the axillary border of the scapula more anteriorly, and external rotation turns the border more posteriorly. The shape of the thorax can enhance this motion. As the scapula translates laterally on the thorax in scapular abduction, the scapula rotates internally. Conversely, as the scapula adducts, it tends to rotate externally.

Anterior and posterior tilt of the scapula occur about a ML axis. Anterior tilt moves the superior portion of the scapula anteriorly while moving the inferior angle of the scapula posteriorly. Posterior tilt reverses the motion. Again, the shape of the thorax can enhance these motions. As the scapula elevates it tends to tilt anteriorly, and as it depresses it tends to tilt posteriorly (*Fig. 8.23*).

The motions of the scapulothoracic joint depend upon the motions of the sternoclavicular and acromioclavicular joints and under normal conditions occur through movements at both of these joints. For example, elevation of the scapulothoracic joint occurs with elevation of the sternoclavicular joint. Therefore, an important limiting factor for scapulothoracic elevation excursion is sternoclavicular ROM. Similarly, limits to scapulothoracic abduction and adduction as well as rotation include the available motions at the sternoclavicular and acromioclavicular joints. Tightness of the muscles of the scapulothoracic joint—particularly the trapezius, serratus anterior, and rhomboid muscles—may limit excursion of the scapula. The specific effects of individual muscle tightness are discussed in Chapter 9.

Although excursion of the scapulothoracic joint is not typically measured in the clinic and few studies exist that have investigated the normal movement available at this joint, it is useful to have an idea of the magnitude of excursion possible at the scapulothoracic joint. Excursions of 2–10 cm of scapular elevation and no more than 2 cm of depression are found in the literature [46,50]. Ranges of up to 10 cm are reported for abduction and 4–5 cm for adduction [46,50].

Upward rotation of the scapula is more thoroughly investigated than other motions of the scapulothoracic joint. The joint allows at least 60° of upward rotation of the scapula, but the full excursion depends upon the sternoclavicular joint elevation and acromioclavicular joint excursion available [40,63,80]. Tightness of the muscles that downwardly rotate the scapula may prevent or limit normal excursion of the scapula as well. Downward rotation on the scapula, on the other hand, is poorly studied. There are no known studies that

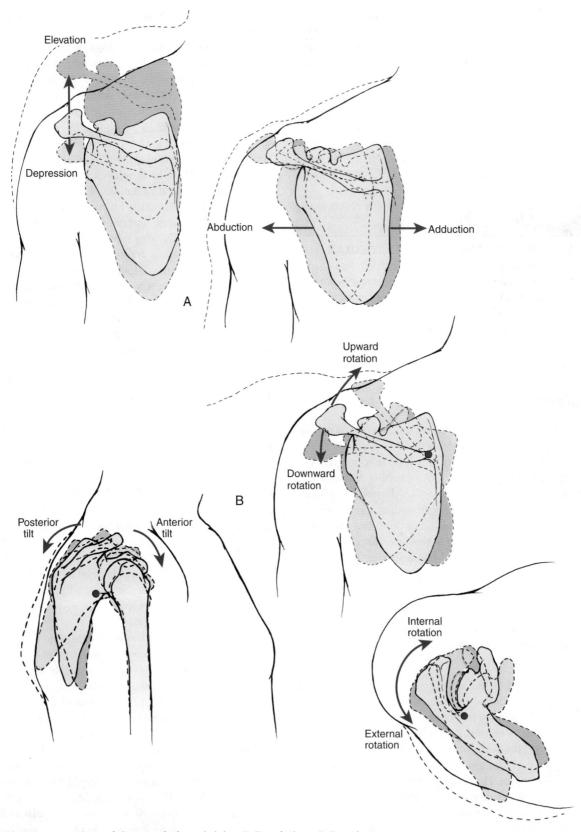

Figure 8.22: Primary motions of the scapulothoracic joint. **A.** Translations. **B.** Rotations.

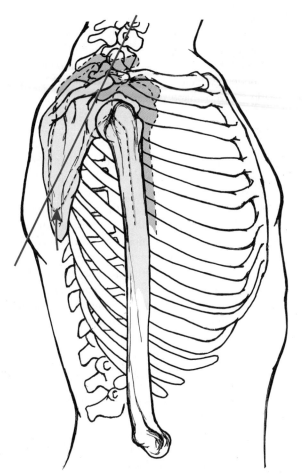

Figure 8.23: Scapular motion on the elliptical thorax. The shape of the thorax causes the scapula to tilt anteriorly as it elevates on the thorax.

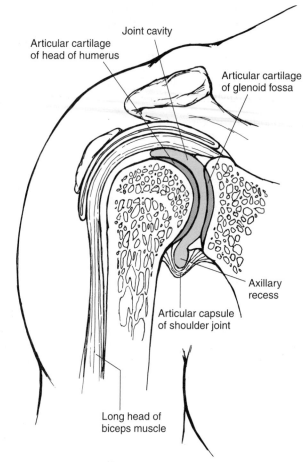

Figure 8.24: Articular surfaces of the glenohumeral joint. The humeral head and the glenoid fossa possess similar curvatures.

describe its excursion. However, downward rotation is greatly reduced compared with upward rotation. Although full potential excursions are not reported, the scapula reportedly tilts posteriorly and rotates externally approximately 30° and 25°, respectively, during shoulder elevation.

Glenohumeral Joint

Although the glenohumeral joint is frequently referred to as the *shoulder joint*, it must be emphasized that the "shoulder" is a composite of four joints, of which the glenohumeral joint is only a part, albeit a very important part. The glenohumeral joint is a classic ball-and-socket joint that is the most mobile in the human body [18]. Yet its very mobility presents serious challenges to the joint's inherent stability. The interplay between stability and mobility of this joint is a major theme that must be kept in mind to understand the mechanics and pathomechanics of the glenohumeral joint.

The two articular surfaces, the head of the humerus and the glenoid fossa, are both spherical (*Fig. 8.24*). The curve of their surfaces is described as their **radius of curvature.** As detailed in Chapter 7, the radius of curvature quantifies the amount of curve in a surface by describing the radius of the circle from which the surface is derived. Although the bony

surfaces of the humeral head and glenoid fossa may have slightly different curvatures, their cartilaginous articular surfaces have approximately the same radius of curvature [39,89,99]. Because these surfaces have similar curvatures, they fit well together; that is, there is a high degree of congruence. Increased congruence spreads the loads applied to the joint across a larger surface area and thus reduces the stress (force/area) applied to the articular surface. However, the amount of congruence is variable, even in healthy glenohumeral joints [4]. In cadavers, decreased congruence leads to an increase in the gliding motions between the humeral head and the glenoid fossa [4,48]. Thus decreased congruence may be a contributing factor in glenohumeral joint instability.

Although the articular surfaces of the glenohumeral joint are similarly curved, the actual areas of the articular surfaces are quite different from one another. While the head of the humerus is approximately one half of a sphere, the surface area of the glenoid fossa is less than one half that of the humeral head [45,52]. This disparity in articular surface sizes has dramatic effects on both the stability and mobility of the glenohumeral joint. First, the difference in the size of the articular surfaces allows a large degree of mobility since there is no bony limitation to the excursion. The size of the articular surfaces is an important factor in making the glenohumeral joint the most mobile in the body. However, by allowing tremendous mobility, the articular surfaces provide little or no stability for the glenohumeral joint [58]. The stability of the glenohumeral joint depends upon nonbony structures.

SUPPORTING STRUCTURES OF THE GLENOHUMERAL JOINT

The supporting structures of the glenohumeral joint consist of the

- Labrum
- Capsule
- Three glenohumeral ligaments
- Coracohumeral ligament
- Surrounding musculature

The noncontractile supporting structures of the glenohumeral joint are discussed in this section. The role of muscles in supporting the joint is discussed in Chapter 9.

The shallow glenoid fossa has already been identified as a contributing factor in glenohumeral joint instability. The stability is improved by deepening the fossa with the labrum (*Fig. 8.25*). The labrum is a ring of fibrous tissue and fibrocartilage surrounding the periphery of the fossa, approximately doubling the depth of the articular surface of the fossa [38,70]. Besides increasing the depth of the articular surface,

the ring increases the articular contact area, which also decreases the stress (force/area) on the glenoid fossa. The labrum provides these benefits while being deformable, thereby adding little or no restriction to glenohumeral movement. Magnetic resonance imaging (MRI) shows considerable variation in the shape of the labrum in asymptomatic shoulders, including notches and separations, particularly in the anterior aspect of the ring. A small percentage of individuals lack portions of the labrum [77].

Labral tears are well described in the clinical literature [16,76]. Mechanical tests of the ring demonstrate that it is weakest anteriorly and inferiorly, which is consistent with the clinical finding that anterior tears are the most common [31]. However, the functional significance of a torn labrum in the absence of other pathology remains controversial [17,76,79]. The amount of dysfunction that results from a labral tear probably depends upon the severity of the lesion. Small tears may have little or no effect, while large tears that extend to other parts of the joint capsule produce significant instability. The normal variability of the labrum in asymptomatic shoulders lends strength to the concept that small isolated labral tears do not result in significant dysfunction. However, additional studies are needed to clarify the role of labral tears in glenohumeral dysfunction.

The remaining connective tissue supporting structures of the glenohumeral joint are known collectively as the **capsuloligamentous complex.** It consists of the joint capsule and reinforcing ligaments. It encircles the entire joint and provides protection against excessive rotation and translation in all directions. It is important to recognize that the integrity of the complex depends on the integrity of each of its components.

The fibrous capsule of the glenohumeral joint is intimately related to the labrum. The capsule attaches distally to the anatomical neck of the humerus and proximally to the periphery of the glenoid fossa and/or to the labrum itself. Inferiorly, it is quite loose, forming folds (*Fig. 8.26*). These folds must open, or unfold, as the glenohumeral joint elevates in abduction or flexion.

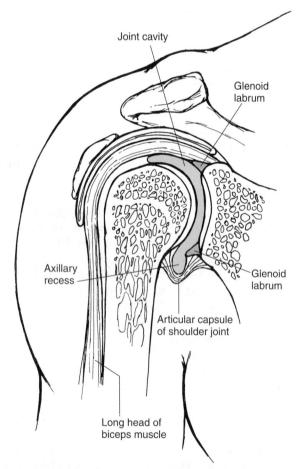

Figure 8.25: Glenoid labrum. The glenoid labrum deepens the glenoid fossa.

Clinical Relevance

ADHESIVE CAPSULITIS: *In adhesive capsulitis, fibrous adhesions form in the glenohumeral joint capsule. The capsule then is unable to unfold to allow full flexion or abduction, resulting in decreased joint excursion. Onset is frequently insidious, and the etiology is unknown. However, the classic physical findings are severe and painful limitations in joint ROM [30,73].*

The normal capsule is quite lax and, by itself, contributes little to the stability of the glenohumeral joint. However, it is reinforced anteriorly by the three glenohumeral ligaments and superiorly by the coracohumeral ligament. It also is supported anteriorly, superiorly, and posteriorly by the rotator cuff muscles that attach to it. Only the most inferior portion of the capsule is without additional support.

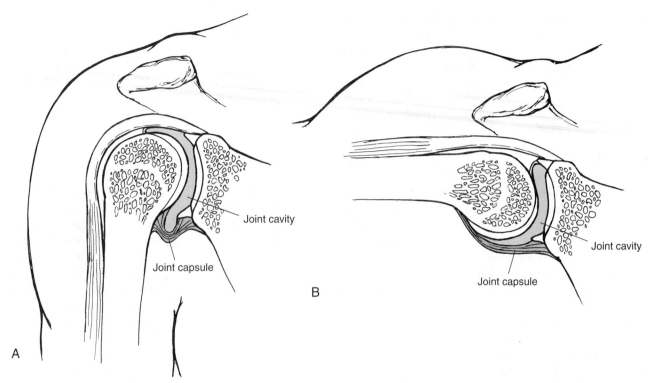

Figure 8.26: Glenohumeral joint capsule. **A.** When the shoulder is in neutral, the inferior portion of the capsule is lax and appears folded. **B.** In abduction the folds of the inferior capsule are unfolded, and the capsule is pulled more taut.

The three glenohumeral ligaments are thickenings of the capsule itself (*Fig. 8.27*). The superior glenohumeral ligament runs from the superior portion of the labrum and base of the coracoid process to the superior aspect of the humeral neck. The middle glenohumeral ligament has a broad attachment on the anterior aspect of the labrum inferior to the superior glenohumeral ligament and passes inferiorly and laterally, expanding as it crosses the anterior aspect of the glenohumeral joint. It attaches to the lesser tubercle deep to the tendon of the subscapularis. The superior glenohumeral ligament along with the coracohumeral ligament and the tendon of the long head of the biceps lies in the space between the tendons of the supraspinatus and subscapularis muscles. This space is known as the **rotator interval.**

The inferior glenohumeral ligament is a thick band that attaches to the anterior, posterior, and middle portions of the glenoid labrum and to the inferior and medial aspects of the neck of the humerus. The coracohumeral ligament attaches to the lateral aspect of the base of the coracoid process and to the greater tubercle of the humerus. It blends with the supraspinatus tendon and with the capsule.

These reinforcing ligaments support the glenohumeral joint by limiting excessive translation of the head of the humerus on the glenoid fossa. Tightness of these ligaments actually contributes to increased translation of the humeral head in the opposite direction [34]. The coracohumeral ligament provides protection against excessive posterior glides of the humerus on the glenoid fossa [7]. All three of the glenohumeral ligaments help to prevent anterior displacement of the humeral head on the glenoid fossa, especially when they are pulled taut by lateral

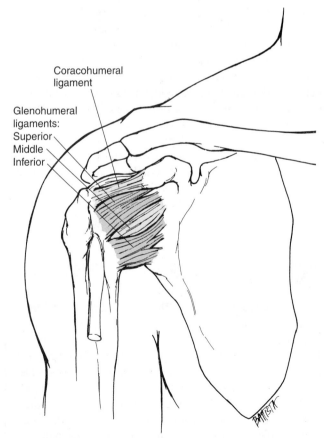

Figure 8.27: Glenohumeral joint. The glenohumeral joint capsule is reinforced by the superior, middle, and inferior glenohumeral ligaments. The joint is also supported by the coracohumeral ligament.

rotation of the glenohumeral joint [68]. The position of the glenohumeral joint in the frontal plane influences what parts of these ligaments are pulled taut [18]. In neutral and in moderate abduction, the superior and middle glenohumeral ligaments are pulled tight. However in more abduction, the inferior glenohumeral ligament provides most of the resistance to anterior displacement [5,37,78,81]. The three glenohumeral ligaments also limit excessive lateral rotation of the glenohumeral joint [54,75]. As with anterior displacement, increasing abduction increases the role the inferior glenohumeral ligament plays in limiting lateral rotation [43].

Although the posterior capsule is reinforced passively only by a portion of the inferior glenohumeral ligament, it too provides resistance to excessive glide of the glenohumeral joint. The posterior capsule functions as a barrier to excessive posterior glide of the humeral head. It also limits excessive medial rotation of the joint. In certain positions of the glenohumeral joint, the anterior and posterior portions of the glenohumeral joint capsule are under tension simultaneously, demonstrating how the function of the capsule and its reinforcing ligaments is complex and interdependent [10,95].

There are opposing views regarding the support of the glenohumeral joint against inferior glide. The weight of the upper extremity in upright posture promotes inferior glide of the humeral head on the glenoid fossa. Some authors suggest that inferior glide of the humeral head is resisted by the pull of the coracohumeral ligament and to a lesser degree by the superior glenohumeral ligament, particularly when the joint is laterally rotated [18,34,42]. However, another cadaver study reports little support from the superior glenohumeral ligament against inferior subluxation [90]. This study, which suggests that the inferior glenohumeral ligament provides more support in the inferior direction, with additional support from the coracohumeral ligament, examines smaller displacements than the preceding studies. The individual contributions from these supporting structures may depend on the position of the glenohumeral joint and the magnitude of the humeral displacements. Additional research is needed to elucidate the roles the glenohumeral joint capsule and ligaments play in supporting the glenohumeral joint. Subtle changes in joint position also appear to alter the stresses applied to the capsuloligamentous complex.

Clinical Relevance

EXAMINING OR STRETCHING THE GLENOHUMERAL JOINT LIGAMENTS: *Altering the position of the glenohumeral joint allows the clinician to selectively assess specific portions of the glenohumeral capsuloligamentous complex. For example, lateral rotation of the glenohumeral joint reduces the amount of anterior translation of the humeral head by several millimeters. If the clinician assesses anterior glide of the humeral head with the joint laterally rotated and does not observe a reduction in the anterior glide excursion, the clinician may suspect injury to the anterior capsuloligamentous complex.*

Similarly, by altering the position of the glenohumeral joint, the clinician can direct treatment toward a particular portion of the complex. Anterior glide with the glenohumeral joint abducted applies a greater stretch to the inferior glenohumeral ligament than to the superior and middle glenohumeral ligaments. The clinician can also use such knowledge to reduce the loads on an injured or repaired structure.

One of the factors coupling the support of the glenohumeral ligaments and capsule to each other is the **intraarticular pressure** that also helps to support the glenohumeral joint [41,42]. Puncturing, or **venting,** the rotator interval in cadavers results in a reduction of the inferior stability of the humeral head, even in the presence of an otherwise intact capsule [42,102]. Isolated closure of rotator interval defects appears to restore stability in young subjects who have no additional glenohumeral joint damage [23]. This supports the notion that tears in this part of the capsule can destabilize the joint not only by a structural weakening of the capsule itself but also by a disruption of the normal intraarticular pressure.

Thus the capsule with its reinforcing ligaments acts as a barrier to excessive translation of the humeral head and limits motion of the glenohumeral joint, particularly at the ends of glenohumeral ROM. It also contributes to the normal glide of the humerus on the glenoid fossa during shoulder motion. However, this complex of ligaments still is insufficient to stabilize the glenohumeral joint, particularly when external loads are applied to the upper extremity or as the shoulder moves through the middle of its full ROM. The role of the muscles in stabilization of the glenohumeral joint is discussed in Chapter 9.

MOTIONS OF THE GLENOHUMERAL JOINT

As a ball-and-socket joint, the glenohumeral joint has three axes of motion that lie in the cardinal planes of the body. Therefore the motions available at the glenohumeral joint are

- Flexion/extension
- Abduction/adduction
- Medial/lateral (internal/external) rotation

Abduction and flexion sometimes are each referred to as **elevation.** Authors also distinguish between elevation of the glenohumeral joint in the plane of the scapula and that in the sagittal and frontal planes.

Flexion and abduction in the sagittal and frontal planes of the body, respectively, occur with simultaneous rotation of the glenohumeral joint about its long axis. Rotation of the humerus during shoulder elevation is necessary to maximize the space between the acromion and proximal humerus. This space, known as the **subacromial space,** contains the subacromial bursa, the muscle and tendon of the supraspinatus, the superior portion of the glenohumeral joint capsule, and the intraarticular tendon of the long head of the biceps brachii

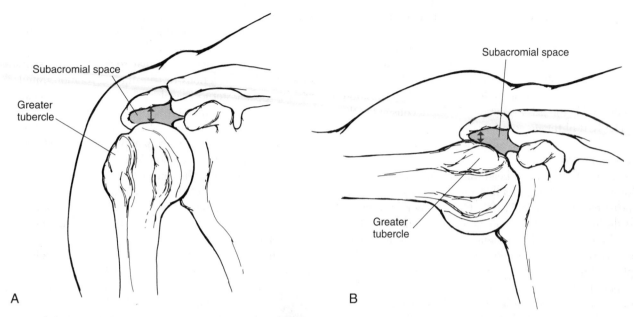

Figure 8.28: Subacromial space during abduction. **A.** The subacromial space is large when the shoulder is in neutral. **B.** During shoulder abduction the greater tubercle moves closer to the acromion, narrowing the subacromial space.

(*Fig. 8.28*). Each of these structures could sustain injury with the repeated or sustained compression that would occur without humeral rotation during shoulder elevation.

Determining the exact direction and pattern of humeral rotation during shoulder elevation has proven challenging. The traditional clinical view is that lateral rotation of the humerus accompanies shoulder abduction, and medial rotation occurs with shoulder flexion [6,86,93]. Consistent with this view is that little or no axial rotation occurs with shoulder elevation in the plane of the scapula [86]. Data to support these concepts come from cadaver and two-dimensional analysis of humeral motion in vivo.

More recently three-dimensional studies of arm-trunk motion call these data into question. Most of these reports agree that the humerus undergoes lateral rotation during shoulder abduction [63,94]. However, these studies also suggest that lateral rotation may occur in shoulder flexion as well. In order to interpret these differing views regarding axial rotation and shoulder flexion, it is essential to note that these more recent studies use three-dimensional analysis and employ euler angles to describe these motions. Euler angles are extremely sensitive to the order in which they are determined and are not comparable to two-dimensional anatomical measurements.

Despite the confusion regarding the exact anatomical rotations that occur with shoulder elevation, it remains clear that axial rotation of the humerus is an essential ingredient of shoulder elevation. Large compressive forces are reported on the coracohumeral ligament in healthy individuals who actively medially rotate the shoulder through the full ROM while maintaining 90° of shoulder abduction [103]. Such forces would also compress the contents of the subacromial space, thereby creating the potential for an impingement syndrome.

Clinical Relevance

SHOULDER IMPINGEMENT SYNDROME IN COMPETITIVE SWIMMERS: *Impingement syndrome is the cluster of signs and symptoms that result from chronic irritation of any or all of the structures in the subacromial space. Such irritation can come from repeated or sustained compression resulting from an intermittent or prolonged narrowing of the subacromial space. Symptoms of impingement are common in competitive swimmers and include pain in the superior aspect of the shoulder beginning in the midranges of shoulder elevation and worsening with increasing excursion of flexion or abduction.*

Most competitive swimming strokes require the shoulder to actively and repeatedly assume a position of shoulder abduction with medial rotation. This position narrows the subacromial space and consequently increases the risk of impingement. Some clinicians and coaches suggest that to prevent impingement, swimmers must strengthen their scapular muscles so that scapular position can enhance the subacromial space even as the humeral position tends to narrow it.

Although flexion, abduction, and rotation of the glenohumeral joint imply pure rotational movements, the asymmetrical articular areas of the humeral head and glenoid fossa, the pull of the capsuloligamentous complex, and the forces from the surrounding muscles result in a complex combination of rotation and gliding motions at the glenohumeral joint. If the motion of the glenohumeral joint consisted entirely of pure rotation, the motion could be described as a rotation about a fixed axis. When rotation is accompanied by gliding, the rotation can be described as occurring about a moving axis. As described in Chapter 7, the degree of mobility of the axis of rotation in the two-dimensional case is described by the **instant center of rotation** (ICR). The ICR is the location of the axis of motion at a given joint position. The more stable the axis of motion, the more constant is the ICR. The ICR of the glenohumeral joint moves only slightly during flexion or abduction of the shoulder, indicating only minimal translation [100].

The amount of humeral head translation during shoulder motion has received considerable attention among clinicians and researchers [28,33,34,52,100]. Glenohumeral translation is less during active shoulder motions when muscle contractions help to stabilize the humeral head than during passive motions [28]. In active elevation of the glenohumeral joint in the plane of the scapula, the humeral head undergoes minimal superior glide (≤3 mm) and then remains fixed or glides inferiorly no more than 1 mm [11,21,28,50,80,89]. Individuals with muscle fatigue or glenohumeral instability, however, consistently exhibit excessive superior glide during active shoulder elevation [10,18,21,46].

The humeral head glides posteriorly in shoulder extension and in lateral rotation; it translates anteriorly during abduction and medial rotation [28,33,68,70,75,89]. These data contradict the so-called **concave–convex rule,** which states that the convex humeral head glides on the concave glenoid fossa in directions opposite the humeral roll. For example, the concave–convex rule predicts that inferior glide of the humerus accompanies its superior roll in flexion or abduction, and lateral rotation occurs with anterior glide [86,93]. Direct measurements reveal otherwise, showing repeatedly that the concave–convex rule does *not* apply to the glenohumeral joint.

Although slight, joint glides appear to accompany glenohumeral motions. This recognition supports the standard clinical practice of restoring translational movement to restore full ROM at the glenohumeral joint. The concept of joint glide at the glenohumeral joint also forms the theoretical basis for many mobilization techniques used in the clinic. Reporting the amount of available passive humeral head glide as a percentage of the glenoid diameter in the direction of the glide, a study of anesthetized subjects without shoulder pathology reports that the humeral head can glide 17, 26, and 29% in the anterior, posterior, and inferior directions, respectively, with the glenohumeral joint in neutral [35]. Passive glides of almost 1.5 cm are reported in subjects without shoulder impairments [9,65]. Patients with anterior instabilities demonstrate significant increases in both anterior and inferior directions. Patients with multidirectional instabilities exhibit significantly increased excursions in all three directions [11,21]. It is essential for the clinician to understand that slight translation occurs in normal glenohumeral joint motion. Yet excessive translation may contribute to significant dysfunction.

Total glenohumeral joint elevation is most frequently described as a percentage of shoulder complex motion. Glenohumeral flexion and abduction are reported to be 100–120° [40,80,98]; however, shoulder rotation comes solely from the glenohumeral joint. Although protraction of the sternoclavicular joint and abduction and internal rotation of the scapulothoracic joint cause the humerus to face medially, these are substitutions for medial rotation of the shoulder rather than contributions to true medial rotation. Similarly, retraction of the sternoclavicular joint and adduction, posterior tilting, and external rotation of the scapulothoracic joint can substitute for lateral rotation of the shoulder. True shoulder rotation ROM values range from approximately 70 to 90° for both medial and lateral rotation. There are no known studies that identify the contribution of the glenohumeral joint to shoulder extension, but the glenohumeral joint is the likely source of most extension excursion, with only a minor contribution from adduction, downward rotation and anterior tilt of the scapulothoracic joint.

In summary, this section reviews the individual joints that constitute the shoulder complex. Each joint has a unique structure that results in a unique pattern of mobility and stability. The overall function of the shoulder complex depends on the individual contributions of each joint. A patient's complaints to the clinician usually are focused on the function of the shoulder as a whole, such as an inability to reach overhead or the presence of pain in throwing a ball. The clinician must then determine where the impairment is within the shoulder complex. A full understanding of the role of each joint in the overall function of the shoulder complex is essential to the successful evaluation of the shoulder complex. The following section presents the role of each joint in the production of normal motion of the shoulder complex.

TOTAL SHOULDER MOVEMENT

The term *shoulder* means different things to different people (i.e., the shoulder complex or the glenohumeral joint). Therefore, motion in this region is perhaps more clearly presented as **arm–trunk motion,** since motion of the shoulder complex generally is described by the angle formed between the arm and the trunk (*Fig. 8.29*). However, the literature and clinical vocabulary commonly use **shoulder motion** to mean arm–trunk motion. Therefore, both terms, *arm–trunk motion* and *shoulder motion,* are used interchangeably in the rest of this chapter. For the purposes of clarity, the terms **arm–trunk elevation** and **shoulder elevation** are used to mean abduction or flexion of the shoulder complex. These can occur in the cardinal planes of the body or in the plane of the scapula. When the distinction is important, the plane of the motion is identified. It is essential to recognize the distinction between *shoulder elevation,* which involves all of the joints of the shoulder complex, and *scapular elevation,* which is motion of the scapulothoracic joint and indirectly produces elevation at the sternoclavicular joint but does not include glenohumeral joint motion. The following section describes the individual contributions of the four joints of the shoulder complex to the total arm-trunk motion. In addition, the timing of these contributions and the rhythmic interplay of the joints are discussed.

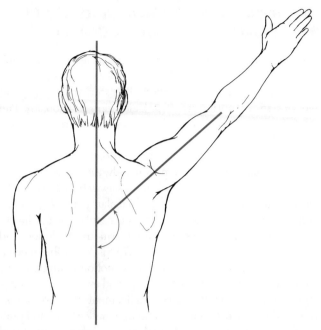

Figure 8.29: Arm–trunk motion. Shoulder motion is described by the orientation of the mechanical axis of the arm with respect to the trunk.

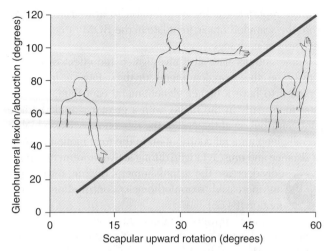

Figure 8.30: Contribution of the glenohumeral and scapulohumeral joints to arm–trunk motion. There is approximately 2° of glenohumeral motion to every 1° of scapulothoracic motion during shoulder flexion or abduction.

Movement of the Scapula and Humerus during Arm–Trunk Elevation

During arm–trunk elevation the scapula rotates upward as the glenohumeral joint flexes or abducts. In addition, the scapula tilts posteriorly about a medial–lateral axis and rotates externally about a vertical axis during shoulder elevation [29,47,60,63]. Upward rotation is the largest scapulothoracic motion in shoulder elevation. It has long been recognized that the upward rotation of the scapula and the flexion or abduction of the humerus occur synchronously throughout arm–trunk elevation in healthy individuals [66]. In the last 50 years, several systematic studies have been undertaken to quantify this apparent rhythm, known as **scapulohumeral rhythm.** The vast majority of these studies have examined the relationship of movement at the joints of the shoulder complex during voluntary, active shoulder movement. In addition, some of these investigations examine arm–trunk movement in the cardinal planes of the body, while others report motions in the plane of the scapula. Some of the differences in the results of the studies discussed below may be attributable to these methodological differences.

The classic study of the motion of the shoulder is by Inman et al. in 1944 [40]. Although some of the data reported in this study have been refuted, the study continues to form the basis for understanding the contributions made by the individual joints to the total movement of the shoulder complex. These investigators report on the active, voluntary motion of the shoulder complex in the sagittal and frontal planes of the body in individuals without shoulder pathology. They state that for every 2° of glenohumeral joint abduction or flexion there is 1° of upward rotation at the scapulothoracic joint, resulting in

a 2:1 ratio of glenohumeral to scapulothoracic joint movement in both flexion and abduction (*Fig. 8.30*). Thus these authors suggest that the glenohumeral joint contributes approximately 120° of flexion or abduction and the scapulothoracic joint contributes approximately 60° of upward rotation of the scapula, yielding a total of about 180° of arm–trunk elevation. The authors state that the ratio of glenohumeral to scapulothoracic motion becomes apparent and remains constant after approximately 30° of abduction and approximately 60° of flexion. McClure et al. also found a 2:1 ratio for scapulohumeral rhythm during active shoulder flexion [63]. In contrast these authors and others report mostly smaller ratios for shoulder elevation in the scapular plane [1,25,29,63,80]. In other words, these authors report more scapular (or less glenohumeral) contribution to the total movement.

These results are presented in *Table 8.1.* McQuade and Smidt do not report average ratios [66]. However, in contrast to the data reported in Table 8.1, their data suggest even more contribution to the total movement by the glenohumeral joint than is suggested by Inman et al., with ratios varying from approximately 3:1 to 4:1 through the range. In addition, several authors report a variable ratio rather than the constant ratio reported by Inman et al. [1,29,66,80]. Although there is little agreement in the actual change in the ratios, most

TABLE 8.1: Reported Average Ratios of Glenohumeral to Scapulothoracic Motion during Active Arm–Trunk Elevation in the Plane of the Scapula

Authors	Ratio
Freedman and Munro [25]	1.58:1
Poppen and Walker [80]	1.25:1
Bagg and Forrest [1]	1.25:1 to 1.33:1
Graichen et al. [29]	1.5:1 to 2.4:1
McClure [63]	1.7:1

authors report a greater contribution to arm–trunk motion from the scapulothoracic joint late in the ROM rather than in the early or midrange.

Some authors have also investigated the effect of muscle activity on the scapulohumeral rhythm. Passive motion is reported to have a higher glenohumeral contribution to the movement early in the range, with a greater scapulothoracic joint contribution at the end of the motion as well as a higher overall glenohumeral contribution to the total motion [29,66]. Resistance and muscle fatigue during active movement reportedly decrease the scapulohumeral rhythm, resulting in an increased scapulothoracic contribution to the motion [64,66].

In addition to upward rotation, the scapula also exhibits slight external rotation until at least 90° of shoulder elevation [19,22,63]. The scapula also exhibits a few degrees of posterior tilt through at least the first 90° of shoulder elevation.

Despite the differences reported in the literature, some very important similarities exist. Conclusions to be drawn from these studies of healthy shoulders are

- The scapulothoracic and glenohumeral joints move simultaneously through most of the full range of shoulder elevation.
- Both the glenohumeral and scapulothoracic joints contribute significantly to the overall motion of flexion and abduction of the shoulder.
- The scapula and humerus move in a systematic and coordinated rhythm.
- The exact ratio of glenohumeral to scapulothoracic motion may vary according to the plane of motion and the location within the ROM.
- The exact ratio of glenohumeral to scapulothoracic motion during active ROM is likely to depend on muscle activity.
- There is likely to be significant variability among individuals.

The clinician can use these observations to help identify abnormal movement patterns and to help understand the mechanisms relating shoulder impairments to dysfunction.

Clinical Relevance

ANOTHER POSSIBLE MECHANISM PRODUCING SHOULDER IMPINGEMENT SYNDROME: *Shoulder, or subacromial, impingement syndrome results from a persistent or repeated compression of the structures within the subacromial space, the space between the acromion process and humeral head. As noted earlier in the chapter, abnormal humeral axial rotation may contribute to the compressive forces leading to impingement. Another possible source of impingement is abnormal scapulothoracic motion during shoulder elevation. Either excessive scapular internal rotation or anterior tilt could narrow the subacromial space and produce compression of the subacromial contents. Repeated or prolonged compression could cause an inflammatory response resulting in pain.*

Sternoclavicular and Acromioclavicular Motion during Arm–Trunk Elevation

With the upward rotation of the scapula during arm–trunk elevation, there must be concomitant elevation of the clavicle to which the scapula is attached. The sternoclavicular joint elevates 15–40° during arm–trunk elevation [1,40,59,98]. The joint also retracts and upwardly rotates during arm-trunk elevation [40,63,59].

Note that the total scapular upward rotation is 60° and the total clavicular elevation is approximately 40°. This disparity of motion suggests that the scapula moves away from the clavicle, causing motion at the acromioclavicular joint (*Fig. 8.31*). Although the motion at the acromioclavicular joint is inadequately studied, its motion during arm–trunk flexion and abduction appears undeniable [82,87,98]. A possible mechanism to control the acromioclavicular motion is proposed by Inman et al. [40]. As the scapula is pulled away from the clavicle by upward rotation, the conoid ligament (the vertical portion of the coracoclavicular ligament) is pulled tight and pulls on the conoid tubercle situated on the inferior surface of the crank-shaped clavicle. The tubercle is drawn toward the coracoid process, causing the clavicle to be pulled into upward rotation (Fig. 8.31). The crank shape of the clavicle allows the clavicle to remain close to the scapula as it completes its lateral rotation, without using additional elevation ROM at the sternoclavicular joint. The sternoclavicular joint thus elevates

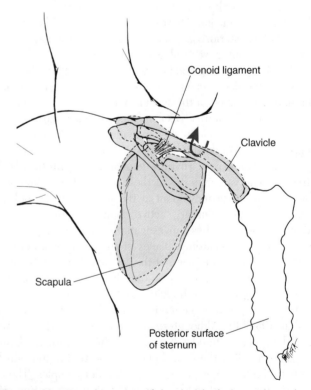

Figure 8.31: Upward rotation of the clavicle during arm–trunk motion. As the scapula moves away from the clavicle during arm–trunk elevation, the conoid ligament is pulled taut and causes the clavicle to rotate upwardly.

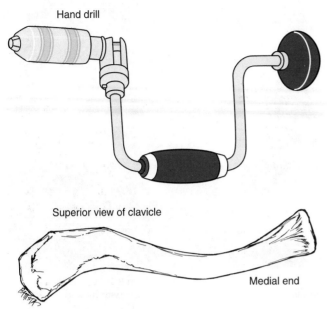

Hand drill

Superior view of clavicle

Medial end

Figure 8.32: Crank shape of clavicle. The shape of the clavicle allows the conoid tubercle to rotate toward the scapula while the medial and lateral ends of the clavicle stay relatively fixed.

less than its full available ROM, which is approximately 60°. Therefore, full shoulder flexion or abduction can still be augmented by additional sternoclavicular elevation in activities that require an extra-long reach, such as reaching to the very top shelf. This sequence of events demonstrates the significance of the crank shape of the clavicle and the mobility of the acromioclavicular joint to the overall motion of the shoulder complex (*Fig. 8.32*). The coordinated pattern of movement at the sternoclavicular and scapulothoracic joints during normal shoulder flexion and abduction also reveals the role of the conoid ligament in *producing* movement, unlike most ligaments that only limit movement.

This description of sternoclavicular and acromioclavicular motion reveals the remarkable synergy of movement among all four joints of the shoulder complex necessary to complete full arm–trunk flexion and abduction. The scapulothoracic joint must rotate upward to allow full glenohumeral flexion or abduction. The clavicle must elevate and upwardly rotate to allow scapular rotation. This extraordinary coordination occurs in activities as diverse and demanding as lifting a 20-lb child overhead and throwing a 95-mph fastball. However, the rhythm certainly is interrupted in some individuals. Any of the four joints can be impaired. The following section considers the effects of impairments of the individual joints on overall shoulder movement.

Impairments in Individual Joints and Their Effects on Shoulder Motion

The preceding section discusses the intricately interwoven rhythms of the four joints of the shoulder complex during arm–trunk motion. This section focuses on the effects of

alterations in the mechanics of any of these joints on shoulder motion. Common pathologies involving the glenohumeral joint include capsular tears, rheumatoid arthritis, and inferior subluxations secondary to stroke. The sternoclavicular joint can be affected by rheumatoid arthritis or by ankylosing spondylitis. The acromioclavicular joint is frequently dislocated and also is susceptible to osteoarthritis. Scapulothoracic joint function can be compromised by trauma such as a gunshot wound or by scarring resulting from such injuries as burns. These are just examples to emphasize that each joint of the shoulder complex is susceptible to pathologies that impair its function. Each joint is capable of losing mobility and thus affecting the mobility of the entire shoulder complex. It is not possible to consider all conceivable pathologies and consequences. The purpose of this section is to consider the altered mechanics and potential substitutions resulting from abnormal motion at each of the joints of the shoulder complex. Such consideration illustrates a framework from which to evaluate the function of the shoulder complex and the integrity of its components.

LOSS OF GLENOHUMERAL OR SCAPULOTHORACIC JOINT MOTION

As discussed earlier in this chapter, the data from studies of scapulohumeral rhythm suggest that the glenohumeral joint provides more than 50% of the total shoulder flexion or abduction. Therefore, the loss of glenohumeral motion has a profound effect on shoulder motion. However, it must be emphasized that shoulder motion is not lost completely, even with complete glenohumeral joint immobility. The scapulothoracic and sternoclavicular joints with the acromioclavicular joint combine to provide the remaining one third or more motion. In the absence of glenohumeral movement these joints, if healthy, may become even more mobile. Thus without glenohumeral joint motion and in the presence of intact scapulothoracic, sternoclavicular, and acromioclavicular joints, an individual should still have at least one third the normal shoulder flexion or abduction ROM.

Complete loss of glenohumeral joint motion, however, results in total loss of shoulder rotation. Yet even under these conditions scapulothoracic motion can provide some substitution. Forward tipping of the scapula about a medial–lateral axis is a common substitution for decreased medial rotation of the shoulder.

Clinical Relevance

MEASUREMENT OF MEDIAL ROTATION ROM OF THE SHOULDER: *Goniometry manuals describe measurement of medial rotation of the shoulder with the subject lying supine and the shoulder abducted to 90° [74]. In this position the shoulder is palpated to identify anterior tilting of the scapula as the shoulder is medially rotated. Firm manual stabilization is usually necessary to prevent the scapula from tilting anteriorly to substitute for medial rotation* (Fig. 8.33).

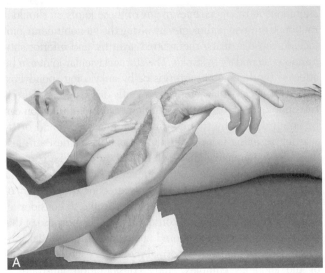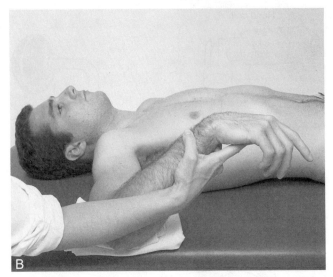

Figure 8.33: Scapular substitutions in shoulder ROM. **A.** Standard goniometric measurement of medial rotation ROM of shoulder requires adequate stabilization of the scapula. **B.** Inadequate stabilization allows anterior tilting of the scapula with an apparent increase in medial rotation ROM of the shoulder.

Conversely, the loss of scapulothoracic motion results in a loss of at least one third of full shoulder elevation ROM. Although this appears to be roughly true in passive ROM, Inman et al. report that in the absence of scapulothoracic joint motion, active shoulder abduction is closer to 90° of abduction rather than the expected 120° [40]. These authors hypothesize that upward rotation of the scapula is essential to maintaining

an adequate contractile length of the deltoid muscle. Scapular upward rotation lengthens the deltoid even as the muscle contracts across the glenohumeral joint during abduction (*Fig. 8.34*). In the absence of upward scapular rotation, the deltoid contracts and reaches its maximal shortening, approximately 60% of its resting length, by the time the glenohumeral joint reaches about 90° of abduction. (See Chapter 4 for details

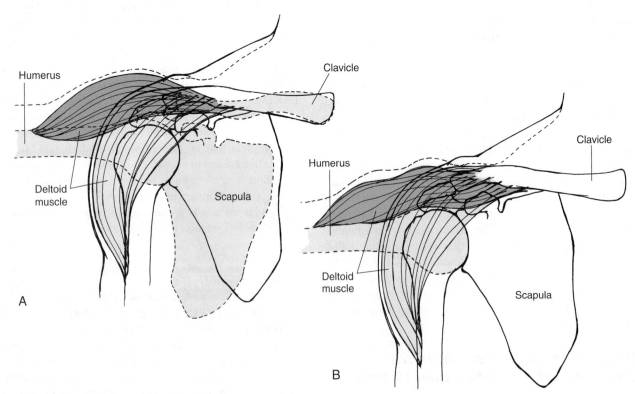

Figure 8.34: Scapular motion and deltoid muscle function. **A.** During normal active shoulder abduction, the upward rotation of the scapula lengthens the deltoid, maintaining an adequate contractile length. **B.** During shoulder abduction without scapular rotation, the deltoid reaches its maximal shortening and is unable to pull the glenohumeral joint through its full abduction ROM.

on muscle mechanics.) Thus without the contributions of the scapulothoracic joint motion, passive ROM of shoulder flexion and abduction are reduced by at least one third. However, active ranges in these two directions appear to be even more severely affected.

In addition to the overall loss of passive and active excursion, decreased scapulothoracic joint motion impairs the synergistic rhythm between the scapulothoracic and glenohumeral joints. This may contribute directly to abnormal glenohumeral joint motion and result in an impingement syndrome.

Clinical Relevance

NO WONDER SHOULDER IMPINGEMENT IS SO COMMON!: *Shoulder impingement syndrome is the most common source of shoulder complaints, and the complicated and finely coordinated mechanics of the shoulder complex help explain the frequency of complaints [67]. Earlier clinical relevance boxes demonstrate the possible contributions to impingement syndromes from dysfunction within individual components of the shoulder complex, such as abnormal axial rotation of the humerus or abnormal scapular positions [50,53,61]. Abnormal scapulothoracic rhythm during shoulder flexion or abduction is also associated with impingement syndromes, although it is unclear whether the abnormal rhythm is a cause or an effect of the impingement [12,60].*

The multiple mechanical dysfunctions that can lead to symptoms of impingement demonstrate the importance of understanding the normal mechanical behavior of each individual component of the shoulder complex as well as the behavior of the complex as a whole. With such an understanding the clinician will be able to thoroughly and accurately evaluate the movements and alignments of the individual parts of the shoulder as well as the coordinated function of the entire complex in order to develop a sound strategy for intervention.

LOSS OF STERNOCLAVICULAR OR ACROMIOCLAVICULAR JOINT MOTION

For the scapulothoracic joint to rotate upwardly 60°, the sternoclavicular joint must elevate, and the acromioclavicular joint must glide or rotate slightly. If the clavicle is unable to elevate but the acromioclavicular joint can still move, the scapulothoracic joint may still be able to contribute slightly to total shoulder motion but is likely to have a significant reduction in movement. The effects of lost or diminished scapulothoracic joint motion noted in the preceding section would then follow. If acromioclavicular joint motion is lost, disruption of scapulothoracic joint motion again occurs, although perhaps to a lesser degree than with sternoclavicular joint restriction.

It is important to recognize the potential plasticity of the shoulder complex. Decreased motion at the acromioclavicular joint appears to result in increased sternoclavicular motions, and decreased motion at the sternoclavicular joint results in increased motion at the acromioclavicular joint [82].

Inman et al. report that one subject with the acromioclavicular joint pinned had only 60° of shoulder elevation remaining [40]. However, others report far less dysfunction with loss of motion at the acromioclavicular joint [51]. Perhaps the effects of the loss of acromioclavicular motion depend upon the viability of the remaining structures or the presence of pain.

Case reports suggest that total resection of the clavicle secondary to neoplastic disease and chronic infection have no negative effects on passive ROM of the shoulder [57]. However, scapulohumeral rhythms are not reported. Similarly in another study, 71% of the individuals who underwent distal resection of the clavicle to decrease acromioclavicular pain returned to recreational sports [24]. These data suggest that while there is clear interplay among the four joints of the shoulder complex, there also appears to be a remarkable capacity to compensate for losses by altering the performance of the remaining structures. However, an important consequence of such alterations may be the overuse of remaining joints or the development of hypermobility elsewhere in the system. Therefore, diagnosis of mechanical impairments of the shoulder requires careful assessment of overall shoulder function but also identification of each joint's contribution to the shoulder's total motion.

Clinical Relevance

IDENTIFYING LINKS BETWEEN A PATIENT'S COMPLAINTS AND ABNORMAL JOINT MOBILITY: *A 60-year-old male patient came to physical therapy with complaints of shoulder pain. He reported a history of a severe "shoulder" fracture from a motorcycle accident 30 years earlier. He noted that he had never regained normal shoulder mobility. However, he reported that he had good functional use of his shoulder. He owned a gas station and was an auto mechanic and was able to function fully in those capacities, but he reported increasing discomfort in his shoulder during and after activity. He noted that the pain was primarily on the "top" of his shoulder.*

Active and passive ROM were equally limited in the symptomatic shoulder: 0–80° of flexion, 0–70° of abduction, 0° medial and lateral rotation. Palpation during ROM revealed a 1:1 ratio of scapular to arm–trunk motion, revealing that all of the arm–trunk motion was coming from the scapulothoracic joint. Palpation revealed tenderness and crepitus at the acromioclavicular joint during shoulder movement.

These findings suggested that in the absence of glenohumeral joint motion, the sternoclavicular and acromioclavicular joints developed hypermobility as the patient maximized shoulder function, ultimately resulting in pain at the acromioclavicular joint. This impression was later corroborated by radiological findings of complete fusion of the glenohumeral joint and osteoarthritis of the acromioclavicular joint. Since there was no chance of increasing glenohumeral joint mobility, treatment was directed toward decreasing the pain at the acromioclavicular joint.

It should be clear that because shoulder motion originates from several locations and normally occurs in a systematic and coordinated manner, evaluation of total shoulder function depends on the ability to assess the individual components and then consider their contributions to the whole. The evaluation requires consideration of the shoulder movement as a whole as well. The following section presents a review of normal arm–trunk ROM.

SHOULDER RANGE OF MOTION

Values of "normal" ROM reported in the literature are presented in *Table 8.2*. Examination of this table reveals large differences among the published values of normal ROM, particularly in extension, abduction, and lateral rotation of the shoulder complex. Unfortunately, many authors offer no information to explain how these normal values were determined. Consequently, it is impossible to explain the disparity displayed in the literature.

All but one of the references report that lateral rotation is greater than medial rotation. The two studies that report empirical data also suggest that abduction ROM may be slightly greater than flexion ROM, although direct comparisons are not reported [8,71]. In addition, these two studies indicate that gender and age may have significant effects on these values. Thus at the present time, values of "normal" ROM must be used with caution to provide a perspective for the clinician without serving as a precise indicator of the presence or absence of pathology. The clinician must also consider the contributions to the total motion made by the individual components as well as the sequencing of those contributions.

Clinical Relevance

SHOULDER MOTION IN ACTIVITIES OF DAILY LIVING:
Magermans et al. report the shoulder mobility required in diverse activities of daily living (ADL) [62]. Activities such as combing one's hair use an average of 90° of glenohumeral flexion or abduction, 70° of lateral rotation of the shoulder, and approximately 35° of concomitant scapular upward rotation. In contrast personal hygiene activities such as perineal care use glenohumeral hyperextension and essentially full medial rotation ROM. As the clinician strives to help a patient regain or maintain functional independence, the clinician must work to ensure that the mobility needed for function is available and that all four components of the shoulder complex contribute to the mobility appropriately.

SUMMARY

This chapter examines the bones and joints of the shoulder complex, which allow considerable mobility but possess inherent challenges to stability. The bones provide little limitation to the motion of the shoulder under normal conditions. The primary limits to normal shoulder motion are the capsuloligamentous complex and the surrounding muscles of the shoulder. The normal function of the shoulder complex depends on the integrity of four individual joint structures and their coordinated contributions to arm–trunk motion. The glenohumeral joint is the sole contributor to medial and lateral rotation of the shoulder and contributes over 50% of

TABLE 8.2: Normal ROM Values from the Literature (in Degrees)

	Flexion	Extension	Abduction	Medial Rotation	Lateral Rotation	Abduction in Scapular Plane
Steindler [93]	180	30–40	150			
US Army/Air Force [20]	180	60	180	70	90	
Boone and Azin [8][a]	165.0 ± 5.0	57.3 ± 8.1	182.7 ± 9.0	67.1 ± 4.1	99.6 ± 7.6	
Hislop and Montgomery [36][b]	180	45	180	80	60	170
Murray, et al [71]	170 ± 2[c]	57 ± 3[c]	178 ± 1[c]	49 ± 3[c]	94 ± 2[c]	
	172 ± 1[d]	58 ± 3[d]	180 ± 1[d]	53 ± 3[d]	101 ± 2[d]	
	165 ± 2[e]	55 ± 2[e]	178 ± 1[e]	59 ± 2[e]	82 ± 4[e]	
	170 ± 1[f]	61 ± 2[f]	178 ± 1[f]	56 ± 2[f]	94 ± 2[f]	
Gerhardt and Rippstein [27]	170	50	170	80	90	
Bagg and Forrest [1]						168.1
Freedman and Munro [25]						167.17 ± 7.57

[a]Data from 56 adult males. These values are also used as "normal" values by the American Academy of Orthopedic Surgeons.
[b]Reported wide ranges from the literature.
[c]Data from 20 young adult males.
[d]Data from 20 young adult females.
[e]Data from 20 male elders.
[f]Data from 20 female elders.

the motion in arm–trunk elevation. The remaining arm–trunk elevation comes from upward rotation of the scapula. The scapula also undergoes posterior tilting and lateral rotation about a vertical axis during arm–trunk elevation. In addition to glenohumeral and scapulothoracic contributions to arm–trunk elevation, the sternoclavicular and acromioclavicular joints contribute important motions to allow full, pain-free arm–trunk elevation. Impairments in the individual joints of the shoulder complex produce altered arm–trunk movement and are likely contributors to complaints of pain in the shoulder complex.

Throughout this chapter the importance of muscular support to the shoulder is emphasized. The following chapter presents the muscles of the shoulder complex and discusses their contributions to the stability and mobility of the shoulder.

References

1. Bagg SD, Forrest WJ: A biomechanical analysis of scapular rotation during arm abduction in the scapular plane. Am J Phys Med Rehabil 1988; 238–245.
2. Basmajian JV, DeLuca CJ: Muscles Alive. Their Function Revealed by Electromyography. Baltimore: Williams & Wilkins, 1985.
3. Bearn JG: Direct observations on the function of the capsule of the sternoclavicular joint in clavicular support. J Anat 1967; 101: 159–170.
4. Bigliani L, Morrison DS, April EW: The morphology of the acromion and its relationship to rotator cuff tears. Orthop Trans 1986; 10: 228 (Abstract).
5. Bigliani LU, Kelkar R, Flatow EL, et al.: Glenohumeral stability biomechanical properties of passive and active stabilizers. Clin Orthop 1996; 330: 13–30.
6. Blakely RL, Palmer ML: Analysis of rotation accompanying shoulder flexion. Phys Ther 1984; 64: 1214–1216.
7. Blasier RB, Soslowsky LJ, Malicky DM, Palmer ML: Posterior glenohumeral subluxation: active and passive stabilization in a biomechanical model. J Bone Joint Surg 1997; 79A: 433–440.
8. Boone DC, Azen SP: Normal range of motion of joints in male subjects. J Bone Joint Surg 1979; 61-A: 756–759.
9. Borsa PA, Sauers EL, Herling DE, Manzour WF: In vivo quantification of capsular end-point in the noninjured glenohumeral joint using an instrumented measurement system. J Orthop Sports Phys Ther 2001; 31: 419–431.
10. Branch TP, Lawton RL, Iobst CA, Hutton WC: The role of glenohumeral capsular ligaments in internal and external rotation of the humerus. Am J Sports Med 1995; 23: 632–637.
11. Chen SK, Simonian PT, Wickiewicz TL, et al.: Radiographic evaluation of glenohumeral kinematics: a muscle fatigue model. J Shoulder Elbow Surg 1999; 8: 49–52.
12. Cohen RB, Williams GR Jr: Impingement syndrome and rotator cuff disease as repetitive motion disorders. Clin Orthop 1998; 95–101.
13. Costic RS, Vangura A, Fenwick JA, et al.: Viscoelastic behavior and structural properties of the coracoclavicular ligaments. Scand J Med Sci Sports 2003; 13: 305–310.
14. Couteau B, Mansat P, Darmana R, et al.: Morphological and mechanical analysis of the glenoid by 3D geometric reconstruction using computed tomography. Clin Biomech 2000; 15: S8–S12.
15. Crenshaw AH: Campbell's Operative Orthopaedics. Vol 2. St. Louis: Mosby Year Book, 1992.
16. Crenshaw AH: Campbell's Operative Orthopaedics. Vol 3. St. Louis: Mosby Year Book, 1992.
17. Culham E, Peat M: Functional anatomy of the shoulder complex. JOSPT 1993; 18: 342–350.
18. Curl LA, Warren RF: Glenohumeral joint stability selective cutting studies on the static capsular restraints. Clin Orthop 1996; 54–65.
19. Dayanidhi S, Orlin M, Kozin S, et al.: Scapular kinematics during humeral elevation in adults and children. Clin Biomech 2005; 20: 600–606.
20. Departments of the U.S. Army and Air Force. US Army Goniometry Manual: Technical Manual No. 8-640. Air Force Pamphlet No. 160-14. 1-8-1968. Washington, DC: Departments of the Army and Air Force.
21. Deutsch A, Altchek DW, Schwartz E, et al.: Radiologic measurement of superior displacement of the humeral head in the impingement syndrome. J Shoulder Elbow Surg 1996; 5: 186–193.
22. Ebaugh DD, McClure PW, Karduna AR: Three-dimensional scapulothoracic motion during active and passive arm elevation. Clin Biomech 2005; 20: 700–709.
23. Field LD, Warren RF, O'Brien SJ, et al.: Isolated closure of rotator interval for shoulder instability. Am J Sports Med 1995; 23: 557–563.
24. Flatow EL, Duralde XA, Nicholson GP, et al.: Arthroscopic resection of the distal clavicle with a superior approach. J Shoulder Elbow Surg 1995; 4: 41–50.
25. Freedman L, Munro RR: Abduction of the arm in the scapular plane: scapular and glenohumeral movements a roentgenographic study. J Bone Joint Surg 1966; 48A: 1503–1510.
26. Fukuda K, Craig EV, An K, et al.: Biomechanical study of the ligamentous system of the acromioclavicular joint. J Bone Joint Surg 1986; 68A: 434–440.
27. Gerhardt JJ, Rippstein J: Measuring and Recording of Joint Motion Instrumentation and Techniques. Lewiston, NJ: Hogrefe & Huber, 1990.
28. Graichen H, Stammberger T, Bonel H, et al.: Glenohumeral translation during active and passive elevation of the shoulder—a 3D open-MRI study. J Biomech 2000; 33: 609–613.
29. Graichen H, Stammberger T, Bonel H, et al.: Magnetic resonance based motion analysis of the shoulder during elevation. Clin Orthop 2000; 370: 154–163.
30. Grubbs N: Frozen shoulder syndrome: a review of literature. JOSPT 1993; 18: 479–487.
31. Hara H, Ito N, Iwasaki K: Strength of the glenoid labrum and adjacent shoulder capsule. Shoulder Elbow Surg 1996; 5: 263–268.
32. Harrington MA Jr, Keller TS, Seiler JGI, et al.: Geometric properties and the predicted mechanical behavior of adult human clavicles. J Biomech 1993; 26: 417–426.
33. Harryman DT II, Sidles JA, Clark JM, et al.: Translation of the humeral head on the glenoid with passive glenohumeral motion. J Bone Joint Surg 1990; 72-A: 1334–1343.
34. Harryman DT II, Sidles JA, Harris SL, Matsen FA III: The role of the rotator interval capsule in passive motion and stability of the shoulder. J Bone Joint Surg [AM] 1992; 74: 53–66.
35. Hawkins R, Schutte J, Janda D, Huckell G: Translation of the glenohumeral joint with the patient under anesthesia. J Shoulder Elbow Surg 1996; 5: 286–292.

36. Hislop HJ, Montgomery J: Daniel's and Worthingham's Muscle Testing: Techniques of Manual Examination. Philadelphia: WB Saunders, 1995.

37. Hjelm R, Draper C, Spencer S: Anterior-inferior capsular length insufficiency in the painful shoulder. JOSPT 1996; 23: 216–222.

38. Howell SM, Galinat BJ: The glenoid-labral socket. A constrained articular surface. Clin Orthop 1989; 243: 122–125.

39. Iannotti JP, Gabriel JP, Scheck SL, et al.: The normal glenohumeral relationships an anatomical study of one hundred and forty shoulders. J Bone Joint Surg 1992; 74A: 491–500.

40. Inman VT, Saunders JB, Abbott LC: Observations of the function of the shoulder Joint. J Bone Joint Surg 1944; 42: 1–30.

41. Inokuchi W, lsen B, Ojbjerg J, Neppen O: The relation between the position of the glenohumeral joint and the intraarticular pressure: an experimental study. J Shoulder Elbow Surg 1997; 6: 144–149.

42. Itoi E, Berglund LJ, Grabowski JJ, et al.: Superior-inferior stability of the shoulder: role of the coracohumeral ligament and the rotator interval capsule. Mayo Clin Proc 1998; 73: 508–515.

43. Jansen JHW, de Gast A, Snijders CJ: Glenohumeral elevation-dependent influence of anterior glenohumeral capsular lesions on passive axial humeral rotation. J Biomech 2006; 39: 1702–1707.

44. Jobe CM: Superior glenoid impingement. Orthop Clin North Am 1997; 28: 137–143.

45. Jobe CM, Iannotti JP: Limits imposed on glenohumeral motion by joint geometry. J Shoulder Elbow Surg 1995; 4: 281–285.

46. Kapandji IA: The Physiology of the Joints. Vol 1, The Upper Limb. Edinburgh: Churchill Livingstone, 1982.

47. Karduna AR, McClure PW, Michener L: Scapular kinematics: effects of altering the Euler angle sequence of rotations. J Biomech 2000; 33: 1063–1068.

48. Karduna AR, Williams GR, Williams JL, Iannotti JP: Glenohumeral joint translations before and after total shoulder arthroplasty. J Bone Joint Surg 1997; 79–A: 1166–1174.

49. Kebaetse M, McClure P, Pratt NA: Thoracic position effect on shoulder range of motion, strength, and three-dimensional scapular kinematics. Arch Phys Med Rehabil 1999; 80: 945–950.

50. Kelley MJ: Biomechanics of the shoulder. In: Orthopedic Therapy of the Shoulder. Kelley MJ, Clark WA, eds. Philadelphia: JB Lippincott, 1995.

51. Kennedy JC, Cameron H: Complete dislocation of the acromio-clavicular joint. J Bone Joint Surg 1954; 36: 202–208.

52. Kent BE: Functional anatomy of the shoulder complex a review. Phys Ther 1971; 51: 867–888.

53. Kibler WB: The role of the scapula in athletic shoulder function. Am J Sports Med 1998; 26: 325–337.

54. Kuhn JE, Huston LJ, Soslowsky LJ, et al.: External rotation of the glenohumeral joint: ligament restraints and muscle effects in the neutral and abducted positions. J Shoulder Elbow Surg 2005; 14: 39S–48S.

55. Lee K, Debski RE, Chen C, et al.: Functional evaluation of the ligaments at the acromioclavicular joint during anteroposterior and superoinferior translation. Am J Sports Med 1997; 25: 858–862.

56. Levinsohn EM, Santelli ED: Bicipital groove dysplasia and medial dislocation of the biceps brachii tendon. Skeletal Radiol 1991; 20: 419–423.

57. Lewis MM, Ballet FL, Kroll PG, Bloom N: En bloc clavicular resection: operative procedure and postoperative testing of function case reports. Clin Orthop 1985; 214–220.

58. Lucas D: Biomechanics of the shoulder joint. Arch Surg 1973; 107: 425–432.

59. Ludewig PM, Behrens SA, Meyer SM, et al.: Three-dimensional clavicular motion during arm elevation: reliability and descriptive data. JOSPT 2004; 34: 140–149.

60. Ludewig PM, Cook TM: Alterations in shoulder kinematics and associated muscle activity in people with symptoms of shoulder impingement. Phys Ther 2000; 80: 276–291.

61. Lukasiewicz AM, McClure P, Michener L, et al.: Comparison of 3-dimensional scapular position and orientation between subjects with and without shoulder impingement. J Orthop Sports Phys Ther 1999; 29: 574–586.

62. Magermans DJ, Chadwick EKJ, Veeger HEJ, van der Helm FCT: Requirements for upper extremity motions during activities of daily living. Clin Biomech 2005; 20: 591–599.

63. McClure PW, Michener LA, Sennett BJ, Karduna AR: Direct 3-dimensional measurement of scapular kinematics during dynamic movements in vivo. J Shoulder Elbow Surg 2001; 10: 269–277.

64. McQuade KJ, Dawson J, Smidt GL: Scapulothoracic muscle fatigue associated with alterations in scapulohumeral rhythm kinematics during maximum resistive shoulder elevation. JOSPT 1998; 28: 74–80.

65. McQuade KJ, Murthi AM: Anterior glenohumeral force/translation behavior with and without rotator cuff contraction during clinical stability testing. Clin Biomech 2004; 19: 10–15.

66. McQuade KJ, Smidt GL: Dynamic scapulohumeral rhythm: the effects of external resistance during elevation of the arm in the scapular plane. JOSPT 1998; 27: 125–133.

67. Michener LA, McClure PW, Karduna AR: Anatomical and biomechanical mechanisms of subacromial impingement syndrome. Clin Biomech 2003; 18: 369–379.

68. Moore SM, Musahl V, McMahon PJ, Debski RE: Multidirectional kinematics of the glenohumeral joint during simulated simple translation tests: impact on clinical diagnoses. J Orthop Res 2004; 22: 889–894.

69. Moseley H: The clavicle: its anatomy and function. Clin Orthop 1968; 58: 17–27.

70. Moseley H, Övergaard B: The anterior capsular mechanism in recurrent anterior dislocation of the shoulder. J Bone Joint Surg 1962; 44 B: 913–927.

71. Murray MP, Gore DR, Gardner GM, Mollinger LA: Shoulder motion and muscle strength of normal men and women in two age groups. Clin Orthop 1985; 268–273.

72. Nettles JL, Linscheid RL: Sternoclavicular dislocations. J Trauma 1968; 8: 158–164.

73. Neviaser TJ: Adhesive capsulitis. Orthop Clin North Am 1987; 18: 439–443.

74. Norkin CC, White DJ: Measurement of Joint Motion. A Guide to Goniometry. Philadelphia: FA Davis, 1995.

75. Novotny JE, Beynnon BD, Nichols CE: Modeling the stability of the human glenohumeral joint during external rotation. J Biomech 2000; 33: 345–354.

76. Novotny JE, Nichols CE, Beynnon BD: Kinematics of the glenohumeral joint with Bankart lesion and repair. J Bone Joint Surg 1998; 16: 116–121.

77. Nuemann CH, Petersen SA, Jahnke AH: MR imaging of the labral-capsular complex: normal variations. Am J Roentgenol 1991; 157: 1015–1021.

78. O'Connell PW, Nuber GW, Mileski RA, Lautenschlager E: The contribution of the glenohumeral ligaments to anterior stability of the shoulder joint. Am J Sports Med 1990; 18: 579–584.

79. Pagnani MJ, Deng XH, Warren RF, et al.: Effect of lesions of the superior portion of the glenoid labrum on glenohumeral translation. J Bone Joint Surg 1995; 77A: 1003–1010.

80. Poppen NK, Walker PS: Normal and abnormal motion of the shoulder. J Bone Joint Surg 1976; 58A: 195–201.

81. Pratt NE: Anatomy and biomechanics of the shoulder. J Hand Ther 1994; 7: 65–76.

82. Pronk GM, van der Helm FCT, Rozendaal LA: Interaction between the joints in the shoulder mechanism: the function of the costoclavicular, conoid and trapezoid ligaments. Proc Inst Mech Eng 1993; 207: 219–229.

83. Roberts D: Structure and function of the primate scapula. In: Primate Locomotion. Jenkins FA Jr., ed. New York: Academic Press, 1974; 171–200.

84. Romanes GJE: Cunningham's Textbook of Anatomy. Oxford: Oxford University Press, 1981.

85. Saha AK: Mechanics of elevation of glenohumeral joint, its application in rehabilitation of flail shoulder in upper brachial plexus injuries and poliomyelitis and in replacement of the upper humerus by prosthesis. Acta Orthop Scand 1973; 44: 668–678.

86. Saha AK: The classic mechanism of shoulder movements and a plea for the recognition of "zero position" of glenohumeral joint. Clin Orthop 1983; 3–10.

87. Sahara W, Sugamoto K, Murai M, et al.: 3D kinematic analysis of the acromioclavicular joint during arm abduction using vertically open MRI. J Orthop Res 2006; 24: 1823–1831.

88. Soslowsky LJ, An CH, Johnston SP, Carpenter JE: Geometric and mechanical properties of the coracoacromial ligament and their relationship to rotator cuff disease. Clin Orthop 1994; 10–17.

89. Soslowsky LJ, Flatow EL, Bigliani L, et al.: Quantitation of in situ contact areas at the glenohumeral joint: a biomechanical study. J Orthop Res 1992; 10: 524–534.

90. Soslowsky LJ, Malicky DM, Blasier RB: Active and passive factors in inferior glenohumeral stabilization: a biomechanical model. J Shoulder Elbow Surg 1997; 6: 371–379.

91. Spencer EE, Valdevit A, Kambic H, et al.: The effect of humeral component anteversion on shoulder stability with glenoid component retroversion. J Bone Joint Surg 2005; 87: 808–814.

92. Stanley D, Trowbridge EA, Norris SH: The mechanism of clavicular fracture: a clinical and biomechanical analysis. J Bone Joint Surg 1988; 70B: 461–464.

93. Steindler A: Kinesiology of the Human Body under Normal and Pathological Conditions. Springfield, IL: Charles C. Thomas, 1955.

94. Stokdijk M, Eilers PHC, Nagels J, Rozing PM: External rotation in the glenohumeral joint during elevation of the arm. Clin Biomech 2003; 18: 296–302.

95. Terry GC, Hammon D, France P, Norwood LA: The stabilizing function of passive shoulder restraints. Am J Sports Med 1991; 19: 26–34.

96. Thomas CB Jr, Friedman RJ: Case report ipsilateral sternoclavicular dislocation and clavicle fracture. J Orthop Trauma 1989; 3: 353–357.

97. van der Helm FCT: A finite element musculoskeletal model of the shoulder mechanism. J Biomech 1994; 27: 551–569.

98. van der Helm FCT, Pronk G: Three-dimensional recording and description of motions of the shoulder mechanism. J Biomech Eng 1995; 117: 27–40.

99. van der Helm FCT, Veeger HEJ, Pronk GM: Geometry parameters for musculoskeletal modelling of the shoulder mechanism. J Biomech 1992; 25: 129–144.

100. Veeger HEJ: The position of the rotation center of the glenohumeral joint. J Biomech 2000; 33: 1711–1715.

101. Williams P, Bannister L, Berry M, et al: Gray's Anatomy, The Anatomical Basis of Medicine and Surgery, Br. ed. London: Churchill Livingstone, 1995.

102. Wuelker N, Korell M, Thren K: Dynamic glenohumeral joint stability. J Shoulder Elbow Surg 1998; 7: 43–52.

103. Yanai T, Fuss FK, Fukunaga T: In vivo measurements of subacromial impingement: substantial compression develops in abduction with large internal rotation. Clin Biomech 2006; 21: 692–700.

Mechanics and Pathomechanics of Muscle Activity at the Shoulder Complex

The preceding chapter describes the bones and joints of the shoulder complex as well as the interaction among these structures. The present chapter presents the muscles that support and move this complex (*Fig. 9.1*). The purpose of this chapter is to

- Describe the characteristics of the individual muscles
- Discuss how these muscles work together to provide both mobility and stability to the shoulder complex
- Discuss how impairments of these muscles contribute to the pathomechanics of the shoulder

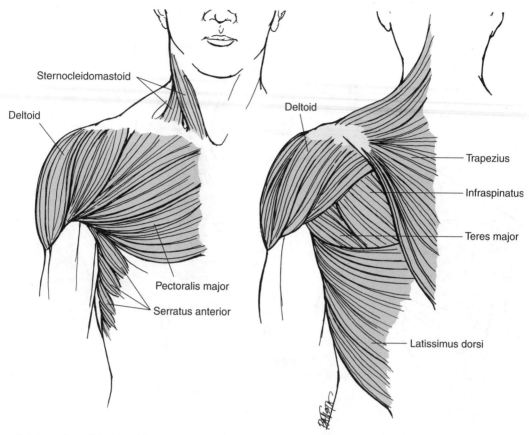

Figure 9.1: Superficial muscles of the shoulder complex. The muscles of the shoulder are grouped by their functions to move the scapulothoracic joint, move the glenohumeral joint, or add additional force to the whole complex. **A.** Anterior view. **B.** Posterior view.

It is important to recognize that many muscles of the shoulder have actions on the axioskeleton as well. These actions are addressed in the appropriate chapters on the head, vertebral column, and trunk. The present chapter focuses on the shoulder muscles' contribution to shoulder function.

The muscles of the shoulder can be divided into three groups according to their attachments and the joints they affect. These groups are

- **Axioscapular and axioclavicular**
- **Scapulohumeral**
- **Axiohumeral**

Each group is discussed separately so that the clinician can recognize the primary function of each group as well as the functions of the individual muscles that compose each group.

AXIOSCAPULAR AND AXIOCLAVICULAR MUSCLES

The muscles of the axioscapular and axioclavicular group all possess an attachment on the axioskeleton as well as on the shoulder girdle, that is, on the scapula or clavicle (*Fig. 9.2*). The primary role of these muscles is to position the scapula and clavicle by moving the sternoclavicular and scapulothoracic joints, with resulting motion at the acromioclavicular joint. To understand fully the role of these muscles, it is important to recall that the scapula's only bony attachment is at the small acromioclavicular joint. Thus the scapula floats freely on the thorax, supported primarily by muscles. The muscles of the axioscapular group frequently work in teams to hold the scapula stable as it moves on the thorax. The axioscapular and axioclavicular group includes the following muscles: trapezius, serratus anterior, levator scapulae, rhomboid major and minor, pectoralis minor, subclavius, and

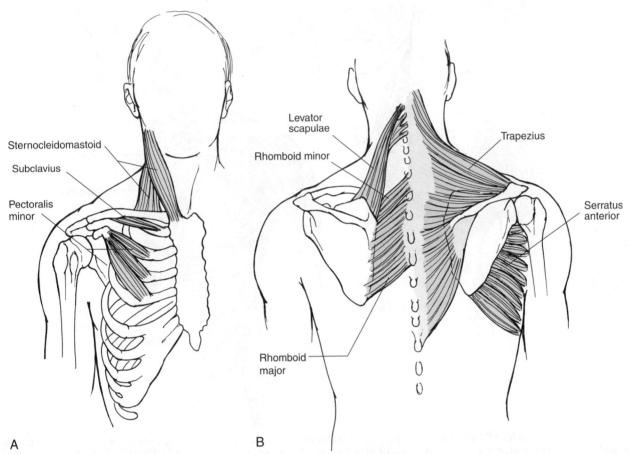

Figure 9.2: Axioscapular and axioclavicular muscles. The axioscapular and axioclavicular muscles **(A)** on the anterior surface of the trunk are the subclavius, pectoralis minor, and sternocleidomastoid muscles. The posterior axioscapular muscles **(B)** are the trapezius, rhomboid major and minor, levator scapulae, and serratus anterior.

sternocleidomastoid. Each is discussed separately below. The muscles that function together as teams are also discussed.

Trapezius

The trapezius is composed of three distinct bellies: upper, middle, and lower (*Fig. 9.3*) (*Muscle Attachment Box 9.1*). Each of these has its unique function, and each contributes significantly to the function of the trapezius as a whole. The muscle's attachments on both the clavicle and scapula indicate that it acts at both the sternoclavicular and scapulothoracic joints. The actions and effects of weakness and tightness of each belly of the muscle are discussed below. Then the role of the whole muscle is presented.

ACTIONS OF THE UPPER TRAPEZIUS

MUSCLE ACTION: UPPER TRAPEZIUS

Action	Evidence
Elevation of sternoclavicular joint	Supporting
Scapular elevation	Supporting
Scapular adduction	Supporting
Scapular upward rotation	Supporting

Careful cadaver dissection of individual fascicles of the trapezius reveals that the upper trapezius actually has much smaller muscle bundles than the other two portions of the trapezius [31]. This study also suggests that the fibers of the upper trapezius attach only to the clavicle, with no direct attachment on the scapula.

Electromyography (EMG) reveals considerable activity in the upper trapezius during active elevation of the shoulder girdle as in a shoulder shrug (*Fig. 9.4*) [8,11,12]. Gradual descent of the scapula from the elevated position in the upright position also is accompanied by contraction of the upper trapezius, presumably as an eccentric control of the action [11,12]. Similarly, scapular adduction in the erect standing position elicits significant upper trapezius activity. Thus EMG data support the notion that the upper trapezius actively elevates and adducts the shoulder girdle. Although there are no known studies that directly examine the upper trapezius muscle's contribution to upward rotation of the scapulothoracic joint, its attachment on the lateral clavicle is consistent with that function, since elevation of the clavicle must accompany normal scapulothoracic joint upward rotation. EMG studies reporting activity of the upper trapezius during shoulder abduction indirectly support its role as an

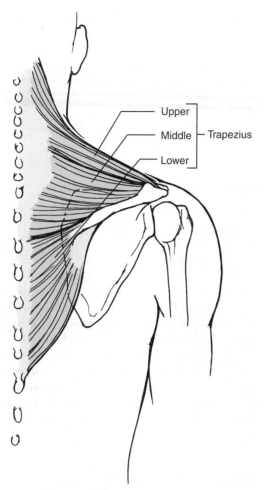

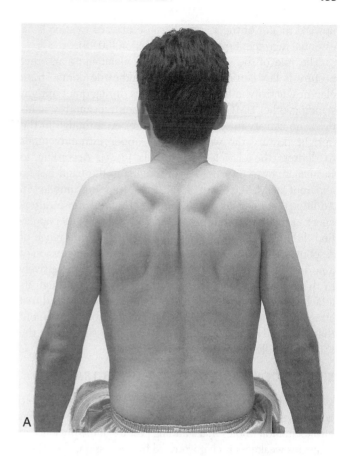

Figure 9.3: Trapezius muscle. The trapezius is divided into upper, middle, and lower parts.

MUSCLE ATTACHMENT BOX 9.1

ATTACHMENTS AND INNERVATION OF THE TRAPEZIUS

Proximal attachment: Medial third of the superior nuchal line, external occipital protuberance, ligamentum nuchae, the tips of the spinous processes, and the supraspinous ligaments from C7 through T12.

Distal Attachment: Posterior aspect of the lateral one third of the clavicle, medial aspect of the acromion, superior lip of the crest of the scapular spine, and the medial aspect and tubercle of the scapular spine.

Innervation: Spinal accessory nerve (11th cranial nerve, spinal portion). It also receives sensory fibers from the ventral rami of C3 and C4.

Palpation: The trapezius is superficial, and all three portions of the trapezius are easily palpated and distinguished from one another.

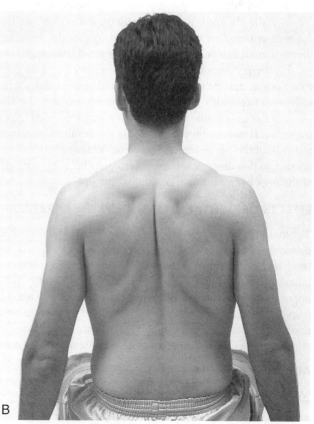

Figure 9.4: Function of the upper trapezius. The upper trapezius is active during a shoulder shrug **(A)** and during scapular adduction **(B)**.

upward rotator of the scapula because upward rotation is an essential ingredient of shoulder abduction (30,49).

The role of the upper trapezius in maintaining an erect posture is less certain. While some studies do demonstrate electrical activity in the upper trapezius during quiet upright standing, other EMG studies of the upper trapezius reveal little or no activity in quiet erect posture, even though in the upright posture the weight of the upper extremity tends to depress the clavicle and scapula [3,27]. According to Basmajian, even the addition of weights in the hand has no apparent facilitating effect on the upper trapezius muscle [3]. Additional studies are needed to determine if these differences in the literature represent methodological and population differences in the various investigations or the range of responses seen in a normal population. The resting tension of a normal upper trapezius probably does contribute passively to the upward support of the shoulder complex through its attachment on the clavicle [5,27]. Thus even without a direct attachment on the scapula, there remains broad agreement that the upper trapezius plays some role in supporting the shoulder girdle in erect posture [5,27,31].

EFFECTS OF WEAKNESS OF THE UPPER TRAPEZIUS

Isolated upper trapezius weakness is unusual but is likely to contribute to diminished strength in elevation of the shoulder girdle. Steindler notes that standing posture in the presence of trapezius weakness is characterized by depression, abduction, and forward tilting of the scapula [75]. Bearn notes that although the clavicle is depressed with trapezius paralysis, the depression is not as great as expected, nor is the resulting depression all that is available [5]. Even though some studies cited in the previous section deny active upper trapezius contributions to upright posture, the postural abnormalities typically associated with upper trapezius weakness may be the result of the loss of sufficient resting tone in a weakened upper trapezius. However, they may also be the result of weakness throughout the whole trapezius muscle. Additional studies are needed to demonstrate a clear relationship between strength of the upper trapezius and postural alignment.

EFFECTS OF TIGHTNESS OF THE UPPER TRAPEZIUS

Tightness of the upper trapezius is associated with elevated shoulders or asymmetrical head positions as well as restricted head and neck ranges of motion (ROM). However because other scapular elevators exist, it is difficult to identify pure upper trapezius tightness. If the upper trapezius alone is tight, scapular elevation is likely to be accompanied by upward rotation of the scapula. Therefore, careful assessment of scapular position is essential to distinguish among the scapular elevators.

ACTIONS OF THE MIDDLE TRAPEZIUS

MUSCLE ACTION: MIDDLE TRAPEZIUS

Actions	Evidence
Scapular adduction	Supporting
Scapular elevation	Supporting

The middle trapezius is regarded as a pure scapular adductor because of its horizontally aligned fibers. In cadaver specimens, the middle trapezius has the largest cross-sectional area of the three trapezius muscle segments [31]. Thus the middle trapezius provides considerable strength in scapular adduction and plays an important role in stabilizing the scapula. EMG studies report activity during shoulder shrugs, suggesting its upper fibers may assist the smaller upper trapezius in scapular elevation [30].

WEAKNESS OF THE MIDDLE TRAPEZIUS

Weakness of the middle trapezius results in a significant decrease in strength of scapular adduction. Isolated weakness of the middle trapezius is unusual, although some authors suggest that it can occur from prolonged stretch of the muscle as might occur in a posture characterized by scapular abduction [35]. However, attempts to correlate scapular position with middle trapezius strength have been unsuccessful thus far [14]. Loss of middle trapezius strength also presents difficulties when contracting the scapulohumeral muscles. For example, the lateral rotators of the shoulder, including the infraspinatus and posterior deltoid muscles, require a stable scapula to exert their force at the glenohumeral joint. Decreased scapular adduction strength can allow these muscles to pull the scapula toward the humerus instead of pulling the humerus toward the scapula.

TIGHTNESS OF THE MIDDLE TRAPEZIUS

Tightness of the middle trapezius alone is rare because the weight of the entire upper extremity pulls the scapula toward abduction.

ACTIONS OF THE LOWER TRAPEZIUS

MUSCLE ACTION: LOWER TRAPEZIUS

Actions	Evidence
Scapular depression	Supporting
Scapular adduction	Inadequate
Scapular upward rotation	Supporting

Careful inspection of the line of pull of the lower trapezius explains its potential contributions to all these actions. Such inspection also suggests that the muscle is best suited for depression and upward rotation. The line of pull of the lower trapezius is ideal for depression of the scapula. However, in the upright posture, the weight of the upper extremity already pulls the scapula toward depression. Additional depression by activity of the lower trapezius is not required. In contrast, when the subject is prone, manual resistance against scapular depression does elicit electrical activity of the lower trapezius [8]. The importance of the scapular depression force provided by the lower trapezius is most apparent with simultaneous contraction of the upper trapezius. This combined activity is discussed when the trapezius is discussed as a whole.

Clinical Relevance

MANUAL MUSCLE TESTING OF THE LOWER TRAPEZIUS: *In the prone position with the shoulder flexed, the weight of the upper extremity tends to pull the scapula into elevation. Consequently, the lower trapezius is used to stabilize the scapula (Fig. 9.5). Thus the resistance in the "Fair" test of the lower trapezius is the weight of the upper extremity.*

EMG activity of the lower trapezius during isometric shoulder adduction from the abducted position may also support the role of the lower trapezius as a scapular adductor [30].

To understand the lower trapezius muscle's contribution to upward rotation of the scapula, it is essential to recall the location of the axis for upward and downward scapular rotation (Chapter 8). Although the precise location of the axis remains controversial, it is clear that the axis lies lateral to the scapular attachment of the lower trapezius on the root of the spine of the scapula. Therefore, as the lower trapezius pulls the medial aspect of the scapular spine inferiorly, the scapula rotates upwardly (*Fig. 9.6*). Like the upper trapezius, the activity of the lower trapezius during shoulder elevation supports its role as an upward rotator of the scapula.

WEAKNESS OF THE LOWER TRAPEZIUS

Isolated weakness of the lower trapezius has been suggested to be the consequence of prolonged stretch resulting from an elevated and downwardly rotated scapula [35]. However, there are no known studies that verify such a relationship. Weakness of the lower trapezius may lead to difficulty in

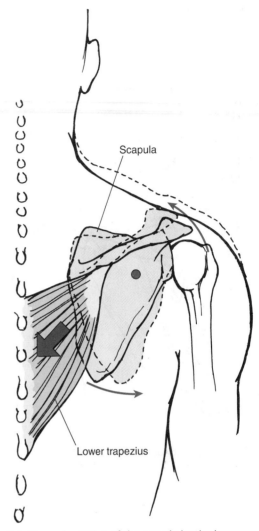

Figure 9.6: Upward rotation of the scapula by the lower trapezius. The attachment of the lower trapezius on the medial aspect of the spine of the scapula causes upward rotation of the scapula.

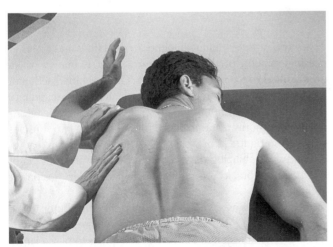

Figure 9.5: MMT position for the lower trapezius. The lower trapezius stabilizes the scapula as the weight of the upper extremity tends to elevate the scapula on the thorax when the subject lies prone.

stabilizing the scapula during contraction of the other upward rotators of the scapula.

TIGHTNESS OF THE LOWER TRAPEZIUS

Tightness of the lower trapezius theoretically results in decreased elevation and downward rotation ROM of the scapulothoracic joint and perhaps a depressed and posteriorly tilted shoulder girdle in quiet standing. However, there are no known reports of isolated lower trapezius tightness, although a difference in shoulder height is often reported in healthy adults. This difference reportedly is associated with hand dominance [35,72]. The absence of identified lower trapezius tightness despite the apparent scapular depression in some individuals has several possible explanations. The depression may be accompanied by concomitant scapular downward rotation and/or abduction, which may balance or indeed overcome the shortening effect of the depression (*Fig. 9.7*). There may be no adaptive change in the lower trapezius

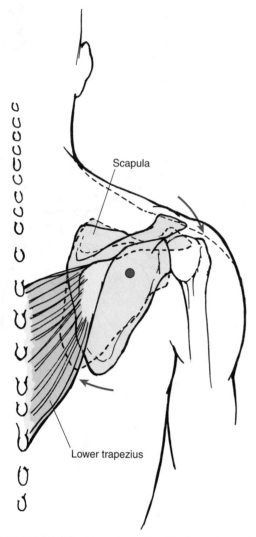

Figure 9.7: Length of the lower trapezius. The lower trapezius may actually be stretched in a subject when the scapula is abducted and downwardly rotated, producing a posture in which the shoulder appears lowered.

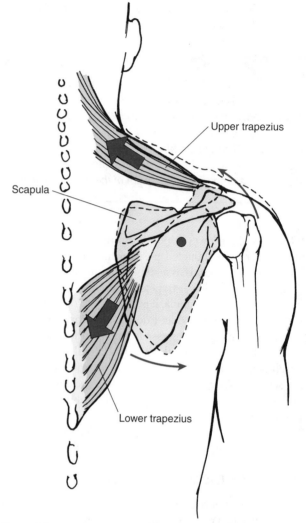

Figure 9.8: Force couple composed of upper and lower trapezius. The elevation and depression pulls by the upper and lower trapezius, respectively, are balanced out while both rotate the scapula upwardly.

despite the prolonged scapular depression because it is interrupted enough by scapular elevation during upper extremity use. In addition, since there is no accepted standard of scapular position in healthy individuals, what appears as scapular depression actually may be contralateral elevation. Thus impairments resulting from lower trapezius tightness are unclear and may be nonexistent.

ACTIONS OF THE ENTIRE TRAPEZIUS

The actions of the whole trapezius can be considered the vector sum of the forces from the upper, middle, and lower trapezius muscles. As a whole the trapezius adducts and upwardly rotates the scapula. The elevation and depression motions of the upper and lower components, respectively, balance each other out. In fact it is this balancing by two opposing forces that is essential to the stability of the scapula.

These two muscles pulling in opposite directions and together causing rotation of the scapula form what is known as an **anatomical force couple** (*Fig. 9.8*). The combined action of the upper and lower trapezius muscles allows the scapula to rotate upwardly without being displaced superiorly or inferiorly on the thorax. An imbalance between these two muscles either from tightness or weakness of one of them can lead to difficulty in stabilizing the scapula during upward rotation of the scapulothoracic joint (i.e., during shoulder flexion or abduction).

The trapezius as a whole is an important contributor to the scapular upward rotation that is a necessary ingredient of normal arm–trunk flexion or abduction. It appears to play a larger role in shoulder abduction than in shoulder flexion [27,49]. Its greater role in shoulder abduction is consistent with the fact that the muscle lies primarily in the frontal plane. Acting by itself, the entire trapezius upwardly rotates the scapula and adducts it. Yet normal arm–trunk elevation occurs without significant scapular adduction. Thus the whole trapezius requires another muscle to balance its adduction component. This balance is provided by the serratus anterior, described next.

Clinical Relevance

SPINAL ACCESSORY NERVE INJURY: *Weakness of any or all of the trapezius can result from an injury to the spinal accessory nerve, which lies superficially in the posterior triangle of the neck, formed by the anterior border of the upper trapezius muscle, the posterolateral border of the sternocleidomastoid muscle, and the middle third of the clavicle. The nerve can be injured during neck surgery, such as a lymph node biopsy, or by a blow or laceration to the top of the shoulder.*

*A patient with a spinal accessory nerve palsy typically reports weakness in activities overhead. The individual's posture may be characterized by a drooping shoulder and the scapula may be pulled into abduction. The abducted position of the scapula is accentuated during active shoulder abduction and is sometimes known as **lateral winging.** Assessment of shoulder strength reveals decreased strength in shoulder elevation, particularly in shoulder abduction as well as in weakness in the discrete movements of the scapula attributable to the trapezius.*

Serratus Anterior

The serratus anterior is a large muscle described by some as a single muscle uniformly distributed along the costal attachments (*Muscle Attachment Box 9.2*) (*Fig. 9.9*) [63]. Others describe the serratus anterior as consisting of a small upper and a larger lower bundle, each having its separate role [27,31,84].

MUSCLE ATTACHMENT BOX 9.2

ATTACHMENTS AND INNERVATION OF THE SERRATUS ANTERIOR

Proximal attachment: Anterolateral surfaces and superior borders of the first 8 to 10 ribs and the intercostal muscles in between.

Distal attachment: Medial border of the ventral surface of the scapula from the superior to the inferior angles.

Innervation: Long thoracic nerve, C5-7.

Palpation: The serratus anterior is most easily palpated at its attachment on the lateral thorax as it interdigitates with the external oblique abdominal muscle.

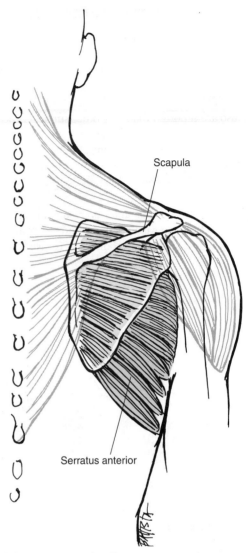

Figure 9.9: Serratus anterior. The serratus anterior passes over the anterior surface of the scapula to attach to its medial border.

ACTIONS OF THE SERRATUS ANTERIOR

MUSCLE ACTION: SERRATUS ANTERIOR

Actions	Evidence
Scapular abduction	Supporting
Scapular upward rotation	Supporting
Scapular elevation	Supporting

Textbooks often name the action of the serratus anterior *protraction*. However, as discussed in Chapter 8, *protraction* can mean abduction of the scapula with either upward or downward rotation. Therefore, to avoid ambiguity, this text lists the actions specifically. When the serratus anterior is described as two parts, the role of elevation is ascribed to the upper portion and that of abduction and upward rotation to the larger lower portion [12,27,84].

WEAKNESS OF THE SERRATUS ANTERIOR

Weakness of the serratus anterior usually results from injury to its nerve supply, the long thoracic nerve. The long thoracic nerve lies on the ventral surface of much of the muscle and can be injured during surgical procedures such as mastectomies in which tumors close to the nerve must be excised. Injuries also are reported following other surgical procedures and during the administration of local anesthesia [32]. Direct traction injuries to the nerve in young athletes are reported as well [20]. In all reports of injury, the resulting impairments are reported to be severe, although recovery is possible [32,78,80].

Weakness of the serratus anterior results in weakness of scapular abduction, upward rotation, and, to some extent, scapular elevation. Scapular abduction is used to reach forward. So weakness of the serratus anterior is apparent when pushing forward against a resistance, as in pushing a revolving door forward (*Fig. 9.10*). In this situation the door exerts a reaction force on the upper extremity (including the shoulder girdle) that tends to adduct the scapula. In the absence of sufficient serratus anterior strength, the scapula slides medially on the thorax. Because the serratus anterior attaches to the medial aspect of the ventral surface of the scapula, the serratus anterior holds the scapula firmly onto the thorax. Consequently, in the presence of serratus anterior weakness, forces that adduct the scapula also tend to cause the medial aspect of the scapula to protrude posteriorly from the thorax. This is known as **medial winging** and is a sign of weakness of the serratus anterior prominent during abduction of the scapula against resistance (*Fig. 9.11*). Medial winging due to weakness of the serratus anterior also is apparent during active shoulder flexion and abduction.

To understand fully the mechanics of this winging during active shoulder elevation, the role of the serratus anterior with the trapezius muscle in shoulder elevation must be understood. Recall that the trapezius adducts and upwardly rotates the scapula while the serratus anterior abducts and upwardly rotates the scapula. Recall also that the scapula is

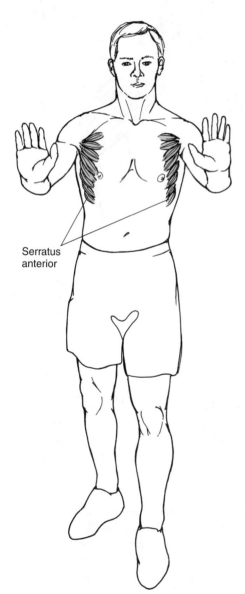

Figure 9.10: Function of the serratus anterior. The serratus is active as an individual pushes forward on a revolving door.

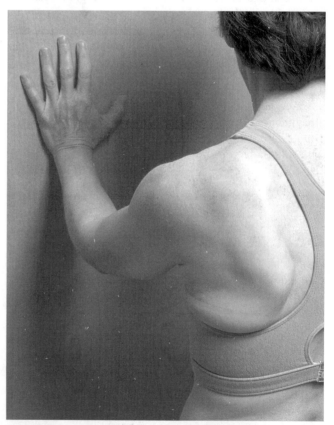

Figure 9.11: Medial winging of the scapula due to serratus anterior weakness. The scapula is pushed into adduction and wings medially as an individual pushes forward against a wall in the presence of serratus anterior weakness.

free to slide on the posterior thorax. Finally, recall that flexion and abduction of the shoulder require approximately 60° of upward rotation of the scapula. The trapezius and serratus anterior form another force couple that rotates the scapula upwardly while counteracting the adduction and abduction components of the respective muscles (*Fig. 9.12*). This combined activity is essential to stabilize the scapula during arm–trunk flexion and abduction [2]. In contrast to the trapezius, the serratus anterior plays a greater role in shoulder flexion in keeping with its orientation closer to the sagittal plane [27,49].

Since both the trapezius and serratus anterior muscles contribute to scapular rotation during shoulder elevation, distinguishing between weakness of one or the other is critical to choosing an appropriate treatment. As noted above, weakness of the serratus anterior is manifested by a classic physical sign called **medial winging of the scapula.** This winging is apparent during upper extremity activities requiring serratus anterior contraction including *active*

shoulder elevation, particularly shoulder flexion. Scapular winging secondary to serratus anterior weakness is a protrusion of the medial border of the scapula away from the thorax, visible during active shoulder elevation, especially flexion. It results from the residual imbalance of muscle pull on the scapula. The serratus anterior is attached to the ventral surface of the scapula, while the trapezius is attached to the dorsal surface. During normal cocontraction of these muscles, the dorsal pull of the trapezius tends to adduct the scapula and to pull it slightly dorsally. However, the simultaneous ventral pull of the serratus anterior muscle holds the vertebral border of the scapula firmly to the thorax (*Fig. 9.13*). With weakness of the serratus anterior muscle, there is loss of this ventral pull, and the scapula's medial border protrudes posteriorly from the thorax; that is, it **wings.**

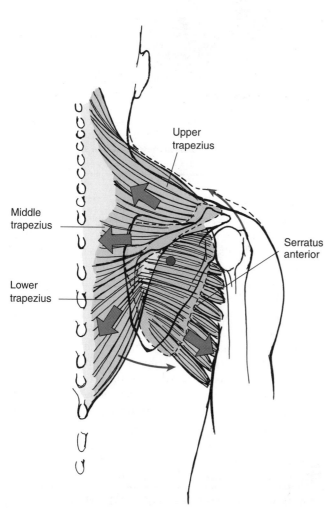

Figure 9.12: Force couple formed by trapezius and serratus anterior. The adduction and abduction pulls of the trapezius and serratus anterior counteract each other while the two muscles produce upward rotation of the scapula.

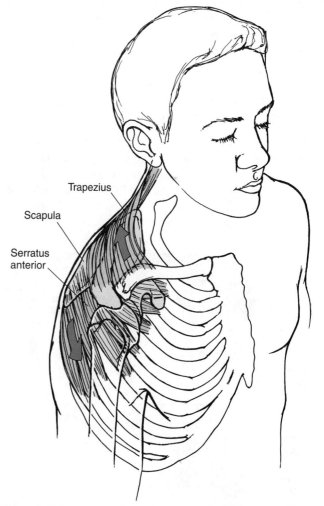

Figure 9.13: Transverse plane view of the scapula. A transverse view of the scapula on the thorax reveals how the pull of the serratus anterior on the medial border of the scapula stabilizes the scapula against the pull of the trapezius on the lateral aspect of the scapula.

Clinical Relevance

SCAPULAR WINGING DUE TO SERRATUS ANTERIOR WEAKNESS: *Medial winging of the sapula during arm–trunk elevation is a classic sign of weakness of the serratus anterior muscle. Scapular winging due to serratus anterior weakness is visible during activities requiring active contraction of the serratus anterior. Such activities include active shoulder flexion or abduction or resisted scapular abduction (Fig. 9.14). In contrast, winging of the scapula at rest or during passive motion of the shoulder can be the sign of restricted ROM at the glenohumeral joint or postural abnormalities. For example, as described in the previous chapter, anterior tilting of the scapula is an effective substitute for inadequate medial rotation of the glenohumeral joint. The position of the scapula when it is tilted anteriorly is similar to that seen with serratus weakness (Fig. 9.15). However, in the case of glenohumeral joint restriction, the prominence of the scapula occurs during activities such as reaching into a back pocket, when no serratus anterior contraction is required. Thus the scapular prominence in this case cannot be the result of serratus anterior muscle weakness. This is a critical distinction for the clinician to make.*

CONSEQUENCES OF WEAKNESS OF THE SERRATUS ANTERIOR AND TRAPEZIUS MUSCLES

Chapter 8 describes the contribution the scapulothoracic joint makes to shoulder motion. Passively, upward rotation of the scapulothoracic joint contributes at least one third of the shoulder's total flexion and abduction ROM. However, loss of scapulothoracic joint motion appears to have a more dramatic

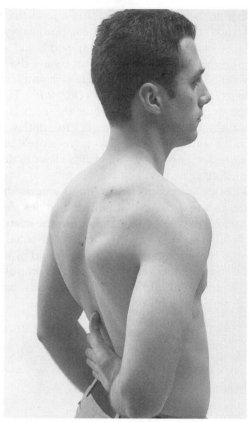

Figure 9.15: Apparent medial winging due to decreased ROM. An individual with decreased medial rotation ROM of the shoulder can use anterior tilting of the scapula to reach behind the back. The scapula appears to be winging; however, this position is not the result of serratus anterior weakness, since the serratus anterior is not required to perform the activity.

effect on active ROM of the shoulder. Weakness of the trapezius and/or the serratus anterior hampers active shoulder elevation in two ways. First, weakness in either or both of these muscles limits, and perhaps eliminates, active upward rotation of the scapulothoracic joint and thereby reduces the active shoulder flexion or abduction ROM by at least one third. Additionally, however, the normal upward rotation of the scapula helps maintain adequate contractile length of the deltoid and rotator cuff muscles to permit full movement of the glenohumeral joint. Thus weakness of either or both of the upward rotators of the scapula not only impairs the motion of the scapula but also disrupts the actions of the muscles at the glenohumeral joint. Weakness of the serratus anterior and or trapezius muscles can result in profound disability at the shoulder complex.

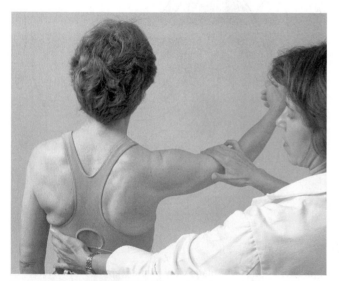

Figure 9.14: Medial winging due to serratus anterior weakness during resisted shoulder flexion. With serratus anterior weakness, the scapula wings medially during shoulder flexion when upward rotation of the scapula is required.

Clinical Relevance

WEAKNESS OF THE SERRATUS ANTERIOR OR TRAPEZIUS MUSCLE: *Weakness of either the serratus anterior or the trapezius results in impaired function in both*
(continued)

(Continued)

flexion and abduction of the shoulder [20,50]. Regardless of whether the serratus anterior, the trapezius, or both are weak, the weakness impairs the active motion of the scapulothoracic joint. Abnormal scapulothoracic joint rotation during shoulder elevation may contribute to impingement of the contents of the subacromial space. Consequently, a patient's complaints originating from weakness of the scapular rotators usually consist of complaints of weakness and difficulty reaching overhead but also may include complaints of pain when attempting overhead activities. Similarly, an evaluation of an individual with a shoulder impingement syndrome must include a careful assessment of the muscles that rotate the scapula upward.

Su et al. [76] assessed 20 competitive swimmers with complaints and signs consistent with subacromial impingement syndrome and 20 matched swimmers without complaints or signs of impingement. Scapular movements during shoulder elevation were similar in both groups prior to swim practice. However, after a hard practice, those swimmers with complaints exhibited significantly less upward rotation of the scapula. These data suggest the importance of active scapular control during repetitive shoulder elevation activities in protecting against impingement syndromes.

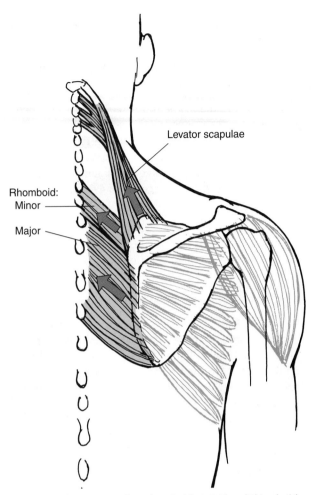

Figure 9.16: Levator scapulae, rhomboid major, and rhomboid minor muscles. The line of pull is approximately the same for the levator scapulae and the rhomboid major and minor.

TIGHTNESS OF THE SERRATUS ANTERIOR

Although tightness of the serratus anterior muscle is rarely described, tightness of the upper portion can conceivably occur with tightness of the upper trapezius. Such tightness may result in a posture characterized by elevated shoulders and upwardly rotated scapulae.

Levator Scapulae, Rhomboid Major, and Rhomboid Minor

The levator scapulae, rhomboid major, and rhomboid minor are almost parallel to each other, running superiorly and medially from the vertebral border of the scapula to the vertebral column (*Fig. 9.16*) (*Muscle Attachment Boxes 9.3 and 9.4*). These three muscles produce essentially the same motions at the scapulothoracic joint. However, their attachments on the vertebral column result in differing actions at the spine. The rhomboid muscles cause contralateral rotation of the cervical spine, and the levator scapulae produces ipsilateral rotation of the cervical spine. These differences allow the careful clinician to distinguish between the rhomboid muscles and the levator scapulae. Actions of these muscles at the spine are detailed in Chapter 27. The actions of these three muscles on the scapula as well as the effects of their weakness and tightness are very similar and are discussed together.

MUSCLE ATTACHMENT BOX 9.3

ATTACHMENTS AND INNERVATION OF THE LEVATOR SCAPULAE

Proximal attachment: Posterior tubercles of the transverse processes of the first four cervical vertebrae.

Distal attachment: Medial border of the scapula between the superior angle and scapular spine.

Innervation: Spinal nerves C3-5. The contribution from C5 is by way of the dorsal scapular nerve.

Palpation: The levator scapulae is palpated between the upper trapezius and the sternocleidomastoid, particularly with elevation and downward rotation of the scapula.

MUSCLE ATTACHMENT BOX 9.4

ATTACHMENTS AND INNERVATION OF THE RHOMBOID MAJOR AND MINOR

Proximal attachment: The rhomboid major is attached proximally to the spines and supraspinous ligaments of the second through fifth thoracic vertebrae. The rhomboid minor muscle has a more superior attachment on the inferior portion of the ligamentum nuchae and the spinous processes of C7 and T1.

Distal attachment: The rhomboid major attaches to the medial border of the scapula from the root of the spine to the inferior angle. The rhomboid minor attaches to the medial aspect of the scapula at the level of the scapular spine.

Innervation: Dorsal scapular nerve, C4 and 5.

Palpation: The fibers of the rhomboid major and minor are approximately parallel to one another. These two muscles lie deep to the trapezius but can be palpated through the trapezius during motions combining active downward rotation and adduction of the scapula.

ACTIONS OF THE LEVATOR SCAPULAE, RHOMBOID MAJOR, AND RHOMBOID MINOR

MUSCLE ACTION: LEVATOR SCAPULAE, RHOMBOID MAJOR, AND RHOMBOID MINOR

Actions	Evidence
Scapular elevation	Supporting
Scapular adduction	Supporting
Scapular downward rotation	Supporting

Inman demonstrates active contraction of the levator scapulae along with the upper trapezius and upper portion of the serratus anterior muscles in quiet standing, suggesting that these muscles are providing upward support for the shoulder girdle and upper extremity [27]. However, Johnson notes that only the levator scapulae and the rhomboid major and minor muscles can directly suspend the scapula [31]. EMG studies show that in the presence of voluntary relaxation of the upper trapezius in quiet standing, there is an increase in EMG activity of the two rhomboid muscles but a decrease in activity in the levator scapulae [56]. These data support the notion that the rhomboid muscles can and do support the upright position of the shoulder girdle, at least under certain circumstances. Whether the levator scapulae contributes additional support remains debatable.

Inspection of the lines of pull of these three muscles suggests that the rhomboid muscles are better aligned to adduct the scapula than is the levator scapulae. EMG activity in the rhomboids increases with resisted adduction of the scapulae,

supporting their role as adductors [68]. One study shows the rhomboid major and minor muscles active with the middle trapezius during shoulder flexion and abduction, with more activity in the latter motion [27]. However, most authors agree that the trapezius and serratus anterior muscles are the primary scapulothoracic muscles needed for shoulder flexion and abduction.

Downward rotation of the scapula may be used as an individual reaches into a back hip pocket or scratches the middle of the back (*Fig. 9.17*). These activities elicit considerable EMG activity in the rhomboid muscles (greater than 50% of the EMG elicited during a manual muscle test) [74]. The attachment of the levator scapulae, rhomboid major, and rhomboid minor along the vertebral border of the scapula allows them to rotate the scapula downwardly about its axis located lateral to the root of the spine. As they contract to downwardly rotate the scapula, they cause simultaneous elevation and adduction of the scapula. Therefore, to obtain more-isolated downward rotation these muscles require the contraction of another muscle to provide a balance. The muscle that forms an anatomical **force couple** with the levator scapulae, rhomboid major, and rhomboid minor to produce isolated downward rotation of the scapulothoracic joint is the pectoralis minor. It is discussed later in this chapter.

WEAKNESS OF THE LEVATOR SCAPULAE, RHOMBOID MAJOR, AND RHOMBOID MINOR

Pulling actions such as pulling open doors and rowing can be impaired by weakness of the levator scapulae, rhomboid

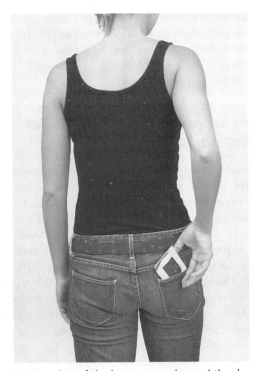

Figure 9.17: Function of the levator scapulae and the rhomboid major and minor. Reaching to a back pocket typically requires the rhomboid major and minor and the levator scapulae.

major, and rhomboid minor. Weakness of these muscles also is cited as a cause of a posture characterized by rounded shoulders. Some suggest that the muscles are needed for erect posture and thus their weakness allows the scapulae to abduct and depress [14]. However, no studies have successfully identified a relationship between the strength of these muscles and postural alignment. Nor has the incidence of weakness of these muscles been described. Consequently, while there is a widespread belief that weakness of these muscles may contribute to postural impairment of the shoulder girdle, this relationship has yet to be established.

TIGHTNESS OF THE LEVATOR SCAPULAE, RHOMBOID MAJOR, AND RHOMBOID MINOR

Like weakness of the levator scapulae, rhomboid major, and rhomboid minor, tightness in these muscles has been described as the basis for the rounded-shoulders posture [35]. Adaptive shortening of these muscles results in elevation, adduction, and downward rotation of the scapula. This position turns the glenoid fossa downward and causes the scapula to tilt anteriorly, thus lowering and *rounding* the shoulder. Consequently, tightness of these three muscles results theoretically in a complex three-dimensional positional change of the scapula. However, no direct link between tightness of these muscles and postural abnormalities has been established. The difficulty in establishing the link between tightness of these muscles and postural abnormalities lies in the difficulty in quantifying the exact position of the scapula and the muscles' true length. Until results of studies using more precise measurement tools are available, a clear understanding of the postural impact of tightness or weakness of the levator scapulae, rhomboid major, and rhomboid minor muscles will remain elusive.

Clinical Relevance

PAIN IN THE LEVATOR SCAPULAE, RHOMBOID MAJOR, AND RHOMBOID MINOR: *Pain and tenderness in the levator scapulae, rhomboid major, and rhomboid minor are common clinical findings [56,77]. Both weakness and tightness have been described as the explanation for pain along the medial aspect of the scapula and at its superior angle. At the present time, although there are widespread beliefs regarding the contributions of weakness and tightness to these complaints, there are no clear findings supporting or refuting these beliefs. Therefore, it is essential that more precise means of assessing strength and tightness of these muscles become available.*

Pectoralis Minor

The pectoralis minor muscle is an unusual axioscapular muscle because it lies entirely on the anterior surface of the thorax and attaches to the coracoid process, an anterior projection of the scapula (*Muscle Attachment Box 9.5*) (*Fig. 9.18*).

MUSCLE ATTACHMENT BOX 9.5

ATTACHMENTS AND INNERVATION OF THE PECTORALIS MINOR

Proximal attachment: The anterior surfaces and superior borders of the third through fifth ribs close to the costal cartilages but may include the second or sixth rib as well. Attachment is also provided by the fascia covering the external intercostal muscles in the area.

Distal attachment: Medial border and superior surface of the coracoid process of the scapula.

Innervation: Medial and lateral pectoral nerves, C5-T1.

Palpation: This muscle lies deep to the pectoralis major and consequently is difficult to palpate. However, it may be palpated just inferior to the coracoid process of the scapula during activities that elicit active contractions of the muscles in the force couple for downward rotation of the scapula.

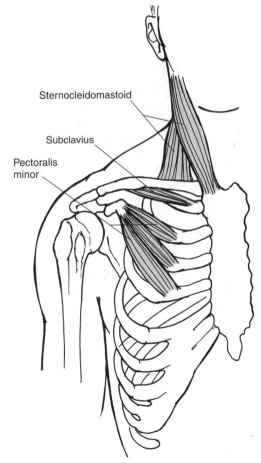

Figure 9.18: Pectoralis minor, subclavius, and sternocleidomastoid muscles. The pectoralis minor, subclavius, and sternocleidomastoid muscles lie on the anterior aspect of the thorax.

Even the serratus anterior, which has an anterior attachment on the thorax, attaches posteriorly on the scapula. The anterior location of the pectoralis minor has a rather dramatic effect on the actions resulting from contraction of the pectoralis minor. Its location also produces confusing contradictions in its reported actions.

ACTION

MUSCLE ACTION: PECTORALIS MINOR

Actions	Evidence
Scapular anterior tilt	Supporting
Scapular elevation	Inadequate
Scapular depression	Inadequate
Scapular adduction	Inadequate
Scapular abduction	Inadequate
Scapular upward rotation	Inadequate

Isolated contraction of the pectoralis minor pulls the coracoid process anteriorly, tipping the scapula anteriorly (*Fig. 9.19*). However, because the scapula lies on the posterior aspect of the thorax, for it to tip forward, it also must elevate. Thus the pectoralis minor elevates the scapula as it tips it anteriorly. Yet inspection of the line of pull of the pectoralis minor reveals that it is aligned to pull the coracoid process down. When other muscles contract to prevent the anterior tilting of the scapula caused by the pull on the coracoid process by the pectoralis minor, the pectoralis minor with these other muscles contributes to scapular depression. Chapter 8 notes that there is very little ROM of scapulothoracic joint depression available. Thus active contraction of the pectoralis minor muscle along with other scapular depressors is most important when the upper extremity is exposed to an upwardly directed external load such as the reaction force from a crutch that applies an elevation force on the scapula through the upper extremity. Under this circumstance the pectoralis minor and other shoulder depressor muscles provide a depressive force to stabilize the scapula and shoulder girdle against the force of elevation (*Fig. 9.20*) [24]. Therefore, the pectoralis minor elevates the

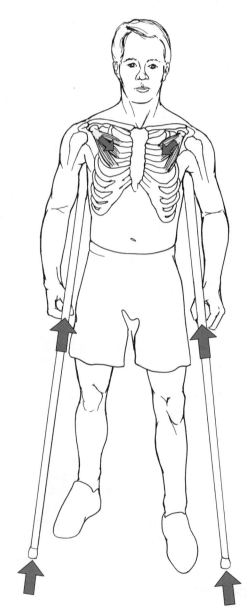

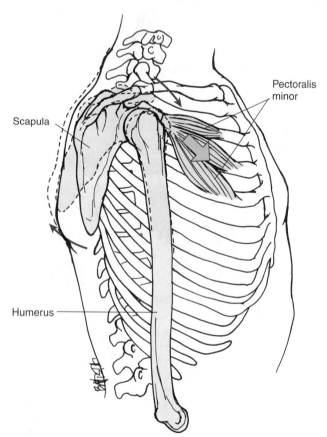

Figure 9.19: Function of the pectoralis minor. Contraction of the pectoralis minor pulls the coracoid process anteriorly, causing the scapula to tilt anteriorly and to elevate.

Figure 9.20: Function of the pectoralis minor to depress the shoulder. The pectoralis minor exerts a downward force on the scapula to stabilize it against the reaction force of a crutch that is directed upward and tends to elevate the shoulder.

scapula when contracting alone and depresses the shoulder girdle when contracting with other shoulder depressors.

Similarly, inspection of the line of pull of the pectoralis minor creates confusion regarding its role in abduction and adduction of the scapula [24,89]. The muscle certainly pulls medially on the coracoid process, which is interpreted by some as scapular adduction. However, the muscle's position on the anterior aspect of the thorax means that its anterior pull on the coracoid process causes the scapula to slide anteriorly on the thorax, causing the scapula to abduct. Hence the pectoralis minor abducts the scapula despite its medial pull on the coracoid process.

The ability of the pectoralis minor to abduct the scapula makes it a suitable partner with the levator scapulae, rhomboid major, and rhomboid minor muscles in an anatomical force couple for downward rotation of the scapula. The pectoralis minor's action of abduction balances the adduction component of the levator scapulae, rhomboid major, and rhomboid minor, while together they contribute to the scapula's downward rotation (*Fig. 9.21*) [63,84]. The action of these muscles in scapular downward rotation creates a confusing clinical picture in which the inferior angle of the scapula is elevated but the acromion is depressed. Inspection of only one of these landmarks can lead a clinician to conclude that the scapula is elevated or depressed when it is merely downwardly rotated. Clinicians must use caution when analyzing the position of the scapula.

WEAKNESS OF THE PECTORALIS MINOR

Weakness may contribute to difficulty in controlling the shoulder girdle, particularly during upper extremity weight-bearing activities such as crutch walking. It may also decrease the stability of the scapula during activities requiring downward rotation of the scapulothoracic joint, since weakness of the pectoralis minor disrupts the force couple for scapular downward rotation.

TIGHTNESS OF THE PECTORALIS MINOR

Tightness of the pectoralis minor will pull the scapula into an anterior tilt (*Fig. 9.22*). Additionally tightness of the pectoralis minor may, with the other muscles of its force couple, contribute to the "rounded shoulder" posture [6]. Individuals with shortened pectoralis minor muscles exhibit less posterior tilting and more internal rotation of the scapula during shoulder elevation [7]. The alterations in scapular motions during shoulder elevations reported in individuals with shortened pectoralis minor muscles may increase the risk of impingement syndromes in these individuals.

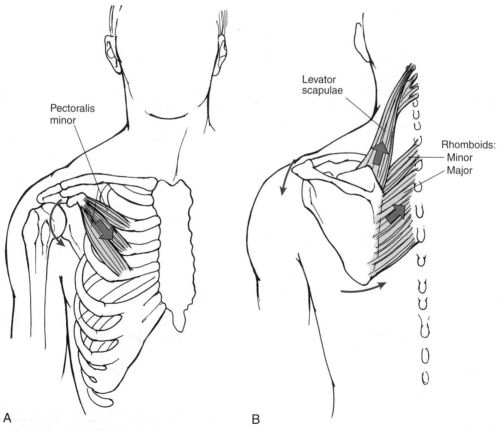

Figure 9.21: Force couple formed by the rhomboid muscles, the levator scapulae, and the pectoralis minor. The pectoralis minor abducts the scapula and balances the adduction pull of the rhomboid major and minor and levator scapulae as all four muscles rotate the scapula downward.

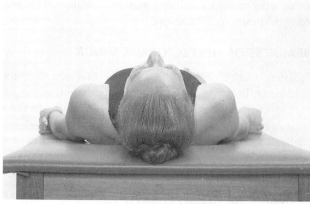

Figure 9.22: Tightness of the pectoralis minor. Tightness of the pectoralis minor muscle pulls the scapula into an anterior tilt. In supine the shoulder with tightness looks more forward than the opposite side.

MUSCLE ATTACHMENT BOX 9.6

ATTACHMENTS AND INNERVATION OF THE SUBCLAVIUS

Proximal attachment: Junction of the first rib and first costal cartilage, anterior to the costoclavicular ligament.

Distal attachment: Inferior surface of the middle one third of the clavicle.

Innervation: Subclavian branch of the upper trunk of the brachial plexus, C5 and C6.

Palpation: This muscle cannot be palpated directly.

Clinical Relevance

TIGHTNESS OF THE PECTORALIS MINOR: *The brachial plexus and axillary blood vessels lie deep to the pectoralis minor muscle. Therefore, a stretch of a tightened pectoralis minor muscle can compress these sensitive structures and cause symptoms radiating distally into the upper extremity. Impingement of the brachial plexus or axillary blood vessels by a tight pectoralis minor muscle is one form of thoracic outlet syndrome (TOS) [44]. Neurological symptoms typically include tingling and perhaps numbness in the hand. Vascular symptoms may include blanching of the skin and a diminished pulse. Exercises to stretch the pectoralis minor muscle must proceed carefully to avoid exacerbating the symptoms.*

Subclavius

The subclavius is a small muscle binding the clavicle to the first rib (*Muscle Attachment Box 9.6*). Because of its size and location it is not well studied. It lies too deep to be palpated.

ACTIONS OF THE SUBCLAVIUS

MUSCLE ACTION: SUBCLAVIUS

Actions	Evidence
Sternoclavicular joint depression	Inadequate

The subclavius is believed to depress the clavicle. Since there is actually little ROM of the sternoclavicular joint in the direction of depression, this muscle, like the pectoralis minor, is more likely a stabilizer of the clavicle against forces that tend to elevate the sternoclavicular joint, such as weight bearing on

the upper extremity. There are many other muscles that also depress the shoulder. Their role in stabilizing the shoulder during weight-bearing activities is discussed at the end of this chapter. The one known EMG study of the subclavius suggests that the muscle contracts to stabilize the sternoclavicular joint, reinforcing the ligamentous supports [62].

EFFECTS OF WEAKNESS AND TIGHTNESS OF THE SUBCLAVIUS

Because the subclavius has not been studied in detail, effects of weakness and tightness can only be theorized. Weakness is unlikely to have significant effects on strength, since there are many other larger muscles to depress the sternoclavicular joint. However, this muscle's contribution to dynamic stabilization of the joint would be lost in the presence of subclavius weakness. Tightness is likely to bind the clavicle onto the first rib, thus limiting elevation at the sternoclavicular joint. The effects of diminished sternoclavicular joint elevation are discussed in detail in Chapter 8. That discussion reveals that inadequate sternoclavicular joint elevation is likely to impair shoulder elevation ROM either by limiting scapulothoracic joint upward rotation and thus restricting total shoulder ROM or by causing excessive acromioclavicular joint excursion and pain during shoulder elevation.

Sternocleidomastoid

The sternocleidomastoid is regarded generally as a muscle of the head and neck (*Muscle Attachment Box 9.7*). However, its attachment to the clavicle allows it to participate with other axioscapular and axioclavicular muscles to position the shoulder girdle.

MUSCLE ACTION: STERNOCLEIDOMASTOID

Actions	Evidence
Sternoclavicular joint elevation	Conflicting

MUSCLE ATTACHMENT BOX 9.7

ATTACHMENTS AND INNERVATION OF THE STERNOCLEIDOMASTOID

Proximal attachment: Lateral surface of the mastoid process and lateral half or one third of the superior nuchal line of the occiput.

Distal attachment: By two heads to the manubrium of the sternum and the superior surface of the medial one third of the clavicle.

Innervation: Spinal accessory nerve and from the ventral rami of C2-3.

Palpation: This muscle is easy to palpate at its distal attachments. However, contraction of the sternoclavicular is elicited best with side bending and contralateral rotation of the head. These movements are discussed again in Chapter 27.

The sternocleidomastoid purportedly can assist in elevating the clavicle. However, because the axes of the sternoclavicular joint are lateral to the joint itself, the sternocleidomastoid's attachment on the clavicle is very close to the axes of motion of the sternoclavicular joint. Therefore, the muscle has a very short moment arm and a poor mechanical advantage for sternoclavicular joint elevation [5]. Its actions and impairments are more readily observed at the head and neck. It is discussed in greater detail in Chapter 27 with other muscles of the head and neck.

Summary of Axioscapular and Axioclavicular Muscles

The muscles of the axioscapular and axioclavicular group position and stabilize the shoulder girdle. Movement of the scapulothoracic and sternoclavicular joints is essential to the full and normal motion of the shoulder complex. For example, a complex three-dimensional model of the shoulder apparatus suggests that the scapulothoracic muscles provide up to 45% of the energy to flex the shoulder rapidly through small excursions [22]. Therefore, weakness of these muscles can disrupt the motion of the shoulder complex by preventing or limiting the essential contribution from the shoulder girdle and seriously altering the mechanics of the whole shoulder complex.

The scapulothoracic muscles' role in stabilizing the scapula also is critical to the proper function of the shoulder. Because the scapula is free to glide across the posterior thorax, muscles of the axioscapular and axioclavicular group frequently contract in pairs, creating anatomical force couples. These force couples are composed of muscles that exert opposing forces to stabilize the scapula while providing similar forces to

produce a rotation. The ability of the scapulohumeral muscles to move the glenohumeral joint depends upon their contraction from a stable scapula. If the scapula is not fixed adequately, pull from any of the scapulohumeral muscles may move the scapula instead of the humerus. Recognition of these general principles dictating the function of the muscles in this group provides the clinician with the tools to identify the abnormal mechanics contributing to a patient's complaints of shoulder pain or dysfunction.

SCAPULOHUMERAL MUSCLES

The scapulohumeral muscles provide motion and dynamic stabilization to the glenohumeral joint (*Fig. 9.23*). The glenohumeral joint provides over 50% of the ROM of arm–trunk elevation. Therefore, these muscles are critical to the active mobility of the shoulder as a whole. The muscles of the scapulohumeral group are the deltoid, teres major, coracobrachialis, and the four muscles of the rotator cuff, which are the supraspinatus, infraspinatus, teres minor, and subscapularis. The functions of these muscles are intimately related to each other, particularly those of the deltoid and rotator cuff muscles. The deltoid and the rotator cuff muscles are first presented individually; then their functional interplay is presented. The remaining two scapulohumeral muscles are then discussed.

Deltoid

The deltoid exhibits substantial change from the deltoid of lower primates and other mammals (*Muscle Attachment Box 9.8*) [27]. It has greatly increased in size in keeping with the increased breadth of the scapula, described in Chapter 8. The expansion of the acromion in humans increases the mechanical advantage of the deltoid as the distal migration of the deltoid tuberosity effectively increases the deltoid's contractile length [27]. These changes improve the deltoid's ability to move the glenohumeral joint through its large available ROM.

The deltoid is divided into three parts: anterior, middle, and posterior (*Fig. 9.24*). Like some of the axioscapular muscles, the deltoid's individual components have unique actions that are presented first, followed by the effects of impairments of each component. The muscle's actions and impairments as a whole are then discussed.

ACTIONS OF THE ANTERIOR DELTOID

MUSCLE ACTION: ANTERIOR DELTOID

Actions	Evidence
Shoulder flexion	Supporting
Shoulder medial rotation	Conflicting
Shoulder abduction	Conflicting
Shoulder horizontal adduction	Inadequate

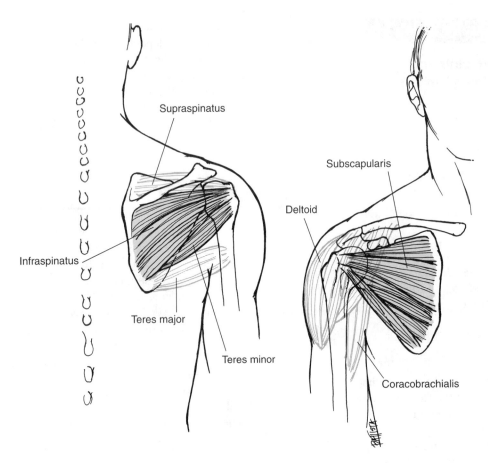

Figure 9.23: Scapulohumeral muscles. The scapulohumeral muscles consist of the deltoid, supraspinatus, infraspinatus, teres minor, subscapularis, teres major, and coracobrachialis.

There is general agreement regarding the anterior deltoid muscle's contribution to flexion of the shoulder [3,24,35,39, 63,82,84]. However, there is less agreement about its role in the other actions. Some EMG studies report activity of the anterior deltoid muscle in medial rotation, while others deny activity [3,39]. Analysis of its moment arm supports its role as a medial rotator in most positions [41].

MUSCLE ATTACHMENT BOX 9.8

ATTACHMENTS AND INNERVATION OF THE DELTOID

Proximal attachment: The anterior and superior surfaces of the lateral one third of the clavicle, the lateral border and superior surface of the acromion, and the lower lip of the crest of the scapular spine. It is a multipennate muscle.

Distal attachment: Deltoid tuberosity.

Innervation: Axillary nerve, C5-6.

Palpation: Each part of the deltoid muscle is easily identified over the superior aspect of the shoulder.

Brandell and Wilkinson demonstrate selective contraction of the anterior deltoid during isometric contraction with resistance in the combined direction of abduction and flexion with the shoulder slightly rotated laterally (*Fig. 9.25*) [8]. This position represents a standard position to test the strength of the anterior deltoid muscle in manual muscle testing, and these data support the view that the position selectively recruits the anterior deltoid without the other two portions of the deltoid [35]. Although there are no known studies denying the anterior deltoid's activity in horizontal adduction, only a few authors mention the action at all [3,24,82].

Most of the EMG studies in the literature report data collected from only a few subjects and assess a relatively small group of muscles [8,39]. Therefore, the normal variation in recruitment patterns exhibited in a healthy population is probably underrepresented. In addition, clearly certain actions have multiple muscles contributing to the motion. The recruitment order may be individual. For example, Jackson et al. report that during shoulder flexion, the anterior deltoid is generally recruited before the clavicular portion of the pectoralis major muscle, but some individuals reverse that order [28]. Thus continued investigation is required to clarify the role of the anterior deltoid in actions of the shoulder. It undoubtedly contributes to shoulder flexion, but its contribution to other actions remains unclear.

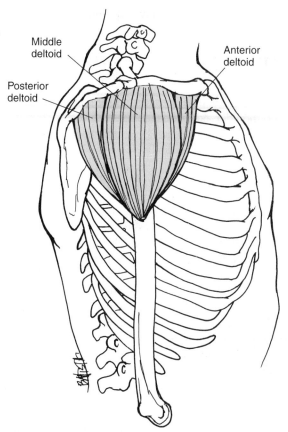

Figure 9.24: Deltoid muscle. The deltoid muscle consists of an anterior, middle, and posterior portion.

EFFECTS OF WEAKNESS OF THE ANTERIOR DELTOID

The effects of weakness of the anterior deltoid muscle depend, of course, upon the role it plays in the actions listed above.

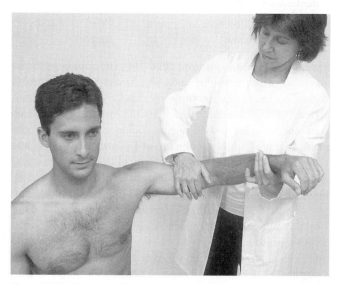

Figure 9.25: The manual muscle test (MMT) position for the anterior deltoid muscle. EMG studies show that the MMT position of flexion, abduction, and slight lateral rotation of the shoulder isolates the anterior deltoid better than other suggested positions.

Weakness of the anterior deltoid muscle is likely to produce weakness in shoulder flexion. However, weakness may also result in diminished strength of shoulder medial rotation, shoulder abduction, and horizontal adduction.

EFFECTS OF TIGHTNESS OF THE ANTERIOR DELTOID

Like the effects of weakness, the effects of tightness of the anterior deltoid depend on its actions. However, it is commonly accepted that tightness of the anterior deltoid can contribute to diminished shoulder extension and lateral rotation ROM.

ACTIONS OF THE POSTERIOR DELTOID

MUSCLE ACTION: POSTERIOR DELTOID

Actions	Evidence
Shoulder extension	Supporting
Shoulder lateral rotation	Conflicting
Shoulder abduction	Conflicting
Shoulder adduction	Conflicting
Shoulder horizontal abduction	Supporting

As with the anterior deltoid, there is confusion and disagreement regarding the actions of the posterior deltoid. There is widespread agreement that the posterior deltoid muscle contributes to shoulder extension [3,8,82]. In one study, shoulder hyperextension isolates posterior deltoid activity from the rest of the deltoid muscle better than lateral rotation, abduction, or combined movements [8]. Lateral rotation also is reported by some to elicit activity of the posterior deltoid muscle, but others deny its contribution [3,39]. Its moment arm for rotation is small but could produce lateral rotation with the shoulder in neutral [41].

Several studies demonstrate that horizontal abduction activates the posterior deltoid [2,3,8,71,82]. Finally, some authors report activity in the posterior deltoid during abduction, while others find it active during adduction [3,39]. Analysis of the moment arm of the posterior deltoid supports its role as an adductor of the shoulder in both the plane of the scapula and in the frontal plane, especially with the shoulder laterally rotated [4,40,55]. It is clear from this discussion that the full role of the posterior deltoid in shoulder motion remains to be elucidated. It is also likely that the position of the shoulder can alter the line of pull of the posterior deltoid with respect to the axes of motion of the shoulder. Such alteration may allow the posterior deltoid to produce an action in one shoulder position and the opposite action in another shoulder position where the line of pull of the muscle has crossed the axis of motion. Additional EMG studies combined with thorough analyses of the muscle's line of pull are required to define clearly the role of the posterior deltoid muscle.

EFFECTS OF WEAKNESS OF THE POSTERIOR DELTOID

The effects of weakness of the posterior deltoid depend on its roles listed above but surely include decreased shoulder extension strength. Identification of additional effects requires further study.

EFFECTS OF TIGHTNESS OF THE POSTERIOR DELTOID

As in weakness, the most likely effects of tightness of the posterior deltoid muscle are restricted shoulder flexion and horizonal adduction ROM. Additional effects may include reduced medial rotation ROM, but additional study is needed to determine this conclusively.

ACTIONS OF THE MIDDLE DELTOID

The middle deltoid is the only head of the deltoid that is multipennate [63,84]. In addition, it has a larger proximal attachment and a larger cross-sectional area than the other two parts of the deltoid muscle [43,45]. These findings suggest that the middle portion of the deltoid muscle is specialized for force production.

MUSCLE ACTION: MIDDLE DELTOID

Actions	Evidence
Shoulder abduction	Supporting
Shoulder flexion	Supporting
Shoulder extension	Inadequate

There is little doubt that the middle deltoid is an abductor of the shoulder. Although some authors suggest that the anterior and posterior deltoid muscles also contribute to shoulder abduction [39], Brandell and Wilkinson state that maximally resisted abduction with neutral shoulder rotation or with slight medial rotation yielded consistent isolated middle deltoid muscle activity compared to the other parts of the deltoid muscle in three individuals without shoulder pathology [8]. Regardless of the contributions of the anterior and posterior segments, the middle deltoid muscle is a major contributor to shoulder abduction. It contracts throughout active abduction but is most active in the middle of the ROM [39]. However, the role of the deltoid muscle as an abductor is intimately related to the roles of the rotator cuff muscles. Therefore, the action of the deltoid muscle (particularly the middle deltoid) in abduction is revisited following the presentation of the rotator cuff muscles.

EMG studies reveal activity of the middle deltoid during shoulder flexion [2,3]. Analysis of the muscle's moment arm also supports its capacity to assist in shoulder flexion [40]. In contrast, there is less evidence supporting a role in shoulder extension [39].

EFFECTS OF WEAKNESS OF THE MIDDLE DELTOID

Loss of the middle deltoid weakens, but does not eliminate, active abduction of the shoulder [25,82]. Case reports suggest that deltoid paralysis results in only a moderate decrease in abduction strength [82]. Effects of weakness in the abductor component of the deltoid muscle is discussed again following the discussion of the rotator cuff muscles. Weakness of the

middle deltoid muscle probably also contributes to decreased strength in shoulder flexion.

EFFECTS OF TIGHTNESS OF THE MIDDLE DELTOID

It is unlikely that tightness of the middle deltoid muscle actually can restrict shoulder adduction ROM. However, the position of shoulder adduction applies tension to the middle deltoid and may cause pain or additional disruption to the tendon of the deltoid or the bursa lying deep to it.

Supraspinatus

The supraspinatus is part of the rotator cuff, which also includes the infraspinatus, teres minor, and subscapularis. All of these muscles play an essential role in stabilizing the glenohumeral joint. EMG data demonstrate activity in these muscles throughout most active shoulder elevation [27,39,65]. Some of this activity reflects the muscles' function as prime movers and some likely reflects their roles as dynamic stabilizers. This section presents the individual muscles and their specific roles as prime movers. Following the discussion of the individual muscles, their group function as dynamic stabilizers during shoulder motion is presented.

The supraspinatus muscle is the most superior muscle of the rotator cuff group (*Fig. 9.26*) (*Muscle Attachment Box 9.9*). It lies deep to the subacromial (subdeltoid) bursa, the coracoacromial ligament, and the deltoid muscle and acromion process [47].

ACTIONS OF THE SUPRASPINATUS

MUSCLE ACTION: SUPRASPINATUS

Actions	Evidence
Shoulder abduction	Supporting
Shoulder lateral rotation	Supporting
Shoulder medial rotation	Supporting
Shoulder stabilization	Supporting

There is general consensus that the supraspinatus is an abductor of the shoulder [3,63,84]. Analysis of the muscle's abduction moment arm supports this view [55]. Maximum activity of the supraspinatus with minimal activity in surrounding muscles is seen during shoulder abduction in the plane of the scapula accompanied by lateral rotation [34]. However, a classic test of the integrity of the supraspinatus is resisted shoulder abduction in the plane of the scapula with medial rotation of the shoulder [44,85]. These positions suggest that the supraspinatus may contribute to either medial or lateral rotation of the shoulder. Analysis of the moment arms of the supraspinatus suggests that the posterior portion of the muscle is capable of lateral rotation; the anterior portion has a slight medial rotation moment arm when the shoulder is in neutral or in flexion but can cause a lateral rotation moment when the shoulder is moderately abducted [41,55]. EMG activity supports the role of the supraspinatus in shoulder lateral rotation [61].

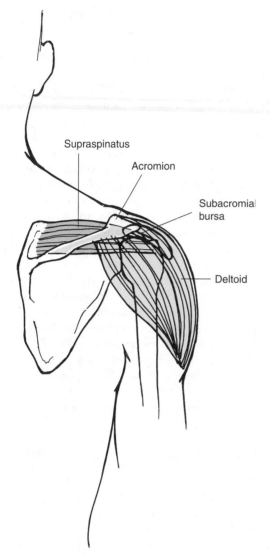

Figure 9.26: Supraspinatus muscle. The supraspinatus lies deep to the acromion, the deltoid, and the subacromial bursa.

MUSCLE ATTACHMENT BOX 9:9

ATTACHMENTS AND INNERVATION OF THE SUPRASPINATUS

Proximal attachment: Medial two thirds of the supraspinous fossa and the overlying supraspinous fascia.

Distal attachment: Superior facet of the greater tubercle of the humerus and the glenohumeral joint capsule.

Innervation: Suprascapular nerve, C5-6.

Palpation: The superficial portion of the supraspinatus muscle belly can be palpated in the supraspinous fossa through a relaxed trapezius. The tendon of the supraspinatus muscle also can be palpated at its insertion through a relaxed deltoid muscle with the shoulder in extension and adduction. Data from cadavers reveal that a position combining maximal adduction, 80–90° of medial rotation, and 30–40° of hyperextension gives best exposure of the tendon [46].

pull to hold the humeral head against the glenoid process [3]. This role may be enhanced by the upward tilt of the glenoid fossa in upright posture, because descent of the humeral head on the upwardly turned glenoid fossa requires simultaneous lateral movement of the humeral head (*Fig. 9.27*).

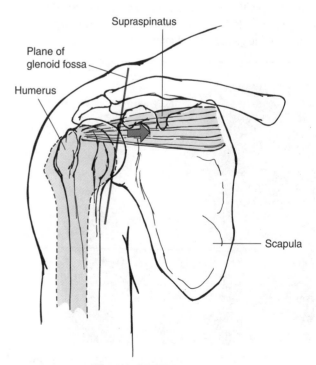

Figure 9.27: Pull of the supraspinatus. The medial pull of the supraspinatus helps prevent inferior displacement of the humeral head, since in an upwardly turned glenoid fossa, the humeral head must move laterally as it slides inferiorly on the fossa.

Some references state that the supraspinatus "initiates" shoulder abduction [63]. However EMG data clearly reveal activity in all of the rotator cuff muscles and the deltoid muscle throughout the range of active abduction [27,39]. A study in which the supraspinatus muscle was temporarily paralyzed by a neural block demonstrates full active shoulder abduction range even in the absence of any supraspinatus force [79]. These studies demonstrate that the supraspinatus muscle is *not* solely responsible for the initiation of shoulder abduction.

The supraspinatus muscle also is reported to participate specifically in stabilizing the glenohumeral joint in the inferior direction [3,73]. Although the deltoid muscle is well aligned to prevent descent of the humeral head in the glenoid fossa in quiet standing [21], some individuals show no activity in the deltoid in upright posture [3]. In contrast, the supraspinatus in some individuals exhibits EMG activity during erect standing, particularly as the upper extremity is pulled inferiorly by a weight in the hand. The supraspinatus helps stabilize the glenohumeral joint by exerting a horizontal

A force that prevents lateral movement, such as the one applied by the supraspinatus, also prevents descent. However, since some authors suggest that the glenoid fossa is actually turned downward in normal alignment, the role of the supraspinatus in preventing inferior instability of the glenohumeral joint remains unresolved.

Clinical Relevance

INFERIOR SUBLUXATION OF THE GLENOHUMERAL JOINT: *The proposed function of the supraspinatus in preventing the inferior subluxation of the glenohumeral joint is facilitated by the upward tilt of the glenoid fossa. Thus weakness of the muscles that suspend the scapula may contribute to inferior subluxations of the joint. Such inferior subluxations of the shoulder are frequently found in patients with diffuse upper extremity weakness following stroke (Fig. 9.28). Weakness of the trapezius is reportedly characterized by depression of the acromion process demonstrating downward rotation of the scapula. Thus the inferior subluxation of the glenohumeral joint may be the result of the combined effects of weakness of the supraspinatus and trapezius muscles. Splints that provide an upward force on the humerus to stabilize an inferiorly subluxed glenohumeral joint are generally unsuccessful in reducing the subluxation. Current treatment approaches include exercises to restore an upward tilt of the glenoid fossa while facilitating the activity of the rotator cuff muscles [13,64]. Additional study is required to clarify the mechanism of inferior subluxation and to optimize treatment. However, the position of the scapula should be considered when developing strategies to stabilize the glenohumeral joint.*

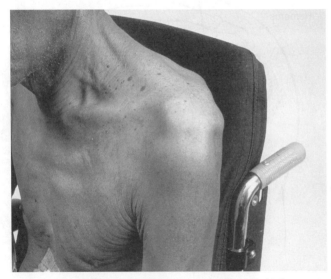

Figure 9.28: Inferior subluxation of the glenohumeral joint. Inferior subluxation of the glenohumeral joint is seen frequently in individuals following a stroke. Downward rotation of the scapula may decrease the stabilizing forces of the horizontally aligned muscles and ligaments.

EFFECTS OF WEAKNESS OF THE SUPRASPINATUS

Weakness of the supraspinatus muscle is rather common. It can result from denervation secondary to an entrapment of the suprascapular nerve [36,51]. However, it more commonly results from mechanical disruption of the muscle's tendon or its insertion into the glenohumeral joint capsule. Weakness may also result from inhibition of muscle contraction caused by pain secondary to such disorders as tendinitis. Degeneration of the tendons of the rotator cuff with age is well documented and is particularly evident in the supraspinatus [9,66,67]. Inherent in this process of degeneration is a decrease in the vascularity of the supraspinatus tendon, predisposing the tendon to further damage. Degeneration of the supraspinatus tendon is correlated with a decrease in the material strength of the tendon. Consequently, degeneration of the supraspinatus tendon may be a causative factor in rotator cuff tears, particularly since rotator cuff tears most frequently involve the supraspinatus [84]. Thus there are many factors to consider to explain the presence of supraspinatus weakness.

Weakness of the supraspinatus is manifested by a significant decrease in the strength and endurance of shoulder abduction [79]. However, it must be emphasized that active shoulder abduction is still possible, albeit significantly weakened, even in the presence of complete supraspinatus paralysis or disruption.

EFFECTS OF TIGHTNESS OF THE SUPRASPINATUS

Although spontaneous tightness of the supraspinatus tendon is unlikely, it can be present following surgical repair of a rotator cuff tear. Consideration should be given to positions that could stretch the supraspinatus since they should be avoided in the presence of a rotator cuff tear or following repair of the supraspinatus tendon. Adduction or medial rotation, particularly with shoulder hyperextension, stretches the supraspinatus [53]. Shoulder adduction across the plane of the body also may stretch the supraspinatus. Kelley advises care when exercising in the position of shoulder medial rotation and adduction in the presence of supraspinatus pathology [33].

Infraspinatus

The infraspinatus is described in most anatomy textbooks as a single muscle belly (*Muscle Attachment Box 9.10*) [63,84]. However, in biomechanical literature the muscle is described with two or three separate portions (*Fig. 9.29*) [31,55].

ACTIONS OF THE INFRASPINATUS

MUSCLE ACTION:

Actions	Evidence
Shoulder lateral rotation	Supporting
Shoulder horizontal abduction	Supporting
Shoulder abduction	Supporting
Shoulder stabilization	Supporting

MUSCLE ATTACHMENT BOX 9.10

ATTACHMENTS AND INNERVATION OF THE INFRASPINATUS

Proximal attachment: Medial two thirds of the infraspinous fossa and overlying infraspinous fascia.

Distal attachment: Middle facet on the greater tubercle of the humerus and the glenohumeral joint capsule.

Innervation: Suprascapular nerve, C5-6.

Palpation: The infraspinatus muscle belly is palpable in the infraspinous fossa lateral to the trapezius and inferior to the deltoid muscle. The tendon also can be palpated with the shoulder flexed, adducted, and medially rotated [46].

The infraspinatus muscle is regarded by most authors as an important and powerful lateral rotator muscle [24,35,63,84]. This is consistent with the muscle's large attachment on the scapula and its large lateral rotation moment arm. Kuechle

describes it as the most efficient lateral rotator of the shoulder [41]. EMG data and analysis of its moment arms also support the role of the infraspinatus in horizontal abduction [2,3,40]. Although not typically described as an abductor of the shoulder, careful analysis of the moment arms of the individual parts of the infraspinatus suggests that the infraspinatus also is positioned to contribute to the total abductor moment [26,40,55]. Selective ablation of the infraspinatus decreases the abduction moment produced by simulated activity of the remaining muscles in cadaver specimens [52].

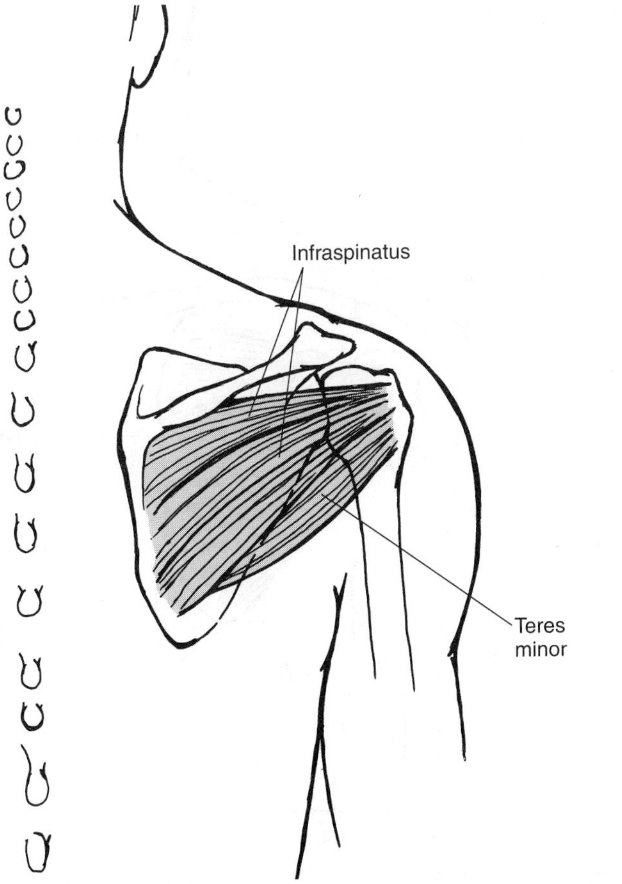

EFFECTS OF WEAKNESS OF THE INFRASPINATUS

Isolated weakness of the infraspinatus is unusual but has been reported [36,42]. It is manifested clinically by a significant reduction in the strength of lateral rotation of the shoulder. More frequently, the infraspinatus is weakened together with other muscles of the rotator cuff through a mechanical disruption of the cuff itself.

EFFECTS OF TIGHTNESS OF THE INFRASPINATUS

Tightness of the infraspinatus contributes to decreased ROM of shoulder medial rotation and may also contribute to decreased horizontal adduction ROM. However, Muraki et al. suggest that the posterior deltoid and posterior glenohumeral joint capsule are more likely limiters [53].

Teres Minor

Some describe the teres minor as a distal belly of the deltoid muscle, noting both their common innervation and the attachment of the teres minor muscle distal to the glenohumeral joint capsule (*Muscle Attachment Box 9.11*) [27,31]. It also has the smallest physiological cross-sectional area of the rotator cuff muscles, although it is substantially larger than in other mammals.

MUSCLE ATTACHMENT BOX 9.11

ATTACHMENTS AND INNERVATION OF THE TERES MINOR

Proximal attachment: Superior two thirds of the lateral aspect of the dorsal surface of the scapula, lateral to the infraspinatus.

Distal attachment: Inferior facet of the greater tubercle of the humerus and distally onto the shaft of the humerus. It also attaches to the capsule of the glenohumeral joint.

Innervation: Axillary nerve, C5-6.

Palpation: The teres minor muscle can be palpated with the infraspinatus muscle.

Figure 9.29: Infraspinatus and the teres minor. The infraspinatus and teres minor are important lateral rotators of the shoulder.

ACTIONS OF THE TERES MINOR

MUSCLE ACTION: TERES MINOR

Actions	Evidence
Shoulder lateral rotation	Supporting
Shoulder adduction	Supporting
Shoulder stabilization	Supporting

The role of the teres minor as a lateral rotator of the shoulder is well established [24,35,63,84]. However, its physiological cross-sectional area is approximately one third that of the infraspinatus [31]. Therefore, the teres minor can contribute only a small additional amount of force to lateral rotation. Although adduction is not mentioned as an action of the teres minor in most anatomy texts, analysis of its moment arm supports its ability to produce an adduction moment [55].

EFFECTS OF WEAKNESS OF THE TERES MINOR

Weakness of the teres minor can contribute to a decrease in the strength of shoulder lateral rotation. However, since the physiological cross-sectional area of the teres minor is so much smaller than that of the other lateral rotators, the decrease in lateral rotation strength is unlikely to be significant.

EFFECTS OF TIGHTNESS OF THE TERES MINOR

Isolated tightness of the teres minor is unlikely. The size of the teres minor also suggests that tightness of the teres minor by itself has little functional significance. However, tightness of the teres minor is likely to be accompanied by tightness of the infraspinatus. Together they limit medial rotation ROM.

Subscapularis

The subscapularis muscle is the largest of the rotator cuff muscles (*Muscle Attachment Box 9.12*) (*Fig. 9.30*) [27,31,43].

ACTIONS OF THE SUBSCAPULARIS

MUSCLE ACTION:

Actions	Evidence
Shoulder medial rotation	Supporting
Shoulder flexion	Inadequate
Shoulder extension	Inadequate
Shoulder abduction	Supporting
Shoulder adduction	Supporting
Shoulder horizontal adduction	Inadequate
Shoulder stabilization	Supporting

There is broad agreement regarding the role of the subscapularis in medial rotation of the shoulder [24,35,63,84]. The remaining actions are reported infrequently. The role of the subscapularis in abduction and adduction may depend on the position of the glenohumeral joint [71]. Analysis of the moment arms of the subscapularis muscle suggest that it may adduct when the shoulder is medially rotated but may abduct

MUSCLE ATTACHMENT BOX 9.12

ATTACHMENTS AND INNERVATION OF THE SUBSCAPULARIS

Proximal attachment: Subscapularis fossa and the lateral border of the ventral surface of the scapula. It also attaches to tendinous intramuscular septa and the aponeurosis that covers the muscle ventrally.

Distal attachment: Lesser tubercle of the humerus and the anterior aspect of the glenohumeral joint capsule.

Innervation: Upper and lower subscapular nerves, C5-6 and perhaps C7.

Palpation: This muscle is difficult to palpate but can be felt in the axilla by palpating the ventral surface of the scapula when the scapula is abducted. Cadaver data also suggest that the tendon is palpable in the deltopectoral triangle with the upper extremity against the thorax and the shoulder in neutral [46].

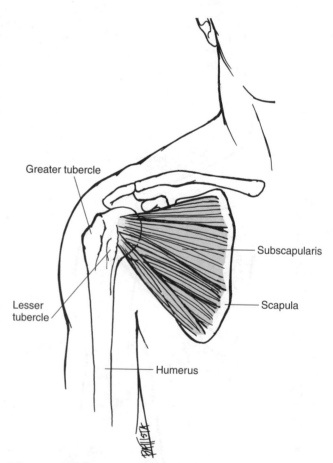

Figure 9.30: Subscapularis muscle. The subscapularis is the only rotator cuff muscle on the anterior aspect of the glenohumeral joint.

when the shoulder is in neutral or is laterally rotated [26,40,55].

One explanation for the confusion about the actions of the subscapularis may be the fact that the subscapularis contracts during most active motions of the glenohumeral joint [39]. However, that recorded activity may be the activity of the subscapularis to stabilize the glenohumeral joint. Distinguishing its role as a dynamic stabilizer of the shoulder from prime mover of the shoulder is difficult and requires concerted effort combining EMG data and careful analysis of the muscle's line of pull.

EFFECTS OF WEAKNESS OF THE SUBSCAPULARIS

Weakness of the subscapularis results in a significant decrease in strength of shoulder medial rotation [19]. Weakness of the subscapularis may also contribute to anterior instability of the glenohumeral joint.

Clinical Relevance

SUBSCAPULARIS WEAKNESS: *Decreased activation of the subscapularis is reported in some individuals who can sublux their glenohumeral joints spontaneously using lateral rotation [10,29,33]. Muscle re-education to facilitate the subscapularis and other medial rotators is an important component of the rehabilitation program to increase stability [48].*

EFFECTS OF TIGHTNESS OF THE SUBSCAPULARIS

Tightness of the subscapularis causes decreased lateral rotation ROM at the shoulder. Tightness of the subscapularis muscle sometimes is induced deliberately to improve joint stability surgically in individuals with chronic anterior dislocations of the glenohumeral joints.

DYNAMIC STABILIZATION BY THE ROTATOR CUFF

Chapter 8 presents the role of the noncontractile supporting structures of the glenohumeral joint in stabilizing the joint. While these structures provide some stability, they are insufficient to stabilize the joint against large forces and in all joint positions. EMG and cadaver studies as well as mathematical models consistently indicate the importance of the rotator cuff in stabilizing the glenohumeral joint [2,22]. The rotator cuff muscles provide critical additional support to the joint. One study demonstrates that contraction of the rotator cuff prevents visible instability of the glenohumeral joint during shoulder movement, even in the presence of large anterior disruptions of the joint capsule [1]. This same study suggests that contraction of the rotator cuff muscles even prevents dislocation after complete anterior–posterior disruption of the capsule. Conversely, decreased contraction force of the rotator cuff results in increased anterior and posterior gliding of the glenohumeral joint during abduction in the plane of the

scapula [86]. Weakness may also allow increased superior glide of the humeral head during shoulder elevation.

Clinical Relevance

ROTATOR CUFF MUSCLES AND REHABILITATION OF THE UNSTABLE GLENOHUMERAL JOINT: *Studies demonstrating the importance of rotator cuff activity in stabilizing the glenohumeral joint suggest that these muscles should be evaluated carefully in the presence of glenohumeral joint instability. Additionally, exercises to strengthen the rotator cuff muscles are an important element of the treatment of the unstable shoulder [17,38].*

COORDINATED ACTIVITY OF DELTOID AND ROTATOR CUFF MUSCLES DURING SHOULDER ELEVATION

The roles of the deltoid and rotator cuff muscles in producing shoulder flexion and abduction are well studied. These studies grew out of the clinical observation that individuals with rotator cuff weakness, particularly of the supraspinatus, had severe difficulty elevating the shoulder. These observations led to the myth that the supraspinatus is responsible for initiating shoulder abduction, which has subsequently been refuted although not completely abandoned. Clinical evidence supported, but did not explain, the integral role of the rotator cuff in arm–trunk elevation. Careful anatomical and biomechanical studies have now provided firm evidence for, and a clear explanation of, the integrated function of the deltoid and the rotator cuff during these motions.

When the glenohumeral joint is in the neutral position, the deltoid muscle has a small angle of application, or moment arm, for abduction, while the supraspinatus has a larger abduction moment arm (1.42 vs. 2.6 cm) (*Fig. 9.31*) [55]. In this position the line of pull of the middle deltoid, the primary abductor of the shoulder, is directed mostly superiorly, so that contraction of the middle deltoid muscle tends to produce superior translation of the humeral head on the glenoid fossa rather than an abduction rotation. The supraspinatus has a mechanical advantage by virtue of its larger moment arm, so contraction by the supraspinatus tends to produce abduction while simultaneously compressing the glenohumeral joint. Thus the deltoid and supraspinatus muscles form another anatomical force couple to produce abduction. However, the physiological cross-sectional area of the supraspinatus muscle is considerably smaller that that of the deltoid muscle, and consequently, the supraspinatus is incapable of generating large abduction moments. Thus powerful abduction requires the simultaneous activity of both the deltoid and supraspinatus muscles.

Unrestricted superior glide of the humeral head results in compression of the contents of the subacromial space. However, as the deltoid contracts at the beginning of elevation, all of the

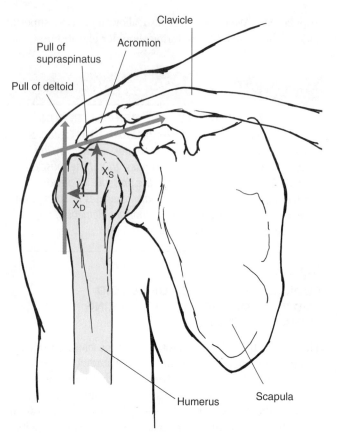

Figure 9.31: Moment arms of the deltoid and supraspinatus for abduction. The abduction moment arm of the supraspinatus muscle is slightly greater than that of the deltoid muscle with the shoulder in neutral. However, the deltoid's moment arm improves in the midrange of abduction.

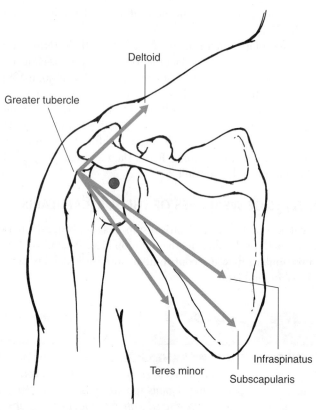

Figure 9.32: Force couple formed by the deltoid and the infraspinatus, teres minor, and subscapularis. The upward pull of the deltoid is balanced by the downward pull of the infraspinatus, teres minor, and subscapularis muscles.

rotator cuff muscles also contract and exert a compressive force on the proximal humerus holding the head of the humerus firmly against the glenoid fossa. Simultaneously, the teres minor, the lower portion of the infraspinatus, and the subscapularis apply an inferior force on the humeral head, providing additional protection against superior glide of the humeral head (*Fig. 9.32*) [27,58]. The contraction of the teres minor, infraspinatus, and subscapularis with the deltoid is another example of an anatomical force couple in which the upward and downward pulls of the muscles are balanced, and the forces contribute to abduction.

By midrange of abduction the mechanical advantage of the deltoid improves, its abduction moment arm exceeding that of the supraspinatus [55]. Thus as the moments required to abduct the upper extremity increase, the large deltoid muscle is better able to perform the task. However, the entire rotator cuff continues contracting throughout the full range of abduction, providing continued stabilizing forces to the glenohumeral joint [27,39]. Details of the forces involved in this function are presented in Chapter 10.

Thus abduction and flexion of the glenohumeral joint depend on three factors: the deltoid, the supraspinatus, and the depressors of the humeral head, including the infraspinatus, teres minor, and subscapularis muscles. The deltoid provides strength to the movement; the supraspinatus provides mechanical advantage early in the ROM and, with the rest of the rotator cuff, joint compression throughout the movement; and the infraspinatus, teres minor, and subscapularis muscles stabilize the humeral head inferiorly. Loss of any of these elements results in significant impairment in the ability to elevate the shoulder.

Clinical Relevance

ROTATOR CUFF WEAKNESS: ANOTHER POSSIBLE CAUSE OF IMPINGEMENT SYNDROME: *The rotator cuff muscles seem to be particularly susceptible to fatigue and overuse, especially in middle-aged adults. Thus it is not surprising to see middle-aged patients who report a history of acute onset of shoulder pain following unusual and prolonged overhead activity such as three sets of tennis at the beginning of the tennis season or an afternoon of window washing. A likely scenario to explain the complaints is (a) prolonged overhead activity; (b) fatigue of the rotator cuff muscles; (c) inadequate stabilization of the humeral head; and (d) superior glide of the humerus causing compression of the contents of the subacromial space, including the subacromial*

(continued)

(Continued)

bursa and supraspinatus tendon; with (e) resulting bursitis or tendinitis. Successful treatment of the patient's complaints must include interventions to reduce inflammation of the bursa or tendon. These interventions include medication, rest, and ice. However, treatment should also address the underlying pathomechanics, with particular focus on strength and endurance training for the rotator cuff muscles. Patient education explaining the relationship between fatigue and pathomechanics also may help the patient avoid a recurrence.

Teres Major

ACTIONS OF THE TERES MAJOR

MUSCLE ACTION:

Actions	Evidence
Shoulder medial rotation	Supporting
Shoulder extension	Supporting
Shoulder adduction	Supporting

The teres major is not well studied (*Muscle Attachment Box 9.13*) (*Fig. 9.33*). However, available EMG data reveal activity of the teres major muscle during all three of these actions in the presence of resistance but no activity without resistance unless the shoulder is hyperextended [3]. The teres major appears to be recruited without resistance during shoulder hyperextension and during adduction in the hyperextended position. Moment arm analysis supports its potential as a medial rotator in most shoulder positions [41].

The teres major also exhibits EMG activity with the shoulder held in static positions of flexion or abduction [27]. This contradicts the classic view of the actions of the teres major. However, the teres major is also able to pull on the scapula when the humerus is held fixed. Perhaps the reported activity of the teres major during isometric shoulder flexion or abduction is to assist in stabilizing the scapulothoracic joint rather than to move or hold the glenohumeral joint (*Fig. 9.34*). Additional study is needed to clarify its role in shoulder movements.

MUSCLE ATTACHMENT BOX 9.13

ATTACHMENTS AND INNERVATION OF THE TERES MAJOR

Proximal attachment: Dorsal surface of the inferior angle of the scapula and surrounding fascia.

Distal attachment: Medial lip of the intertubercular groove of the humerus.

Innervation: Lower subscapular nerve, C6-7 and perhaps C5.

Palpation: This muscle is easily identified at the inferior angle of the scapula.

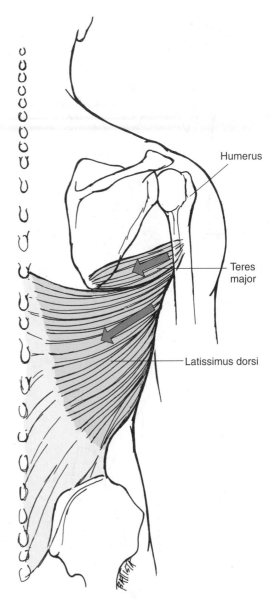

Figure 9.33: Teres major and latissimus dorsi. The teres major and latissimus dorsi have similar directions of pull on the shoulder.

EFFECTS OF WEAKNESS OF THE TERES MAJOR

Because few studies exist investigating the role of the teres major muscle, the effects of weakness can only be hypothesized. It is logical to expect weakness in shoulder medial rotation, extension and hyperextension, and adduction with weakness of the teres major. However data are needed to substantiate these expectations.

EFFECTS OF TIGHTNESS OF THE TERES MAJOR

Again, in the absence of detailed data, tightness of the teres major can be expected to result in restricted ROM in shoulder lateral rotation, flexion, and abduction. The tightness could also influence the resting position and mobility of the scapulothoracic joint. Specifically, tightness of the teres major

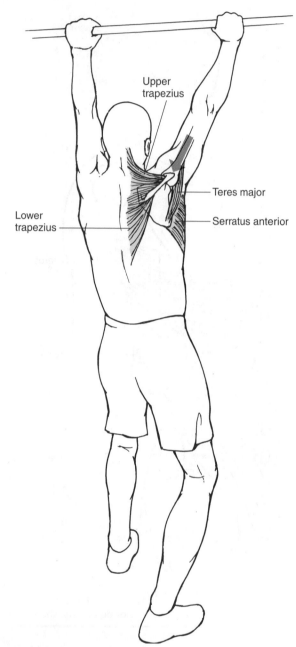

Figure 9.34: Role of the teres major during overhead lifts. A heavy overhead load tends to adduct the scapula, and the contracting teres major may help to stabilize the scapula.

could pull the scapula into a position of abduction and upward rotation, contributing to another variant of the rounded-shoulders posture (*Fig 9.35*).

Coracobrachialis

ACTIONS OF THE CORACOBRACHIALIS

MUSCLE ACTION:

Actions	Evidence
Shoulder flexion	Inadequate
Shoulder adduction	Inadequate

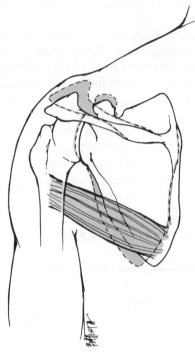

Figure 9.35: Tightness of the teres major. Tightness of the teres major can pull the scapula into upward rotation if the humerus is fixed.

The coracobrachialis is even more poorly studied than the teres major (*Muscle Attachment Box 9.14*) (*Fig. 9.36*). An examination of the moment arm of the coracobrachialis in cadaver shoulders positioned in 90° of abduction and lateral rotation supports its role as a shoulder flexor [4]. In this position the muscle has almost negligible moment arms for shoulder adduction and lateral rotation.

MUSCLE ATTACHMENT BOX 9.14

ATTACHMENTS AND INNERVATION OF THE CORACOBRACHIALIS

Proximal attachment: Tip of the coracoid process of the scapula.

Distal attachment: Middle of the medial aspect of the shaft of the humerus between the attachments of the triceps brachii and the brachialis muscles.

Innervation: Musculocutaneous nerve, C6-7 and perhaps C5.

Palpation: The coracobrachialis is palpable in the proximal arm just distal to the attachment of the pectoralis major and medial to the tendon of the short head of the biceps muscle.

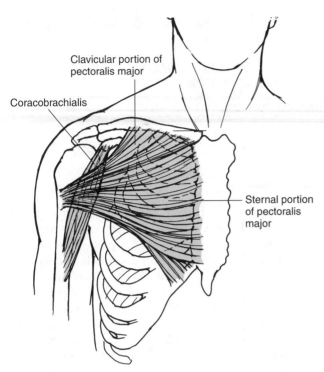

Figure 9.36: Coracobrachialis and pectoralis major. The coracobrachialis and pectoralis major contribute to shoulder flexion.

EFFECTS OF WEAKNESS OR TIGHTNESS OF THE CORACOBRACHIALIS

Effects of weakness must be hypothesized and include diminished strength in flexion and adduction of the shoulder. Effects of tightness also must be hypothesized and presumably include decreased ROM in abduction and extension of the shoulder. Isolated tightness of the coracobrachialis is unlikely.

Summary of the Scapulohumeral Muscles

The scapulohumeral muscles are responsible for positioning the glenohumeral joint as well as providing dynamic stability to the joint. Weakness of these muscles can seriously decrease the strength of shoulder motions. Additionally, weakness can impair the stability of the glenohumeral joint, contributing to a variety of movement dysfunctions ranging from glenohumeral subluxations to shoulder impingement disorders. Careful analysis of each of these muscles is essential to identify the basis of glenohumeral joint dysfunction.

AXIOHUMERAL MUSCLES

The axiohumeral muscles include the pectoralis major and the latissimus dorsi. These muscles attach to the thorax and to the humerus. Thus their fibers cross and consequently affect all four joints of the shoulder complex. The muscles described in the previous two sections, axioscapular, axioclavicular, and scapulohumeral, are capable of moving all four joints of the

shoulder complex through their full ROM. The two muscles of the axiohumeral group are redundant for the purposes of providing full ROM of the shoulder complex. Rather, these two muscles are characterized by their massive attachment sites and large physiological cross-sectional areas. These characteristics suggest that the roles of the pectoralis major and the latissimus dorsi are to provide additional strength to the movements of the shoulder. Between them, the pectoralis major and the latissimus dorsi assist in all motions of the shoulder except lateral rotation. Their combined role in shoulder depression is discussed specifically at the end of this section.

Pectoralis Major

The pectoralis major has two distinct bellies, a smaller clavicular portion and a much larger sternal portion, each named for its proximal attachment (*Muscle Attachment Box 9.15*). These two portions can function together or independently of one another. The following discusses the muscle as a whole and then presents the individual components of the pectoralis major.

ACTIONS OF THE PECTORALIS MAJOR

MUSCLE ACTION:

Actions	Evidence
Shoulder medial rotation	Supporting
Shoulder adduction	Inadequate
Shoulder horizontal adduction	Inadequate
Shoulder depression	Supporting

MUSCLE ATTACHMENT BOX 9.15

ATTACHMENTS AND INNERVATION OF THE PECTORALIS MAJOR

Proximal attachment: Anterior surface of medial one half or two thirds of the clavicle, one half of the anterior surface of the sternum from the sternal notch to the level of about the sixth or seventh costal cartilage, the first through sixth or seventh costal cartilages, and the aponeurosis of the external oblique abdominal muscle.

Distal attachment: Lateral lip of the intertubercular groove of the humerus.

Innervation: Medial and lateral pectoral nerves. The clavicular portion receives innervation from C5-6 and perhaps C7. The sternal portion receives innervation from C8 through T1 and perhaps also from C6 and C7.

Palpation: The clavicular and sternal portions of the pectoralis major are palpated individually anterior to the axilla.

Although there is general agreement that the pectoralis major medially rotates the shoulder, there is less agreement about the conditions under which this occurs. Moment arm analysis supports its potential as a medial rotator with its greatest potential with the shoulder in the neutral position [41]. Some investigators note that it participates in medial rotation only against resistance, while others report activity particularly in the clavicular portion regardless of resistance [3]. These differences may represent individual variability in recruitment patterns, as has been reported with the anterior deltoid [24]. The subscapularis and pectoralis major appear to have the greatest medial rotation potential of all the medial rotators regardless of shoulder position [41]. However, additional studies are needed to clarify the pectoralis major muscle's role in medial rotation as well as in the other purported actions. EMG studies verify that the pectoralis major, including both its bellies, plays an important role in shoulder depression along with the latissimus dorsi [18,59]. This role is described in more detail with the latissimus dorsi. EMG data also demonstrate activity of the pectoralis major muscle during forced inspiration [3]. Its role as a muscle of respiration is discussed again in Chapter 30.

EFFECTS OF WEAKNESS OF THE PECTORALIS MAJOR

Weakness of the pectoralis major affects the combined actions of the whole muscle and the actions of each part in isolation. Weakness of the whole pectoralis major may result in decreased strength in medial rotation, adduction, horizontal adduction of the shoulder, and shoulder depression.

Clinical Relevance

RADICAL MASTECTOMY, A CASE REPORT: *Surgical procedures for the treatment of breast cancer include removal of breast tissue and sometimes underlying musculature. The radical mastectomy, rarely performed any longer, involved the removal of all or part of the pectoralis major. Although weakness was demonstrated following surgery, in some individuals surprisingly little dysfunction followed. A 62-year-old female had undergone bilateral radical mastectomies and total resection of the pectoralis major muscle bilaterally in the 1960s. Yet 10 years later she was the reigning female champion of her local tennis club. The absence of profound loss of function is consistent with the fact that the pectoralis major provides additional strength to the shoulder but no additional motions that are not available from contractions of other muscles.*

EFFECTS OF TIGHTNESS OF THE PECTORALIS MAJOR

Tightness of the pectoralis major is often detected following thoracic surgery or breast surgery [72]. Tightness limits ROM of the shoulder in lateral rotation and horizontal abduction. It may limit shoulder flexion ROM as well. This is explained in

greater detail in the discussion of the individual components of the pectoralis major.

ACTIONS OF THE PECTORALIS MAJOR— CLAVICULAR PORTION

MUSCLE ACTION:

Actions	Evidence
Shoulder flexion	Supporting
Shoulder medial rotation	Supporting
Shoulder depression	Supporting

These actions are widely accepted and substantiated by EMG studies [3,27]. The clavicular head of the pectoralis major and the anterior deltoid muscles are the prime flexors of the shoulder (*Fig. 9.37*) [27,28]. The anterior deltoid muscle was recruited first, followed by the clavicular head of the pectoralis major in seven of eight healthy male subjects during isotonic shoulder flexion. The order was reversed in the remaining subject [28]. These data support the notion that these two muscles work synchronously throughout the ROM of shoulder flexion, although the exact pattern of recruitment may vary.

EFFECTS OF WEAKNESS OF THE CLAVICULAR PORTION OF THE PECTORALIS MAJOR

Weakness of the clavicular portion of the pectoralis major causes significant reduction in the strength of shoulder flexion

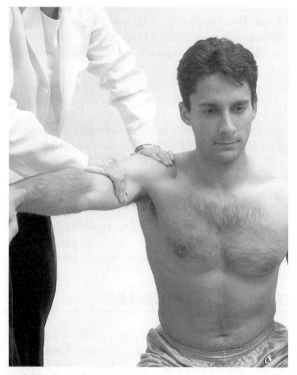

Figure 9.37: Clavicular portion of the pectoralis major. Contraction of the clavicular portion of the pectoralis major is visible during resisted shoulder flexion.

and may contribute to a decrease in the strength of medial rotation of the shoulder.

EFFECTS OF TIGHTNESS OF THE CLAVICULAR PORTION OF THE PECTORALIS MAJOR

Because the weight of the upper extremity tends to keep the shoulder in a neutral sagittal plane position, tightness of only the clavicular head of the pectoralis major is unlikely. However, as a part of the whole pectoralis major, tightness of the clavicular head may contribute to decreased ROM of lateral rotation of the shoulder.

ACTIONS OF THE PECTORALIS MAJOR—STERNAL PORTION

MUSCLE ACTION:

Actions	Evidence
Shoulder extension	Supporting
Shoulder flexion	Supporting
Shoulder adduction	Inadequate
Shoulder medial rotation	Inadequate
Shoulder depression	Supporting

Most authors report that the sternal portion of the pectoralis major extends the shoulder *against resistance*. Note that in the upright position the weight of the upper extremity tends to extend the shoulder, and no additional muscle force is needed. However, when the subject pushes down onto a piece of furniture with the shoulder flexed to 90° the sternal portion is active (*Fig. 9.38*).

Only Inman and colleagues report any activity of the pectoralis major, sternal portion, during flexion, and they note

that the activity is found in the most superior portion and generally through the midrange of flexion only [27]. The remaining activities of the sternal portion of the pectoralis major muscle appear to be widely accepted but apparently untested [24,35,63,71,84].

EFFECTS OF WEAKNESS OF THE STERNAL PORTION OF THE PECTORALIS MAJOR

Weakness of the sternal portion of the pectoralis major causes a loss of strength in shoulder extension from the flexed position and perhaps in medial rotation and adduction.

EFFECTS OF TIGHTNESS OF THE STERNAL PORTION OF THE PECTORALIS MAJOR

Tightness of the sternal portion of the pectoralis major is likely to restrict shoulder abduction and flexion ROM as well as lateral rotation ROM of the shoulder.

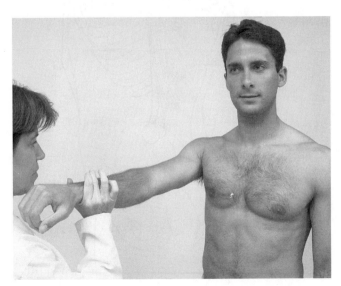

Figure 9.38: Sternal portion of the pectoralis major. Contraction of the sternal portion of the pectoralis major is apparent during resisted shoulder extension.

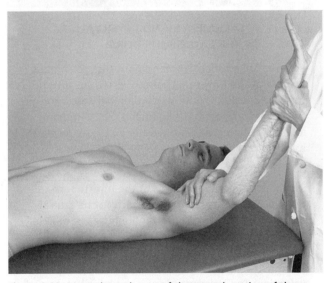

Figure 9.39: Manual muscle test of the sternal portion of the pectoralis major. When the individual is supine with the shoulder flexed, the weight of the upper extremity tends to flex the shoulder. Extension of the shoulder from this position requires a concentric contraction of the sternal portion of the pectoralis major.

Latissimus Dorsi

The latissimus dorsi is a broad flat muscle with an extensive attachment on the spine and pelvis, suggesting that this muscle is capable of generating large forces (*Muscle Attachment Box 9.16*).

ACTIONS OF THE LATISSIMUS DORSI MUSCLE

MUSCLE ACTION:

Actions	Evidence
Shoulder extension	Supporting
Shoulder adduction	Supporting
Shoulder medial rotation	Supporting
Shoulder depression	Supporting

EMG studies confirm the role of the latissimus dorsi in all of these motions with and without resistance, unlike the teres major that appears to participate in extension, adduction, and medial rotation activities only when resistance is present [3,57]. EMG studies verify the latissimus dorsi's role with the pectoralis major in shoulder depression [18,59]. EMG studies also suggest that the latissimus dorsi is active in both forced inspiration and forced expiration [84].

EFFECTS OF WEAKNESS OF THE LATISSIMUS DORSI

Weakness of the latissimus dorsi contributes to decreased strength in the motions listed above.

MUSCLE ATTACHMENT BOX 9.16

ATTACHMENTS AND INNERVATION OF THE LATISSIMUS DORSI

Proximal attachment: By tendinous slips to spinous process of the lower six thoracic vertebrae, anterior to the trapezius, by the thoracolumbar fascia to the spines and supraspinous ligaments of the lumbar and sacral vertebrae, to the outer lip of the posterior aspect of the iliac crest lateral to the erector spinae, and to the lower three or four ribs.

Distal attachment: The floor of the intertubercular groove. The muscle may also attach to the lateral aspect of the scapula's inferior angle as the muscle passes over the scapula.

Innervation: Thoracodorsal nerve, C6-8.

Palpation: The latissimus dorsi is most easily palpated along its lateral border on the axillary line of the trunk. With the teres major muscle, the latissimus dorsi muscle forms the posterior axillary wall.

Clinical Relevance

LATISSIMUS DORSI PEDICLE FOR RECONSTRUCTIVE SURGERY: *Because of its size and vascular supply from multiple arteries, the latissimus dorsi is a frequent source of grafting material for reconstructive surgery, including wound closures and breast reconstruction. Such surgery can significantly impair the strength of the shoulder from which the latissimus dorsi is taken [16].*

EFFECTS OF TIGHTNESS OF THE LATISSIMUS DORSI

The latissimus dorsi is an important muscle in swimming and is very strong and perhaps overdeveloped in competitive swimmers. Tightness of the latissimus dorsi limits shoulder ROM in flexion, lateral rotation, and perhaps abduction. Attached to the pelvis and lumbar spine posteriorly and to the anterior aspect of the humerus, the latissimus dorsi crosses from the posterior to the anterior surface of the trunk. Consequently, tightness of the latissimus dorsi also may contribute to flexion of the upper thoracic spine (*Fig 9.40*).

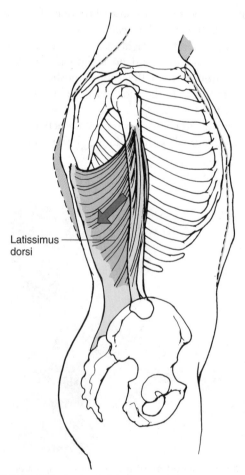

Latissimus dorsi

Figure 9.40: Latissimus dorsi tightness. A tight latissimus dorsi may contribute to increased thoracic kyphosis.

Shoulder Depression

Although there is little movement available in the direction of shoulder depression, the muscular forces in the direction of shoulder depression are exceedingly important. The force of shoulder depression is particularly important when the upper extremity is used in weight-bearing activities. For example, as a person uses a cane, the arm is bearing weight (*Fig. 9.41*). The reaction force of the cane tends to elevate the shoulder. Active contraction of the shoulder depressors stabilizes the shoulder, preventing elevation.

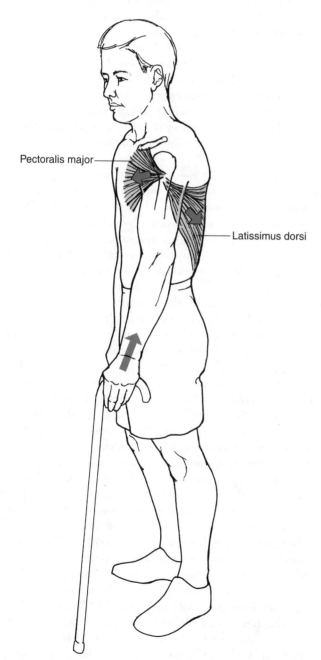

Figure 9.41: Function of the latissimus dorsi and pectoralis major. The latissimus dorsi and pectoralis major help stabilize the shoulder against the upward reaction force from a cane.

Clinical Relevance

UPPER EXTREMITY WEIGHT BEARING: *Upper extremity weight bearing is extremely important in rehabilitation and also in athletic events. An individual who uses a wheelchair must lift himself off the seat to relieve pressure on the buttocks or to transfer to another seat. Without the use of the lower limbs, such as occurs following some spinal cord injuries, the individual lifts almost the entire weight of the body with the upper extremities, pushing down with the hands (Fig. 9.42). The wheelchair exerts a reaction force on the upper extremities in an upward direction. This force tends to elevate the shoulders, therefore, the shoulder depressor muscles are required to "depress" the shoulder, or, more accurately, "fix" the shoulder, preventing it from being elevated by the reaction force. By stabilizing the shoulder girdle, the shoulder depressor muscles allow the upward chair reaction force to be transmitted to the rest of the body to lift it from the chair. Similarly, a gymnast supports the weight of the body through the upper extremities during many gymnastic movements (Fig. 9.43). In both cases the pectoralis major and latissimus dorsi muscles are the primary muscles lifting the body weight by "depressing the shoulder." These two muscles can be assisted by additional shoulder depressors, including the pectoralis minor and subclavius muscles.*

Summary of the Axiohumeral Muscles

These two muscles, the pectoralis major and the latissimus dorsi, are large, powerful muscles that cross all of the joints of the shoulder complex. Yet the actions they cause at the

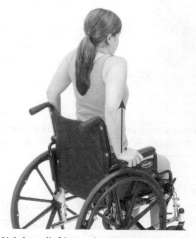

Figure 9.42: Weight relief in a wheelchair. A person who uses a wheelchair and has the inability to use the lower extremities uses the upper extremities to lift the body weight up off the buttocks, relieving pressure. The wheelchair pushes up on the upper extremities, tending to raise the shoulders. Shoulder depressor muscles fix the shoulder to transfer the force to lift the body.

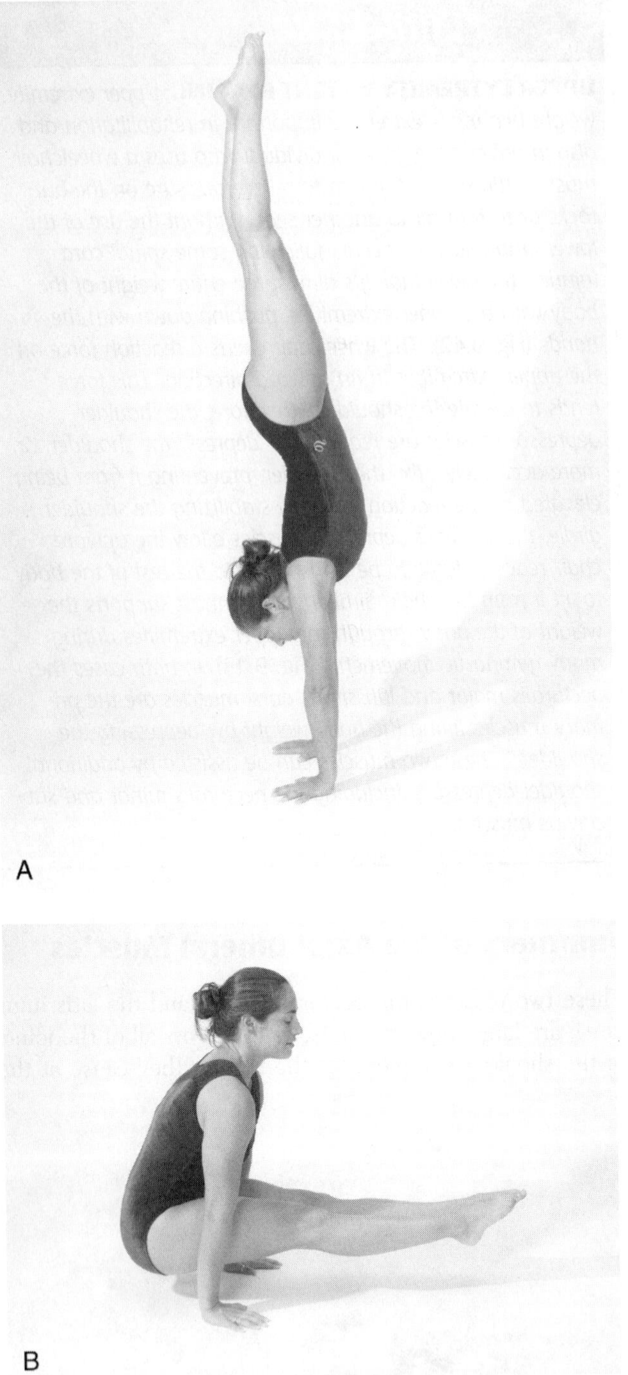

A

B

Figure 9.43: Floor exercises in gymnastics. The gymnast lifts body weight with the upper extremities in many floor exercises.

shoulder are also provided by other muscles of the shoulder. These two muscles have no unique actions at the shoulder. However, these two muscles add significant strength to all motions of the shoulder except lateral rotation. In addition, they are the primary shoulder depressors that provide essential strength and stability in activities when the upper extremity bears weight. Weakness of these muscles is most likely manifested in forceful activities such as weight bearing or in sporting activities such as gymnastics and golf [60].

Tightness of these muscles may limit all but medial rotation ROM of the shoulder complex. Therefore, impairment of either of these muscles may significantly affect some functions of the shoulder.

MUSCLE STRENGTH COMPARISONS

An understanding of the relative strength of the muscles of the shoulder in individuals with no shoulder pathology provides insight into the functional requirements of the shoulder during daily life. It also provides a perspective for the clinician who is trying to judge the functional significance of weakness in the shoulder musculature. Several studies examine the strength of various muscle groups of the shoulder and assess the factors affecting those strengths. While two studies report a trend toward increased strength in the shoulder on the dominant side, these studies deny any statistically significant differences in shoulder strength between the dominant and nondominant sides [54,70]. Not surprisingly, shoulder strengths in men are substantially larger than those in women.

Shklar and Dvir list the strength of the shoulder muscle groups in descending order: extensors, adductors, flexors, abductors, medial rotators, and lateral rotators [70]. These authors note that in men this order is unchanged by direction of contraction (concentric or eccentric). However, in the women studied, the concentric strength of the flexors is greater than that of the adductors. Two other studies report that the strength of the shoulder flexors exceeds that of the extensors in men, while the two are essentially equal in women [54]. The differences in the results from these studies demonstrate an important aspect of muscle comparisons. The study by Shklar and Dvir examines peak torque during concentric and eccentric contractions throughout the shoulder's ROM from neutral to the flexed position. The study by Murray and colleagues examines isometric strength with the shoulder in the neutral position [54,70]. Williams and Stutzman report isometric strength in various shoulder positions and demonstrate the effect of shoulder position on the isometric strength of the shoulder flexors and extensors [83]. These data support the notion that peak isometric force is greater in the flexor than in the extensor muscles. This peak occurs when the shoulder is hyperextended (i.e., when the flexor muscles are stretched). Neither of the previously cited studies report strength in this position. With the shoulder at neutral, the shoulder flexors produce a larger force than the extensors, supporting the conclusions by Murray et al. [54]. However, when the shoulder is flexed, the extensors produce more force than the flexors, as reported by Shklar and Dvir. Thus joint position and the mode of contraction are likely to affect comparative muscle strengths. The clinician must consider all of the factors influencing muscle force when interpreting the results of muscle strength tests (Chapter 4).

Several studies compare the strengths of the medial and lateral rotator muscle groups of the shoulder and consistently find the medial rotators stronger than the lateral rotators regardless of the speed of contraction or the position of the shoulder [15,37,46,54,69,70]. These findings are quite understandable when the number and total physiological cross-sectional area of the medial rotator muscles is compared with the number and total physiological cross-sectional area of the lateral rotator muscles.

It is frequently suggested that the strength of the shoulder is greater when tested in the plane of the scapula. Although few studies have assessed this directly, two studies report no difference in strength of abduction or rotation when tested in the frontal plane and in the plane of the scapula [23,81]. Although there may be issues of stability and comfort that are optimized by measuring strength of the shoulder in the plane of the scapula, there is no support at the present time for the notion that this position enhances strength. These studies serve to remind the clinician of the complexities affecting muscle performance. Evaluation of muscle performance at the shoulder and an understanding of a muscle's contribution to shoulder impairment requires the clinician to have a broad understanding of the normal performance of these muscles and the factors that influence their output.

SUMMARY

This chapter discusses the individual muscles of the shoulder. They are presented in the functional groups of axioscapular and axioclavicular, scapulohumeral, and axiohumeral. These groups, named according to the attachments of the muscles in the respective group, have unique functional responsibilities at the shoulder. The axioscapular and axioclavicular muscles position the scapulothoracic and sternoclavicular joints. Similarly, the muscles of the scapulohumeral group position the glenohumeral joint. Finally, the axiohumeral muscles add power to the motions of the shoulder.

Impairments of muscles within these groups produce predictable effects on shoulder function. Impairments within the axioclavicular and axioscapular groups impair the ability to position the scapula during active shoulder elevation. Impairments in the scapulohumeral muscle group impair the ability to position the glenohumeral joint, and impairments in the axiohumeral muscles impair the ability to exert large muscle forces on the shoulder, particularly during upper extremity weight-bearing activities. An understanding of the functional role of each muscle allows the clinician to evaluate the contribution of individual muscles to function and dysfunction of the shoulder. Comparisons of group muscle strengths reveal how joint position and contraction mode affect muscle force production at the shoulder. Peak shoulder flexion strength is greater than peak extension strength, and medial rotation strength is greater than lateral rotation strength.

The following chapter discusses the forces sustained by the shoulder joints and the surrounding muscles during daily activities as well as during more vigorous activities such as sports.

References

1. Apreleva M, Hasselman CT, Debski RE, et al.: A dynamic analysis of glenohumeral motion after simulated capsulolabral injury, a cadaver model. J Bone Joint Surg 1998; 80A: 474–480.
2. Arwert HJ, de Groot J, Van Woensel WWLM, Rozing PM: Electromyography of shoulder muscles in relation to force direction. J Shoulder Elbow Surg 1997; 6: 360–370.
3. Basmajian JV, DeLuca CJ: Muscles Alive. Their Function Revealed by Electromyography. Baltimore: Williams & Wilkins, 1985.
4. Bassett RW, Browne AO, Morrey BF, An KN: Glenohumeral muscle force and moment mechanics in a position of shoulder instability. J Biomech 1990; 23: 405–415.
5. Bearn JG: Direct observations on the function of the capsule of the sternoclavicular joint in clavicular support. J Anat 1967; 101: 159–170.
6. Borstad JD: Resting position variables at the shoulder: evidence to support a posture-impairment association. Phys Ther 2006; 86: 549–557.
7. Borstad JD, Ludewig PM: The effect of long versus short pectoralis minor resting length on scapular kinematics in healthy individuals. JOSPT 2005; 35: 227–238.
8. Brandell BR, Wilkinson DA: An electromyographic study of manual testing procedures for the trapezius and deltoid muscles. Physiother Can 1991; 43: 33–39.
9. Brewer BJ: Aging of the rotator cuff. Am J Sports Med 1979; 7: 102–110.
10. Brostrom L, Kronberg M, Nemeth G: Muscle activity during shoulder dislocation. Acta Orthop Scand 1989; 60: 639–641.
11. Bull ML, Vitti M, De Freitas V: Electromyographic study of the trapezius (upper portion) and levator scapulae muscles in some movements. Anat Anz [Jena] 1985; 159: 21–27.
12. Bull ML, Vitti M, De Freitas V: Electromyographic study of the trapezius (pars superior) and serratus anterior (pars inferior) muscles in free movements of the shoulder. Electromyogr Clin Neurophysiol 1989; 29: 119–125.
13. Davies PM: Steps to Follow. A Guide to the Treatment of Adult Hemiplegia. Berlin: Springer-Verlag, 1985.
14. DiVeta J, Walker M, Skibinski B: Relationship between performance of selected scapular muscles and scapular abduction in standing subjects. Phys Ther 1990; 70: 470–476.
15. Ellenbecker TS, Mattalino AJ: Concentric isokinetic shoulder internal and external rotation strength in professional baseball pitchers. JOSPT 1997; 25: 323–328.
16. Elliott LF, Raffel B, Wade J: Segmental latissimus dorsi free flap: Clin Appl Ann Plast Surg 1989; 23: 231–238.
17. Engle RP, Canner GC: Posterior shoulder instability: approach to rehabilitation. J Orthop Sports Phys Ther 1989; 488–494.
18. Gagnon D, Nadeau S, Gravel D et al.: Biomechanical analysis of a posterior transfer maneuver on a level surface in individuals with high and low-level spinal cord injuries. Clin Biomech 2003; 18: 319–331.
19. Gerber C, Krushell RJ: Isolated rupture of the tendon of the subscapularis muscle, clinical features in 16 cases. J Bone Joint Surg [Br] 1991; 73: 389–394.
20. Gregg JR, Labosky D, Harty M, et al: Serratus anterior paralysis in the young athlete. J Bone Joint Surg 1979; 61A: 825–832.
21. Halder AM, Halder CG, Zhao KD, et al.: Dynamic inferior stabilizers of the shoulder joint. Clin Biomech 2001; 16: 138–143.

22. Happee R, van der Helm FCT: The control of shoulder muscles during goal directed movements, an inverse dynamic analysis. J Biomech 1995; 28: 1179–1191.

23. Hartsell HD, Forwell L: Postoperative eccentric and concentric isokinetic strength for the shoulder rotators in the scapular and neutral planes. JOSPT 1997; 25: 19–25.

24. Hislop HJ, Montgomery J: Daniel's and Worthingham's Muscle Testing: Techniques of Manual Examination. Philadelphia: WB Saunders, 1995.

25. Howell SM, Imobersteg AM, Seger DH, Marone PJ: Clarification of the role of the supraspinatus muscle in shoulder function. J Bone Joint Surg [AM] 1986; 68: 398–404.

26. Hughes RE, Niebur G, Liu J, An K: Comparison of two methods for computing abduction moment arms of the rotator cuff. J Biomech 1998; 31: 157–160.

27. Inman VT, Saunders JB, Abbott LC: Observations of the function of the shoulder joint. J Bone Joint Surg 1944; 42: 1–30.

28. Jackson KM, Joseph J, Wyard SJ: Sequential muscular contraction. J Biomech 1977; 10: 97–106.

29. Jobe FW, Moynes DR, Brewster CE: Rehabilitation of shoulder joint instabilities. Orthop Clin North Am 1987; 18: 473–482.

30. Johnson GR, Pandyan AD: The activity in the three regions of the trapezius under controlled loading conditions—an experimental and modeling study. Clin Biomech 2005; 20: 155–161.

31. Johnson GR, Spalding D, Nowitzke A, Bogduk N: Modelling the muscles of the scapula morphometric and coordinate data and functional implications. J Biomech 1996; 29: 1039–1051.

32. Kauppila LI, Vastamaki M: Iatrogenic serratus anterior paralysis long-term outcome in 26 patients. Chest 1996; 109: 31–34.

33. Kelley MJ: Biomechanics of the Shoulder. In: Orthopedic Therapy of the Shoulder. Kelley MJ, Clark WA, eds. Philadelphia: JB Lippincott, 1995.

34. Kelly BT, Kadrmas WR, Speer KP: The manual muscle examination of rotator cuff strength. An electromyographic investigation. Am J Sports Med 1996; 24: 581–588.

35. Kendall FP, McCreary EK, Provance PG: Muscle Testing and Function. Baltimore: Williams & Wilkins, 1993.

36. Kiss G, Komar J: Suprascapular nerve compression at the spinoglenoid notch. Muscle Nerve 1990; 13: 556–557.

37. Kramer JF, Ng LR: Static and dynamic strength of the shoulder rotators in healthy, 45- to 75-year-old men and women. JOSPT 1996; 24: 11–18.

38. Kronberg M, Brostrom L, Nemeth G: Differences in shoulder muscle activity between patients with generalized joint laxity and normal controls. Clin Orthop 1991; 26: 181–192.

39. Kronberg M, Nemeth G, Brostrom L: Muscle activity and coordination in the normal shoulder, an electromyographic study. Clin Orthop 1990; 76–85.

40. Kuechle DK, Newman SR, Itoi E, et al.: Shoulder muscle moment arms during horizontal flexion and elevation. J Shoulder Elbow Surg 1997; 6: 429–439.

41. Kuechle DK, Newman SR, Itoi E, et al.: The relevance of the moment arm of shoulder muscles with respect to axial rotation of the glenohumeral joint in four positions. Clin Biomech 2000; 15: 322–329.

42. Kukowski B: Suprascapular nerve lesion as an occupational neuropathy in a semiprofessional dancer. Arch Phys Med Rehabil 1993; 74: 768–769.

43. Langenderfer J, Jerabek SA, Thangamani VB, et al.: Musculoskeletal parameters of muscles crossing the shoulder and elbow and the effect of sarcomere length sample size on

estimation of optimal muscle length. Clin Biomech 2004; 19: 664–670.

44. Magee DA: Orthopedic Physical Assessment. Philadelphia: WB Saunders, 1998.

45. Makhsous M, Hogfors C, Siemien'ski A, Peterson B: Total shoulder and relative muscle strength in the scapular plane. J Biomech 1999; 32: 1213–1220.

46. Malerba JL, Adam ML, Harris BA, Krebs DE: Reliability of dynamic and isometric testing of shoulder external and internal rotators. JOSPT 1993; 18: 543–552.

47. Mattingly GE, Mackarey PJ: Optimal methods for shoulder tendon palpation: a cadaver study. Phys Ther 1996; 76: 166–174.

48. McQuade KJ, Murthi AM: Anterior glenohumeral force/translation behavior with and without rotator cuff contraction during clinical stability testing. Clin Biomech 2004; 19: 10–15.

49. Meskers CGM, de Groot JH, Arwert HJ, et al.: Reliability of force direction dependent EMG parameters of shoulder muscles for clinical measurements. Clin Biomech 2004; 19: 913–920.

50. Moore KL: Clinically Oriented Anatomy. Baltimore: Williams & Wilkins, 1980.

51. Moskowitz E, Rashkoff ES: Suprascapular nerve palsy. Conn Med 1989; 53: 639–640.

52. Mura N, O'Dirscoll SW, Zobitz ME, et al.: The effect of supraspinatus disruption on glenohumeral torque and superior migration of the humeral head: a biomechanical study. J Shoulder Elbow Surg 2003; 12: 179–184.

53. Muraki T, Aoki M, Uchiyama E, et al.: The effect of arm position on stretching of the supraspinatus, infraspinatus, and posterior portion of deltoid muscles: a cadaveric study. Clin Biomech 2006; 21: 474–480.

54. Murray MP, Gore DR, Gardner GM, Mollinger LA: Shoulder motion and muscle strength of normal men and women in two age groups. Clin Orthop 1985; 268–273.

55. Otis JC, Jiang C, Wickiewicz TL, et al.: Changes in the moment arms of the rotator cuff and deltoid muscles with abduction and rotation. J Bone Joint Surg 1994; 76A: 667–676.

56. Palmerud G, Sporrong H, Herberts P, Kadefors R: Consequences of trapezius relaxation on the distribution of shoulder muscle forces: an electromyographic study. J Electromyogr Kinesiol 1998; 8: 185–193.

57. Paton ME, Brown JMM: Functional differentiation within latissimus dorsi. Electromyogr Clin Neurophysiol 1995; 35: 301–309.

58. Payne LZ, Deng XH, Craig EV, et al.: The combined dynamic and static contributions to subacromial impingement. Am J Sports Med 1997; 25: 801–808.

59. Perry J, Gronley JK, Newsam CJ, et al.: Electromyographic analysis of the shoulder muscles during depression transfers in subjects with low-level paraplegia. Arch Phys Med Rehabil 1996; 77: 350–355.

60. Pink M, Jobe FW, Perry J: Electromyographic analysis of the shoulder during the golf swing. Am J Sports Med 1990; 18: 137–140.

61. Reinold MM, Wilk KE, Fleisig GS, et al.: Electromyographic analysis of the rotator cuff and deltoid musculature during common shoulder external rotation exercises. JOSPT 2004; 34: 385–394.

62. Reis FP, deCamargo AM, Vitti M, de Carvalho CA: Electromyographic study of the subcalvius muscle. Acta Anat [Basel] 1979; 105: 284–290.

63. Romanes GJE: Cunningham's Textbook of Anatomy. Oxford: Oxford University Press, 1981.

64. Ryerson S, Levit K: Functional Movement Reeducation. New York: Churchill Livingstone, 1997.

65. Saha AK: Mechanics of elevation of glenohumeral joint: its application in rehabilitation of flail shoulder in upper brachial plexus injuries and poliomyelitis and in replacement of the upper humerus by prosthesis. Acta Orthop Scand 1973; 44: 668–678.

66. Sano H, Ishii H, Yeadon A, et al.: Degeneration at the insertion weakens the tensile strength of the supraspinatus tendon: a comparative mechanical and histologic study of the bone-tendon complex. J Orthop Res 1997; 15: 719–726.

67. Sano H, Uhthoff HK, Backman DS, et al.: Structural disorders at the insertion of the supraspinatus tendon. J Bone Joint Surg 1998; 80B: 720–725.

68. Schüldt K, Harms-Ringdahl K: Activity levels during isometric test contractions of neck and shoulder muscles. Scand J Rehab Med 1988; 20: 117–127.

69. Scoville CR, Arciero RA, Taylor DC, Stoneman PD: End range eccentric antagonist/concentric agonist strength ratios: a new perspective in shoulder strength assessment. JOSPT 1997; 25: 203–207.

70. Shklar A, Dvir Z: Isokinetic strength relationships in shoulder muscles. Clin Biomech 1995; 10: 369–373.

71. Smith LK, Weiss EL, Lehmkuhl LD: Brunnstrom's Clinical Kinesiology. Philadelphia: FA Davis, 1996.

72. Sobush DC, Simoneau GG, Dietz KE, et al.: The Lennie test for measuring scapular position in healthy young adult females: a reliability and validity study. JOSPT 1996; 23: 39–50.

73. Soslowsky LJ, Malicky DM, Blasier RB: Active and passive factors in inferior glenohumeral stabilization: a biomechanical model. J Shoulder Elbow Surgery 1997; 6: 371–379.

74. Stefko JM, Jobe FW, VanderWilde RS, et al.: Electromyographic and nerve block analysis of the subscapularis liftoff test. J Shoulder Elbow Surg 1997; 6: 347–355.

75. Steindler A: Kinesiology of the Human Body under Normal and Pathological Conditions. Springfield, IL: Charles C Thomas, 1955.

76. Su KPE, Johnson MP, Gracely EJ, Karduna AR: Scapular rotation in swimmers with and without impingement syndrome: practice effects. Med Sci Sports Exerc 2004; 36: 1117–1123.

77. Travell J: Myofascial Pain and Dysfunction: The Trigger Point Manual. Baltimore: Williams & Wilkins, 1982.

78. Truong XT, Rippel DV: Orthotic devices for serratus anterior palsy: some biomechanical considerations. Arch Phys Med Rehabil 1979; 60: 66–69.

79. Van Linge B, Mulder JD: Function of the supraspinatus muscle and its relation to the supraspinatus syndrome. An experimental study in man. J Bone Joint Surg 1963; 45B: 750–754.

80. Watson C, Schenkman M: Physical therapy management of isolated serratus anterior muscle paralysis. Phys Ther 1995; 75: 194–202.

81. Whitcomb LJ, Kelley MJ, Leiper CI: A comparison of torque production during dynamic strength testing of shoulder abduction in the coronal plane and the plane of the scapula. JOSPT 1995; 21: 227–232.

82. Williams M: Action of the deltoid muscle. Phys Ther Rev 1949; 29: 154–157.

83. Williams M, Stutzman L: Strength variation through the range of joint motion. Phys Ther Rev 1959; 39: 145–152.

84. Williams P, Bannister L, Berry M, et al.: Gray's Anatomy, The Anatomical Basis of Medicine and Surgery, Br. ed. London: Churchill Livingstone, 1995.

85. Worrell TW, Corey BJ, York SL, Santiestaban J: An analysis of supraspinatus EMG activity and shoulder isometric force development. Med Sci Sports Exerc 1992; 744–748.

86. Wuelker N, Korell M, Thren K: Dynamic glenohumeral joint stability. J Shoulder Elbow Surg 1998; 7: 43–52.

Analysis of the Forces on the Shoulder Complex during Activity

CHAPTER CONTENTS

The preceding two chapters describe the structure of the bones, joints, and muscles of the shoulder complex. The purpose of the present chapter is to discuss the mechanical demands placed on these structures during daily activities. This discussion helps the clinician comprehend the daily loads sustained by the articular structures of the shoulder complex and the forces that must be generated by the muscles of the shoulder under normal conditions of activity. By understanding the demands placed on the shoulder complex under normal conditions, the clinician can appreciate how various pathological conditions can affect the loads to which the shoulder complex is subjected.

Specifically, the goals of this chapter are to

- Review a simplified two-dimensional analysis used to estimate the forces sustained by the glenohumeral joint while maintaining a static position
- Examine the forces sustained by structures throughout the shoulder complex
- Use mechanical analyses to consider the effects of discrete joint and muscle impairments on the loads sustained by the unimpaired structures
- Consider the loads on the shoulder when the upper extremity is used for propulsive activities

TWO-DIMENSIONAL ANALYSIS OF THE FORCES ON THE GLENOHUMERAL JOINT

Examining the Forces Box 10.1 outlines a classic two-dimensional model to calculate the forces generated at the glenohumeral joint during abduction of the shoulder and presents a free-body diagram identifying the forces present in this activity. It also provides the two-dimensional analysis used to determine the loads on the head of the humerus during isometric contractions at a given position of abduction.

This analysis yields the loads required of the abductor muscles to support the upper extremity at that position. By repeating the analysis at different positions, the loads through the entire range of motion (ROM) can be approximated. *Figure 10.1* presents estimates of such analyses based on data by Inman et al. [7].

The analysis presented in Examining the Forces Box 10.1 uses several simplifications. First, only the glenohumeral joint is examined. Yet upward rotation of the scapula may allow the glenoid fossa to support the inferior aspect of the joint,

EXAMINING THE FORCES BOX 10.1

TWO-DIMENSIONAL ANALYSIS OF THE FORCES ON THE HEAD OF THE HUMERUS WITH THE SHOULDER ABDUCTED TO 90° AND THE ELBOW EXTENDED

The following dimensions are based on a well-conditioned male who is 6 feet tall and weighs 180 lb. The limb segment parameters are extrapolated from the anthropometric data of Braune and Fischer [2].

L is the length of the upper extremity, 0.8 m

W is the weight of the upper extremity

The weight of the upper extremity is located at the center of gravity of the limb, located approximately 48% of the limb's length from the shoulder, 0.38 m

F is the force of the abductor muscles

The moment arm of the abductor muscles is 0.05 m

The muscles' angle of application is 30°

J is the joint reaction force

Solve for abductor force (F):

$$\Sigma M = 0$$

$$(F \times 0.05 \text{ m}) - (W \times 0.38 \text{ m}) = 0$$

$$(F \times 0.05 \text{ m}) = (W \times 0.38 \text{ m})$$

$$F = 7.6 \text{ W}$$

Calculate the forces on the head of the humerus

$$\Sigma F_X: \quad F_X + J_X = 0$$

$$J_X = -F_X \qquad \text{where } F_X = -F(\cos 30°)$$

$$J_X = F(\cos 30°)$$

$$J_X = 6.6 \text{ W}$$

$$\Sigma F_Y: \quad F_Y - W + J_Y = 0$$

$$J_Y = W - F_Y \qquad \text{where } F_Y = F(\sin 30°)$$

$$J_Y = -2.8 \text{ W}$$

Using the pythagorean theorem:

$$J^2 = J_X{}^2 + J_Y{}^2$$

$$\mathbf{J \approx 7.2 \text{ W}}$$

Assuming the weight of the upper extremity is 0.05 times body weight (BW), $J \approx 0.4$ BW

Using trigonometry, the direction of J can be determined:

$$\cos \alpha = J_X/J$$

$$\alpha \approx 24° \text{ from the horizontal}$$

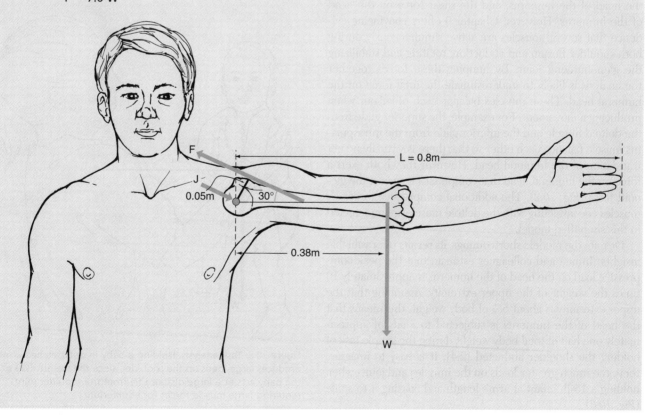

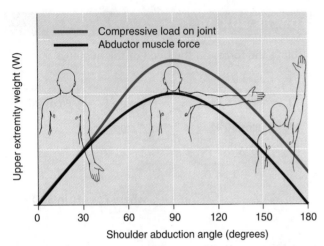

Figure 10.1: Muscle and joint reaction forces during abduction of the shoulder. These forces are largest when the shoulder is abducted to 90°.

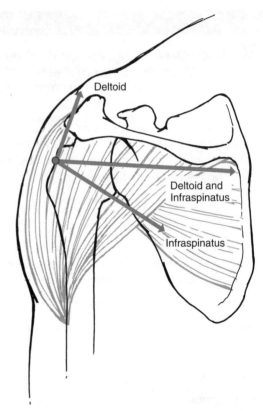

Figure 10.2: The effect of cocontraction on the joint reaction force. The vector sum of the deltoid and infraspinatus muscle forces increases the load on the joint.

particularly later in the joint's ROM. By ignoring the position of the scapula, the shear forces on the head of the humerus may be overestimated. On the other hand, the analysis also lumps all of the muscle and ligament forces into one, the deltoid muscle force. This simplification is necessary to decrease the number of "unknowns," so that the number of unknowns is equal to the number of equations available. As described in Chapter 1, a two-dimensional analysis provides only three equations to analyze the relevant forces: $\Sigma F_x = 0$, $\Sigma F_y = 0$, and $\Sigma M = 0$. Thus only three unknown quantities can be determined, the deltoid force, the compressive force on the head of the humerus, and the shear force on the head of the humerus. However, Chapter 9 offers convincing evidence that several muscles are active simultaneously during both shoulder flexion and abduction, rotating and stabilizing the glenohumeral joint. By lumping these forces together the analysis is likely to underestimate the total force on the humeral head. These muscles balance each other out when producing a movement. For example, the superior glide from the deltoid muscle and the inferior glide from the infraspinatus muscle balance each other so that there is virtually no net translation of the humeral head. However they both exert a force on the humeral head that compresses it against the glenoid fossa (*Fig. 10.2*). The additional compressive forces by muscles cocontracting with the deltoid muscle are undetected in this simplified model.

Despite the model's shortcomings, its results offer valuable insights. Inman and colleagues estimate that the peak compressive load on the head of the humerus is approximately 10 times the weight of the upper extremity. Assuming that the upper extremity is about 5% of body weight, this means that the head of the humerus is subjected to loads of approximately one half of total body weight during the simple task of holding the shoulder abducted [2,4]. It is easy to imagine, then, the much greater loads on the muscles and joints when holding a 15-lb infant at arm's length and coaxing it to smile (*Fig. 10.3*).

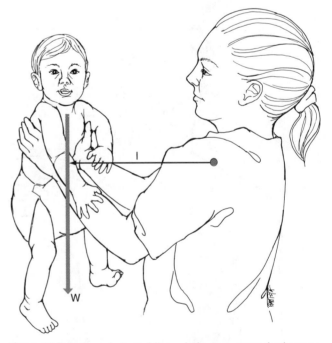

Figure 10.3: Task analysis. Holding a baby in outstretched arms produces large loads on the shoulder, since the weight (*W*) of the baby acts at a large distance (*l*) from the shoulder joint, requiring large muscle forces for equilibrium.

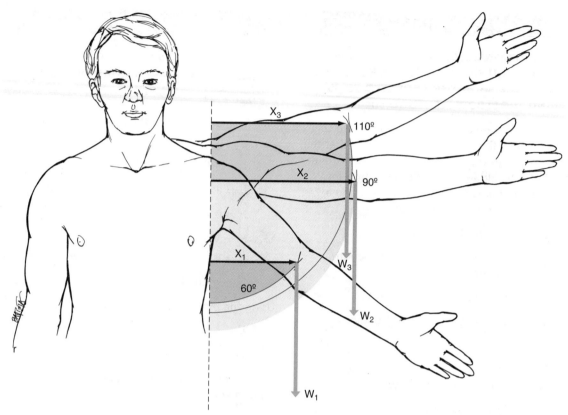

Figure 10.4: The moment arm of the weight of the upper extremity. Comparing these three positions, the moment arm of the weight of the upper extremity *(W)* is smallest when the shoulder is abducted to 60° and largest at 90°.

Peak joint reaction force occurs when the shoulder is abducted to 90°, which is not surprising, since at 90° of abduction, the adduction moment due to the weight of the upper extremity is at its maximum *(Fig. 10.4)*. Therefore, the abductor muscle force must be greatest to generate a moment to counteract the adduction moment created by the weight of the upper extremity. This large abduction muscle force, estimated to be approximately eight times the weight of the upper extremity, is the major factor influencing the joint reaction force. Maximum shear forces of slightly less than 50% of body weight are also reported but occur earlier in the ROM, at approximately 60° of abduction [7].

Examining the Forces Box 10.2 demonstrates the effect of flexing the elbow to 90°, shortening the moment arm of the weight of the upper extremity. Similarly, holding the infant with flexed elbows decreases the moment arm of the weight of the baby *(Fig. 10.5)*. The results of these analyses, based on a significant oversimplification of the mechanical reality manifested by the shoulder complex, still challenge the traditional view that the shoulder is "non-weight-bearing." While under normal circumstances humans do not walk on their hands, these data clearly suggest that the shoulder complex must bear large and repeated forces during everyday activity.

More recent mechanical analyses have been used to improve on the classic analysis of Inman et al. These results suggest that the shoulder is subjected regularly to even larger forces than suggested by Inman et al. [17]. These increased estimates reflect the greater sophistication of the modeling process. A model with a more accurate representation of the rotator cuff muscles suggests that the maximum compressive load on the humeral head during abduction of the shoulder in the plane of the scapula is almost 90% of total body weight, almost twice the estimates in the earlier study, and maximum shear is almost 50% of body weight! The addition of only a 1-kg load in the hand results in a 60% increase in joint reaction forces. It is not surprising then that activities of the upper extremities can result in large joint forces and pain in individuals with arthritis. Many activities of daily living (ADL) require considerable shoulder motion. Many of these activities occur with simultaneous elbow flexion, effectively decreasing the external moment on the shoulder [12]. Consequently, the reported forces on the shoulder during activities such as drinking from a mug or lifting a low-weight block to shoulder height range from only 8–50 newtons (approximately 2–11 pounds) in the superior direction. Teaching the patient ways to reduce loads on the shoulder during daily activities is an important part of effective treatment [3].

EXAMINING THE FORCES BOX 10.2

TWO-DIMENSIONAL ANALYSIS OF THE FORCES ON THE HEAD OF THE HUMERUS WITH THE SHOULDER ABDUCTED TO 90° AND THE ELBOW FLEXED TO 90°

The free body diagram of the shoulder abducted to 90° and the elbow flexed to 90° demonstrates that the moment arm due to the weight of the upper extremity is shorter with the elbow flexed. Consequently, less muscle force is required to support the limb, and a smaller joint reaction force is produced.

Length of arm (shoulder to elbow): 0.4 m

Center of gravity of the arm is 44% of the length of the arm from the proximal end: 0.18 m

Weight of the arm: 0.028 body weight (BW)

Weight of the forearm and hand: 0.022 body weight (BW)

Moment arm of the deltoid: 0.05 m

Angle of application of the deltoid muscle: 30°

Solve for the abductor force (F):

$$\Sigma M = 0$$
$$(F \times 0.05\,m) - (0.028\,BW \times 0.18\,m)$$
$$- (0.022\,BW \times 0.4\,m) = 0$$

$$(F \times 0.05\,m) = (0.028\,BW \times 0.18\,m)$$
$$+ (0.022\,BW \times 0.4\,m)$$

$$F = 0.28\,BW$$

Calculate the forces on the head of the humerus

$$\Sigma F_X:\ F_X + J_X = 0$$
$$J_X = -F_X \qquad\qquad \text{where } F_X = -F(\cos 30°)$$
$$J_X = F(\cos 30°)$$
$$J_X = 0.24\,BW$$

$$\Sigma F_Y:\ F_Y - W_A - W_F + J_Y = 0$$
$$J_Y = W_A + W_F - F_Y \qquad \text{where } F_Y = F(\sin 30°)$$
$$J_Y = -0.09\,BW$$

Using the pythagorean theorem:

$$J^2 = J_X{}^2 + J_Y{}^2$$

$$\mathbf{J \approx 0.26\,BW}$$

Using trigonometry, the direction of J can be determined:

$$\cos \alpha = J_X/J$$
$$\alpha \approx 23° \text{ from the horizontal}$$

MECHANICAL DEMANDS PLACED ON STRUCTURES THROUGHOUT THE SHOULDER COMPLEX

Investigators have vigorously pursued models that more accurately portray the morphology and behavior of the whole shoulder complex [1,5,9,13,14,21]. As stated earlier, the classical approach to the analysis of forces in a joint has been to use simplifying assumptions that reduce the number of unknowns to a number equal to the number of equations available to describe the phenomenon. However, the reality is that at any joint in the human body, there are far more unknowns than available equations. This is known as **redundancy,** and the system with these unknowns is said to be **indeterminate,** possessing an infinite number of solutions to the equations. However, sophisticated mathematical algorithms are available that allow investigators to determine the "best" or optimal solution, based on some predetermined optimization criteria. By using this approach, numerous models have been developed to calculate the forces in the muscles and ligaments of the glenohumeral joint as well as in the other joints of the shoulder complex. The following briefly presents data from some of these models. These results remain mere approximations of the real loads sustained by the shoulder structures. However, they can provide the clinician with at least a perspective on the requirements and consequences of activity and exercise on discrete structures of the shoulder complex.

In a greatly more complex model of the shoulder, van der Helm [20] reports peak medial-lateral joint reaction forces at the glenohumeral joint of approximately 300 N (67 lb) and 100 N (22.5 lb) for abduction and flexion, respectively. (One kilogram equals 9.81 newtons (N), or 1 lb equals 4.45 N.) The anterior–posterior and longitudinal joint reaction forces are slightly smaller. Unlike the joint reaction forces estimated by previous studies, this study presents the separate three-dimensional components rather than the total reaction force. Therefore the magnitudes cannot be compared directly. However, like the previous studies, the peaks appear at approximately 90°, when the moment due to the upper extremity weight is greatest. In this same study, reported peak joint reaction forces in the sternoclavicular and acromioclavicular joints are approximately 50 and 120 N (11 and 27 lb), respectively, and are in the medial–lateral direction. This study provides analytical evidence for the integral role of the scapulothoracic joint in the mobility and stability of the whole shoulder complex. It also is one of the few studies to provide any estimate of the loads sustained at the other joints of the shoulder. A similar, albeit less detailed, model predicts muscle loads up to 150 N (34 lb) in the deltoid muscle and over 100 N (22.5 lb) in the supraspinatus during abduction with a 1-kg weight in the hand [9]. This study also reports peak joint reaction forces of approximately 80% of body weight in the middle of the ROM.

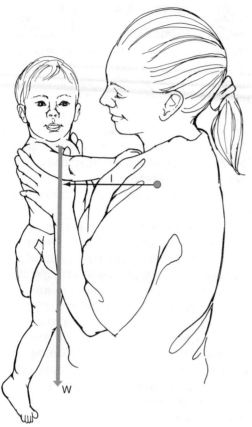

Figure 10.5: Application of the principles to a patient problem. An individual with shoulder pain should be instructed to avoid holding a baby at arm's length (*l*). Holding the child with shoulders less flexed and elbows more bent reduces the load on the shoulder by reducing the moment created by the weight (*W*) of the child.

Clinical Relevance

ARTHRITIC CHANGES IN THE GLENOHUMERAL JOINT: *Rheumatoid arthritis frequently affects the glenohumeral joint, resulting in significant pain and disability [10]. The large joint loads sustained by the humeral head during simple active ROM provide ample justification for the patient's complaints of pain. The benefits of exercise to maintain mobility and to increase strength must be weighed against the risks of increasing the joint loads and pain as well as perhaps hastening joint destruction. The clinician must investigate joint positions and modes of exercise that minimize the risks to the joint while maximizing the physiological benefits. For example, active ROM activities performed in the supine position or in water decrease the moment generated by the weight of the upper extremity. Therefore, less muscle force is needed to move the shoulder. Consequently, the joint reaction force is smaller. The decrease in joint reaction force is one reason why patients with arthritis tolerate these exercises more readily.*

The studies described so far have used mathematical analyses with standard Newtonian mechanics to estimate the loads on the joints and soft tissues of the shoulder complex. Another approach uses anatomically based models that mimic muscle behaviors. By creating realistic physical models of muscles of the shoulder or investigating the relative activity of muscles of the shoulder, these studies provide insight into the comparative difficulty of tasks as well as contributions of individual muscles to certain activities. One such study reports that the average peak force of the deltoid muscle required to abduct the shoulder in the plane of the scapula is approximately 250 N (±34.5), approximately 56 lb [25]. The effects of the absence of the supraspinatus, the whole rotator cuff, and the deltoid muscles also are recorded. Total active shoulder elevation decreases by 6, 16, and 25%, respectively, with selective cutting of the supraspinatus, the other rotator cuff muscles, or the deltoid. A similar model using a physical model of the muscles of the shoulder reports that the force required of the deltoid to elevate the upper extremity in the absence of the rotator cuff muscles increases by 17% [16]. Another study uses electromyography (EMG) and intramuscular pressure to examine the relative activity of the supraspinatus and verifies what is reported in mathematical analyses, that is, that the activity of the supraspinatus muscle increases as the shoulder is abducted from 0° to 90° [8]. These studies help identify the relative contributions and importance of given structures to the overall function of the shoulder. They consistently demonstrate that the loss of function in one muscle results in either impaired motion or an increased load in the remaining muscles. These results provide a theoretical basis to explain such clinical observations as a patient's complaints of shoulder weakness and fatigue in the presence of a rotator cuff tear.

Two additional studies serve as useful examples of how studies investigating the loads on muscles can provide insight that may help the clinician understand the mechanical basis for a patient's complaints. The first study uses a mathematical model of the shoulder and EMG recordings of the shoulder muscles to determine the fatigability of some of these muscles [14]. These authors suggest that the deltoid, infraspinatus, and supraspinatus are the first to show signs of fatigue during prolonged isometric contraction of the shoulder at 90° of flexion against a 4-kg weight. The trapezius appears more resistant to fatigue in this study. The second study investigates the level of EMG activity in shoulder muscles at different shoulder and elbow positions with and without performing a low-resistance manual task [19]. The presence of a manual task results in increased EMG activity in almost all positions and muscles. While neither of these studies provides a direct measurement of the forces generated in the muscles of the shoulder, together they suggest that even small increases in the loads carried by the upper extremity may significantly increase the loads sustained by muscles.

Clinical Relevance

CASE REPORT: *A thirty-something female came to physical therapy complaining of a gradual onset of shoulder pain. She was an artist whose primary art form was oil painting. She was working on a new project using a very large canvas that required prolonged elevation of her painting hand above the level of her head. The patient began to notice shoulder pain while working. She reported that the pain began in the first week of the new project and generally appeared only after a few hours of work. However, the pain was growing more intense and lasting longer after each painting session.*

The patient's initial evaluation occurred on a Monday morning. She had not painted for 3 days. She denied pain at the time of the evaluation, and no tests elicited pain. She was instructed to return to physical therapy after several days of painting. She was also instructed to schedule the visit after a full day of painting. At the time of the patient's second visit she had slight pain with palpation at the superior aspect of the greater tubercle. ROM was full and pain free, and isometric contractions of the shoulder in the neutral position were strong but slightly painful. Resisted shoulder abduction was mildly painful, especially in midrange. The pain increased with repetitions.

These findings were consistent with mild impingement or with irritation of the supraspinatus tendon. The therapist hypothesized that the task of painting on such a large canvas was fatiguing the rotator cuff muscles, which gradually lost their ability to stabilize the glenohumeral joint. As stability decreased, superior glide of the glenohumeral joint increased and gradually allowed impingement of the tendon. This hypothesis is consistent with the findings reported in the literature. The patient's history revealed that the job required prolonged periods of increased shoulder elevation, which was a new activity for her, so the muscles were untrained for this strenuous activity. (The patient had not recognized this as a new or strenuous activity.) She was treated with strengthening and endurance exercises for the rotator cuff muscles and was instructed to take frequent rests while painting, to avoid excessive fatigue. The patient reported decreased pain in 1 week and denied any pain while painting after 4 weeks.

FORCES ON THE SHOULDER COMPLEX WHEN THE UPPER EXTREMITY IS USED FOR PROPULSION

In Chapter 9 the role of the muscles that depress the shoulder is discussed. These muscles are particularly important in activities in which the upper extremity bears weight, such as pushing up from a chair or crutch walking. The upper extremity is particularly important as a weight-bearing structure when the function of the lower extremities is impaired. It is reasonable to hypothesize that the task of using crutches or propelling a wheelchair subjects the muscles, ligaments, and articular surfaces of the shoulder to considerably larger forces than tasks such as holding the upper extremity flexed. However, only a few studies actually offer any analysis of the loads sustained during these activities. Several studies provide analyses of the loads sustained during wheelchair activities. Investigators report average peak contact forces on the glenohumeral joint ranging from approximately 110–200 N (25–45 pounds) during wheelchair propulsion by individuals with spinal cord injuries [11,22]. Average peak moments of 20–35 Nm are also reported during propulsion [11,18].

The weight relief maneuver wheelchair users employ to lift their buttocks off the wheelchair seat and avoid pressure sores on the sacrum generates loads on the shoulder of approximately 1,000–1,500 N (225–337 pounds) [22,23]. These data demonstrate the burden the shoulder sustains in habitual wheelchair users and may explain why complaints of shoulder pain are common in these individuals. Careful analysis of the task and the wheelchair itself will help researchers, clinicians and wheelchair uses to develop strategies and equipment to protect the shoulders of wheelchair users.

In a study of crutch walking using a swing-through gait, peak flexor moments at the shoulder normalized by body weight were reported to be an average of 0.4 N-m/kg in five individuals with paraplegia, compared with average peak moments of slightly more than 0.2 N-m/kg in eight individuals without paraplegia [15]. The moments reported during these activities are approximately three times the moments reported during isometric shoulder abduction at 90° with the elbow extended [6]. None of these studies report actual calculations of joint reaction forces, but it is probable that the moments during weight bearing, which are more than three times the moments generated during static postures without resistance, result in similarly large increases in joint reaction forces. Despite such apparently large loads sustained during crutch walking, a study of 10 subjects with a mean duration of crutch-aided ambulation of 8.7 years reveals no degenerative changes at the shoulder bilaterally [24]. These data emphasize the remarkable resilience of the shoulder complex.

CONNECTIONS BETWEEN ANALYSES OF JOINT AND MUSCLE FORCES AND CLINICAL PRACTICE

This chapter presents the results of several studies investigating the forces sustained by the joints and muscles of the shoulder complex. The analyses use simplifying assumptions or uncomplicated physical representations of complex anatomical structures. Consequently, these results are at best an estimation of the real loads to which the shoulder is subjected. Comparing the absolute values of forces reported by these studies with the maximum sustainable loads for

cartilage, bone, and muscle can help the clinician assess the potentially detrimental effects of an activity or exercise. Similarly, such knowledge is essential in the design of suitable joint replacement devices. However, in the broader sense, these studies offer the clinician a theoretical framework from which to analyze any patient's complaints. Even a simplistic model representing the forces involved in an activity allows the clinician to ask the question, How much muscle force is required to lift this 20-lb baby? and perhaps more importantly, Is there another way to lift the baby so that less muscle force is required? Similarly, the clinician can ask, What is the load on this inflamed joint during this strengthening exercise? Can the exercise be performed differently to reduce the force on the joint? Although few clinicians have the opportunity to answer these questions quantitatively, an understanding of the basic approach to the analysis enables the clinician to generate hypothetical answers to these questions. Clinical observations can then support or refute these estimates.

SUMMARY

In this chapter the basic two-dimensional approach to calculating muscle forces and joint reaction forces is presented. A simplified model demonstrates that the shoulder sustains loads of approximately 50% of body weight during unresisted active abduction. Results from more-sophisticated analyses predict even higher loads, and weight-bearing activities can be expected to generate still larger loads on the shoulder. Impairments within the shoulder complex also are likely to alter the direction and magnitude of the loads on the shoulder. Although the published data offer only estimates of the forces in the shoulder, the clinical use of the theoretical framework used in these analyses is discussed, and a patient example demonstrates the clinical relevance of some of the data presented.

The preceding two chapters present the structure and functions of the bones, joints, and muscles of the shoulder complex. The effects of impairments of these structures are also discussed. The current chapter presents a scheme to conceptualize the shoulder as a mechanical system that sustains variable loads that depend on the nature of the activity. Such a framework offers the clinician a method for identifying the underlying mechanisms that cause the abnormal performance of the bones, joints, and muscles of the shoulder and the theoretical basis for prescribing treatment regimens to improve or restore normal function. This same framework of mechanical analysis is repeated in the rest of the anatomical regions presented in this book.

References

1. Bassett RW, Browne AO, Morrey BF, An KN: Glenohumeral muscle force and moment mechanics in a position of shoulder instability. J Biomech 1990; 23: 405–415.
2. Braune W, Fischer O: Center of gravity of the human body. In: Human Mechanics; Four Monographs Abridged AMRL-TDR-63-123. Krogman WM, Johnston FE, eds. Wright-Patterson Air

Force Base, Ohio: Behavioral Sciences Laboratory, 6570th Aerospace Medical Research Laboratories, Aerospace Medical Division, Air Force Systems Command, 1963; 1–57.

3. Cordery J, Rocchi M: Joint protection and fatigue management. In: Rheumatologic Rehabilitation Series. Melvin M, Jensen GM, eds. Bethesda: American Occupational Therapy Association, 1998; 279–322.

4. Dempster WT: Space requirements of the seated operator. In: Human Mechanics; Four Monographs Abridged AMRL-TDR-63-123. Krogman WM, Fischer O, eds. Wright-Patterson Air Force Base, Ohio: Behavioral Sciences Laboratory, 6570th Aerospace Medical Research Laboratories, Aerospace Medical Division, Air Force Systems Command, 1963; 215–340.

5. Hogfers C, Karlsson D, Peterson B: Structure and internal consistency of a shoulder model. J Biomech 1995; 28: 767–777.

6. Hughes RE, An K: Force analysis of rotator cuff muscles. Clin Orthop 1996; 330: 75–83.

7. Inman VT, Saunders JB, Abbott LC: Observations of the function of the shoulder joint. J Bone Joint Surg 1944; 42: 1–30.

8. Jarvholm U, Palmerud G, Herberts P, et al.: Intramuscular pressure and electromyography in the supraspinatus muscle at shoulder abduction. Clin Orthop 1989; 245: 102–109.

9. Karlsson D, Peterson B: Towards a model for force predictions in the human shoulder. J Biomech 1992; 25: 189–199.

10. Klippel JH: Primer on the Rheumatic Diseases. Atlanta: Arthritis Foundation, 2001.

11. Koontz AM, Cooper RA, Boninger ML, et al.: Shoulder kinematics and kinetics during two speeds of wheelchair propulsion. J Rehab Res Dev 2002; 39: 635–650.

12. Murray IA, Johnson GR: A study of the external forces and moments at the shoulder and elbow while performing every day tasks. Clin Biomech 2004; 19: 586–594.

13. Niemi J, Nieminen H, Takala EP, Viikari-Juntura E: A static shoulder model based on a time-dependent criterion for load sharing between synergistic muscles. J Biomech 1996; 29: 451–460.

14. Nieminen H, Takala EP, Viikari-Juntura E: Load-sharing patterns in the shoulder during isometric flexion tasks. J Biomech 1995; 28: 555–566.

15. Noreau L, Comeau F, Tardif D, Richards CL: Biomechanical analysis of swing-through gait in paraplegic and non-disabled individuals. J Biomech 1995; 28: 689–700.

16. Payne LZ, Deng XH, Craig EV, et al.: The combined dynamic and static contributions to subacromial impingement. Am J Sports Med 1997; 25: 801–808.

17. Poppen N, Walker PS: Forces at the glenohumeral joint in abduction. Clin Orthop 1978; 135: 165–170.

18. Robertson RN, Boninger ML, Cooper RA, Shimada SD: Pushrim forces and joint kinetics during wheelchair propulsion. Arch Phys Med Rehabil 1996; 77: 856–864.

19. Sporrong H, Palmerud G, Kadefors R, Herberts P: The effect of light manual precision work on shoulder muscles—an EMG analysis. J Electromyogr Kinesiol 1998; 8: 177–184.

20. van der Helm FCT: A finite element musculoskeletal model of the shoulder mechanism. J Biomech 1994; 27: 551–569.

21. van der Helm FCT: Analysis of the kinematic and dynamic behavior of the shoulder mechanism. J Biomech 1994; 27: 5: 527–569.

22. van Drongelen S, van der Woude LH, Janssen TW, et al.: Glenohumeral contact forces and muscle forces evaluated in wheelchair-related activities of daily living in able-bodied subjects versus subjects with paraplegia and tetraplegia. Arch Phys Med Rehabil 2005; 86: 1434–1440.

23. van Drongelen S, van der Woude LHV, Janssen TWJ, et al.: Glenohumeral joint loading in tetraplegia during weight relief lifting: a simulation study. Clin Biomech 2006; 21: 128–137.

24. Wing PC, Tredwell SJ: The weightbearing shoulder. Paraplegia 1983; 21: 107–113.

25. Wuelker N, Wirth CJ, Plitz W, Roetman B: A dynamic shoulder model: reliability testing and muscle force study. J Biomech 1995; 28: 489–499.

UNIT 2   ELBOW UNIT

*I*n the previous unit, the structure and function of the shoulder are presented. It is shown that the purpose of the shoulder, to position the upper extremity in space, requires that the shoulder complex possess remarkable flexibility. Such flexibility is provided by the unique coordination of four separate joints as well as by the extreme flexibility available at the glenohumeral joint itself. However, such mobility comes at a cost to stability. The glenohumeral joint has several unique anatomical features and structures to enhance stability, particularly the rotator cuff muscles.

In contrast, the function of the elbow is simpler. The role of the elbow is primarily to shorten or lengthen the upper extremity, allowing the hand to move away from and toward the body during such activities as reaching into the refrigerator and bringing a snack to the mouth. In addition, the elbow assists in turning the hand toward or away from the body. These simplified functional demands are paralleled by decreased structural complexity. A reduction in available motion is accompanied by a significant increase in inherent stability. The following three chapters review the structure and the functional requirements of the elbow joint and demonstrate how issues of mobility and stability at the elbow differ from those of the shoulder.

The purposes of this three-chapter unit on the elbow are to

- Present the structure of the elbow joint and discuss its effects on the mobility and stability of the joint
- Discuss the role of muscles in the mechanics and pathomechanics of the elbow joint
- Analyze the forces to which the elbow is subjected and the factors that influence those forces

Structure and Function of the Bones and Noncontractile Elements of the Elbow

CHAPTER CONTENTS

The focus of this chapter is the bony architecture and supporting structures of the elbow joint and their contributions to function. Specifically, the purposes of the present chapter are to

- Discuss the structure of the bones that constitute the elbow and their effect on joint mobility and stability.
- Present the functional units of the elbow and the noncontractile structures that support them.
- Examine the normal movement of the elbow joint.
- Compare the structure and function of the elbow with those of the shoulder.

STRUCTURE OF THE BONES OF THE ELBOW

The elbow joint consists of the articulations among the distal humerus, the proximal ulna, and the proximal radius (*Fig. 11.1*). The relevant details of each bone are presented below. As in the preceding unit on the shoulder complex, only the details of each bone that apply to the elbow are presented. Thus the current chapter provides a discussion of the distal humerus and proximal radius and ulna. Chapter 8 presents a detailed discussion of the structure of the proximal humerus

because it is directly associated with the shoulder. Similarly, the distal radius and ulna are discussed in Chapter 14, which presents the bones and joints of the wrist and hand.

Distal Humerus

Chapter 8 describes the humerus to the level of the deltoid tuberosity and radial groove, which are located in the midshaft of the humerus. The shaft of the humerus is approximately round in cross section proximally but gradually flattens anteriorly and posteriorly and widens medially and laterally as

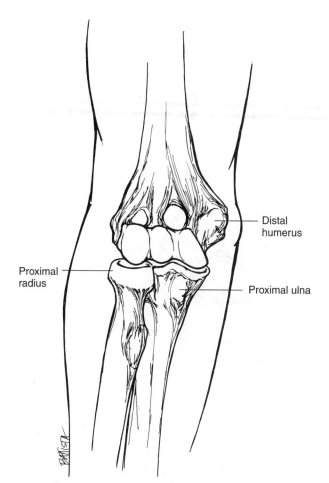

Figure 11.1: The elbow joint complex is composed of the distal humerus, proximal ulna, and proximal radius.

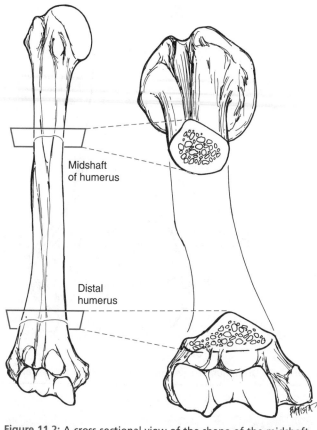

Figure 11.2: A cross-sectional view of the shape of the midshaft of the humerus and of the distal humerus reveals how the distal humerus flattens anteriorly and posteriorly.

the shaft continues distally (*Fig. 11.2*). The distal shaft also curves slightly anteriorly, directing its articular surfaces more anteriorly, thus positioning the articular surfaces in a way that favors flexion mobility (*Fig. 11.3*). The flattening of the distal shaft of the humerus gives rise to the medial and lateral supracondylar ridges.

The distal end of the humerus consists of the articular surface, including the trochlea and the capitulum, and the nonarticulating surfaces, the medial and lateral epicondyles, as well as the olecranon fossa and the coronoid and radial fossae (*Fig. 11.4*). The medial and lateral epicondyles are prominent projections that are distal culminations of the medial and lateral supracondylar ridges. Although both epicondyles are palpable, the medial epicondyle is more prominent than the lateral. It encompasses approximately one third of the distal humerus. It is grooved posteriorly by a shallow sulcus for the ulnar nerve. As the ulnar nerve travels in this groove it lies directly against the bone and is susceptible to compression against the humerus by a blow to the medial elbow. The groove is covered by a fascial roof running from the medial epicondyle to the proximal end of the ulna's olecranon process. This roof forms the cubital tunnel for the ulnar nerve [53].

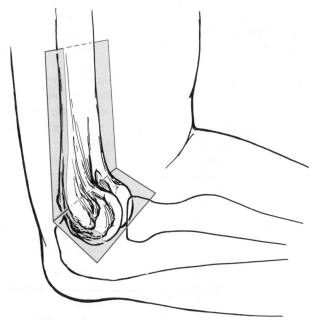

Figure 11.3: A sagittal view of the humerus reveals the anterior curvature of its distal end.

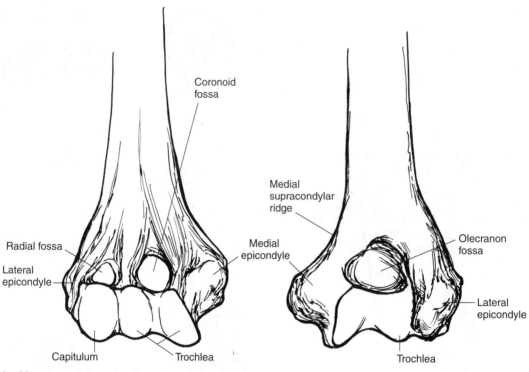

Figure 11.4: Distal humerus. A. Anterior view. B. Posterior view.

Clinical Relevance

THE "CRAZY BONE" OF THE ELBOW: *Nerves are most susceptible to injury in locations where they lie against rigid structures or in rigid spaces. The radial nerve is particularly vulnerable as it travels along the humerus in the radial (spiral) groove. Similarly, the ulnar nerve is at risk as it wraps around the medial epicondyle at the elbow. Few individuals have escaped the characteristic pain and tingling that radiate distally through the medial aspect of the forearm and hand when the medial aspect of the elbow (the crazy bone) hits a door or piece of furniture (Fig. 11.5). More serious and lasting injuries to the ulnar nerve also occur as the nerve travels through the restricted space of the cubital tunnel. Preliminary studies suggest that the cubital tunnel narrows during elbow flexion, as a result of a stretch to the fascial covering. This narrowing apparently is accompanied by a stretch to the nerve itself. The combination of tunnel narrowing and nerve stretch may contribute to some ulnar nerve neuropathies at the elbow.*

The medial epicondyle provides important attachments for the joint capsule and medial (ulnar) collateral ligament of the elbow as well as for the superficial flexor muscles of the forearm. The lateral epicondyle is prominent posteriorly, particularly in elbow flexion. It gives rise to the lateral collateral ligament and to the superficial extensor muscles of the forearm.

The radial and coronoid fossae of the humerus are shallow depressions on the anterior surface of the distal humerus just proximal to the articular surfaces of the capitulum and trochlea, respectively. These depressions allow close

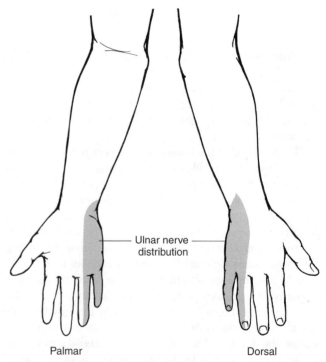

Figure 11.5: Sensory distribution of the ulnar nerve. A. Palmar view. B. Dorsal view.

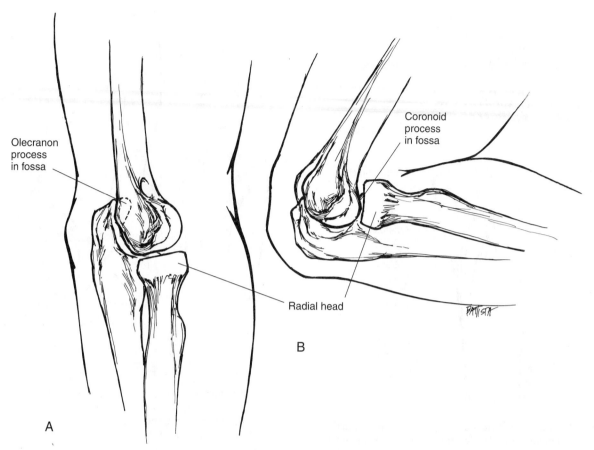

Figure 11.6: The role of the olecranon, radial and coronoid fossae of the humerus. **A.** The elbow joint reveals the olecranon in the olecranon fossa in extension. **B.** The radial head and the coronoid process in the radial and coronoid fossae, respectively, in flexion.

approximation between the humerus and the radius and ulna during maximum elbow flexion (*Fig. 11.6*). The olecranon fossa is a deep depression on the posterior surface of the distal humerus, proximal to the trochlea. The proximal aspect of the ulna's olecranon process fits into this notch when the elbow is extended.

The articular surfaces of the distal humerus form the lateral two thirds of its distal aspect. The trochlea lies in the middle third, and the capitulum lies in the lateral one third. The capitulum forms approximately a hemisphere and is situated on the anterior and distal aspects of the humerus but does not extend onto the posterior surface (Fig. 11.4). The trochlea is a pulley-shaped surface that extends over the anterior, distal, and posterior aspects of the humerus, forming almost 330° of a circle [59,60]. The medial portion of the trochlea expands farther distally than the lateral, which helps to explain the lateral orientation of the ulna with respect to the humerus. This orientation, described as the **carrying angle,** is discussed in greater detail later in this chapter.

The articular surfaces of both the trochlea and capitulum are covered by hyaline cartilage. Average cartilage thickness on the capitulum from 12 cadaver specimens ranges from 1.06 to 1.42 mm (± 0.24–0.30 mm) [51]. Mineralization and density of the subchondral bone appear to be greatest anteriorly on the capitulum and distally and anteriorly on the trochlea

[16,18,19] (*Fig. 11.7*). According to Wolff's law, the mineralization and density of the distal humerus suggests that the distal humerus sustains its largest loads anteriorly and distally. (See Chapter 3 for more details about Wolff's law.)

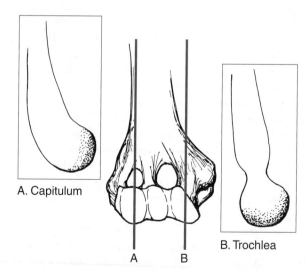

Figure 11.7: Areas of increased mineralization on the distal humerus. The areas of greatest bone mineralization on the distal humerus are (*A*) anterior on the capitulum and (*B*) anterior and distal on the trochlea.

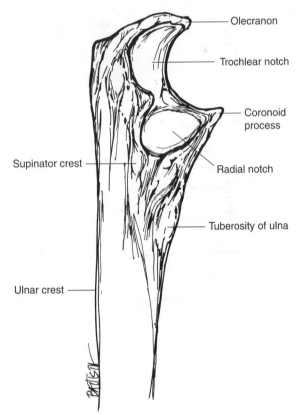

Figure 11.8: Anterolateral view of the proximal ulna reveals the relevant landmarks and articular surfaces of the proximal ulna.

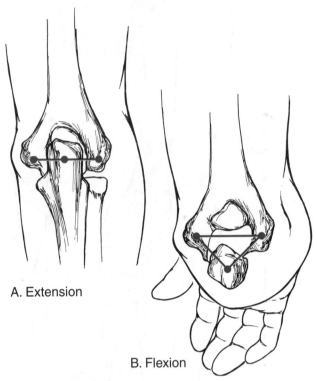

A. Extension

B. Flexion

Figure 11.9: Relationship of the olecranon process to the humeral epicondyles. A posterior view of the elbow joint reveals the relationships among the olecranon process and the medial and lateral condyles in (A) elbow extension and (B) elbow flexion.

Proximal Ulna

The proximal end of the ulna is considerably larger than the distal end. Like the distal end of the humerus, the proximal ulna is curved anteriorly. It consists primarily of the olecranon and coronoid processes and the trochlear notch they create (*Fig. 11.8*). The notch articulates with the trochlea of the humerus. The olecranon is a hooklike projection extending proximally and then anteriorly. It is smooth and easily palpated posteriorly when the elbow is extended, positioned between the two humeral epicondyles. When the elbow is flexed, the pointed junction between the posterior and superior surfaces of the olecranon process is found distal to the two epicondyles, forming a triangle with these two bony landmarks (*Fig. 11.9*). The olecranon is continuous distally with the posterior border of the ulna, also known as the ulnar crest, which is palpable the length of the ulna.

The coronoid process lies on the anterior aspect of the proximal ulna, and its superior surface forms the floor of the trochlear notch. The distal aspect of the anterior surface of the process is known as the tuberosity of the ulna. On the lateral aspect of the coronoid process is a smooth oval facet. This facet, the radial notch, is the site for articulation with the head of the radius. Just distal to this facet is a fossa that provides attachment for the supinator muscle. This fossa is limited posteriorly by the supinator crest.

The trochlear notch is formed by the anterior surface of the olecranon process and the superior surface of the coronoid process. The trochlear notch itself is covered with articular cartilage and has a central ridge running proximally and distally through the length of the notch. It fits into the deepest part of the trochlea on the humerus. The junction of olecranon and coronoid processes in the trochlear notch is somewhat narrowed medially and laterally. The articular surface of the trochlear notch frequently is separated into two distinct articular surfaces proximally and distally, divided by a nonarticular roughened area [19,62,69] (*Fig. 11.10*). The hyaline cartilage covering the trochlear notch is thinnest medially and laterally, thickening toward the midline of the surface, with an average maximum thickness of approximately 2 mm in 14 cadaver specimens [38]. However, the pattern of cartilage thickness appears to vary proximally and distally along the surface and seems to depend on whether the articular surface of the trochlear notch is continuous or separated into individual articular surfaces. As in the humerus, the degree of subchondral bone mineralization also varies across the trochlear notch, greater in the proximal and distal regions than centrally, again suggesting that the bone's architecture depends on the loads it sustains [38].

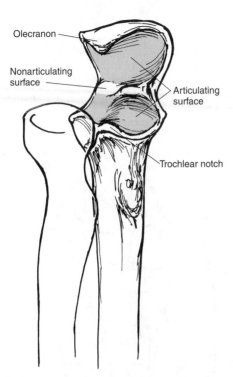

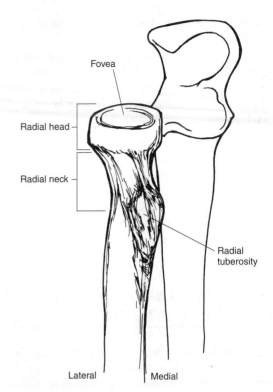

Figure 11.10: Articular surface of the trochlear notch. An anterior view of the trochlear notch demonstrates two sites of contact, with no contact in the deepest part of the notch, a common pattern of contact with the trochlea.

Figure 11.11: An anterior view of the proximal radius reveals the articular surfaces and important landmarks of the proximal radius.

Proximal Radius

The proximal radius includes the radial head, neck, and tuberosity (*Fig. 11.11*). The radial head is a disc-shaped expansion of the proximal end of the radius. The proximal surface of the head is concave and known as the fovea of the radius, which articulates with the capitulum [61]. The peripheral surface, or rim, of the head is also articular, rotating in the radial fossa of the ulna. In the transverse view, the rim of the radial head can be either circular or ellipsoid [9,65]. The exact shape of the rim dictates the path of the distal radius during pronation and supination. The rim is highest medially and more shallow laterally [1,69]. The rim of the radial head is palpable at the lateral aspect of the elbow, just distal to the lateral epicondyle of the humerus.

Like that of the humerus and ulna, the articular surface of the proximal radius, including the head and rim, is covered with hyaline cartilage, with thicknesses in the foveae of cadaver specimens ranging from about 0.9 to 1.10 mm [38]. The mineralization of the subchondral bone reportedly is thickest in the central part of the fovea [19].

Distal to the head of the radius, the diameter of the radius decreases, forming the neck of the radius. In adults the head of the radius is expanded beyond the circumference of the neck, creating a constriction at the neck into which the annular ligament fits. The radial tuberosity is distal to the radial neck, on the medial aspect of the radius. The shaft of the radius is slightly bowed, with the maximum bend found approximately midshaft where the pronator teres attaches (*Fig. 11.12*). The radius can

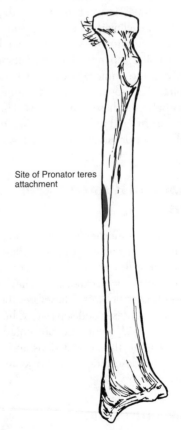

Figure 11.12: Bow shape of the radius. The bowing of the radius effectively increases the moment arm of the pronator teres that attaches at the peak of the bow.

then function as a crank to alter the moment arm of the pronator teres (Chapter 12) [6].

The bones of the elbow possess several landmarks that are identifiable with palpation. Reliable identification of these structures is an essential ingredient of a valid physical examination. The following bony structures are identifiable through palpation:

- Medial epicondyle of the humerus
- Lateral epicondyle of the humerus
- Medial supracondylar ridge of the humerus
- Lateral supracondylar ridge of the humerus
- Olecranon process
- Olecranon fossa of the humerus
- Crest of the ulna
- Radial head

ARTICULATIONS AND SUPPORTING STRUCTURES OF THE ELBOW

Although the elbow is enclosed by a single joint capsule, there are three distinct articulations within that capsule: the **humeroulnar, humeroradial,** and **superior radioulnar** joints. The term *elbow* refers to the humeroulnar and humeroradial articulations. However, because the superior radioulnar joint is so intimately related to the other articulations, the term sometimes is used to include the superior radioulnar joint. So the clinician must take care to clarify whether elbow also refers to the superior radioulnar joint. The following discussion separates the presentation of the articulations involving the humerus from that between only the radius and ulna. This separation results from the functional distinctions between these two systems. The humeral articulations with the ulna and radius are the source of flexion and extension. The superior radioulnar joint allows pronation and supination.

Humeroulnar and Humeroradial Articulations

The humeroulnar and humeroradial articulations are distinct from one another. However, together they form the elbow articulation that is described as a hinge joint, producing the motion of flexion and extension. They also share some of the supporting structures. Therefore, the articular surfaces of each unit are described separately, but the supporting structures for both joints are presented together. The motions allowed at the articulations are described together following the descriptions of the joints and supporting structures.

HUMEROULNAR ARTICULATION

The humeroulnar articulation consists of the trochlear notch of the ulna surrounding the trochlea of the humerus. The reciprocal articular surfaces are generally congruent, with the

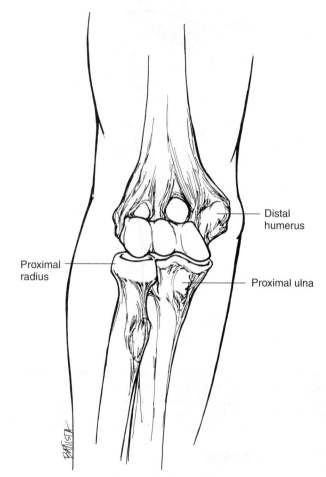

Figure 11.13: Congruence of the articular surfaces of the elbow. An anterior view of the elbow complex reveals that the articular surfaces of the humerus, radius, and ulna fit very well together.

ridge of the trochlear notch of the ulna fitting well into the groove of the trochlea (*Fig. 11.13*). However, close examination reveals that the fit is not perfect. Assessment of 15 cadaver specimens sustaining a load of 10 N (approximately 2.25 lb) suggests that the joint space varies from 0.5 to 1.0 mm in the depth of the trochlear notch and may reach 3.0 mm medially and laterally [17]. In these same specimens, much smaller joint spaces are reported anteriorly and posteriorly (*Fig. 11.14*). The joint congruity increases with increasing joint load as the articular cartilage deforms.

The anterior curve of the distal humerus and the similar bend in the proximal ulna help define the relative amounts of flexion and extension motion at the humeroulnar joint. The forward bend of both bones positions the articular surfaces to favor flexion excursion over extension excursion (*Fig. 11.15*). A more superior orientation of these surfaces would allow more extension range of motion (ROM) by increasing the distance the ulna could travel before the olecranon enters the olecranon fossa. However, flexion would be limited earlier by the coronoid process entering the coronoid fossa.

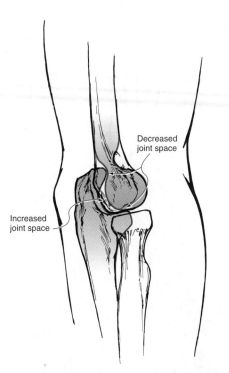

Figure 11.14: Humeroulnar articular surfaces. A sagittal view of the humeroulnar articulation reveals an asymmetrical joint space, deeper in the middle and narrower at the superior and inferior limits of the joint.

Clinical Relevance

CHANGES IN BONY ALIGNMENT FOLLOWING FRACTURE: *Fractures of the distal humerus or proximal ulna can alter the normal orientation of the articular surfaces of the humeroulnar articulation. Changes in the relative alignment of these surfaces can have a significant influence on the available ROM at the elbow following the fracture. Of course, stretching exercises cannot ameliorate motion restrictions due to bony malalignments. Therefore, clinicians must distinguish between restrictions secondary to soft tissue limitations and those due to bony blocks.*

The alignment of the ulna and humerus in the frontal plane also is related to the shape of their articulation. The medial flare of the trochlea extends more distally than the lateral flare. This expansion places the medial aspect of the trochlear notch of the ulna farther distally as well, resulting in a lateral deviation of the ulna with respect to the humerus (*Fig. 11.16*). Although this orientation is typically described as the carrying angle, a more generic term for the alignment is **valgus**. Valgus is defined as a lateral deviation of a distal segment with respect to the segment proximal to it. **Varus** is the opposite, that is, a medial deviation of a limb segment

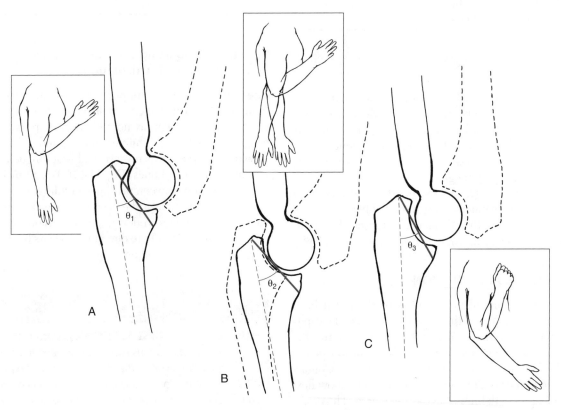

Figure 11.15: The effect of the curves of both the distal humerus and the proximal ulna on elbow ROM. **A.** The mutual anterior curves of the distal humerus and proximal ulna allow flexion ROM but limit extension ROM. **B.** A hypothetical increase in the superior orientation of the trochlear notch increases extension ROM and decreases flexion ROM. **C.** A theoretical increase in anterior orientation of the ulna decreases extension ROM and increases flexion ROM.

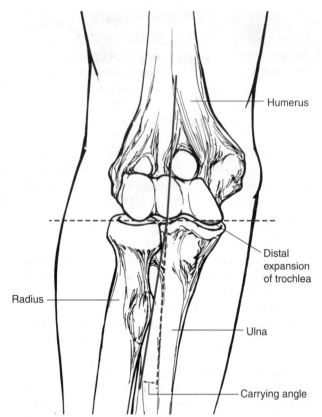

Figure 11.16: Carrying angle of the elbow. The distal expansion of the humeral trochlea contributes to the lateral deviation of the ulna defined as the normal carrying angle.

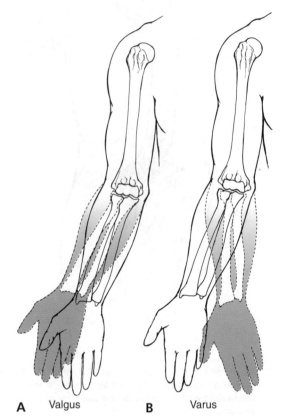

Figure 11.17: Alignment of the elbow in the frontal plane. **A.** Valgus. **B.** Varus.

with respect to the proximal segment. The neutral position between varus and valgus is achieved when the angle between the proximal and distal segments is 180° (usually described as 0°) (*Fig. 11.17*). The valgus alignment, or carrying angle, of the elbow has been the focus of considerable study. Average carrying angles of 10–15° are reported [27,60]. Although texts frequently report that the carrying angle is greater in women than in men [49,59], careful measurements suggest that there is no statistically significant difference in carrying angle between the sexes [27,68].

HUMERORADIAL ARTICULATION

The humeroradial articulation consists of the radial head resting on the capitulum of the humerus. Because the capitulum lies on the anterior surface of the distal humerus, the head of the radius articulates with only a portion of the capitulum when the elbow is extended (*Fig. 11.18*). Contact between the humerus and radius increases with elbow flexion [68]. Chapter 2 defines *stress* as force/area. Thus for a given load at the humeroradial joint, the stress at the joint is less when the elbow is flexed than when it is in maximum extension because the contact between the bones is greater with flexion.

Structures Stabilizing the Humeroulnar and Humeroradial Articulations

The first source of support to the humeroulnar and humeroradial articulations consists of the bony surfaces themselves. Although, as noted above, there is not perfect congruency among the humerus, ulna, and radius, a frontal view of the three bones reveals an almost tongue-and-groove fit among the three bones (Fig. 11.13). This fit makes medial and lateral glide between proximal and distal surfaces almost impossible. Conversely, the reciprocal concave–convex surfaces serve as guides to flexion and extension much like the rails of a train track, where derailment occurs by the train tipping to one side or another.

Clinical Relevance

HUMEROULNAR DISLOCATIONS: *Dislocations of the humeroulnar articulations can occur posteriorly where there is little bony limitation to the trochlear notch being pushed off the trochlea. More frequently, dislocations occur in a combination of lateral and posterior movement of the forearm resulting from a force directed laterally on the distal forearm [27] (Fig. 11.19). Such dislocations are usually accompanied by tears of the supporting ligaments, described below.*

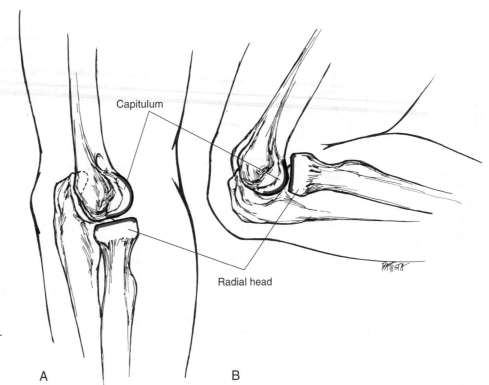

Figure 11.18: Sagittal view of the elbow. **A.** In extension, the capitulum articulates with only the anterior half of the head of the radius. **B.** In flexion, the capitulum articulates with the entire radial head.

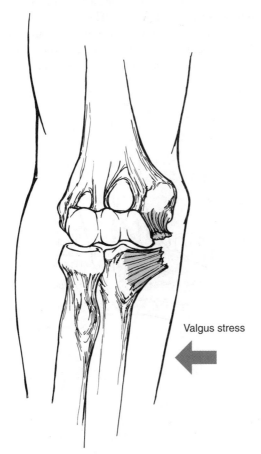

Figure 11.19: Lateral dislocations of the elbow occur as the ulna rotates laterally because lateral translation is prevented by the congruent surfaces of the humerus, ulna, and radius.

The primary supports to the elbow joint are the capsule; the medial, or ulnar, collateral ligament (MCL); and the lateral collateral ligament (LCL). The annular ligament supports the superior radioulnar joint and is described with that joint. The capsule of the elbow joint surrounds all three articulations, the humeroulnar, humeroradial, and superior radioulnar joint (*Fig. 11.20*). The capsule is attached proximally to the humerus at the margins of the olecranon and coronoid and radial fossae as well as to the anterior and posterior surfaces of the medial epicondyle. It also attaches to the posterior surface of the capitulum. Distally, the capsule attaches to the border of the olecranon and coronoid processes and to the annular ligament.

The capsule is by necessity somewhat loose anteriorly and especially posteriorly. Like the capsule of the glenohumeral joint, the elbow joint capsule has folds that unfold and refold during flexion and extension to allow full ROM. In flexion, the posterior capsule unfolds to allow full excursion; in extension, the anterior capsule unfolds as the posterior capsule refolds. These folds allow large flexion and extension excursions but provide little joint stability. Cadaver dissection reveals no increase in joint laxity with isolated transection of the elbow joint capsule [43]. Data collected from 13 cadaver specimens suggest that the entire elbow joint capsule is most lax in 80° of elbow flexion [44]. The tension on the joint capsule in the presence of joint effusion appears to be minimized in this position.

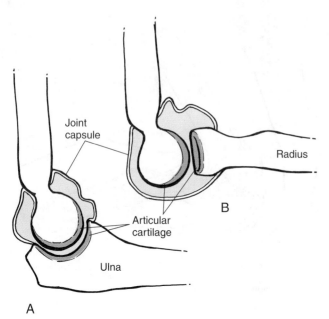

Figure 11.20: Elbow joint capsule. **A.** Medial view. **B.** Lateral view.

Clinical Relevance

JOINT SWELLING AND ELBOW FLEXION CONTRACTURES: *Patients with inflammation of the elbow joint frequently find that the position of comfort is significant elbow flexion. This clinical finding is consistent with*

the evidence suggesting that the tension in the joint capsule is minimized with the elbow flexed to 80° [44]. It is likely that patients seek a position that minimizes the tension on the joint capsule, thus relieving pain associated with a stretch of the capsular ligament. However, prolonged positioning in flexion in the presence of inflammation may result in adaptive changes in the surrounding musculature as well as structural changes in the capsule itself, resulting in a flexion contracture. Treatment to reduce the inflammation is critical to maintaining joint function.

The MCL and LCL reinforce the capsule medially and laterally, respectively. The MCL is the larger of the two collateral ligaments. It consists of distinct anterior and posterior parts and a smaller transverse portion (*Fig. 11.21*). The MCL is attached proximally to the distal surface of the medial epicondyle. The anterior portion of the MCL attaches distally to the coronoid process, and the posterior portion attaches to the olecranon process. The transverse portion actually spans the medial aspect of the trochlear notch, with no attachment on the humerus. The MCL as a whole resists valgus forces that tend to deviate the forearm laterally.

The normal valgus alignment of the elbow predisposes it to valgus stress. Overhead and throwing activities increase the valgus stresses even more (*Fig. 11.22*). Thus it is not surprising that the MCL is a more extensive and complex ligament than the LCL. The organization of the MCL provides protection against excessive valgus throughout the range of flexion and extension.

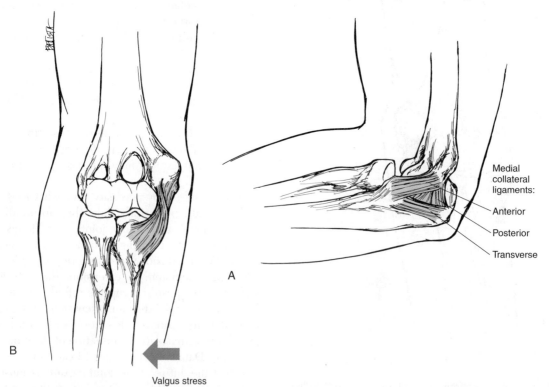

Figure 11.21: Medial collateral ligament. **A.** The medial collateral ligament consists of an anterior, posterior, and transverse section. **B.** The medial collateral ligament resists valgus stresses.

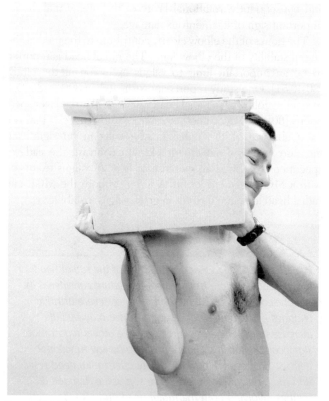

Figure 11.22: Valgus stress on the elbow. Many everyday activities produce large loads that tend to push the elbow into valgus.

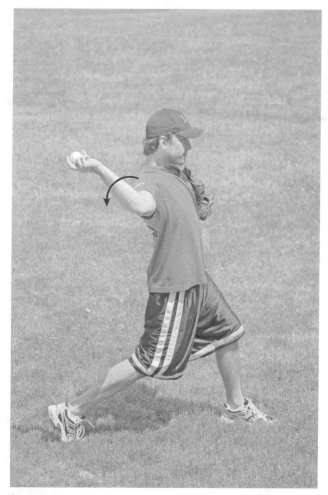

Figure 11.23: Valgus stress on the elbow while pitching. The large shoulder lateral rotation used by most baseball pitchers produces large valgus stresses on the pitching elbow.

Studies repeatedly demonstrate that the posterior portion of the MCL (PMCL) is taut when the elbow is flexed [8,24,48]. Similarly, the anterior portion of the MCL (AMCL) is taut in extension [8,24,40,48,55]. Closer inspection of the AMCL suggests that it has three separate portions, which provide support through distinct regions of joint excursion [24,48]. The anteriormost segment of the AMCL is tight in extension, the middle portion is taut in midrange of flexion, and the posteriormost portion of the AMCL is taut with the PMCL in the later stages of flexion. Studies suggest that the AMCL is the main protection against excessive valgus through extension and moderate flexion ROM [8,21,47]. This complex organization of the MCL ensures that the elbow is protected from valgus displacement throughout its entire ROM.

Clinical Relevance

PITCHERS' ELBOW: *The throwing motion puts a significant valgus stress on the elbow and consequently on the medial collateral ligament (MCL) (Fig. 11.23). The repetitive stresses sustained by baseball pitchers from Little League players to Major League baseball pitchers can and frequently do lead to injuries to the MCL. When the injury includes tears of the MCL, surgical repair may be indicated. The most common, known as Tommy John surgery, named for the major league pitcher whose career was saved by the surgery, reconstructs the torn MCL with a tendon, usually*

from the palmaris longus or the plantaris muscles, small muscles from the forearm or leg, respectively. The best way to prevent such injuries in children is to limit the number of pitches the child throws.

The LCL attaches to the lateral epicondyle of the humerus and can be divided into three discrete bundles (*Fig. 11.24*). One portion, known as the lateral ulnar collateral ligament (LUCL), inserts on the proximal portion of the supinator crest of the ulna. The radial portion of the LCL is known as the radial collateral ligament (RCL) and extends from the lateral epicondyle to the annular ligament in a fan-shaped arrangement with anterior, middle, and posterior segments [48]. The third component of the LCL, known as the accessory LCL (ALCL), runs from the annular ligament to the supinator crest [60]. These three portions of the LCL provide stability against excessive varus deviation. Like those of the MCL, the distinct segments appear to have individual roles in providing stability. Specifically, the middle portion of the RCL is taut throughout the range of flexion and extension, while the anterior and

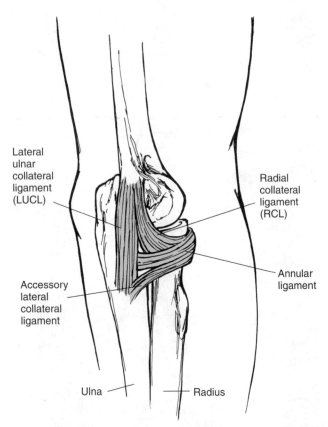

Lateral
ulnar
collateral
ligament
(LUCL)

Radial
collateral
ligament
(RCL)

Accessory
lateral
collateral
ligament

Annular
ligament

Ulna   Radius

Figure 11.24: The lateral collateral ligament consists of the radial collateral, lateral ulnar collateral, and the accessory lateral collateral ligament.

posterior segments are taut in extension and flexion, respectively. The LUCL is taut in the extremes of elbow flexion but is pulled tight with an additional varus stress anywhere in the range of flexion or extension. A study of 30 cadaver specimens suggests that the RCL provides the primary support to the lateral aspect of the elbow [45]. However, in a study of only four cadaver specimens, Morrey and An suggest that the LCL's contribution to elbow stability was less than that provided by the bony articulations themselves [40]. However, these authors tested the elbow specimens only in 0° and 90° of flexion. Additional studies are needed to clarify the functional significance of each ligamentous element to the overall stability of the elbow joint. Regardless of the outcomes of future studies in this area, the elbow appears to be protected from excessive varus and valgus excursions by ligamentous and bony support throughout the ROM.

The collateral ligaments also appear to limit medial and lateral rotation of the ulna on the humerus. In a study of 10 elbows from five cadavers, average maximal lateral rotation at the humeroulnar articulation is almost 10°, and average peak medial rotation is less than 5° [63]. This same study demonstrates that sudden high-velocity loads to the elbow in hyperextension and supination lead to tears of the anterior capsule and to both collateral ligaments. These lesions result in increased hyperextension and valgus and rotational laxity. The rotational laxity is more apparent than the valgus laxity,

and consequently, rotational laxity of the elbow may be an important sign of ligamentous damage.

The bones of the elbow clearly contribute to the medial and lateral stability of the elbow joint. The radial head is reported to be an important limit to valgus excursion at the elbow [30,40,51]. One study reports approximately a 30% reduction in stability following a radial head resection in 30 cadaver specimens [30]. However, another cadaver study suggests that isolated absence of the radial head results in no significant increase in elbow movement [42]. In contrast, the cadaver specimens exhibited an increase of 6–8° of valgus excursion with a MCL ligament lesion. A lesion to both the MCL and radial head appears to result in gross valgus instability.

Thus the humeroulnar and humeroradial articulations, which compose the elbow joint proper, are supported by the bony surfaces involved as well as by ligamentous structures including the capsule and the collateral ligaments.

Superior Radioulnar Joint

The superior radioulnar joint is mechanically quite distinct from the humeral articulations despite its enclosure within the capsule of the elbow joint (*Fig. 11.25*). The articulation is described as a pivot joint with a single axis of motion. Unlike the humeral articulations, the bony architecture of the superior radioulnar joint, which includes the rim of the radial head and the radial facet on the ulna, provides little or no support to the joint. Therefore, the support of the superior radioulnar joint comes from the surrounding connective tissue, including the capsule and LCL, the annular ligament, the interosseous membrane, and the oblique cord. The capsule and LCL have been described and need no further review. The following presents the structure and function of the remaining ligaments.

ANNULAR LIGAMENT

The annular ligament is a broad, tough, fibrous band surrounding the neck of the radius, attaching to the anterior and posterior margins of the radial notch on the ulna. Thus it forms a loop encircling the radius, with its primary attachments on the ulna, although there are some loose attachments to the capsule as well as to the posterior aspect of the

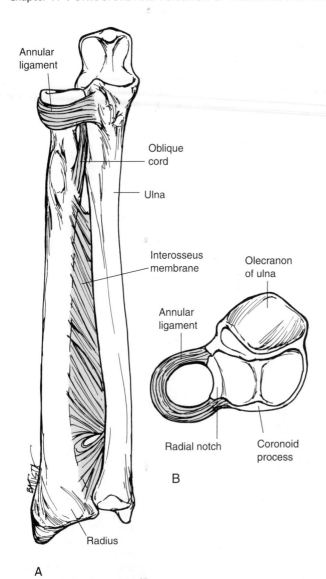

Figure 11.25: The superior radioulnar joint is supported by the annular ligament that surrounds the neck of the radius and by the oblique and interosseous membrane. **A.** Anterior view shows all three of the supporting structures. **B.** Superior view reveals how the annular ligament surrounds the head of the radius.

trochlea and to the radial neck. The deep surface of the annular ligament is lined with fibrocartilage, providing additional stiffness and resilience. The increased mechanical stiffness is important because unlike most ligaments, which attach directly to the bones they support, the annular ligament functions primarily as a sling, acting as a barrier to slippage of the radius. It has little or no limiting effect on the normal motion of the superior radioulnar joint.

The annular ligament binds the radius to the ulna, serving as an effective check to lateral subluxation. In addition, the annular ligament is the primary protection against distal subluxation or dislocation of the superior radioulnar joint. Such an injury typically occurs from a traction force pulling the forearm distally from the elbow, such as that applied when lifting or swinging a child by the hands (*Fig. 11.26*).

Clinical Relevance

"PULLED ELBOW" INJURIES: *Inferior dislocations of the superior radioulnar joint most frequently occur in preschool children and often result from swinging the child by the hands in play [46,54,57]. Consequently, the injury is known as the "pulled elbow" or "nursemaid's elbow." The radial head is pulled through the ring of the annular ligament by the tensile force applied to the forearm. A common explanation for this dislocation has been that at this stage of development the radial head is inadequately formed and is no wider than the neck of the radius; thus the annular ligament cannot serve as a satisfactory noose to prevent slippage of the radial head. More-recent data suggest that the radial head is larger than the radial neck throughout development. However, in young children, the annular ligament is weaker and more easily torn [50]. In addition, it appears that the more narrow lateral aspect of the radial head slips out easily when the elbow is extended and the forearm pronated [1]. The injury may also be more prevalent in children with hypermobility. As the child develops, the annular ligament becomes stronger as does the surrounding musculature. The injury rarely occurs after age six or seven. The incidence of injury can be reduced by cautioning parents and other caregivers to avoid swinging or pulling young children by their hands.*

OBLIQUE CORD AND INTEROSSEOUS MEMBRANE

The oblique cord is a thin bundle of fibers running distally from the tuberosity of the ulna to the radius, just distal to its tuberosity (Fig. 11.25). Its functional significance is unclear. The interosseous membrane attaches to the length of the medial surface of the shaft of the radius and passes medially and distally to the interosseous border of the ulna. The fibers of the interosseous border run perpendicular to the fibers of the oblique cord. One clear role of the interosseous membrane is to bind the radius and ulna together through the length of the forearm. Another role, directly related to the membrane's fiber orientation, has also been identified [4,14]. At the elbow the ulna transmits most of the load to or from the humerus. At the wrist, the radius transmits most of the load (approximately two thirds) to or from the hand [56]. The interosseous membrane plays a role in distributing to the ulna the loads applied to the distal radius [22]. Such loads are applied during weight bearing on the hand or during a fall on the outstretched hand.

Clinical Relevance

LOAD DISTRIBUTION AT THE ELBOW: *When an individual falls on an outstretched hand, the radius sustains large axial loads that could be transmitted directly to the distal humerus (Fig. 11.27). However, the orientation of the*
(continued)

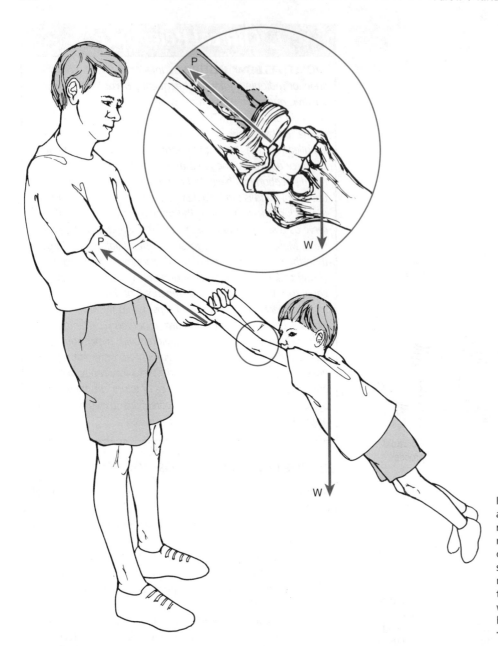

Figure 11.26: Typical mechanism of a distal dislocation of the superior radioulnar joint. The classic mechanism producing a distal dislocation of the superior radioulnar joint is a strong quick pull (*P*) on the distal radius, pulling the head of the radius through the annular ligament as the weight of the body (*W*) pulls the humerus away from the radius.

(Continued)

interosseous membrane allows it to disperse some of the load to the ulna, thus decreasing the load directed onto the capitulum [4,14,37,68]. The load on the radius tends to push it proximally into the humerus. However, as the radius tends to move proximally, the interosseous membrane pulls the ulna proximally as well, thus distributing the axial load to the ulna and ultimately to the trochlea. Consequently, the load is spread over a larger area of the humerus, and the stress (force/area) is decreased, perhaps decreasing the risk of fracture. However, ulnar head resection as the result of severe arthritis or fracture effectively eliminates the load-sharing ability of the ulna when loads are applied through the hand [56].

In conclusion, all of the articulations of the elbow depend on the support of noncontractile soft tissue. The humeral articulations gain additional support from the congruency of the bones themselves. How these bony surfaces and ligamentous structures affect joint mobility is presented in the following section.

Motion of the Elbow Joint

The elbow joint complex contains both a hinge and a pivot joint. Therefore, it is described sometimes as a **trochoginglymus** joint. However, the motions of flexion and extension involve the humeral articulations, and the motions of pronation and supination occur at the superior radioulnar joint. The motions are quite independent of one another and are discussed separately below.

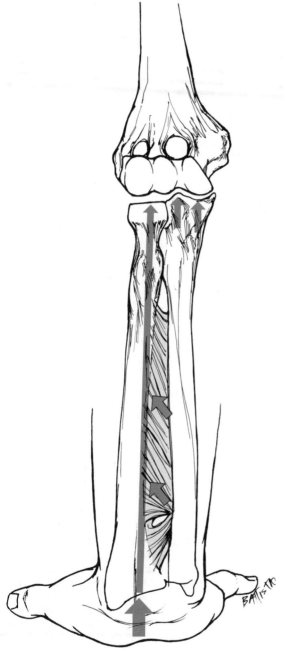

Figure 11.27: Role of the interosseous membrane in transmitting a load on the radius onto the ulna. During weight bearing on the upper extremity, the radius is loaded initially, but the orientation of the fibers of the interosseous membrane allows the load to be transmitted to the ulna.

FLEXION AND EXTENSION

Flexion and extension occur about an axis that passes through the centers of the trochlea and capitulum [34,39]. Chapter 7 presents the concept of the **instant center of rotation (ICR),** which is a two-dimensional method to describe the amount of translation that occurs at a joint during rotation. The ICR changes very little throughout the elbow's range of

flexion and extension, indicating that these motions occur about an almost fixed axis [10,34,68]. However, there has been considerable study of the change in the carrying angle during flexion and extension. Some suggest that the angle decreases as the elbow flexes [10,31,37,70]. This has been attributed to the large distal expansion of the medial aspect of the trochlea as well as to the purported spiral shape of the groove of the trochlea. However, careful study reveals that the change in carrying angle depends on the way it is measured and reconfirms the notion of a relatively fixed axis of rotation during normal flexion and extension [2,34].

The humeral articulations have slight medial and lateral mobility as well as medial and lateral rotation mobility totaling perhaps 10° [59,68]. These motions are apparent during flexion and extension when a varus or valgus stress is applied. They may also be important during pronation and supination [3]. Recognition of the existence of this nonhingelike mobility has been crucial in the development of viable total elbow prostheses.

Clinical Relevance

ELBOW JOINT TOTAL ARTHROPLASTY: *Early total elbow replacements used strict hinge joint devices. Such devices frequently failed because the device began to loosen. More recent developments include unlinked and "semiconstrained" elbow joint implants that allow slight frontal and transverse plane joint mobility during flexion and extension [29]. These devices have exhibited fewer problems with loosening [53].*

PRONATION AND SUPINATION

Pronation and supination occur at the superior radioulnar joint but also involve the distal radioulnar joint. The axis of pronation and supination is a line that runs from close to the center of the fovea of the radial head to the head of the ulna [68,70]. Like the axis of flexion and extension, the axis of pronation and supination appears fixed, with the distal radius gliding about a relatively immovable distal ulna. During pronation and supination with a fixed ulna, the axis of motion is located in the head of the ulna [10,70]. When pronation occurs with the radius moving about a fixed ulna, the hand must move in space (*Fig. 11.28*). However, it is possible to pronate the hand while keeping it fixed in space without compensation at the shoulder or wrist. This ability suggests that the ulna moves radially as the radius rotates around it, thus keeping the hand in the same location. Evidence for the existence of movement by the ulna during pronation and supination is found during forearm movement with the hand fixed, such as turning a screwdriver. Several studies demonstrate that pronation and supination involves slight radial deviation of the ulna [3,20,30–33,67,70]. In this case the axis of motion lies more laterally in the ulna [33]. This complex

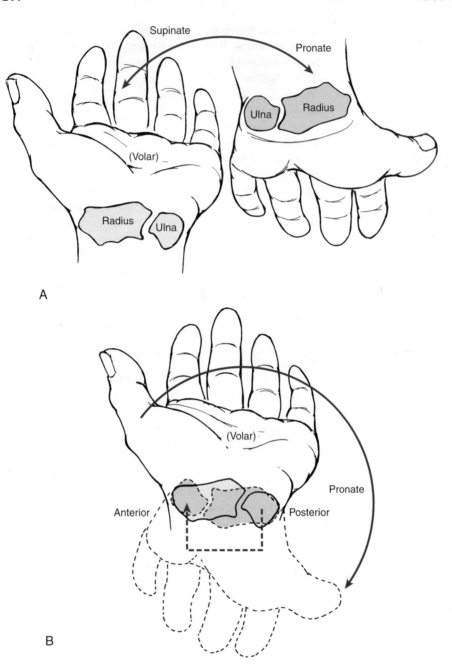

Figure 11.28: The motion of the distal radius and ulna during pronation. **A.** Pronation produced by motion of the radius about a fixed ulna causes the hand to move in space. **B.** Pronation with the hand fixed in space requires movement of the ulna posteriorly, laterally, and then anteriorly.

movement of both the radius and ulna during pronation and supination provides further evidence that the elbow joint complex has more elaborate motion than generally believed. This awareness also supports the need for carefully designed prosthetic devices that are less rigidly constrained than simple hinge joints.

RANGES OF ELBOW MOTION REPORTED IN THE LITERATURE

Ranges of elbow motion reported in the literature are found in *Table 11.1*. Like many of the joint ranges of motion reported in the literature, values frequently are reported without supporting data. Often the values that are based on controlled population studies differ from those values commonly accepted as "normal." Such is the case at the elbow. Although elbow hyperextension ROM is commonly noted, studies that actually measure it report little or no available hyperextension ROM [5,64,66]. There also is wide variability among the reported values for normal pronation and supination flexibility. The large standard deviations reported for pronation and supination by Schoenmarklin and Marras suggest that some of the differences in reported ranges of motion may result from individual differences [52].

TABLE 11.1: Normal Passive Range of Motion Values from the Literature (in Degrees)

	Flexion	Hyperextension	Pronation	Supination
Steindler [59]	135–140	10–20		
US Army/Air Force [15]	150	0	80	80
Boone and Azin [5][a]	140.59 ± 4.9	0.3 ± 2.7	75.0 ± 5.3	88.1 ± 4.0
American Academy of Orthopaedic Surgeons [26]	150	10	[b]	
Walker et al [66][c]	143 ± 11	−4 ± 5[d]	71 ± 11	74 ± 14
Youm et al [70][e]	140 ± 5		70 ± 5	85 ± 4
Schoenmarklin and Marras [52][f]			80 ± 20	100 ± 19
Gerhardt and Rippstein [25]	150	0	80	90
Solveborn and Olerud [58][g]	143 (141–145)	4 (1–6)		

[a]Based on 56 male subjects greater than 20 years of age (x = 34.9 ± 3.4 years).
[b]Reported data from Boone and Azin.
[c]Based on 30 male and 30 female subjects 60 to 84 years old (x = 75.6 ± 7.4 years).
[d]Negative numbers indicate inability to reach an extension position.
[e]Based on eight fresh frozen cadaver specimens.
[f]Based on 39 industrial workers, 22 men and 17 women. Mean age was 41.7 ± 10.5 years.
[g]Based on the right elbows of 16 subjects, 12 men and 4 women. Mean age was 46 years. Reported as mean and 95% CI.

Clinical Relevance

CLINICAL JUDGMENTS FROM ROM MEASUREMENTS:

When making judgments about the quality of a patient's ROM, the clinician must remember the possibility of large intersubject differences. The difference between an individual's right and left sides may be more important than the difference between an individual's ROM and the "normal" value found in the literature. The clinician must evaluate the uninvolved side to help establish the patient's "normal" excursion.

The differences among the studies that report data from described measurements also may result from differences in populations studied [5,52,66]. Boone and Azin present data from only males, and the mean age of the subjects is considerably lower than the age of the subjects studied by Walker et al. [5,66]. Walker et al. note significantly more elbow flexion, extension, and supination in women than in men. Although these authors deny any age effects on elbow ROM in their population of subjects, the study examines only a small spectrum of elderly subjects. Schoenmarklin and Marras report pronation and supination from men and women whose jobs require very repetitive hand activities that may influence their ROM [52]. They do not report comparisons based on sex or age. The differences among the values reported by Walker et al., by Boone and Azin, and by Schoenmarklin and Marras may be the result of age, gender, and occupational differences.

Investigations into the elbow excursions that occur during functional activities help put these ROM values in perspective [7,11,41]. Studies report that most activities of daily living use the middle ranges of joint excursion for elbow flexion and extension from about 30° to 130° [11,36,41]. Personal care tasks such as feeding and personal hygiene may use up to 150° of flexion but little extension. Activities such as rising from a chair and tying a shoelace use less flexion and more extension.

 Similarly, these studies suggest that most activities use the midranges of pronation and supination from approximately 50° of one to 50° of the other.

Clinical Relevance

COMPENSATIONS FOR RESTRICTED ELBOW ROM:

Compensations for restricted elbow ROM during functional activities include increased shoulder motions [12]. Shoulder pain can then develop in patients with limited elbow mobility, as a result of overuse of the shoulder. Therefore, clinicians 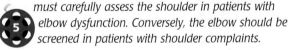 *must carefully assess the shoulder in patients with elbow dysfunction. Conversely, the elbow should be screened in patients with shoulder complaints.*

In conclusion, these data suggest that the commonly accepted ROM of the elbow requires verification by careful studies. The effects of age and gender must also be examined. In the meantime, the clinician should draw conclusions carefully regarding the functional implications of altered joint ROM at the elbow.

STRUCTURES LIMITING NORMAL ROM AT THE ELBOW

Discussion of the elbow joint capsule earlier in this chapter reveals that the capsule is somewhat loose anteriorly and posteriorly to allow full flexion and extension ROM. The collateral ligaments however are taut in flexion and extension. These collateral ligaments have some effect on normal joint excursion; however, their primary role is to prevent excessive ROM. Elbow flexion is limited most by the soft tissue contact of the forearm and arm muscles. The elbow provides an opportunity to learn to recognize the structure responsible for stopping a motion by assessing the **end-feel** of a joint. End-feel is the tactile sensation provided at the end of passive ROM. Bony contact that stops a movement yields a hard end-feel.

The stretch of a ligament produces a hard but springy end-feel. Soft tissue approximation causes a soft end-feel [35].

Clinical Relevance

ELBOW MOTION AND END-FEELS: *Normal elbow flexion range has a characteristic soft end-feel resulting from the contact of the forearm muscles against the relaxed elbow flexors. Elbow extension has a springier end-feel, suggesting limits from the ligaments and stretch of the elbow flexors. Bony contact is sometimes reported as the limiting factor in elbow extension. However, nerve blocks to the elbow flexors in healthy individuals have resulted in increased extension ROM, suggesting that muscles provide the initial limits to normal elbow extension ROM in most individuals [13]. It is important to recall the wide range of variability within the healthy population, as suggested by the standard deviations presented in Table 11.1. Perhaps individuals with little muscle mass and generalized hypermobility do have bony limitations in elbow ROM, particularly extension. Assessment of end-feel can help determine the structures responsible for stopping the joint motion.*

Elbow pronation and supination ROM also is limited primarily by the reciprocal stretch of antagonist muscles. The LCL may contribute some limitation to pronation ROM, and the interosseous membrane may restrict both pronation and supination. However, normal pronation and supination excursions are limited by muscle stretch.

Comparison of the Shoulder and the Elbow

The links between structure and function are particularly apparent when regions as diverse as the elbow and shoulder are compared. The elbow has tightly fitting articular surfaces that guide and restrict elbow motion. The elbow also possesses collateral ligaments that serve as important stabilizing structures in the mediolateral direction and contribute to the limits of elbow extension. Although the muscles of the elbow play some role in stabilizing the joint, their primary responsibility is to move the elbow. In contrast, the shoulder, the most mobile unit in the body, depends heavily on muscles for its stability. In fact, the bony shape of the glenohumeral joint provides remarkable mobility but offers little assistance in stability. The ligaments of the glenohumeral joint provide support but only at the end ranges of motion. Thus the elbow and shoulder provide dramatic contrasts in functional requirements and in the architectures that fulfill those requirements.

SUMMARY

This chapter presents the structure of the bones and supporting elements of the elbow joint and the movements available. The bones offer congruent articular surfaces that provide

significant stability to the elbow complex. The MCL and LCL provide the primary ligamentous support to the humeroulnar and radiohumeral articulation. The MCL and LCL resist valgus and varus stresses, respectively, throughout the full range of flexion and extension. The annular and interosseous ligaments support the superior radioulnar joint.

The variety and magnitude of motion available at the elbow are much less than at the shoulder, reflecting the difference in the elbow's structure, which consists of less-complex articulations and a simpler ligamentous organization contributing to a joint complex that is inherently more stable and less mobile. Considerable variability exists in the reported mobility of the elbow and may indicate effects of gender, age, and use. The role of the muscles in propelling this joint is presented in the following chapter.

References

1. Amir D, Frankl U, Pogrund H: Pulled elbow and hypermobility of joints. Clin Orthop 1990; 257: 94–99.
2. An KN, Morrey BF, Chao EY: Carrying angle of the human elbow joint. J Orthop Res 1984; 1: 369–378.
3. Basmajian JV, DeLuca CJ: Muscles Alive. Their Function Revealed by Electromyography. Baltimore: Williams & Wilkins, 1985.
4. Birkbeck DP: The interosseous membrane affects load distribution in the forearm. J Hand Surg [Am] 1997; 22: 975–980.
5. Boone DC, Azen SP: Normal range of motion of joints in male subjects. J Bone Joint Surg 1979; 61-A: 756–759.
6. Bremer AK, Sennwald GR, Favre P, Jacob HAC: Moment arms of forearm rotators. Clin Biomech 2006; 21: 683–691.
7. Buckley MA, Yardley A, Johnson GR, Carus DA: Dynamics of the upper limb during performance of the tasks of everyday living—a review of the current knowledge base. Proc Inst Mech Eng 1996; 210: 241–247.
8. Callaway GH, Field LD, Deng XH, et al: Biomechanical evaluation of the medial collateral ligament of the elbow. J Bone Joint Surg 1997; 79-A: 1223–1231.
9. Captier G, Canovas F, Mercier N, et al.: Biometry of the radial head: biomechanical implications in pronation and supination. Surg Radiol Anat 2002; 24: 295–301.
10. Chao EY: Three-dimensional rotation of the elbow. J Biomech 1978; 11: 57–73.
11. Chao EY, An KN, Askew LJ, Morrey BF: Electrogoniometer for the measurement of human elbow joint rotation. J Biomech Eng 1980; 102: 301–310.
12. Cooper JE, Shweddyk E, Quanbury AO, et al.: Elbow joint restrictions: effect on functional upper limb motion during performance of three feeding activities. Arch Phys Med Rehabil 1993; 74: 805–808.
13. Cummings GS: Comparison of muscle to other joint soft tissue in limiting elbow extension. J Orthop Sports Phys Ther 1984; 5: 170–174.
14. Defrate LE, Li G, Zayontz SJ, Herndon JH: A minimally invasive method for the determination of force in the interosseous ligament. Clin Biomech 2001; 16: 895–900.
15. Departments of the U.S. Army and Air Force. US Army Goniometry Manual: Technical Manual no. 8-640. Air Force Pamphlet no. 160-14. 1-8-1968. Washington, DC: Departments of the Army and Air Force, 1968.

16. Eckstein F, Jacobs CR, Merz BR: Mechanobiological adaptation of subchondral bone as a function of joint incongruity and loading. Med Eng Phys 1997; 19: 720–728.

17. Eckstein F, Lohe F, Schulte E, et al.: Physiological incongruity of the humero-ulnar joint: a functional principle of optimized stress distribution acting upon articulating surfaces? Anat Embryol 1993; 188: 449–455.

18. Eckstein F, Merz B, Schon M, et al.: Tension and bending, but not compression alone determine the functional adaptation of subchondral bone in incongruous joints. Anat Embryol (Berl) 1999; 199: 85–97.

19. Eckstein F, Muller-Gerbl M, Steinlechner M, et al.: Subchondral bone density in the human elbow assessed by computed tomography osteoabsorptiometry: a reflection of the loading history of the joint surfaces. J Orthop Res 1995; 13: 268–278.

20. Ekenstam FA: Anatomy of the distal radioulnar joint. Clin Orthop 1992; 275: 14–18.

21. Eygendaal D, Olsen BS, Jensen SL, et al.: Kinematics of partial and total ruptures of the medial collateral ligament of the elbow. J Shoulder Elbow Surg 1999; 8: 612–616.

22. Fischer KJ, Bastidas JA, Pfaeffle HJ, Towers JD: A method for estimating relative bone loads from CT data with application to the radius and the ulna. CMES 2003; 4: 397–403.

23. Fuchs S, Chylarecki C: Do functional deficits result from radial head resection? J Shoulder Elbow Surg 1999; 8: 247–251.

24. Fuss FK: The ulnar collateral ligament of the human elbow joint. Anatomy, function and biomechanics. J Anat 1991; 175: 203–212.

25. Gerhardt JJ, Rippstein J: Measuring and Recording of Joint Motion Instrumentation and Techniques. Lewiston, NJ: Hogrefe & Huber, 1990.

26. Greene WB, Heckman JDE: The Clinical Measurement of Joint Motion. Rosemont, IL: American Academy of Orthopaedic Surgeons, 1994.

27. Habernek H, Ortner F: The influence of anatomic factors in elbow joint dislocation. Clin Orthop 1992; 274: 226–230.

28. Hall JA, McKee MD: Posterolateral rotatory instability of the elbow following radial head resection. J Bone Joint Surg Am 2005; 87: 1571–1579.

29. Hargreaves D, Emery R: Total elbow replacement in the treatment of rheumatoid arthritis. Clin Orthop 1999; 366: 61–71.

30. Hotchkiss RN: Valgus stability of the elbow. J Orthop Res 1987; 5: 372–377.

31. Kapandji IA: The Physiology of the Joints. Vol 1, The Upper Limb. Edinburgh: Churchill Livingstone, 1982.

32. Kasten P, Krefft M, Hesselbach J, Weinberg AM: Kinematics of the ulna during pronation and supination in a cadaver study: implications for elbow arthroplasty. Clin Biomech 2004; 19: 31–35.

33. Linscheid RL: Biomechanics of the distal radioulnar joint. Clin Orthop 1992; 275: 46–55.

34. London JT: Kinematics of the elbow. J Bone Joint Surg 1981; 63-A: 529–534.

35. Magee DA: Orthopedic Physical Assessment. Philadelphia: WB Saunders, 1998.

36. Magermans DJ, Chadwick EKJ, Veeger HEJ, van der Helm FCT: Requirements for upper extremity motions during activities of daily living. Clin Biomech 2005; 20: 591–599.

37. Markolf KL, Lamey D, Yang S, et al.: Radioulnar load-sharing in the forearm. A study in cadavera. J Bone Joint Surg [Am] 1998; 80-A: 879–888.

38. Milz S, Eckstein F, Putz R: Thickness distribution of the subchondral mineralization zone of the trochlear notch and its correlation with the cartilage thickness: an expression of functional adaptation to mechanical stress acting on the humeroulnar joint? Anat Rec 1997; 248: 189–197.

39. Morrey BF: Passive motion of the elbow joint. J Bone Joint Surg [Am] 1976; 58: 501–508.

40. Morrey BF, An KN: Articular and ligamentous contributions to the stability of the elbow joint. Am J Sports Med 1983; 11: 315–319.

41. Morrey BF, Askew LJ, An KN, Chao EY: A biomechanical study of normal functional elbow motion. J Bone Joint Surg 1981; 63-A: 872–876.

42. Morrey BF, Tanaka S, An KN: Valgus stability of the elbow: a definition of primary and secondary constraints. Clin Orthop 1991; 265: 187–195.

43. Nielsen KK, Olsen BS: No stabilizing effect of the elbow joint capsule. A kinematic study. Acta Orthop Scand 2000; 70: 6–8.

44. O'Driscoll SW, Morrey BF, An KN: Intraarticular pressure and capacity of the elbow. Arthroscopy 1990; 6: 100–103.

45. Olsen BS, Sojbjerg JO, Dalstra M, Sneppen O: Kinematics of the lateral ligamentous constraints of the elbow joint. J Shoulder Elbow Surg 1996; 5: 333–341.

46. Prendergast M: Hysteria or pulled elbow? Lancet 1994; 343: 926.

47. Pribyl CR, Hurley DK, Wascher DC, et al.: Elbow ligament strain under valgus load; a biomechanical study. Orthopedics 1999; 22: 607–612.

48. Regan WD, Korinek SL, Morrey BF, An KN: Biomechanical study of ligaments around the elbow joint. Clin Orthop 1991; 271: 170–179.

49. Romanes GJE: Cunningham's Textbook of Anatomy. Oxford: Oxford University Press, 1981.

50. Salter RB: Textbook of Disorders and Injuries of the Musculoskeletal System. 3rd ed. Baltimore: Williams & Wilkins, 1999.

51. Schenck RC Jr, Athanasiou KA, Constantinides G, Gomez E: A biomechanical analysis of articular cartilage of the human elbow and a potential relationship to osteochondritis dissecans. Clin Orthop 1994; 299: 305–312.

52. Schoenmarklin RW, Marras WS: Dynamic capabilities of the wrist joint in industrial workers. Int J Ind Ergonom 1993; 11: 207–224.

53. Schuind FA, Goldschmidt D, Bastin C, Burny F: A biomechanical study of the ulnar nerve at the elbow. J Hand Surg 1995; 20B: 623–627.

54. Schunk JE: Radial head subluxation: epidemiology and treatment of 87 episodes. Ann Emerg Med 1990; 19: 1019–1023.

55. Schwab GH: Biomechanics of elbow instability: the role of the medial collateral ligament. Clin Orthop 1980; 146: 42–52.

56. Shaaban H, Giakas G, Bolton M, et al.: The load-bearing characteristics of the forearm: pattern of axial and bending force transmitted through ulna and radius. J Hand Surg [Br] 2006; 31B: 274–279.

57. Snyder HS: Radiographic changes with radial head subluxation in children. J Emerg Med 1990; 8: 265–269.

58. Solveborn SA, Olerud C: Radial epicondylalgia (tennis elbow): measurement of range of motion of the wrist and the elbow. J Orthop Sports Phys Ther 1996; 23: 251–257.

59. Steindler A: Kinesiology of the Human Body under Normal and Pathological Conditions. Springfield, IL: Charles C Thomas, 1955.

60. Stroyan M, Wilk KE: The functional anatomy of the elbow complex. JOSPT 1993; 17: 279–288.

61. Swieszkowski W, Skalski K, Pomianowski S, Kedzior K: The anatomic features of the radial head and their implication for prothesis design. Clin Biomech 2001; 16: 880–887.

62. Tillmann B: A contribution to the functional morphology of articular surfaces. Norm Pathol Anat (Stuttg) 1978; 34: 1–50.

63. Tyrdal S, Olsen BS: Combined hyperextension and supination of the elbow joint induces lateral ligament lesions: an experimental study of the pathoanatomy and kinematics in elbow ligament injuries. Knee Surg Sports Traumatol Arthrosc 1998; 6: 36–43.

64. Tyrdal S, Olsen BS: Hyperextension trauma to the elbow joint induced through the distal ulna or the distal radius: pathoanatomy and kinematics: an experimental study of the ligament injuries. Scand J Med Sci Sports 1998; 8: 177–182.

65. van Riet RP, Van Glabbeek F, Neale PG, et al.: The noncircular shape of the radial head. J Hand Surg [Am] 2003; 28: 972–978.

66. Walker JM, Sue D, Miles-Elkousy N, et al.: Active mobility of the extremities in older subjects. Phys Ther 1984; 64: 919–923.

67. Weinberg AM, Pietsch IT, Helm MB, et al.: A new kinematic model of pro- and supination of the human forearm. J Biomech 2000; 33: 487–491.

68. Werner FW, An KN: Biomechanics of the elbow and forearm. Hand Clin 1994; 10: 357–373.

69. Williams P, Bannister L, Berry M, et al: Gray's Anatomy, The Anatomical Basis of Medicine and Surgery, Br. ed. London: Churchill Livingstone, 1995.

70. Youm Y, Dryer RF, Thambyrajah K, et al.: Biomechanical analyses of forearm pronation-supination and elbow flexion-extension. J Biomech 1979; 12: 245–255.

Mechanics and Pathomechanics of Muscle Activity at the Elbow

CHAPTER CONTENTS

T he preceding chapter presents the bones and articulations that constitute the elbow joint complex. Although it is clear that the structure and function of the elbow joint complex are simpler than those of the shoulder, the musculature has its own unique specializations. The elbow joint complex consists of two mechanically distinct articulations, the humeral articulations that allow flexion and extension and the superior radioulnar articulation that contributes to pronation and supination of the forearm and hand. Therefore, the muscles of the elbow are organized in a way that allows the elbow to function in virtually any combination of elbow and forearm position.

The purposes of this chapter are to

- Discuss the architecture and action of each of the primary muscles of the elbow
- Examine the individual functional roles of each of the elbow muscles
- Discuss the contributions to functional deficits from impairments of individual muscles
- Compare the relative strengths of the flexor and extensor muscle groups of the elbow

For the purposes of this chapter, the primary muscles of the elbow are defined as those that cross the elbow and attach on the forearm with no attachment across the wrist. Most of the muscles acting at the elbow can be characterized as muscles that flex or extend the elbow. These muscles are the biceps brachii, brachialis, brachioradialis, pronator teres, triceps brachii, and anconeus. The supinator also is a muscle of the elbow. Although it makes no contributions to flexion or extension of the elbow, it is an essential muscle of the elbow, functioning solely at the superior radioulnar joint.

The brachioradialis, pronator teres, and supinator muscles actually have their proximal attachments with the forearm muscles. Although the rest of the forearm muscles also affect the elbow, their primary actions are at the wrist. The brachioradialis, pronator teres, and supinator muscles function at the elbow rather than at the wrist. The current chapter focuses on all of the muscles whose primary actions are at the elbow. The rest of the forearm muscles are described in Chapter 15. In that chapter, the role of the remaining forearm muscles is presented, including their effects on the motions at the humeral and radioulnar articulations.

ELBOW FLEXOR MUSCLES

The primary flexors of the elbow are the biceps brachii, brachialis, and brachioradialis (*Fig. 12.1*). The pronator teres also contributes to active elbow flexion and is included in this group. The actions attributable to each muscle are presented below. After each muscle is discussed individually, the current understanding of their contributions to the coordinated movement of elbow flexion is presented. This understanding is based on electromyographic (EMG) data as well as on mathematical models of the region.

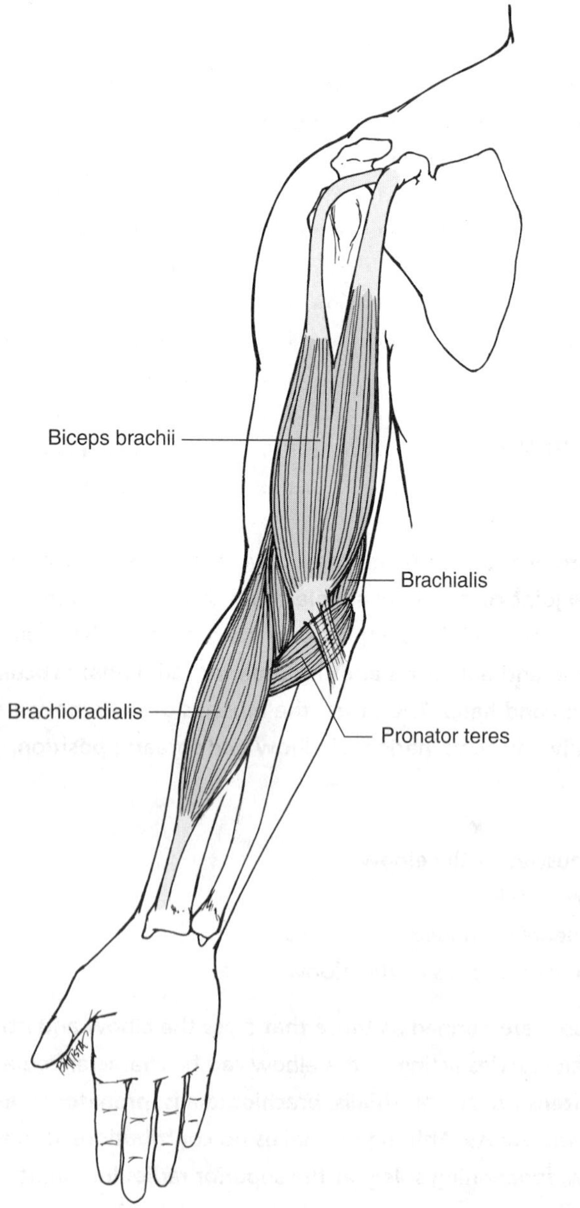

Biceps Brachii

The biceps brachii is a fusiform muscle with two heads (*Muscle Attachment Box 12.1*). Its attachments span both the shoulder and the elbow, and at the elbow it crosses both the humeral and radioulnar articulations. Thus contractions of the biceps brachii affect the glenohumeral, humeroulnar, and humeroradial articulations as well as the superior radioulnar joint.

Biceps brachii

Brachialis

Brachioradialis

Pronator teres

Figure 12.1: The primary flexor muscles of the elbow include the biceps brachii, brachialis, brachioradialis, and pronator teres.

MUSCLE ATTACHMENT BOX 12.1

ATTACHMENTS AND INNERVATION OF THE BICEPS BRACHII

Proximal attachment: The long head attaches to the supraglenoid tubercle of the scapula. It is intracapsular and covered by a synovial sheath. It may also have a direct attachment to the anterosuperior part of the glenoid labrum [4]. The short head of the biceps brachii attaches to the coracoid process of the scapula.

Distal attachment: The two tendons merge and attach together as the biceps tendon onto the tuberosity of the radius. The tendon has a medial expansion, the bicipital aponeurosis, which fuses with the deep fascia of the flexor muscles of the wrist.

Innervation: Musculocutaneous nerve, C5 and C6.

Palpation: The belly of the biceps brachii is easily palpated on the volar surface of the arm. The distal tendon and aponeurosis are also palpable. The tendon of the long head often can be discerned in the intertubercular groove.

ACTIONS

MUSCLE ACTION: BICEPS BRACHII

Action	Evidence
Elbow flexion	Supporting
Elbow supination	Supporting
Shoulder flexion	Supporting
Shoulder abduction	Supporting
Stabilization of the glenohumeral joint	Supporting

There is no doubt that the biceps brachii flexes the elbow and supinates the forearm [6,10,33,41,44,53]. Although both heads of the biceps brachii contribute to these actions, their relative contributions are unclear. Basmajian and De Luca suggest that the long head is more active than the short head during concentric elbow flexion and during unresisted supination in most subjects [6]. However, Stewart et al. find no difference in the activity of the two heads during elbow flexion, regardless of forearm position or contractile speed [47]. A study of 10 people with longstanding (an average of 3.2 years) ruptures of the tendon of the long head of the biceps reveals strength deficits of 10–15% for elbow flexion and less than 2% for supination compared with the unaffected side [49]. EMG data suggest that the muscles of the elbow have specific individual roles in elbow motion depending on forearm position, the amount of resistance during the movement, and the speed of the motion. The activity of the biceps brachii during elbow motion depends on these conditions. The specific conditions under which the biceps brachii participates in elbow flexion and forearm supination are reviewed following the discussion of the rest of the elbow flexors.

The biceps brachii frequently is reported as a shoulder flexor [44,50]. Basmajian and De Luca report EMG data supporting this commonly held view [6]. These authors note activity in both heads of the biceps brachii during shoulder flexion but more in the long head in most subjects. However, a study of five cadaver shoulders suggests that the short head of the biceps brachii has a substantial moment arm for shoulder flexion, while the long head has a negligible one [7].

Because the biceps brachii crosses both the shoulder and the elbow, muscle length is affected by position changes at either joint. Passive elbow flexion puts the muscle in a shortened position, thus putting the muscle on slack. Passive shoulder flexion does the same. Passive elbow and shoulder extension put the muscle in a lengthened position, thus stretching the muscle.

The length–tension relationship suggests that as a muscle is stretched, its force of contraction is increased, and as a muscle is shortened, its force of contraction is decreased. (Details of this relationship are presented in Chapter 4.) Because the biceps brachii is a two-joint muscle, isolated contraction causes elbow and shoulder flexion together. However, if sufficient elbow and shoulder flexion occur together, the biceps brachii may be so shortened that it can generate little force. This is known as **active insufficiency**

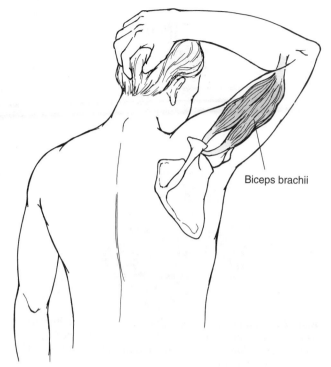

Biceps brachii

Figure 12.2: Active insufficiency of the biceps brachii occurs as the result of combined elbow and shoulder flexion putting the muscle in an excessively shortened position.

(*Fig. 12.2*). In contrast, shoulder extension lengthens the biceps brachii and increases the biceps contractile force during elbow flexion.

Contraction of the biceps brachii with simultaneous contraction of a shoulder extensor muscle produces elbow flexion and shoulder extension, thus maintaining sufficient length of the biceps brachii muscle. Allen et al. note the presence of slight shoulder hyperextension during a maximum voluntary contraction (MVC) of the elbow flexors (*Fig. 12.3*) [1]. These authors interpret this finding as a means of increasing the force of contraction by stretching the biceps in accordance with the length–tension relationship of a muscle. Clinicians can use this effect of positioning to facilitate a patient's elbow flexion strength.

Clinical Relevance

CHANGING SHOULDER POSITION TO AFFECT BICEPS BRACHII CONTRACTILE FORCE AT THE ELBOW:
Clinicians affect a patient's elbow flexion strength by varying the position of the elbow or shoulder joint. To correctly identify a change in strength as the result of intervention or disease, a clinician must standardize the position of both the shoulder and elbow when testing elbow strength. On the other hand, shoulder hyperextension is a useful position in which to exercise a patient with weakness of the biceps brachii, since the resulting muscle stretch enhances the muscle's force output.

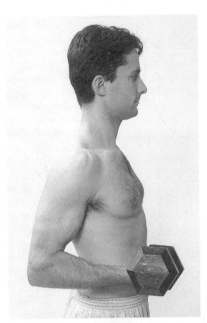

Figure 12.3: Lengthening the biceps brachii to increase its contraction force. Slight hyperextension of the shoulder during heavily resisted elbow flexion lengthens the biceps brachii and increases its force output.

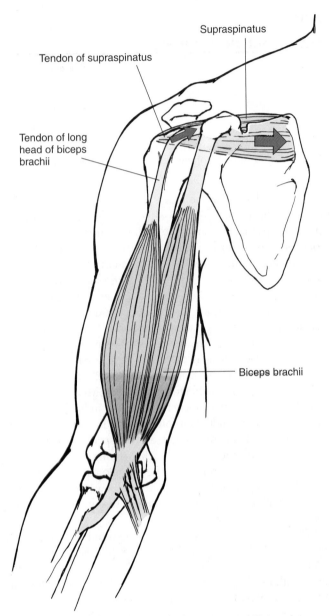

Figure 12.4: The role of the biceps brachii in stabilizing the glenohumeral joint. The pull of the tendon of the long head of the biceps brachii is almost parallel to the pull of the supraspinatus, allowing the biceps brachii to contribute to the stability of the glenohumeral joint.

A few reports describe the biceps brachii as an abductor of the shoulder [6,41]. Sturzenegger et al. [49] report an average 8% reduction in shoulder abduction strength in the presence of longstanding ruptures of the tendon of the long head of the biceps brachii. A study of five cadaver shoulders suggests that both heads of the biceps brachii have abduction moment arms, implying that the muscle is capable of producing abduction at the shoulder. However, there are no known studies examining the EMG activity of the biceps brachii during shoulder abduction. The cadaver study also suggests that the long head of the biceps can produce a lateral rotation moment. However, EMG data show no biceps brachii activity in lateral rotation but occasional activity of the short head during medial rotation [6]. These studies support the notion that the biceps brachii may contribute to shoulder abduction and rotation. Additional research is necessary to clarify these roles.

Many authors identify the long head of the biceps brachii as an important dynamic stabilizer of the glenohumeral joint [4,8,37,45]. The proximal end of the tendon of the long head of the biceps brachii is almost parallel to the supraspinatus muscle and probably functions similarly to stabilize the glenohumeral joint by compressing the joint [8,37] (*Fig. 12.4*). A detailed study of cadavers suggests that the biceps can provide important protection against both anterior and posterior dislocation of the glenohumeral joint, depending on the joint's rotation [8]. Additional cadaver studies support the role of the biceps in stabilizing the glenohumeral joint in the anterior–posterior (AP) and in the superior and inferior directions [29,37,45]. However, EMG data reveal no activity of the biceps brachii to stabilize the glenohumeral joint against loads

to sublux the joint inferiorly in individuals without shoulder pathology [6].

Although these studies appear to contradict one another, it is important to recognize the difficulty in comparing these studies. The cadaver studies demonstrate the potential of the biceps brachii to stabilize the glenohumeral joint. The EMG data are from a study of subjects with normal joint stability that examined movement of the humerus in the inferior direction only. Additional studies are needed to examine the role of the biceps brachii in stabilizing the glenohumeral joint in each direction in live subjects with and without stable shoulders.

Until those data are available, the role of the biceps brachii in stabilizing the glenohumeral joint in specific directions remains unclear. However, there is ample evidence to support its role as a glenohumeral joint stabilizer when other stabilizers are impaired.

EFFECTS OF WEAKNESS

Weakness of the biceps brachii causes a loss of strength in elbow flexion and supination. However, a case report of an individual with an isolated lesion of the musculocutaneous nerve with complete denervation of the biceps brachii reveals an individual with excellent function because of the compensations provided by other elbow muscles [12]. It must be noted that "excellent function" is not defined in the report, nor are strength measures reported. While the elbow has several muscles that produce flexion, the biceps brachii is a primary flexor, and weakness in it results in a substantial decrease in strength. However, the remaining elbow flexor muscles apparently preserve considerable function. Similarly, weakness of the biceps brachii produces a significant decrease in supination strength, although the remaining muscles that supinate the forearm limit the functional loss [40].

Weakness of the biceps brachii may also be manifested by slight weakness in shoulder flexion. However, the primary shoulder flexors are so large and strong that isolated weakness of the biceps muscle is unlikely to produce a functionally significant loss of shoulder flexion strength. Still, decreased biceps brachii strength in the presence of rotator cuff pathology may contribute to even more glenohumeral joint instability.

EFFECTS OF TIGHTNESS

Tightness of the biceps brachii muscle may cause a reduction in elbow extension and pronation range of motion (ROM) and, perhaps even shoulder extension ROM. However as a two-joint, or biarticular, muscle, the effects of tightness at one joint are altered by the position of the other joint. The interrelationship between shoulder and elbow positions and the effect this relationship has on the biceps brachii can assist the clinician in differentiating among various structures that may limit the extension ROM of the elbow joint.

Clinical Relevance

IDENTIFYING TIGHTNESS OF THE BICEPS BRACHII:
An elbow flexion contracture is the loss of full passive elbow extension ROM. This may be the result of tightness of the anterior joint capsule and collateral ligaments or one or all of the elbow flexor muscles. Appropriate treatment to reduce the contracture requires correct identification of the offending structure. Identification of tightness of the biceps brachii muscle is based on an understanding of its actions at both the elbow and the shoulder joints and the clinician's ability to manipulate the muscle length by changing the position

of the shoulder and elbow. If the elbow joint capsuloligamentous complex is tight, elbow joint ROM is restricted, regardless of shoulder and forearm position. However, if the biceps brachii is tight and limiting elbow joint extension ROM, flexion of the shoulder joint puts the muscle in a slackened position that can allow an increase in elbow joint extension ROM. Similarly, pronation of the forearm stretches the biceps brachii and may decrease the elbow extension ROM available (Fig. 12.5). The biceps brachii muscle is maximally stretched by shoulder extension combined with elbow extension and forearm pronation. It is maximally shortened by shoulder and elbow flexion with forearm supination. Combinations of these motions can be used to identify any contribution from the biceps brachii to an elbow flexion contracture (Fig. 12.6).

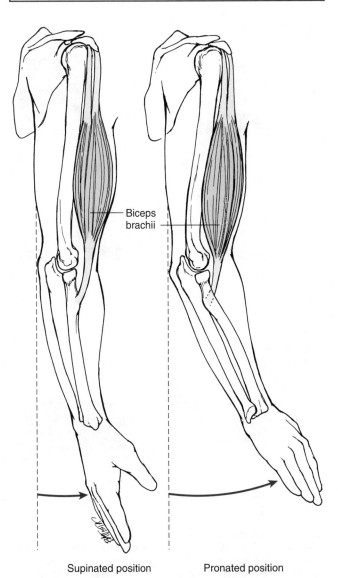

Biceps brachii

Supinated position   Pronated position

Figure 12.5: Passive pronation of the forearm stretches the biceps brachii. **A.** Tightness of the biceps brachii limits elbow extension with the forearm supinated. **B.** An additional pull on the biceps brachii exerted when the forearm is moved passively into pronation causes the biceps brachii to pull the elbow into additional flexion.

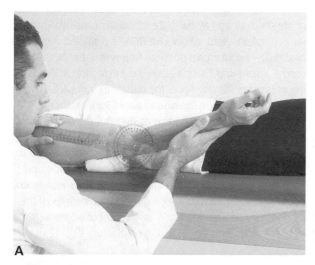

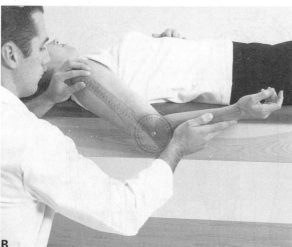

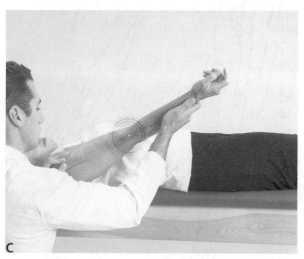

Figure 12.6: An individual with tightness of the biceps brachii. The positions of the shoulder and elbow including flexion–extension and supination–pronation all affect the length of the biceps brachii. **A.** The elbow flexion contracture is assessed with the shoulder in neutral and the forearm supinated. **B.** With the shoulder hyperextended and the forearm still supinated, the elbow flexion contracture appears greater. **C.** With the shoulder flexed and the forearm still supinated, the elbow flexion contracture appears decreased.

Brachialis

The brachialis is a pennate muscle with a broad attachment to the distal humerus (*Muscle Attachment Box 12.2*). This extensive attachment indicates that the muscle is large and capable of generating significant force [22].

ACTIONS

MUSCLE ACTION: BRACHIALIS

Action	Evidence
Elbow flexion	Supporting

The brachialis is a one-joint, or monarticular, muscle. Consequently, its actions are at the elbow only. The reported action of the brachialis is elbow flexion. The role of the brachialis as an elbow flexor is widely accepted and unchallenged [6,22,36,41,44,47,53]. The muscle's attachment to the ulna explains why it has no apparent participation in forearm pronation or supination, since the ulna remains relatively fixed during pronation and supination. The brachialis has essentially no moment arm for pronation or supination regardless of elbow and forearm position and can generate no moment for either pronation or supination [15,36]. Thus the sole action of the brachialis muscle is elbow flexion.

EFFECTS OF WEAKNESS

Weakness of the brachialis results in decreased elbow flexion strength in all forearm positions.

MUSCLE ATTACHMENT BOX 12.2

ATTACHMENTS AND INNERVATION OF THE BRACHIALIS

Proximal attachment: Distal one half to two thirds of the volar surface of the humerus and the medial and lateral intermuscular septa.

Distal attachment: Ulnar tuberosity and distal aspect of the coronoid process.

Innervation: Musculocutaneous nerve, C5 and C6. A branch from the radial nerve innervates a small portion of the muscle, but this may provide only sensory input [38].

Palpation: The brachialis lies deep to the biceps brachii but can be palpated on the medial and lateral aspects of the biceps tendon as the biceps brachii tapers toward its insertion. Palpation is facilitated during elbow flexion with the forearm pronated, decreasing the activity of the biceps brachii.

EFFECTS OF TIGHTNESS

Unlike tightness of the biceps brachii muscle, tightness of the brachialis causes diminished elbow extension ROM regardless of shoulder and forearm position.

Clinical Relevance

IDENTIFYING TIGHTNESS OF THE BRACHIALIS MUSCLE: *As a one-joint muscle, tightness of the brachialis produces a flexion contracture similar to the effects of capsular tightness at the elbow, that is, unchanged by shoulder or forearm position (Fig. 12.7). Therefore, tightness of the brachialis can be distinguished from tightness of the biceps brachii by examining the effects of shoulder position on elbow extension ROM. However, the clinician must then distinguish between brachialis and capsular tightness. The only way to make this distinction is by identifying the end-feel. End-feel, described in Chapter 11, is the tactile sensation the examiner receives when a joint is moved passively to the end of its available ROM. A joint motion limited by tight muscular tissue feels rubbery or springy at the end range. A joint with an abnormally tight capsule produces a harder, less springy end-feel. Of course at the elbow, the restriction could be the result of tightness in both the brachialis and the capsule, perhaps from chronic joint inflammation with concomitant elbow flexion positioning for comfort.*

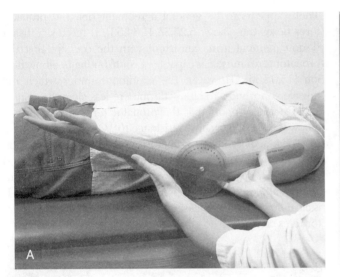
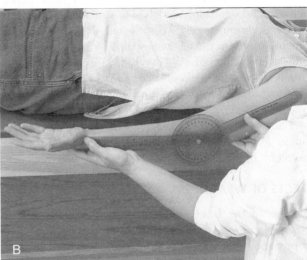
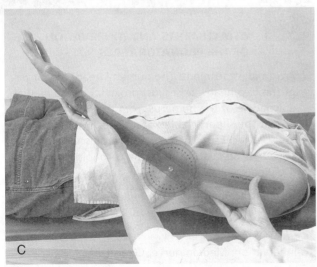
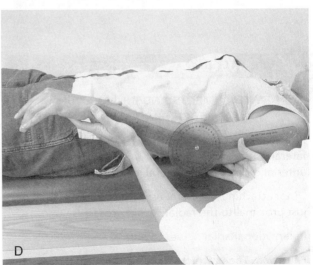

Figure 12.7: An individual with tightness of the brachialis and elbow joint capsule. Shoulder and forearm positions have no effect on the elbow flexion contracture. Elbow extension ROM is the same with (**A**) the shoulder in neutral and the forearm supinated; (**B**) the shoulder hyperextended and the forearm supinated; (**C**) the shoulder flexed and the forearm supinated; and (**D**) the shoulder in neutral and the forearm pronated.

Brachioradialis

The brachioradialis is positioned with the superficial extensor muscles of the wrist and shares an innervation with them from the radial nerve (*Muscle Attachment Box 12.3*). Despite these shared characteristics, the brachioradialis is, indeed, a muscle of the elbow.

ACTIONS

MUSCLE ACTION: BRACHIORADIALIS

Action	Evidence
Elbow flexion	Supporting
Elbow supination	Supporting
Elbow pronation	Supporting

There is virtually complete acceptance of the role of the brachioradialis as a flexor of the elbow [6,41,44,47,53]. However, its role in forearm movements is less well understood. Computer and simulation models of the moment arms of the brachioradialis muscle reveal that the muscle has a pronation moment arm when the elbow is supinated and a supination moment arm when the elbow is pronated [10,36]. Yet anatomical studies reveal only very small moment arms and also demonstrate significant variability among individuals [15,33]. EMG data suggest that the brachioradialis muscle may contribute to pronation and supination to the neutral position against heavy resistance but not during unresisted movement [6].

EFFECTS OF WEAKNESS

Weakness of the brachioradialis contributes to decreased elbow flexion strength. It may also result in decreased resisted pronation and supination force output as the forearm moves toward the neutral position.

EFFECTS OF TIGHTNESS

Tightness of the brachioradialis muscle results in decreased elbow extension ROM and may contribute to decreased pronation and supination ROM. However, these latter consequences are only conjecture and need to be verified by careful study.

Pronator Teres

The pronator teres is situated with the superficial flexors of the wrist (*Muscle Attachment Box 12.4*). However, it functions solely at the elbow and superior radioulnar joint.

ACTIONS

MUSCLE ACTION: PRONATOR TERES

Action	Evidence
Elbow flexion	Supporting
Elbow pronation	Supporting

There appears to be general agreement that the pronator teres flexes the elbow [6,25,36,41,44,53]. It has a significant flexion moment arm, consistent with the concept that the pronator teres muscle is capable of contributing to elbow flexion [15,35,36]. However, the conditions under which the muscle contributes to elbow flexion are less clear. Basmajian and De Luca report that the pronator teres contributes to elbow flexion only against resistance [6]. Other studies reveal electrical activity in the pronator teres during elbow flexion with minimal resistance, even when the forearm is supinated [43,47]. These differences may reflect normal variations among subjects or differences in data collection and analysis. It is clear however that at least under some conditions, the pronator teres contributes to elbow flexion in healthy individuals.

MUSCLE ATTACHMENT BOX 12.4

ATTACHMENTS AND INNERVATION OF THE PRONATOR TERES

Proximal attachment: The humeral head, the larger of the two heads, arises just proximal to the medial epicondyle of the humerus from the common tendon of the superficial flexor muscles of the forearm. It also attaches to the medial intermuscular septum. The ulnar head attaches to the coronoid process of the ulna.

Distal attachment: The two heads attach together on the lateral aspect of the radius midway along the shaft.

Innervation: Median nerve, C6 and C7.

Palpation: The pronator teres is palpable on the volar surface of the forearm as it traverses diagonally from the medial epicondyle to the mid shaft of the radius.

MUSCLE ATTACHMENT BOX 12.3

ATTACHMENTS AND INNERVATION OF THE BRACHIORADIALIS

Proximal attachment: Proximal two thirds of the lateral supracondylar ridge of the humerus and the anterior surface of the lateral intermuscular septum.

Distal attachment: Lateral aspect of the distal radius just proximal to the radial styloid process.

Innervation: Radial nerve, C5 and C6.

Palpation: The brachioradialis is easily palpated on the lateral aspect of the volar surface of the proximal forearm, particularly during resisted elbow flexion with the forearm in neutral.

It also is well accepted that the pronator teres participates in pronation of the forearm. However, as in elbow flexion, there are other muscles that also pronate the forearm, particularly the pronator quadratus, which is presented in Chapter 15. Thus careful analysis is required to identify the exact role the pronator teres plays in elbow flexion. Unfortunately few controlled studies of the pronator muscles exist. Bremer et al. report that the moment arm of the pronator teres is greatest with the elbow in neutral pronation and supination and is almost zero with the forearm maximally supinated [10]. The crank shape of the radius described in Chapter 11 explains the variation in moment arms. Basmajian and De Luca report that the pronator teres muscle is held in reserve during pronation, being recruited only with resistance or during rapid active pronation [6]. They also note that the position of the elbow has no effect on the recruitment of the pronator teres muscle. This latter finding needs careful consideration because elbow position is an important variable in the assessment of strength of the pronator muscles. Basmajian and De Luca investigated the level of recruitment of the muscle, which may be quite different from the level of force generated by a muscle contraction. (A full discussion of the relationship between electrical activity of a muscle and force output is presented in Chapter 4.) However, Kendall uses elbow flexion to help discern the difference in strength between the pronator teres and the other pronators [25].

Clinical Relevance

MANUAL MUSCLE TESTING (MMT) THE MUSCLES THAT PRONATE THE FOREARM: *The standard position to perform a MMT of the pronators of the forearm is with the elbow partly flexed. However, to assess the strength of the pronator quadratus alone, the elbow is flexed maximally [25] (Fig. 12.8). Although according to Basmajian and De Luca this elbow position does not alter the recruitment pattern of the pronator teres muscle, it puts the pronator teres in a very shortened position and alters the muscle's moment arm [15]. Thus although it may remain electrically active, the elbow position shortens the pronator teres enough that it can no longer effectively generate a pronation force. The pronator teres apparently exhibits active insufficiency as described earlier in the biceps brachii with shoulder and elbow flexion. The force of pronation with the elbow maximally flexed presumably comes from the pronator quadratus muscle.*

EFFECTS OF WEAKNESS

From the discussion above, it is clear that weakness of the pronator teres may contribute to weakness of both elbow flexion and forearm pronation. However, the role of the pronator teres in both motions is to provide additional force against resistance. Thus functional limitations due to weakness of this muscle alone may only be apparent during activities requiring additional force, such as loosening a screw with the right hand.

EFFECTS OF TIGHTNESS

Tightness of the pronator teres may contribute to a loss of ROM in elbow extension and forearm supination. However, the pronator teres is essentially a two-joint muscle, crossing the humeroulnar and humeroradial articulations (the elbow joint proper) and the superior radioulnar joint. Therefore, manifestation of tightness of the pronator teres depends on the relative position of these articulations. Elbow extension

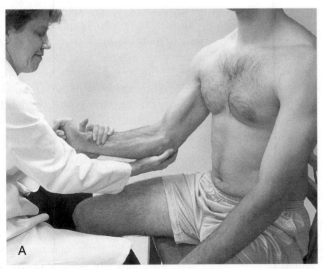
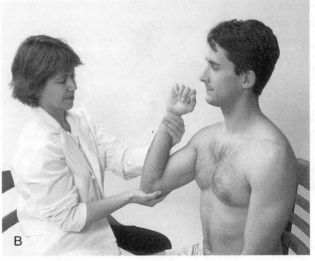

Figure 12.8: Standard manual muscle testing procedures to assess the strength of forearm pronation. **A.** With the elbow slightly flexed, both the pronator teres and pronator quadratus contribute to the strength of pronation. **B.** With the elbow maximally flexed, the pronator teres is in such a shortened position that it cannot exert an effective pronation force.

and forearm supination together apply a maximum stretch to the pronator teres. If the muscle is tight, ROM in supination is most limited when the elbow is extended. Similarly, when the pronator teres is tight, supination ROM may increase as the elbow is flexed (*Fig. 12.9*). So, like the biceps brachii, the pronator teres demonstrates that understanding the interplay of joint position and muscle length allows the clinician to identify the contributions of specific tissues to joint ROM restrictions.

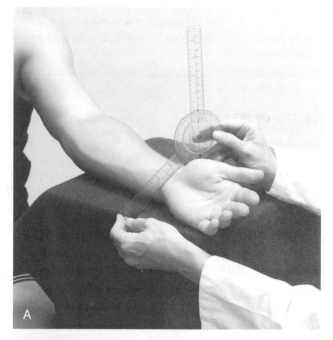

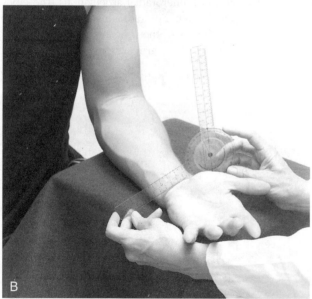

Figure 12.9: The use of elbow flexion position to distinguish between tightness of the pronator teres muscle and other structures. **A.** ROM of elbow supination measured with the pronator teres stretched by elbow extension. **B.** ROM of elbow supination measured with the pronator teres slackened by elbow flexion. Supination ROM is greater in (**B**) than in (**A**) if the pronator teres is limiting supination ROM.

Comparisons among the Elbow Flexors

Chapter 4 presents the parameters of muscle performance, force output, and the production of movement. It also discusses the factors that influence a muscle's performance, including a muscle's size, angle of application, and level of recruitment. It is these factors that distinguish the elbow flexors from one another. Although there are four primary elbow flexors, each appears to make its own unique contribution to elbow function. In this section, data are presented comparing the structural characteristics of these muscles, specifically their physiological cross-sectional areas (PCSAs), moment arms, and muscle lengths. Then EMG data are discussed to provide an understanding of the role each muscle appears to play in the function of the elbow.

STRUCTURAL COMPARISONS OF THE ELBOW FLEXORS

PCSA is a measure of the number and size of the muscle fibers available in a muscle and thus is an indicator of a muscle's potential for force production. The larger the PCSA, the greater the potential for force production. The brachialis has the largest PCSA (approximately 5.5–8.0 cm^2). The biceps brachii is next (approximately 4.5 cm^2), followed closely by the pronator teres (approximately 4.0 cm^2). The brachioradialis has the smallest PCSA (approximately 1.3 cm^2) [2,11,30,32,35].

In addition to the force of contraction, a muscle's mechanical output depends on its moment arm and its muscle length. The moment arm ($M = r \times F$) a muscle applies to the joint is a function of its force of contraction (F) and its moment arm (r). The brachioradialis, attaching distally on the radius, has the largest moment arm, followed by the biceps brachii and then the brachialis [36,51] (*Fig. 12.10*). The pronator teres has the smallest moment arm [35,36].

Thus while the brachialis is the largest elbow flexor, it is at a mechanical disadvantage because of its moment arm. It is impossible to measure directly the contribution each muscle makes to the total flexion moment applied to the elbow. However biomechanical models suggest that the brachialis and the biceps brachii make the largest contributions to the elbow flexion torque during elbow flexion with the forearm in neutral, although their relative contributions remain debatable [3,35]. Models also suggest that the relative contribution of the elbow flexor muscles varies through the range of elbow flexion [3,11].

The varying contributions to the total moment made by these muscles can be explained partially by their moment arms, which vary through the joint excursion. Anatomical studies and computer models demonstrate that the moment arms of the elbow flexors change significantly through the range of flexion and extension as well as through pronation and supination [36,39,51]. The angles of application reach their maxima in the second half of the range of elbow flexion. The biceps brachii reaches a maximum moment arm between about 90° and 110° of elbow flexion. The brachialis moment

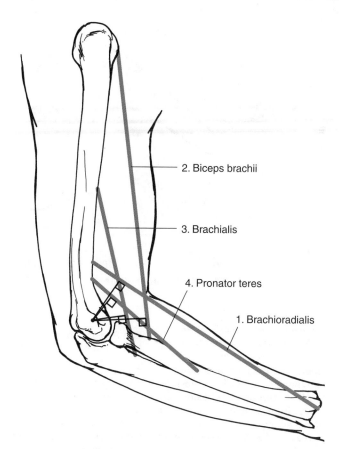

Figure 12.10: The moment arms of the primary flexor muscles of the elbow. A muscle's moment arm is measured as the perpendicular distance from the point of rotation to the muscle pull. In order of longest to shortest moment arms, the muscles are *1*, brachioradialis; *2*, biceps brachii; *3*, brachialis; and *4*, pronator teres.

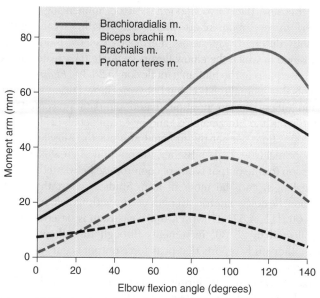

Figure 12.11: A comparison of the moment arms of the four primary elbow flexors as they change through the flexion ROM of the elbow. The moment arms of the elbow flexors peak in the midrange of flexion. The pronator teres reaches its peak first, at approximately 75°. The brachioradialis reaches its peak last, at between 100 and 120°of flexion.

arm also peaks at about 90° of flexion. The pronator teres appears to peak earlier, at about 75°, and the brachioradialis reaches a maximum moment arm between 100° and 120° of elbow flexion. *Figure 12.11* graphs the approximate moment arms of these four muscles as the elbow moves through its ROM. The data in Figure 12.11 are based on data from Pigeon et al. [39] and Murray et al. [36]. Estimates of the change in moment arm from complete extension to complete flexion vary from 30 to 85%. The moment generated by a muscle contraction is proportional to the muscle's moment arm. Thus for a given level of contraction, a muscle generates a larger moment when its moment arm is large. Therefore, the capacity of the elbow flexors to generate a moment varies dramatically through the range by virtue of their changing moment arms.

The length of each elbow flexor also changes significantly through the ROM, increasing in length as the elbow is extended and decreasing in length as the elbow is flexed. According to the length–tension relationship, a muscle's ability to produce force improves as the muscle is lengthened and diminishes as the muscle is shortened. Thus when the elbow is extended, the elbow flexors are lengthened, facilitating force production. *Figure 12.12* presents estimates of muscle lengths of the elbow

flexor muscles through the ROM, based on data reported by Pigeon et al. [39]. However, in the extended position, the moment arms for the flexors are quite small thereby decreasing the muscles' capacity to generate a torque. Thus the effect of elbow joint position on the length of the elbow flexors is quite different from its effect on muscle moment arm.

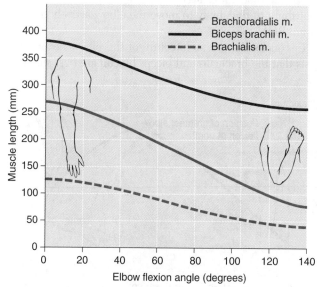

Figure 12.12: A comparison of the muscle lengths of the brachioradialis, biceps brachii, and brachialis as they change through the flexion ROM of the elbow. Muscle length decreases steadily through most of the range from elbow extension to complete elbow flexion. No data are available for the pronator teres.

Because these two important factors influencing muscle performance, moment arm and muscle length, vary in significantly different ways across the range of elbow motion, the position in which the elbow flexors generate the greatest flexion torque is in the midrange of flexion [5,28,38]. *Figure 12.13* plots the general relationship between elbow flexion strength and elbow flexion position, based on data presented by Williams and Stutzman [52] and by Knapik et al. [27]. In the midposition, neither the moment arm nor the muscle length is optimal (*Fig. 12.14*). Rather, the position of greatest elbow flexion torque output is one of compromise between the muscle length and the moment arm. Studies report that peak elbow flexion isometric strength occurs with the elbow flexed to 90° [11,14,52]. However, this conclusion is based on data collected in 25–30° increments through the elbow ROM. Another study reports that peak force output occurs at 70° of elbow flexion in women during isometric and isokinetic contractions and in men during isokinetic contractions [27]. This study reports that isometric contraction force peaks at 90° in men and that the actual location of the peak force varies considerably among subjects. Despite these disagreements, the central point is clear: elbow flexion strength peaks somewhere in the middle of elbow flexion ROM where neither the muscles' moment arms nor their lengths are optimal for force production.

The length of a muscle's moment arm and its fiber length also influence the amount of excursion caused by a contraction. As noted in Chapter 4, a muscle with a short moment arm can cause a large joint excursion for a given amount of shortening, while a muscle with a large moment arm produces less joint excursion for the same amount of shortening. Thus the brachialis with the shortest moment arm is well designed to move the elbow through a large excursion. The biceps and brachioradialis possess long muscle fibers that also contribute to the ability to move the elbow actively through its full ROM [35].

In conclusion, the architecture of the elbow flexors suggests that the brachialis and biceps brachii are best suited to

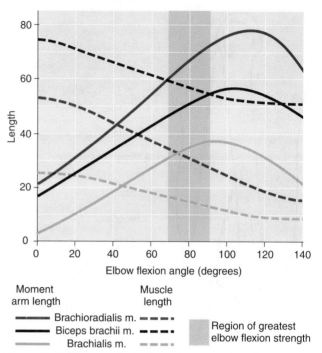

Figure 12.14: A comparison of the changes in muscle lengths and moment arms of the brachioradialis, biceps brachii, and brachialis through the flexion ROM of the elbow. As the elbow moves from complete extension to maximum flexion, the length of the elbow flexors decreases. However, their moment arms increase as flexion increases until midrange flexion, at least. Thus the advantage of increasing moment arms is counteracted by the disadvantage of decreasing muscle length.

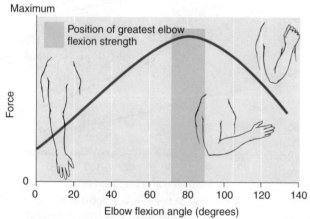

Figure 12.13: Maximum isometric elbow flexion force as it changes through the flexion ROM of the elbow. Elbow flexion force peaks in midrange between 75 and 90° of flexion.

generate large flexor moments at the elbow. The elbow flexors also exhibit architectural patterns that facilitate active elbow movement through its full arc. Although understanding the output potential of each muscle is helpful, a thorough understanding of the role of the elbow flexors requires an appreciation of the available data describing their recruitment patterns during elbow motion. The following reports the available data regarding activity of these muscles during movement of the elbow.

COMPARISONS OF FLEXOR MUSCLE ACTIVITY DURING ELBOW MOTION USING EMG DATA

Few controlled EMG studies have been carried out to determine the individual contributions to motion of each of the elbow flexors. The classic studies are those described by Basmajian and De Luca [6]. The following is a brief synopsis of their conclusions. The data they report suggest that the biceps brachii, brachialis, and brachioradialis function in a finely coordinated manner with each muscle having its unique role. However, the authors also emphasize that there is significant variety in the behavior of these muscles among the healthy population. Despite this caveat, the data suggest functional patterns for each muscle.

The biceps brachii is activated in most individuals during elbow flexion with the forearm supinated, regardless of flexion speed or resistance. When the forearm is partially pronated, the biceps brachii appears to be recruited only with resistance. When the forearm is fully pronated, the muscle is recruited only with resistance, and even then it appears to be only partially activated. Similarly, the biceps is active during resisted forearm supination when the elbow is flexed. However, when the elbow is extended, only vigorously resisted supination activates the biceps brachii and is often accompanied by slight elbow flexion.

These data suggest that the biceps brachii is most active when the elbow is moving in both flexion and supination. This finding is quite logical, since these are the motions directly attributed to the biceps brachii. Since a muscle's function is to shorten and the resulting motion is a function of the line of pull of the muscle, it is to be expected that a muscle is most active performing the motions for which it is aligned. When one of those motions is undesirable, the choice is to recruit another muscle whose precise action is desired or to inhibit from full activity the muscle with multiple actions while using another muscle to stabilize the joint in the desired direction. This latter choice appears to operate during heavily resisted elbow flexion with the forearm pronated as well as in resisted supination of the forearm with the elbow extended. In each case the biceps contributes to the desired motion but also adds a pull in an undesired direction. In resisted elbow flexion with pronation, the biceps brachii, while active, is inhibited from full activity so that its supination role does not interfere with the pronation position. Resisted supination with elbow extension similarly inhibits the activity of the biceps brachii to avoid interference with elbow extension. In both examples, the biceps brachii is recruited, but only partially.

In contrast, the brachialis is active whenever the elbow is flexed, regardless of forearm position, resistance, or speed of movement. The brachialis attaches to the ulna, which moves very little during pronation or supination of the forearm. Thus the brachialis is unaffected by forearm position. The constancy of its activity is efficient, since it has the largest PCSA and therefore has a potentially large contractile force. It also is able to move the elbow through its full excursion because of the muscle's short moment arm. The consistent activity of the brachialis during any elbow flexion has led to its nickname, the "workhorse" of elbow flexion.

The brachioradialis appears to be activated with resisted elbow flexion, particularly in the partially pronated and fully

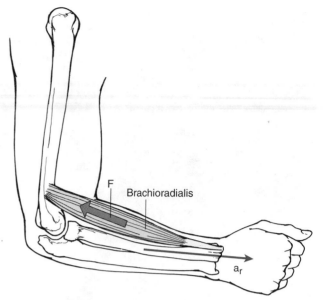

Figure 12.15: The hypothetical role of the brachioradialis. The hypothetical explanation for the activity of the brachioradialis during rapid elbow flexion is to exert a stabilizing force (*F*) on the elbow joint against the forces resulting from the radial acceleration (*a$_r$*) of the forearm during high-velocity elbow flexion.

pronated positions but also even when the forearm is supinated. It is also active during rapid elbow flexion. This latter activity is somewhat surprising because of the muscle's long moment arm. However, it is hypothesized that the muscle's alignment along the length of the forearm provides an important stabilizing force for the elbow against the centrifugal force tending to distract the elbow during rapid movements (*Fig. 12.15*). Finally, as noted earlier, the pronator teres appears to be recruited for either elbow flexion or pronation only when resistance is added.

These findings are summarized in *Table 12.1*. Resisted elbow flexion with the forearm slightly pronated elicits the greatest electrical activity from the biceps brachii, brachialis, and brachioradialis. Although the authors do not report data collected during elbow flexion with a neutral forearm position, their report does not contradict the finding that elbow flexion is strongest with the forearm in neutral [5,52]. Resisted elbow flexion with the forearm pronated vigorously activates the brachialis and the brachioradialis but elicits only partial activity from the biceps, supporting the observation

TABLE 12.1: Summary of EMG Data for the Elbow Flexor Muscles

	Elbow Flexion in Supination	Elbow Flexion in Semipronated Position	Elbow Flexion with Pronation
Biceps brachii	+	With resistance	Slightly active with resistance
Brachialis	+	+	+
Brachioradialis	With resistance	With resistance	With resistance
Pronator teres	Not active	With resistance	With resistance

Data from Basmajian JV, De Luca CJ: Muscles Alive. Their Function Revealed by Electromyography. Baltimore: Williams & Wilkins, 1985.

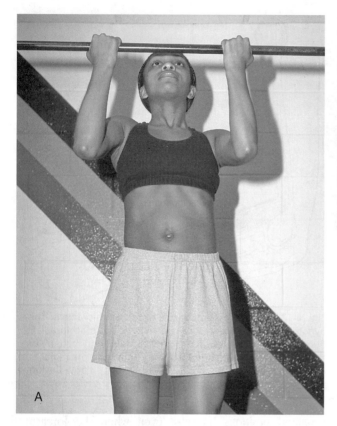
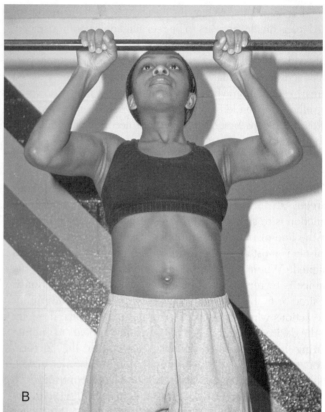

Figure 12.16: Chin-up exercises. The difficulty of a chin-up exercise changes with the position of the forearms. **A.** Forearms are supinated, allowing recruitment of the three large elbow flexor muscles. **B.** Forearms are pronated, partially inhibiting the biceps brachii, thus reducing the strength of elbow flexion.

that elbow flexion with the forearm pronated is the weakest. To test this observation one need only compare the difficulty of a chin-up exercise with the forearm supinated with one with the forearm pronated (*Fig. 12.16*).

There are no known studies that fully replicate the studies reviewed above. However, some studies provide partial corroboration. Stewart et al. also demonstrate brachialis activity in elbow flexion, regardless of forearm position [47]. Studies show lower biceps brachii activity and higher brachioradialis activity during elbow flexion with forearm pronation than in supination [43,47]. However, in one of these studies, brachioradialis activity occurs without resistance [43]. Another study suggests that the brachioradialis is not fully activated when the biceps brachii is fully recruited during a maximal voluntary contraction, suggesting that the brachioradialis functions as a reserve for additional force, as purported by Basmajian and De Luca [1,6]. Finally, in a study of well-trained competitive rowers, the partially pronated grip generates a larger force than the traditional fully pronated position [9]. While this study provides no direct EMG data, it offers important functional evidence supporting the belief that the elbow flexors are more fully recruited when the forearm is only partially pronated than when it is fully pronated.

These data support the original contention by Basmajian and De Luca that there is very precise coordination among the elbow flexors during movement of the elbow and forearm. An understanding of the interplay among these muscles allows

the clinician to perform a precise evaluation of the muscles flexing the elbow to develop a specific intervention strategy that can focus the treatment most effectively on the specific impairment.

Clinical Relevance

IDENTIFYING INDIVIDUAL WEAKNESS IN THE ELBOW FLEXORS: *The EMG data for the elbow flexor muscles reveal that no single motion isolates any of the elbow flexors. Consequently, identification of weakness in an individual elbow flexor muscle requires measurement of elbow flexion strength in several forearm positions combined with careful palpation (Fig. 12.17). Isolated weakness of the biceps affects elbow flexion strength most when the forearm is supinated or in neutral and to a lesser degree with forearm pronation. In contrast, weakness of the brachioradialis has little effect on elbow flexion strength with the forearm supinated but a larger effect when the forearm is pronated maximally. Isolated weakness of the brachialis causes decreased elbow strength in all forearm positions. However, it may be most evident when the forearm is pronated, since in this position, the biceps has a smaller role and consequently provides less compensation for brachialis*

(continued)

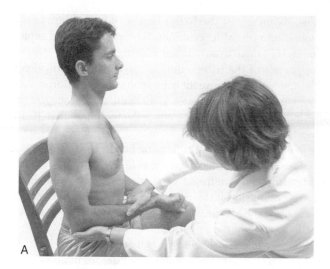

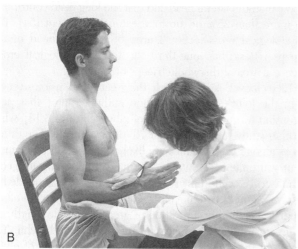

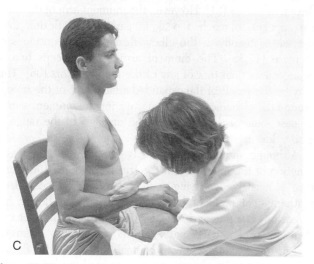

Figure 12.17: Assessing the strength of the three elbow flexors, biceps brachii, brachialis, and brachioradialis. Three forearm positions are needed to fully assess the contribution of the three large elbow flexor muscles to isometric elbow flexion strength. **A.** With the forearm supinated, the biceps and brachialis are recruited. Additional resistance recruits the brachioradialis. **B.** With the forearm in neutral, all three muscles are active. The brachioradialis is readily seen and palpated. **C.** With the forearm pronated, the biceps is partially inhibited and the brachialis is more easily palpated.

(Continued)
weakness. Measurement of supination strength with the elbow flexed and extended also helps to identify weakness of the biceps brachii.

ELBOW EXTENSORS

The primary extensors of the elbow are the triceps brachii and the anconeus muscles (*Fig. 12.18*). As in elbow flexion, muscles of the forearm may also contribute to elbow extension.

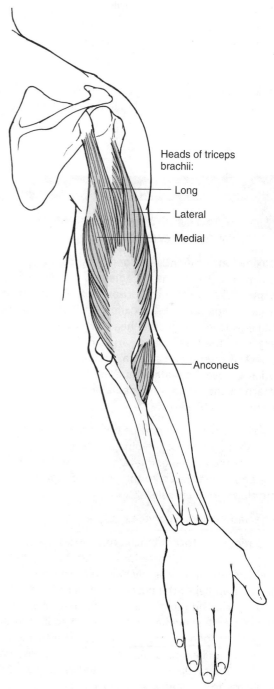

Heads of triceps brachii:
- Long
- Lateral
- Medial

Anconeus

Figure 12.18: The primary extensor muscles of the elbow. The elbow extensors include the triceps brachii and the anconeus.

However, these muscles exert their primary function at the wrist and hand and therefore are discussed in Chapter 15.

Triceps Brachii

The triceps brachii is the large muscle that constitutes the entire muscle mass on the posterior aspect of the arm (*Muscle Attachment Box 12.5*).

ACTIONS

MUSCLE ACTION: TRICEPS BRACHII

Action	Evidence
Elbow extension	Supporting
Shoulder extension	Inadequate
Shoulder adduction	Inadequate

The role of the triceps brachii as an extensor of the elbow is uncontested. The muscle attaches to the ulna. Consequently,

MUSCLE ATTACHMENT BOX 12.5

ATTACHMENTS AND INNERVATION OF THE TRICEPS BRACHII

Proximal attachment: The long head of the triceps brachii attaches to the infraglenoid tubercle of the scapula. The lateral head arises from the posterior aspect of the humerus, proximal and lateral to the radial groove. The medial head, which is the largest of the three heads, arises on the posterior aspect of the humerus, distal and medial to the radial groove. The lateral and medial heads also attach to the lateral and medial intermuscular septa, respectively.

Distal attachment: The three heads attach to the olecranon process of the ulna and to the deep fascia of the medial and lateral forearm. The medial head also sends fibers to the posterior aspect of the elbow joint capsule.

Innervation: Radial nerve, C6, C7, and C8.

Palpation: The triceps brachii constitutes the entire muscle mass of the posterior arm distal to the deltoid and therefore is easily palpated. The lateral head is parallel to the posterior border of the deltoid muscle and is prominent on the lateral aspect of the arm. Just medial to the lateral head is the belly of the long head. It can also be identified as it enters the axilla inferior and anterior to the posterior deltoid. The medial head is palpated distally on the arm close to the medial epicondyle.

unlike its antagonist the biceps brachii, it contributes only to elbow extension, with no influence on pronation and supination. EMG data from surface electrodes suggest that the three heads of the triceps muscle are recruited individually, although individual variation in recruitment patterns exists among the healthy population [18]. Some studies suggest that the medial head is more frequently recruited first [6,18]. These reports suggest that increased resistance appears to activate the muscle's long and lateral heads. However, another study, using both surface and indwelling electrodes, demonstrates similar recruitment of all three heads, even during contractions with little resistance [31]. Like that of the brachialis, the EMG activity of the triceps brachii is unaffected by the position of the forearm.

Biomechanical analysis suggests that the medial head of the triceps brachii contributes more to the extensor moment at the elbow than the lateral head and that the long head contributes no more than 25% of the total extensor moment [54]. The physiological cross-sectional area of the long head of the triceps is less than one-third the total physiological cross-sectional area of the whole triceps brachii [35].

Like elbow flexion strength, the greatest extension strength is in the joint's midrange. Some authors report that peak extension torque occurs at 90° of elbow flexion [5,13], while another study reports peaks at 70° of flexion [27]. The differences among these studies are likely the result of differences in measurement techniques. Normal variation may also contribute to the differences, and further research is needed to resolve them. Like the elbow flexors, midrange of elbow excursion is neither a position of greatest muscle length nor of greatest angle of application for the triceps brachii. The length of the triceps brachii increases as the angle of elbow flexion increases [31]. However, the moment arm of the muscle appears to reach a peak in early elbow flexion then decreases steadily as the elbow flexion angle continues to increase [17,36]. The moment arm of the triceps brachii changes less than that of any of the elbow flexors [36]. This may be the result of the expanded attachment of the triceps around the olecranon process maximizing the moment arm of at least some of the triceps brachii throughout the range of elbow flexion.

Although shoulder extension is generally accepted as a function of the long head of the triceps brachii, little literature is available verifying such a role [23,25,41,44]. In a mathematical model of the shoulder during rapid flexion and extension, Happee and van der Helm provide indirect evidence of triceps participation in active shoulder extension and in the braking action to control rapid shoulder flexion [20]. However, there are no known studies that provide EMG data to identify the conditions under which the triceps brachii is activated during shoulder motion. Similarly, there are no known studies that confirm the ability of the triceps brachii to adduct the shoulder, although several references report adduction as an action of the muscle's long head [25,41,46]. It is clear that further study is needed to clarify the action of the triceps brachii at the shoulder.

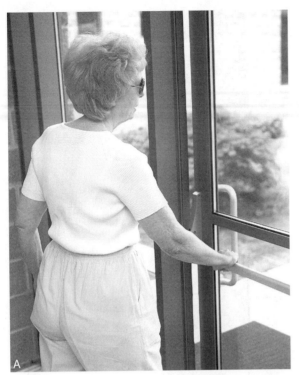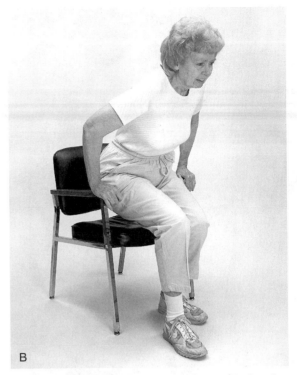

Figure 12.19: Functional activities requiring contraction of the extensor muscles of the elbow. Pushing activities recruit the triceps brachii. **A.** The individual pushes the door with active elbow extension. **B.** Active elbow extension is used to assist an individual in rising from a chair.

EFFECTS OF WEAKNESS

Weakness of the triceps brachii has a profound effect on the strength of elbow extension. Although other muscles contribute slightly to elbow extension, no other muscle has the capacity to generate as much force in elbow extension. Loss of the triceps muscle results in almost complete loss of extension strength. The functional implications of zero elbow extension strength must be considered carefully. In the upright posture, the weight of the forearm and hand cause the elbow to extend. Picking up and putting down an object require concentric and eccentric contractions of the elbow flexors. However, pushing an object or using the upper extremity to assist in rising from a chair requires the active contraction of the triceps brachii (*Fig. 12.19*).

Clinical Relevance

TRICEPS WEAKNESS IN INDIVIDUALS WITH TETRAPLEGIA: *Individuals with tetraplegia at the level of C6 lack active control of the triceps brachii (mmT ≤ 3), innervated at the level of C7 and C8. Yet these individuals generally have control of the elbow flexors and the shoulder muscles. This remaining motor control allows most to perform independent sliding transfers such as to and from*

wheelchairs. Despite the absence of elbow extension strength, the individual is able to bear weight on the upper extremity by locking the elbow in extension. The elbow can be maintained in extension passively by placing the elbow in hyperextension and supporting it by the bones and ligaments of the joint or by keeping the weight of the head and trunk posterior to the elbow joint, thereby creating an extension moment at the joint (Fig. 12.20). However, the presence of a flexion contracture prevents the individual from supporting the elbow passively by locking the elbow and may compromise function [21]. Grover et al. demonstrate that an elbow flexion contraction of approximately 25° prevents a patient with C6 tetraplegia and complete loss of triceps brachii strength from performing a sliding transfer [19]. Thus the prevention of elbow flexion contractures is an essential element in the goal of independent function for individuals with C6 tetraplegia.

EFFECTS OF TIGHTNESS

Tightness of the triceps brachii limits elbow flexion ROM and may contribute to diminished shoulder elevation ROM. Chapter 11 notes that most activities of daily living can be performed with a total elbow flexion excursion of about 100° [34]. Thus significant tightness of the triceps could result in

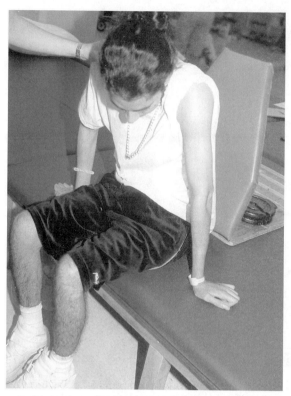

Figure 12.20: Locking the elbow allows stable elbow extension during weight bearing on the upper extremity, even in the absence of elbow extension strength.

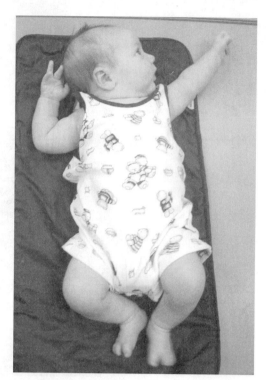

Figure 12.21: Asymmetrical tonic reflex. The infant demonstrates the typical posture assumed by a healthy child exhibiting an asymmetrical tonic reflex (ATNR).

serious functional impairments, especially in personal care activities such as feeding and hygiene.

Clinical Relevance

ASYMMETRICAL TONIC NECK REFLEX (ATNR) IN A CHILD WITH A DEVELOPMENTAL DISORDER: *The ATNR is a normally occurring motor reflex in infants. The reflex is manifested in the upper extremities by a change in muscle tone in each upper extremity, determined by the rotation of the head and neck. As the head is turned to one side, there is an increase in motor tone in the extensor muscles of the upper extremity to which the head is turned. There is a concomitant increase in flexor tone in the opposite extremity (Fig. 12.21). Increased muscle tone in the extensor muscles creates an increased resistance to flexion. This reflex usually is integrated as normal motor development unfolds during the first year, before the child can perform many independent activities of daily living. However, in some children with developmental delays and impaired motor control, the reflex may continue to be evident even as the child becomes ready for some functional independence. In this case, the abnormal presence of an ATNR may interfere with the child's ability to gain independence in activities*

such as self-feeding. As the child looks at the hand with the food in it, the extensor tone increases in that limb, increasing the difficulty of flexing the elbow and bringing the food to the mouth.

Anconeus

The anconeus is a short, small muscle that lies slightly distal to the triceps brachii (*Muscle Attachment Box 12.6*).

ACTIONS

The actions and functional significance of the anconeus remain elusive.

MUSCLE ACTION: ANCONEUS

Action	Evidence
Elbow extension	Supporting
Lateral deviation of the ulna	Inadequate

Authors consistently report that the anconeus assists the triceps brachii in elbow extension [23,25,41,44,53]. Bozec et al. use EMG data to conclude that the anconeus is a "true extensor muscle," particularly when a subject generates small levels of extension torque [31]. However, inspection

MUSCLE ATTACHMENT BOX 12.6

ATTACHMENTS AND INNERVATION OF THE ANCONEUS

Proximal attachment: Posterior surface of the lateral epicondyle of the humerus and adjacent joint capsule.

Distal attachment: Lateral aspect of the olecranon process and posterior surface of the proximal ulna.

Innervation: Radial nerve, C6, C7, and C8.

Palpation: The anconeus can be palpated distal to the triceps brachii on the lateral aspect of the elbow. It must be carefully distinguished from the nearby extensor carpi ulnaris [41].

of the anconeus reveals that the muscle is considerably smaller in PCSA than the triceps. Therefore, its potential strength is much less. In addition, its moment arm is smaller than that of the triceps brachii, which attaches to the olecranon process of the ulna. Consequently, while the anconeus may contribute to elbow extension, it is unlikely to add significant strength to the movement or to be able to compensate for the loss of the triceps brachii. It is estimated that it may contribute no more than 10–15% to a total extensor muscle moment [31,54]. As the extensor muscle activity increases, the relative contribution of the anconeus decreases [54].

However, the attachment of the anconeus to the posterior joint capsule of the elbow may explain another role for the anconeus in active elbow extension. The capsule is lax posteriorly, allowing the joint its large flexion ROM. However, this laxity could permit a portion of the capsule to be caught between the olecranon process and olecranon fossa during extension. Such impingement would be very painful, since joint capsules possess large sensory innervations. The function of the anconeus may be to assist in pulling the posterior joint capsule of the elbow out of harm's way during active extension.

The role of the anconeus in moving the ulna laterally continues to be debated. Pronation of the forearm is classically described as the radius rotating around a fixed ulna. However, to keep the hand fixed in space, pronation occurs with slight lateral deviation of the ulna as the radius turns around it. Some authors suggest that the anconeus contributes to the lateral deviation, or abduction of the ulna, during pronation of the forearm when the hand must remain fixed in space, such as when turning a screwdriver [24,53]. EMG studies report activity in the anconeus during pronation. However, the muscle appears active during supination as well [6]. Therefore, its role in ulnar abduction has been neither verified nor refuted, requiring further study to resolve the issue.

EFFECTS OF WEAKNESS

Reports of isolated weakness of the anconeus have not been found in the literature. As noted above, the triceps brachii remains the primary extensor of the elbow joint. Therefore, weakness of the anconeus may have little effect on extension strength. However, weakness may impair the ability to prevent impingement of the posterior joint capsule during elbow extension. In addition, perhaps weakness of the anconeus impairs the ability to pronate the forearm while maintaining the hand in the same location. These latter two functional deficits are merely conjecture. Additional study and clinical evidence are needed to clarify the impact of weakness of the anconeus muscle.

EFFECTS OF TIGHTNESS

Isolated tightness of the anconeus is unrealistic, since the factors leading to its tightness would also affect the triceps brachii as well as other nearby structures. Therefore, the effects of the tightness in the other structures would override impairments from anconeus tightness.

SUPINATOR MUSCLES

The primary supinator muscles of the forearm are the biceps brachii and the supinator. Other forearm muscles that are discussed in Chapter 15 may contribute to supination, but their primary actions are at the wrist and hand. The biceps brachii is discussed earlier in the current chapter. Only the supinator is presented below.

Supinator

The supinator muscle is usually presented with the other forearm muscles innervated by the radial nerve. It is presented here because its action is focused at the superior radioulnar joint (*Muscle Attachment Box 12.7*). It lies deep to the wrist and finger extensor muscles in the proximal forearm (*Fig. 12.22*).

ACTIONS

MUSCLE ACTION: SUPINATOR

Action	Evidence
Elbow supination	Supporting

The reported action of the supinator is, as its name suggests, supination. There appears to be no doubt among authors regarding the muscle's role as a supinator [23,25,41,44,53]. However, fewer data are available regarding its coordination with the biceps brachii, the other essential supinator of the forearm. The most conclusive EMG data available examining the functions of these two muscles are presented by Basmajian and De Luca [6]. EMG data suggest that the supinator is responsible for slow unresisted

MUSCLE ATTACHMENT BOX 12.7

ATTACHMENTS AND INNERVATION OF THE SUPINATOR

Proximal attachment: The lateral epicondyle of the humerus with attachments on the lateral aspect of the joint capsule, the annular ligament and supinator fossa and crest of the ulna.

Distal attachment: Lateral, anterior and posterior surfaces of the proximal one third of the radius.

Innervation: Nerve supply to the supinator muscle may arise from the posterior interosseus nerve or from the main trunk of the radial nerve [50]. Thus authors report spinal innervation from C6 and C7 [50] or from C5 and C6 [31,38].

Palpation: The muscle lies deep to the superficial extensor muscles of the forearm and is difficult to palpate. Palpation may be possible just posterior to the extensor muscle mass if the latter remains relaxed [41].

supination, regardless of elbow position. The biceps brachii appears to be held in reserve until supination is resisted. The supinator remains particularly important during supination when the elbow is extended, even in the presence of resistance, since, as noted above in the chapter, the biceps brachii is inhibited during supination when the elbow is extended. Additionally, elbow flexion or extension position appears to have little effect on the supinator's supination moment arm [10]. In contrast, elbow extension appears to significantly reduce the supination moment arm of the biceps brachii.

Clinical Relevance

MANUAL MUSCLE TESTING (MMT) OF THE SUPINATOR MUSCLE: *Standard MMT procedures for the supinator muscle are described with the elbow extended and with the elbow and shoulder flexed [25] (Fig. 12.23). EMG data and an understanding of the mechanics of muscle action demonstrate the theories underlying these two positions. EMG data suggest that with the elbow extended, the biceps brachii is inhibited. Its contribution to supination strength also may be reduced because of its decreased supination moment arm in elbow extension. Therefore, supination in that position presumably results from activity of the supinator muscle. However, aggressively resisted supination with the elbow extended does appear to elicit biceps brachii activity, usually resulting in some*

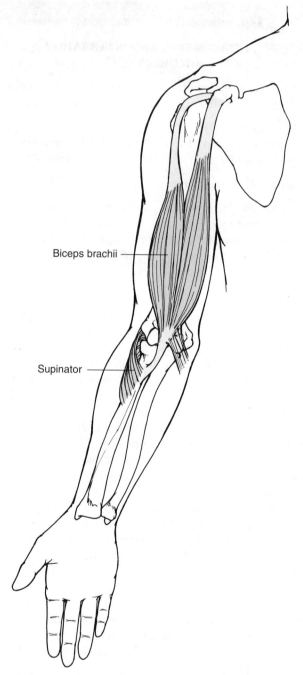

Figure 12.22: Primary supinator muscles of the elbow. The primary supinator muscles of the elbow are the biceps brachii and the supinator muscles.

elbow flexion. Since MMT is designed to resist the patient maximally, it is likely that the biceps is recruited in this test, at least in the phase when maximum resistance is applied.

On the other hand, the MMT position with the elbow and shoulder flexed is likely to recruit both the supinator and biceps brachii muscles. However, in this position the biceps brachii is shortened almost maximally. As noted

(continued)

(Continued)

earlier in this chapter and in detail in Chapter 4, shortening a muscle reduces its contractile force. Therefore, although the biceps brachii is most likely active during this MMT of supination, the force that it can generate in supination is greatly reduced, and the force of supination measured is primarily the force of the supinator muscle. It is important for the clinician to recognize that either test may be suitable under certain circumstances. However, it is essential to keep in mind the factors influencing the results of each test.

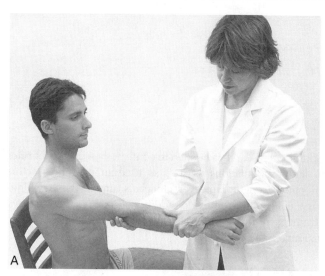

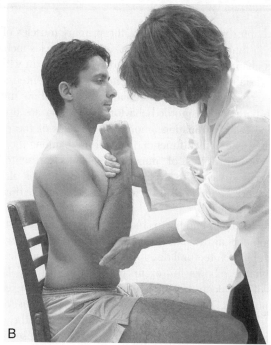

Figure 12.23: Standard manual muscle testing (MMT) positions to assess supination strength without the contribution of the biceps brachii. **A.** Resisted supination with the elbow extended inhibits the biceps brachii. **B.** Although the biceps brachii muscle is active during resisted supination with the elbow maximally flexed, the muscle is so short that it is unable to generate significant supination strength.

EFFECTS OF WEAKNESS

Weakness of the supinator weakens the strength of supination. Of course if the biceps brachii remains intact, the individual continues to have considerable supination strength. However, forceful supination and the ability to supinate with the elbow extended are impaired.

EFFECTS OF TIGHTNESS

Isolated tightness of the supinator muscle is unlikely. However, it may be tight along with the biceps brachii. Tightness of the supinator can be distinguished from tightness of the biceps brachii by applying an understanding of two joint muscles. As described in the discussion of tightness of the biceps brachii, shoulder position affects the length of the biceps and thus can alter the manifestations of biceps tightness at the elbow. Shoulder position has no effect on the supinator muscle's length.

COMPARISONS OF THE STRENGTH OF ELBOW FLEXION AND EXTENSION

Determining the functional significance of weakness of elbow muscles is an essential element of a valid evaluation. An understanding of the relative strength of muscle groups can help provide a perspective on the extent of weakness that a patient exhibits. Several studies report the strength of either the flexor muscle group or the extensor muscle group [13,42,48,52]. However, only a few studies directly compare

TABLE 12.2: Strength of Elbow Flexor and Extensor Muscle Groups Reported in the Literature

	Gallagher et al. [16][a]	Askew et al. [5][b]	Sale et al. [42][c]	Currier [13][d]	Williams and Stutzman [52][e]
Flexion, males dominant side	40.0 Nm	725 ± 154 kg-cm	60 Nm	NT[f]	80 lb
Flexion, males nondominant	NT	708 ± 156 kg-cm	NT	NT	NT
Flexion, females dominant side	NT	336 ± 80 kg-cm	30 Nm	NT	NT
Flexion, females nondominant	NT	323 ± 78 kg-cm	NT	NT	NT
Extension, males dominant side	27.1 Nm	421 ± 109 kg-cm	NT	48.8 lb	NT
Extension, males nondominant	NT	406 ± 106 kg-cm	NT	NT	NT
Extension, females dominant side	NT	210 ± 61 kg-cm	NT	NT	NT
Extension, females nondominant	NT	194 ± 50 kg-cm	NT	NT	NT

[a]N = 30 males, 2–30 years old.
[b]N = 50 males, 41.0 ± 12.3 years; 54 females, 45.1 ± 16.1 years.
[c]Torque values estimated from graphs. N = 13 males, 22.5 ± 1.6 years; 8 females, 21.0 ± 0.6 years.
[d]N = 41 males, 20–40 years old
[e]Torque values estimated from graphs. N = 10 "college men."
[f]NT, authors did not test that factor.

the strength of the elbow flexors and extensors in individuals without elbow pathology [5,16,26]. Absolute measures of strength reported in the literature are difficult to compare because they are reported in different units of force and torque. Values of isometric strength collected at 90° of elbow flexion are presented in *Table 12.2*. Askew et al. report that mean isometric extension strength is 61% of mean isometric flexion strength in 104 male and female subjects [5]. However, Knapik and Ramos report isometric elbow extension strength is approximately 82% of isometric elbow flexion strength in 352 males [26]. Although no direct comparison is presented, Gallagher et al. consistently report greater flexion strength than extension strength during concentric isokinetic contractions at various speeds [16]. Comparison of data across studies supports the conclusion that flexion strength is greater than extension strength at the elbow [30].

Men demonstrate significantly greater flexion and extension strength than women, regardless of contraction mode [5,16,27,42]. Flexion and extension strengths also appear to decrease with age. A small but significant increase in elbow flexion strength is reported on the dominant side [5,16]. However, there is disagreement about the effect of hand dominance on elbow extension strength, with one study reporting small but significant increases on the dominant side, similar to that found in flexion strength [5]. Another study finds no effect of dominance on extension strength [16].

Although the data are scanty and direct comparisons are not easily made, certain principles begin to emerge from these studies:

• Mean elbow flexion strength is greater than mean extension strength.
• Mean elbow strength is greater in men than in women.
• Elbow strength appears to decrease with age.
• Hand dominance may explain only a small difference in strength between the left and right elbows.

Additional research is needed to confirm these apparent rules in larger populations as well as to examine other factors affecting strength. However, clinicians can use these preliminary concepts to provide additional perspective as they attempt to interpret strength measures acquired from patients in the clinic.

SUMMARY

This chapter reviews the role of the primary muscles of the elbow in function and in dysfunction. The muscles included in this chapter are those that insert in the forearm with no effect distally at the wrist. Each muscle is presented separately to examine its specific contribution to elbow motion and to pathological motor behavior. EMG data are used to examine the coordination among the muscles of the elbow and the way in which function is distributed among the muscles. The principles of muscle mechanics presented in Chapter 4 are used to explain the individual roles of each muscle and the methods used to isolate each muscle during a clinical examination.

The brachialis and biceps brachii generate the largest flexion moments at the elbow, and all three primary elbow flexors exhibit architectural designs to provide active movements through the elbow's full excursion. The medial and lateral heads of the triceps brachii generate the largest elbow extension moments. The pronator teres and supinator muscles are tested by positioning the subject's elbow so that the other muscles are rendered ineffective. Several wrist muscles also affect the elbow. These muscles and their effects on the wrist and elbow are presented in Chapter 15. In the following chapter, the issues of joint structure and muscle performance presented in the previous and current chapters are examined in combination by studying their effects on the forces at the elbow joint and loads in the elbow muscles during activity.

References

1. Allen GM, McKenzie DK, Gandevia SC: Twitch interpolation of the elbow flexor muscles at high forces. Muscle Nerve 1998; 21: 318–328.
2. An KN, Hui FC, Morrey BF, et al.: Muscles across the elbow joint: a biomechanical analysis. J Biomech 1981; 14: 659–669.
3. An KN, Kaufman KR, Chao EYS: Physiological considerations of muscle force through the elbow joint. J Biomech 1989; 22: 1249–1256.
4. Andrews JR: Glenoid labrum tears related to the long head of the biceps. Am J Sports Med 1985; 13: 337–341.
5. Askew LJ, An KN, Morrey BF, Chao EYS: Isometric elbow strength in normal individuals. Clin Orthop 1987; 261–266.
6. Basmajian JV, De Luca CJ: Muscles Alive. Their Function Revealed by Electromyography. Baltimore: Williams & Wilkins, 1985.
7. Bassett RW, Browne BF, Morrey BF, An KN: Glenohumeral muscle force and moment mechanics in a position of shoulder instability. J Biomech 1990; 23: 405–415.
8. Blasier RB, Soslowsky LJ, Malicky DM, Palmer ML: Posterior glenohumeral subluxation: active and passive stabilization in a biomechanical model. J Bone Joint Surg 1997; 79A: 433–440.
9. Bompa TO, Borms J, Hebbelinck M: Mechanical efficiency of the elbow flexors in rowing. Am J Phys Med Rehabil 1990; 69: 140–143.
10. Bremer AK, Sennwald GR, Favre P, Jacob HAC: Moment arms of forearm rotators. Clin Biomech 2006; 21: 683–691.
11. Chang YW, Su F-C, Wu HW, An KN: Optimum length of muscle contraction. Clin Biomech 1999; 14: 537–542.
12. Corner NB, Milner SM, MacDonald R, Jubb M: Isolated musculocutaneous nerve lesion after shoulder dislocation. J R Army Med Corps 1990; 136: 107–108.
13. Currier DP: Maximal isometric tension of the elbow extensors at varied positions. Part 1. Assessment by cable tensiometer. Phys Ther 1972; 52: 1043–1049.
14. Downer AH: Strength of the elbow flexor muscles. Phys Ther Rev 1953; 33: 68–70.
15. Ettema GJC, Styles G, Kippers V: The moment arms of 23 muscle segments of the upper limb with varying elbow and forearm positions: implications for motor control. Hum Mov Sci 1998; 17: 201–220.
16. Gallagher MA, Cuomo F, Polonsky L, et al.: Effects of age, testing speed, and arm dominance on isokinetic strength of the elbow. J Shoulder Elbow Surg 1997; 6: 340–346.
17. Gerbeaux M, Turpin E, Lensel-Corbeil G: Musculo-articular modelling of the triceps brachii. J Biomech 1996; 29: 171–180.
18. Grabiner MD, Jaque V: Activation patterns of the triceps brachii muscle during sub-maximal elbow extension. Med Sci Sports Exerc 1987; 19: 616–620.
19. Grover J: The effect of a flexion contracture of the elbow on the ability to transfer in patients who have quadriplegia at the sixth cervical level. J Bone Joint Surg [Am] 1996; 78: 1397–1400.
20. Happee R, van der Helm FCT: The control of shoulder muscles during goal directed movements, an inverse dynamic analysis. J Biomech 1995; 28: 1179–1191.
21. Harvey LA, Crosbie J: Weight bearing through flexed upper limbs in quadriplegics with paralyzed triceps brachii muscles. Spinal Cord 1999; 37: 780–785.
22. Herbert RD, Gandevia SC: Changes in pennation with joint angle and muscle torque: in vivo measurements in human brachialis muscle. J Physiol 1995; 484: 523–532.
23. Hislop HJ, Montgomery J: Daniel's and Worthingham's Muscle Testing: Techniques of Manual Examination. Philadelphia: WB Saunders, 1995.
24. Kapandji IA: The Physiology of the Joints. Vol 1, The Upper Limb. Edinburgh: Churchill Livingstone, 1982.
25. Kendall FP, McCreary EK, Provance PG: Muscle Testing and Function. Baltimore: Williams & Wilkins, 1993.
26. Knapik JJ: Isokinetic and isometric torque relationships in the human body. Arch Phys Med Rehabil 1980; 61: 64–67.
27. Knapik JJ, Wright JE, Mawdsley RH, Braun J: Isometric, isotonic, and isokinetic torque variations in four muscle groups through a range of joint motion. Phys Ther 1983; 63: 938–947.
28. Kulig K, Andrews JG, Hay JG: Human strength curves. Exerc Sport Sci Rev 1984; 12: 417–466.
29. Kumar VP: The role of the long head of biceps brachii in the stabilization of the head of the humerus. Clin Orthop 1989; 172–175.
30. Langenderfer J, Jerabek SA, Thangamani VB, et al.: Musculoskeletal parameters of muscles crossing the shoulder and elbow and the effect of sarcomere length sample size on estimation of optimal muscle length. Clin Biomech 2004; 19: 664–670.
31. Le Bozec S, Maton B, Cnockaert JC: The synergy of elbow extensor muscles during static work in man. Eur J Appl Physiol 1980; 43: 57–68.
32. Lemay MA, Crago PE: A dynamic model for simulating movements of the elbow, forearm, and wrist. J Biomech 1996; 29: 56–52.
33. Moore KL: Clinically Oriented Anatomy. Baltimore: Williams & Wilkins, 1980.
34. Morrey BF, Askew LJ, An KN, Chao EY: A biomechanical study of normal functional elbow motion. J Bone Joint Surg 1981; 63-A: 872–876.
35. Murray WM, Buchanan TS, Delp SL: The isometric functional capacity of muscles that cross the elbow. J Biomech 2000; 33: 943–952.
36. Murray WM, Delp SL, Buchanan TS: Variation of muscle moment arms with elbow and forearm position. J Biomech 1995; 28: 513–525.
37. Pagnani MJ, Deng XH, Warren RF, et al.: Effect of lesions of the superior portion of the glenoid labrum on glenohumeral translation. J Bone Joint Surg 1995; 77A: 1003–1010.
38. Petrofsky JS: The effect of elbow angle on the isometric strength and endurance of the elbow flexors in men and women. J Hum Ergol (Tokyo) 1980; 9: 125–131.
39. Pigeon P, Yahia L, Feldman AJ: Moment arms and lengths of human upper limb muscles as functions of joint angles. J Biomech 1996; 29: 1365–1370.
40. Rokito AS, McLaughlin JA, Gallagher MA, Zuckerman JD: Partial rupture of the distal biceps tendon. J Shoulder Elbow Surg 1996; 5: 73–75.
41. Romanes GJE: Cunningham's Textbook of Anatomy. Oxford: Oxford University Press, 1981.
42. Sale DG, MacDougall JD, Alway SE, Sutton JR: Voluntary strength and muscle characteristics in untrained men and women and male bodybuilders. J Appl Physiol 1987; 62: 1786–1793.
43. Sergio LE, Ostry SJ: Coordination of multiple muscles in two degree of freedom elbow movements. Exp Brain Res 1995; 105: 123–137.
44. Smith LK, Weiss EL, Lehmkuhl LD: Brunnstrom's Clinical Kinesiology. Philadelphia: FA Davis, 1996.

45. Soslowsky LJ, Malicky DM, Blasier RB: Active and passive factors in inferior glenohumeral stabilization: a biomechanical model. J Shoulder Elbow Surg 1997; 6: 371–379.

46. Steindler A: Kinesiology of the Human Body under Normal and Pathological Conditions. Springfield, IL: Charles C Thomas, 1955.

47. Stewart OJ, Peat M, Yaworski GR: Influence of resistance, speed of movement, and forearm position on recruitment of the elbow flexors. Am J Phys Med 1981; 60: 165–179.

48. Stratford PW, Balsor BE: A comparison of make and break tests using a hand-held dynamometer and the kin-com. J Orthop Sports Phys Ther 1994; 19: 28–32.

49. Sturzenegger M, Beguin D, Grunig B, Jakob RP: Muscular strength after rupture of the long head of the biceps. Arch Orthop Trauma Surg 1986; 105: 18–23.

50. van Bolhuis BM, Gielen CCAM: The relative activation of elbow-flexor muscles in isometric flexion and in flexion/extension movements. J Biomech 1997; 30: 803–811.

51. van Zuylen EJ, van Velzen A, van der Gon JJD: A biomechanical model for flexion torques of human arm muscles as a function of elbow angle. J Biomech 1988; 21: 183–190.

52. Williams M, Stutzman L: Strength variation through the range of joint motion. Phys Ther Rev 1959; 39: 145–152.

53. Williams P, Bannister L, Berry M, et al: Gray's Anatomy, The Anatomical Basis of Medicine and Surgery, Br. ed. London: Churchill Livingstone, 1995.

54. Zhang LQ, Nuber GW: Moment distribution among human elbow extensor muscles during isometric and submaximal extension. J Biomech 2000; 33: 145–154.

Analysis of the Forces at the Elbow during Activity

CHAPTER CONTENTS

*I*n the preceding two chapters the structure of the elbow joint and its supporting elements is described and the roles of the primary muscles of the elbow are presented. The purpose of the present chapter is to discuss the loads to which the elbow joint and surrounding structures are subjected. Specifically the aims of this chapter are to

- Present a two-dimensional analysis of the loads on the elbow during a simple lifting task
- Present a two-dimensional analysis of the loads on the elbow during upper extremity weight bearing
- Review the loads the elbow sustains during a variety of activities
- Discuss the stresses (load/area) applied to the humeroulnar and humeroradial articulations

ANALYSIS OF THE FORCES EXERTED AT THE ELBOW

Forces on the Elbow during Simple Upper Extremity Lifting Techniques

Elbow flexion is a basic element of countless activities of daily living as diverse as eating an apple and lifting a bag of groceries or an anatomy textbook. *Examining the Forces Box 13.1* presents the free-body diagram depicting the task of holding a 5-lb bag of sugar [5,18]. It also provides the simple two-dimensional analysis of the required flexor force and resulting joint reaction force at the elbow generated during the activity. By lumping the flexor force all into the brachialis muscle, the calculation reveals that the flexor force needed to hold a 5-lb load in an outstretched limb is greater than 1 times body weight! Calculation of the joint reaction force suggests compressive loads of almost 1.2 times body weight.

The solution presented in *Examining the Forces Box 13.1* requires the rather large and inaccurate assumption that all of the flexor forces can be ascribed to the brachialis muscle, whose moment arm is known. In reality, it is most likely that the brachialis and biceps are both participating, and under enough resistance, the brachioradialis and pronator teres may

EXAMINING THE FORCES BOX 13.1

TWO-DIMENSIONAL ANALYSIS OF THE FORCES IN THE ELBOW WHILE HOLDING A FIVE-POUND LOAD WITH THE ELBOW FLEXED TO 30°

The following dimensions are based on a well-conditioned male who is 6 feet tall (1.83 m) and weighs 180 lb (800 N). The limb segment parameters are extrapolated from the anthropometric data of Braune and Fischer [5]. The flexion force is assumed to be provided entirely by the brachialis muscle (B).

Length of forearm and hand (L): 0.4 m
Center of gravity (c.g.) of forearm and hand is 47% of length of forearm and hand from proximal end (l)
Weight of forearm and hand (W): 3% of body weight (BW)
Weight in the hand: 5 lb (3% BW)
Moment arm of brachialis (ma): 0.015 m

Solve for brachialis force (B):

$\Sigma M = 0$

$(B \times 0.015 \text{ m}) - (0.03 \text{ BW} \times 0.47 \times 0.4 \text{ m})$
$\qquad\qquad - (0.03 \text{ BW} \times 0.4 \text{ m}) = 0$

$(B \times 0.015 \text{ m}) = (0.03 \text{ BW} \times 0.47 \times 0.4 \text{ m})$
$\qquad\qquad + (0.03 \text{ BW} \times 0.4 \text{ m})$

B = 1.18 BW

Calculate the joint reaction forces (J) on the ulna. Assume that the brachialis is applied to the ulna at an angle of 25°.

$\Sigma F_X: \ J_X - B_X = 0$

$\qquad J_X = B_X$, where $B_X = B \ (\cos 25°)$

$\qquad J_X = B \ (\cos 25°)$

$\qquad J_X = 1.07 \text{ BW}$

$\Sigma F_Y: \ J_Y + B_Y - 0.03 \text{ BW} - 0.03 \text{ BW} = 0$, where the weight of the forearm and hand is 0.03 BW and the 5-lb weight = 0.03 BW

$\qquad J_Y = 0.06 \text{ BW} - B_Y$, where $B_Y = B \ (\sin 25°)$

$\qquad J_Y = -0.45 \text{ BW}$

Using the pythagorean theorem:

$J^2 = J_X{}^2 + J_Y{}^2$

J ≈ 1.16 BW

Using trigonometry, the direction of J can be determined:

$\qquad \sin \theta = \dfrac{J_x}{J}$

θ ≈ 67° from the vertical

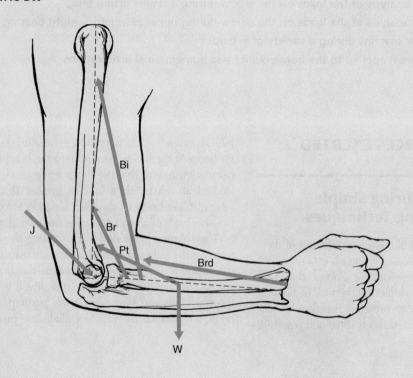

Free-body diagram of the elbow for the task of lifting a 5-lb load identifies all of the forces acting on the forearm.

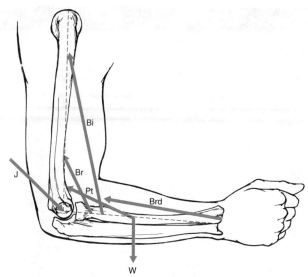

Figure 13.1: Free-body diagram of the elbow during flexion. The free-body diagram shows the forces from all of the elbow flexors, demonstrating that there are more unknown forces than can be determined using the static equilibrium equations. The system is described as statically indeterminate. *Bi*, biceps brachii; *Br*, brachialis; *Pt*, pronator teres; *Brd*, brachioradialis.

also contribute to the flexor force. However, the real situation of multiple muscles contracting simultaneously has more unknowns than equations to solve and is known as **statically indeterminate** [4] (*Fig.13.1*).

A problem that is indeterminate has an infinite number of possible solutions. Chapter 1 briefly describes methods used to solve the indeterminate problem by choosing the *best* solution on the basis of some rather arbitrary optimizing criterion. Another approach to managing the case of more unknowns than equations is to solve only for the **internal moment** that must be exerted by the surrounding muscles and ligaments. The internal moment is the moment generated by muscles and ligaments to resist the **external moment** generated by the weight of the limb and any additional weights or forces applied from the environment. Such forces include additional weights such as the bag of sugar, resistance applied by a therapist, and ground reaction forces. By solving only for the internal moment, there is no attempt to distribute that moment to the muscles or other surrounding tissue. Therefore, there is no need for erroneous simplifying assumptions such as lumping the force into a single muscle. However, the solution provides no estimates of muscle or joint forces. *Examining the Forces Box 13.2* presents the free-body diagram and the calculation of the internal moment using the same case described in Box 13.1.

The internal moment needed from the flexor muscles to hold a 5-lb (22.24 N) bag is 13.4 Nm. In a published biomechanical analysis of lifting, the reported peak internal

moment needed to lift a 38-lb (170 N) dumbbell through the range of elbow flexion is approximately 45 Nm [7]. These results offer enough similarity between the model presented in Examining the Forces Box 13.2 and the published model to provide at least face validity to the model in Box 13.2.

Although the solution in Examining the Forces Box 13.1 is based on a clearly erroneous simplification, it does offer the clinician a useful perspective on the magnitude of the loads required of the muscles of the elbow during such a simple task as lifting a relatively small load. The reason for such large muscular loads is the mechanical disadvantage of the muscles compared with the advantage of the 5-lb load and the weight of the forearm and hand. The moment arm of the brachialis is approximately 8% of the moment arm of the weight of the forearm and hand and less than 4% of the moment arm of the 5-lb load (*Fig. 13.2*). Consequently, the muscle must generate large forces to create a moment to balance the moments exerted by the weight of the limb and the 5-lb load.

A muscle's contraction force has a direct impact on the joint reaction force. The solution seen in Examining the Forces Box 13.1, albeit only a rough estimate, demonstrates that the elbow joint sustains large loads even during simple tasks such as lifting small loads. Several more elaborate biomechanical models examine the elbow joint forces during elbow function. Loads of up to 1,600 N (360 lb) and 800 N (180 lb) are reported at the humeroulnar and radiohumeral articulations, respectively, during simple lifting tasks, lifting loads of only 2–4 kg (4.4–8.8 lb) [6]. The elbow forces vary significantly with the type of hand grip used. High-speed flexion and extension movements generate even larger loads at the humeroulnar and radio-humeral joints, 1,910 N (approximately 430 lb) and 2,680 N (approximately 602 lb), respectively [2]. Maximum isometric flexion efforts generate still larger loads, over 3,000 N (675 lb) at each joint [1]. Peak compressive forces parallel to the forearm and directed into the humerus are estimated to be approximately 45% of body weight during two-handed push-ups and approximately 65% of body weight in a one-handed push-up [9,10].

Similar loads on the elbow are reported in falls on an outstretched limb from a low height (3–6 cm) [8]. It seems surprising that lifting activities could generate larger elbow joint forces than push-ups. Differences in models may explain some of the differences in solutions, but differences in the moment arms of the external loads on the elbow may also contribute to the larger elbow loads during lifting activities. The effects of moment arms are discussed in more detail in the next section. These data, although only estimates, reveal that the elbow articulations sustain very large loads during activity. A clinician must remain aware of these loads when establishing an intervention strategy for an individual with joint disease and modify the intervention in ways to reduce the loads on the joint.

EXAMINING THE FORCES BOX 13.2

CALCULATION OF THE INTERNAL MOMENT (M$_i$) GENERATED IN THE EXAMPLE PRESENTED IN EXAMINING THE FORCES BOX 13.1

Dimensions presented in Examining the Forces Box 13.1 remain the same.

Length of forearm and hand *(L):* 0.4 m
c.g. of forearm and hand is 47% of length of forearm and hand from proximal end, *(l)*
Weight of forearm and hand *(W):* 3% of body weight
Body weight: 180 lb (800 N)
Weight in the hand: 5 lb (22.24 N)

$\Sigma M = 0$

$M_{internal} + M_{external} = 0$, where $M_{internal}$ is the moment created by the muscles and ligaments of the elbow and $M_{external}$ is the moment generated by the weights of the forearm and hand and the 5-lb load

$M_{internal} = -M_{external}$

$M_{internal} = (0.03 \times 800\ N \times 0.47 \times 0.4\ m)$
$\qquad\qquad\qquad + (22.24\ N \times 0.4\ m) = 0$

$M_{internal} = 13.4\ Nm$

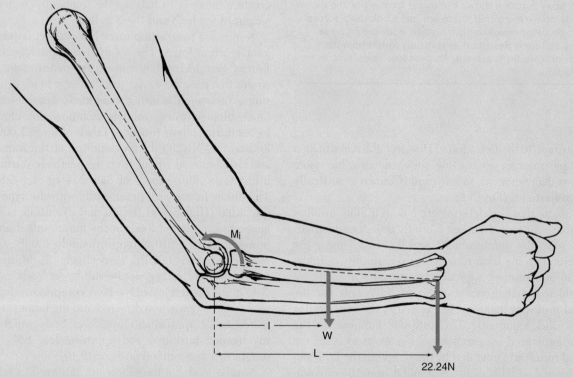

Free-body diagram of the elbow for the task of lifting a 5-lb load, indicating the external loads and the internal moments. The free-body diagram reduces the muscle forces and their moment arms to a single internal moment (*M$_i$*).

Clinical Relevance

ELBOW LOADS IN BASEBALL PITCHERS: *External valgus moments (frontal plane moments tending to rotate the elbow into valgus) of approximately 18 Nm are reported in 11- and 12-year-old male baseball pitchers [23]. Professional baseball pitchers reportedly sustain valgus moments of approximately*

65 Nm [15]. Contrast these moments that are balanced by the elbow's medial collateral ligament with perhaps additional support from forearm muscles with the flexion moment of 28 Nm balanced by the elbow extensor muscles during crutch walking. It should not be a surprise that elbow injuries are common in baseball pitchers. These data support the need to limit the number of pitches thrown by skeletally immature athletes.

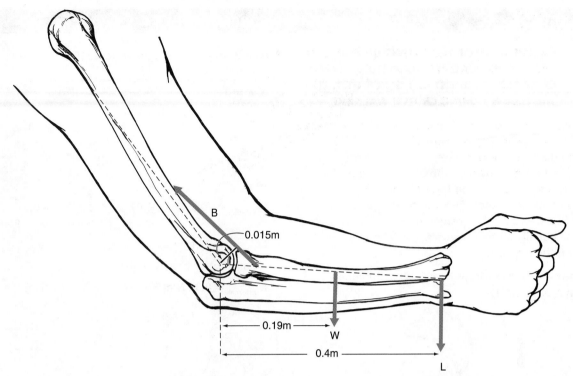

Figure 13.2: Comparison of the brachialis muscle's moment arm with the moment arms of the external loads. The moment arms of the external loads are much greater than the moment arm of the brachialis (*B*), increasing the mechanical advantage of the weight of the forearm and hand (*W*) and the weight in the hand (*L*).

Forces on the Elbow during Upper Extremity Weight Bearing

Although the upper extremity is typically described as having non-weight-bearing joints, discussions regarding the shoulder in Chapters 9 and 10 clearly indicate that even in healthy individuals, the upper extremity frequently participates in weight-bearing activities such as rising from a chair. When an individual has a lower extremity impairment, the upper extremities may become even more involved in weight bearing by actual participation in locomotion, as in crutch walking and wheelchair propulsion. Increased bone mineral density is reported in the shaft of the radius in 10 subjects with a mean duration of 8.7 years of crutch use [25]. These data provide an indirect indication of the increased stress applied to the elbow region as a result of the additional weight-bearing responsibility of the upper extremity in individuals who ambulate with assistive devices. This report also demonstrates the application of Wolff's law as the structures of the bones of the elbow respond to their altered function. *Examining the Forces Box 13.3* presents the basic two-dimensional analysis of the loads on the elbow joint during the swing phase of crutch ambulation.

The solution in Examining the Forces Box 13.3 is presented as the estimated force of the triceps brachii (1.4 times body weight) and as a net internal moment

(28 Nm). It is useful to compare the estimated force of the triceps brachii in the crutch walking example to the flexor force in the lifting example in Examining the Forces Box 13.1. Although the resistance in the crutch walking task (one half body weight) is several times the resistance in the lifting task, the required force of the triceps brachii is only 30% greater than that of the flexors. The reason for the difference in the mechanical requirements of these two tasks is the difference in the length of the moment arms between the resistances and between the muscles (*Fig. 13.3*). In the crutch walking example, the moment arm of the body weight is 0.07 m, but in the lifting task, the moment arm of the 5-lb weight is 0.4 m. Similarly, the moment arm of the brachialis is 0.015 m, while the moment arm of the triceps brachii is 0.025 m.

Clinical Relevance

THE IMPACT OF CRUTCH HEIGHT ON ELBOW JOINT MOMENTS: *Although the clinician can rarely alter a muscle's moment arm, the moment arm of the resistance is easily manipulated. Reisman et al. report an almost 100% increase in internal moment in subjects ambulating with*

(continued)

EXAMINING THE FORCES BOX 13.3

CALCULATION OF THE EXTENSION FORCE OF THE TRICEPS BRACHII (T) AND THE INTERNAL EXTENSION MOMENT (Mᵢ) GENERATED AT THE ELBOW DURING CRUTCH WALKING

The subject's anthropometric measures are the same as those used in Examining the Forces Boxes 13.1 and 13.2. Assume that the elbow is flexed to 10° [7]. Note that the subject pushes down on the crutch and therefore the crutch exerts a reaction force (F_c) on the hand and forearm. That force (F_c) is assumed to be equal to 1/2 BW, based on the presumption that the weight is borne equally on two crutches. The joint reaction force on the ulna is (J).

Moment arm of the triceps brachii (T) at 10° elbow flexion is 0.025 m [17]

Moment arm (l) of the crutch force (F_c) = 0.4 m
(sin 10°) = 0.07 m

$\Sigma M = 0$

$F_c \times 0.07\ m - T \times 0.025\ m = 0$

$0.5\ BW \times 0.07\ m = T \times 0.025\ m$

T = 1.4 BW

$M_{internal} + M_{external} = 0$

$M_{internal} = (0.5\ BW \times 0.07\ m) = 0.035\ BW\ m,$
$\qquad\qquad\qquad\qquad\qquad\qquad$ where BW = 800 N

$M_{internal}$ = 28 Nm

Normalizing for body weight:

$M_{internal}$ = 0.34 N m/kg, where BW = 81.6 kg

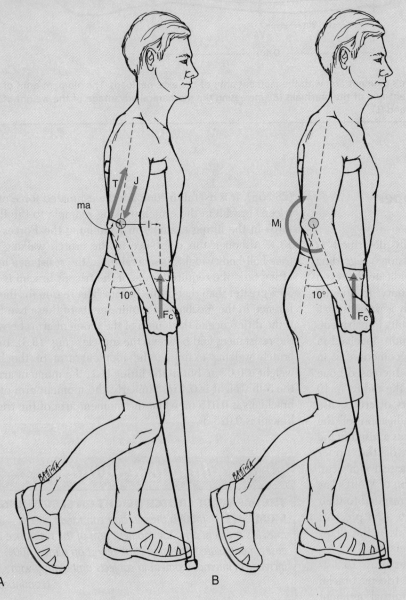

Free-body diagram of the elbow during crutch walking. **A.** The external load and the internal forces exerted by the triceps muscle and the joint reaction force. **B.** The external load and the internal moment to balance it.

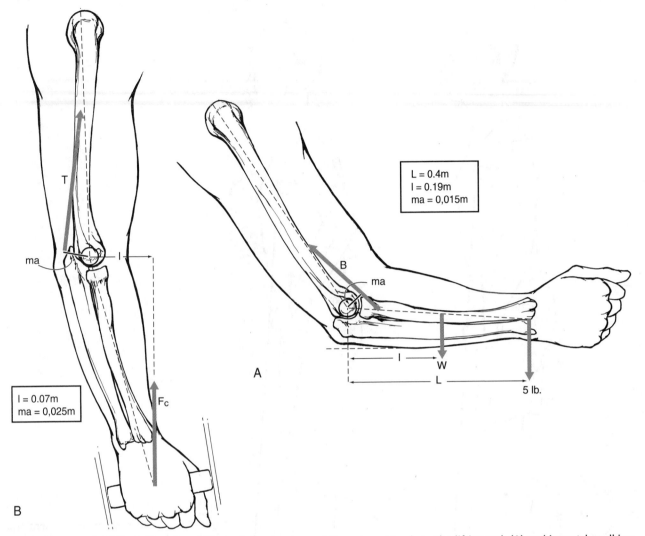

Figure 13.3: Comparisons of the moment arms of the muscles and the external loads on the lifting task (**A**) and in crutch walking (**B**). Although the resistances are smaller in the lifting task, their moment arms are much larger than the moment arm of the crutch force.

(Continued)

axillary crutches when the crutch handle is raised 1–2 in from its optimal height [21]. This remarkable increase in the muscles' requirements is the result of increased elbow flexion and, consequently, an increase in the moment arm of the resistance (Fig. 13.4). Similar changes in joint loads are reported in exercises such as the push-up and bench press [10,14]. These examples provide a powerful example of how an understanding of joint moments can guide the clinician in altering the requirements of a joint's muscles and the load on a patient's joint by altering the moment applied by the external load.

The net moment of 28 Nm in the crutch walking example also can be compared with other reports in the literature. Robertson et al. calculate mean peak internal moments at the elbow of 12.3 Nm during wheelchair propulsion by regular wheelchair users and even larger mean peak moments in those who are not wheelchair users [22]. In Examining the Forces Box 13.3, the internal moment is normalized for body weight to compare the results of this model with additional results from published studies [19,20]. Nordau et al. report normalized internal moments of about 0.2 Nm/kg in a careful and thorough analysis of individuals, with and without paraplegia, ambulating with forearm crutches. Although the agreement is not perfect, the solution from the current example is close enough to be a reasonable reflection of the biomechanical task. An analysis of the forces sustained by muscles and joints during a task such as wheelchair propulsion or crutch walking helps the clinician appreciate the wear and tear that the upper extremity sustains during activity.

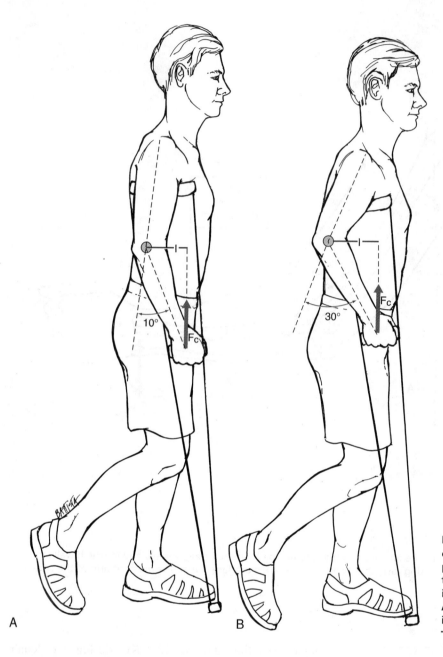

Figure 13.4: Comparison of the moment arm of the crutch force with different elbow positions. Increased elbow flexion increases the moment arm of the crutch force, creating a larger flexion moment on the elbow. **A.** The elbow is flexed to 10°. **B.** The elbow is flexed to 30°.

STRESSES APPLIED TO THE ARTICULAR SURFACES OF THE ELBOW

The studies described above reveal that the elbow sustains very large loads during everyday activities. However, how these loads are applied to the articular surfaces is also an important factor in understanding the mechanics and patho-mechanics of the elbow. The shape and relative fit of the articular surfaces of the humerus, ulna, and radius are described in Chapter 11. That presentation reveals that in many elbows, contact between the humerus and ulna occurs only at the proximal and distal extents of the articular surface of the trochlear notch [12,17,24]. In fact, measurements of the joint space reveal that there is greater space

between the humerus and ulna in the center of the trochlear notch than at the proximal and distal aspects [11].

The joint reaction forces at the elbow are dispersed across only the contacting surfaces of the humerus and ulna. Stress is the measure of how a force is distributed over an area (stress = force/area). Thus the stress at the elbow is concentrated at the proximal and distal extremes of the humeroulnar articulation. A study using both mathematical analysis and experimental tests on a single cadaver specimen assessed the stresses on the humeroulnar joint resulting from simulated isometric extension forces of up to 500 N. (approximately 112 lb) [16]. Stresses of up to 3.6 MPa (MN/m²) (approximately 522 lb/in², psi) are reported at the proximal aspect of the trochlear notch and up to 2.3 MPa

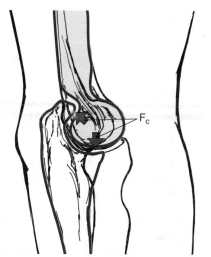

Figure 13.5: Compressive forces on the trochlea. Compressive forces *(F_c)* on the trochlea are exerted on the proximal and distal aspects of the trochlear notch.

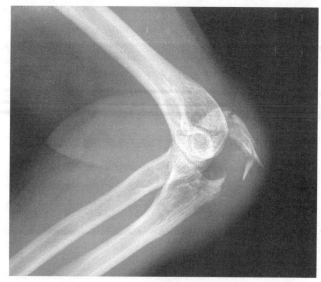

Figure 13.7: Radiograph of a fracture of the olecranon. An X-ray film of a fracture of the olecranon reveals that it occurred through the middle of the trochlear notch at its deepest point, where the bone mineralization is reduced and the notch sustains tensile forces. (Courtesy of S. Kozin, MD, Shriner's Hospital for Children, Philadelphia, PA.)

(approximately 334 psi) in the distal aspect of the notch, with only 0.45 MPa (approximately 65 psi) at the deepest part of the notch (*Fig. 13.5*). This same study suggests that the subchondral bone in the deepest portion of the notch sustains tensile forces, while the proximal and distal aspects undergo compressive loading (*Fig. 13.6*). Since Wolff's law states that the structure of bone responds to the loads applied to it, an understanding of the loading pattern of the joint helps explain the bony architecture of the ulna. Studies demonstrate increased mineralization in the subchondral bone in the proximal and distal aspects of the trochlear notch [13]. These data provide evidence that Wolff's law is applicable to the architecture of the elbow.

Clinical Relevance

OLECRANON FRACTURES: *Olecranon fractures can occur from an aggressive pull of the triceps causing an avulsion fracture or from a direct blow to the tip of the olecranon. In vitro experiments with 40 cadaver limbs reveal that olecranon fractures through the deepest part of the trochlear notch are easily produced by direct impacts to the proximal olecranon [3] (Fig. 13.7). The average impact producing the fracture is 4100 N (approximately 920 lb). Such an impact simulates a fall onto the tip of the elbow. It is significant that the fractures occur in the deepest part of the trochlear notch where there is less mineralization in the subchondral bone. Thus an awareness of the bony architecture of the elbow helps explain a common injury.*

Summary

This chapter examines the forces that are likely to be sustained by the elbow musculature during activity. Simple examples used to determine muscle and joint forces demonstrate that the elbow sustains loads equal to at least body weight during simple lifting tasks and may sustain loads several times body weight during more vigorous activities. The examples demonstrated that the forces required of the muscles, and consequently the loads on the joints, can be altered readily by manipulation of the magnitude or location of the external loads.

The joint reaction force at the elbow is spread unevenly across the joint surface of the humeroulnar articulation,

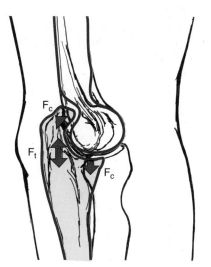

Figure 13.6: Tensile forces on the trochlear notch. Tensile forces *(F_t)* are exerted in the deepest aspect of the trochlear notch.

resulting in two areas of concentrated stress in the trochlear notch. Data are presented demonstrating uneven bone mineralization consistent with Wolff's law. The clinician can use the understanding of joint forces gained from this chapter to guide interventions to optimize the positive outcomes while minimizing the deleterious effects of joint loading. This understanding will also heighten the clinician's appreciation of the hurdles to overcome in the design of prosthetic devices for even one of the simplest joints, the elbow.

References

1. Amis AA: The derivation of elbow joint forces, and their relation to prosthesis design. J Med Eng Technol 1979; 3: 229–234.

2. Amis AA, Dowson D, Wright V: Analysis of elbow forces due to high-speed forearm movements. J Biomech 1980; 13: 825–831.

3. Amis AA, Miller JH: The mechanisms of elbow fractures: an investigation using impact tests in vitro. Injury 1995; 26: 163–168.

4. Andrews JR: Glenoid labrum tears related to the long head of the biceps. Am J Sports Med 1985; 13: 337–341.

5. Braune W, Fischer O: Center of gravity of the human body. In: Human Mechanics; Four Monographs Abridged AMRL-TDR-63-123. Krogman WM, Johnston FE, eds. Wright-Patterson Air Force Base, Ohio: Behavioral Sciences Laboratory, 6570th Aerospace Medical Research Laboratories, Aerospace Medical Division, Air Force Systems Command, 1963; 1–57.

6. Chadwick EKJ, Nicol AC: Elbow and wrist joint contact forces during occupational pick and place activities. J Biomech 2000; 33: 591–600.

7. Challis JH, Kerwin DG: Quantification of the uncertainties in resultant joint moments computed in a dynamic activity. J Sports Sci 1996; 14: 219–231.

8. Chou P-H, Chou Y-L, Lin C-J, et al.: Effect of elbow flexion on upper extremity impact forces during a fall. Clin Biomech 2001; 16: 888–894.

9. Chou PH, Lin CJ, Chou YL, et al.: Elbow load with various forearm positions during one-handed pushup exercise. Int J Sports Med 2002; 23: 457–462.

10. Donkers MJ, An K, Chao EYS, Morrey BF: Hand position affects elbow joint load during push-up exercise. J Biomech 1993; 26: 625-632.

11. Eckstein F, Lohe F, Hillebrand S, et al.: Morphomechanics of the humero-ulnar joint: I. Joint space width and contact areas as a function of load and flexion angle. Anat Rec 1995; 243: 318–326.

12. Eckstein F, Lohe F, Schulte E, et al.: Physiological incongruity of the humero-ulnar joint: a functional principle of optimized stress distribution acting upon articulating surfaces? Anat Embryol 1993; 188: 449–455.

13. Eckstein F, Muller-Gerbl M, Steinlechner M, et al.: Subchondral bone density in the human elbow assessed by computed tomography osteoabsorptiometry: a reflection of the loading history of the joint surfaces. J Orthop Res 1995; 13: 268–278.

14. Elliott BC, Wilson GJ, Kerr GK: A biomechanical analysis of the sticking region in the bench press. Med Sci Sports Exerc 1989; 21: 450–462.

15. Fleisig GS, Barrentine SW, Zheng N, et al.: Kinematic and kinetic comparison of baseball pitching among various levels of development. J Biomech 1999; 32: 1371–1375.

16. Merz B, Eckstein F, Hillebrand S, Putz R: Mechanical implications of humero-ulnar incongruity-finite element analysis and experiment. J Biomech 1997; 30: 713–721.

17. Milz S, Eckstein F, Putz R: Thickness distribution of the subchondral mineralization zone of the trochlear notch and its correlation with the cartilage thickness: an expression of functional adaptation to mechanical stress acting on the humeroulnar joint? Anat Rec 1997; 248: 189–197.

18. Murray WM, Delp SL, Buchanan TS: Variation of muscle moment arms with elbow and forearm position. J Biomech 1995; 28: 513–525.

19. Noreau L, Comeau F, Tardif D, Richards CL: Biomechanical analysis of swing-through gait in paraplegic and non-disabled individuals. J Biomech 1995; 28: 689–700.

20. Opila KA: Upper limb loadings of gait with crutches. J Biomech Eng 1987; 109: 285–290.

21. Reisman M, Burdett RG, Simon SR, Norkin C: Elbow moment and forces at the hands during swing-through axillary crutch gait. Phys Ther 1985; 65: 601–605.

22. Robertson RN, Boninger ML, Cooper RA, Shimada SD: Pushrim forces and joint kinetics during wheelchair propulsion. Arch Phys Med Rehabil 1996; 77: 856–864.

23. Sabick MB, Torry MR, Lawton RL, Hawkins RJ: Valgus torque in youth baseball pitchers: a biomechanical study. J Shoulder Elbow Surg 2004; 13: 349–355.

24. Tillmann B: A contribution to the functional morphology of articular surfaces. Norm Pathol Anat (Stuttg) 1978; 34: 1–50.

25. Wing PC, Tredwell SJ: The weightbearing shoulder. Paraplegia 1983; 21: 107–113.

he preceding chapters discuss the structure and function of the shoulder and elbow. The shoulder is remarkably mobile, and that mobility creates a huge potential space through which the hand can be moved (Figure). In contrast, the elbow is much less mobile but allows the hand to approach and move away from the body. The ultimate functional application for both of these joint complexes is to position the hand. The hand is responsible for carrying out the work of the upper extremity.

The functions that can be accomplished by the hand are as varied as kneading bread dough and sculpting a masterpiece, as diverse as meat cutting and neurosurgery. The hand is a manipulator and a communicator. Hands are thrown up in disgust or laid tenderly on a baby's cheek. The hand is powerful enough to be a weapon and gentle enough to be a tool of art and love.

Such diversity requires a wide range of positions and forces, as well as remarkable sensitivity. This broad spectrum of performances demands structural complexity with relative ease of operation. The hand represents a significant increase in architectural complexity compared with the more proximal joints of the upper extremity. Yet the organization of the hand offers remarkable synergy among its structures, which allows efficient completion of a task.

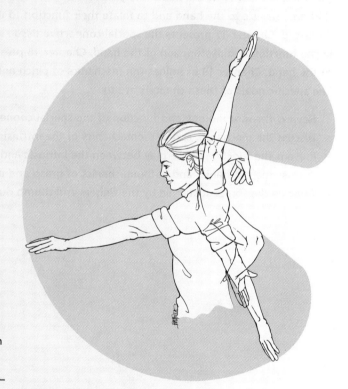

The approximate space through which the hand can move. Motion of the shoulder and elbow can position the hand anywhere in a huge volume in front of, beside, and behind the body.

The focus of the next six chapters is the structure and function of the hand and all of its components. These chapters demonstrate how the components function individually and together, so that the clinician can appreciate how pathology in one element affects the entire complex. These six chapters are divided into two interrelated groups. Chapters 14, 15, and 16 present the linkage between the hand and the rest of the upper extremity, focusing on the wrist and the muscles of the forearm. Since many of the muscles of the forearm affect the hand, this section includes the bones and joints of the hand. As in the preceding units on the shoulder and elbow, the first chapter in this unit (Chapter 14) presents the bones and joints of the region. The second chapter (Chapter 15) provides a discussion of the mechanics and pathomechanics of the muscles, and the third chapter (Chapter 16) furnishes an analysis of the forces sustained by the region. The specific purposes of Chapters 14–16 on the wrist and forearm are to

- Present the structure and function of the bones and joints of the wrist and hand
- Discuss the muscles of the forearm and their contribution to the function and dysfunction of the hand
- Analyze the forces that are transmitted through the wrist

Chapters 17, 18, and 19 present the morphology and function of the structures that are specific to the hand, including the intrinsic muscles of the hand. The purposes of Chapters 17 through 19 are to discuss the soft tissue structures that are intrinsic to the hand and to relate their function to the function of the joints and extrinsic muscles already discussed. Chapter 17 presents the special connective tissue structures of the hand and discusses their participation in the function and dysfunction of the hand. Chapter 18 presents the structure and function of the intrinsic muscles of the hand. Chapter 19 examines the mechanics of pinch and grasp and then explores the forces applied to the digits. The specific goals of these chapters are to

- Review the morphology and function of the special connective tissue structures found within the hand
- Discuss the mechanics and pathomechanics of the intrinsic muscles of the hand
- Present the functional interplay between the intrinsic and extrinsic muscles of the hand
- Discuss the mechanics and pathomechanics of grasp and pinch
- Analyze the forces sustained by the fingers and thumb during activity

Structure and Function of the Bones and Joints of the Wrist and Hand

CHAPTER CONTENTS

This chapter focuses on the skeleton and joints of the wrist and hand. All of these structures are considered together, since many of the muscles of the forearm extend into the fingers. Understanding the role of these muscles in the fingers requires a thorough knowledge of the joints and movements of the fingers. The specific purposes of this chapter are to

- Describe the structure of the bones of the wrist and hand to understand how they contribute to movements of the hand
- Discuss the ligaments and supporting structures of the joints of the wrist and hand and their contribution to the stability of the hand
- Demonstrate the clinical relevance of some of the specific anatomical details of the bones and ligaments of the region
- Review the normal ranges of motion in the wrist and hand

Details of the bony structures in the wrist and hand are presented first to demonstrate how the shapes of the bones influence the mechanics and pathomechanics of the wrist and hand. The structure of the joints and their supporting structures are discussed next. An understanding of the joints and surrounding structures forms the basis for the presentation of the motions that occur at the wrist and within the hand.

STRUCTURE OF THE BONES OF THE WRIST AND HAND

A partial explanation for the precision movements available in the hand is the presence of so many bones and joints that can move in concert with, or independently of, one another. The shoulder and elbow complexes each consist of three bones, although the shoulder complex also involves a fourth bone, the sternum. The hand, however, contains 27 primary bones with an important, albeit indirect, association with a twenty-eighth, the ulna, and a variable number of sesamoid bones! The relevant characteristics of the bones that influence the mechanics and pathomechanics of the wrist and hand are presented below.

Distal Radius and Shaft

The proximal radius is described in Chapter 11 with the elbow. The shaft of the radius is somewhat triangular in the transverse plane, with a sharp medial edge that provides attachment for the interosseous membrane, also known as the interosseous ligament. The radial shaft is largely covered by muscles of the forearm, and only the proximal and distal ends of the radius are readily palpated. The radius widens distally in the medial and lateral directions so that the distal end is the widest part of the radius.

The distal end of the radius has five important surfaces: dorsal (posterior), volar (anterior), radial (lateral), ulnar (medial), and distal (*Fig. 14.1*). The dorsal surface is characterized by a palpable prominence known as the dorsal tubercle, with grooves on either side of it for the extensor pollicis longus tendon on its ulnar side and for the extensor digitorum and the extensor indicis tendons radially. The dorsal tubercle serves as a pulley to redirect the pull of the extensor pollicis longus.

The radial surface of the radius is roughened and terminates in the distal projection, the styloid process, which is easily palpated on the radial aspect of the wrist joint in the anatomical snuffbox. The volar surface of the radius is slightly concave in the radioulnar direction and terminates distally in a distinct ridge to which the capsule of the wrist attaches. This ridge is palpable about 2.5 cm proximal to the thenar eminence. It serves as a reliable identifying landmark of the radiocarpal joint.

The ulnar surface of the distal radius is composed of the ulnar notch, providing an articular surface for the distal radioulnar joint. This notch is generally described as concave from its volar to its dorsal borders [77,141]; however, its shape

is quite variable. It may be concave, flat, and even S-shaped, or sigmoid [38]. Consequently, clinical literature frequently refers to the ulnar notch as the **sigmoid notch** [34,77]. Because of its use in the clinical literature, this text employs the term *sigmoid notch* rather than the anatomical term, *ulnar notch*. The notch is variable in its proximal-to-distal orientation [34,77] and appears to be influenced by the relative length of the ulna [29,65] (*Fig. 14.2*). Like all joints, the mobility and stability of the distal radioulnar joint are influenced significantly by the shape of the articular surfaces, including the sigmoid notch.

The distal surface of the radius is the proximal articular surface of the wrist. It articulates with the scaphoid and lunate. It is biconcave, concave in both the volar–dorsal and the ulnar–radial directions (*Fig. 14.3*). Although the articular surface is continuous, there is a ridge that separates the surface into distinct surfaces for the scaphoid radially and the lunate on the ulnar side of the ridge. The distal articular surface is tilted in a volar direction approximately 10–15° and faces in an ulnar direction approximately 15–25° [12,127] (*Fig. 14.4*). Karnezis suggests that the volar tilt decreases the shear forces on the distal radius during lifting tasks and is positively correlated with the wrist joint reaction force [64]. The tilt and inclination of the distal radius also helps explain the direction of carpal subluxation, ulnar and volar, in the unstable wrists of patients with rheumatoid arthritis.

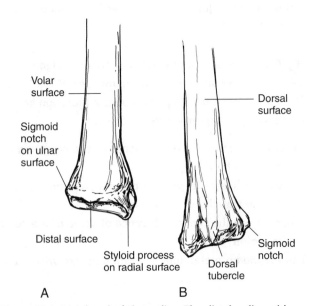

Figure 14.1: Distal end of the radius. The distal radius widens and displays five distinct surfaces: dorsal, volar, radial, ulnar, and distal. **A.** Volar view. **B.** Dorsal view.

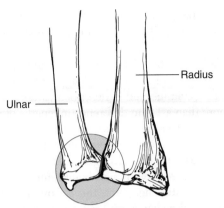

Figure 14.2: Tilt of the sigmoid notch. The proximal–distal tilt of the sigmoid notch is influenced by the relative length of the articulating ulna. When the ulna is relatively short, the notch is often tilted proximally as demonstrated in this figure.

Clinical Relevance

DISTAL RADIUS FRACTURE: *Fractures of the distal radius are the most common fractures in adults over 50 years of age, more than three times more common in women than in men [74,78,79,107]. The most common type of distal radius fracture is the Colles' fracture, an extraarticular fracture in which the distal fragment of the radius undergoes dorsal displacement accompanied by dorsal tilting [99]. A close approximation of the original alignment of the radius is essential to restore normal movement and load distribution across the wrist [64,94,103,126,145]. Malalignment of the fragment can lead to significant reductions in the resulting range of motion (ROM) at the wrist and at the distal radioulnar joint. Limited ROM secondary to bony malalignment does not respond to exercise. The clinician must be able to distinguish between range limitations resulting from bony blocks and those caused by soft tissue restrictions, which can respond to conservative treatment.*

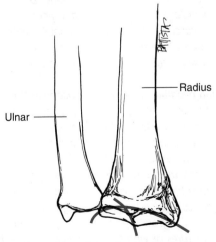

Figure 14.3: The surface of the distal radius is biconcave, concave in the radioulnar and dorsal–volar directions.

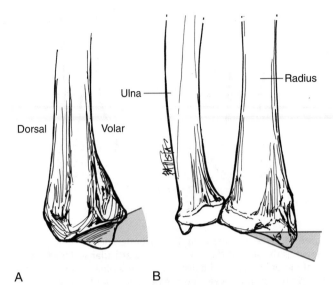

Figure 14.4: Tilt of the articular surface of the distal radius. The articular surface of the distal radius is tilted **(A)** volarly (anteriorly) and **(B)** in an ulnar direction.

Distal Ulna and Shaft

Although the ulna is separated from the wrist proper by a fibrocartilaginous disc, the ulna is an important functional element of the wrist, integral to the normal function of the forearm and hand [38]. The proximal aspect of the ulna is described in Chapter 11. The shaft of the ulna is triangular for most of its length and narrows from proximal to distal. The posterior border of the shaft of the ulna is subcutaneous and palpable along its entire length. The distal end of the ulnar shaft expands slightly into the head of the ulna that articulates with the distal radius and with the triangular fibrocartilage between the ulna and the carpal bones. The rounded head of the ulna is easily palpated dorsally when the forearm is pronated.

The head of the ulna has two articular surfaces (*Fig. 14.5*). The articular surface for articulation with the radius is known as the seat of the ulna and lies on the circumference of the head of the ulna. The seat of the ulna encompasses two thirds to three quarters of the perimeter of the ulnar head and is covered with articular cartilage [38,77]. Like the radius's articular surface for the ulna, the ulna's articular surface for the radius varies in shape and curvature [65,77]. The ulna is generally flatter than the reciprocating surface of the radius in the anterior–posterior direction, allowing gliding motions between the two bones and providing little inherent stability [34,77].

The distal aspect of the ulna consists of three parts, the ulnar styloid process, the fovea, and the pole (Fig. 14.5). The ulnar styloid process is a medial bony projection, easily palpated on the ulnar aspect of the wrist with the forearm supinated. The fovea is a roughened depression at the base of the styloid process on its radial aspect. It provides attachment for the apex of the fibrocartilaginous disc. The pole is

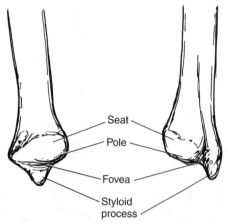

Figure 14.5: Head of the ulna. The circumference of the head is known as the *seat of the ulna* and is the articular surface for the distal radioulnar joint. The distal end of the ulna consists of the styloid process, the fovea, and the pole, which articulates with the fibrocartilaginous disc.

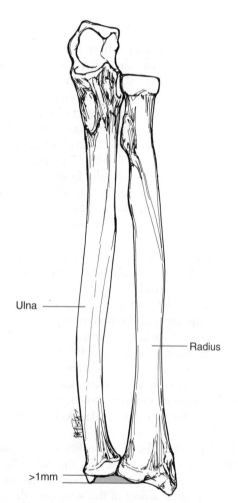

Figure 14.6: Ulnar variance is a greater than 1.0-mm difference between the articular surfaces of the distal radius and distal ulna.

a U-shaped articular surface for articulation with the fibrocartilaginous disc. It lies radial to both the styloid process and fovea.

The relative lengths of the radius and ulna are variable [29]. The difference between the lengths of these bones is called **ulnar variance** and is described as abnormal when there is more than a 1-mm difference in lengths of the distal radius and ulna measured at their distal articular surfaces (*Fig. 14.6*). Ulnar variance is determined by an individual's age and genetic traits as well as by external forces at the wrist or pathology at the elbow. Although ulnar variance is described as a static alignment, the relative lengths of the radius and ulna also change with forearm position. Pronation results in a functional shortening of the radius as the ulna moves distally, and supination causes a functional lengthening of the radius as the ulna moves proximally [38,61]. This change in relative lengths of the radius and ulna affects the tension in the interosseous membrane during pronation and supination [38]. Supination generates greater tension in the interosseous membrane than pronation as the radius moves distally [30]. Individuals with a negative ulnar variance (a shorter ulna) exhibit increased ulnar deviation range of motion (ROM) at the wrist compared with those with a radius and ulna of equal length [128].

Clinical Relevance

ULNAR VARIANCE: *A positive ulnar variance in which the distal articular surface of the ulna extends more than 1 mm beyond the radius is associated with degenerative changes of the ulna, the fibrocartilaginous disc, and some carpal bones [29]. The increased relative length of the ulna may produce abnormal loading of the ulnar aspect of the wrist joint (ulnocarpal impaction) since the ulna projects distally beyond the radius. Conversely, a decrease in the relative length of the ulna (negative ulnar variance) is likely to decrease the stability of the lunate, leading to an increase in shear forces, microtrauma, and perhaps eventually to avascular necrosis of the lunate (Kienböck's disease) (Fig. 14.7). Negative ulnar variance may also result in increased loading on the radial side of the wrist [113,127].*

Positive and negative ulnar variance alignments in individuals with no history of wrist trauma are associated with differences in mineralization of the subchondral bone of the distal radius, supporting the notion of altered loading patterns with ulnar variance deformities [42].

Positive ulnar variance is reported in young female gymnasts who subject their wrists to repeated loading, apparently inducing microtrauma leading to premature closure of the radial growth plate. Similarly, patients with distal radial fractures or who have undergone radial head

(continued)

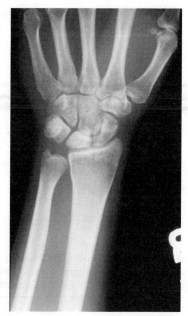

Figure 14.7: Negative ulnar variance. Negative ulnar variance increases the shear forces on the lunate.

(Continued)
resections may exhibit positive ulnar variance as the radius migrates proximally [29]. These patients may be prone to more degenerative changes in the ulna, the medial carpal bones, and the intervening disc. In cases of ulnar variance, the patient may need to learn joint protection strategies to reduce the magnitude of the loads sustained at the wrist.

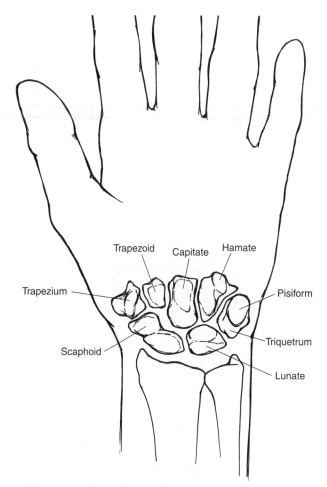

Figure 14.8: The eight carpal bones. An exploded view of the volar aspect of the eight carpal bones reveals their positions in the proximal and distal rows of the carpus.

Carpal Bones

The carpus is composed of eight bones that are arranged roughly into two rows, proximal and distal (*Fig. 14.8*). The proximal row contains the scaphoid, lunate, triquetrum, and pisiform. The distal row consists of the trapezium, trapezoid, capitate, and hamate. The scaphoid appears to extend across both rows, giving the appearance of the proximal row curving around the capitate. As a whole, the carpal bones form an arch, convex dorsally and concave volarly (*Fig. 14.9*). The arch is transformed to an enclosed carpal tunnel by the transverse carpal ligament, also known as the flexor retinaculum. This ligament spans the carpal arch, attaching to the scaphoid and trapezium on the radial side and to the pisiform and hamate on its ulnar aspect.

The proximal surface of the carpus is biconvex, articulating with the reciprocal biconcavity of the radius and triangular fibrocartilage (*Fig. 14.10*). The distal surface of the carpus is much more irregular, forming multiple articular surfaces for

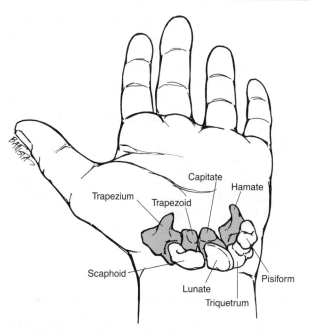

Figure 14.9: View of the carpus from its proximal end. The carpal bones form an arch with an anterior concavity. This arch is the carpal arch of the hand.

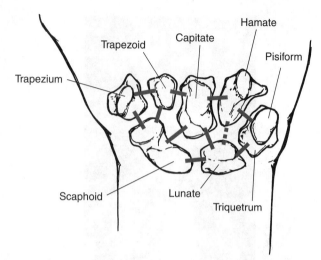

Figure 14.11: The articular surfaces between adjacent carpal bones vary considerably among the carpal bones and influence the direction and magnitude of movement between adjacent carpal bones.

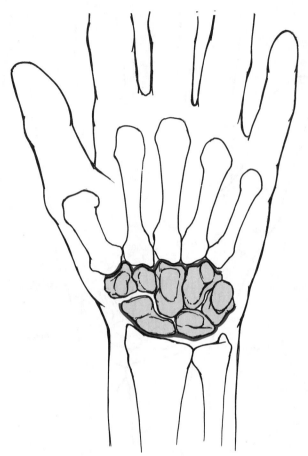

Figure 14.10: The proximal and distal articular surfaces of the carpus exhibit two very different types of surfaces. The proximal surface is biconvex, and the distal surface is irregular with many different articular facets.

are varied. Its articular surface for the radius is convex, while its articular surface for the capitate is concave. These articulations allow significant mobility between the articulating surfaces. However, the surfaces for articulation with the lunate, trapezium, and trapezoid are generally flat. These surfaces provide considerably less mobility, since they allow mostly translation between adjacent surfaces. The scaphoid tubercle lies on the radial side of the volar surface of the scaphoid and provides attachment for the transverse carpal ligament as well as for some of the intrinsic muscles of the thumb. It is palpable just proximal to the thenar eminence when the wrist is extended.

the proximal surfaces of the articulating metacarpal bones. These variations in articular surfaces result in considerable variety in the motion and stability available throughout the carpus. The articular surfaces and surrounding ligaments provide the essential support of the carpal arch and individual articulations. The tendons of the forearm muscles crossing the wrist also provide substantial indirect support to the carpus [82,136].

Although the eight bones of the carpus may function together as units, each bone possesses unique characteristics that help explain the normal mechanics of the wrist and hand as well as some of the abnormal mechanics that result from trauma or disease. The articulations among the carpal bones are depicted in *Fig. 14.11*. Each bone has a unique position within the carpus, with articulations that contribute to the stability and mobility of each bone.

SCAPHOID (ALSO KNOWN AS THE NAVICULAR)

The scaphoid is the largest carpal bone of the proximal row. It is somewhat elongated, with its long axis projecting radially, distally, and volarly. The scaphoid articulates with five other bones, although the shapes of its articular surfaces

Clinical Relevance

SCAPHOID FRACTURE AND AVASCULAR NECROSIS:
*The proximal and distal portions of the scaphoid, known as the **proximal** and **distal poles** are joined together by a slightly narrowed region known as the waist of the scaphoid. This is the site of most scaphoid fractures, the most common fracture of the carpal bones [40]. Fractures of the scaphoid usually occur as a result of impact between the dorsal surface of the scaphoid and the dorsal border of the distal radius. Such impacts result from forceful hyperextension of the wrist. As with distal radius fractures, the typical mechanism for a scaphoid fracture is a fall on an outstretched hand [142]. Reports suggest that impacts with the wrist in more than 95° of hyperextension result in scaphoid fractures, while impacts with less wrist hyperextension are more likely to result in distal radial fractures [137,138].*

The dorsal nonarticular aspect of the scaphoid is also the primary location of the nutrient foramina through which the scaphoid receives its blood supply. However, in approximately 13–14% of individuals the nutrient foramina are located distal to the waist of the scaphoid [40,141]. A scaphoid fracture at

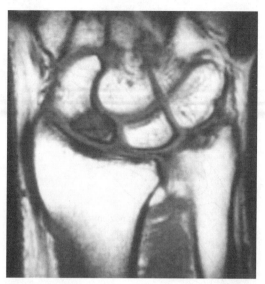

Figure 14.12: Avascular necrosis of the scaphoid following fracture. Coronal magnetic resonance imagery (MRI) of the wrist (T1-weighted) shows a dark signal replacing the normal bright marrow signal of the proximal pole of the scaphoid, indicating necrosis of the proximal pole. (Reprinted with permission from Chew FS, Maldjian C, Leffler SG: Musculoskeletal Imaging, A Teaching File. Philadelphia: Lippincott Williams & Wilkins, 1999.)

*the waist of the scaphoid in an individual whose nutrient foramina are located only in the distal pole of the scaphoid leaves the proximal fragment without a blood supply. **Avascular necrosis** of the proximal fragment is a common complication of scaphoid fractures, delaying or preventing union of the fracture (Fig. 14.12). The scaphoid is palpable in the floor of the anatomical snuffbox (Fig. 14.13). Tenderness on palpation here in the presence of a history of trauma to the thumb or wrist indicates the need for further assessment to rule out a scaphoid fracture or avascular necrosis from a previously undiagnosed fracture [138].*

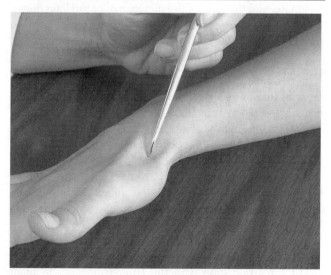

Figure 14.13: Palpation of the scaphoid. The scaphoid is palpable in the floor of the snuff box.

LUNATE

The lunate receives its name from its crescent shape, convex proximally to articulate with the radius and triangular fibrocartilage and concave distally to articulate with the head of the capitate. Its other articular surfaces are relatively flat, allowing mostly translation between the articular surfaces. The lunate is located in the center of the proximal row of carpal bones and plays an important role in stabilizing the entire carpus. Palpation is possible just distal and slightly ulnar to the dorsal tubercle of the radius with the wrist slightly flexed [55,127]. The dorsal tubercle is just proximal to the scapholunate joint line, or interval. Tenderness in the interval suggests an injury to the scapholunate ligament.

Since no muscles attach to it, stability of the lunate within the carpal arch depends primarily upon the shape of the articular surfaces and upon the surrounding ligamentous structures [123]. Unlike most of the carpal bones, the volar surface of the lunate is broader than its dorsal surface.

Clinical Relevance

LUNATE DISLOCATION: *The shape of the lunate may explain why dislocations of the lunate typically occur in the volar direction. The narrower dorsal surface can slip volarly with little obstruction, while the broader volar surface is less likely to protrude dorsally. The lunate is the second most frequently injured carpal bone [40]. The lunate is particularly susceptible to avascular necrosis (Kienböck's disease) (Fig. 14.14). One study reports that about 8% of the 75 cadaver limbs examined had a lunate that received its blood supply only from the volar surface [40]. The authors suggest that such a supply can be disrupted easily by injury.*

TRIQUETRUM

The triquetrum is small, and much of its surface is covered by ligaments [12]. It articulates with the fibrocartilaginous disc on its proximal and ulnar surface during ulnar deviation of the wrist. It attaches to the hamate by a concave–convex surface, allowing significant movement between the two bones. The triquetrum is palpable on the ulnar side of the wrist during radial deviation.

PISIFORM

The pisiform is named for its pealike shape. It sits anteriorly on the triquetrum and provides attachment for the tendon of the flexor carpi ulnaris muscle, improving the mechanical advantage of this muscle. The pisiform also provides attachment for the distal continuation of the flexor carpi

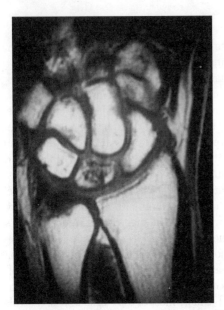

Figure 14.14: MRI reveals avascular necrosis of lunate (Kienböck's disease).

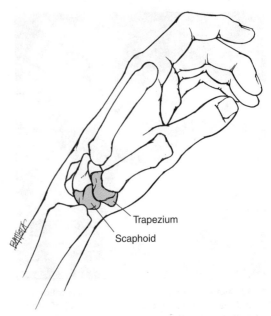

Figure 14.15: Position of the thumb. The thumb is positioned slightly anterior to the palm because the trapezium articulates anteriorly on the scaphoid.

ulnaris, the pisohamate ligament [100,141]. It provides attachments for many other important ligamentous and muscular structures of the wrist and hand, including the transverse carpal ligament. The pisiform is easily palpated in the heel of the hand just distal to the distal wrist crease.

TRAPEZIUM (FORMERLY KNOWN AS THE GREATER MULTANGULAR)

The trapezium boasts a saddle-shaped facet for articulation with the base of the metacarpal bone of the thumb. However, its remaining articular surfaces are flat or only slightly curved. The tubercle of the trapezium is located proximally on the anterior surface and provides attachment for the transverse carpal ligament. It is palpable at the base of the thenar eminence, distal to the distal wrist crease. It is important to note that the trapezium articulates volarly with the scaphoid. This articulation places the trapezium out of the plane of the other carpal bones of the distal row. Consequently, the thumb lies at about a 45° angle with the index finger [25,127] (Fig. 14.15). The trapezium is palpated radially and dorsally at the articulation of the trapezium and the metacarpal of the thumb.

TRAPEZOID (FORMERLY KNOWN AS THE LESSER MULTANGULAR)

The trapezoid is one of the smallest carpal bones and is covered almost entirely by flat articular surfaces. It provides the primary articulation for the metacarpal bone of the index finger, and it is surrounded by bones on all sides. Therefore, it contributes to the stable base of the index finger [138]. This stable base is critical to the role of the index finger

during powerful pinch, which is discussed in greater detail in Chapter 19. The trapezoid is not palpable.

CAPITATE

The capitate is the largest carpal bone and is located in the center of the carpus, acting as a keystone of the carpal arch, with many of the ligaments supporting the wrist attaching to it. The capitate is divided into a proximal head and a distal body, joined by a neck. The head is approximately half a sphere and projects into the concavity created by the lunate and scaphoid. The other articular surfaces for the carpal and metacarpal bones are flat [12,104] or slightly curved [141]. The capitate is in line with the dorsal tubercle of the radius, the lunate, and the base of the metacarpal of the long finger. It is palpable proximal to the metacarpal bone, with the wrist flexed slightly.

HAMATE

The hamate also is a large carpal bone and is characterized by a large projection or hook on its distal anterior surface. The hook, or hamulus, gives this carpal bone its name. The hook projects volarly and radially so that its tip points toward the radial side of the hand. The tip is palpated easily by placing the interphalangeal joint (IP) of the palpating thumb on the pisiform, pointing toward the subject's thumb web space. The hook of the hamate lies directly under the tip of the palpating thumb [55] (Fig. 14.16). This hook provides the fourth and final attachment of the transverse carpal ligament (Fig. 14.17). The proximal segment of the hamate is convex for articulation with the triquetrum and, in ulnar deviation, with the ulnar side of the lunate. The distal facets are flatter, allowing translation between adjacent surfaces.

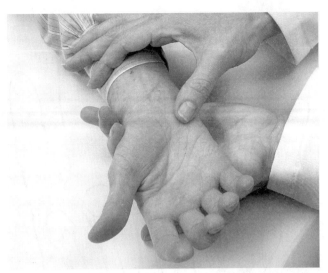

Figure 14.16: Palpation of the hook of the hamate. To palpate the hook of the hamate, place the interphalangeal joint of the palpating thumb on the subject's pisiform, pointing toward the subject's thumb web space. The hook of the hamate lies directly under the tip of the thumb.

Metacarpals

The metacarpal bones are miniature long bones with common characteristics among all of the digits. Each metacarpal consists of a proximal base, a shaft, and a distal head. The bases are the most varied of the metacarpals' characteristics among the five digits (*Fig. 14.18*). Their shapes reflect the

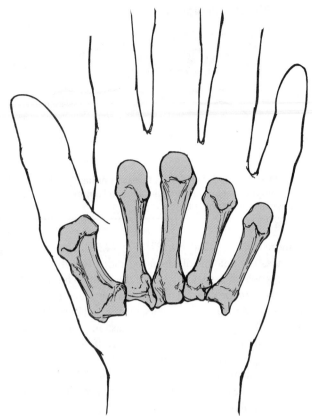

Figure 14.18: The shapes of the fingers' metacarpal bases are quite varied and influence the amount of motion that is available at each articulation.

articulations between each metacarpal and corresponding carpal bone(s). The base of the metacarpal of the thumb is characterized by its saddle-shaped articular surface allowing the distinctive opposition motion available in the human thumb [138]. The base of the metacarpals of the index and long fingers have rather flattened facets for articulation with their respective carpal bones. However, the metacarpal of the ring finger has a slightly more curved facet for the hamate, and the base of the metacarpal of the little finger has a somewhat saddle-shaped facet for articulation with the hamate. This variation in the bases of the metacarpal bones of the fingers produces distinct differences in the mobility of their carpometacarpal (CMC) articulations. The CMC articulations of the index and long fingers exhibit almost no motion, while the articulation between the metacarpal bone of the little finger and hamate is quite mobile.

The heads of the metacarpals of the fingers are almost perfectly round from volar to dorsal and are more curved than the bases of phalanges to which they attach [9] (*Fig. 14.19*). The articular cartilage on the heads of the metacarpals covers the volar and distal surfaces and extends slightly onto the dorsal surface, providing an articular surface for a small amount of hyperextension at the metacarpophalangeal (MCP) joints.

In the ulnar and radial directions, the articular surfaces of the metacarpal heads are convex but somewhat asymmetrical

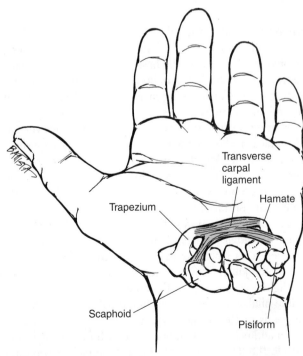

Figure 14.17: The transverse carpal ligament attaches on the four "pillars" of the carpus: the scaphoid, trapezium, pisiform, and hamate.

Base of proximal phalanx

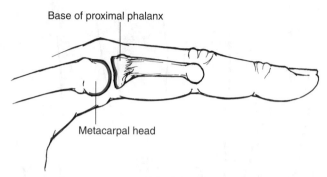

Metacarpal head

Figure 14.19: A sagittal view of a metacarpal head and articulating phalangeal base. The metacarpal head is more curved than its respective phalangeal base.

and more variable [45,48,86,127] (*Fig. 14.20*). This asymmetry influences the amount of ulnar and radial deviation that can occur at each of the MCP joints of the digits. The metacarpal heads also are broader in the radioulnar direction on their volar surfaces than on their dorsal surfaces [138]. This variation in width contributes to the decrease in radioulnar mobility of the MCP joints when the joints are flexed.

The head of the thumb's metacarpal is flatter and broader in the radioulnar direction than those of the other metacarpals [63] (*Fig. 14.21*). This flattening reduces the radioulnar motion available at the thumb's MCP joint. However, the shape of the head of the thumb's metacarpal is quite variable, which may help to explain the wide variation of available motion at this joint reported in the literature [17,138,141].

Phalanges

The phalanges, like the metacarpals, possess bases, heads, and shafts (*Fig. 14.22*). There are 14 phalanges in each hand, 3 in each finger (proximal, middle, and distal), and 2 in the

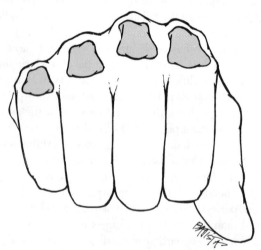

Figure 14.20: A frontal view of the metacarpal heads of the fingers reveals asymmetry among the fingers. The view also demonstrates that the width of the metacarpal heads is narrower at their dorsal borders than at their volar surfaces. This difference contributes to the decrease in mobility in radial and ulnar deviation when the MCP joints are flexed.

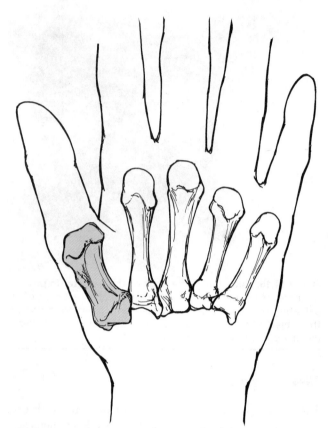

Figure 14.21: The head of the thumb's metacarpal is broader and flatter in the radial and ulnar direction than the metacarpal heads of the fingers.

thumb (proximal and distal). The phalanges decrease in size from proximal to distal. The bases of the proximal phalanges are biconcave, although the base of the proximal phalanx of the thumb is flatter in the radioulnar direction than those of the fingers. The articulating surface of each base of the middle and distal phalanges is almost a mirror image of the articulating head of the respective phalanx. However, as in the metacarpal bones, the bases of the phalanges are slightly flatter than the articular surfaces of the heads of the adjacent phalanx [1]. The heads of the proximal and middle phalanges are convex in a dorsal–volar direction, with a prominent central groove so that each head takes on a pulley, or trochlear, shape similar to that of the elbow [17]. The ulnar and radial aspects of the trochlea are also known as condyles. This trochlear shape limits the radioulnar movement at the joints. The two condyles of the proximal phalanx are slightly asymmetrical; the condyles of the heads of the middle phalanges are more symmetrical [76]. The shapes of the heads of the phalanges affect the precise direction of flexion and extension that occurs at each finger [72,138]. As a result, the fingers converge toward the base of the thumb during finger flexion. The heads of the distal phalanges narrow to a nonarticulating point distally and provide an anchor for the fingernails.

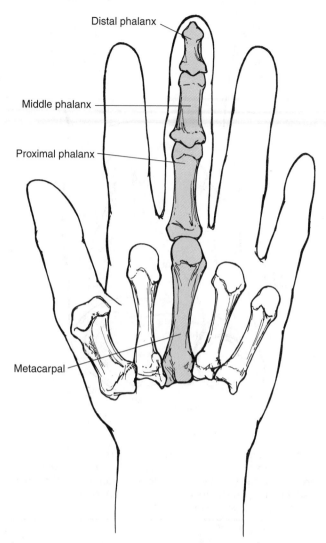

Distal phalanx

Middle phalanx

Proximal phalanx

Metacarpal

Figure 14.22: Dorsal view of the phalanges. Like the metacarpal bones, the phalanges possess a base, a shaft, and a head. The heads of the proximal and middle phalanges have a distinct trochlear shape.

Sesamoid Bones

Typically there are two sesamoid bones, one in each of the tendons of the flexor pollicis brevis and the adductor pollicis. Similar sesamoid bones are frequently found in the tendons anterior to the MCP joint of the little finger, less frequently at the index finger, and only infrequently at the other fingers [141]. These bones alter the lines of pull of the tendons in which they insert, thus improving the muscles' mechanics.

Bony Landmarks

The wrist and hand are composed of more than 27 bones, each with its own unique characteristics. The bony landmarks that can be palpated in the forearm and hand are listed below:

- Radial styloid process
- Volar ridge of distal radius

- Dorsal tubercle of radius
- Ulnar crest
- Ulnar head
- Styloid process of ulna
- Dorsal surface of the scaphoid
- Scaphoid tubercle
- Dorsal surface of lunate
- Triquetrum
- Trapezium
- Dorsal surface of capitate
- Pisiform bone
- Hook of the hamate
- Shafts and the margins of the bases and heads of the metacarpal bones and phalanges

As demonstrated already in the preceding chapters on the shoulder and elbow, the shape of each bone and its articular surfaces directly affects the motion and stability of the joints of the hand. The following section presents the joints, their supporting structures, and the available motion of the wrist and hand.

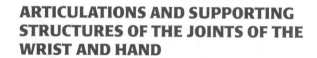

ARTICULATIONS AND SUPPORTING STRUCTURES OF THE JOINTS OF THE WRIST AND HAND

The wrist and hand possess multiple articulations that together provide the dexterity of movement exhibited by the hand. Each of the joints is presented below with a full discussion of the articulations, supporting mechanism, and motion available. Although the carpus is involved in four distinct joints, the radiocarpal, midcarpal, and the two CMC joints, it represents a distinct functional unit as well. A discussion is presented on the stability and mobility of the carpus as a whole and those structures that contribute to its support.

Distal Radioulnar Joint

The distal radioulnar joint has been described as part of a compound joint with the proximal radioulnar joint [46]. Together these two joints are the source of pronation and supination of the forearm [38,46,65]. The distal radioulnar joint [33,65] allows the large excursions of forearm pronation and supination as well as ulnar deviation of the wrist that enhance the manipulating skills of the hand [2]. The distal radioulnar joint also allows transmission of loads from the hand and radius onto the ulna [115]. Resection of the head of the ulna eliminates most of the load transmission so that most of the axial load is borne through the radius. Although the distal radioulnar joint is not part of the wrist joint proper, it is important to the normal function of the wrist and frequently is implicated in wrist pathology [33,34,38,61,68]. A thorough awareness of the joint and surrounding tissues is essential for a complete understanding of both the elbow and the wrist.

The distal radioulnar joint is a synovial joint, and the contributing surfaces of the radius and ulna are both covered by articular cartilage. It is classified as a pivot joint. However, there also is considerable gliding between the head of the ulna and the sigmoid notch on the radius [61,77]. One reason for the extensive gliding that occurs between the radius and ulna at the distal radioulnar joint is the differences in the curvatures of each articular surface. The radius of curvature of the ulnar head is shorter than that of the sigmoid notch, indicating that the ulnar head is more curved than the sigmoid notch [34,68,77] (*Fig. 14.23*). The difference in curvatures between these two surfaces encourages gliding motion at the joint.

Clinical Relevance

ULNAR HEAD RESECTION AND ARTHROPLASTY:
Patients with rheumatoid arthritis and wrist involvement sometimes develop pain and even instability at the distal radioulnar joint, making hand function difficult and painful. In a painful but stable wrist, resection of the ulnar head (a Darrach procedure) may reduce the pain and restore function. However, in unstable wrists the patient may have better pain relief and functional improvement with an ulnar head arthroplasty.

SUPPORTING STRUCTURES OF THE DISTAL RADIOULNAR JOINT

The shapes of the articular surfaces of the distal radioulnar joint contribute little to the stability of the distal radioulnar joint [112]. The stability of the joint comes from the surrounding soft tissue structures. The nonmuscular supporting structures of the distal radioulnar joint are the joint capsule and the triangular fibrocartilage complex (TFCC), which consists of the triangular fibrocartilage, dorsal radioulnar ligament, volar radioulnar ligament, ulnar collateral ligament complex, and the meniscus homologue. Although the ulnar collateral ligament plays an important role in stabilizing the distal radioulnar joint, it also contributes to the support of the wrist [33,61]. Therefore, it is discussed later in this chapter as part of the supporting structure for the radiocarpal joint and carpus as a whole. The interosseous membrane and annular ligaments also provide support to the distal radioulnar joint and are described in detail in Chapter 11 with the bones and joints of the elbow. They bind the radius and ulna together proximally and along their shafts, supporting both the superior and inferior radioulnar joints [135].

The capsule of the distal radioulnar joint attaches to the periphery of the sigmoid notch of the radius, the proximal and lateral borders of the seat of the ulna, and the borders of the triangular fibrocartilage (*Fig. 14.24*). The capsule projects a small pocket proximally between the radius and the ulna, creating an L-shaped joint space [104]. The distal aspect of the capsule is more robust and may help stabilize the radioulnar

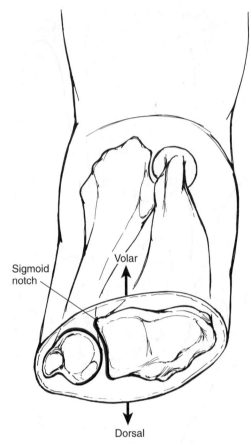

Figure 14.23: Curvature of the sigmoid notch. A view of the distal surface of the radius and ulna reveals that the radius of curvature of the sigmoid notch is longer than that of the ulnar head. In other words, the ulnar head is more curved than its articular surface on the radius.

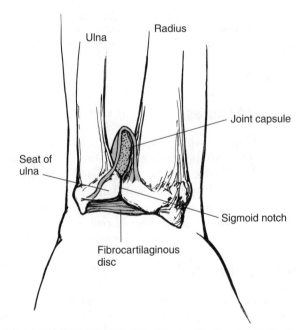

Figure 14.24: The capsule of the distal radioulnar joint attaches to the periphery of the sigmoid notch, the seat of the ulna, and the borders of the fibrocartilaginous disc.

articulation in an axial direction [68]. Isolated sectioning of the joint capsule produces significant distal radioulnar joint instability in cadaver models [134]. The capsule is quite thin anteriorly but has folds that unfold during supination to allow full ROM. Although the capsule is thicker posteriorly, it has fewer folds than its anterior counterpart.

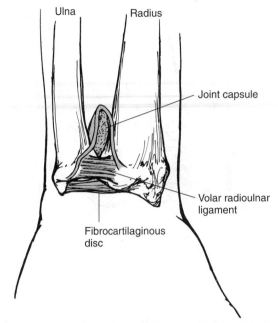

Figure 14.25: The volar radioulnar ligament blends with the capsule of the distal radioulnar joint on the volar surface of the joint. The dorsal radioulnar ligament does the same on the dorsal surface.

Clinical Relevance

TIGHTNESS OF THE DISTAL RADIOULNAR JOINT CAPSULE AND LIMITED PRONATION AND SUPINA-TION ROM: *The capsule of the distal radioulnar joint is frequently described as weak, providing little resistance to the normal limits of pronation and supination ROM [34]. However, a clinical study of nine patients suggests that an abnormal joint capsule may contribute to pathological limitations of ROM [68]. The study reports that capsulectomies in these patients with limited pronation and supination without any pathology of the TFCC resulted in increased pronation and supination ROM. The authors note that scarring of the capsule and adhesions in the volar (anterior) folds were visible in the capsules of these patients and may have contributed to the limited ROM. The adhesions are probably similar to those that can form in the folds of the glenohumeral joint in adhesive capsulitis (Chapter 8). These data suggest that the capsule of the distal radioulnar joint may play a part in decreased pronation and supination ROM in some patients. Treatments to stretch or release the capsule may prove beneficial in some patients.*

The TFCC is critical to the function of the distal radioulnar joint [112]. It performs several functions including

- Stabilizing the distal radioulnar joint
- Cushioning the ulna on the carpus
- Allowing axial loading of the ulnar aspect of the forearm
- Increasing the articular surface for the carpus
- Stabilizing the ulnar side of the carpus itself

The dorsal and volar radioulnar ligaments of the TFCC blend with the joint capsule but are histologically distinct from it [68]. They attach to the dorsal and volar surfaces of the sigmoid notch, respectively, and both have some attachment to the triangular fibrocartilage (*Fig. 14.25*). These two ligaments provide critical support to the distal radioulnar joint, but the role each plays in limiting normal pronation and supination remains controversial [34,46,61,77,112]. Some authors report that the volar radioulnar ligament is tight in pronation and the dorsal radioulnar ligament is tight in supination [34,46]. Others report exactly the opposite; that is, the dorsal radioulnar ligament is tight in pronation, and the volar radioulnar ligament is tight in supination [77,112,133]. The complex nature of the movement between the radius and the ulna during pronation and supination may

actually justify both conclusions. As explained in Chapter 11, during pronation with the hand fixed in space, the ulna glides radially as the radius rolls into pronation [30]. It appears that both ligaments participate together to stabilize the distal radioulnar joint in both pronation and supination by limiting both the rotation and the translation of the radius and ulna [32,38].

The triangular fibrocartilaginous disc fills the space between the ulna and the carpus. As its name indicates, the disc is shaped like a triangle, with its base attached to the distal border of the sigmoid notch of the radius (*Fig. 14.26*). The apex of the disc is attached by loose connective tissue to the base of the ulna's styloid process and fovea. The disc is concave on both its proximal and distal surfaces for articulation with the pole of the ulna proximally and with the lunate and triquetrum distally. The central portion of the disc is quite thin and actually may be perforated in older adults, creating a communication between the distal radioulnar and the radiocarpal joints. The triangular fibrocartilage serves as a shock absorber between the ulna and the carpus. It helps distribute any load transmitted by the hand to the ulna and may contribute to the axial and medial–lateral stability of the distal radioulnar joint [116]. However, excision of up to two thirds of the disc in cadavers seems to have little effect on the stability of the distal radioulnar joint [87].

The meniscus homologue is the soft tissue that runs from the dorsal border of the radius medially to the volar surface of the medial aspect of the triquetrum [61]. Histological examination reveals that the meniscus homologue is vascularized loose connective tissue rather than fibrocartilage or ligamentous tissue [38]. Its functional significance is unclear.

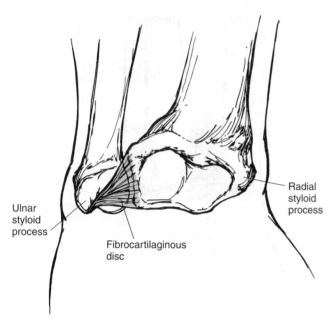

Figure 14.26: The fibrocartilaginous disc between the ulna and the carpus. A distal view of the radius and ulna reveals that the fibrocartilaginous disc between the ulna and the carpus is triangular and attaches to the distal border of the sigmoid notch of the radius and to the base of the ulna's styloid process and fovea.

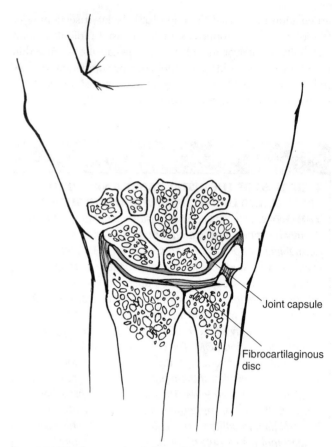

Figure 14.27: The capsule of the radiocarpal joint attaches to the distal radius, the fibrocartilaginous disc, and the proximal row of carpal bones.

In conclusion, there are several supporting structures that are essential to the stability of the distal radioulnar joint [67,112]. Despite the relative absence of stability imparted by the articular surfaces, the connective tissue surrounding the joint confers considerable stability to the distal radioulnar joint. Dislocation of the distal radioulnar joint appears to occur only with complete disruption of the TFCC [112,133].

MOTIONS OF THE DISTAL RADIOULNAR JOINT

The motion of the distal radioulnar joint is intimately tied to the motion of the proximal radioulnar joint, the two joints essentially acting as a single compound joint. Thus pronation and supination occur simultaneously at the two joints. Values of normal pronation and supination ROM found in the literature are presented in Table 11.1 in Chapter 11. However, the motion at the distal radioulnar joint is more complex than a simple pivot around a fixed point. As noted in Chapter 11, pronation can occur around a hand fixed in space or around a hand that moves to a new location in space (see *Fig. 11.28*). In the latter case, the radius rotates about the ulna, with an axis close to the fovea of the ulna. However, when the hand is fixed in space as when the hand is grasping a doorknob or turning a screwdriver, both the ulna and radius move during pronation. In this instance, the axis of rotation is located more laterally in the ulna. As the radius rotates about the ulna during pronation with the hand fixed, the ulna moves dorsally and radially about the radius [30,127,139] (see video in Chapter 11). This gliding motion is allowed by the incongruities of the joint surfaces of the distal radioulnar joint.

Joints of the Wrist

The wrist is the junction of the hand and forearm. Although the radiocarpal joint is the most familiar joint of the wrist, motion of the wrist also comes from the midcarpal and intercarpal joints. Each of the joints is described below, including a discussion of the articular surfaces and individual joint capsules. The stability and mobility of the joints are so interdependent that discussion of the extracapsular supports and the motions of the joints can occur together. The joint surfaces and the individual joint capsules are presented first. The extracapsular supports for the region are discussed as a unit. Individual joint contributions to overall wrist motions are discussed after all of the joints are reviewed.

RADIOCARPAL JOINT

The radiocarpal joint is the articulation between the radius and the proximal row of carpal bones, but only the scaphoid and the lunate articulate directly with the radius. The triquetrum articulates with the distal surface of the triangular fibrocartilage. The capsule of the radiocarpal joint encloses all of these surfaces.

The distal surface of the radius with the adjoining triangular fibrocartilage is biconcave; the proximal surface of the proximal row of carpal bones is biconvex. The bony articulating surfaces are covered by articular cartilage. Although the reciprocal articulating surfaces appear congruent, contact between the scaphoid and lunate and the radius is neither constant nor uniform [94]. Contact involves approximately 20% of the surface area when a load of less than 25 lb is applied. A load of almost 50 lb across the wrist increases the contact area to a maximum of 40% by causing deformation of the articular cartilage. In addition, the area of contact is greater between the scaphoid and radius than between the lunate and radius. Thus the radiocarpal joint demonstrates less congruency between the articulating surfaces than is expected of a classic biaxial joint. While the overall shape of the surfaces of the radiocarpal joint are consistent with a simple biaxial unit, there is significant evidence that the individual carpal bones play unique individual roles in the mechanics of the radiocarpal joint [28,60,69,96].

The radiocarpal joint has little inherent stability imparted by the shapes of the articular surfaces. Instead it is supported on all four sides of the joint by a fibrous capsule and ligaments. The capsule of the radiocarpal joint surrounds and attaches to the dorsal, radial, and volar borders of the articular surface of the radius and to the dorsal, ulnar, and volar edges of the triangular fibrocartilage. Thus the triangular fibrocartilage forms the floor of the distal radioulnar joint and the roof of the ulnar aspect of the radiocarpal joint. The capsule attaches distally to the periphery of the proximal articular surfaces of the scaphoid, lunate, and triquetrum (*Fig. 14.27*).

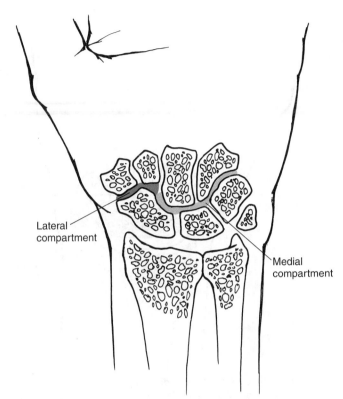

Figure 14.28: The midcarpal joint has two distinct regions, the medial and lateral compartments.

MIDCARPAL JOINT

The midcarpal joint is the junction between the proximal and distal rows of carpal bones. All of the articular surfaces are covered with typical articular cartilage. The joint has two distinct regions encased by a single joint capsule (*Fig. 14.28*). The medial compartment is composed mainly of a proximal concavity formed by the scaphoid, lunate, and triquetrum and a distal convexity formed by the capitate and hamate. This portion of the joint functions as a biaxial or condyloid structure [62]. The lateral portion of the joint is composed of the flatter articular facets of the distal scaphoid and the trapezium and trapezoid bones. This lateral portion is described as either a saddle joint [141] or a plane joint [62]. Regardless of the classification of the joint, the motions between adjacent carpal bones of the two rows are complex and are discussed later in this chapter.

The irregular surface of the midcarpal joint leads to an uneven distribution of the loads across the joint surface [94]. Data collected on cadaver specimens suggest that the greatest load is transmitted through the scaphoid–capitate articulation, and the least is through the triquetrum–hamate connection. As in the radiocarpal joint, light loads appear to be distributed through only a small area of the articular surface (slightly more than 25%). The area of contact increases to approximately 35% with heavy loads.

The irregularity of the articular surfaces of the midcarpal joint provides some inherent stability to the joint, but ligamentous support remains the primary source of stability. The midcarpal joint is supported by its capsule as well as by the extrinsic and intrinsic ligaments of the wrist and carpus. It is important to recognize that although the midcarpal joint is anatomically distinct from the radiocarpal joint, these two joints are structurally and functionally interdependent, so that if one structure fails, the effects are felt throughout the wrist. The capsule of the midcarpal joint is irregular because it encloses the joint space between the proximal and distal rows of carpal bones and also sends projections proximally and distally between the adjacent carpal bones of each row (*Fig. 14.29*). Therefore, the capsule of the midcarpal joint creates joint spaces for each of the intercarpal articulations except the triquetropisiform articulation, which usually has its own joint capsule and joint space [141].

INTERCARPAL JOINTS

The intercarpal joints are the articulations between adjacent carpal bones within each row. These articulations are synovial and are encapsulated by extensions of the capsule of the midcarpal joint. They are regarded as plane joints. These articulations are stabilized by the joint capsule and by the extrinsic and intrinsic ligaments described in the next section. The

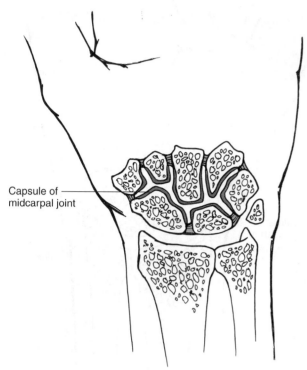

Figure 14.29: The capsule of the midcarpal joint is very irregular, extending proximally and distally into the intercarpal articulations.

Capsule of midcarpal joint

[37,39]. Changes in the dimensions of the carpal tunnel after CTR are particularly apparent during activities against a load [39]. The clinical importance of these changes in the carpal tunnel is unknown. Although CTR often provides substantial relief of pain in patients with CTS, the altered transverse carpal ligament may contribute to instability of the hand and pain, creating functional difficulties. The clinician needs to appreciate the mechanical and functional implications of this surgical intervention.

EXTRACAPSULAR SUPPORTING STRUCTURES OF THE WRIST

Although there is considerable variation in the literature in the names used to identify the extracapsular supporting structures of the wrist, there is a broad acceptance of their general organization. The ligaments of the wrist can be divided into two large categories: extrinsic and intrinsic. The extrinsic

transverse carpal ligament, or flexor retinaculum, is an accessory ligament that supports the entire carpal arch. It attaches medially to the pisiform bone and hook of the hamate. The lateral portion of the transverse carpal ligament attaches to the tubercles of the trapezium and scaphoid. The entire transverse carpal ligament bridges the carpal arch, creating the carpal tunnel helping to stabilize the arch and the contents of the tunnel. It is pulled taut in both maximum pronation and maximum supination [37]. Surgical release of the transverse carpal ligament is a common treatment for **carpal tunnel syndrome (CTS),** in which the contents of the carpal tunnel including the median nerve are compressed by swelling within the carpal tunnel.

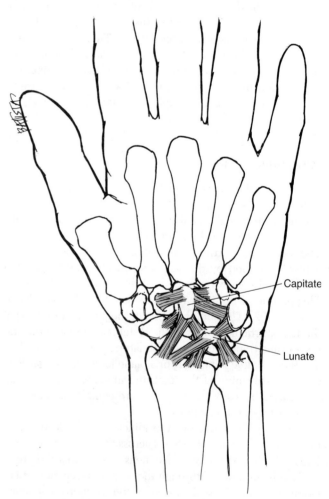

Figure 14.30: General organization of the ligaments of the wrist. Most of the proximal ligaments of the wrist converge on the lunate, and most of the distal ligaments of the wrist converge on the capitate.

Capitate

Lunate

Clinical Relevance

CARPAL TUNNEL RELEASE (CTR): *One treatment to relieve the pressure on the median nerve is a carpal tunnel release performed by cutting the transverse carpal ligament. Surgical approaches include complete transection of the ligament, Z-plasties that retain some continuity, and complete transection with ligamentous reconstruction [18]. Authors report an increase in the width of the carpal arch at rest following CTR and also an increase in maximum width of the arch when a supination torque is applied to the hand* ligaments have attachments to the radius, ulna, or the TFCC, as well as to the carpal bones. The intrinsic ligaments are contained entirely within the carpus. Most of the ligaments of the wrist are found on either the palmar (volar) or dorsal surfaces, although the radial and ulnar collateral ligaments lie slightly more laterally and medially, respectively. The palmar ligaments are thicker, stronger, and more critical to the stability of the wrist than are the dorsal ligaments [19,125].

Examination of the overall system of ligaments of the wrist reveals that the radius and four of the carpal bones—the scaphoid, lunate, triquetrum, and capitate—have extensive ligamentous attachments. The ligaments also form a pattern of convergence in the midline of the hand, with the proximal ligaments converging on the lunate and the distal ligaments converging on the capitate (*Fig. 14.30*). The following presents a closer examination of the individual ligaments of the wrist to illuminate the role each plays in stabilizing the wrist complex.

The extrinsic ligaments of the wrist reinforce the radiocarpal joint capsule on the palmar, dorsal, radial, and ulnar surfaces (*Fig. 14.31*). These ligaments serve to support both the radiocarpal and midcarpal joints. The palmar are the thickest and most extensive of the extrinsic ligaments [19,125]. Anatomical texts describe five large extrinsic ligaments, the palmar radiocarpal ligament, the ulnocarpal complex (which is also on the palmar side), the dorsal radiocarpal ligament, and the radial and ulnar collateral ligaments [104,141].

The extrinsic ligaments also can be described as more discrete bundles of fibers to individual carpal bones, with distinct functional roles [102,118,130]. The names of the individual ligamentous bundles, based on their bony attachments, vary slightly among authors (*Table 14.1*). Despite the slight variations among the names applied to the wrist ligaments, the basic organization remains the same throughout the literature [12,102,118,125,130].

The collateral ligaments are reportedly weaker than the other extrinsic ligaments of the wrist [141]. A comparison of the cross-sectional area of the radial collateral ligament with

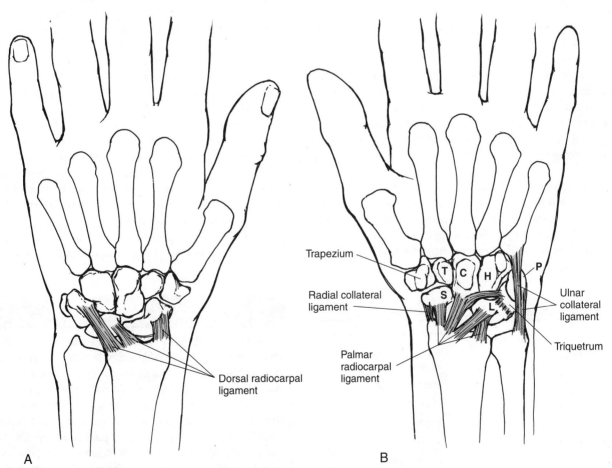

Figure 14.31: Extrinsic ligaments of the wrist. **A.** Dorsal extrinsic ligaments of the wrist. The dorsal radiocarpal ligament arises from the dorsal surface of the distal border of the radius. It projects distally onto the lunate and triquetrum, although attachments to the scaphoid are also described. **B.** Palmar extrinsic ligaments of the wrist. The palmar radiocarpal ligament extends from the radius to the proximal row of carpal bones including the scaphoid, lunate, and triquetrum and onto the capitate in the distal row. The radial and ulnar collateral ligaments project from the radial and ulnar styloid processes, respectively. The radial collateral ligament extends to the radial aspect of the scaphoid and onto the capitate as part of the radioscaphocapitate ligament. It lies more on the palmar surface and sometimes is described as part of the palmar radiocarpal complex. The ulnar collateral ligament projects to the triquetrum and the metacarpal of the little finger and sends a slip to the pisiform.

TABLE 14.1: Extrinsic Ligaments of the Wrist

Surface	Ligament	Individual Fiber Bundles
Palmar	Palmar radiocarpal	Radioscaphocapitate
		Radioscapholunate
		Short radiolunate
		Long radiolunate
Palmar	Ulnocarpal complex	Ulnocapitate
		Ulnotriquetral
		Ulnolunate
Palmar and radial	Radial collateral	
Palmar and ulnar	Ulnar collateral	
Dorsal	Dorsal radiocarpal	

other dorsal and palmar radiocarpal ligaments in seven cadaver specimens reveals that the collateral ligament has no more than half the cross-sectional area of the other extrinsic ligaments of the wrist [109].

Although the role of the extrinsic wrist ligaments has been extensively studied [100,110,125,136], questions remain regarding their individual roles in stabilizing and guiding the movement of the wrist complex. In general, the palmar ligaments limit excessive extension ROM, while the dorsal ligaments resist excessive flexion ROM. The radial ligaments assist in limiting ulnar deviation, and the ulnar ligaments help limit radial deviation. The extrinsic ligaments function with the intrinsic ligaments to stabilize the wrist complex and limit its mobility.

The intrinsic ligaments of the wrist have attachments solely in the carpus. They are classified as dorsal and palmar midcarpal ligaments and interosseous ligaments [12,19,141] (*Table 14.2*). Like the extrinsic ligaments, the palmar midcarpal ligaments are thicker and stronger than the dorsal midcarpal ligaments [123]. The interosseous ligaments are

TABLE 14.2: Intrinsic Ligaments of the Wrist

Ligament	Individual Fiber Bundles
Palmar midcarpal	Palmar scaphotrapezium-trapezoid
	Scaphocapitate
	Triquetrocapitate
	Triquetrohamate
Dorsal midcarpal	Dorsal scaphotriquetral
	Dorsal intercarpal
Interosseous	Scapholunate
	Lunotriquetral
	Pisotriquetral
	Trapezium-trapezoid
	Trapeziocapitate
	Capitohamate

thick, strong, horseshoe-shaped ligaments that run between adjacent carpal bones of each row. They are named according to their attachments. For example, the scapholunate ligament attaches to the scaphoid and lunate bones of the proximal row. The proximal portions of the interosseous ligaments of the proximal row consist mainly of fibrocartilage rather than fibrous material, giving them unique mechanical properties [12,102].

The mechanical properties of some of the ligaments of the wrist have been examined. There is general agreement that the interosseous ligaments are much stronger than the other intrinsic and extrinsic ligaments of the wrist [12,102,112]. Loads to failure of more than 300 N (67 lb) are reported for the interosseous ligaments and of less than 200 N (45 lb) for extrinsic ligaments, although individual ligaments vary [12,102]. In contrast, the interosseous ligaments [92] are significantly less stiff than other wrist ligaments sustaining more elongation before failure [109]. However, all of the wrist ligaments tested sustain more elongation before failure than ligaments elsewhere in the body, such as the anterior cruciate ligament of the knee [92,93]. Wrist ligaments also behave viscoelastically, exhibiting higher loads to failure with increasing loading rate. As noted in Chapter 2, viscoelasticity may provide protection, allowing ligaments to sustain the high, rapidly applied loads generated by accidents such as falling on an outstretched arm.

These mechanical properties suggest that the individual ligaments of the wrist are highly specialized. At least two classes of ligaments seem to be present in the wrist, one that is stiff but able to sustain only moderate loads or large deformations and another that is less stiff but stronger in both load and deformation to failure. Despite the unique mechanical characteristics of these wrist ligaments, however, patients commonly sprain the ligaments of the wrist resulting in considerable impairment and disability.

Clinical Relevance

LUNATE INSTABILITY—A CASE REPORT: *A 30+-year-old mechanic for a car dealership visited a therapist complaining of wrist pain, particularly with motion. He reported that he had been changing a tire when the tire unexpectedly bounced and forcefully flexed his wrist. Evaluation revealed that the patient had limited and painful wrist flexion. Flexion combined with ulnar deviation was particularly painful. ROM was 0–30° of flexion, with pain at the end of the range. However, in a slightly reduced range the patient was able to function without pain and exhibited strength within normal limits. The patient was unable to return to his job, which requires full wrist mobility. Evaluation revealed that the patient had torn the scapholunate interosseous ligament, producing malalignment of the lunate. Radiographs revealed that*

(continued)

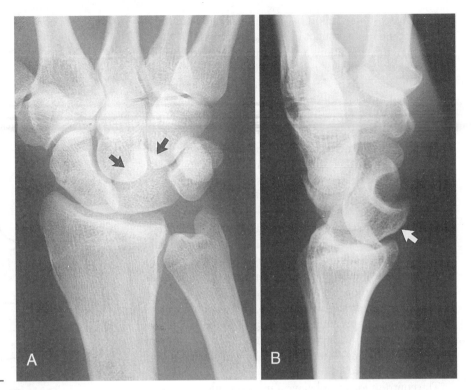

Figure 14.32: Posteroanterior **(A)** and lateral **(B)** radiographs show dorsal tilt of the lunate with respect to the scaphoid.

(Continued)
the lunate was tilted dorsally with respect to the scaphoid (Fig. 14.32). The patient's wrist was treated by pinning the lunate to the capitate and scaphoid and immobilizing it for 4 weeks. After the cast was removed, the patient resumed active and passive exercise. Pain-free mobility was restored, although passive ROM remained slightly diminished. He was able to return to full-time work as a car mechanic. This case study demonstrates that a tear in a single interosseous ligament can produce serious impairments and functional deficits.

Movements of the Wrist

The wrist as a whole is a condyloid or biaxial joint allowing flexion, extension, radial deviation (abduction), and ulnar deviation (adduction) *(Fig. 14.33)*. Like any biaxial joint, the wrist also combines these motions to perform circumduction, a circular movement of the hand on the forearm. These motions often are referred to as **global motions** of the wrist. However, the motion at the wrist is much more complex than these movements suggest. To understand the movements available at the wrist, the movements of the individual components must be appreciated. The following reviews the individual movements of the bones of the wrist. Then their contribution to overall wrist motion is presented.

MOVEMENT IN THE PROXIMAL ROW OF CARPAL BONES

Considerable effort has been exerted to define the relative motion of the carpal bones [22,28,60,69,96,105,108,110,124].

Despite over 20 years of study, however, disagreements continue about the direction and magnitude of relative motion among the carpal bones during wrist movements. There are at least two important reasons for the continued confusion. First, accurate methods to assess small, three-dimensional motions have become available only recently [22,59,60,69,96,110].

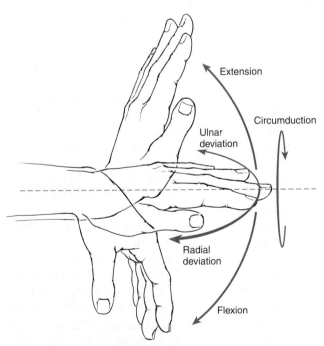

Figure 14.33: Total, or global, motions of the wrist include flexion, extension, radial and ulnar deviation, and circumduction.

Second, many studies report on such a small number of specimens that the results cannot be generalized [60,110].

Despite the limitations of the studies of carpal movement, there are some accepted concepts. There is now a consensus that each of the carpal bones is capable of three-dimensional motion, flexion, extension, radial and ulnar deviation, and even pronation and supination [12,22,60,69]. Most studies suggest that the distal row moves almost as a single unit, and its motion reflects the motion of the hand, specifically the motion of the metacarpal of the long finger [12,95,110,140]. In contrast, the scaphoid, lunate, and triquetrum appear to move more independently of one another. They flex on the radius during wrist flexion and extend during wrist extension [12,69,140], with the scaphoid moving through the greatest excursion in both directions [22,108]. These findings reveal that there is relative flexion between the scaphoid and lunate during wrist flexion and relative extension during wrist extension [12,69]. There are also reports that during wrist flexion, the scaphoid and triquetrum undergo pronation with respect to the lunate, and supination during wrist extension [69,117]. The motions that occur in a plane different from the global wrist motion are known as **out-of-plane motions.**

The contribution to global wrist motion made by each row of carpal bones also is important in understanding the mechanics of wrist movement. In wrist flexion and extension, the distal row of carpal bones moves as a unit and undergoes simple flexion and extension on the proximal row of bones [12,110]. Several studies using the capitate to represent the motion of the distal row report that in flexion, the capitate is more mobile than any of the bones of the proximal row [12,22,69,108]. Estimates of the capitate's (and thus the distal row's) contribution to total wrist flexion range from 60 to 70% [69,108]. Yet others report that the radiocarpal joint contributes more to flexion than the midcarpal joint [96] or that the contributions from radiocarpal and midcarpal joints are equal [13,124]. Similarly, there are differences in the reports of the distal row's relative contributions to extension, some indicating that the midcarpal joint contributes most of the extension [22,95,124] and others saying that most comes from the radiocarpal joint [108]. Finally, some studies suggest that the capitate (and therefore, the midcarpal joint) contributes more motion to both flexion and extension of the wrist than the lunate, representing the radiocarpal joint [12,22,69,140]. The differences in these reported data may be the result of differences in measurement techniques or subject variation [120]. Jackson et al. report that their two specimens exhibited virtually opposite results from one another [60]. Another study suggests that the relative contributions made by the radiocarpal and midcarpal joints to total wrist motion vary depending upon where in the range the measurements are taken [95]. Although there is no consensus about the relative contributions of the two rows to wrist flexion and extension, there is clear recognition that normal global motion of the wrist requires substantial movement at both the radiocarpal joint and the midcarpal joint (*Fig. 14.34*).

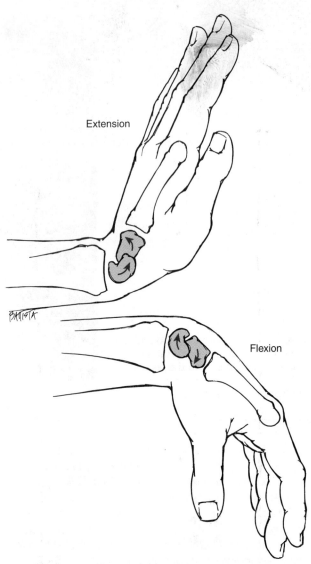

Figure 14.34: Source of total wrist motion. Total wrist motion is the combined result of motion from both the radiocarpal and midcarpal joints.

Radial and ulnar deviations of the wrist appear to include more complex, out-of-plane motions of the carpal bones. Radial deviation of the wrist appears to be accompanied by flexion of the proximal row of carpal bones, which helps the scaphoid avoid impingement on the radial styloid process [22,123,127]. At the same time, the distal row of carpal bones undergoes extension [12,22,69,70]. The reverse appears true in ulnar deviation of the wrist. Similarly, radial deviation is reported to occur with relative pronation of the proximal row, while ulnar deviation reportedly is accompanied by supination of the proximal row [12,22,70]. Reports suggest that the distal row also demonstrates out-of-plane motions that are nearly the reverse of the proximal row during radial and ulnar deviation: pronation with ulnar deviation, supination with radial deviation [22,70]. Most studies agree that the distal row contributes most of the ROM in ulnar and radial deviation [12,69,105,140,144]. Finally, carpal bone motions may be altered by forearm position [13,28] and by wrist movements that combine flexion, extension, and radial or ulnar deviation [110,140].

Clinical Relevance

MOBILIZATION TECHNIQUES FOR THE WRIST:
An understanding of the individual contributions to wrist motion made by the carpal bones provides the biomechanical rationale for the many manual techniques developed to evaluate and restore motion to individual bones in the carpus. Appropriate assessments and interventions depend on a clear understanding of how carpal movement accompanies each global wrist motion.

It is clear from the results presented above that continued research is needed to clarify the precise movements of the individual motions of the carpal bones as well as the factors that affect those motions. However, certain conclusions can be drawn:

- The carpus functions primarily as two separate rows.
- The distal row functions more as a unit.
- The bones of the proximal row demonstrate significant independent movement.
- The motions of the carpal bones are three-dimensional even when the wrist movement occurs in a single plane.
- All wrist motions are composed of significant contributions from both the radiocarpal and midcarpal joints.

The movement of the carpal bones is primarily the result of ligamentous pull and/or the push and pull of adjacent carpal bones [12,27,114]. It is likely that patients who have even small instabilities or subluxations of a single carpal bone may exhibit significant dysfunction of the wrist as a whole [81,118].

Global Wrist Motions

While an understanding of the relative motions of the individual bones of the carpus is essential to understanding the mechanics of the wrist, measurement of total, or global, wrist motion remains a standard clinical assessment tool. Such an assessment describes the motion of the wrist as the relative orientation of the hand with respect to the forearm, typically represented by the metacarpal of the long finger and the long axis of the radius or ulna [91,108] (*Fig. 14.35*). This measurement assumes that the motion of the wrist can be described by motion around a single fixed axis. The data describing the individual contributions of the carpal bones to wrist motion demonstrate that this assumption is untrue. However, studies show that such an assumption allows a reasonable approximation of the *total* wrist movement [3,144]. Several studies have attempted to identify the axis or axes of rotation of the wrist [3,81,110,144], but there is little agreement on the precise location [108]. Many authors suggest that the theoretical

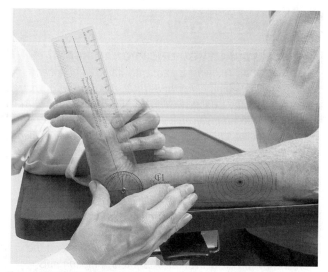

Figure 14.35: Assessment of total wrist motion. Total wrist motion is approximated typically by assessment of the position of the metacarpal of the long finger with respect to the long axis of the forearm.

axis or axes, if existent, lie within or very close to the proximal capitate [3,12,60,96,144]. There is some evidence that the location of the theoretical axis of wrist motion changes with wrist position, suggesting that wrist motion includes considerable translation of the carpal bones in addition to rotation [95].

Clinical Relevance

WRIST ROM: *Because global wrist motion is a composite of motions between the radius and proximal row of carpal bones, between the proximal and distal rows, and among the individual carpal bones, a thorough clinical assessment of global motion includes assessment of global motion through the use of a goniometric device as well as evaluation of the component motions performed by palpation and discrete passive movements. Similarly, treatment includes mobilization techniques to restore the discrete carpal movements and active and passive ROM exercises to increase the total wrist motion.*

Total wrist motion consists of flexion, extension, radial and ulnar deviation, and the combined motion of circumduction. The wrist also allows a limited and generally unquantified amount of pronation and supination. When the wrist is relaxed, the wrist can be passively rotated on the forearm. To transmit forearm pronation and supination to the hand during tasks such as turning a light bulb or a doorknob, the wrist is stabilized by muscles, allowing little pronation and supination between the hand and forearm [12]. Pronation and supination available at the wrist can amplify forearm pronation and supination in tasks in which increased ROM is required. Gupta and Moosawi report an average of approximately 15° pronation and supination at the wrist in healthy male subjects [44].

Clinical Relevance

WRIST INSTABILITY DURING PRONATION AND SUPINATION: *The wrist is frequently involved in patients with juvenile rheumatoid arthritis (JRA). A patient with wrist involvement may exhibit swelling and instability at the wrist and hand with no involvement of the elbow. Clinical inspection may reveal little difficulty with forearm movement when the hand is free to move in space. Yet this patient may have severe functional deficits associated with an inability to pronate and supinate. For example, the patient may be unable to turn a doorknob. The difficulty arises as the patient fixes the hand on the doorknob and then attempts to transmit forearm motion to the hand through the wrist. This transmission requires the wrist to be stabilized on the forearm by muscle activation. This forearm motion puts stress on the wrist and produces pain.*

Clinical Relevance

WRIST POSITIONS DURING FUNCTION: *Because there is such diversity in the wrist ROM reported, the clinician must use additional criteria to determine the adequacy of a patient's ROM. Comparison with the uninvolved limb, when possible, is critical in determining whether an individual's ROM is normal. Another standard useful in judging a patient's ROM is the ROM needed for pain-free, efficient function. Studies of the wrist positions and motions of healthy individuals during functional activities reveal that personal hygiene activities are accomplished with the wrist positioned between 50° of flexion and 40° of extension [20] (Fig. 14.36). Other activities studied—using a fork, holding a newspaper, opening a jar, pouring from a pitcher—typically use up to 35–40° of extension. Typing at a standard computer terminal uses approximately 10° of wrist extension [119]. Rising from a chair with upper extremity assistance uses 50 to 60° of extension ROM [4,20,88,106]. In individuals with spinal cord injuries, the level of spinal cord injury influences upper extremity joint positions used during wheelchair propulsion; those with higher injuries use more wrist extension (>40°) [90]. Such data can assist the clinician in judging the adequacy of a patient's ROM as well as in establishing appropriate treatment goals.*

WRIST ROM REPORTED IN THE LITERATURE

Normal passive ranges of motions reported for the wrist in the literature are presented in *Table 14.3*. Some of the studies cited provide descriptions of the populations on which the data are based [14,15,106,111,121,131]. There are differences in the reported data, but general trends in the values are apparent. All of the sources report that ulnar deviation ROM is greater than radial deviation ROM. Similarly, the reports suggest that wrist flexion ROM is equal to, or greater than, wrist extension ROM. Age and gender seem to have only slight effects on ROM [14,91,106].

Although wrist motions are typically assessed in the sagittal (flexion-extension) and frontal (ulnar and radial deviation) planes, observation of common daily activities demonstrates that the wrist normally functions in a diagonal plane, combining extension with radial deviation and flexion

TABLE 14.3: Normal ROM Values for Wrist Movement from the Literature

	Flexion (°)	Extension (°)	Radial Deviation (°)	Ulnar Deviation (°)
Steindler [122]	84	64	30	30–50
US Army/Air Force [31]	80	70	20	30
Boone and Azin [15][a]	74.8 ± 6.6	74.0 ± 6.6	21.1 ± 4.0	35.3 ± 3.8
Walker et al. [131][b]	64 ± 10	63 ± 9	19 ± 6	26 ± 7
Schoenmarklin and Marras [111][c]	62 ± 10	57 ± 9	20 ± 7.5	28 ± 7
Gerhardt and Rippstein [41]	60	50	20	30
Bird and Stowe [14]	96.2[d]	60.0[d]	31.5[d]	36.7[d]
	98.2[e]	66.5[e]	34.1[e]	37.2[e]
Ryu et al [106][f]	79.1	59.3	21.1	37.2
Spilman and Pinkston [121][g]	—	—	16.7 ± 5.5	32 ± 5.0
	—	—	18.6 ± 5.8	32.4 ± 6.2
	—	—	18.9 ± 6.2	35 ± 5.3

[a]Data from 56 men over 19 years of age.
[b]Data from 30 men and 30 women aged 60–84 years.
[c]Data from 39 industrial workers, 22 men and 17 women. Mean age was 41.7 ± 10.5 years.
[d]Data from 8 males and 5 females aged 40–49 years.
[e]Data from 5 males and 6 females aged 50–80+ years.
[f]Data from 20 males and 20 females.
[g]Data from 63 males and 37 females aged 18–28 years in three test positions.

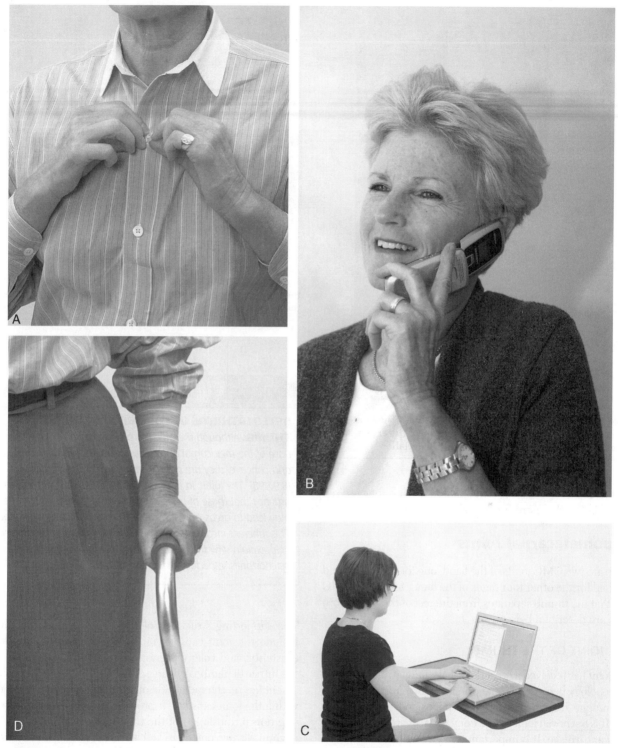

Figure 14.36: Wrist positions in various activities of daily living. Activities of daily living demonstrate the varied positions of the wrist. Buttoning a shirt **(A)**, holding a telephone **(B)**, and typing at a computer **(C)** use less wrist extension than is required when using the upper extremity for weight bearing, such as with a cane **(D)**.

with ulnar deviation (*Fig. 14.37*) Li et al. show a strong coupling of ulnar and radial deviation with flexion and extension, respectively, during active unlar and radial deviation, with somewhat less coupling during active flexion and extension [76]. These authors also report that maximum total excursion in flexion/extension

and radial/ulnar deviation occurs when the wrist is in the neutral position with respect to the other plane of motion. For example maximum flexion/extension excursion occurs with the wrist in neutral radial/ulnar deviation. The clinician must take care to maintain the neutral alignment when taking standard ROM measurements. The clinician may also

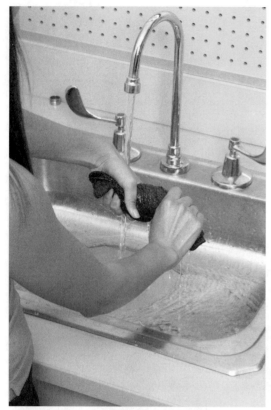

Figure 14.37: Wrist function in diagonal patterns. The wrist usually functions in diagonal patterns, combining wrist extension with radial deviation and flexion with ulnar deviation.

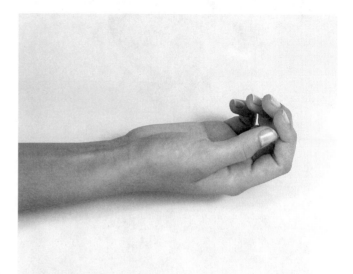

Figure 14.38: The resting position of the thumb is anterior to the plane of the palm, with the thumb rotated slightly toward the fingers.

need to consider assessing wrist motion in both the cardinal planes and in the more functional diagonal patterns.

Carpometacarpal Joints

There are two CMC joints of the hand, one for the thumb and a second for the other four digits of the hand. It is at the CMC joint that the thumb separates from the rest of the hand. Both joints are described below.

CMC JOINT OF THE THUMB

This joint has received a great deal of attention in anatomy and anthropology because it is the primary source of the purportedly unique human movement of opposition of the thumb [50]. It is a synovial joint whose bony surfaces are covered with articular cartilage. It is important to note that because the trapezium is positioned anteriorly out of the plane of the hand, the metacarpal of the thumb also lies out of the plane of the hand. The volar surface of the thumb is turned slightly toward the little finger, and the radial aspect of the thumb is directed slightly toward the volar surface of the forearm [25] (*Fig. 14.38*). This position facilitates opposition of the thumb.

The joint's proximal articular surface on the trapezium is saddle-shaped, concave in the plane of the thumb's abduction and adduction motion and convex in the plane of its flexion and extension motion [24,47,104,141]. The articulating surface on the base of the metacarpal is reciprocally convex and concave.

Clinical Relevance

OSTEOARTHRITIS OF THE CMC JOINT OF THE THUMB: *Although the articular surfaces of the trapezium and base of the metacarpal of the thumb are reciprocally convex and concave, they are not mirror images of each other [8,97,98]. The joints in female specimens demonstrate less congruency that those of males. Less congruent articular surfaces may lead to areas of high stress (force/area) in the joint surface. This inherent incongruency at the CMC joint of the thumb may help explain why the CMC joint is so commonly affected by osteoarthritis, especially in women [7,10,97].*

The supporting structures of the CMC joint of the thumb include the joint capsule, radial CMC ligament, the dorsal (posterior) and volar (anterior) oblique CMC ligaments, and the intraarticular beak ligament [47,57,97,129]. The beak ligament lies on the radial side of the palmar aspect of the joint, within the joint capsule. It provides protection against excessive dorsal translation of the thumb's metacarpal on the trapezium during pinch [97]. It is considered by many as the primary ligamentous stabilizer of the carpometacarpal joint of the thumb. All of these ligaments support the joint but also serve an important role in guiding the motion of the CMC joint of the thumb [47,138]. In addition, there are two intermetacarpal ligaments connecting the proximal ends of the metacarpals of the thumb and index fingers.

The joint is described typically as a saddle joint [24,47,58,104,141] but is described by some as a ball-and-socket joint [21] or as a condyloid joint [52,53,57]. Despite the various classifications of the joint, there is little disagreement about the motions available at this joint. The saddle-shaped articular surfaces allow flexion, extension, abduction, and adduction as well as some rotation about the long axis of the metacarpal.

The classic and most common classification of the CMC joint of the thumb is as a saddle joint. However, the real issue for the clinician is to understand the basis for, and quality of, the movement at this joint. The names of the motions of the CMC joint of the thumb vary considerably among clinicians and anatomists. This book uses the widely used terms, *flexion,*

extension, abduction, and *adduction.* It is useful for the reader also to appreciate that many hand specialists use *radial abduction* in place of extension and *palmar abduction* in place of abduction of the thumb's CMC joint. Flexion and extension of the CMC joint of the thumb are defined as movements of the metacarpal of the thumb in the plane of the palm toward and away from the ulnar side of the hand, respectively (*Fig. 14.39*). Abduction and adduction occur as

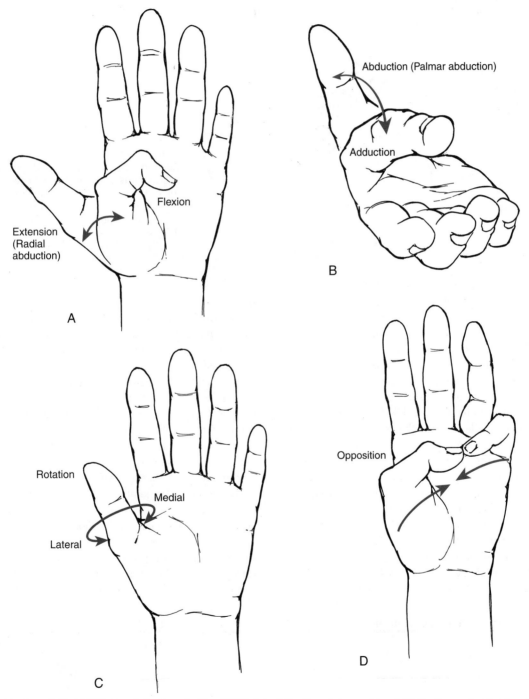

Figure 14.39: Motion of the CMC joint of the thumb. The CMC joint of the thumb is capable of **(A)** flexion and extension (radial abduction), which occur in the plane of the palm; **(B)** abduction (palmar abduction) and adduction, which occur perpendicular to the plane of the palm; **(C)** medial and lateral rotation about the long axis of the thumb; and **(D)** opposition, which is a combination of flexion, abduction, and medial rotation.

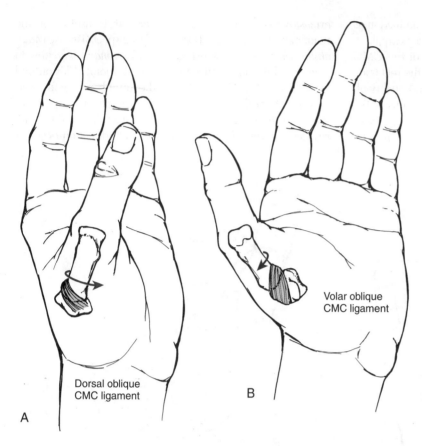

Dorsal oblique
CMC ligament

Volar oblique
CMC ligament

A

B

Figure 14.40: Rotation of the CMC joint of the thumb produced by the pull of the dorsal and volar oblique carpometacarpal ligaments. **A.** The pull of the dorsal oblique CMC ligament rotates the metacarpal in the ulnar direction during flexion and abduction. **B.** The pull of the volar oblique CMC ligament rotates the metacarpal radially during extension and adduction.

the thumb moves away from and toward the palm, respectively, in a plane perpendicular to the palm. Adduction beyond the palm is known as *retropulsion*. Medial rotation (pronation) of the CMC joint of the thumb is the rotation of the pulp of the thumb toward the palm, and lateral rotation (supination) is the rotation of the pulp away from the pulp of the other fingers. Opposition of the CMC joint is defined as simultaneous flexion, abduction, and medial rotation.

Medial rotation of the thumb's CMC joint occurs concomitantly with either flexion or abduction, while lateral rotation occurs with extension or adduction. Once the joint is flexed or when the muscles crossing the joint contract and increase the compression between the trapezium and the head of the metacarpal of the thumb, independent rotation at the CMC joint is impossible. Under these circumstances, the thumb's CMC joint behaves as a biaxial, or condyloid joint [25,47,53]. However, when the joint is in the neutral position, up to 45° of passive rotation of the joint is available [47].

Because rotation of the thumb's CMC joint depends on the amount of flexion or abduction present, it appears to

result from ligamentous tension, specifically from the pull of the oblique CMC ligaments of the thumb. The attachment of these two ligaments on the ulnar side of the head of the metacarpal explains their contributions to rotation of the CMC joint of the thumb [47]. Flexion of the CMC joint pulls the dorsal oblique CMC ligament taut, which then pulls the thumb's metacarpal into medial rotation (*Fig. 14.40*). Abduction of the CMC joint produces the same effect on the dorsal oblique CMC ligament, resulting in medial rotation of the thumb. Conversely, the volar oblique CMC ligament pulls the metacarpal back into lateral rotation as it is stretched during extension or adduction of the thumb's CMC joint. Thus the oblique ligaments of the CMC joint of the thumb contribute to the motion of the joint just as the coracoclavicular ligament contributes to the motion of the sternoclavicular and acromioclavicular joints of the shoulder complex (Chapter 8).

Ranges of motion of the thumb's CMC joint reported in the literature are presented in *Table 14.4*. Reports of retropulsion ROM are not found in the literature because it is rarely if ever assessed. There are only a few reports of the

TABLE 14.4: Normal ROM Values from the Literature for Motion of the CMC of the Thumb

	Flexion (°)	Extension (°)	Abduction (°)
Steindler [122]	[a]		25
American Academy of Orthopaedic Surgeons [43]		80	70
Gerhardt and Rippstein [41]	15	20	40
US Army/Air Force [31]	15	70	70

[a]Reports 35–40° combined flexion and extension excursion.

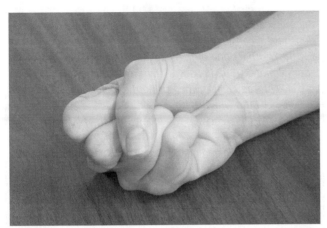

Figure 14.41: Thumb rotation in a closed fist. The thumb appears to have a large amount of rotation when positioned in full opposition, as in a closed fist.

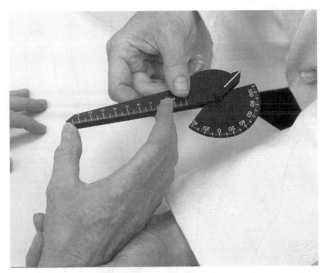

Figure 14.42: Linear measurements of the distance between the tips of the thumb and fingers may be more convenient in the clinic to assess changes in thumb mobility.

normal ROM of the CMC joint of the thumb and no known reports in which the methods used to obtain the ranges are reported. Although rotations of the CMC joint of the thumb are not measured separately, Haines reports that passive medial rotation of approximately 30° and passive lateral rotation of about 15° are available [47]. The rotation ROM available at the CMC joint of the thumb does not appear to match the rotation of the whole thumb that occurs during grasping activities of the whole hand (*Fig. 14.41*). Disagreements remain regarding the source of the total rotation, or *circumduction,* mobility of the thumb [23]. Perhaps rotation also occurs at the MCP and IP joints of the thumb. Or, more likely, the axes of flexion and extension of these joints are aligned so that flexion turns the distal segments toward the palm and extension turns them away. The data presented in Table 14.4 reveal considerable variations in reported values for the ROM of the CMC joint of the thumb. Population studies are needed to clarify the ranges of motion of the CMC joint and the normal variability in a healthy population.

Clinical Relevance

ROM OF THE THUMB: *In the absence of reliable normative values of ROM for the thumb and because ROM measures are difficult to perform, clinicians frequently assess the excursions of the joints of the thumb by examining the ability of the thumb to oppose the fingers. This is readily evaluated by taking a linear measurement of the distance between the tip of the thumb and the tip of the opposing finger (Fig. 14.42). Such a measurement may be very useful to monitor the progress of a single patient. However, these measures are affected by the length of the digits and cannot be used to compare subjects.*

CMC AND INTERMETACARPAL JOINTS OF THE FINGERS

Although the CMC articulations of the fingers are enclosed by a single joint capsule creating a single synovial joint space, the individual articulations between the carpal bones and the metacarpals of the fingers are each unique, resulting in important functional differences. The respective articular surfaces are covered with articular cartilage. The supporting structures include the capsule that surrounds the entire common CMC joint and sends extensions distally between the adjacent metacarpals of the fingers. These projections create the intermetacarpal joints of the fingers. The CMC and intermetacarpal articulations are reinforced by dorsal and palmar CMC and intermetacarpal ligaments and by interosseous ligaments. Strong ligaments extend from the capitate to the metacarpals of the index, long, and ring fingers. The metacarpal of the little finger receives strong ligamentous support from the hamate and pisiform bones.

The CMC articulations are typically characterized as a common gliding joint [104]. The metacarpal of the index finger articulates with the trapezium, trapezoid, capitate, and metacarpal of the long finger. Consequently, it is wedged in securely and is the least mobile of all CMC articulations [104] (*Fig. 14.43*). The mobility of the CMC articulations of the fingers increases from radial to ulnar sides of the hand as the articular surfaces become more curved. The metacarpal of the little finger articulates only with the hamate and the adjacent metacarpal of the ring finger. The articulation between the little finger and the hamate is characterized by reciprocally concave–convex surfaces and is sometimes described as a saddle articulation [62,104]. Consequently, the CMC articulation of the little finger exhibits considerable mobility, second only to the thumb's CMC joint.

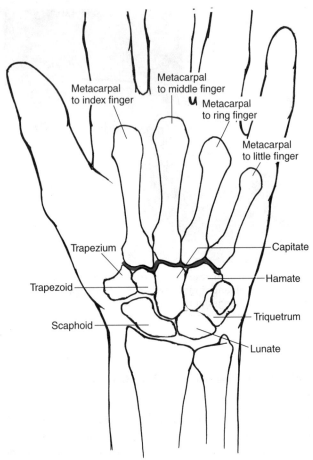

Figure 14.43: CMC joint of the fingers. The mobility of the CMC joint of the fingers is least at the index finger because its metacarpal is wedged in among the trapezium, trapezoid, capitate, and metacarpal of the long finger. Mobility increases ulnarly as the articulations become more curved, with fewer bony attachments.

Clinical Relevance

THE EFFECT OF CMC JOINT MOTION ON WRIST FLEXION AND EXTENSION ROM MEASURES: *Texts describing ROM measurements of the wrist direct the clinician to align the movable arm of the goniometer along the metacarpal of the long finger [43] or along the metacarpal of the little finger [91]. In both cases the goniometer crosses the radiocarpal, midcarpal, and CMC joints, but the specific CMC articulation varies between the two methods. Use of the long finger means that the wrist ROM measurement reflects the wrist motion and the motion between capitate and the metacarpal of the long finger. Several studies demonstrate that there is little or no motion between the metacarpal of the long finger and capitate during wrist motions [12,95,110,140].*

Use of the little finger as the reference for alignment of the goniometer means that the measurement reflects radio-carpal and midcarpal joint motion and the motion between

the metacarpal of the little finger and the hamate. Observations reveal considerable motion between the hamate and the metacarpal bone of the little finger, particularly in the sagittal plane [138]. Consequently, wrist flexion ROM values are likely to be greater when using the metacarpal of the little finger than when using the long finger's metacarpal (Fig. 14.44). Differences in the location of the reference, or movable, arm of the goniometer on the metacarpals may contribute to the differences in wrist ROM measures reported in the literature and demonstrated in Table 14.3 [43]. When possible, use of the metacarpal bone of the long finger as the reference is recommended to assess wrist motion, particularly for flexion and extension. Use of the metacarpal of the little finger does provide information about the mobility of the CMC articulation that may be clinically useful in some circumstances. Clinicians must recognize that both measures are used clinically but are not interchangeable.

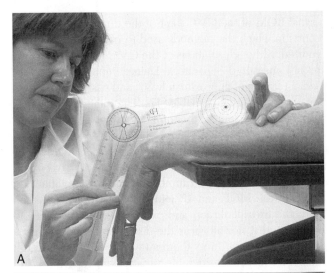

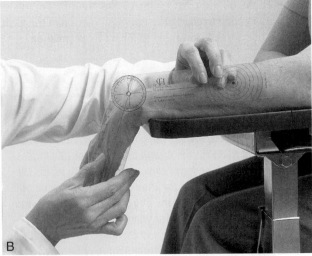

Figure 14.44: Wrist flexion ROM measurements using **(A)** the metacarpal of the long finger and **(B)** the little finger. Measured wrist flexion or extension ROM may vary depending upon whether the metacarpal to the long or little finger is used.

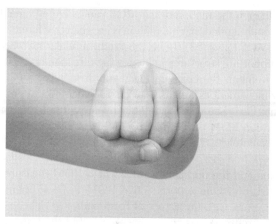

Figure 14.45: The volar arch of the hand is apparent during a forceful grasp.

The intermetacarpal articulations are gliding joints, but most of their movements are so small that they are not measured. Since there is more mobility at the articulation between the hamate and the metacarpal bone of the little finger than between the CMC articulation of the ring finger, there also is simultaneous gliding between the metacarpal bones of the little and ring fingers. The motions at these CMC and intermetacarpal articulations allow the formation of the second transverse arch of the hand, distal to the first transverse arch, the carpal arch. This second arch, known as the **volar arch,** is essential for powerful grasp (*Fig. 14.45*).

Clinical Relevance

LOSS OF THE VOLAR ARCH: *There are several reasons for an individual to be unable to form the volar arch including weakness in the intrinsic muscles of the hand, severe scarring of the skin on the dorsal surface of the hand subsequent to a severe burn, and ligamentous tightening following immobilization with a flattened arch. If the skin or ligaments are allowed to tighten enough to prevent the formation of the transverse arch, the patient may be unable to perform a powerful grasp. The clinician must take care to maintain the arches of the hand during immobilization and healing, to preserve function. The mechanics of powerful grasp are discussed in greater detail in Chapter 19.*

MCP Joints of the Digits

The structure and function of the MCP joints are similar throughout the five digits. However, the joint of the thumb and those of the fingers are discussed separately because they exhibit small but important differences in structure that affect their function.

MCP JOINT OF THE THUMB

The MCP joint is the synovial joint between the head of the metacarpal of the thumb and the base of the thumb's proximal phalanx. Although the head of the thumb's metacarpal bone is convex in the volar–dorsal and radioulnar directions, it is flatter in the radioulnar than in volar–dorsal direction [63]. The degree of curvature in the radioulnar direction is quite variable and leads to considerable variation in available mobility and to differences in joint classification [71,138]. When the radioulnar curvature is notable, abduction and adduction mobility is present, and the MCP joint of the thumb is described as a biaxial joint, reflecting its ability to flex and extend and to abduct and adduct [54,62,141]. As the radioulnar curvature decreases, the ability to abduct and adduct decreases. Some authors report very limited abduction mobility, and others describe the joint as a simple hinge joint allowing only flexion and extension [11,51].

The supporting structures of the MCP joint of the thumb include the capsule, the collateral ligaments, and a volar (palmar) plate (*Fig. 14.46*). The capsule itself is somewhat thin, particularly dorsally, where it is reinforced by the tendon of the extensor pollicis longus [138]. The collateral ligaments are thick bands running obliquely from the head of the metacarpal to the volar aspects of the ulnar and radial

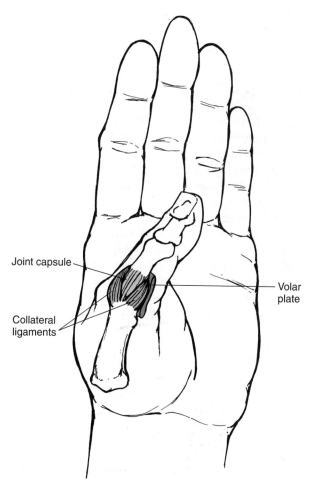

Joint capsule

Volar plate

Collateral ligaments

Figure 14.46: The supporting structures of the MCP joint of the thumb include the capsule, collateral ligaments, and the volar plate.

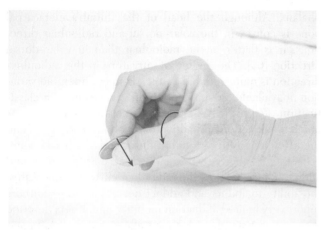

Figure 14.47: Forces on the thumb's MCP joint during pinch. Lateral pinch applies a valgus stress on the thumb's MCP joint which is resisted by the ulnar collateral ligament.

surfaces of the base of the phalanx and to the volar plate [71]. The volar plate consists of fibrous connective tissue and fibrocartilage, the latter providing additional articular surface for the head of the metacarpal bone. It covers the volar surface of the joint and is firmly attached with the capsule to the proximal border of the head of the metacarpal. Distally, the plate is attached loosely just distal to the base of the proximal phalanx.

Clinical Relevance

SKIER'S THUMB (ALSO KNOWN AS GAMEKEEPER'S THUMB): *Injuries to the ulnar collateral ligament of the thumb's MCP joint are common and potentially debilitating. A common mechanism is a fall on the outstretched hand while skiing. If the skier keeps the strap of the ski pole wrapped around the thumb, the fall and the pull on the pole strap can apply an extension and valgus stress to the thumb's MCP joint, loading the ulnar collateral ligament. A rupture of the ligament produces valgus laxity, making it difficult and painful to stabilize the thumb during lateral pinch (Fig. 14.47). New ski pole designs have emerged to minimize the risk of such injuries.*

Although the motion of the MCP joint is highly variable, it is generally agreed that the motion is less than that found at the other MCP joints [63,104,141]. Both the articular surfaces and the supporting structures influence the direction and quantity of movement, the collateral ligaments restraining radial and ulnar movement as well as volar displacement of the proximal phalanx [71]. The volar plate limits hyperextension excursion.

Flexion ROM of the thumb's MCP joint is reported to be approximately 0–50° [31,43], although ranges of up to 80° are also reported [122]. Few studies describe a data collection method and the population from which ROM measures are derived [56]. One reports active ROM from 35 men aged 26–28 years, with no history of hand pathology. The average flexion excursion was 56° in 30 subjects, but the remaining 5 subjects exhibited a mean flexion excursion of less than 30°, despite the absence of any evidence or history of pathology. A report on seven cadaver specimens notes that all specimens exhibited approximately 10° of hyperextension [49]. Maximum flexion ranged from 40° to 80°. Although more studies are required, clinicians must recognize that there may be a broad range of mobility found in thumb MCP joint flexion, even in individuals without pathology.

Only one known source offers any magnitudes for abduction and adduction. Kapandji suggests that there are only "a few degrees" of adduction [62]. Abduction is described as greater than adduction but is not quantified. Clinicians are cautioned to use these data carefully. Research is needed to establish normal values based on population studies and to determine the clinical significance of abnormal joint movement at the thumb's MCP joint.

MCP JOINTS OF THE FINGERS

The MCP joints of the fingers usually are described as condyloid or biaxial joints but also are known as ellipsoid joints [62,86]. The term *ellipsoid* reflects the difference in the dorsal–volar and radioulnar diameters of the articular surfaces. As noted in Chapter 7, both condyloid and ellipsoid joints are biaxial, so both terms reflect the available motion at the joints.

The supporting structures of the MCP joints of the fingers are similar to those of the MCP joint of the thumb, including the capsule, collateral ligaments, and the volar (palmar) plates (*Fig. 14.48*). In addition, the joints are supported by the

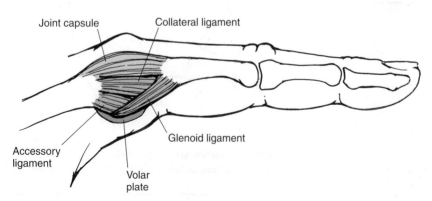

Figure 14.48: The supporting structures of the MCP joints of the fingers include the capsule, collateral ligaments, the accessory and glenoid ligaments, and the volar plate.

accessory collateral ligaments and the phalangioglenoid [83] or metacarpoglenoid [138] ligaments, the transverse intermetacarpal ligaments, and the surrounding tendons and associated soft tissue [83,138]. Studies demonstrate that the collateral, accessory, and glenoid ligaments help support the MCP joints of the fingers throughout the ROM [73,83,84]. However, the collateral ligaments are the primary support of the MCP joints of the fingers [84].

Careful analysis of the collateral ligaments reveals that they are complex structures with deep and superficial parts. The radial collateral ligaments are thicker and wider than the ulnar ligaments [83]. The radial and ulnar collateral ligaments have broad attachments on the sides of the metacarpal heads and proximal phalanges [73,83]. Their broad attachments on the metacarpals help to explain why abduction and adduction mobility is present when the joint is extended but virtually disappears when MCP joint flexion approaches 90° [83]. As the joints go from extension to flexion, the ligament is drawn taut, thus limiting mediolateral displacement. In addition, because the metacarpal heads are broader volarly than dorsally, the collateral ligaments are stretched more as they lie over the expanded head during MCP flexion when the phalanx is in contact with the volar portion of the metacarpal head (*Fig. 14.49*). The stretch is relieved in extension when the proximal phalanx is in contact with the narrower more dorsal surface [127].

Clinical Relevance

FUNCTIONAL IMPAIRMENT RESULTING FROM TIGHTNESS IN THE COLLATERAL LIGAMENTS:
Flexion of the MCP joints pulls the collateral ligaments taut. Full MCP flexion through the normal excursion requires

compliance of the collateral ligaments. If a patient's hand is immobilized with the MCP joints extended, the collateral ligaments may shorten, thus preventing MCP joint flexion mobility once immobilization is discontinued. Therefore, a hand that requires immobilization must be positioned with the MCP joints flexed to maintain adequate length of the collateral ligaments.

As in the thumb, the volar plates add articular surface for the metacarpal head and limit hyperextension mobility of the MCP joints. The volar plates also serve an important protective role by providing a protective fibrocartilaginous covering for the articular surfaces during grasp. Grasping a large object such as a baseball or soda can uses only slight flexion excursion of the MCP joints of the fingers [75,89]. Since articulation between the proximal phalanx and metacarpal head moves progressively more distally on the surface of the metacarpal head as flexion decreases, slight MCP flexion leaves the volar surfaces of the heads of the metacarpal bones exposed to the structures being held in the hand. The volar plates protect this surface of the metacarpal heads from abrasion by the object in the hand. A more forceful grasp increases the risk of injury. Activities involving powerful grasp of a large object such as hammering or chopping wood could be very painful and damaging to the metacarpal heads without the protection of the volar plates.

Ranges of motion of the MCP joints of the fingers are slightly better studied than the MCP joint of the thumb. The joints are biaxial joints, allowing flexion and extension as well as abduction and adduction. The shapes of the metacarpal bones differ among the four fingers, producing differences in the motion available at each MCP joint. Although these joints

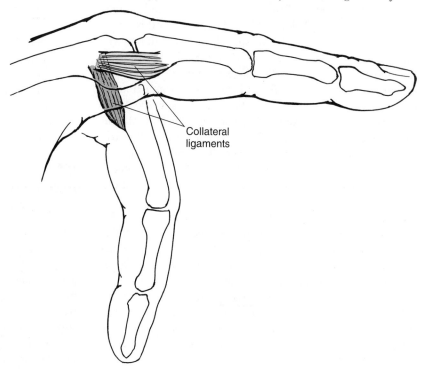

Collateral ligaments

Figure 14.49: Effects of flexion and extension on the collateral and accessory ligaments of the MCP joints of the fingers. In extension, the collateral and accessory ligaments are slightly slack and allow abduction and adduction at the MCP joints of the fingers. In flexion, the collateral and accessory ligaments are stretched and allow little abduction and adduction at the MCP joints of the fingers.

are biaxial, there is some disagreement about whether the axis of flexion and extension is fixed or moving. Some studies report that the axis remains fixed in the center of the metacarpal head [45,143]. Others suggest that the axis moves in a volar direction during flexion and in a dorsal direction during extension [36,73]. The clinical importance of this controversy is its relationship to the motion at the MCP joint. Those who suggest that the axis of flexion and extension moves report significant volar and dorsal translation of the proximal phalanx on the metacarpal during flexion and extension of the joint.

Clinical Relevance

JOINT MOBILIZATIONS TO RESTORE MCP FLEXION AND EXTENSION: *A common treatment in therapy to restore MCP flexion and extension ROM is to glide the proximal phalanx passively in an anterior and posterior direction on the head of the metacarpal. The theoretical basis for this approach is the need to restore the translatory motion that purportedly occurs in normal flexion and extension. Yet there is some evidence that MCP flexion and extension involve little or no translation. The manual gliding techniques may still be beneficial in restoring normal motion by reducing joint stress and improving lubrication, even if significant translation does not occur in the normal movement of these joints. Additional research is needed to explain the benefits of manual therapy at the joints of the fingers.*

Reports also suggest that in the fingers, MCP flexion, extension, abduction, and adduction are accompanied by slight rotation [9,35,45,73,75,84,127]. The complexity of the motion of the MCP joints of the fingers can be appreciated by noting the position of the fingers when the hand is open and when it is closed (*Fig. 14.50*). When the hand is open, the extended fingers are slightly spread, and the difference in finger lengths is readily apparent. However, when the fingers flex and the hand closes, the fingers converge toward the thenar eminence, and the finger lengths appear much more equal. The convergence of the fingers begins at the MCP joints by combining flexion with radial deviation and rotation toward the thumb [26,127]. This combination is particularly apparent in the little and ring fingers. The combined movements of flexion, radial deviation, and rotation are facilitated by the shape of the metacarpal heads and by the pull of the collateral ligaments [73].

Available radial deviation excursion is less than ulnar deviation excursion at the MCP joints, particularly in the index and long fingers. The ring finger exhibits approximately equal excursions in radial and ulnar deviation, and the little finger may have slightly more radial than ulnar deviation [127].

Ranges of flexion and extension motions of the MCP joints of the fingers found in the literature are reported in *Table 14.5*. There is only one known study reporting passive ROM data collected from a described population of healthy individuals [80]. This study, based on 60 men and 60 women

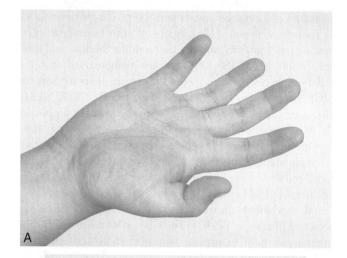

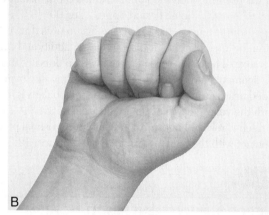

Figure 14.50: Comparison of the position of the fingers when the hand is open and fingers extended and the closed hand with flexed fingers. **A.** When the hand is open, the fingers are slightly spread, and the varied length of the fingers is apparent. **B.** In a fist, the fingers converge toward the thenar eminence, and the fingertips are nearly aligned with each other.

aged 18 to 35 years, reveals that women exhibit significantly greater hyperextension ROM than men at the MCP joints of the fingers. The data also demonstrate an increase in mobility from the radial to the ulnar fingers. This variation in flexion excursion allows the finger tips to come into line with one another when the hand is closed. The authors deny any effect of hand dominance on the mobility of the MCP joints.

Interphalangeal Joints of the Fingers and Thumb

There are nine interphalangeal joints in the fingers and thumb, four proximal interphalangeal (PIP) and four distal interphalangeal (DIP) joints in the fingers and a single interphalangeal (IP) joint in the thumb. The structure of these joints is similar. Each is a hinge joint with trochlear articular surfaces. The joint surfaces are covered by articular cartilage typical of most synovial joints. The capsules surround the joint surfaces and attach to the margins of the articular surfaces.

The condyles of the proximal phalanges are slightly asymmetrical creating what some describe as a slight **carrying**

TABLE 14.5: Normal ROM Values (°) from the Literature for Motion of the MCP of the Fingers

		Mallon et al. [80][a]		US Army/Air Force [31]	Hume [56][b]
		60 Men	**60 Women**	**US Army/Air Force [31]**	**Hume [56][b]**
Flexion	Index	94	95	90[c]	100[c]
	Long	98	100		
	Ring	102	103		
	Little	107	107		
Extension	Index	29	56	45[c]	Not measured
	Long	34	54		
	Ring	29	60		
	Little	48	62		

[a]Mean passive ROM measurements from 60 men and 60 women, aged 18–35 years. No standard deviations reported.
[b]Mean active ROM measurement from 35 men, aged 26–28 years. No standard deviations reported.
[c]No separate values for individual fingers.

angle at the PIP joints of all the fingers except the long finger and at the IP joint of the thumb [6,54]. The consequence of these slight asymmetries is that the axes of motion are slightly tilted, and the resulting flexion and extension motions occur at a slight angle with respect to the long axes of the digits (Fig. 14.50). This slight out-of-plane flexion and extension motion assists the convergence of the fingers and thumb toward the thenar eminence during hand closure [54] (*Fig. 14.51*). In contrast, the articular surfaces of the DIP joints are more symmetrical, and motion at these joints occurs in planes parallel to the long axes of the fingers.

The primary noncontractile supporting structures of the interphalangeal joints of the thumb and fingers are similar. They consist of a capsule, collateral ligaments, and a volar (palmar) plate (*Fig. 14.52*). The collateral ligaments include a cord-like portion that attaches to the proximal and distal segments of the joint and another fan-shaped section, or accessory ligament, that attaches to the proximal segment and to the volar plate. These collateral ligaments provide the primary support to the joints in a radioulnar direction throughout the range of flexion and extension excursion [66,85,101,127]. The articular surfaces and the accessory ligaments also contribute to radioulnar stability, particularly when the joints are extended.

The volar plate at each joint is similar to those at the MCP joints. The proximal border of the volar plate is attached at its ulnar and radial margins to the proximal phalanx. The volar plates of the interphalangeal joints serve purposes similar to those at the MCP joints, limiting hyperextension excursion and protecting the volar surface of the head of each phalanx [16]. The interphalangeal joints also receive considerable support from the surrounding tendons and from the connective tissue structures related to these tendons. The dorsal aspects of the joints receive reinforcement from the extensor digitorum tendons.

Classified as hinge joints, these interphalangeal joints allow only flexion and extension excursion. However, slight radioulnar movement and rotation also occur at these joints, particularly at the IP joint of the thumb [26,85]. These motions help direct the fingers toward the thenar eminence

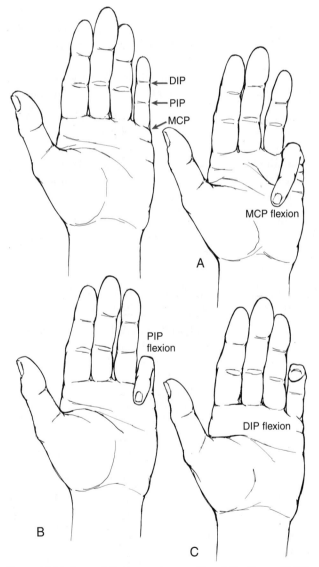

Figure 14.51: Axes of flexion and extension of the fingers' MCP, PIP, and DIP joints. Flexion about the oblique axes of the fingers' MCP **(A)** and PIP **(B)** joints contribute to the convergence of the fingers toward the thumb during finger flexion. Flexion about the medial–lateral axis **(C)** of the DIP joint produces sagittal plane motion.

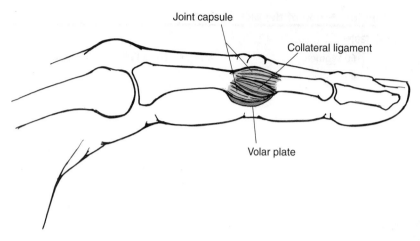

Figure 14.52: The supporting structures of the IP joints of the fingers include the capsule, collateral ligaments, and the volar plate.

and the thumb toward the fingers as the digits flex. The ranges of motion reported in the literature are presented in *Tables 14.6* and *14.7*.

There is considerable variability in the ranges presented, but certain trends are consistent throughout the literature:

- The IP joint of the thumb exhibits less mobility than the interphalangeal joints of the fingers [91].
- The PIP joints of the fingers exhibit more flexion mobility than the MCP or DIP joints of the fingers [80].
- The DIP joints of the fingers allow more extension excursion than the PIP joints [26,127].

Few authors report extension excursion of the IP joint of the thumb, and the values vary widely [5,56]. Extension may be

present, particularly in the presence of abnormal mobility or stability of the more proximal joints of the thumb. The presence of extension of the thumb's IP joint affects the mechanics of pinch, which is discussed in more detail in Chapter 19.

Clinical Relevance

MEASURES OF FINGER MOBILITY IN THE CLINIC:
ROM assessment for all of the joints of the hand is extremely time consuming. Consequently, linear measurements of finger motions are frequently performed in the clinic. These measures are convenient, are relatively quick,

TABLE 14.6: Normal ROM Values (°) from the Literature for Motion of the Interphalangeal Joint of the Thumb and the Proximal Interphalangeal Joints of Fingers

	Mallon et al. [80][a]		AAOS[b] [43]	US Army/Air Force [31]	Hume et al. [56][c]	Apfel [5][d]	
	Men	Women				Men	Women
Flexion							
Thumb			80	90	73	78.6 ± 9.5	83.5 ± 10.9
Index	106	107	[e]	100[f]	105[f]		
Long	110	112					
Ring	110	108					
Little	111	111					
Extension							
Thumb			0	Not reported	5	35.2 ± 16.4	25.8 ± 14.4
Index	11	19	[e]	0[f]	Not measured		
Long	10	20					
Ring	14	20					
Little	13	21					

[a]Mean passive ROM measurements from 60 men and 60 women, aged 18–35 years. No standard deviations reported.
[b]American Academy of Orthopaedic Surgeons
[c]Mean active ROM measurement from 35 men, aged 26–28 years. No standard deviations reported.
[d]Mean passive ROM based on the right hands of 19 men, mean age 35.7 ± 13.9 years, and 12 women, mean age 33.7 ± 6.0 years.
[e]Reported data from Mallon et al. [80].
[f]Not reported for individual fingers.

TABLE 14.7: Normal ROM Values (°) from the Literature for Motion of the Distal Interphalangeal Joints of Fingers

	Mallon et al. [80][a]		AAOS[b] [43]	US Army/Air Force [31]	Hume et al. [56][c]
	Men	**Women**			
Flexion					
Index	75	75	[d]	90[e]	85[e]
Long	80	79			
Ring	74	76			
Little	72	72			
Extension					
Index	22	24	[d]	0[e]	Not measured
Long	19	23			
Ring	17	18			
Little	15	21			

[a]Mean passive ROM measurements from 60 men and 60 women, aged 18–35 years. No standard deviations reported.
[b]American Academy of Orthopaedic Surgeons.
[c]Mean active ROM measurement from 35 men, aged 26–28 years. No standard deviations reported.
[d]Reported data from Mallon et al. [80].
[e]Not reported for individual fingers.

and can be reliable, but they reflect the total mobility of a digit and are a function of the size of the hand. They may be quite appropriate in some clinical situations; for example, linear measures may be useful to monitor weekly changes in hand mobility in a patient with hand burns. Precise ROM measures of individual joints of the fingers remain useful to assess changes in individual joints and to compare subjects. For example, to compare the results of two types of PIP joint arthroplasties, discrete ROM measures may be necessary.

Summary

This chapter presents a discussion of the bones and joints that compose the wrist and hand. The architecture of this region is more intricate than the more proximal elbow and shoulder complexes by virtue of the large number of bones and joints. The bony architecture throughout the region allows substantial mobility but provides minimal stability. Each joint is stabilized by an intricate system of ligaments.

The distal radioulnar joint is supported primarily by the TFCC and, with the proximal radioulnar joint, allows pronation and supination. The wrist, composed of the radiocarpal, midcarpal, and intercarpal joints, is supported by extrinsic and intrinsic ligaments. The radiocarpal and midcarpal joints both contribute to global wrist motion. The CMC joint of the thumb separates the thumb from the hand and allows the thumb to oppose the fingers. The CMC joints of the fingers help form the volar arch that contributes to powerful grasp. The MCP joints of the thumb and fingers are supported by a capsule, collateral ligaments, and a volar plate, but the thumb is less mobile than the fingers. The interphalangeal joints of

the thumb and fingers exhibit similar supportive structures, but their articular surfaces allow only uniaxial motion.

This complex of joints with its considerable mobility provides the hand with the potential for remarkably varied and precise movements as long as the surrounding muscles provide adequate dynamic control. The following chapter presents the muscles of the forearm, the primary movers of the wrist and significant contributors to motion of the digits.

References

1. Aleksandrowicz R, Pagowski S: Functional anatomy and bioengineering of the third finger of the human hand. Folia Morphol (Warsz) 1981; 40: 181–192.
2. Almquist EE: Evolution of the distal radioulnar joint. Clin Orthop 1992; 275: 5–13.
3. Andrews JG, Youm Y: A biomechanical investigation of wrist kinematics. J Biomech 1979; 12: 83–93.
4. Anglin C, Wyss UP: Arm motion and load analysis of sit-to-stand, stand-to-sit, cane walking and lifting. Clin Biomech 2000; 15: 441–448.
5. Apfel E: The effect of thumb interphalangeal joint position on strength of key pinch. J Hand Surg [Am] 1986; 11: 87–91.
6. Ash HE, Unsworth A: Proximal interphalangeal joint dimensions for the design of a surface replacement prosthesis. Proc Inst Mech Eng [H] 1996; 210: 95–108.
7. Ateshian GA, Ark JW, Rosenwasser MP, et al.: Contact areas in the thumb carpometacarpal joint. J Orthop Res 1995; 13: 450–458.
8. Ateshian GA, Rosenwasser MP, Mow VC: Curvature characteristics and congruence of the thumb carpometacarpal joint: differences between female and male joints. J Biomech 1992; 25: 591–607.
9. Backhouse KM: Mechanical factors influencing normal and rheumatoid metacarpophalangeal joints. Ann Rheum Dis 1969; 28: 15–19.

10. Barden GA: Trapezial resection arthroplasty for osteoarthritis, use of abductor pollicis longus tendoplasty with interpositional material. J South Orthop Assoc 1999; 9: 1–7.

11. Barmakian JT: Anatomy of the joints of the thumb. Hand Clin 1992; 8: 683–691.

12. Berger RA: The anatomy and basic biomechanics of the wrist joint. J Hand Ther 1996; 9: 84–93.

13. Berger RA, Crowninshield RD, Flatt AE: The three-dimensional rotational behaviors of the carpal bones. Clin Orthop 1982; 167: 303–310.

14. Bird HA, Stowe J: The Wrist. In: Clinics in Rheumatic Diseases. Wright V, ed. London: WB Saunders, 1982; 559–569.

15. Boone DC, Azen SP: Normal range of motion of joints in male subjects. J Bone Joint Surg 1979; 61-A: 756–759.

16. Bowers WH, Wolf JW, Nehil JL, Bittinger S: The proximal interphalangeal joint volar plate. I. An anatomical and biomechanical study. J Hand Surg [Am] 1980; 5: 79–88.

17. Brand PW, Hollister A: Clinical Mechanics of the Hand. St. Louis, MO: Mosby-Year Book, 1999.

18. Brooks JJ, Schiller JR, Allen SD, Akelman E: Biomechanical and anatomical consequences of carpal tunnel release. Clin Biomech 2003; 18: 685–693.

19. Brown RR, Fliszar E, Cotten A, et al.: Extrinsic and intrinsic ligaments of the wrist: normal and pathologic anatomy at MR arthrography with three-compartment enhancement. Radiographics 1998; 18: 667–674.

20. Brumfield RH, Champoux JA: A biomechanical study of normal functional wrist motion. Clin Orthop 1984; 187: 23–25.

21. Buchholz B, Armstrong TJ: A kinematic model of the human hand to evaluate its prehensile capabilities. J Biomech 1992; 25: 149–162.

22. Camus EJ, Millot F, Lariviere J, et al.: Kinematics of the wrist using 2D and 3D analysis: biomechanical and clinical deductions. Surg Radiol Anat 2004; 26: 399–410.

23. Coert JH, Hoek van Dijke GA, Hovius SER, et al.: Quantifying thumb rotation during circumduction utilizing a video technique. J Orthop Res 2003; 21: 1151–1155.

24. Cooney WP III, Chao EYS: Biomechanical analysis of static forces in the thumb during hand function. J Bone Joint Surg 1977; 59A: 27–36.

25. Cooney WP III, Lucca MJ, Chao EYS, Inscheid RL: The kinesiology of the thumb trapeziometacarpal joint. J Bone Joint Surg 1981; 63A: 1371–1381.

26. Craig SM: Anatomy of the joints of the fingers. Hand Clin 1992; 8: 693–700.

27. de Lange A, Huiskes R, Kauer JMG: Wrist-joint ligament length changes in flexion and deviation of the hand: an experimental study. J Orthop Res 1990; 8: 722–730.

28. de Lange A, Kauer JMG, Huiskes R: Kinematic behavior of the human wrist joint: a roentgen-stereophotogrammetric analysis. J Orthop Res 1985; 3: 56–64.

29. De Smet L: Ulnar variance: facts and fiction review article. Acta Orthop Belg 1994; 60: 1–9.

30. Defrate LE, Li G, Zayontz SJ, Herndon JH: A minimally invasive method for the determination of force in the interosseous ligament. Clin Biomech 2001; 16: 895–900.

31. Departments of the U.S. Army and Air Force. US Army Goniometry Manual.: Technical Manual no. 8-640. Air Force Pamphlet no. 160-14. 1-8-1968. Washington, DC: Departments of the Army and Air Force.

32. DiTano O, Trumble TE, Tencer AF: Biomechanical function of the distal radioulnar and ulnocarpal wrist ligaments. J Hand Surg [Am] 2003; 28: 622–627.

33. Drobner WS, Hausman MR: The distal radioulnar joint. Hand Clin 1992; 8: 631–644.

34. Ekenstam FA: Anatomy of the distal radioulnar joint. Clin Orthop 1992; 275: 14–18.

35. Fioretti S, Germani A, Leo T: Stereometry in very close-range stereophotogrammetry with non-metric cameras for human movement analysis. J Biomech 1985; 18: 831–842.

36. Fioretti S, Jetto L, Leo T: Reliable in vivo estimation of the instantaneous helical axis in human segmental movements. IEEE Trans Biomed Eng 1990; 37: 398–409.

37. Fuss FK, Wagner TF: Biomechanical alterations in the carpal arch and hand muscles after carpal tunnel release: a further approach toward understanding the function of the flexor retinaculum and the cause of postoperative grip weakness. Clin Anat 1996; 9: 100–108.

38. Garcia-Elias M: Soft-tissue anatomy and relationships about the distal ulna. Hand Clin 1998; 14: 165–176.

39. Garcia-Elias M, Sanchez-Freijo JM, Salo JM, Lluch AL: Dynamic changes of the transverse carpal arch during flexion-extension of the wrist: effects of sectioning the transverse carpal ligament. J Hand Surg [Am] 1992; 17A: 1017–1019.

40. Gelberman RH, Gross MS: The vascularity of the wrist. Identification of arterial patterns at risk. Clin Orthop 1986; 202: 40–49.

41. Gerhardt JJ, Rippstein J: Measuring and Recording of Joint Motion Instrumentation and Techniques. Lewiston, NJ: Hogrefe & Huber, 1990.

42. Giunta RE, Biemer E, Muller-Gerbl M: Ulnar variance and subchondral bone mineralization patterns in the distal articular surface of the radius. J Hand Surg 2004; 24A: 835–840.

43. Greene WB, Heckman JDE: The Clinical Measurement of Joint Motion. Rosemont, IL: American Academy of Orthopaedic Surgeons, 1994.

44. Gupta A, Moosawi NA: How much can carpus rotate axially? An in vivo study. Clin Biomech 2005; 20: 172–176.

45. Hagert CG: Anatomical aspects on the design of metacarpophalangeal implants. Reconstr Surg Traumatol 1981; 18: 92–110.

46. Hagert CG: The distal radioulnar joint in relation to the whole forearm. Clin Orthop 1992; 275: 56–64.

47. Haines RW: The mechanism of rotation at the first carpometacarpal joint. J Anat 1944; 78: 44–46.

48. Hakstian RW, Tubiana R: Ulnar deviation of the fingers. The role of joint structure and function. J Bone Joint Surg 1967; 49A: 299–316.

49. Harley BJ, Werner FW, Green JK: A biomechanical modeling of injury, repair, and rehabilitation of ulnar collateral ligament injuries of the thumb. J Hand Surg 2004; 29A: 915–920.

50. Harty M: The hand of man. Phys Ther 1971; 51: 777–781.

51. Hirsch D, Page D, Miller D, et al.: A biomechanical analysis of the metacarpophalangeal joint of the thumb. J Biomech 1974; 7: 343–348.

52. Hollister A, Buford WL, Myers LM, et al.: The axes of rotation of the thumb carpometacarpal joint. J Orthop Res 1992; 10: 454–460.

53. Hollister A, Giurintano DJ: Thumb movements, motions, and moments. J Hand Ther 1995; 8: 106–114.

54. Hollister A, Giurintano DJ, Buford WL, et al.: The axes of rotation of the thumb interphalangeal and metacarpophalangeal joints. Clin Orthop 1995; 320: 188–193.

55. Hoppenfeld S: Physical Examination of the Spine and Extremities. New York: Appleton-Century-Crofts, 1976.

56. Hume MC, Gellman H, McKellop H, Brumfield RH Jr: Functional range of motion of the joints of the hand. J Hand Surg [Am] 1990; 15A: 240–243.

57. Imaeda T, An KN, Cooney WP III: Functional anatomy and biomechanics of the thumb. Hand Clin 1992; 8: 9–15.

58. Imaeda T, Cooney WP, Niebur GL, et al.: Kinematics of the trapeziometacarpal joint: a biomechanical analysis comparing tendon interposition arthroplasty and total-joint arthroplasty. J Hand Surg [Am] 1996; 21A: 544–553.

59. Ishikawa J, Niebur GL, Uchiyama S, et al.: Feasibility of using a magnetic tracking device for measuring carpal kinematics. J Biomech 1997; 30: 1183–1186.

60. Jackson WT, Hefzy MS, Guo H: Determination of wrist kinematics using a magnetic tracking device. Med Eng Phys 1994; 16: 123–133.

61. Jaffe R, Chidgey LK, LaStayo PC: The distal radioulnar joint: anatomy and management of disorders. J Hand Ther 1996; 9: 129–138.

62. Kapandji IA: The Physiology of the Joints. Vol 1, The Upper Limb. Edinburgh: Churchill Livingstone, 1982.

63. Kaplan EB: Anatomy and Kinesiology of the Hand. In: Hand Surgery. Flynn JE, ed. Baltimore: Williams & Wilkins, 1982; 14–24.

64. Karnezis IA: Correlation between wrist loads and the distal radius volar tilt angle. Clin Biomech 2005; 20: 270–276.

65. Kauer JMG: The distal radioulnar joint. Anatomic and functional considerations. Clin Orthop 1992; 275: 37–45.

66. Kiefhaber TR, Stern PJ, Grood ES: Lateral stability of the proximal interphalangeal joint. J Hand Surg [Am] 1986; 11A: 661–669.

67. Kihara H, Short WH, Werner FW, et al.: The stabilizing mechanism of the distal radioulnar joint during pronation and supination. J Hand Surg [Am] 1995; 20A: 930–936.

68. Kleinman WB, Graham TJ: The distal radioulnar joint capsule: clinical anatomy and role in posttraumatic limitation of forearm rotation. J Hand Surg [Am] 1998; 23A: 588–599.

69. Kobayashi M, Berger RA, Linscheid RL, An KN: Intercarpal kinematics during wrist motion. Hand Clin 1997; 13: 143–149.

70. Kobayashi M, Berger RA, Nagy L, et al.: Normal kinematics of carpal bones: a three-dimensional analysis of carpal bone motion relative to the radius. J Biomech 1997; 30: 787–793.

71. Kozin SH, Bishop AT: Gamekeeper's thumb. Early diagnosis and treatment. Orthop Rev 1994; 23: 797–804.

72. Kuczynski K: Less known aspects of the proximal interphalangeal joints of the human hand. Hand 1975; 7: 31–33.

73. Landsmeer JMF: Anatomical and functional investigations of the articulation of the human fingers. Acta Anat 1955; 25: 1–69.

74. Larsen CF, Lauritsen J: Epidemiology of acute wrist trauma. Int J Epidemiol 1993; 22: 911–916.

75. Lee JW, Rim K: Measurement of finger joint angles and maximum finger forces during cylinder grip activity. J Biomed Eng 1991; 13: 153–162.

76. Li ZM, Kuxhaus L, Fisk JA, Christophel TH: Coupling between wrist flexion-extension and radial-ulnar deviation. Clin Biomech 2005; 20: 177–183.

77. Linscheid RL: Biomechanics of the distal radioulnar joint. Clin Orthop 1992; 275: 46–55.

78. Mallmin H, Ljunghall S: Incidence of Colles' fracture in Uppsala; a prospective study of a quarter-million population. Acta Orthop Scand 1992; 63: 213–215.

79. Mallmin H, Ljunghall S, Persson I, Bergstrom R: Risk factors for fractures of the distal forearm: a population-based case-control study. Osteoporos Int 1994; 4: 298–304.

80. Mallon WJ, Brown HR, Nunley JA: Digital ranges of motion: normal values in young adults. J Hand Surg [Am] 1991; 16A: 882–887.

81. McMurtry RY, Youm Y, Flatt AE, Gillespie TE: Kinematics of the wrist. Clinical applications. J Bone Joint Surg 1978; 60A: 955–961.

82. Melling M, Reihsner R, Steindl M, et al.: Biomechanical stability of abductor pollicis longus muscles with variable numbers of tendinous insertions. Anat Rec 1998; 250: 475–479.

83. Minami A, An KN, Cooney WP III, et al.: Ligamentous structures of the metacarpophalangeal joint: a quantitative anatomic study. J Orthop Res 1984; 1: 361–368.

84. Minami A, An KN, Cooney WP III, et al.: Ligament stability of the metacarpophalangeal joint: a biomechanical study. J Hand Surg [Am] 1985; 10A: 255–260.

85. Minamikawa Y, Horii E, Amadio PC, et al.: Stability and constraint of the proximal interphalangeal joint. J Hand Surg [Am] 1993; 18A: 198–204.

86. Moran CA: Anatomy of the hand. Phys Ther 1989; 69: 1007–1013.

87. Munk B, Jensen SL, Olsen BS, et al.: Wrist stability after experimental traumatic triangular fibrocartilage complex lesions. J Hand Surg 2005; 30A: 43–49.

88. Murgia A, Kyberd PJ, Chappell PH, Light CM: Marker placement to describe the wrist movements during activities of daily living in cyclical tasks. Clin Biomech 2004; 19: 248–254.

89. Napier JR: The prehensile movements of the human hand. J Bone Joint Surg 1956; 38B: 902–913.

90. Newsam CJ, Rao SS, Mulroy SJ, et al.: Three dimensional upper extremity motion during manual wheelchair propulsion in men with different levels of spinal cord injury. Gait Posture 1999; 10: 223–232.

91. Norkin CC, White DJ: Measurement of Joint Motion. A Guide to Goniometry. Philadelphia: FA Davis, 1995.

92. Nowalk MD, Logan SE: Distinguishing biomechanical properties of intrinsic and extrinsic human wrist ligaments. J Biomech Eng 1991; 113: 85–93.

93. Noyes FS, Grood ES: The strength of the anterior cruciate ligament in humans and rhesus monkeys. J Bone Joint Surg 1976; 58A: 1074–1082.

94. Patterson R, Viegas SF: Biomechanics of the wrist. J Hand Ther 1995; 8: 97–105.

95. Patterson RM, Nicodemus CL, Viegas SF, et al.: Normal wrist kinematics and the analysis of the effect of various dynamic external fixators for treatment of distal radius fractures. Hand Clin 1997; 13: 129–141.

96. Patterson RM, Nicodemus CL, Viegas SF, et al.: High-speed, three-dimensional kinematic analysis of the normal wrist. J Hand Surg [Am] 1998; 23A: 446–453.

97. Pellegrini VD Jr: The ABJS 2005 Nicolas Andry Award: osteoarthritis and injury at the base of the human thumb: survival of the fittest? Clin Orthop Relat Res 2005; 438: 266–276.

98. Pellegrini VD Jr, Olcott CW, Hollenberg G: Contact patterns in the trapeziometacarpal joint: the role of the palmar beak ligament. J Hand Surg [Am] 1993; 18A: 238–244.

99. Peltier LF: Fractures of the distal end of the radius. Clin Orthop 1984; 187: 18–22.

100. Pevny T, Rayan GM, Egle D: Ligamentous and tendinous support of the pisiform: anatomic and biomechanical study. J Okla State Med Assoc 1995; 88: 205–210.

101. Rhee RY, Reading G, Wray RC: A biomechanical study of the collateral ligaments of the proximal interphalangeal joint. J Hand Surg [Am] 1992; 17A: 157–163.

102. Ritt MJPF, Bishop AT, Berger RA, et al.: Lunotriquetral ligament properties: a comparison of three anatomic subregions. J Hand Surg [Am] 1998; 23A: 425–431.

103. Rodriguez-Merchan EC: Management of comminuted fractures of the distal radius in the adult; conservative or surgical? Clin Orthop 1998; 353: 53–62.

104. Romanes GJE: Cunningham's Textbook of Anatomy. Oxford: Oxford University Press, 1981.

105. Ruby LK, Cooney WP III, An KN, et al.: Relative motion of selected carpal bones: a kinematic analysis of the normal wrist. J Hand Surg [Am] 1988; 13A: 1–10.

106. Ryu JR, Cooney WP III, Askew LJ, et al.: Functional ranges of motion of the wrist joint. J Hand Surg 1991; 16A: 409–419.

107. Salter RB: Textbook of Disorders and Injuries of the Musculoskeletal System. 3rd ed. Baltimore: Williams & Wilkins, 1999.

108. Sarrafian SK, Melamed JK, Goshgarian GM: Study of wrist motion in flexion and extension. Clin Orthop 1977; 126: 153–159.

109. Savelberg HH, Kooloos JGM, Huiskes R, Kauer JMG: Stiffness of the ligaments of the human wrist joint. J Biomech 1992; 25: 369–376.

110. Savelberg HH, Otten JDM, Kooloos JGM, et al.: Carpal bone kinematics and ligament lengthening studied for the full range of joint movement. J Biomech 1993; 26: 1389–1402.

111. Schoenmarklin RW, Marras WS: Dynamic capabilities of the wrist joint in industrial workers. Int J Ind Ergonomics 1993; 11: 207–224.

112. Schuind F, An KN, Berglund L, et al.: The distal radioulnar ligaments: a biomechanical study. J Hand Surg [Am] 1991; 16A: 1106–1114.

113. Schuind F, Cooney WP, Linscheid RL, et al.: Force and pressure transmission through the normal wrist. A theoretical two-dimensional study in the posteroanterior plane. J Biomech 1995; 28: 587–601.

114. Sennwald GR, Zdravkovic V, Kern HP, Jacob HAC: Kinematics of the wrist and its ligaments. J Hand Surg 1993; 18A: 805–814.

115. Shaaban H, Giakas G, Bolton M, et al.: The load-bearing characteristics of the forearm: pattern of axial and bending force transmitted through ulna and radius. J Hand Surg [Br] 2006; 31: 274–279.

116. Shaw JA, Bruno A, Paul EM: Ulnar styloid fixation in the treatment of posttraumatic instability of the radioulnar joint: a biomechanical study with clinical correlation. J Hand Surg [Am] 1990; 15A: 712–720.

117. Short WH, Werner FW, Fortino MD, Mann KA: Analysis of the kinematics of the scaphoid and lunate in the intact wrist joint. Hand Clin 1997; 13: 93–108.

118. Short WH, Werner FW, Fortino MD, et al.: A dynamic biomechanical study of scapholunate ligament sectioning. J Hand Surg [Am] 1995; 20: 986–999.

119. Simoneau GG, Marklin RW, Berman JE: Effect of computer keyboard slope on wrist position and forearm electromyography of typists without musculoskeletal disorders. Phys Ther 2003; 83: 816–830.

120. Small CF, Bryant JT, Pichora DR: Rationalization of kinematic descriptors for three-dimensional hand and finger motion. J Biomed Eng 1992; 14: 133–141.

121. Spilman HW, Pinkston D: Relation of test positions to radial and ulnar deviation. Phys Ther 1967; 49: 837–844.

122. Steindler A: Kinesiology of the Human Body under Normal and Pathological Conditions. Springfield, IL: Charles C Thomas, 1955.

123. Stuchin SA: Wrist anatomy. Hand Clin 1992; 8: 603–609.

124. Sun J, Shih TT, Ko C, et al.: In vivo kinematic study of normal wrist motion: an ultrafast computed tomographic study. Clin Biomech 2000; 15: 212–216.

125. Taleisnik J: The ligaments of the wrist. J Hand Surg [Am] 1976; 1: 110–118.

126. Tang JB, Jaiyoung R, Omokawa S, et al.: Biomechanical evaluation of wrist motor tendons after fractures of the distal radius. J Hand Surg [Am] 1999; 24A: 121–132.

127. Tubiana R, Thomine JM, Mackin E: Examination of the Hand and Wrist. Philadelphia: WB Saunders, 1996.

128. Unver B, Gocen Z, Sen A, et al.: Normal ranges of ulnar and radial deviation with reference to ulnar variance. J Int Med Res 2004; 32: 337–340.

129. Van Brenk B, Richards RR, Mackay MB, Boynton EL: A biomechanical assessment of ligaments preventing dorsoradial subluxation of the trapeziometacarpal joint. J Hand Surg [Am] 1998; 23A: 607–611.

130. Viegas SF, Patterson RM, Ward K: Extrinsic wrist ligaments in the pathomechanics of ulnar translation instability. J Hand Surg [Am] 1995; 20: 312–318.

131. Walker JM, Sue D, Miles-Elkousy N, et al.: Active mobility of the extremities in older subjects. Phys Ther 1984; 64: 919–923.

132. Walker PS, Poppen NK: Biomechanics of the shoulder joint during abduction in the plane of the scapula. Bull Hosp Jt Dis 1977; 38: 107–111.

133. Ward L, Ambrose C, Masson M, Levaro F: The role of the distal radioulnar ligaments, interosseous membrane and joint capsule in distal radioulnar joint stability. J Hand Surg 2000; 25A: 341–351.

134. Watanabe H, Berger RA, An KN, et al.: Stability of the distal radioulnar joint contributed by the joint capsule. J Hand Surg 2004; 29A: 1114–1120.

135. Watanabe H, Berger RA, Berglund LJ, et al.: Contribution of the interosseous membrane to distal radioulnar joint constraint. J Hand Surg 2005; 30A: 1164–1171.

136. Weaver L, Tencer AF, Trumble TE: Tensions in the palmar ligaments of the wrist. I. The normal wrist. J Hand Surg [Am] 1994; 19: 464–474.

137. Weber ER, Chao EY: An experimental approach to the mechanism of scaphoid wrist fractures. J Hand Surg [Am] 1978; 3: 142–148.

138. Weeks PM, Gilula LA, Manske PR, et al.: Acute Bone and Joint Injuries of the Hand and Wrist; a Clinical Guide to Management. St. Louis, MO: CV Mosby, 1981.

139. Weinberg AM, Pietsch IT, Helm MB, et al.: A new kinematic model of pro- and supination of the human forearm. J Biomech 2000; 33: 487–491.

140. Werner FW, Short WH, Fortino MD, Palmer AK: The relative contribution of selected carpal bones to global wrist motion

during simulated planar and out-of-plane wrist motion. J Hand Surg [Am] 1997; 22A: 708–713.

141. Williams P, Bannister L, Berry M, et al.: Gray's Anatomy, The Anatomical Basis of Medicine and Surgery, Br. ed. London: Churchill Livingstone, 1995.

142. Yanni D, Lieppins P, Laurence M: Fractures of the carpal scaphoid. A critical study of the standard splint. J Bone Joint Surg 1991; 73B: 600–602.

143. Youm Y: Instantaneous center of rotation by least square method. J Bioeng 1978; 2: 129–137.

144. Youm Y, McMurtry RY, Flatt AE, Gillespie TE: Kinematics of the wrist I. An experimental study of radial-ulnar deviation and flexion-extension. J Bone Joint Surg 1978; 60A: 423–431.

145. Zmurko MG, Eglseder Jr. WA, Belkoff SM: Biomechanical evaluation of distal radius fracture stability. J Orthop Trauma 1998; 12: 46–50.

Mechanics and Pathomechanics of the Muscles of the Forearm

CHAPTER CONTENTS

The preceding chapter presents the bones and joints of the wrist and hand. That chapter discusses the influence of the articular surfaces and surrounding ligaments on the available motion and resulting stability at each joint. The current chapter presents the muscles of the forearm, which not only serve as the motors for the wrist and hand but also contribute to the stability of the entire complex.

Many of the forearm muscles cross some or all of the joints of the thumb or fingers. These muscles are known as the *extrinsic muscles of the hand*. Their effects on the hand are intimately related to the intrinsic muscles of the hand and to supporting structures that are unique to the hand. Consequently, a full understanding of the influence of these extrinsic muscles on the mechanics and pathomechanics of the hand can be complete only after presentation of the special structures of the hand. The special connective tissue structures found in the hand are discussed in Chapter 17. The intrinsic muscles of the hand are presented in Chapter 18.

Although more than one half of the muscles of the forearm are positioned to have some effect on the elbow, only the pronator teres and supinator muscles function primarily at the elbow. The other forearm muscles act primarily at the wrist and hand. Their roles at the elbow are discussed in this chapter, although these actions are inadequately studied and poorly understood. Since the normal elbow possesses other large muscles dedicated to moving it, these forearm muscles may have little functional significance at the elbow except in individuals lacking normal elbow musculature. In these individuals, the forearm muscles crossing the elbow may be functionally important.

Manifestation of weakness in many of the forearm muscles differs somewhat from that of more proximal muscles. Weakness of a muscle alters the normal balance of forces crossing any joint. As a result of such an imbalance, the stronger, opposing muscle forces tend to pull the joint in the opposite direction. For example, in the presence of weakness of the triceps brachii, the elbow flexors tend to pull the elbow into flexion, but in the upright position, the weight of the forearm and hand helps resist the flexion force of the stronger elbow flexors. The weights of the distal segments in the wrist and hand are less significant and thus are less able to resist the deforming forces of muscle imbalances. Consequently, weakness or tightness of muscles of the wrist and hand are more directly associated with deformities than elsewhere in the upper extremity. In the following presentations of the forearm muscles, discussions of weakness and tightness of these muscles include discussions of the potential deformities. It is important to recognize that muscle balance in the hand depends on the balance among the extrinsic muscles presented in this chapter and also on a balance between these extrinsic muscles and the intrinsic muscles presented in Chapter 18. Additional details of many of these deformities are found in Chapter 18.

One characteristic common to most of the muscles in the forearm is the proximity of each muscle to the axes of motion of the joints they cross. The moment arms of muscles at the shoulder and the elbow are typically a few centimeters or more. In contrast, the moment arms of muscles in the forearm range from approximately 0.1 to 3.0 cm. Because the moment arms are so small and most of the tendons can migrate slightly around a joint, many of the forearm muscles have variable actions. Such variability stems from a change in the muscle's moment arm from, for example, extension to flexion. The flexor carpi radialis provides a good example *(Fig. 15.1)*. This muscle attaches to the medial epicondyle of the humerus, lying very close to the elbow's axis of flexion and extension. Reports suggest that the muscle lies anterior to the axis when the elbow is flexed and consequently produces a flexion moment at the elbow [1]. When the elbow is extended, the muscle apparently slides to the posterior side of the elbow's axis and produces an extension moment. The presence of small moment arms and the ability of the tendons to slide from one side of a joint axis to another help explain disagreements presented in this chapter regarding muscle actions.

The purposes of the present chapter are to

- Describe the architecture and action of each of the muscles of the forearm
- Discuss the functional roles of each of the forearm muscles at the elbow, wrist, and hand
- Begin to examine the contributions to functional deficits in the wrist and hand made by impairments of individual muscles

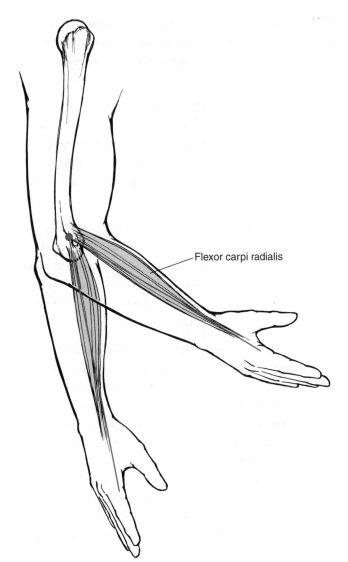

Flexor carpi radialis

Figure 15.1: Effect of joint position on the moment arm of a muscle. The flexor carpi radialis (FCR) lies so close to the axis of flexion and extension at the elbow that the muscle may be anterior to the axis and thus act to flex the elbow when the elbow is flexed, and may slide to the posterior side of the axis and act to extend the elbow when the elbow is extended.

■ Describe the necessary interplay between the wrist and hand muscles of the forearm required for optimal hand function
■ Compare the relative strengths of opposing muscle groups of the forearm

The muscles of the forearm are readily divided into four distinct groups, two on the volar surface and two on the dorsal surface of the forearm. There are deep and superficial muscle groups on each surface. The four forearm muscle groups are

■ Superficial muscles of the volar surface
■ Superficial muscles of the dorsal surface
■ Deep muscles of the volar surface
■ Deep muscles of the dorsal surface

Each muscle group is presented below. After all of the muscles of the forearm are discussed, the synergistic activity between the wrist and extrinsic hand muscles is presented. Finally, the relative strengths of the forearm muscles are reviewed.

SUPERFICIAL MUSCLES ON THE VOLAR SURFACE OF THE FOREARM

There are five superficial forearm muscles on the volar surface: pronator teres, flexor carpi radialis, palmaris longus, flexor digitorum superficialis, and flexor carpi ulnaris (*Fig. 15.2*). Each of these muscles has a common origin on the medial epicondyle of the humerus by way of the common

flexor tendon. These muscles have additional proximal attachments that are presented with each muscle.

Pronator Teres

The pronator teres is presented in Chapter 12 with the other flexor muscles of the elbow. Its actions consist of elbow flexion and pronation [34,75]. Electromyographic (EMG) data suggest that its role is to provide additional force in these motions against heavy resistance [5]. It is readily palpated in the middle of the volar aspect of the forearm. Weakness of the pronator teres contributes to decreased strength in elbow flexion and pronation. If the other elbow flexors remain unaffected, resulting elbow flexion weakness is minimal. Similarly, if the pronator quadratus (presented later in this chapter) remains intact, the disability associated with pronator teres weakness is restricted to activities requiring forceful pronation.

Tightness of the pronator teres can result in decreased supination range of motion (ROM). However, the effect of the muscle's tightness depends on the position of elbow flexion, since the pronator teres affects both pronation and flexion. The interrelationship of these two joint positions is discussed in detail in Chapter 12, but elbow flexion puts the pronator teres in a slackened position and consequently allows more supination ROM (see Fig. 12.9). Conversely, increasing the stretch on the pronator teres by extending the elbow decreases flexibility in the direction of supination.

Flexor Carpi Radialis

The flexor carpi radialis is fusiform and lies just medial to the pronator teres (*Muscle Attachment Box 15.1*). It is one of six dedicated wrist muscles of the forearm whose distal function

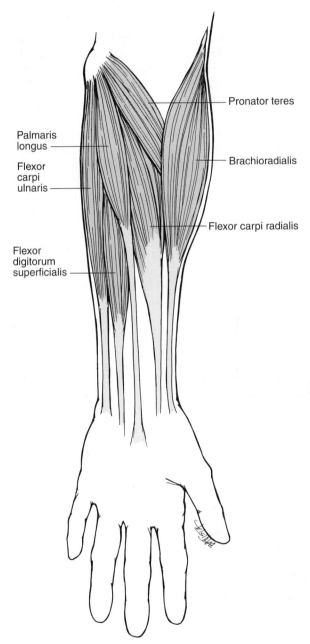

Palmaris longus

Flexor carpi ulnaris

Flexor digitorum superficialis

Pronator teres

Brachioradialis

Flexor carpi radialis

Figure 15.2: The five superficial muscles on the volar surface of the forearm. From radial to ulnar the five superficial muscles on the volar surface of the forearm are pronator teres (PT), flexor carpi radialis (FCR), palmaris longus (PL), flexor digitorum superficialis (FDS), and flexor carpi ulnaris (FCU).

MUSCLE ATTACHMENT BOX 15.1

ATTACHMENTS AND INNERVATION OF THE FLEXOR CARPI RADIALIS

Proximal attachment: The medial epicondyle of the humerus by way of the common flexor tendon and from the surrounding fascia. It lies medial to the pronator teres.

Distal attachment: The palmar surfaces of the bases of the metacarpals to the index and long fingers.

Innervation: Median nerve, C6 and C7.

Palpation: The tendon of the flexor carpi radialis is readily palpated in the distal forearm just medial to the radial artery.

is directed solely at the wrist. The other dedicated wrist muscles are the palmaris longus, flexor carpi ulnaris, extensor carpi radialis longus and brevis, and extensor carpi ulnaris. Other muscles of the forearm affect the wrist too but have important functions at the digits as well.

ACTIONS

MUSCLE ACTION: FLEXOR CARPI RADIALIS

Action	Evidence
Wrist flexion	Supporting
Wrist radial deviation	Supporting
Elbow flexion	Conflicting
Elbow pronation	Conflicting

The role of the flexor carpi radialis in wrist flexion and radial deviation is supported by EMG data and analysis of the muscle's moment arms [5,8,50,55,67,75]. It has moment arms of approximately 1.0 cm for both wrist flexion and radial deviation [8,12] (Fig. 15.3).

Contraction of the flexor carpi radialis results in simultaneous flexion and radial deviation of the wrist. For the muscle to participate in only wrist flexion or only radial deviation, at least one other muscle must contract at the same time to prevent the undesired movement. For example, the flexor carpi radialis participates in pure wrist flexion by contracting with the flexor carpi ulnaris, whose ulnar deviation pull provides a counterbalance to the radial deviation pull from the flexor carpi radialis (Fig. 15.4). EMG analysis suggests that recruitment of the flexor carpi radialis is greatest when the subject exerts a force in the direction of both flexion and radial deviation [12]. This finding is similar to the findings regarding biceps brachii recruitment. The biceps brachii's participation in elbow flexion is reduced when the forearm is pronated (Chapter 12).

The role of the flexor carpi radialis at the elbow is controversial. Most reports suggest it flexes the elbow [1,8,34,51], although one study reports that it both flexes and extends the elbow, depending on the elbow's position [1]. Most biomechanical studies report that it possesses a pronation moment arm [1,10,28,38,42], although the limited EMG data available show no active contraction during pronation [1,5,46,51]. Biomechanical studies suggest that the flexor carpi radialis has the mechanical potential to exert moments at the elbow; however, its functional activity at the elbow is unverified. The clinician is cautioned to recognize that the flexor carpi radialis may have little function at the elbow under normal conditions, but the muscle has the potential to participate in the absence of other muscle

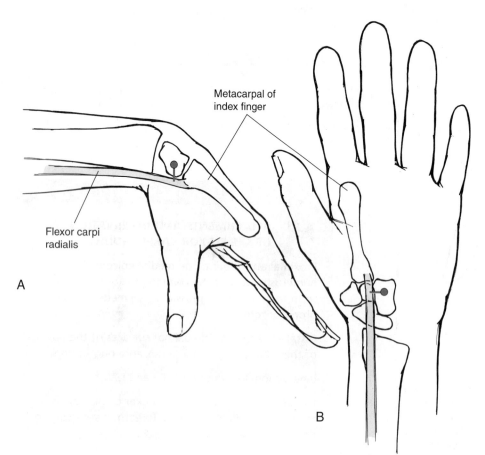

Metacarpal of
index finger

Flexor carpi
radialis

A

B

Figure 15.3: The moment arms of the flexor carpi radialis for both flexion **(A)** and radial deviation **(B)** are approximately 1.0 cm.

ATTACHMENTS AND INNERVATION OF THE PALMARIS LONGUS

Proximal attachment: The medial epicondyle of the humerus by way of the common flexor tendon and from the surrounding fascia. It lies medial to the flexor carpi radialis.

Distal attachment: The superficial surface of the flexor retinaculum and to the proximal portion of the palmar aponeurosis.

Innervation: Median nerve, C8 and perhaps C7.

Palpation: The muscle is readily palpated superficial to the transverse carpal ligament during wrist flexion with simultaneous opposition of the thumb and little finger.

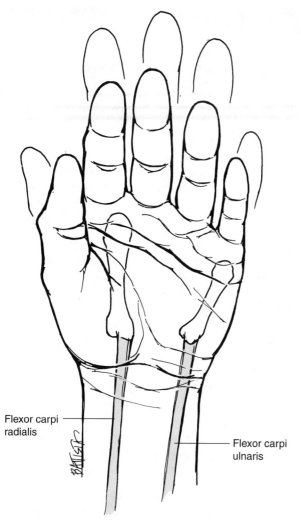

Flexor carpi radialis

Flexor carpi ulnaris

Figure 15.4: Wrist flexion without radial deviation requires the combined contraction of the flexor carpi radialis (FCR) and the flexor carpi ulnaris (FCU).

control at the elbow. Such potential may be realized in individuals with profound loss of the primary elbow musculature, for example, individuals with polio.

EFFECTS OF WEAKNESS

Discrete weakness of the flexor carpi radialis is uncommon. However, tendinitis of the flexor carpi radialis does occur, producing pain with contraction. Consequently, the patient may avoid contraction and function as though there is weakness. The obvious impairment from reduced activity of the flexor carpi radialis is weakness in the combined movements of wrist flexion and radial deviation. The resulting functional deficit at the wrist stems from the muscular imbalance that ensues from weakness of this wrist muscle. This same effect is seen whenever one or a combination of wrist muscles is impaired. A more detailed discussion of the role of muscle balance and the effects of muscle imbalances at the wrist is presented after all of the dedicated wrist muscles are discussed.

EFFECTS OF TIGHTNESS

Like weakness, isolated tightness of the flexor carpi radialis, although unusual, upsets the balance of muscles at the wrist. Tightness results in diminished flexibility in the direction of extension and ulnar deviation.

Palmaris Longus

The palmaris longus is a small fusiform muscle medial to the flexor carpi radialis (*Muscle Attachment Box 15.2*). It has a long tendon that is particularly prominent at the wrist because the tendon remains superficial to the transverse carpal ligament (*Fig. 15.5*). However, the muscle is absent in approximately 10% of the population [8].

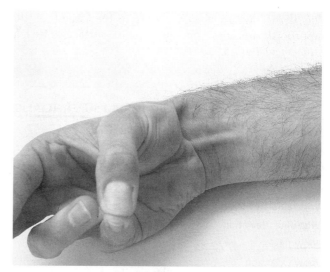

Figure 15.5: The palmaris longus is very prominent because it is superficial to the flexor retinaculum of the wrist.

ACTIONS

MUSCLE ACTION: PALMARIS LONGUS

Action	Evidence
Wrist flexion	Supporting
Hand cupping	Inadequate
Skin anchor	Inadequate

The palmaris longus lies in the center of the wrist and consequently acts as a pure flexor of the wrist. Estimates of its physiological cross-sectional area suggest that the palmaris longus is less than half the size of the flexor carpi radialis and less than one third the size of the flexor carpi ulnaris [1]. Consequently, its contribution to the flexion torque at the wrist is small in most individuals. There are no known EMG studies examining its participation in functional activities.

The functions of the palmaris longus to cup the hand and tighten or support the skin of the hand are the result of the muscle's attachment to the palmar aponeurosis. The functional significance of this aspect of the palmaris longus muscle's action is not known.

EFFECTS OF WEAKNESS

As already noted, the palmaris longus is absent in many individuals. There are no known reports of impairments associated with the absence of the palmaris longus. The muscle's tendon is commonly used by surgeons as graft material for tendon repairs [8,21,68].

EFFECTS OF TIGHTNESS

There are no known reports of discrete tightness of the palmaris longus muscle.

Flexor Digitorum Superficialis (Also Known As Flexor Digitorum Sublimis)

The flexor digitorum superficialis is the largest of the superficial muscles on the volar surface (*Muscle Attachment Box 15.3*).

ACTIONS

MUSCLE ACTION: FLEXOR DIGITORUM SUPERFICIALIS

Action	Evidence
PIP flexion	Supporting
MCP flexion	Supporting
Wrist flexion	Supporting
Wrist radial deviation	Supporting
Wrist ulnar deviation	Supporting
Elbow flexion	Inadequate
Elbow extension	Inadequate
Elbow pronation	Inadequate
Elbow supination	Inadequate

MUSCLE ATTACHMENT BOX 15.3

ATTACHMENTS AND INNERVATION OF THE FLEXOR DIGITORUM SUPERFICIALIS

Proximal attachment: The humeroulnar head attaches to the medial epicondyle of the humerus by way of the common flexor tendon and from the surrounding fascia as well as from the coronoid process of the ulna and the medial collateral ligament of the elbow. The radial portion arises from the anterior surface of the radius from the radial tuberosity to the attachment of the pronator teres.

Distal attachment: A tendon to each finger enters a flexor sheath proximal to the MCP joint. At the MCP joint the tendon splits into two strands through which the tendon of the flexor digitorum profundus travels. The two slips of the flexor digitorum superficialis reunite at the proximal end of the middle phalanx and insert on its palmar surface.

Innervation: Median nerve, C8 and T1, perhaps C7.

Palpation: Tendons of the flexor digitorum superficialis (particularly those to the ring and long fingers) can be palpated in the midline of the wrist as they cross the radiocarpal joint. The muscle belly is palpable along the medial border of the proximal ulna.

The flexor digitorum superficialis is the only muscle that flexes the PIP joints of the fingers without flexing the distal interphalangeal (DIP) joints [5,62,75]. However, contraction of the flexor digitorum superficialis affects each of the joints that the muscle crosses. The tendons of the flexor digitorum superficialis are the most superficial muscles on the volar surface of the MCP joints of the fingers. Consequently, they have the largest moment arms for flexion [2,8] (*Fig. 15.6*). EMG studies reveal activity of the flexor digitorum superficialis during MCP flexion [5]. The flexor digitorum superficialis to the long finger is substantially stronger than that to the index and ring fingers [15], and the flexor digitorum superficialis to the little finger is the weakest [8]. The muscle appears to have no contribution to radial or ulnar deviation of the MCP joints of the fingers under normal conditions [2,7].

The muscle is described as having four separate and distinct muscular slips, each going to a different finger [75], but the tendons to the index, ring, and little finger actually receive muscle fibers from multiple muscle bundles [8]. Only the tendon to the long finger has completely unique muscle fibers. Therefore, only the long finger has completely independent activation of the flexor digitorum superficialis. In contrast, the index and little fingers share some proximal muscle attachments but have independent fiber contributions more distally. As a result, independent activation of the flexor digitorum superficialis at either of these fingers occurs only in low-load

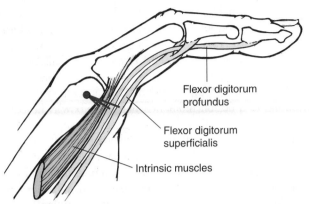

Figure 15.6: The moment arm of the flexor digitorum superficialis. At the MCP joints of the fingers the flexor digitorum superficialis (FDS) lies anterior to all of the other muscles and, therefore, has the largest flexor moment arm of all of these muscles.

activities. More-vigorous contractions recruit the shared musculotendinous units so that the index and little fingers contract together. The tendon to the little finger also may be deficient or completely absent [3,13,29].

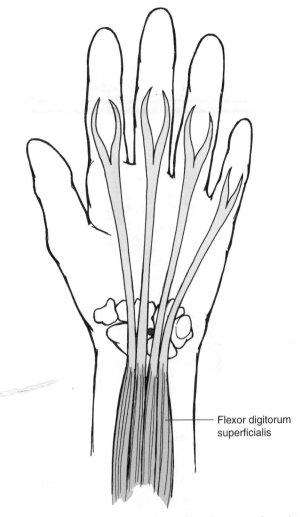

Figure 15.7: The flexor digitorum superficialis crosses the wrist approximately over the capitate, the estimated axis of wrist radial and ulnar deviation. The tendons can slip in a radial and ulnar direction, contributing to radial and ulnar deviation, respectively.

Clinical Relevance

CLINICAL ASSESSMENT OF THE INTEGRITY OF THE FLEXOR DIGITORUM SUPERFICIALIS: *The muscular attachments and variations of the flexor digitorum superficialis are clinically significant for attempting to assess the viability or strength of the flexor digitorum superficialis to individual fingers. Inability to perform the unique flexor digitorum superficialis action of flexion of the PIP joint of the little finger may lead a clinician to conclude that the muscle is impaired, when in fact the muscle is inhibited because it is unable to contract independently of the index finger or perhaps the muscle is absent entirely. The clinician must use additional information including the activation available at other fingers as well as the strength of more-proximal joints of the same digit to draw conclusions regarding the status of the flexor digitorum superficialis. Allowing the patient to flex both the index and little fingers' PIP joints simultaneously may be particularly helpful in assessing the little finger's flexor digitorum superficialis tendon [3].*

The flexor digitorum superficialis crosses the wrist approximately 1.5 cm anterior to the axis of rotation for flexion and extension and has a significant potential for wrist flexion [8]. This role is supported by EMG studies that reveal flexor digitorum superficialis activity during wrist flexion along with activity of the dedicated wrist flexors, the flexor carpi radialis, and flexor carpi ulnaris [5]. At the wrist, the flexor digitorum superficialis tendons cross over the capitate, the approximate location of the axis of radial and ulnar deviation *(Fig. 15.7)*. The tendons of the flexor digitorum superficialis can slide

in either a radial or ulnar direction as they cross the wrist, supporting reports that suggest that the flexor digitorum superficialis is active in both radial and ulnar deviation of the wrist [5,8]. The extent of its contribution to these two motions is not clear.

Clinical Relevance

SUBSTITUTION PATTERNS OBSERVED DURING MANUAL MUSCLE TESTING (MMT) OF WRIST MUSCLES: *Standard MMT procedures to assess the strength of the dedicated wrist flexor muscles call for the fingers to be relaxed [28,34] (Fig. 15.8). Careful observation is essential throughout the test to detect the gradual recruitment of the flexor digitorum superficialis as the resistance to the dedicated wrist flexors muscles overcomes their strength. By allowing the flexor digitorum superficialis to participate in the wrist flexion strength test, the clinician may fail to identify weakness in the dedicated wrist flexor muscles.*

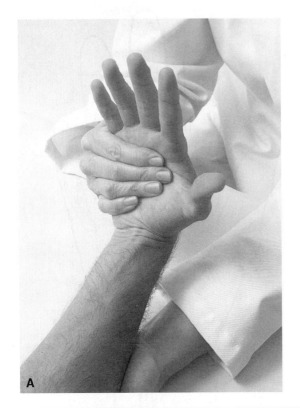

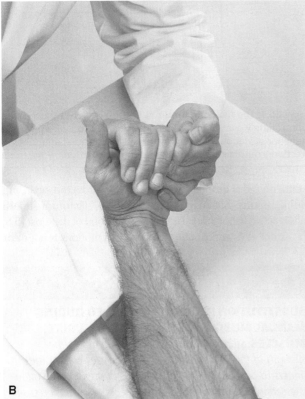

Figure 15.8: The standard manual muscle test (MMT) procedure for wrist flexion. **A.** The standard MMT procedure for wrist flexion strength requires that the fingers remain relaxed. **B.** Flexion of the PIP joints of the fingers during the MMT of wrist flexion demonstrates substitution of the flexor digitorum superficialis during the test.

Few authors mention a role of the flexor digitorum superficialis at the elbow joint. An investigation of the moment arms of muscles that cross the elbow suggests that the flexor digitorum superficialis is similar to the flexor carpi radialis in having a moment arm that results in an extension moment at the elbow when the elbow is extended and a moment arm contributing to a flexion moment when the elbow is flexed [1]. Studies also report that the flexor digitorum superficialis can generate either a pronation or supination moment depending upon the position of the forearm and elbow [1,46]. The moment arms of the flexor digitorum superficialis and flexor carpi radialis at the elbow are less than 1 cm. Whether either muscle contributes significantly to elbow motion remains unclear. As with the flexor carpi radialis, the importance of this potential effect at the elbow may be more apparent in individuals who lack the primary muscles of the elbow.

EFFECTS OF WEAKNESS

The unique effect of weakness of the flexor digitorum superficialis is weakness in PIP flexion while the DIP remains relaxed. Weakness of the flexor digitorum superficialis also can have an impact on all of the joints that it crosses, including the wrist and the MCP joints. Because the flexor digitorum superficialis adds force to finger flexion, flexor digitorum superficialis weakness may result in hyperextension of the PIP and flexion of the DIP during forceful pinch [8]. Functionally, weakness of the flexor digitorum superficialis leads to a reduction in grip strength.

EFFECTS OF TIGHTNESS

Although individual tightness of the flexor digitorum superficialis is unusual, tightness of the flexor digitorum superficialis along with the flexor digitorum profundus is a common consequence of a loss of muscle balance between the extrinsic and intrinsic muscles, resulting in a clawhand deformity. A detailed discussion of the deformities resulting from imbalance of the intrinsic and extrinsic muscles of the hand is presented in Chapter 18.

Flexor Carpi Ulnaris

The flexor carpi ulnaris is a large pennate muscle that has the largest physiological cross-sectional area of the dedicated wrist muscles [8,40,42] (*Muscle Attachment Box 15.4*). Consequently, it is a very powerful muscle, responsible for stabilizing the wrist during such activities as slicing meat and using a hammer [56] (*Fig. 15.9*).

ACTIONS

MUSCLE ACTION: FLEXOR CARPI ULNARIS

Action	Evidence
Wrist flexion	Supporting
Wrist ulnar deviation	Supporting
Elbow flexion	Conflicting
Elbow extension	Conflicting
Elbow pronation	Conflicting
Elbow supination	Conflicting

ATTACHMENTS AND INNERVATION OF THE FLEXOR CARPI ULNARIS

Proximal attachment: The humeral head attaches to the medial epicondyle of the humerus by way of the common flexor tendon and from the surrounding fascia. The larger ulnar portion arises from the medial aspect of the olecranon and from the posterior surface of the proximal two thirds of the ulna and from the adjacent intermuscular septum.

Distal attachment: The pisiform bone and ultimately to the hook of the hamate and the base of the metacarpal bone of the little finger by way of the pisohamate and pisometacarpal ligaments.

Innervation: Ulnar nerve, C7, C8, T1.

Palpation: The tendon of the flexor carpi ulnaris is palpable as it crosses the wrist toward the pisiform bone.

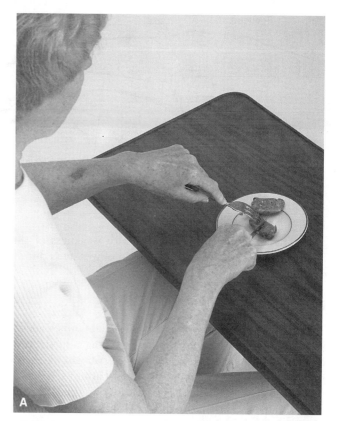

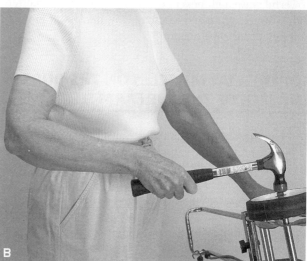

Figure 15.9: The wrist position in some forceful activities. The wrist is positioned in flexion with ulnar deviation during many forceful activities such as **(A)** cutting a piece of meat and **(B)** hammering.

Wrist flexion and ulnar deviation are actions of the flexor carpi ulnaris verified by EMG analysis [5,12,34,55,75]. The moment arm of the flexor carpi ulnaris for wrist flexion is very similar to that of the flexor carpi radialis, approximately 1.0 cm. The moment arm is enhanced by the muscle's attachment on the pisiform bone, effectively lifting the muscle anteriorly and improving its flexion moment arm *(Fig. 15.10)*. By the same token, the muscle's attachment on the pisiform prevents much change in the flexion moment arm as the wrist flexes [8,43].

The effect of the flexor carpi ulnaris at the elbow is controversial. Studies support its participation in both elbow flexion [51] and elbow extension [1]. Similarly, studies suggest that the flexor carpi ulnaris contributes to pronation [1,46] and supination of the forearm [46], while other studies suggest there is no contribution to either [5,51]. These data reveal a need for additional research to resolve the role of the flexor carpi ulnaris at the elbow. Like the other muscles of the forearm discussed so far, the flexor carpi ulnaris is unlikely to be an important participant in elbow function in individuals with normal elbow function. However, this muscle may provide small but useful elbow function in the absence of normal elbow musculature.

EFFECTS OF WEAKNESS

Weakness of the flexor carpi ulnaris weakens the strength of wrist flexion with ulnar deviation. In many activities the wrist moves in a diagonal pattern from extension and radial deviation to flexion and ulnar deviation as force is transmitted from the forearm to the wrist and hand, such as in chopping or hammering. In the pounding phase of hammering, the hand holding the hammer moves into wrist flexion and ulnar deviation [56]. When contact is made with the nail, the nail pushes the hammer and wrist back toward extension and radial deviation, requiring the flexor carpi ulnaris to control the hammer and avoid

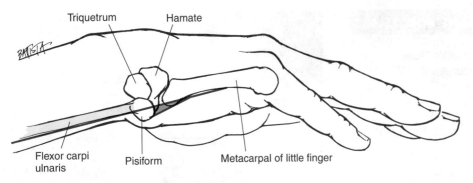

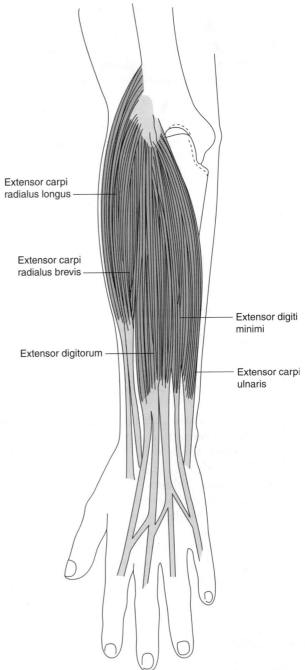

Figure 15.10: Attachment of the flexor carpi ulnaris (FCU) into the pisiform increases the angle of application and therefore the flexion moment arm of the FCU at the wrist.

a rebound from the nail. Patients with weakness of the flexor carpi ulnaris may report a sense of weakness during such activities [8].

Effects of Tightness

Tightness of the flexor carpi ulnaris is found in some patients with central nervous system disorders resulting in spasticity of the flexor carpi ulnaris. It also is seen in patients with wrist instability, such as those with rheumatoid arthritis. In these cases, the wrist is pulled into and held in a position of flexion and ulnar deviation. Since wrist extension is important for powerful grasp, tightness of the flexor carpi ulnaris interferes with powerful grasp and, consequently, may result in significant functional impairment.

SUPERFICIAL MUSCLES ON THE DORSAL SURFACE OF THE FOREARM

The superficial muscles on the dorsal surface of the forearm include the remaining muscles dedicated to wrist function, the extensor carpi radialis longus and brevis and the extensor carpi ulnaris *(Fig. 15.11)*. The other muscles found in the superficial dorsal group include the extensor digitorum and extensor digiti minimi. All of these muscles have a common proximal attachment on the lateral epicondyle of the humerus by way of the common extensor tendon. Their individual attachments and actions are presented below.

Extensor Carpi Radialis Longus and Extensor Carpi Radialis Brevis

The extensor carpi radialis longus and extensor carpi radialis brevis lie so close together at the elbow and follow such similar paths to the hand that they have similar actions at the wrist *(Muscle Attachment Boxes 15.5 and 15.6)*. However, they are distinct muscles and have unique roles at the wrist and elbow, presented here. The extensor carpi radialis longus is the most proximal muscle of those attaching to the common extensor tendon. It is covered proximally by the brachioradialis muscle. The extensor carpi radialis brevis is covered anteriorly by the extensor carpi radialis longus.

Figure 15.11: The superficial muscles on the dorsal surface of the forearm from radial to ulnar are the extensor carpi radialis longus (ECRL), extensor carpi radialis brevis (ECRB), extensor digitorum (ED), extensor digiti minimi (EDM), and extensor carpi ulnaris (ECU).

MUSCLE ATTACHMENT BOX 15.5

ATTACHMENTS AND INNERVATION OF THE EXTENSOR CARPI RADIALIS LONGUS

Proximal attachment: Distal one third of the lateral supracondylar ridge and intramuscular septum and from the common extensor tendon attached to the lateral epicondyle of the humerus.

Distal attachment: Radial aspect of the dorsal surface of the base of the index finger's metacarpal bone.

Innervation: Radial nerve, C6 and C7.

Palpation: The tendon of the extensor carpi radialis longus is palpable on the dorsolateral aspect of the wrist joint just proximal to the base of metacarpal bone of the index finger.

ACTIONS

MUSCLE ACTION: EXTENSOR CARPI RADIALIS LONGUS AND BREVIS

Action	Evidence
Wrist extension	Supporting
Wrist radial deviation	Supporting
Elbow flexion	Inadequate
Elbow pronation	Supporting
Elbow supination	Supporting

The actions of wrist extension and radial deviation by both of these muscles are well accepted in the literature [34,55,75]. EMG data also support their roles in these movements [5,12].

MUSCLE ATTACHMENT BOX 15.6

ATTACHMENTS AND INNERVATION OF THE EXTENSOR CARPI RADIALIS BREVIS

Proximal attachment: Lateral epicondyle of the humerus by way of the common extensor tendon.

Distal attachment: Radial aspect of the dorsal surface of the base of the long finger's metacarpal bone.

Innervation: Radial nerve, C7 and C8, perhaps C6.

Palpation: The tendon of the extensor carpi radialis brevis is palpable on the dorsolateral aspect of the wrist joint just proximal to the base of the metacarpal bone of the long finger and ulnar to the extensor carpi radialis longus tendon.

Although the extensor carpi radialis longus and extensor carpi radialis brevis are anatomically similar, they are not identical. Reports suggest that they make unique contributions to the wrist [8,12,39]. The extensor carpi radialis brevis has a larger extension moment arm and a larger physiological cross-sectional area than the extensor carpi radialis longus [40] *(Fig. 15.12)*. Evidence suggests that the extensor carpi radialis brevis contributes the most to wrist extension strength [37] and is the main wrist extensor, although individual variability exists [5,8,24]. The moment arm for radial deviation is greater in the extensor carpi radialis longus than in the extensor carpi radialis brevis, but their participation in radial deviation appears more equal [8,67], although the extensor carpi radialis longus may play a larger role than the extensor carpi radialis brevis in radial deviation [8,12,43,65] *(Fig. 15.13)*.

The roles of the extensor carpi radialis longus and extensor carpi radialis brevis at the elbow are somewhat less clear. The proximity of the extensor carpi radialis longus to the brachioradialis, an elbow flexor, suggests that the extensor carpi radialis longus has the potential to flex the elbow [8]. Studies of their moment arms at the elbow suggest that both the extensor carpi radialis longus and extensor carpi radialis brevis have the mechanical potential to flex the elbow [20,41,42,45]. However there are no known in vivo studies supporting this role [1,8,39].

Direct electrical stimulation studies of the extensor carpi radialis longus and extensor carpi radialis brevis suggest that each can generate a small supination moment when the forearm is pronated and a more significant pronation moment when the forearm is supinated, particularly with the elbow flexed [10,46]. As with the other wrist muscles that cross the elbow, the contribution of the extensor carpi radialis longus (and perhaps the extensor carpi radialis brevis) at the elbow may be significant only in the absence of the primary muscles of the elbow.

EFFECTS OF WEAKNESS

Weakness of both of these muscles results in a substantial loss of strength in both wrist extension and radial deviation. The loss of the extensor carpi radialis brevis alone results in more impairment than the singular loss of the extensor carpi radialis longus, since the former plays a larger role in wrist extension. Weakness in wrist extension produces difficulty in forceful grasp and pinch because of the necessary interaction between wrist extension and finger flexion. This interaction is explained later in this chapter.

Effects of Tightness

Tightness of these two muscles is not common but results in decreased flexibility in the directions of flexion and ulnar deviation. Such restriction may cause difficulty in performing some personal hygiene tasks that typically require wrist flexion with ulnar deviation [56].

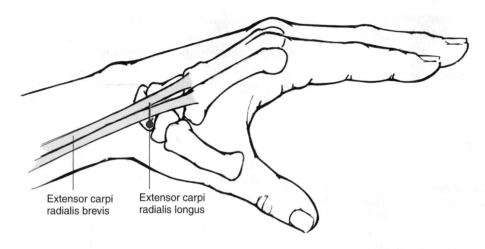

Figure 15.12: Extension moment arms of the extensor carpi radialis longus and brevis. A sagittal view of the wrist demonstrates that the extensor carpi radialis brevis (ECRB) has a larger extension moment arm at the wrist than the extensor carpi radialis longus (ECRL).

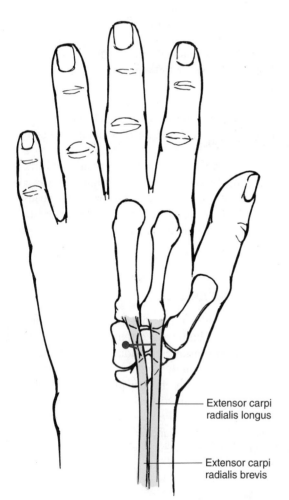

Figure 15.13: Moment arms of the extensor carpi radialis longus and brevis for radial deviation. A frontal view of the wrist demonstrates that the extensor carpi radialis longus (ECRL) has a larger moment arm for radial deviation than the extensor carpi radialis brevis (ECRB).

Clinical Relevance

FUNCTIONAL SIGNIFICANCE OF LIMITED WRIST FLEXION ROM (CASE REPORT): *The position of function of the forearm and wrist in most activities is wrist extension [11,56]. Thus loss of flexion ROM may seem less important. However, one patient's disability reveals the significance of wrist flexion ROM in normal daily function. This patient underwent bilateral wrist and distal radioulnar fusions because of painful instability secondary to rheumatoid arthritis. Both wrists were fused in extension for the purpose of facilitating activities of daily living. The patient functioned well in most activities but was unable to perform one simple yet essential task, that of cleaning herself after using the toilet. This example is a warning to all clinicians to recognize the diversity of movements required to perform the normal spectrum of daily activities. Careful analysis of a patient's daily tasks is needed to appreciate the functional impact of many impairments.*

Extensor Digitorum (Also Known As Extensor Digitorum Communis)

The tendons of the extensor digitorum fan out to the four fingers after crossing the dorsal surface of the wrist (*Muscle Attachment Box 15.7*). The extensor tendons of all the fingers are interconnected by fibrous bands between adjacent fingers known as **juncturae tendinae** (*Fig. 15.14*). The extensor digitorum tendon to the little finger is frequently deficient or even absent [31,70,73] and often receives a slip from the ring finger by way of the juncturae tendinae.

The juncturae tendinae affect both active and passive movements of the fingers. Actively, these interconnections allow an increase in extension force to individual fingers during extensor digitorum contraction by increasing the number of muscle fibers pulling on a single tendon [8]. Passively, flexion of the MCP joint of one or two fingers pulls the extensor tendons of the remaining fingers distally via the juncturae tendinae (*Fig. 15.15*). This distal migration puts the extensor tendons to

MUSCLE ATTACHMENT BOX 15.7

ATTACHMENTS AND INNERVATION OF THE EXTENSOR DIGITORUM

Proximal attachment: Lateral epicondyle of the humerus by way of the common extensor tendon and from the surrounding fascia and intermuscular septum.

Distal attachment: A tendon to each finger broadens into a flat expansion, the extensor hood, at the level of the MCP joint. Distal to the MCP joint, the hood receives attachments from the intrinsic muscles. At the distal end of the proximal phalanx, the hood splits into a central tendon and two lateral bands. The central tendon, or slip, inserts into the base of the middle phalanx on its dorsal surface. The lateral bands pass along the medial and lateral borders of the dorsal surface of the middle phalanx and converge at the DIP joint. The two bands reunite and attach together on the dorsal surface of the base of the distal phalanx.

Innervation: Radial nerve, C7 and C8.

Palpation: The tendons of the extensor digitorum are palpated as they cross the wrist and along the metacarpals of each finger.

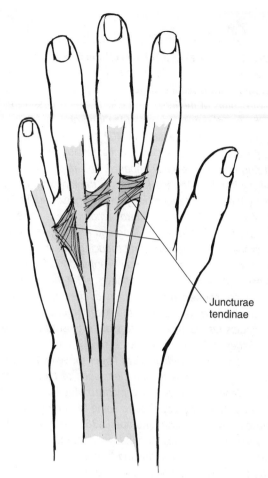

Figure 15.14: Juncturae tendinae of the extensor digitorum. The tendons of the extensor digitorum to the fingers are connected to one another by the juncturae tendinae.

all the fingers on slack, allowing the fingers to flex [50]. The juncturae tendinae also may provide important medial and lateral stabilizing forces to the MCP joints while the fingers are flexed during forceful grip. However, these fibrous interconnections also can impede independent finger movement [38].

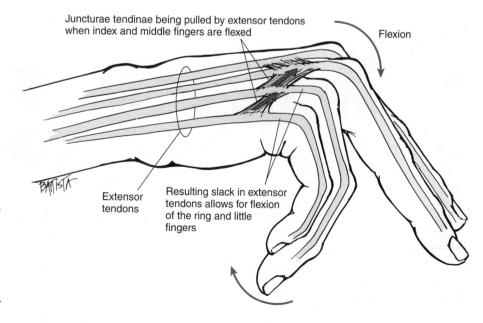

Figure 15.15: Effect of finger flexion on the juncturae tendinae and on flexion excursion of the other fingers. Flexion of the MCP joints of the index or long finger pulls on the juncturae tendinae of the ring and little fingers, putting the extensor tendons to the ring and little fingers on slack and allowing full flexion excursion.

Clinical Relevance

INDEPENDENT FINGER MOVEMENT: *With the fingers relaxed in slight flexion, independent active extension of each MCP joint is readily achieved. Independent extension at the MCP joints of the index and little fingers is possible even with flexion of the MCP joints of the long and ring fingers (Fig. 15.16). However, when the MCP joints of the index and little fingers are flexed, independent extension of the long and ring fingers is severely impaired. This impairment results from the distal pull on the tendons of the long and ring fingers by the juncturae tendinae from the index and little fingers. A distal pull by the juncturae tendinae puts the extensor digitorum tendons to the long and ring fingers on slack and renders them ineffective in producing active extension [62]. At the same time there may be inhibition of any active extension at the ring and long fingers, since the index and little fingers, connected to the others by the juncturae tendinae, are kept flexed. Independent extension at the index and little fingers results from the accessory extensor muscle to each finger.*

The difficulty in independent finger movement presents a particular challenge to musicians such as pianists, who need independent finger movement to play intricate compositions. This difficulty has led some to undergo surgical release of the juncturae tendinae [8,38]. Yet a study of 21 cadaveric limbs reveals that independent movement is only slightly improved following transection of the juncturae tendinae [73]. The study lists other structures, including the skin in the web spaces of the fingers, which also contribute to the functional interdependence of the fingers.

ACTIONS

MUSCLE ACTION: EXTENSOR DIGITORUM

Action	Evidence
Finger MCP extension	Supporting
Finger PIP extension	Supporting (only with intrinsic activity)
Finger DIP extension	Supporting (only with intrinsic activity)
Wrist extension	Supporting
Wrist radial deviation	Refuting
Wrist ulnar deviation	Inadequate
Elbow flexion	Conflicting
Elbow extension	Conflicting
Elbow pronation	Inadequate
Elbow supination	Inadequate

The extensor digitorum is the primary extensor of the MCP joints of the fingers. The muscle to the long finger is the strongest of the four [7,8]. The extensor digitorum contributes to the extension of the PIP and DIP joints of the fingers, although it is unable to accomplish extension at the PIP and DIP joints without the simultaneous activity of the lumbricals or interossei [62,73]. EMG studies consistently reveal activity of the extensor digitorum during MCP extension with the interphalangeal (IP) joints flexed, but combined extensor digitorum and intrinsic muscle activity when the IP joints are extended [13,41]. The coordinated interplay of the extensor digitorum and the intrinsic muscles in producing extension at the IP joints is discussed in Chapter 18.

The extensor digitorum also has been implicated in abduction of the fingers and extension and abduction at the

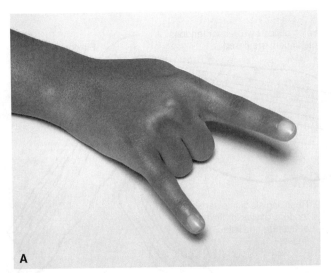
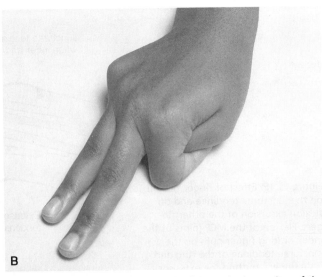

Figure 15.16: Effect of the juncturae tendinae on active extension of the long and ring fingers. **A.** Independent active extension of the index and little fingers is possible even with simultaneous flexion of the MCP joints of the long and ring fingers. **B.** Active extension of the long and ring fingers is difficult when the MCP joints of index and little fingers are flexed.

wrist [34,75], but there are no known studies verifying these actions. The role of the extensor digitorum in abduction of the fingers is complicated by the complex movement of the MCP joints during flexion and extension. As noted in the previous chapter, the fingers converge on the thenar eminence during finger flexion and return to a spread position during extension. This movement gives the appearance of active abduction at the MCP joint but probably is the consequence of the articular shapes, with no need for active abduction from any muscle.

Studies of the extensor digitorum's moment arms at the wrist reveal a potential for wrist extension and ulnar deviation [8,51]. Despite the extensor digitorum's mechanical capacity to extend the wrist, the extensor carpi radialis longus and brevis and the extensor carpi ulnaris remain the primary wrist extensors. However, the clinician must recognize that substitutions from the extensor digitorum can mask weakness in the primary extensor muscles of the wrist.

Although the extensor digitorum crosses the elbow, there are no known reports verifying its participation in elbow motion. Studies of the muscle's moment arms at the elbow are conflicting, reporting both an extension moment arm [51] and a flexion moment [1]. Isolated stimulation of the extensor digitorum in three subjects produced a small supination moment with the forearm pronated and a larger pronation moment with the forearm in supination [46]. Like the other muscles of the forearm, the extensor digitorum appears to have the potential to affect the elbow, but its effects may be negligible unless the normal musculature of the elbow is so compromised that the small contributions from the extensor digitorum are more important.

EFFECTS OF WEAKNESS

Isolated weakness of the extensor digitorum may result from trauma such as tendon lacerations. Such injuries result in weakness or loss of extension of the MCP joints of the fingers. However, if the accessory extensors to the index and little fingers remain, some function can be maintained.

EFFECTS OF TIGHTNESS

Prior to considering the effects of tightness, it is necessary to appreciate the role the distal attachment of the extensor digitorum plays in normal finger flexion ROM. It is the elegant arrangement of this attachment that allows a finger to flex at all of the joints simultaneously, as in making a fist *(Fig. 15.17)*. The central tendon of the extensor digitorum attaches to the middle phalanx and is pulled taut during PIP flexion. Tension on the central tendon pulls the extensor digitorum distally. This distal migration of the extensor digitorum puts its lateral bands on slack, thus allowing flexion mobility of the DIP *(Fig. 15.18)*. Conversely, flexion of the DIP joint tightens the lateral bands, producing a distal pull on the extensor digitorum tendon. In this case the distal migration of the extensor digitorum puts the central tendon on slack and allows full flexion ROM at the PIP *(Fig. 15.19)*.

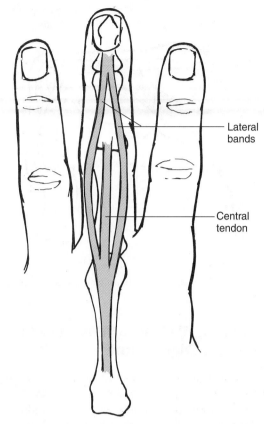

Figure 15.17: Extensive distal attachment of the extensor digitorum. Just distal to the MCP joint the tendon splits into the central tendon that attaches to the base of the middle phalanx and into the lateral bands that pass distally along the radial and ulnar sides of the dorsal surface until they rejoin and insert on the base of the distal phalanx.

Clinical Relevance

FLEXION ROM AT THE PIP AND DIP JOINTS: *To assess the flexion ROM at the PIP and DIP joints, the extensor digitorum must be put on slack. Thus the PIP joint must be flexed when assessing DIP joint flexion ROM (Fig. 15.20). PIP flexion ROM is maximized by allowing the DIP joint to remain relaxed (Fig. 15.21).*

Tightness of the extensor digitorum limits full flexion ROM of the fingers, but the manifestations of tightness of the extensor digitorum are complex, since the muscle crosses many joints. In the presence of extensor digitorum tightness, extension or hyperextension of the MCP joints is accompanied by flexion of the IP joints. This combination of MCP extension and IP flexion results from the pull of the extensor digitorum and the responding pull of the antagonistic flexor digitorum profundus. Tightness of the extensor digitorum may result from adhesions or loss of muscle extensibility in the forearm or hand. Tightness may also follow from the loss

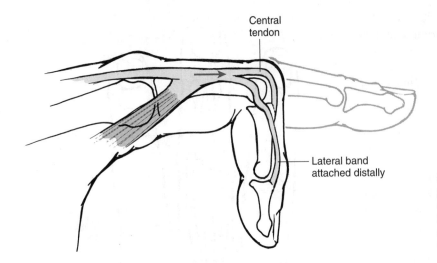

Figure 15.18: Effect of PIP flexion on the extensor mechanism. Flexion of the PIP joint stretches the central tendon, which in turn pulls the lateral bands distally, putting the lateral bands on slack at the level of the DIP joints.

of muscular balance resulting from weakness of the intrinsic muscles.

Extensor Digiti Minimi (Also Known As Extensor Digiti Quinti)

The extensor digiti minimi lies just medial to the extensor digitorum in the forearm (*Muscle Attachment Box 15.8*). It is distinguished from the extensor digitorum tendon in the finger by palpation, lying on the ulnar side of the extensor digitorum tendon crossing the MCP joint of the little finger.

ACTIONS

MUSCLE ACTION: EXTENSOR DIGITI MINIMI

Action	Evidence
Finger MCP extension	Supporting
Finger PIP extension	Supporting (only with intrinsic activity)
Finger DIP extension	Supporting (only with intrinsic activity)
Wrist extension	Inadequate
Wrist ulnar deviation	Inadequate
Elbow flexion	Conflicting

The actions of the extensor digiti minimi are almost identical to those of the extensor digitorum at the fingers. However, if the muscle affects the wrist, it is likely to result in ulnar deviation because the tendon is ulnar to the capitate as it crosses the wrist.

EFFECTS OF WEAKNESS

Weakness or loss of the extensor digiti minimi results in an inability to extend the little finger's MCP joint independently. Because the extensor digitorum to the little finger is frequently deficient and may even be absent, weakness of the extensor digiti minimi is characterized by significant weakness of MCP extension of the little finger.

EFFECTS OF TIGHTNESS

Isolated tightness of the extensor digiti minimi is unlikely. However, the effects of tightness of this muscle mirror the effects of tightness of the extensor digitorum.

Extensor Carpi Ulnaris

The extensor carpi ulnaris is the last of the dedicated wrist muscles (*Muscle Attachment Box 15.9*). It is a pennate muscle, similar in size to the extensor carpi radialis brevis [1,7,40].

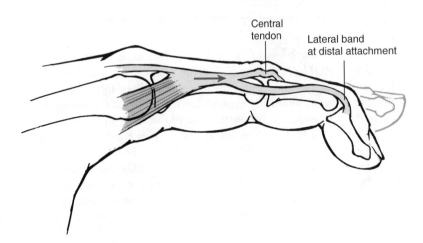

Figure 15.19: Effect of DIP flexion on the extensor mechanism. Flexion of the DIP joint stretches the lateral bands, which pulls the central tendon distally, putting it on slack as it crosses the PIP joint.

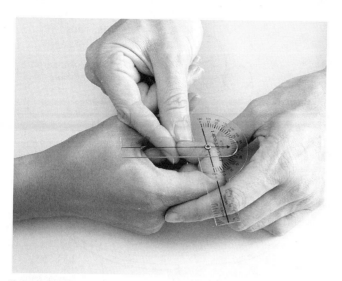

Figure 15.20: Standard position to measure the passive flexion ROM of the DIP joint includes flexion of the PIP joint of the same finger.

ACTIONS

MUSCLE ACTION: EXTENSOR CARPI ULNARIS

Action	Evidence
Wrist extension	Supporting
Wrist ulnar deviation	Supporting
Elbow extension	Inadequate
Elbow pronation	Inadequate

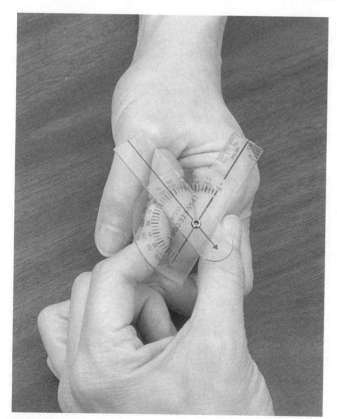

Figure 15.21: Standard position to measure the passive flexion ROM of the PIP joint includes a relaxed position of the DIP joint, which generally assumes a position of slight flexion.

MUSCLE ATTACHMENT BOX 15.8

ATTACHMENTS AND INNERVATION OF THE EXTENSOR DIGITI MINIMI

Proximal attachment: Lateral epicondyle of the humerus by way of the common extensor tendon and from the surrounding fascia.

Distal attachment: The extensor hood of the little finger by two slips. The lateral portion merges with the tendon of the extensor digitorum. Thus the ulnar tendon at the MCP joint of the little finger belongs solely to the extensor digiti minimi.

Innervation: Radial nerve, C7 and C8.

Palpation: The tendon of the extensor digiti minimi is palpable on the ulnar side of the extensor digitorum tendon to the little finger as it crosses the MCP joint.

The role of the extensor carpi ulnaris in wrist extension and ulnar deviation is well accepted and supported by EMG evidence [5,12,34,75]. However, some data suggest that the extensor carpi ulnaris is able to extend the wrist only when the forearm is supinated [8]. Analysis of the extension moment arm of the extensor carpi ulnaris reveals that the moment arm decreases as the forearm moves from supination to pronation [43]. This lends support to the notion that the extensor carpi ulnaris is most effective in extending the wrist when the forearm is supinated. EMG analysis reveals no significant difference in the level of recruitment of the extensor carpi ulnaris during wrist extension with different forearm positions [72]. There is no known report that quantifies the

MUSCLE ATTACHMENT BOX 15.9

ATTACHMENTS AND INNERVATION OF THE EXTENSOR CARPI ULNARIS

Proximal attachment: Lateral epicondyle of the humerus by way of the common extensor tendon and from the surrounding fascia and from the posterior border of the ulna along with the flexor carpi ulnaris.

Distal attachment: Medial aspect of the metacarpal of the little finger.

Innervation: Radial nerve, C7 and C8.

Palpation: The tendon of the extensor carpi ulnaris is palpable on the dorsal and ulnar aspect of the wrist joint during resisted wrist extension with ulnar deviation.

extension moment applied to the wrist by the extensor carpi ulnaris in different forearm positions. Additional research is needed to determine if the extensor role of the extensor carpi ulnaris is altered by forearm position.

The extensor carpi ulnaris has the largest moment arm for ulnar deviation of the dedicated wrist muscles [8,12,43]. The moment arm changes very little with wrist position, making the muscle particularly effective for ulnar deviation. The extensor carpi ulnaris lies just ulnar to the head of the ulna and fibrocartilaginous disc of the triangular fibrocartilage complex (TFCC). It plays an important role in supporting the distal radioulnar joint [19,25,60,74]. In pronation, the muscle is stretched and helps prevent dorsal dislocation; in supination, the muscle may help anterior glide of the ulna.

The extensor carpi ulnaris crosses the elbow and may affect that joint. Measurement of the muscle's moment arms at the elbow reveals substantial extension and pronation moment arms, suggesting that the muscle is at least mechanically capable of elbow extension and forearm pronation [1,50]. Yet EMG data demonstrate no activity of the extensor carpi ulnaris in forearm pronation [5]. Like the other forearm muscles crossing the elbow, additional investigation is needed to determine if the extensor carpi ulnaris does function at the elbow.

EFFECTS OF WEAKNESS

Weakness of the extensor carpi ulnaris results in weakness in wrist extension and ulnar deviation. As noted with the other wrist muscles, the extensor carpi ulnaris participates in the delicate balance exhibited in a healthy wrist. Disruption of this balance resulting from impairments of any of these muscles is likely to produce significant dysfunction. Weakness in wrist extension is particularly disruptive to the ability to produce a strong grip and pinch.

EFFECTS OF TIGHTNESS

Isolated tightness, although uncommon, decreases the available ROM of the wrist in flexion and radial deviation.

COMBINED ACTIONS OF THE FIVE PRIMARY WRIST MUSCLES

From the discussion of each of the dedicated wrist muscles, it is apparent that there is no single muscle that moves the wrist in any of the cardinal planes of motion. Therefore, to produce pure motions of flexion and extension or radial and ulnar deviation, pairs of muscles must contract together (*Fig. 15.22*). For example, the flexor carpi radialis and the flexor carpi ulnaris are both necessary for pure wrist flexion.

During functional activities the wrist commonly moves on a diagonal path from wrist extension with radial deviation to wrist flexion with ulnar deviation [43,56]. It is not surprising

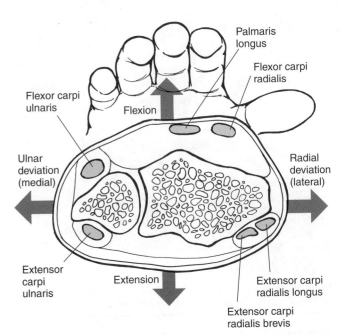

Figure 15.22: Pairs of dedicated wrist muscles that move the wrist in the cardinal planes. A cross-sectional view of the wrist joint demonstrates that pairs of dedicated wrist muscles are needed to produce wrist motion in the cardinal planes of flexion-extension or radial-ulnar deviation. *FCR*, flexor carpi radialis; *FCU*, flexor carpi ulnaris; *PL*, palmaris longus; *ECRL*, extensor carpi radialis longus; *ECRB*, extensor carpi radialis brevis; *ECU*, extensor carpi ulnaris.

to find that the flexor carpi ulnaris has a larger physiological cross-sectional area than the flexor carpi radialis [1]. Similarly, the combined physiological cross-sectional area of the extensor carpi radialis longus and extensor carpi radialis brevis is larger than that of the extensor carpi ulnaris. These wrist muscles appear specialized to support and move the wrist and hand in this diagonal pattern.

Clinical Relevance

IMPAIRMENT OF A SINGLE DEDICATED WRIST MUSCLE: *Impairment of a single wrist muscle results in an impairment of the unique motion provided by that muscle and interferes with the motions in the cardinal planes in which that muscle participates. For example, the extensor carpi ulnaris contracts and produces the combined movement of wrist extension and ulnar deviation. Weakness of that muscle results in weakness of that combined movement as well as in pure wrist extension and pure wrist ulnar deviation, since the extensor carpi ulnaris participates in both of those motions. Consequently, when a clinician identifies a patient's difficulty or inability to perform wrist motion in a cardinal plane, further evaluation is needed to determine the distribution of weakness across the contributing muscles.*

DEEP MUSCLES ON THE VOLAR SURFACE OF THE FOREARM

The deep muscles of the volar surface of the forearm include the flexor digitorum profundus, the flexor pollicis longus, and the pronator quadratus (*Fig. 15.23*).

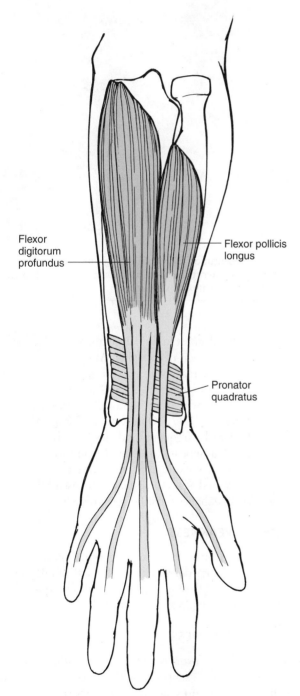

Flexor digitorum profundus

Flexor pollicis longus

Pronator quadratus

Figure 15.23: Deep muscles of the volar surface of the forearm include the flexor digitorum profundus, flexor pollicis longus, and pronator quadratus.

Flexor Digitorum Profundus

The flexor digitorum profundus is a large muscle composed of multiple bundles of unipennate muscles [8], with a large physiological cross-sectional area and a large potential force (*Muscle Attachment Box 15.10*). Based on its physiological cross-sectional area the flexor digitorum profundus is up to 50% stronger than the flexor digitorum superficialis, and both are stronger than the extensor digitorum [7,8,40].

ACTIONS

MUSCLE ACTION: FLEXOR DIGITORUM PROFUNDUS

Action	Evidence
Finger DIP flexion	Supporting
Finger PIP flexion	Supporting
Finger MCP flexion	Supporting
Wrist flexion	Conflicting

The flexor digitorum profundus is the only muscle that can flex the DIP of the fingers. The standard procedure to test the strength and integrity of the muscle is active DIP flexion [28,34]. However, the tendons of the fingers are mechanically linked to one another at the muscle belly and perhaps even in the carpal tunnel, making discrete activation of the flexor digitorum profundus at a single finger difficult if not impossible, except at the index finger, which appears to have more independent control [13,65].

MUSCLE ATTACHMENT BOX 15.10

ATTACHMENTS AND INNERVATION OF THE FLEXOR DIGITORUM PROFUNDUS

Proximal attachment: The proximal two thirds or three quarters of the anterior and medial surfaces of the ulna and the medial half of the interosseous membrane, the medial surface of the coronoid process, and from the posterior border of the ulna by way of the aponeurosis of the flexor carpi ulnaris.

Distal attachment: A tendon to each finger inserts on the palmar surface of the base of distal phalanx.

Innervation: The tendons to the index and long fingers are supplied by the anterior interosseous branch of the median nerve, C8, T1, perhaps C7. The tendons to the little and ring fingers are supplied by the ulnar nerve, C8 and T1.

Palpation: The tendons of the flexor digitorum profundus may be palpable along the volar surface of the middle phalanx of each finger.

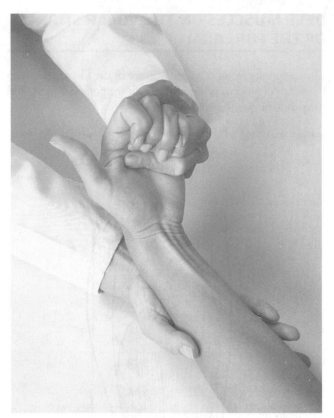

Figure 15.25: Substitution by the flexor digitorum profundus during MMT of the wrist flexors is common and can lead to an overestimate of wrist flexion strength.

Clinical Relevance

MMT OF THE FLEXOR DIGITORUM PROFUNDUS: *The classical MMT procedure for the flexor digitorum profundus is assessment of the strength of flexion of the DIP [28,34,53]. In cases of nerve or tendon injury or in degenerative neuropathies or myopathies, it may be clinically important to determine the strength of the flexor digitorum profundus at each finger. Clinicians must recognize that although the test may be focused on a single finger, the structure of the whole muscle dictates that the subject be allowed to flex all the fingers at once. The mechanical linkage among the muscles to the fingers prevents an individual from isolating DIP flexion of a single finger (Fig. 15.24). Attempts to prevent flexion at the other fingers are likely to inhibit recruitment of the muscle.*

Like the flexor digitorum superficialis, the flexor digitorum profundus has the potential to affect each joint it crosses. Both muscles are capable of producing flexion at the PIP and MCP joints of the fingers and at the wrist. However, EMG studies suggest that the flexor digitorum profundus is the primary flexor of the finger, activated during free, unresisted finger closure [5,13,37]. The flexor digitorum superficialis appears to be held in reserve for additional strength, particularly during forceful pinch and grasp [8,41]. Because the flexor digitorum superficialis has more independent activation of individual fingers, it also is used when individual finger movements are needed [13,37]. Both the flexor digitorum profundus and the flexor digitorum superficialis are strongest at the middle finger [8,15,27,70].

The flexor digitorum profundus crosses the wrist and has the potential to affect it. The tendons of the flexor digitorum

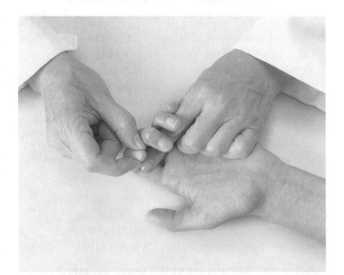

Figure 15.24: The standard MMT procedure to assess the strength of the flexor digitorum profundus allows flexion of all of the fingers, even when a single finger is being assessed.

profundus are the deepest in the carpal tunnel and have small moment arms for flexion of the wrist. Analysis suggests that the moment arms increase with wrist flexion as the tendons bulge anteriorly in the tunnel [8]. EMG studies are conflicting regarding the activity of the flexor digitorum profundus during wrist flexion [5,17]. Observations during MMT of wrist strength reveal a frequent tendency for subjects to flex the fingers in what appears to be an attempt to recruit the flexor digitorum profundus as a wrist flexor (*Fig. 15.25*). Clinicians are warned again to watch for the use of the finger flexor muscles to enhance wrist flexion strength.

EFFECTS OF WEAKNESS

Effects of weakness of the flexor digitorum profundus are manifested directly as a decrease in the strength of DIP flexion, but the overall strength of finger flexion and consequently the strength of pinch and grip also are affected.

EFFECTS OF TIGHTNESS

Tightness of the flexor digitorum profundus leads to decreased extension excursion of the fingers. In extreme cases, usually in the presence of muscle spasticity, the fingers may close into the palm. However, tightness is also the consequence of balance lost across all of the muscles in the hand, resulting from weakness of the intrinsic muscles. In

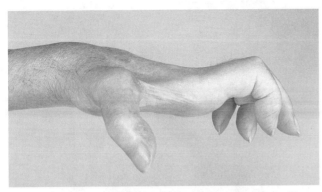

Figure 15.26: Clawhand deformity in an individual with significant weakness of the intrinsic muscles of the hand with concomitant tightness of the flexor digitorum profundus and the extensor digitorum.

MUSCLE ATTACHMENT BOX 15.11

ATTACHMENTS AND INNERVATION OF THE FLEXOR POLLICIS LONGUS

Proximal attachment: The anterior surface of the radius and adjacent interosseous membrane from the radial tuberosity to the attachment of the pronator quadratus. It may also attach to the medial aspect of the coronoid process.

Distal attachment: Palmar surface of the base of the thumb's distal phalanx.

Innervation: Anterior interosseous branch of the median nerve, C7, C8, and perhaps T1.

Palpation: The tendon of the flexor pollicis longus may be palpable on the volar surface of the proximal phalanx of the thumb.

this situation the finger flexors and extensors become tight together, causing the hand to collapse into a claw deformity (*Fig. 15.26*). The factors causing a claw deformity are detailed in Chapter 18.

Flexor Pollicis Longus

The flexor pollicis longus along with the flexor digitorum profundus lies on the floor of the carpal tunnel (*Muscle Attachment Box 15.11*). It is a bipennate muscle crossing the IP, MCP, and carpometacarpal (CMC) joints of the thumb and the wrist joint.

ACTIONS

MUSCLE ACTION: FLEXOR POLLICIS LONGUS

Action	Evidence
Thumb IP flexion	Supporting
Thumb MCP flexion	Conflicting
Thumb CMC flexion	Conflicting
Thumb CMC adduction	Supporting
Wrist flexion	Inadequate
Wrist radial deviation	Inadequate

The flexor pollicis longus is the only muscle able to flex the IP joint of the thumb. Unlike the long flexors to the fingers, the flexor pollicis longus is independent, and isolated IP flexion in the thumb is easily accomplished. The flexor pollicis longus has a smaller moment arm for flexion at the MCP and CMC joints of the thumb than the intrinsic muscles of the thumb. EMG assessment reveals vigorous activation of the flexor pollicis longus with flexion of the IP but zero activation with isolated MCP flexion in the thumb [13]. In fact, activation of the flexor pollicis longus in the absence of other muscle activity at the thumb causes flexion of the IP but hyperextension of the MCP joint of the thumb [8,64]. As is seen throughout the wrist and hand, stable movement of the thumb requires the balanced activation of several muscles.

Few studies examine the flexor pollicis longus muscle's contribution to CMC adduction. Biomechanical analyses reveal very small moment arms generating either abduction (palmar abduction) [63] or adduction moments [47]. EMG analyses reveal activity of the flexor pollicis longus during adduction, with little or no activity during abduction [14,33]. Like the flexor digitorum profundus, the flexor pollicis longus has only a small flexion moment arm at the wrist [8]. It may also produce a slight radial deviation moment [51]. As with other extrinsic muscles to the digits, the contribution of the flexor pollicis longus to these motions may only be apparent with the loss of the primary muscles for these actions.

EFFECTS OF WEAKNESS

Weakness of the flexor pollicis longus results in weakness in flexion at the thumb's IP joint. Isolated weakness of the flexor pollicis longus is unusual but can result from impingement of the anterior interosseous nerve.

Clinical Relevance

A CASE REPORT: *A 45-year-old male reported a sudden onset of difficulty in buttoning his shirt. The difficulty was noted one evening after a day filled by a home-repair job involving prolonged use of a screwdriver in an overhead position. The subject denied pain, noting that his only complaint was difficulty with tasks requiring fine motor manipulation such as buttoning shirts and tying a bow tie. Physical examination revealed full passive ROM throughout the thumb, fingers, and wrist. No active flexion was visible at the IP joint of the thumb or at the DIP joint of the index finger. All other strengths were within normal limits. An evaluation*

(continued)

(Continued)

by a neurologist confirmed impingement of the anterior interosseous nerve, likely precipitated by prolonged repetitive forearm pronation while using the screwdriver. The nerve emerges between the two heads of the pronator teres and was likely compressed against the interosseous membrane during prolonged and repeated contraction of the pronator teres.

One remarkable aspect of this case was how few functional deficits resulted from apparently complete loss of the flexor pollicis longus and the flexor digitorum profundus to the index finger. (Electrodiagnostic tests were not performed to quantify the degree of denervation.) Pinch was characterized by hyperextension of the thumb's IP joint and the index finger's DIP joint. The subject reported only minor inconvenience, particularly with buttoning clothes. The muscles gradually recovered nearly normal strength over a 1-year period.

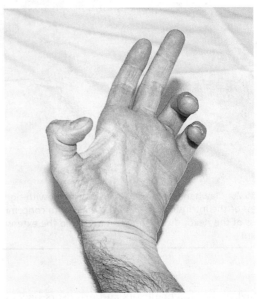

Figure 15.27: Ape thumb deformity. An ape thumb deformity is seen in an individual with significant weakness of the intrinsic muscles of the thumb with concomitant tightness of the flexor pollicis longus and the extensor pollicis longus.

EFFECTS OF TIGHTNESS

Like extrinsic muscles to the fingers, the flexor pollicis longus is rarely tight in isolation. Tightness of the flexor pollicis longus can be seen in cases of upper motor neuron lesions leading to spasticity of the flexor pollicis longus and other muscles of the hand. In cases of severe spasticity, the thumb is pulled into the palm by the combined pull of the flexor pollicis longus, adductor pollicis, and extensor pollicis longus. This thumb-in-palm deformity impairs or even prevents pinch and grasp. In severe cases, the thumb's location in the palm interferes with normal hand hygiene and can lead to skin breakdown [52]. Surgical correction of the deformity may be required to improve function or to facilitate skin care.

The flexor pollicis longus is frequently tight with the extensor pollicis longus in the absence of the intrinsic muscles of the thumb. This loss of balance results in the typical ape thumb deformity *(Fig. 15.27)*. The deformity is discussed in more detail in Chapter 18.

Pronator Quadratus

The pronator quadratus is the second of the primary muscles of pronation *(Muscle Attachment Box 15.12)*. The pronator teres is discussed in Chapter 12 with the elbow flexor muscles.

ACTIONS

MUSCLE ACTION: PRONATOR QUADRATUS

Action	Evidence
Elbow pronation	Supporting

The reported action of the pronator quadratus is pronation of the forearm. As noted in Chapter 12, EMG studies reveal that the pronator quadratus is the primary pronator, participating

in active forearm pronation regardless of condition [5]. The moment arm of the pronator quadratus is at least as large as that of the pronator teres (6–8 mm) and relatively constant through much of the pronation and supination ROM, decreasing slightly at the extreme of pronation and decreasing more at the extreme of supination [10]. The pronator teres appears to have the supportive role in active pronation, contracting only against resistance and during rapid movements.

MUSCLE ATTACHMENT BOX 15.12

ATTACHMENTS AND INNERVATION OF THE PRONATOR QUADRATUS

Proximal attachment: Distal one fourth of the anterior surface of the ulna.

Distal attachment: Distal one fourth of the anterior surface of the radius.

Innervation: Anterior interosseous branch of the median nerve, C7, C8, and perhaps T1.

Palpation: The pronator quadratus may be palpated during unresisted pronation by placing a finger on the volar surface of the distal radius or ulna. The palpating finger must slide deep to the overlying tendons.

Studies also demonstrate that the pronator quadratus plays an essential role in supporting the distal radioulnar joint [35,48,60,61].

EFFECTS OF WEAKNESS

Weakness of the pronator quadratus weakens pronation strength. However, if the pronator teres remains intact, it provides substantial pronation force. Weakness of the pronator quadratus may lead to difficulty in pronation with elbow extension, since the pronator teres flexes the elbow as it pronates. Weakness of the pronator quadratus may also compromise stability of the distal radioulnar joint.

EFFECTS OF TIGHTNESS

Tightness of the pronator quadratus alone is unlikely. However, it is tight in combination with other structures such as the interosseous membrane and ligaments of the distal radioulnar joint, leading to restricted supination ROM.

DEEP MUSCLES ON THE DORSAL SURFACE OF THE FOREARM

The deep muscles of the dorsal surface of the forearm include the supinator, the three "snuff box" muscles (the abductor pollicis longus, the extensor pollicis brevis, and the extensor pollicis longus), and the extensor indicis (*Fig. 15.28*).

Supinator

The supinator muscle is presented in Chapter 12 with the other major supinator of the forearm, the biceps brachii. EMG studies reveal that the supinator is an important supinator of the elbow, particularly when the elbow is extended, effectively inhibiting the biceps brachii. Weakness of the supinator results in significant loss of supination strength when the elbow is extended. The case report presented in Chapter 12 reveals how supinator weakness can be missed if supination strength is evaluated only in the standard MMT position, which is with the elbow flexed [28,53]. In this position the biceps brachii is a powerful supinator and may mask any weakness of the supinator muscle.

Tightness of the supinator alone is improbable but in combination with the biceps brachii limits pronation ROM. Chapter 12 discusses how assessment of pronation ROM with the elbow flexed and extended helps distinguish the contributions of the biceps brachii and the supinator to limited pronation ROM.

Abductor Pollicis Longus

The abductor pollicis longus forms the anterior border of the **anatomical snuffbox,** composed of the abductor

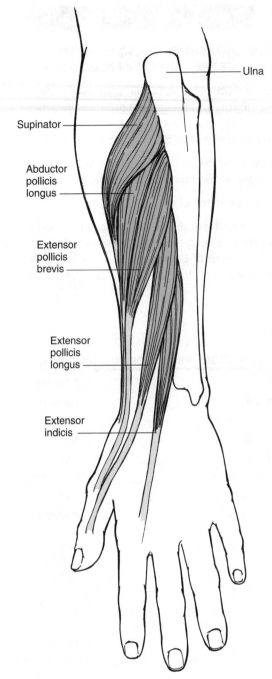

Figure 15.28: Deep muscles of the dorsal surface of the forearm include the supinator, abductor pollicis longus, extensor pollicis brevis, extensor pollicis longus, and extensor indicis.

pollicis longus, the extensor pollicis brevis, and the extensor pollicis longus (*Muscle Attachment Box 15.13*). Investigators report up to seven separate tendons of the abductor pollicis longus as it passes through the first dorsal compartment of the wrist with the extensor pollicis brevis [18,59]. It is a powerful muscle that affects both the thumb and the wrist [8].

MUSCLE ATTACHMENT BOX 15.13

ATTACHMENTS AND INNERVATION OF THE ABDUCTOR POLLICIS LONGUS

Proximal attachment: Posterior surface of the ulna and interosseous membrane distal to the attachment of the anconeus and the middle one third of the posterior radius distal to the supinator muscle.

Distal attachment: Trapezium and radial surface of the base of the thumb's metacarpal bone.

Innervation: Radial nerve, C7 and C8.

Palpation: The abductor pollicis longus tendon is palpated forming the anterior border of the anatomical snuff box of the thumb as it inserts into the base of the thumb's metacarpal bone.

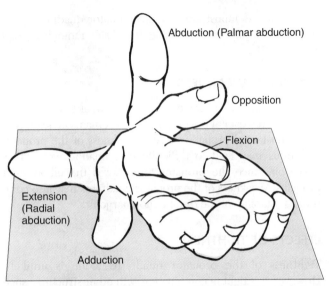

Figure 15.29: Motions available at the CMC joint of the thumb include flexion and extension in a plane parallel to the plane of the palm, abduction and adduction in a plane perpendicular to the plane of the palm, and opposition that combines flexion, abduction, and medial rotation.

ACTIONS

MUSCLE ACTION: ABDUCTOR POLLICIS LONGUS

Action	Evidence
Thumb CMC abduction	Conflicting
Thumb CMC extension	Supporting
Wrist radial deviation	Supporting
Wrist flexion	Supporting
Wrist extension	Supporting
Forearm pronation	Inadequate
Forearm supination	Inadequate

Essential to the understanding of the actions of the abductor pollicis longus is a clear image of the motions of the CMC joint of the thumb. These motions are presented in Chapter 14 and are reviewed in *Fig. 15.29*. Abduction (palmar abduction) of the CMC joint occurs in a plane perpendicular to the plane of the palm. Extension (radial abduction) occurs in a plane parallel to the plane of the palm. Despite the muscle's name, the abductor pollicis longus appears to play only a supportive role in abduction at the CMC joint. Most investigators report some participation of the muscle in abduction of the thumb [5,13,14,33,34], although one report states that the abductor pollicis longus does not participate in abduction at all [8]. Several studies also report that it contributes to extension of the CMC [8,13,14,30,33,34].

Careful analysis of the distal attachments of the abductor pollicis longus and its moment arms helps to explain the role of the abductor pollicis longus at the CMC joint of the thumb. The attachment is both extensive and variable, and this variability may be the source of the variety of interpretations of the muscle's actions [9,63,71]. The primary attachment of the abductor pollicis longus is on the dorsal surface of the base of the thumb's metacarpal (*Fig. 15.30*). Because the thumb lies slightly volar and medially rotated with respect to the rest of

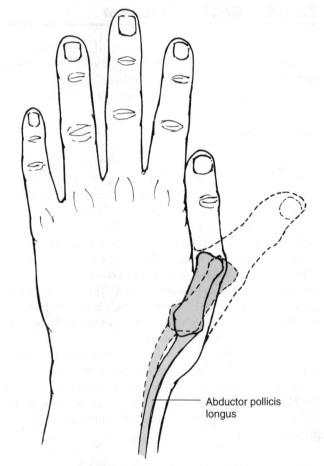

Figure 15.30: Attachment of the abductor pollicis longus on the dorsal aspect of the thumb's metacarpal. Because of the position of the thumb with respect to the hand, attachment of the abductor pollicis longus on the dorsal aspect of the thumb's metacarpal produces extension of the CMC joint.

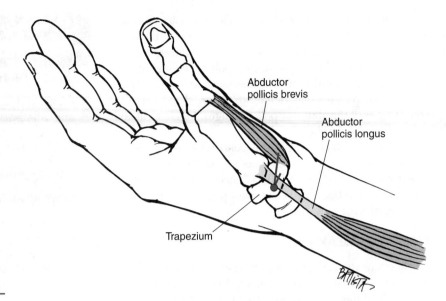

Figure 15.31: Moment arms of the abductor pollicis longus and brevis. The attachment of the abductor pollicis longus on the trapezium may create a slight abduction moment. However, the muscle's moment arm is shorter than the abduction moment arm of the abductor pollicis brevis.

the hand (see Fig. 14.38), attachment of the abductor pollicis longus on the dorsum of the metacarpal is consistent with the action of extension of the CMC. An attachment of the abductor pollicis longus tendon on the lateral aspect of the palmar surface of the trapezium also is described [44,71]. This attachment is consistent with an action of abduction of the CMC joint of the thumb, although the abduction moment arm is much smaller than that of the abductor pollicis brevis [47,63] (*Fig. 15.31*). In fact, the abductor pollicis longus has a larger moment arm for extension than for abduction.

EMG studies demonstrate activity of both the abductor pollicis longus and the intrinsic abductor during active abduction, but these studies demonstrate more activity of the abductor pollicis longus during extension of the CMC joint of the thumb than during abduction [5,9,14,33,72]. Studies of individuals following nerve blocks of the median nerve, which innervates the abductor pollicis brevis, also help clarify the abductor pollicis longus muscle's contribution to abduction of the thumb [6,33]. These subjects demonstrate severe loss of abduction strength at the CMC joint (from 75 to 100%). The variations in response to the nerve blocks are consistent with the anatomical variability already described. Thus it appears that while the abductor pollicis longus participates in abduction of the thumb, the intrinsic abductor is much better at it. The abductor pollicis longus is more important as an extensor of the thumb's CMC joint.

The abductor pollicis longus appears well suited for radial deviation of the wrist. It has one of the largest moment arms for radial deviation of any muscle crossing the wrist [6,8,9]. It also is reported to flex the wrist [6,8,34,55] and to be active during wrist extension [9,72]. Assessment of the muscle's moment arm for wrist flexion and extension suggests that it crosses the wrist through the axis of flexion and extension and thus has neither a flexion nor a extension moment [51]. However, movement of the thumb in the direction of abduction allows the tendon of the abductor pollicis longus to glide anteriorly. In this position it is likely that the muscle

can flex the wrist [9] (*Fig. 15.32*). This is a reported substitution pattern in patients with wrist flexion weakness. Similarly, adduction of the thumb may move the tendon posteriorly so that the muscle is posterior to the wrist's axis

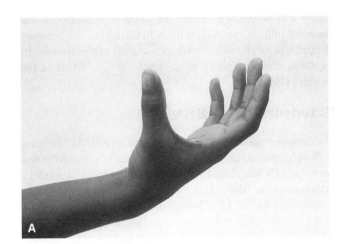

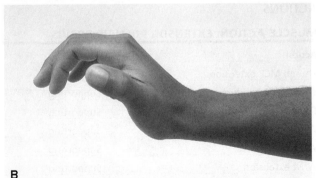

Figure 15.32: Function of the abductor pollicis longus at the wrist. **A.** When the thumb is abducted at the CMC joint, the abductor pollicis may contribute to wrist flexion. **B.** When the thumb is adducted at the CMC joint, the abductor pollicis may contribute to wrist extension.

of flexion and extension and is capable of wrist extension. The large and variable attachment of the muscle at the wrist and thumb may also explain some of the differences in actions attributed to the abductor pollicis longus at the wrist. Clinicians must note that these anatomical variations suggest that patients may demonstrate varied responses to contractions of the abductor pollicis longus. Mechanical and cadaver models of the muscle's moment arm suggest that the abductor pollicis longus can contribute to supination when the forearm is supinated, and to pronation with the forearm in the mid-range [10]. Clinicians need to remain alert for substitutions by the abductor pollicis longus during a variety of wrist movements.

EFFECTS OF WEAKNESS

Weakness of the abductor pollicis longus is manifested primarily in weakness in CMC extension. Extension at the CMC joint of the thumb is an essential component of normal pinch. Therefore, weakness of the abductor pollicis longus compromises an individual's ability to perform a powerful pinch. Details of the mechanics and pathomechanics of pinch are presented in Chapter 19.

EFFECTS OF TIGHTNESS

There are no known reports of isolated tightness of the abductor pollicis longus. It is likely to be tight in the presence of tightness of the other extrinsic muscles of the thumb. Its tightness may contribute to decreased flexion ROM at the thumb's CMC joint.

Extensor Pollicis Brevis

The extensor pollicis brevis travels together with the abductor pollicis longus in the 1st dorsal compartment at the wrist and consequently has almost identical actions except at its distal attachment at the MCP joint of the thumb (*Muscle Attachment Box 15.14*). The extensor pollicis brevis is considerably smaller than the abductor pollicis longus [8].

ACTIONS

MUSCLE ACTION: EXTENSOR POLLICIS BREVIS

Action	Evidence
Thumb MCP extension	Supporting
Thumb CMC abduction	Supporting
Thumb CMC extension	Supporting
Wrist radial deviation	Supporting
Wrist flexion	Supporting
Wrist extension	Supporting

There is little dispute about the ability of the extensor pollicis brevis, lying on the dorsum of the MCP joint, to extend the MCP joint of the thumb [8,34,55,75]. The extensor pollicis longus also can extend the MCP joint, and it is difficult to recruit the extensor pollicis brevis in isolation.

MUSCLE ATTACHMENT BOX 15.14

ATTACHMENTS AND INNERVATION OF THE EXTENSOR POLLICIS BREVIS

Proximal attachment: Posterior surface of the radius and adjacent interosseous membrane distal to the abductor pollicis longus.

Distal attachment: Dorsal surface of the base of the thumb's proximal phalanx.

Innervation: Radial nerve, C7 and C8.

Palpation: The tendon of the extensor pollicis brevis is palpable along with the abductor pollicis longus as the radial side of the anatomical snuff box of the thumb. It lies just dorsal to the tendon of the abductor pollicis longus.

The extensor pollicis brevis and abductor pollicis longus lie in the same tendon sheath and thus have almost identical actions at the wrist and CMC joint of the thumb [8,49,55]. The extensor pollicis brevis lies slightly dorsal and medial to the abductor pollicis longus. It is aligned to extend the CMC joint of the thumb but has only a slight contribution to abduction. It has a similar moment arm for radial deviation of the wrist compared to the abductor pollicis longus has but less ability to flex the wrist [34,51] (*Fig. 15.33*). As with the abductor pollicis longus, movement of the thumb may alter its effect on wrist flexion and extension.

EFFECTS OF WEAKNESS

Weakness of the extensor pollicis brevis weakens MCP and CMC extension of the thumb. However, if the abductor pollicis longus and the extensor pollicis longus remain intact, the functional consequences are small.

EFFECTS OF TIGHTNESS

Tightness of the extensor pollicis brevis alone is unlikely. It may contribute to limited CMC motion along with the larger abductor pollicis longus. It is too small to affect MCP joint motion by itself.

Clinical Relevance

DE QUERVAIN'S DISEASE: *De Quervain's disease* is a thickening and narrowing of the connective tissue compartment containing the extensor pollicis brevis and abductor pollicis longus. It is a disorder commonly found in people who use repetitive thumb flexion and extension, for example, computer keyboard operators [47]. A classic

(continued)

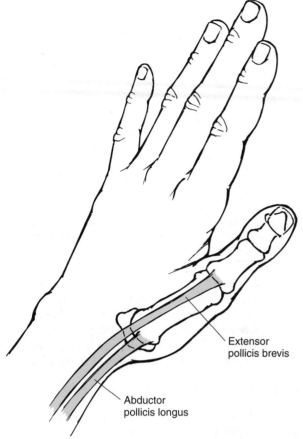

Figure 15.33: The extensor pollicis brevis lies slightly ulnar and dorsal to the abductor pollicis longus and thus has a slightly improved moment arm for extension of the wrist joint.

(Continued)
test for the disorder involves stretching these muscles to reproduce the patient's complaints of pain. The test, known as Finkelstein's test, *places the joints of the thumb in flexion and the wrist in ulnar deviation [58,76]. The test appears to stretch the extensor pollicis brevis more than the abductor pollicis longus, which is consistent with the more distal attachment of the extensor pollicis brevis [36].*

Extensor Pollicis Longus

Another pennate muscle of the forearm, the extensor pollicis longus, takes a circuitous route through the forearm to the thumb (*Muscle Attachment Box 15.15*). It loops around the dorsal tubercle of the radius, which serves as a pulley to redirect the tendon toward the thumb. The muscle's effect on the thumb is influenced directly by the tendon's angle of pull that results from its route around the dorsal tubercle.

MUSCLE ATTACHMENT BOX 15.15

ATTACHMENTS AND INNERVATION OF THE EXTENSOR POLLICIS LONGUS

Proximal attachment: Lateral aspect of the middle one third of the ulna on its posterior surface and the adjacent interosseous membrane.

Distal attachment: Dorsal surface of the base of the thumb's distal phalanx.

Innervation: Radial nerve, C7 and C8.

Palpation: The extensor pollicis longus is palpated as the ulnar border of the anatomical snuff box.

ACTIONS

MUSCLE ACTION: EXTENSOR POLLICIS LONGUS

Action	Evidence
Thumb IP extension	Supporting
Thumb MCP extension	Supporting
Thumb CMC extension	Conflicting
Thumb CMC adduction	Supporting
Thumb retropulsion	Supporting
Wrist radial deviation	Supporting
Wrist extension	Supporting

The extensor pollicis longus is the primary extensor of the IP joint of the thumb. It is the only muscle capable of extending the IP joint through its full range of motion. However, it is important to recognize that other muscles (i.e., the intrinsic muscles to the thumb) also contribute to IP extension [32,66]. The extensor pollicis longus also contributes to extension of the MCP joint along with the extensor pollicis brevis.

The role of the extensor pollicis longus at the CMC joint is more controversial. The muscle is commonly described as an extensor of this joint [8,34,55,75]. However, the extensor pollicis longus crosses on the ulnar side of the CMC as it winds around the dorsal tubercle of the radius (*Fig. 15.34*). Recognition that extension of the CMC occurs in the plane of the palm and adduction occurs in a plane perpendicular to the plane of the palm reveals that the extensor pollicis longus is better aligned to adduct the CMC joint than to extend it [14]. As the thumb adducts, the extensor pollicis longus becomes an even better adductor and less an extensor. It is the only muscle capable of adducting the thumb past the palm of the hand. This action is known as *retropulsion* and can serve as a test of the extensor pollicis longus (*Fig. 15.35*). As the thumb abducts the muscle's moment arm for extension improves [8]. The extensor pollicis longus crosses the wrist dorsally and slightly to the radial side of the capitate and has moment arms for both wrist extension and radial deviation [8,34,51,75].

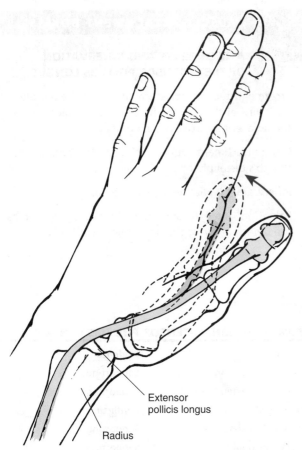

Figure 15.34: The extensor pollicis longus crosses the thumb's CMC dorsally, thus producing a large adduction moment at the CMC joint.

Like the abductor pollicis longus, the extensor pollicis longus may be capable of supination when the forearm is supinated and of pronation when the forearm is in the mid-position [10].

Clinical Relevance

USE OF THE "SNUFF BOX MUSCLES" IN WRIST MOTIONS: *Careful observations are required for a clinician testing wrist strength to notice a subject's use of any of the extrinsic muscles of the thumb for additional strength during wrist motions. However, the capacity of these muscles to contribute to wrist strength may greatly enhance the functional abilities of a patient with wrist weakness (Fig. 15.36).*

EFFECTS OF WEAKNESS

The primary effect of weakness of the extensor pollicis longus is weakness of extension at the IP joint of the thumb. However, some IP extension is preserved if the intrinsic muscles of the thumb remain intact. A study in which a nerve block produced temporary paralysis of the extensor pollicis longus in individuals

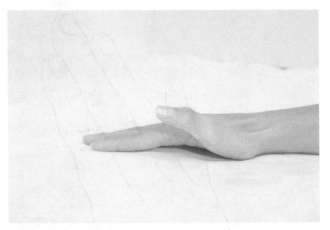

Figure 15.35: Thumb retropulsion. The extensor pollicis longus is the only muscle that is able to pull the thumb into adduction past the palm, or retropulsion.

without hand pathology revealed that most subjects were able to extend the IP joint through at least half its available excursion with the intact intrinsic muscles [66]. This study suggests that the extensor pollicis longus is important for full active extension of the joint, but it is not the only extensor of the IP joint.

EFFECTS OF TIGHTNESS

Tightness of the extensor pollicis longus is seen most commonly in conjunction with tightness of the other extrinsic muscles, particularly the flexor pollicis longus. This combined tightness is often the result of weakness in the intrinsic muscles of the thumb, altering the muscle balance necessary for normal function in the wrist and hand.

Extensor Indicis (Also Known As the Extensor Indicis Proprius)

The extensor indicis is a small muscle that lies deep in the dorsum of the forearm (*Muscle Attachment Box 15.16*).

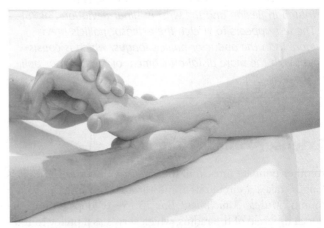

Figure 15.36: Thumb substitutions. The extensor pollicis longus and other snuff box muscles can assist in wrist extension and may substitute for weak dedicated wrist extensor muscles.

MUSCLE ATTACHMENT BOX 15.16

ATTACHMENTS AND INNERVATION OF THE EXTENSOR INDICIS

Proximal attachment: The posterior surface of the ulna and adjacent interosseous membrane just distal to the extensor pollicis longus.

Distal attachment: Extensor hood of the index finger. The tendon lies on the ulnar side of the extensor digitorum tendon.

Innervation: Radial nerve, C7 and C8.

Palpation: The tendon of the extensor indicis is palpable on the ulnar side of the extensor digitorum tendon as the two tendons cross the MCP joint of the index finger.

ACTIONS

MUSCLE ACTION: EXTENSOR INDICIS

Action	Evidence
Index finger DIP extension	Supporting
Index finger PIP extension	Supporting
Index finger MCP extension	Supporting
Index finger MCP ulnar deviation	Inadequate
Wrist extension	Inadequate

The actions of the extensor indicis are virtually identical to those of the extensor digitorum at the index finger.

The role of the extensor indicis at the index finger, like that of the extensor digitorum, is extension of the MCP joint. Extension of all of the joints of the index finger requires the simultaneous contraction of both the extrinsic extensors and the intrinsic muscles to the index finger. The primary functional role of the extensor indicis is to allow independent extension of the index finger. This is essential since the primary extrinsic extensor of the fingers, the extensor digitorum, has interconnections (juncturae tendinae) among the fingers, making independent movement difficult. EMG data suggest that the extensor indicis is more active than the extensor digitorum during unresisted MCP extension in individuals without hand pathology [13]. The tendon of the extensor indicis lies on the ulnar side of the tendon of the extensor digitorum, creating a slight moment arm for ulnar deviation of the index finger.

The extensor indicis is positioned at the center of the wrist on the dorsum and theoretically is capable of contributing to wrist extension. However, it is a small muscle and unable to add much additional force.

EFFECTS OF WEAKNESS

Although weakness of the extensor indicis may produce some weakness in extension of the MCP joint, the primary limitation in the presence of extensor indicis weakness is difficulty in independent movement of the index finger. The functional impairment can be significant in individuals such as computer operators and musicians.

EFFECTS OF TIGHTNESS

Tightness of the extensor indicis alone is unlikely but may accompany tightness of the extensor digitorum. Together they may contribute to hyperextension of the MCP joints of the fingers.

SYNERGISTIC FUNCTION OF THE FOREARM MUSCLES TO THE WRIST AND HAND

Active Coordination of the Dedicated Wrist Muscles and the Finger Muscles

A muscle affects every joint that it crosses. Thus the finger flexor muscles tend to flex the wrist, the MCP joint, and the PIP and DIP joints, while the extensor muscles of the fingers tend to extend these joint. Attempts to make a tight fist with the wrist maximally flexed fail and usually cause discomfort on the volar and/or dorsal surface of the forearm *(Fig. 15.37)*. Conversely, it is difficult to extend the fingers completely

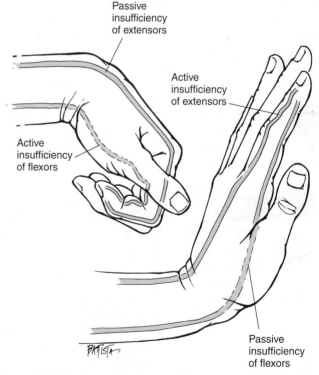

Figure 15.37: Active and passive insufficiency. **A.** Full closure of the fingers with the wrist fully flexed is prevented by active insufficiency of the finger flexors and passive insufficiency of the finger extensors. **B.** Full opening of the fingers with the wrist fully extended is prevented by active insufficiency of the finger extensors and passive insufficiency of the finger flexors.

when the wrist is maximally extended. There are two important factors contributing to the difficulty of these tasks. First in both situations, the agonists of the movement are required to contract while in their shortest position. This results in **active insufficiency** of the finger flexor or extensor muscles. In Chapter 4, active insufficiency is defined as the inability of a muscle to shorten enough to pull the limb through its complete available ROM. Every muscle has a maximum shortening capacity that is defined by the length of its fibers. If the finger flexors are allowed to flex each joint they cross, they reach their maximally shortened length before pulling the joints through their full excursions.

At the same time that the agonists are actively insufficient, the antagonists are being stretched and may produce **passive insufficiency.** Passive insufficiency is defined as the inability to move through the entire available range because of passive restrictions from opposing soft tissue. As the wrist and fingers are flexed, the antagonist finger extensors are stretched and may limit full closure of the fingers. The involved structures are merely reversed in the example of opening the fingers with the wrist extended. The finger extensor tendons exhibit active insufficiency, and the finger flexors may manifest passive insufficiency.

The dedicated wrist muscles are essential in preventing the active and passive insufficiencies that can occur with contraction of the extrinsic muscles of the fingers. Observations of an individual opening and closing a fist reveal the well-programmed pattern of wrist and finger synergy *(Fig. 15.38).* As the fingers actively close in a tight fist, the wrist automatically extends. Similarly the wrist flexes as the fingers actively extend. The dedicated wrist extensor muscles contract with the finger flexor muscles to counteract the flexion moment at the wrist exerted by the finger flexors. Wrist extension occurs during finger flexion, thereby maintaining adequate length of the finger flexors, allowing closure of the fingers. At the same time wrist extension puts the finger extensor tendons on enough slack to allow the necessary finger flexion excursion.

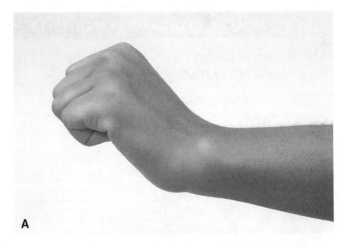

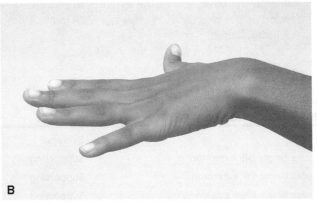

Figure 15.38: Synergists for finger flexion and extension. **A.** The wrist extensors are the synergists to finger flexion. **B.** The wrist flexors are the synergists to finger extension.

of the wrist extensors [23]. The extensor carpi radialis brevis is a common contributor to this pain because it is the primary wrist extensor. Another confusing phenomenon for an individual with tennis elbow is the classic complaint of pain on the lateral aspect of the elbow while shaking hands, an activity that clearly involves the finger flexor muscles. The presence of pain at the lateral epicondyle when shaking hands demonstrates the role of the wrist extensors during activities using the finger flexors.

Clinical Relevance

TENNIS ELBOW": *"Tennis elbow" is a painful condition involving the attachment of the dorsal superficial forearm muscles to the lateral epicondyle of the humerus. It is also known as "lateral epicondylitis," although the role of inflammation is unclear, and as "lateral epicondylosis," based on the notion that it includes degenerative changes in the muscle attachments [22]. The muscles include the dedicated wrist extensors as well as the extensor digitorum and the extensor digiti minimi. Frequently, patients are confused by a diagnosis of tennis elbow when they have never played tennis. Individuals who perform any activity of repeated or heavily resisted finger flexion are at risk for tennis elbow because the activity requires concomitant contraction*

Wrist flexion by contraction of the flexor carpi radialis and ulnaris has a similar effect on the finger extensors. The wrist flexors balance the wrist extension force produced by the finger extension muscles, preventing excessive wrist extension and allowing adequate contractile length in the extensor tendons to the fingers and adequate passive length in the flexor tendons of the fingers. The abductor pollicis longus serves a similar purpose at the thumb. The flexor pollicis longus flexes the CMC, MCP, and IP joints of the thumb as well as the wrist. Yet flexion at all of these joints simultaneously would pull the thumb into the palm. The thumb's CMC joint must be positioned in extension for the thumb to oppose the fingers. Thus the abductor pollicis longus contracts to block the undesired CMC flexion, stabilizing the joint against the pull of the flexor pollicis longus [72].

Passive Interactions between the Dedicated Wrist Muscles and the Finger Muscles

Active contraction of the wrist extensor muscles pulls the wrist into extension, putting the finger extensor muscles on slack and the finger flexor muscles in tension. Passive placement of the wrist in extension has the same effect on the lengths of the finger muscles. Similarly, both active and passive flexion of the wrist loosens the finger flexors and stretches the finger extensors. This passive effect of wrist position on the length and passive tension of the finger muscles is known as **tenodesis** and has very useful applications in rehabilitation.

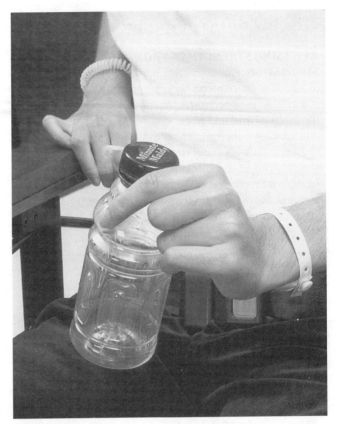

Figure 15.39: Tenodesis. An individual who lacks active finger flexion is able to grasp an object by using wrist extension, which passively flexes the fingers.

Clinical Relevance

TENODESIS: *Patients who lack active finger motion can still demonstrate the opening and closing of the fingers by active or passive movement of the wrist. A patient with a complete C6 tetraplegia lacks control of the extrinsic finger flexor muscles yet has the ability to actively extend the wrist. If the finger flexor muscles are allowed to develop some passive tightness, a functional grasp is possible by active wrist extension resulting in passive closure of the hand (Fig. 15.39). Careful instruction to the patient to avoid stretching the finger flexors is essential to the maintenance of a functional grasp.*

COMPARISONS OF STRENGTHS IN MUSCLES OF THE FOREARM

There are few known studies that examine the force production capabilities of individual muscles or muscle groups at the wrist. The following presents the available data regarding force production capabilities of the forearm musculature. There is only one known study that investigates the effects of age, gender, and hand dominance on wrist and finger strength [54]. This study reports extension strength of the wrist and MCP joints of the fingers and the thumb. It notes significantly greater strength in men than in women, gradual decline in strength with age, and significantly greater strength in the dominant hand. These factors may have similar effects on the other strengths of the forearm muscles, although research is needed to measure them. These factors can be useful when interpreting results of strength measurements in the clinic.

Pronation versus Supination

Results from comparisons of pronation and supination strength are conflicting. In one study of the isometric strengths of pronation and supination in 20 individuals without pathology, the data reveal greater supination strength than pronation strength when the forearm is in the neutral position [69]. Because the forces were collected as the subjects gripped and attempted to turn a handle, these data are likely to reflect force contributions from the primary pronator and supinator muscles and from wrist and finger muscles as well. In other studies that examine the strength of only the primary pronators and supinators, peak pronation strength is slightly greater than peak supination strength [57,62]. These reports also suggest that strength of pronation increases as the forearm supinates, and supination strength increases as the forearm pronates. These data support the view that the performance of the pronators and supinators is dictated primarily by muscle length. As the muscle is stretched, its force output rises. This finding is supported by evidence that elbow flexion tends to decrease pronation strength [57].

Clinical Relevance

ASSESSING STRENGTH OF PRONATION AND SUPINATION: *Pronation and supination strength assessments are common clinical procedures. The clinician is cautioned to use consistent testing positions to control for the effects of wrist and elbow joint position on pronation and supination strength. If testing positions are altered because a patient's status changes (e.g., elbow ROM changes) careful documentation of the position changes will facilitate interpretation of the clinical measures of strength. Similarly, the clinician must be aware of any activity in the finger and thumb muscles that may contribute to the strength of pronation or supination.*

Wrist Flexion versus Extension

Figure 15.40 provides a cross-sectional view of the wrist and the muscles that cross it. This figure is useful in providing an overview of the muscles and their relationships to the axes of motion of the wrist. The figure indicates the number of

muscles capable of causing a given motion at the wrist. It also allows a qualitative comparison of the moment arms of each muscle for the four motions of the wrist: flexion, extension, and radial and ulnar deviation. This figure demonstrates the potential effect that finger and thumb muscles have at the wrist. These effects may help explain the variations in results of studies examining the strength of the wrist flexors and extensors. In addition, *Table 15.1* lists the moment arms of the five dedicated wrist muscles [1,8].

Studies assessing the strength of the dedicated muscles of the wrist—the flexor carpi radialis, flexor carpi ulnaris, palmaris longus, extensor carpi radialis longus, extensor carpi radialis brevis, and extensor carpi ulnaris—consistently suggest that the wrist extensors generate larger peak extension moments than the peak moments exerted by the flexors [1,8,12,43,70]. These results are based on biomechanical models [12] and anatomical studies of muscle size and moment arms [1,8,17,43]. These studies reveal that the total physiological cross-sectional area of the dedicated wrist extensors is slightly greater than that of the dedicated wrist flexors [1,6,40]. Similarly, the extensors have larger moment arms, putting them at a mechanical advantage over the flexors [12]. However, when subjects are allowed to use finger

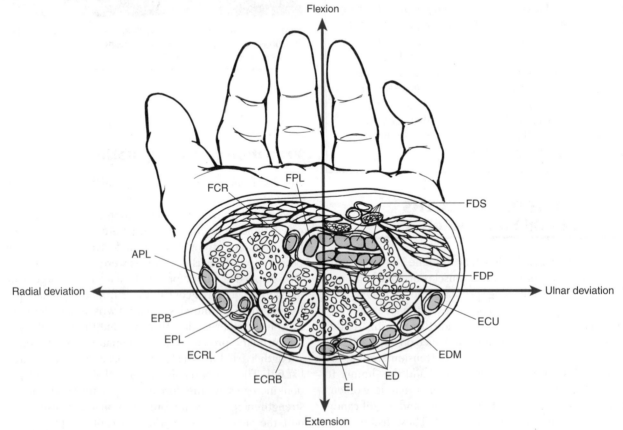

Figure 15.40: A cross section of the distal wrist reveals the number of muscles with the potential to participate in wrist flexion or extension. Flexor carpi ulnaris and palmaris longus (not seen in this view) contribute to wrist flexion. *FCR,* flexor carpi radialis; *FDS,* flexor digitorum superficialis; *FDP,* flexor digitorum profundus; *FPL,* flexor pollicis longus; *ECRL,* extensor carpi radialis longus; *ECRB,* extensor carpi radialis brevis; *ECU,* extensor carpi ulnaris; *ED,* extensor digitorum; *EI,* extensor indicis; *EDM,* extensor digiti minimi; *APL,* abductor pollicis longus; *EPB,* extensor pollicis brevis; *EPL,* extensor pollicis longus.

TABLE 15.1: Approximate Physiological Cross-Sectional Areas (PCSA) and Moment Arms for the Five Primary Dedicated Wrist Muscles

Muscle	Moment Arm for Flexion/Extension (cm)	Moment Arm for Radial/Ulnar Deviation (cm)
Flexor carpi radialis	1.0	1.75
Flexor carpi ulnaris	1.6	1.85
Extensor carpi radialis brevis	2.1	1.0
Extensor carpi radialis longus	1.25	1.35
Extensor carpi ulnaris	2.5	0.6

Data from Brand PW, Hollister A: Clinical Mechanics of the Hand. St. Louis, MO: Mosby-Year Book, 1999.

and thumb muscles as well as the dedicated wrist muscles, a significantly larger flexion moment is generated than extension moment [16,26]. Examination of the total physiological cross-sectional area of all of the muscles with the potential to flex and extend the wrist reveals that the flexors have a larger total cross-sectional area [1,26,40]. The total force capacity of all of the finger extensors is less than 40% of the total capacity of all of the finger flexors. The extensor pollicis longus contributes to active wrist extension, but the abductor pollicis longus and extensor pollicis brevis may contribute to flexion. Consequently, if the muscles to the fingers and thumb are allowed to participate in wrist motion, it is not surprising that wrist flexion strength is greater than wrist extension.

Clinical Relevance

MMT OF THE WRIST: *The studies of wrist strength reveal that measures of strength at the wrist are affected significantly by the presence or absence of activity in the finger muscles. Variations in the muscles participating in the test alter the output. Satisfactory inter- and intrarater reliability of wrist strength requires a consistent method of strength measurement. MMT of wrist flexion with and without finger muscle participation is likely to produce significantly different results.*

Wrist position also affects the force of wrist flexion and extension. Studies based on muscle architecture and biomechanical models suggest that both the wrist flexors and wrist extensors reach their peak forces when the wrist is extended [26,43]. The wrist flexors are on stretch when the wrist is extended, increasing the muscles' force-generating capacity. However, the moment arms of the flexors increase when the wrist is flexed. In contrast, the wrist extensors are shortened when the wrist is extended, but their moment arms increase when the wrist is in extension. These data suggest that force output of the wrist flexors is influenced more by their length, while the force of the dedicated wrist extensors is influenced more by the muscles' moment arms.

These relationships are consistent with the functional demands on these muscle groups. The synergistic activity between the wrist extensors and the finger flexors reveals that the wrist extensors' primary responsibility is to stabilize the wrist against the pull of the finger flexors. It is useful for these muscles to be strongest when the finger flexors are most active, that is, as the wrist is extended. Thus the wrist extensors appear to be architecturally designed to be strong in their most important functional position.

Radial versus Ulnar Deviation of the Wrist

There is only one known study comparing the strengths of radial and ulnar deviation of the wrist, and the finger and thumb muscles were allowed to participate [16]. The study reports that radial deviation is stronger than ulnar deviation because there are many more muscles with the capacity to deviate the wrist radially. Some of these muscles (particularly the snuff box muscles of the thumb) have very large moment arms. Although there are no known studies that compare the strengths of radial and ulnar deviation when only the dedicated wrist muscles are considered, there may be less difference between these strengths. The capacity of these muscles to generate a moment based on both muscle size and mechanical advantage is more similar, although the muscles that deviate the wrist in a radial direction may generate a slightly larger total moment [1,7].

Finger Flexion versus Extension

Few studies are available that assess or compare the strengths of the fingers, and there are no known studies of the strengths across the joints of the thumb. The flexor digitorum profundus is reportedly 50% stronger than the flexor digitorum superficialis, based primarily on muscle mass [8]. An in vivo study of flexion strength at the DIP, PIP, and MCP joints of the fingers reports that PIP flexion is stronger than DIP flexion [15]. The investigator reports that the DIP joints of the fingers were fixed in extension as the strength of PIP flexion was measured. This could allow the flexor digitorum profundus to contract against the fixation. If this occurred, the reported strengths at the PIP joint reflect the force of both the flexor digitorum superficialis and the flexor digitorum profundus.

Assessment of finger extension strength at the MCP joints using both in vivo measurements [4] and anatomical studies [8] reveals that the long finger exerts the greatest extension force, followed by the index and ring fingers. The little finger, which commonly lacks an extensor digitorum tendon, exerts the least force.

Although there is a clear lack of studies characterizing the normal range of strengths of the wrist and hand within a healthy population, studies of functional strengths are available. These studies assess the strengths of pinch and grasp. The results of some of these studies are presented in Chapter 19 following the discussion of the mechanics of normal pinch and grasp.

SUMMARY

This chapter reviews the muscles of the forearm. Each muscle is presented, and its contributions to the function and dysfunction of the wrist and elbow are discussed. Discussions reveal that the functions often depend on the precise position of the joint of interest. Many muscles lie so close to a joint axis that the muscle's effect at the joint changes as the muscle slides back and forth across the axis. In addition, the critical interplay between the dedicated wrist muscles and the muscles of the fingers is analyzed, and a similar interplay between muscles of the thumb is noted.

Although many unresolved issues remain regarding the actions of the muscles of the forearm, several guiding principles can be derived:

- Many forearm muscles cross the elbow and may affect it, particularly in the absence of the primary muscles of the elbow.
- Actions of the forearm muscles at the elbow and wrist may change with changing positions of the elbow and wrist.
- Movements of the wrist in the cardinal planes require pairs of muscles to contract together to accomplish the motion; the muscles composing the pairs vary according to the desired motion.
- Normal movements of the fingers require simultaneous contraction of wrist muscles to block the undesired effects of the finger muscles at the wrist.
- Function of the extrinsic muscles to the fingers is inextricably intertwined with the function of the intrinsic musculature presented in Chapter 18.
- Impairments resulting from dysfunction of the extrinsic muscles of the fingers are also affected by the integrity of the intrinsic muscles.

The clinician must recognize that an evaluation of the wrist also requires an assessment of the structures of the elbow and hand.

Throughout this chapter the function of the extrinsic muscles of the fingers is related to structures unique to the hand, including the intrinsic muscles. Thus the explanation of the functional capability of the hand has just begun.

Before proceeding to these structures, a discussion of the mechanics of the wrist must be completed. The following chapter discusses the loads to which the wrist is subjected during a variety of activities. In addition, the effects of various pathological conditions on the loads at the wrist are considered. An understanding of loads incurred at the wrist will provide a better understanding of the mechanics of loading in the hand.

References

1. An KN, Hui FC, Morrey BF, et al.: Muscles across the elbow joint: a biomechanical analysis. J Biomech 1981; 14: 659–669.
2. An KN, Ueba Y, Chao EY, et al.: Tendon excursion and moment arm of index finger muscles. J Biomech 1983; 16: 419–425.
3. Baker DS, Gaul JS, Williams VK, Graves M: The little finger superficialis-clinical investigations of its anatomic and functional short comings. J Hand Surg [Am] 1981; 6: 374–378.
4. Barnes WJ, Allison JD: Isometric torque of the finger extensors at the metacarpophalangeal joints. Phys Ther 1978; 58: 42–45.
5. Basmajian JV, DeLuca CJ: Muscles Alive. Their Function Revealed by Electromyography. Baltimore: Williams & Wilkins, 1985.
6. Boatright JR, Kiebzak GM: The effects of low median nerve block on thumb abduction strength. J Hand Surg 1997; 22A: 849–852.
7. Brand PW, Beach RB, Thompson DE: Relative tension and potential excursion of muscles in the forearm and hand. J Hand Surg [Am] 1981; 6: 209–219.
8. Brand PW, Hollister A: Clinical Mechanics of the Hand. St. Louis, MO: Mosby-Year Book, 1999.
9. Brandsma JW, Oudenaarde EV, Oostendorp R: The abductores pollicis muscles: clinical considerations based on electromyographical and anatomical studies. J Hand Ther 1996; 9: 218–222.
10. Bremer AK, Sennwald GR, Favre P, Jacob HAC: Moment arms of forearm rotators. Clin Biomech 2006; 21: 683–691.
11. Brumfield RH, Champoux JA: A biomechanical study of normal functional wrist motion. Clin Orthop 1984; 187: 23–25.
12. Buchanan TS, Moniz MJ, Dewald JPA, Rymer WZ: Estimation of muscle forces about the wrist joint during isometric tasks using an EMG coefficient method. J Biomech 1993; 26: 547–560.
13. Close JR, Kidd CC: The functions of the muscles of the thumb, the index, and the long fingers. J Bone Joint Surg 1969; 51A: 1601–1620.
14. Cooney WP III, An KN, Daube JR, Askew LJ: Electromyographic analysis of the thumb: a study of isometric forces in pinch and grasp. J Hand Surg [Am] 1985; 10A: 202–210.
15. Darwin NM: Performance of the finger flexor muscles. Phys Ther Rev 1951; 31: 433–436.
16. Delp SL, Grierson AE, Buchanan TS: Maximum isometric moments generated by the wrist muscles in flexion-extension and radial-ulnar deviation. J Biomech 1996; 29: 1371–1375.
17. Dempster WT, Finerty JC: Relative activity of wrist moving muscles in static support of the wrist joint: an electromyographic study. Am J Physiol 1947; 150: 596–606.
18. DosRemedios C, Chapnikoff D, Wavreille G, Chantelot C et al.: The abductor pollicis longus: relation between innervation, muscle bellies and number of tendinous slips. Surg Radiol Anat 2005; 27: 243–248.

19. Ekenstam FA: Anatomy of the distal radioulnar joint. Clin Orthop 1992; 275: 14–18.

20. Ettema GJC, Styles G, Kippers V: The moment arms of 23 muscle segments of the upper limb with varying elbow and forearm positions: implications for motor control. Hum Mov Sci 1998; 17: 201–220.

21. Fahrer M, Tubiana R: Palmaris longus, anteductor of the thumb. An experimental study. Hand 1976; 8: 287–289.

22. Fedorczyk JM: Tennis elbow: blending basic science with clinical practice. J Hand Ther 2006; 19: 146–153.

23. Finestone H, Helfenstein S: Spray bottle epicondylitis. Diagnosing and treating workers in pain. Can Fam Physician 1994; 40: 336–337.

24. Finsen L, Sogaard K, Graven-Nielsen T, Christensen H: Activity patterns of wrist extensor muscles during wrist extensions and deviations. Muscle Nerve 2005; 31: 242–251.

25. Garcia-Elias M: Soft-tissue anatomy and relationships about the distal ulna. Hand Clin 1998; 14: 165–176.

26. Gonzalez RV, Buchanan TS, Delp SL: How muscle architecture and moment arms affect wrist flexion-extension moments. J Biomech 1997; 30: 705–712.

27. Hazelton FT: The influence of wrist position on the force produced by the finger flexors. J Biomech 1975; 8: 301–306.

28. Hislop HJ, Montgomery J: Daniel's and Worthingham's Muscle Testing: Techniques of Manual Examination. Philadelphia: WB Saunders, 1995.

29. Idler RS: Anatomy and biomechanics of the digital flexor tendons. Hand Clin 1985; 1: 3–11.

30. Imaeda T, An KN, Cooney WP III: Functional anatomy and biomechanics of the thumb. Hand Clin 1992; 8: 9–15.

31. Inoue G, Tamura Y: Dislocation of the extensor tendons over the metacarpophalangeal joints. J Hand Surg [Am] 1996; 21: 464–469.

32. Kaplan EB: Anatomy and Kinesiology of the Hand. In: Hand Surgery. Flynn JE, ed. Baltimore: Williams & Wilkins, 1982; 14–24.

33. Kaufman KR, An KN, Litchy WJ, et al.: In-vivo function of the thumb muscles. Clin Biomech (Bristol, Avon) 1999; 14: 141–150.

34. Kendall FP, McCreary EK, Provance PG: Muscle Testing and Function. Baltimore: Williams & Wilkins, 1993.

35. Kihara H, Short WH, Werner FW, et al.: The stabilizing mechanism of the distal radioulnar joint during pronation and supination. J Hand Surg [Am] 1995; 20A: 930–936.

36. Kutsumi K, Amadio PC, Zhao C, et al.: Finkelstein's test: a biomechanical analysis. J Hand Surg 2005; 30A: 130–135.

37. Leijnse JNAL: The controllability of the unloaded human finger with superficial or deep flexor. J Biomech 1997; 30: 1087–1093.

38. Leijnse JNAL, Snijders CJ, Bonte JE, et al.: The hand of the musician: the kinematics of the bidigital finger system with anatomical restrictions. J Biomech 1993; 10: 1169–1179.

39. Lieber RL, Friden J: Musculoskeletal balance of the human wrist elucidated using intraoperative laser diffraction. J Electromyogr Kinesiol 1998; 8: 93–100.

40. Lieber RL, Jacobson MD, Fazeli BM, et al.: Architecture of selected muscles of the arm and forearm: anatomy and implications for tendon transfer. J Hand Surg [Am] 1992; 17: 787–798.

41. Long C, Brown ME: Electromyographic kinesiology of the hand: muscles moving the long finger. J Bone Joint Surg 1964; 46A: 1683–1706.

42. Loren GJ, Lieber RL: Tendon biomechanical properties enhance human wrist muscle specialization. J Biomech 1995; 28: 791–799.

43. Loren GJ, Shoemaker SD, Burkholder TJ, et al.: Human wrist motors: biomechanical design and application to tendon transfers. J Biomech 1996; 29: 331–342.

44. Melling M, Reihsner R, Steindl M, et al.: Biomechanical stability of abductor pollicis longus muscles with variable numbers of tendinous insertions. Anat Rec 1998; 250: 475–479.

45. Murray WM, Buchanan TS, Delp SL: The isometric functional capacity of muscles that cross the elbow. J Biomech 2000; 33: 943–952.

46. Nathan RH: The isometric action of the forearm muscles. J Biomech Eng 1992; 114: 162–169.

47. Omokawa S, Ryu J, Tang JB, et al.: Trapeziometacarpal joint instability affects the moment arms of thumb motor tendons. Clin Orthop 2000; 372: 262–271.

48. Palmer AK, Werner FW: Biomechanics of the distal radioulnar joint. Clin Orthop 1984; 187: 26–35.

49. Pascarelli EF, Kella JJ: Soft-tissue injuries related to use of the computer keyboard. A clinical study of 53 severely injured persons. J Occup Med 1993; 35: 522–532.

50. Pigeon P, Yahia L, Feldman AJ: Moment arms and lengths of human upper limb muscles as functions of joint angles. J Biomech 1996; 29: 1365–1370.

51. Raikova R: A general approach for modelling and mathematical investigation of the human upper limb. J Biomech 1992; 25: 857–867.

52. Rayan GM, Saccone PG: Treatment of spastic thumb-in-palm deformity: a modified extensor pollicis longus tendon rerouting. J Hand Surg [Am] 1996; 21: 834–839.

53. Reese NB: Muscle and Sensory Testing. Philadelphia: WB Saunders, 1999.

54. Richards RR, Gordon R, Beaton D: Measurement of wrist, metacarpophalangeal joint, and thumb extension strength in a normal population. J Hand Surg [Am] 1993; 18: 253–261.

55. Romanes GJE: Cunningham's Textbook of Anatomy. Oxford: Oxford University Press, 1981.

56. Ryu JR, Cooney WP III, Askew LJ, et al.: Functional ranges of motion of the wrist joint. J Hand Surg 1991; 16A: 409–419.

57. Salter N, Darcus HD: The effect of the degree of elbow flexion on the maximum torques developed in pronation and supination of the right hand. J Anat 1952; 86: 197–202.

58. Salter RB: Textbook of Disorders and Injuries of the Musculoskeletal System. 3rd ed. Baltimore: Williams & Wilkins, 1999.

59. Sarikcioglu L, Yildirim FB: Bilateral abductor pollicis longus muscle variation. Case report and review of the literature. Morphologie 2004; 88: 160–163.

60. Schuind F, An KN, Berglund L, et al.: The distal radioulnar ligaments: a biomechanical study. J Hand Surg [Am] 1991; 16A: 1106–1114.

61. Shaw JA, Bruno A, Paul EM: Ulnar styloid fixation in the treatment of posttraumatic instability of the radioulnar joint: a biomechanical study with clinical correlation. J Hand Surg [Am] 1990; 15A: 712–720.

62. Smith RJ: Balance and kinetics of the fingers under normal and pathological conditions. Clin Orthop 1974; 104: 92–111.

63. Smutz WP, Kongsayreepong A, Hughes RE, et al.: Mechanical advantage of the thumb muscles. J Biomech 2000; 31: 565–570.

64. Srinivasan H, Landsmeer JMF: Internal stabilization in the thumb. J Hand Surg [Am] 1982; 7: 371–375.

65. Strickland JW: Flexor tendon injuries. Part 1. Anatomy, physiology, biomechanics, healing, and adhesion formation around a repaired tendon. Orthop Rev 1986; 15: 632–645.

66. Strong CL, Perry J: Function of the extensor pollicis longus and intrinsic muscles of the thumb: an electromyographic study during interphalangeal joint extension. J Am Phys Ther Assoc 1966; 46: 939–945.

67. Tang JB, Jaiyoung R, Omokawa S, et al.: Biomechanical evaluation of wrist motor tendons after fractures of the distal radius. J Hand Surg [Am] 1999; 24A: 121–132.

68. Terrono AL, Rose JH, Mulroy J, Millender LH: Camitz palmaris longus abductorplasty for severe thenar atrophy secondary to carpal tunnel syndrome. J Hand Surg [Am] 1993; 18A: 204–206.

69. Timm WN, O'Driscoll SW, Johnson ME, An KN: Functional comparison of pronation and supination strengths. J Hand Ther 1993; 6: 190–193.

70. Tubiana R, Valentin P: The anatomy of the extensor apparatus of the fingers. Surg Clin North Am 1964; 44: 897–906.

71. van Oudenaarde E: Structure and function of the abductor pollicis longus muscle. J Anat 1991; 174: 221–227.

72. van Oudenaarde E, Brandsma JW, Oostendorp RAB: The influence of forearm, hand and thumb positions on extensor carpi ulnaris and abductor pollicis longus activity. Acta Anat (Basel.) 1997; 158: 296–302.

73. von Schroeder HP, Botte MJ: The functional significance of the long extensors and juncturae tendinum in finger extension. J Hand Surg [Am] 1993; 18: 641–647.

74. Weaver L, Tencer AF, Trumble TE: Tensions in the palmar ligaments of the wrist. I. The normal wrist. J Hand Surg [Am] 1994; 19: 464–474.

75. Williams P, Bannister L, Berry M, et al: Gray's Anatomy, The Anatomical Basis of Medicine and Surgery, Br. ed. London: Churchill Livingstone, 1995.

76. Yuasa K, Kiyoshige Y: Limited surgical treatment of de Quervain's disease: decompression of only the extensor pollicis brevis subcompartment. J Hand Surg 1998; 23A: 840–843.

Analysis of the Forces at the Wrist during Activity

CHAPTER CONTENTS

Because the hand is the "working end" of the upper extremity, it participates in countless activities that generate large loads in the hand and wrist. Some commonplace examples include twisting the tightened lid from a jar or digging up flower bulbs in a garden. Other activities that involve high loads at the wrist and hand include activities in which the upper extremity is weight bearing. As noted in the chapters on the shoulder and elbow, the upper extremities frequently participate in ambulation through the use of crutches and other assistive devices in the presence of impaired function in the lower extremities. The upper extremities can even replace the propulsion of the lower extremities entirely with the use of a wheelchair. The hand and wrist are also involved in impulsive activities such as hitting a tennis or golf ball, hammering a nail, or handling a jackhammer. Such activities expose the wrist to very large loads. The wrist's ability to withstand such loads is a testament to its remarkable design.

Many impairments involving the structures of the forearm and wrist are directly or indirectly associated with the loads that are generated at the wrist. Such impairments include "tennis elbow" (lateral epicondylitis), carpal tunnel syndrome, and degenerative arthritis. The purpose of this chapter is to examine the loads sustained at the wrist during activity and to discuss the implications of such loads for patients with wrist impairments and for the clinicians who work with these individuals. Specifically the purposes of this chapter are to

- Provide an example of a two-dimensional analysis of the forces at the wrist
- Examine the forces on the wrist joint and surrounding structures during activities
- Review the loading patterns and stresses on specific structures of the wrist complex
- Discuss the clinical implications of the magnitude and locations of loads at the wrist in individuals with and without impairments

ANALYSIS OF FORCES AT THE WRIST

In the analyses of forces generated at the shoulder and elbow (Chapters 10 and 13), simplifying assumptions are made to solve the equations used to calculate the forces and moments at those joints. These assumptions reduce the number of unknown quantities by presuming that only one muscle or muscle group contracts at a time. At the wrist, this is a reasonable assumption for some weight-bearing activities in which the wrist muscles are essential but the finger muscles can be somewhat relaxed. However, in an activity requiring forceful grip, it is clear that the finger flexors and wrist extensor muscles must contract simultaneously. Calculating joint forces under these conditions is more complicated because there are more unknown quantities than there are equations to solve, resulting in a case of static indeterminacy (Chapter 1).

The following example is chosen to review the methods of calculating joint and muscle forces when the simplifying assumptions are valid. Consider an individual who uses a cane for support following a stroke. *Examining the Forces Box 16.1* contains the free-body diagram and analysis of this example. Evaluation reveals that the patient bears approximately 50% of body weight on the weak side during stance on that side. Thus the cane must be supporting the remaining 50%. During the support phase, the cane pushes up on the hand, creating an extension moment at the wrist (*Fig. 16.1*). The finger muscles are not essential at this moment, so the example uses the assumption that only the dedicated wrist flexors are participating in the activity. In addition, the wrist flexors are considered together as one flexor force. These assumptions, while clearly not completely accurate, allow a solution for the equations of motion to determine the muscle and joint reaction forces.

This simplified analysis suggests that the total flexor force needed to balance the extension moment at the wrist generated by the cane is equal to approximately one eighth of body weight. Further analysis estimates the joint reaction force on

EXAMINING THE FORCES BOX 16.1

FREE-BODY DIAGRAM OF THE FORCES ON THE WRIST DURING WEIGHT-BEARING WITH A CANE

A free-body diagram of the forces on the wrist during weight bearing with a cane indicates that approximately 50% of the body weight (BW) is born on the cane (F_C). The flexor muscles generate a force (F_M) to balance the cane force. The joint reaction force (J) is exerted at the wrist.

Assumptions:

X_1 = 2.0 cm, the perpendicular distance from the wrist joint to the pull of the wrist flexors

X_2 = 0.5 cm, the perpendicular distance from the wrist joint to the reaction force of the cane

F_C = ½ BW, the reaction force of the cane

F_M, the total pull of the wrist flexors

$\Sigma M = 0$

$(0.5 \times BW \times 0.005\ m) - (F \times 0.02\ m) = 0$

$(BW \times 0.0025\ m) = (F \times 0.02\ m)$

F = 0.125 BW

Calculate the forces on the wrist. Assume that the reaction force of the cane and the flexor force are parallel and vertical. The weight of the upper extremity is approximately 7% of BW.

ΣF_X: There are no forces in the x direction

ΣF_Y: $J_Y + F_Y - 0.07\ BW + 0.5\ BW = 0$, where F_Y is the force of the wrist flexors

$J_Y = 0.07\ BW - 0.5\ BW - 0.125\ BW$

$J_Y = -0.555\ BW$

Therefore, the joint reaction force at the wrist is approximately 55.5% of body weight in the vertically downward direction.

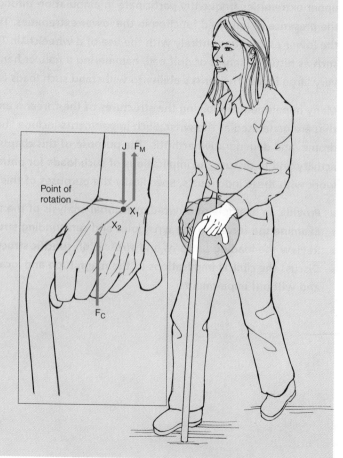

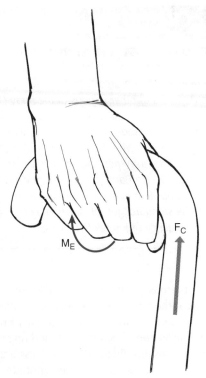

Figure 16.1: Extension moment at the wrist generated by the cane. The reaction force by the cane applied to the hand creates an extension moment (M_E) at the wrist joint.

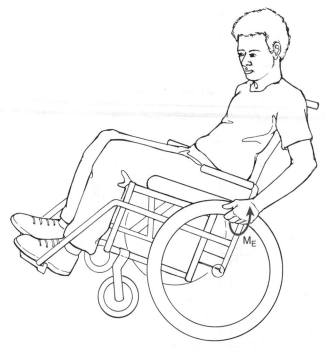

Figure 16.2: Extension moment generated on the wrist by a wheelchair. Propelling a wheelchair creates an extension moment (M_E) at the wrist.

the carpus to be slightly more than 50% of body weight. An important assumption in this example is the location of the reaction force of the cane. The closer the force is to the joint axis, the smaller the extension moment created. However, if the individual bears weight more in the palm of the hand, the extension moment and hence the muscle and joint reaction forces increase accordingly.

The values presented in this example are very rough approximations of reality, but the example demonstrates that the wrist can be subjected to very large loads. A fall onto an outstretched hand can impart an even larger load to the wrist, since the hand may bear more than 50% of body weight. Experimental falls even from low heights (3–6 cm) generate loads on the wrist of 50–55% of body weight [5]. Falls from standing height must generate much larger loads. In addition, the velocity of the body at the instant of impact means that the kinetic energy of the body is transmitted to the wrist. No wonder that the radius fractures or the ligaments rupture!

REVIEW OF THE FORCES ON THE WRIST

There are no known studies that examine the loads on the wrist during crutch walking. Wheelchair propulsion and crutch walking are not exactly analogous, but the tasks have enough similarities that the published data from the wheelchair study can help to put crutch walking into perspective. Neither task requires significant activity of the finger flexor muscles. Both tasks require that the wrist bear a load that

creates an extension moment at the wrist (*Fig. 16.2*). Loads of up to 90 N (approximately 20 lb) applied to the wheelchair rim are reported for manual wheelchair users [2,3,7]. The load applied by the hand onto the crutch may be significantly greater than the load on the wheelchair rim, since the individual may bear as much as 50% of body weight on the crutch [14,16]. Therefore, it is likely that crutch walking generates larger loads at the wrist than does wheelchair propulsion.

Clinical Relevance

USE OF ASSISTIVE DEVICES FOR AMBULATION IN INDIVIDUALS WITH RHEUMATOID ARTHRITIS: *The wrist is commonly affected in individuals with rheumatoid arthritis, which also typically involves the feet, knees, and hips, making ambulation difficult and painful. Assistive devices such as canes, crutches, and walkers can be very useful in reducing the loads on the joints of the lower extremities and improving ambulation. However, the analysis in Examining the Forces Box 16.1 demonstrates that use of these devices can lead to large loads on the wrist as well. The clinician is faced with the dilemma of protecting the joints of the lower extremities while perhaps overloading the joints of the wrist. Special adaptations of the assistive device may provide an alternative. These assistive devices can be fit with special supports that allow the patient to bear weight on the forearm rather than on the hand and wrist (Fig. 16.3). Such modifications provide relief for the lower extremities while minimizing the risk to the wrist.*

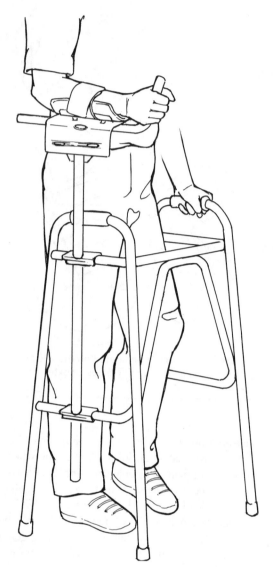

Figure 16.3: Forearm trough crutches are an example of adaptive devices that modify canes and crutches to reduce weight bearing through the wrist joint.

Clinical Relevance

WORK-RELATED WRIST AND HAND INJURIES: *Work-related musculoskeletal disorders of the wrist and hand injuries are associated with greater lost productivity and wages than disorders of other regions of the body [1]. Jobs that require prolonged or high-velocity repetitive wrist positions or high repetitive loads have high risk of wrist and hand problems. Workers with high incidence of such disorders range from data entry personnel to dentists to farm workers milking cows. Job analysis to identify ways to alter or vary the wrist position and employer and employee education about the standards for job safety may help to decrease the frequency of job-related injuries.*

One of the reasons for the scarcity of investigations into the joint forces at the wrist is the complexity of the problem. As noted above, most activities involving the wrist require the simultaneous contraction of several wrist and finger muscles. These cocontractions invalidate the usual assumption that only one muscle or muscle group is acting at any instant in time. Authors use a variety of analytical approaches to investigate the loads sustained by the wrist during cocontractions. Optimization techniques (Chapter 1) to calculate the joint reaction forces in the wrist as subjects pick up a moderate load (2–4 kg) using different grips yield joint reaction forces at the wrist that range from 1200 to 2200 N (270–500 lb) [4]. The cocontractions of the finger and wrist muscles needed to grip the object and stabilize the wrist are apparently responsible for these remarkably large loads.

A theoretical model to estimate the loads at the wrist during light grasp activities (approximately a 1-kg grip) yields estimates of total forces across the wrist of approximately 160 N (36 lb), considerably less than those in the preceding study [19]. Two methodological differences help explain the varied results. The grip force in the theoretical model is one fourth to one half the grip force examined by the optimization technique. In addition, the optimization analysis includes the flexion moment applied to the wrist by the lifted load, while the theoretical model considers only the effects of the compressive loads of the muscles during pinch without applying an additional external moment to the wrist (*Fig. 16.4*). Both analyses demonstrate that cocontraction of opposing muscle groups generate larger joint reaction forces than when only one muscle group is considered. These studies also suggest that even in such mild tasks as gripping and lifting a 2-kg (less than 1 lb) object, the wrist sustains large joint reaction forces.

More-vigorous activities such as some athletic events lead to large increases in loads at the wrist. Peak internal moments as high as 20 Nm are reported at the wrist at the instant of impact in the tennis stroke [6]. This can be compared to 12 Nm reported at the elbow during wheelchair propulsion [21]. Competitive gymnastics includes several events that involve

There are few studies that report direct calculations of loads applied to the wrist joint during common activities of daily living. Chadwick and Nicol report joint reaction forces from 1,200 to over 2,000 N (270–450 lb) when lifting 2–4 kg (4.4–8.8 lb) loads, depending upon the type of grip used [4]. Keir and Wells suggest that more than 25% of the maximum available extensor torque is required to hold the wrist in 30° of extension, a position often assumed by typists and data entry personnel [9]. Such muscle requirements would presumably produce significant joint reaction forces as well. Additionally, since such postures are typically maintained over prolonged periods, it is not surprising that wrist and elbow complaints are common in individuals in these professions.

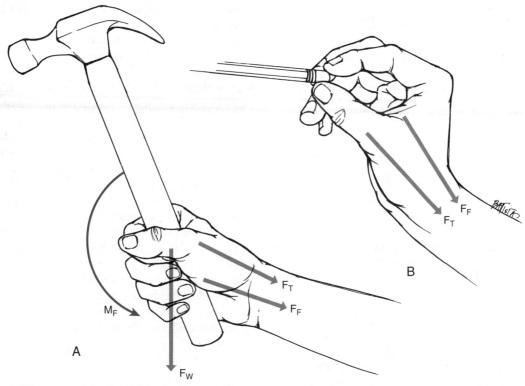

Figure 16.4: Two different models to examine the forces at the wrist during grasp and pinch. **A.** The model includes the muscle forces of the fingers (F_F) and the thumb (F_T) as well as the flexion moment (M_F) created by the load itself. **B.** The model only includes the muscle forces of the fingers (F_F) and the thumb (F_T) needed to pinch an object.

upper extremity weight bearing, usually in ballistic maneuvers involving very high rates of loading. The loads at the wrist during pommel horse and high bar exercises have been examined. Peak joint reaction forces at the wrist of up to twice body weight are reported in elite college-age male gymnasts performing on the pommel horse [11] (*Fig. 16.5*). A study of the kinetics of the high bar exercise reports peak reaction forces on the bar up to 2.2 times body weight in elite male gymnasts during giant swings [12]. These loads on the bar are balanced by tensile forces on the hands and wrist that must, in turn, be countered by large forces in the surrounding ligaments and muscles to stabilize the wrist and prevent dislocation (*Fig. 16.6*). The loads reported in these studies help explain the common complaints of wrist pain reported by gymnasts [11]. Other recreational and occupational activities such as riding dirt bikes over mountainous terrain, doing cartwheels, or driving a jackhammer into concrete may generate similarly high loads and lead to a variety of injuries and complaints at the wrist.

These studies of the joint reaction forces at the wrist suggest that the muscles and ligaments at the wrist also sustain large loads. Direct assessment of tendon loads generated during activity are also reported. Analysis of the peak forces in the extensor carpi radialis brevis during a backhand tennis stroke reveals loads of 90 N (20 lb) in advanced tennis players and 65 N (15 lb) in novice players [15]. Another study based on an anatomical wrist joint simulator examines the muscle

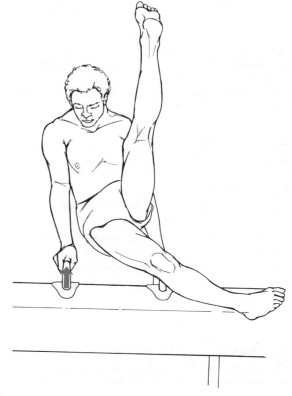

Figure 16.5: Load on the wrist during a pommel horse exercise. The pommel horse exercise produces loads on the wrist that can reach twice body weight.

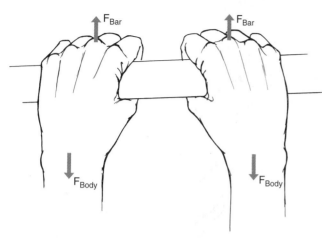

Figure 16.6: Load on the wrists during high bar exercises. The wrist sustains large distraction forces during the high bar exercise and is stabilized by the large forces generated by the surrounding ligaments and muscles.

forces needed to maintain static wrist positions [24]. The reported loads vary from 5 N (1.2 lb) in the flexor carpi radialis to approximately 30 N (6.7 lb) in the flexor carpi ulnaris and extensor carpi ulnaris, depending upon the position. The model supports the view that wrist functions require simultaneous activity of several muscles by predicting cocontraction of the extensor carpi ulnaris, extensor carpi radialis longus, extensor carpi radialis brevis, flexor carpi radialis, flexor carpi ulnaris, and abductor pollicis longus in each of the positions analyzed, 20° of flexion or extension, and 10° of ulnar or radial deviation.

Clinical Relevance

LOADS IN TENDONS AROUND THE WRIST DURING ACTIVITY: *Studies of the loads on the wrist reveal that the muscles surrounding the wrist must sustain substantial loads even in relatively low-load activities and even larger loads during more challenging tasks such as tennis. It is easy to imagine why complaints of pain with tennis elbow become chronic, since even without playing tennis, most individuals perform daily functions requiring large loads in the surrounding muscles. Identification of the loading patterns requires careful analysis of the offending activity. The clinician may be able to recommend modifications in the activity and provide patient education to alter the loads. Supportive devices may also be helpful in reducing the loads in the forearm musculature to allow healing.*

ANALYSIS OF STRESSES APPLIED TO THE WRIST JOINT DURING ACTIVITY

Although analysis of the joint reaction **forces** at the wrist is uncommon, the literature contains several studies that report calculations and direct measurements of the **stresses** applied

to the wrist joint surfaces and surrounding soft tissue. Stress, or pressure, is defined in Chapter 2 as force per unit area (force/area). Direct measurements are performed typically in cadaver specimens by inserting a pressure-sensing device to measure the stress between adjacent articular surfaces during loading [8,20,22]. Larger average stresses are reported at the radioscaphoid articulation than at the radiolunate articulation [8,19,20,22]. Wrist position and joint alignment are among many factors that influence these joint stresses. There is an increase in radioscaphoid pressure when the wrist is in radial deviation and an increase in radiolunate and ulnocarpal stresses when the wrist is in ulnar deviation. Stresses as large as 4.3 MPa, (1 megaPascal = 10^6 N/m², Chapter 1), are reported in single specimens [20]. These stresses can be compared to stresses between 4.0 and 6.0 MPa reported at the hip during ambulation [10]. Other studies demonstrate distinct alterations in loading patterns in the presence of abnormal joint morphology. An abnormally long ulna, described as a *positive ulnar variance,* is accompanied by an increase in the stress on the triangular fibrocartilage complex [8]. Similarly, carpal instability results in changes in stress throughout the carpus [22].

Clinical Relevance

PRESSURE CHANGES WITH CARPAL INSTABILITIES: *Cadaver studies suggest that there is increased pressure between the radius and scaphoid bones in the presence of scaphoid instability [13]. The area of increased pressure is approximately the same area that frequently shows degenerative joint disease in older adults. Pressure studies such as these suggest direct associations among abnormal joint alignment, abnormal loading patterns, and eventual joint destruction. Additional research is needed to clarify these associations, since a better understanding of these links will help guide clinical decisions regarding treatment strategies for joint malalignments.*

CLINICAL IMPLICATIONS OF STUDIES ANALYZING THE FORCES AND STRESSES ON THE WRIST

Osteoarthritis primarily affects the large weight-bearing joints of the body, particularly the hips and knees, but while less common, osteoarthritis does appear at the wrist as well [7]. The most common site of joint degeneration in the wrist is between the scaphoid and the radius [23]. This finding is consistent with the stress data reported earlier. These data support the existence of a relationship between joint pressures and joint degeneration. The altered patterns of loading found in wrist joint malalignments also suggest that wrists with abnormal alignment may be predisposed to degenerative changes.

Some authors suggest that individuals who depend on their upper extremities for weight bearing may be particularly prone to degenerative changes at the wrist [18,25]. A study of 50 individuals who used a single cane for ambulation reports no increased incidence of arthritis in the weight-bearing wrist compared with the non-weight-bearing wrist [25]. The mean duration of cane use among the subjects studied was 4 years. In contrast, another study reports a high incidence of carpal bone instability, usually involving the lunate, in individuals with paraplegia who used wheelchairs exclusively [18]. The mean duration of the spinal cord injury in subjects with wrist joint instability was 30 years.

These two studies seem to have conflicting data, although one study assesses wrist joint instability while the other examines the prevalence of degenerative arthritis. However, the bigger difference in these two studies is the duration of repetitive weight-bearing activity. The population with observed wrist joint pathology had a mean duration of weight-bearing activity approximately seven times the mean duration seen in the population with no pathology. Although additional research is needed to clarify the relationship between prolonged weight-bearing activities and wrist joint pathology, these data suggest the possibility that excessive loading sustained by the wrist for a prolonged period of time may contribute to the development of wrist pathology.

What do these studies mean for the clinician? Avoiding weight-bearing activities to protect the joints is not feasible in a population that depends on upper extremity weight bearing for mobility. Further studies are needed to determine if there are other factors that increase or decrease the risk of eventual degeneration. Perhaps changes in wrist joint flexibility and strength can alter the risks associated with prolonged weight-bearing activities. In addition, modifications to the wheelchairs and ambulation devices can alter the mechanics to lower the loads or redistribute the stresses at the wrist. By being aware of the possible links between loading patterns at the wrist and future joint pathology and by understanding the factors that influence the loads generated during an activity, the clinician may be able to reduce a patient's risk of joint pathology and minimize the impairments resulting from such pathology.

SUMMARY

This chapter examines the forces and stresses to which the wrist is subjected in daily activity. A simple two-dimensional model is used to analyze the forces in the muscles and at the joint during a simple weight-bearing task in which the assumption that only one muscle group is active was valid. The simplified model yielded a joint reaction force on the wrist of 50% of body weight. Data from more-complex models were reviewed, since in many daily activities the wrist requires simultaneous activity from many muscles. Data from these more-complex models revealed that the muscles and the wrist joint can sustain loads of more than twice body weight, particularly during activities requiring upper extremity weight bearing. Studies that report the stresses (force/area) sustained at the wrist were also reported. These data suggest that the wrist withstands stresses similar to those at the hip during ambulation. Stresses on the wrist are altered during normal wrist movement and are directly affected by the mechanics and pathomechanics of the wrist. These studies provide a useful perspective for the clinician to appreciate the mechanical challenges to the wrist during everyday activity.

This chapter completes the discussion of the wrist. However, the function of the hand depends to a large extent on the muscles of the forearm and the integrity of the wrist joint. The following three chapters examine the interaction of forearm structures with the special structures and muscles found within the hand that contribute to the mechanics and the pathomechanics of hand function.

References

1. Barr AE, Barbe MF, Clark BD: Work-related musculoskeletal disorders of the hand and wrist: epidemiology, pathophysiology, and senorimotor changes. J Orthop Sports Phys Ther 2004; 34: 610–627.
2. Boninger ML, Cooper RA, Baldwin MA, et al.: Wheelchair pushrim kinetics: body weight and median nerve function. Arch Phys Med Rehabil 1999; 80: 910–915.
3. Boninger ML, Cooper RA, Robertson RN, Rudy TE: Wrist biomechanics during two speeds of wheelchair propulsion: an analysis using a local coordinate system. Arch Phys Med Rehabil 1997; 78: 364–372.
4. Chadwick EKJ, Nicol AC: Elbow and wrist joint contact forces during occupational pick and place activities. J Biomech 2000; 33: 591–600.
5. Chou P-H, Chou Y-L, Lin C-J, et al.: Effect of elbow flexion on upper extremity impact forces during a fall. Clin Biomech 2001; 16: 888–894.
6. Hatze H: Forces and duration of impact, and grip tightness during the tennis stroke. Med Sci Sports 1976; 8: 88–95.
7. Hochberg MC: Osteoarthritis. B. Clinical features. In: Primer of the Rheumatic Diseases. Klippel JH, ed. Atlanta: Arthritis Foundation, 2001; 289–293.
8. Kazuki K, Kusunoki M, Shimazu A: Pressure distribution in the radiocarpal joint measured with a densitometer designed for pressure-sensitive film. J Hand Surg [Am] 1991; 16A: 401–408.
9. Kier PJ, Wells RP: The effect of typing posture on wrist extensor muscle loading. Hum Factors 2002; 44: 392–403.
10. Krebs DE, Robbins CE, Lavine L, Mann RW: Hip biomechanics during gait. J Orthop Sports Phys Ther 1998; 28: 51–59.
11. Markolf KL, Shapiro MS, Mandelbaum BR, Teurlings L: Wrist loading patterns during pommel horse exercises. J Biomech 1990; 23: 1001–1011.
12. Neal RJ, Kippers V, Plooy D, Forwood MR: The influence of hand guards on forces and muscle activity during giant swings on the high bar. Med Sci Sports Exerc 1995; 27: 1550–1556.
13. Patterson R, Viegas SF: Biomechanics of the wrist. J Hand Ther 1995; 8: 97–105.
14. Reisman M, Burdett RG, Simon SR, Norkin C: Elbow moment and forces at the hands during swing-through axillary crutch gait. Phys Ther 1985; 65: 601–605.

15. Riek S, Chapman AE, Milner T: A simulation of muscle force and internal kinematics of extensor carpi radialis brevis during backhand tennis stroke: implications for injury. Clin Biomech 1999; 14: 477–483.

16. Robertson RN, Boninger ML, Cooper RA, Shimada SD: Pushrim forces and joint kinetics during wheelchair propulsion. Arch Phys Med Rehabil 1996; 77: 856–864.

17. Rodgers MM, Gayle GW, Figoni SF, et al.: Biomechanics of wheelchair propulsion during fatigue. Arch Phys Med Rehabil 1994; 75: 85–92.

18. Schroer W, Lacey S, Frost FS, Keith MW: Carpal instability in the weight-bearing upper extremity. J Bone Joint Surg 1996; 78A: 1838–1843.

19. Schuind F, Cooney WP, Linscheid RL, et al.: Force and pressure transmission through the normal wrist. A theoretical two-dimensional study in the posteroanterior plane. J Biomech 1995; 28: 587–601.

20. Short WH, Werner FW, Fortino MD, Mann KA: Analysis of the kinematics of the scaphoid and lunate in the intact wrist joint. Hand Clin 1997; 13: 93–108.

21. Veeger HEJ, van der Woude LHV, Rozendal RH: Load on the upper extremity in manual wheelchair propulsion. J Electromyogr Kinesiol 1991; 1: 270–280.

22. Viegas SF, Patterson RM: Load mechanics of the wrist. Hand Clin 1997; 13: 109–128.

23. Watson HK, Ryu J: Evolution of arthritis of the wrist. Clin Orthop 1986; 202: 57–67.

24. Werner FW, Palmer AK, Somerset JH, et al.: Wrist joint motion simulator. J Orthop Res 1996; 14: 639–646.

25. Wright V, Hopkins R: Osteoarthritis in weight-bearing wrists? Br J Rheumatol 1993; 32: 243–244.

Mechanics and Pathomechanics of the Special Connective Tissues in the Hand

The preceding three chapters discuss the structure and function of the bones and joints of the wrist and hand, the function of the muscles of the forearm, and the loads that the wrist sustains during certain functional activities. Throughout those chapters the reader is reminded that the function and dysfunction of all of these structures are intimately related to the integrity of the structures found within the hand. The objectives of the next three chapters are to discuss the soft tissue structures that are intrinsic to the hand, to discuss their contribution to the function of the hand, and to present the functional synergies that exist between the intrinsic and extrinsic structures of the hand.

The hand contains several special connective tissue structures that are critical to the normal function of the hand. The purposes of the current chapter are to

- Describe the structure of the special connective tissue elements that are intrinsic to the hand
- Describe how these connective tissue structures contribute to the function and dysfunction of the hand
- Discuss common hand deformities that result from disruption of these connective tissue structures

The primary function of most of the special connective tissue structures presented in this chapter is to stabilize the other soft tissue in the hand, particularly the muscles and tendons. Some structures also are essential for the nutrition, lubrication, and smooth glide of the tendons extending into the digits. Although most of the special connective tissue structures of the hand are subcutaneous, the skin itself plays an important role in the function and mechanics of the hand. In particular, the skin of the web spaces between the digits participates in limiting radial and ulnar deviation of the metacarpophalangeal (MCP) joints of the fingers as well as abduction of the thumb. Loss of the thumb's web space as the result of scarring, for example, can cause significant functional impairment. The skin's folds and sweat glands reduce the chance of slippage between the hand and objects in the hand. The skin also provides useful superficial landmarks to the clinician who is evaluating the hand. Perhaps the most useful and reliable landmarks in the hand are the skin creases that are most prominent on the palmar surface of the hand. The following reviews the relationships between these skin creases in the hand and the underlying structures.

LANDMARKS WITHIN THE HAND

Skin creases form perpendicular to the direction of pull of the underlying muscles. Examination of the skin creases in the hand reveals that they are directed for the most part in a radioulnar direction. These creases are constant, with only slight variations among individuals without hand pathology (*Fig. 17.1*). Inspection of the palmar surface of the hand from proximal to distal reveals

- One to three creases at the wrist
- A crease at the base of the thenar eminence
- A distal palmar crease
- A pair of creases at the base of each finger
- A crease at the base of the thumb
- A pair of creases at the proximal interphalangeal (PIP) joint of each finger
- A single crease at the distal interphalangeal (DIP) joint of each finger and at the IP joint of the thumb

The proximal wrist crease is proximal to the radiocarpal joint. The middle crease passes directly over the radiocarpal joint space, and the distal crease lies just distal to the joint line. These creases provide a reliable means of identifying the radiocarpal joint line. The distal palmar crease lies just proximal to the MCP joints of the middle, long, and little fingers, while the creases at the bases of the fingers lie just distal to the MCP joints. Palpation of the MCP joints occurs between the distal palmar crease and the creases at the base of the fingers. The creases in the fingers and thumb lie directly over, or just proximal to, the underlying joints [14,15]. Similarly, there are creases on the dorsum of the fingers, which lie approximately over the MCP, PIP, and DIP joints of the fingers (*Fig. 17.2*).

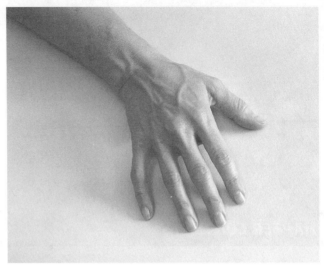

Figure 17.2: Creases on the dorsum of the fingers lie over the joints of the fingers.

Clinical Relevance

EDEMA IN THE HAND: *The creases on the palmar side of the hand are rarely absent and thus are useful to the clinician who is evaluating deeper structures. In contrast, the creases on the dorsal side of the fingers are readily displaced or obscured by swelling in the digits. Swelling is more apparent on the dorsal surface of the hand because the connective tissue structures on the palmar surface prevent distention of the skin and deeper structures. The tissues cannot expand to accommodate increased volume. Consequently, edema accumulates on the dorsal surface where the skin is readily distended. The dorsal creases are unreliable landmarks in the presence of swelling.*

CONNECTIVE TISSUE IN THE HAND

The prevalence of swelling on the dorsum of the hand is a consequence of the unique connective tissue structures found in the hand. These special connective tissue structures consist of the palmar aponeuroses; the retinacular, or pulley, systems of the wrist and fingers; the tendon sheaths; and the special ligaments that anchor the flexor and extensor tendon apparatus in each finger. Each of these structures serves a slightly different purpose and is described separately in the following sections.

Palmar Aponeuroses

There are two layers of aponeuroses in the palm of the hand, the superficial and deep. The superficial palmar aponeurosis has three parts, the thenar, hypothenar, and midpalmar aponeuroses (*Fig. 17.3*). These aponeurotic sheets project fibrous tentacles into the overlying skin, providing essential stabilization of the skin for grasping activities. The ability to pull on a rope or twist off a jar lid requires that the palmar

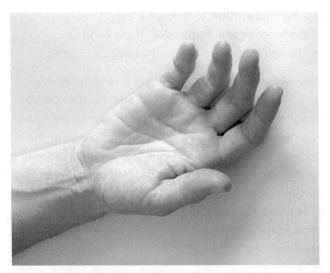

Figure 17.1: Creases on the palmar surface of the hand provide reliable landmarks for palpating the underlying structures.

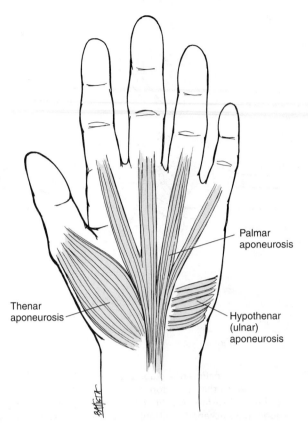

Figure 17.3: The superficial palmar aponeurosis is divided into the thenar, hypothenar, and midpalmar aponeuroses.

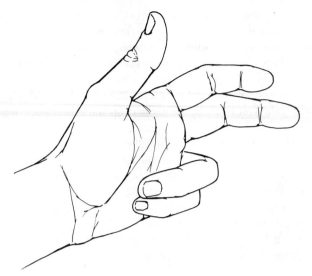

Figure 17.4: Dupuytren's contracture produces flexion of the ulnar fingers.

skin stay fixed to the underlying tissues of the hand. Otherwise the hand would slide inside its skin just as a foot slides in an oversized boot. Connections between an aponeurosis and the skin are absent on the dorsum of the hand allowing the skin to glide freely. It is the absence of these tethers between the skin and the underlying structures that allows swelling to accumulate more readily on the dorsal surface of the hand than on the palmar surface.

Besides the vertical fibers projecting toward the skin, the superficial midpalmar aponeurosis contains transverse and longitudinal fibers that extend toward the fingers. Although most of these fibers end at the web space of the fingers, some fibers extend into the fingers and become continuous with the digital fascia [21].

Clinical Relevance

DUPUYTREN'S CONTRACTURE: *The superficial midpalmar aponeurosis undergoes progressive fibrotic changes in some individuals, particularly in men older than 50 years of age. Although the etiology is unclear, the disorder known as* **Dupuytren's contracture** *is manifested by palpable thickening of the palmar fascia and a progressive flexion contracture of the ulnar two fingers [6,27] (Fig. 17.4). The distal extension of the palmar aponeurosis into the fingers explains the progressive flexion of the fingers.*

The deep palmar aponeurosis lies just anterior to the metacarpal bones and palmar interosseus muscles. There are fascial extensions that run between the deep and superficial palmar aponeuroses, creating compartments within the palm of the hand [21,32] (*Fig. 17.5*). Individual compartments are created to contain the tendons of the flexor digitorum superficialis and profundus to a single finger. Individual compartments also are formed for the lumbricals and for the neurovascular bundles to each finger. Consequently, the structures to each finger are stabilized within their own fascial tunnels as they project toward the fingers.

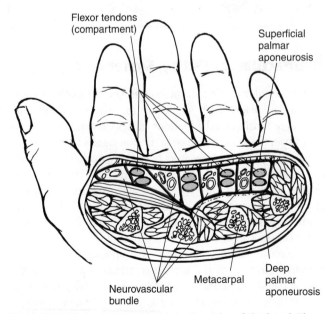

Figure 17.5: Fibrous compartments in the palm of the hand. The deep palmar aponeurosis is connected to the superficial palmar aponeurosis by fascial bands that create compartments in the hand for tendons, nerves, and blood vessels.

The palmar aponeuroses serve several purposes. They anchor the skin to prevent slippage during grasp. They provide protection for the underlying muscles, nerves, and blood vessels. They also create tunnels to stabilize these structures as they travel through the hand. In contrast, the extensor tendons are compartmentalized only as they cross the wrist. They glide relatively freely between the deep and superficial fascial sheaths on the dorsum of the hand.

The fingers also possess fascial compartments containing the neurovascular bundles on the radial and ulnar aspects of each digit as well as fibrous connections to the skin. These include extensions from the palmar aponeurosis as well as specialized supports at the PIP and DIP joints. They serve the same stabilizing function as does the palmar aponeurosis, preventing translation of the neurovascular bundles as well as slippage of the skin during grasp.

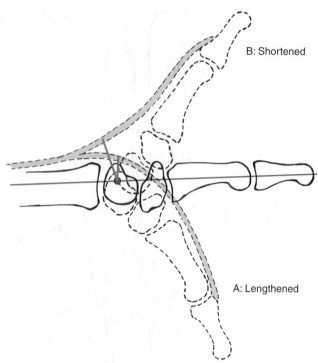

Figure 17.6: The function of a stabilizing retinaculum. (A) When a joint is moved so that a tendon is lengthened, the tendon lies close to the joint surface. (B) When the joint is moved, putting the tendon in a slackened position, the tendon bowstrings away from the joint, increasing the muscle's moment arm.

Clinical Relevance

SWELLING WITHIN THE COMPARTMENTS OF THE HAND OR FINGERS: *The fibrous compartments within the hand and fingers are essential for stabilizing the skin, muscles, and neurovascular supply. However, inflammation within a compartment can produce severe pain and may lead to compression and damage of the neurovascular content. The fibrous walls of these compartments create relatively rigid spaces that cannot accommodate an increase in volume. Consequently, edema within a compartment leads to increased pressure that may compress and impair the sensitive neurovascular structures. The most familiar example of this is compression of the median nerve within the carpal tunnel, but similar examples can occur in the compartments of the fingers as well.*

Retinacular, or Pulley, Systems

The retinacular systems throughout the body function to hold tendons in place. They are found in locations where joint motion or tension on the tendons causes the tendons to move away from the joint. At the wrist, flexion causes the flexor tendons to project anteriorly away from the wrist joint. Similarly, the extensor tendons migrate posteriorly away from the wrist during wrist extension. The flexor and extensor retinacular bands bind the tendons to the wrist to limit their bulging away from the joint. Thus the retinacular bands help maintain a more constant moment arm for each muscle.

The movement of a tendon away from its joint is known as **bowstringing,** since the tendon is stretched away from the joint and limb segments like the string of a bow (*Fig. 17.6*). One of the dangers of bowstringing is that the tendon becomes more prominent and hence more susceptible to injury. This is particularly true in the wrist and fingers, where a protruding tendon is more likely to be crushed or lacerated. Flexor tendons allowed to bowstring in the hand also interfere with the stable contact between hand and object in a firm grasp.

Bowstringing changes the mechanics of the muscle, significantly increasing the muscle's moment arm. This puts the muscle at a mechanical advantage, since a longer moment arm increases a muscle's ability to generate a moment. The improved mechanical advantage is demonstrated by the decrease in force required to flex a digit when the flexor tendon is allowed to bowstring [13]. However, a muscle with a larger moment arm requires more shortening than a muscle with a shorter moment arm to produce the same angular excursion (Chapter 4). When a muscle bowstrings, increasing its moment arm, it must shorten more during contraction to produce the same angular displacement as before the bowstringing. As a result, the muscle is likely to exhibit **active insufficiency,** the inability to contract far enough to pull the joint through its full excursion [30].

RETINACULAR SYSTEMS AT THE WRIST

The transverse carpal ligament (TCL) at the wrist, or flexor retinaculum, functions to stabilize the carpal arch and the tendons that cross the volar surface of the wrist within the carpal tunnel. Wrist flexion causes these tendons to glide in a volar direction, and the TCL prevents excessive volar glide. The TCL sometimes is surgically transected as part of the treatment for carpal tunnel syndrome in the hopes of relieving the pressure on the median nerve within the tunnel. Complete transection allows the flexor tendons to migrate anteriorly, or bowstring, in the carpal tunnel during contraction, decreasing their contraction efficiency. Surgical transection of the TCL decreases the muscle force needed to generate a given pinch load following transection, consistent with the increased muscle moment arms as the tendons bowstring following the release of the flexor retinaculum. However, reported data also reveal a 16–26% increase in shortening required by the finger flexors to pull the fingers through the same excursion [8,9]. Despite the improved moment arm in the finger flexors following TCL release, many patients demonstrate decreased grip and pinch strength [7,9]. This decreased strength may result from the active insufficiency that develops from the bowstringing.

Clinical Relevance

TRANSVERSE CARPAL LIGAMENT RECONSTRUCTION

Patients with carpal tunnel syndrome are frequently treated with a surgical release of the transverse carpal ligament to decrease the pressure within the carpal tunnel, thereby decompressing the median nerve. While the majority of patients report a decrease in pain and improved function, some patients continue to have pain and decreased grip strength. One explanation is that release of the transverse carpal ligament allows increased bowstringing of the flexor tendons to the thumb and fingers with a resultant loss of flexor strength. Reconstruction of the ligament by a "transposition flap" repair using a segment of the palmar aponeurosis appears to stabilize the flexor tendons and improve grip strength [17,18].

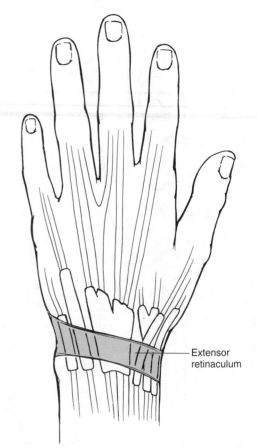

Figure 17.7: The extensor retinaculum at the wrist stabilizes the extensor tendons at the wrist.

The extensor tendons at the wrist are stabilized by a similar extensor retinaculum (*Fig. 17.7*). Yet some extensor tendons still move away from the joint surface during wrist extension, increasing their moment arms. This mobility and the resultant increase in moment arms help explain why the strength of the extensor carpi radialis longus and brevis is greatest when the wrist is extended [10,12]. Active insufficiency is avoided in the extensor carpi radialis longus and brevis because these muscles possess longer muscle fibers producing greater angular excursion during contraction [3,12].

RETINACULAR SYSTEMS AT THE DIGITS

The flexor tendons of the fingers also have an elaborate retinacular, or pulley, system that stabilizes the tendons along the entire length of the fingers on the volar surface (*Fig. 17.8*). This system consists of fibrous bands that attach to the underlying volar plates of the MCP, PIP, and DIP joints or to the bones of the fingers [20]. Some of these bands encircle the flexor tendons much like the annular ligament of the superior radioulnar joint encircles the radius. The five fibrous bands that run circumferentially across the fingers are called annular ligaments [4,32]. They are numbered one to five from proximal to distal. Three pairs of cruciate pulleys are found over the volar surface of the proximal and middle phalanges. Although their typical arrangement is depicted in Figure 17.8,

it is important to recognize that the pulleys exhibit some normal variability within the population [11].

These pulleys are essential to the function of the flexor tendons of the fingers. Studies suggest that the annular ligaments, A2 and A4, are particularly essential to the function of the flexor digitorum profundus [23,30]. The A3 ligament is important to the function of the flexor digitorum superficialis [7]. In addition to affecting the efficiency of the muscles' flexion excursion, the A1 pulley of the fingers provides an important radioulnar stabilizing force on the flexor tendons as they cross the MCP joints [4]. The thumb also has a system of annular and cruciate ligaments to stabilize the tendon of the flexor pollicis longus as it traverses the thumb [33].

Clinical Relevance

PULLEY INJURIES IN ROCK CLIMBERS: *Pulley ruptures in the fingers can occur with hyperextension injuries but also as the result of large forces in the flexor tendons, especially with the fingers flexed. Rock climbers generate huge flexion forces in the fingers as they pull themselves up along vertical rock walls by their fingers. A common hand hold called "crimping" uses considerable flexion at the PIP joints and requires large forces in the flexor tendons. This grip puts the pulleys A2, A3, and A4 at particular risk of rupture [28].*

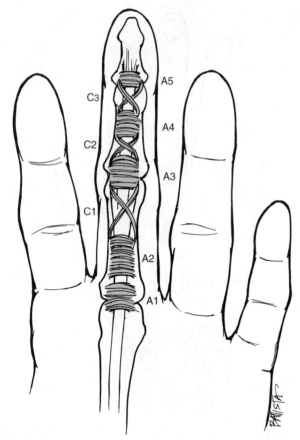

Figure 17.8: The flexor tendons of the fingers are stabilized by an extensive series of fibrous pulleys. Typically there are five circumferential, or annular, ligaments (A1–A5) and three pairs of cruciate ligaments (C1–C3).

The tendons of the extensor digitorum are stabilized by a less elaborate retinaculum as they cross the MCP joints of the fingers. The tendons are secured by the **sagittal bands** that run from the extensor tendons to the volar plate on the volar surface of the joint [22] (*Fig. 17.9*). These bands stabilize the tendons in the radioulnar direction to prevent dislocation of these tendons to either side of the fingers.

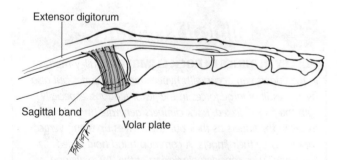

Figure 17.9: The extensor digitorum tendons of the fingers are stabilized at the MCP joints by sagittal bands.

Tendon Sheaths

The tendons of the wrist and fingers are encased in synovial sheaths. The flexor tendons to the radial three fingers have separate sheaths at the wrist, palm, and fingers [25,32] (*Fig. 17.10*). The sheath for the tendons to the little finger is continuous with the palmar sheath. The extensor tendons are enclosed by sheaths only at the wrist. These sheaths reduce the friction of the tendons as they glide over the wrist and along the finger. Reduced friction is critical, since the tendons to the fingers slide several centimeters during full finger motion [1–3].

The synovial sheaths also play an important role in the nutrition of the flexor tendons in the fingers [5,26]. There are three vascular sources to these tendons: (*a*) vessels proceeding distally from the muscle belly through the musculotendinous junction, (*b*) blood vessels proceeding proximally in the tendon from the bone at the tendon's distal attachment, and (*c*) vessels entering the dorsal surface of the tendons via the tiny, fragile **vinculae** [20] (*Fig. 17.11*). These three sources leave some regions of the tendons relatively far from a vascular source. Nutrition, particularly in these regions, depends on diffusion across the synovial sheaths similar to the mechanism for nourishing articular cartilage.

Clinical Relevance

"NO MAN'S LAND": *Hand surgeons refer to the region of the hand that contains the finger flexor tendons within their digital sheaths as Zone II. However, historically this region has been known as "no man's land" because it was believed that primary repairs of the flexor digitorum profundus or superficialis were unsuccessful within this region because nutrition to the tendons was so tenuous and scarring and adhesions were so likely [31] (Fig. 17.12). Disruption of a tendon in this region can easily rupture the nearby vinculae, compromising an already precarious blood supply.*

Over the last several decades, careful examination and clinical trials have demonstrated that primary tendon repairs in this region are not only feasible but desirable over the alternative of tendon grafts [19,29]. Yet the success of such repairs hinges a great deal on the postoperative rehabilitation that occurs. Recognition that synovial fluid diffusing through the tendon sheath contributes to a tendon's nutrition has led to the use of early mobilization in the treatment of tendon repairs. Mobilization assists in bathing the tendon in synovial fluid while reducing the development of adhesions. However, early mobilization also carries the risk of disrupting the repaired tendon. The clinician must avoid excessive active or passive tension in the tendon during the early stages of healing. Chapter 19 discusses the loads sustained by the finger flexor tendons during activity.

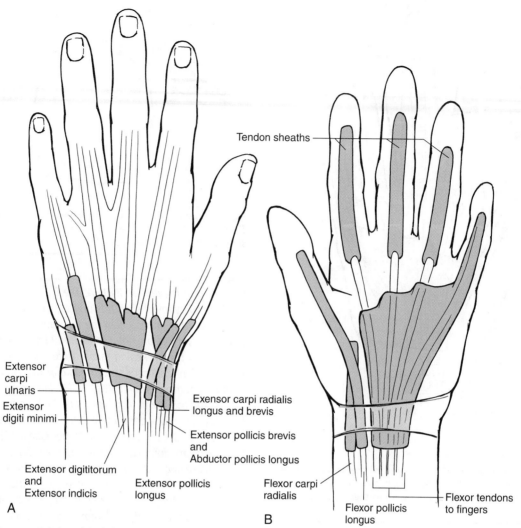

Extensor
carpi
ulnaris

Extensor
digiti minimi

Extensor digititorum
and
Extensor indicis

Extensor pollicis
longus

Exensor carpi radialis
longus and brevis

Extensor pollicis brevis
and
Abductor pollicis longus

Tendon sheaths

Flexor carpi
radialis

Flexor pollicis
longus

Flexor tendons
to fingers

A

B

Figure 17.10: The synovial sheaths of the tendons to the digits. **A.** The extensor tendons are encased in synovial sheaths only at the wrist. **B.** The flexor tendons to the digits are surrounded by synovial sheaths at the wrist and digits.

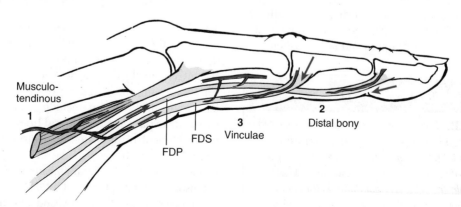

Musculo-
tendinous

1

FDP

FDS

3
Vinculae

2
Distal bony

Figure 17.11: The blood supply to the flexor tendons in the fingers. Flexor tendons (*FDP* and *FDS*) in the fingers receive their blood supply from *(1)* the proximal musculotendinous junction, *(2)* the distal bony attachment, and *(3)* the tiny blood vessels passing through the vinculae.

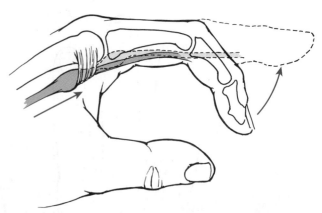

Figure 17.13: A "trigger finger" becomes stuck moving into either flexion or extension as the swollen flexor tendon or sheath tries to squeeze into the fibrous tunnel.

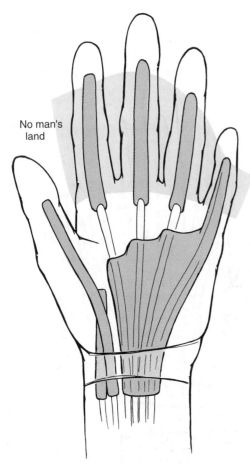

No man's land

Figure 17.12: "No man's land" is the area where healing is most difficult for the fingers' flexor tendons. It encompasses much of the region where the digital tendons are in their synovial sheaths.

Pathology of the synovial sheath itself also contributes to common functional impairments of the fingers. Infection within the sheath can result from trauma such as puncture wounds in the hand and can lead to impaired circulation to, and necrosis of, the flexor tendons and adhesions within the sheath. As a synovial tissue, the tendon sheath also is susceptible to inflammatory processes such as rheumatoid arthritis. Excessive friction within the sheaths and fibrous tunnels also may contribute to overuse syndromes and inflammation.

Clinical Relevance

TRIGGER FINGER: *The tendon sheath complex is suscep-tible to inflammation as the result of disease, overuse, or trauma. The synovial membrane then can exhibit all of the cardinal signs of inflammation including swelling. As the sheath swells within the relatively rigid fibrous tunnel formed by the pulley system, the swelling causes compres-sion of the enclosed tendon. Compression of the tendon can compromise the vascular flow to the tendon and lead to*

swelling of the tendon itself. As the finger is flexed, the thickened synovial sheath is pulled proximally through the pulleys of the finger. Often the thickening can be palpated in the palm just proximal to the MCP joint. As the finger is extended, the thickening must reenter the fibrous tunnel, but the swollen tendon or sheath has difficulty squeezing back into the narrow channel (Fig. 17.13). Finger extension is blocked, and the patient reports that the finger is "stuck." With additional extension force the thickening suddenly snaps into the tunnel, and the finger extends [5,16,27]. Such blocks to motion can occur in either flexion or extension as the thickening slides through any of the individual pulleys. The block to motion releases so suddenly that the finger acts like a "trigger." The mechanical block to movement results from the initial inflammatory process and resultant thickening. Treatments to reduce the inflammation and pre-vent recurrence are most beneficial. These may include anti-inflammatory medications, corticosteroid injections, and the use of splints and patient education to avoid overuse.

Structures That Anchor the Flexor and Extensor Apparatus of the Fingers

The flexor tendons to the fingers are bound firmly to each digit by the synovial sheaths and fibrous pulleys just described. The extensor tendons are stabilized somewhat at the MCP joints by the intersection of the interossei and lum-bricals forming the **extensor hood mechanism,** which is known by many names including **extensor mechanism, extensor expansion,** and **dorsal hood** (*Fig. 17.14*). The dis-tal attachment of the extensor digitorum, composed of the central tendon attached to the middle phalanx, and lateral bands attached to the distal phalanx form the skeleton of the extensor hood (Chapter 15). Distal attachments of the intrin-sic muscles of the fingers expand into a fibrous sheet that encompasses the extensor digitorum tendons forming a fibrous covering over the dorsum of the phalanges of the fingers. A similar fibrous expansion from intrinsic muscles of the thumb

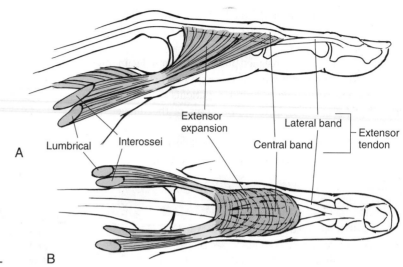

Figure 17.14: The extensor hood mechanism consists of the central tendon and lateral bands of the extensor digitorum and the fibrous sheet that is an extension of the distal attachments of the lumbricals and interossei. **A.** Lateral view. **B.** Dorsal view.

forms a fibrous expansion over the dorsum of the phalanges of the thumb, blending with the tendons of extensor pollicis longus and extensor pollicis brevis.

Careful inspection of each finger reveals additional soft tissue structures that contribute to the stability of the flexor tendons and extensor hood mechanisms as they travel the length of each finger. These additional structures play an integral role in maintaining a balance between the flexor and extensor muscles but also participate in the development of common structural deformities in the hand. A cross-sectional view of a finger at the level of the MCP joint reveals interconnection among the many structures crossing the joint. The interconnection occurs at the lateral borders of the volar surface of the MCP joint [31] (*Fig. 17.15*). The sagittal bands of the extensor digitorum, the flexor tendon sheath, and the collateral ligaments all join with the volar plate and the transverse intermetacarpal ligaments at this intersection. The opposing flexor and extensor muscle groups also are linked at the PIP joints by the oblique and transverse retinacular ligaments that run from the flexor sheath on the volar surface to the extensor expansion on the dorsal side of the finger [31] (*Fig. 17.16*). These ligaments suspend the lateral bands of the extensor hood mechanism over the lateral aspects of the dorsum of the finger. Thus the flexor and extensor muscles are actually connected to one another throughout much of the length of the finger.

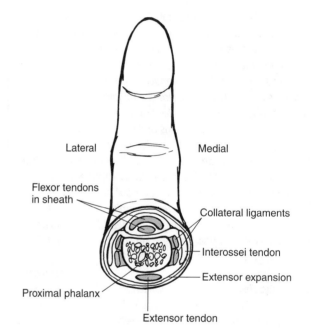

Figure 17.15: Interconnections among the tendons and ligaments at the MCP joint of a finger. A cross section of an MCP joint of a finger reveals the interconnections among the flexor tendon sheath, the extensor tendon, the collateral ligaments, the transverse intermetacarpal ligaments, and the volar plate.

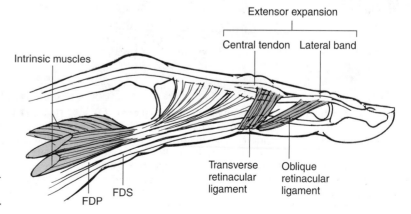

Figure 17.16: The oblique and transverse retinacular ligaments at the PIP joint of a finger connect the flexor tendon sheaths and the extensor hood.

These linkages not only help stabilize the tendons circumferentially on the finger but also contribute to the overall balance of opposing forces within the finger.

The importance of the balance provided by these ligaments is most evident in its absence. The classic hand deformities, swan neck and boutonniere, found in patients with rheumatoid arthritis provide vivid demonstrations of the impact of pathology involving the structures that balance the flexion and extension forces in the fingers [24]. Both deformities are precipitated by synovitis at the PIP joint of any finger.

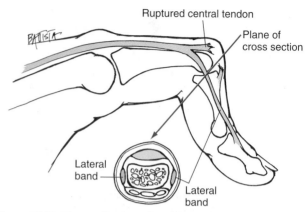

Figure 17.18: The mechanism of a boutonniere deformity. A cross section of a PIP joint of a finger reveals how rupture of the central tendon of the extensor hood allows the lateral bands to slip to the volar side of the joint, producing flexion at the PIP. The intact distal attachment of the lateral bands produces hyperextension of the DIP joint.

Clinical Relevance

BOUTONNIERE AND SWAN NECK DEFORMITIES: *The* ***boutonniere deformity*** *is characterized by flexion of the PIP joint and hyperextension of the DIP joint of the finger (Fig. 17.17). In this deformity, the swelling of the PIP joint resulting from the inflammation of the joint's synovium is located particularly in the dorsum of the joint. This puts prolonged tension on the extensor digitorum tendon, especially the central tendon and the fibrous sheet connecting the lateral bands of the extensor mechanism. Prolonged swelling causes these structures to stretch. As they stretch, the lateral bands gradually slide toward the volar surface of the finger. When the bands slide volarly past the axis of flexion and extension of the joint, they begin to exert a flexion moment on the joint (Fig. 17.18). The resulting PIP flexion puts additional stretch on the central tendon, which can eventually rupture. The PIP joint then protrudes through the extensor hood like a button through a buttonhole, giving the deformity its name. At the same time the volar migration of the lateral bands causes an increased extension pull from the intact extensor tendon at the DIP joint and that joint hyperextends.*

A similar mechanism in reverse is at work in a ***swan neck deformity****. This deformity is characterized by hyperextension of a finger's PIP joint with concomitant flexion of the DIP joint (Fig. 17.19). In this deformity the PIP joint swelling has a greater effect on the sides of the PIP joint capsule. Prolonged swelling in this region puts a prolonged stretch on the lateral joint capsule and the retinacular ligaments. The resulting laxity in the*

retinacular ligaments allows the lateral bands of the extensor hood to migrate dorsally, increasing their extension moment arms and the extension moment at the PIP (Fig. 17.20). The PIP joint is pulled into hyperextension by this increased extension moment stretching the tendon of the flexor digitorum profundus, which responds by pulling the DIP into flexion.

Swan neck deformities are frequently associated with another classic hand deformity, ***ulnar drift*** *of the fingers at the MCP joint. Ulnar drift is also the result of a loss of balance between the flexor and extensor mechanisms at the fingers, but because the external loads on the fingers are important contributing factors, this deformity is described in Chapter 19 within the context of the forces sustained by the fingers and thumb during activity.*

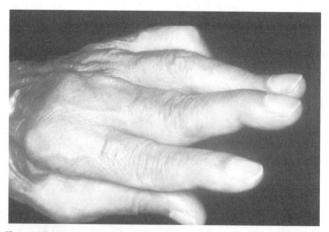

Figure 17.19: A swan neck deformity in an individual with rheumatoid arthritis consists of hyperextension of the PIP joint with flexion of the DIP joint. (Reprinted from the AHPA Teaching Slide Collection Second Edition now known as the ARHP Assessment and Management of the Rheumatic Diseases: The Teaching Slide Collection for Clinicians and Educators. Copyright 1997. Used by permission of the American College of Rheumatology.)

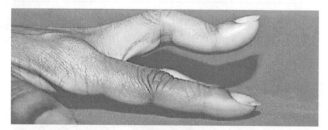

Figure 17.17: A boutonniere deformity in an individual with rheumatoid arthritis exhibits flexion of the PIP joint and hyperextension of the DIP joint. (Reprinted from the AHPA Teaching Slide Collection Second Edition now known as the ARHP Assessment and Management of the Rheumatic Diseases: The Teaching Slide Collection for Clinicians and Educators. Copyright 1997. Used by permission of the American College of Rheumatology.)

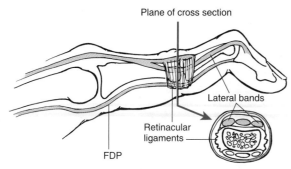

Figure 17.20: The mechanism of a swan neck deformity. A cross section of a PIP joint of a finger reveals how stretch of the retinacular ligaments allows the lateral bands of the extensor hood to slip dorsally, increasing the extension moment at the PIP joint and causing hyperextension. The hyperextension stretches the flexor digitorum profundus, producing flexion at the DIP joint.

SUMMARY

This chapter presents the special connective tissue structures that make critical contributions to the mechanics of the hand. These structures serve several roles that include stabilizing skin, muscles, and neurovascular bundles; protecting underlying structures; and contributing to the balance between the flexor and extensor apparatus. Many common hand deformities and joint impairments result from disruption of these connective tissue structures. A loss of balance between the flexor and extensor mechanisms contributes to the classic hand deformities seen in patients with rheumatoid arthritis. Another system that is essential to the maintenance of balance within the hand is the intrinsic muscle group. These muscles are presented in the following chapter.

References

1. Aleksandrowicz R, Pagowski S: Functional anatomy and bioengineering of the third finger of the human hand. Folia Morphol (Warsaw) 1981; 40: 181–192.
2. An KN, Ueba Y, Chao EY, et al.: Tendon excursion and moment arm of index finger muscles. J Biomech 1983; 16: 419–425.
3. Brand PW, Beach RB, Thompson DE: Relative tension and potential excursion of muscles in the forearm and hand. J Hand Surg [Am] 1981; 6: 209–219.
4. Brand PW, Cranor KC, Ellis JC: Tendon and pulleys at the metacarpophalangeal joint of a finger. J Bone Joint Surg 1975; 57A: 779–784.
5. Ferlic DC: Rheumatoid flexor tenosynovitis and rupture. Hand Clin 1996; 12: 561–572.
6. Gelberman RH, Amiel D, Rudolph RM, Vance RM: Dupuytren's contracture. J Bone Joint Surg 1980; 62-A: 425–432.
7. Hamman J, Ali A, Phillips C, et al.: A biomechanical study of the flexor digitorum superficialis: effects of digital pulley excision and loss of the flexor digitorum profundus. J Hand Surg [Am] 1997; 22A: 328–335.
8. Kang HJ, Lee SG, Phillips CS, Mass DP: Biomechanical changes of cadaveric finger flexion: the effect of wrist position and of the transverse carpal ligament and palmar and forearm fasciae. J Hand Surg [Am] 1996; 21A: 963–968.
9. Kiritsis PG, Kline SC: Biomechanical changes after carpal tunnel release: a cadaveric model for comparing open, endoscopic, and step-cut lengthening techniques. J Hand Surg [Am] 1995; 20: 173–180.
10. Lieber RL, Friden J: Musculoskeletal balance of the human wrist elucidated using intraoperative laser diffraction. J Electromyogr Kinesiol 1998; 8: 93–100.
11. Lin GT, Amadio PC, An KN, Cooney WP: Functional anatomy of the human digital flexor pulley system. J Hand Surg [Am] 1989; 14A: 949–956.
12. Loren GJ, Shoemaker SD, Burkholder TJ, et al.: Human wrist motors: biomechanical design and application to tendon transfers. J Biomech 1996; 29: 331–342.
13. Low CK, Pereira BP, Ng RTH, et al.: The effect of the extent of A1 pulley release on the force required to flex the digits. A cadaver study on the thumb, middle and ring fingers. J Hand Surg [Br] 1998; 23B: 46–49.
14. Magee DA: Orthopedic Physical Assessment. Philadelphia: WB Saunders, 1998.
15. Moore KL: Clinically Oriented Anatomy. Baltimore: Williams & Wilkins, 1980.
16. Mulpruek P, Prichasuk S, Orapin S: Trigger finger in children. J Pediatr Orthop 1998; 18: 239–241.
17. Netscher D, Lee M, Thornby J, Polsen C: The effect of division of the transverse carpal ligament on flexor tendon excursion. J Hand Surg 1997; 22A: 1016–1024.
18. Netscher D, Mosharrafa A, Lee M, et al.: Transverse carpal ligament: its effect on flexor tendon excursion, morphologic changes of the carpal canal, and on pinch and grip strengths after open carpal tunnel release. Plast Reconstr Surg 1997; 100: 636–642.
19. Newmeyer WL 3rd, Manske PR: No man's land revisited: the primary flexor tendon repair controversy. J Hand Surg 2004; 29A: 1–5.
20. Ochiai N, Matsui T, Miyaji N, et al.: Vascular anatomy of flexor tendons. I. Vincular system and blood supply of the profundus tendon in the digital sheath. J Hand Surg [Am] 1979; 4: 321–330.
21. Rayan GM: Palmar fascial complex anatomy and pathology in Dupuytren's disease. Hand Clin 1999; 15: 73–86.
22. Rayan GM, Murray D, Chung KW, Rohrer M: The extensor retinacular system at the metacarpophalangeal joint. Anatomical and histological study. J Hand Surg [Br] 1997; 22B: 585–590.
23. Rispler D, Greenwald D, Shumway S, et al.: Efficiency of the flexor tendon pulley system in human cadaver hands. J Hand Surg [Am] 1996; 21A: 444–450.
24. Rizio L, Belsky MR: Finger deformities in rheumatoid arthritis. Hand Clin 1996; 12: 531–540.
25. Romanes GJE: Cunningham's Textbook of Anatomy. Oxford: Oxford University Press, 1981.
26. Rosenblum NI, Robinson SJ: Advances in flexor and extensor tendon management. In: Moran CA, ed. Hand Rehabilitation. New York: Churchill Livingstone, 1986; 17–44.
27. Salter RB: Textbook of Disorders and Injuries of the Musculoskeletal System. 3rd ed. Baltimore: Williams & Wilkins, 1999.
28. Schoffl VR, Einwag F, Strecker W, Schoffl I: Strength measurement and clinical outcome after pulley ruptures in climbers. Med Sci Sports Exerc 2006; 38: 637–643.

29. Su BW, Solomons M, Barrow A, et al.: Device for zone-II flexor tendon repair. J Bone Joint Surg 2005; 87: 923–935.

30. Tomaino M, Mitsionis G, Basitidas J, et al.: The effect of partial excision of the A2 and A4 pulleys on the biomechanics of finger flexion. J Hand Surg [Br] 1998; 23B: 50–52.

31. Tubiana R, Thomine JM, Mackin E: Examination of the Hand and Wrist. Philadelphia: WB Saunders, 1996.

32. Williams P, Bannister L, Berry M, et al.: Gray's Anatomy, The Anatomical Basis of Medicine and Surgery, Br. ed. London: Churchill Livingstone, 1995.

33. Zissimos AG, Szabo RM, Yinger KE, Sharkey NA: Biomechanics of the thumb flexor pulley system. J Hand Surg [Am] 1994; 19A: 475–479.

Mechanics and Pathomechanics of the Intrinsic Muscles of the Hand

Chapter 15 discusses the muscles of the forearm including the extrinsic muscles of the hand. However, the normal function of the extrinsic muscles is inextricably intertwined with the function of the intrinsic muscles. Few if any normal functional movements of the hand use only the extrinsic or the intrinsic muscle groups. The hand functions by using a delicately balanced combination of muscles from both groups. To understand the integrated activity of these muscle groups, the clinician must first appreciate the potential of the individual muscles. The purposes of this chapter are to

- Describe the structure and function of the individual intrinsic muscles of the hand
- Review the activity of the intrinsic muscles during movements of the hand
- Discuss the contribution to dysfunction in the hand made by impairments of the intrinsic muscles
- Explain the mechanics of the deformities of the hand resulting from weakness of the intrinsic muscles

Although the intrinsic muscles of the hand frequently are classified by muscle attachment, this chapter arranges the muscles into four functional groups: *(a)* the primary intrinsic movers of the thumb, *(b)* the primary intrinsic movers of the little finger, *(c)* the interossei, and *(d)* the lumbrical muscles. This classification scheme helps the clinician recognize the interaction of individual muscles.

PRIMARY INTRINSIC MOVERS OF THE THUMB

The muscles that are the primary intrinsic movers of the thumb are the abductor pollicis brevis, flexor pollicis brevis, opponens pollicis, and adductor pollicis (*Fig. 18.1*). The first three of these muscles are referred to as the thenar muscles, forming the muscle mass overlying the metacarpal of the thumb. These muscles are innervated by the median nerve. The adductor pollicis is critical to the function of the thumb, particularly in pinch, but is distinct from the thenar muscle mass. It lies in the palm of the hand and is innervated by the ulnar nerve. The thenar muscles are rarely tight. Therefore, only impairments associated with weakness of the thenar muscles are discussed below. In contrast, the adductor pollicis exhibits abnormal tightness in some hands, so tightness of the adductor pollicis is discussed as a possible impairment.

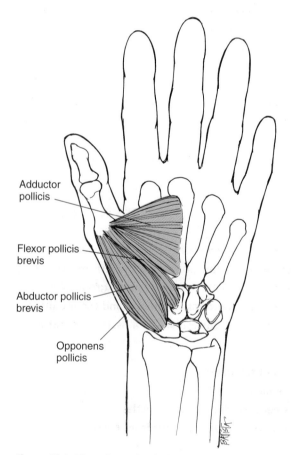

Figure 18.1: The primary intrinsic movers of the thumb include the abductor pollicis brevis, the flexor pollicis brevis, the opponens pollicis, and the adductor pollicis.

Labels on figure:
- Adductor pollicis
- Flexor pollicis brevis
- Abductor pollicis brevis
- Opponens pollicis

Abductor Pollicis Brevis

The abductor pollicis brevis is the most prominent muscle of the thenar muscle mass lying on the volar and radial aspect of the thenar prominence (*Muscle Attachment Box 18.1*).

ACTIONS

MUSCLE ACTION: ABDUCTOR POLLICIS BREVIS

Action	Evidence
Abduction (palmar abduction) of the thumb's CMC joint	Supporting
Medial rotation of the thumb's CMC joint	Supporting
Opposition of the thumb's CMC joint	Supporting
Abduction of the thumb's MCP joint	Inadequate
Flexion of the thumb's MCP joint	Inadequate
Extension of the thumb's IP joint	Supporting

The primary actions of the abductor pollicis brevis are those at the CMC joint. The abductor pollicis brevis is ideally positioned on the volar surface of the CMC joint of the thumb to abduct (palmar abduction) that joint. It has a larger abduction moment arm than the abductor pollicis longus and is optimally positioned to pull the thumb into abduction [7,27,34]. It is approximately only one third the size of the abductor pollicis longus [5] and consequently is limited in force production [15]. However, abduction of the CMC joint rarely occurs against resistance, so large forces are not necessary [5]. Electromyographic (EMG) studies support its role as one of the primary abductors of the CMC of the thumb, with the abductor pollicis longus at best an accessory abductor [7–9,39].

MUSCLE ATTACHMENT BOX 18.1

ATTACHMENTS AND INNERVATION OF THE ABDUCTOR POLLICIS BREVIS

Proximal attachment: Flexor retinaculum and the tubercles of the scaphoid and trapezium

Distal attachment: Radial side of the base of the thumb's proximal phalanx and the extensor expansion of the EPL

Innervation: Median nerve, C8, and T1

Palpation: The abductor pollicis brevis can be palpated on the radial aspect of the thenar eminence during active abduction of the thumb.

There are no known studies that specifically examine the abductor pollicis brevis as a medial rotator of the CMC joint. Medial rotation, also known as pronation, is virtually inseparable from abduction or flexion at the CMC joint [10,14] and is an automatic consequence of the active abduction resulting from contraction of the abductor pollicis brevis [13]. Since abduction and medial rotation are components of opposition, the abductor pollicis brevis also contributes to opposition [32].

The attachment of the abductor pollicis brevis on the radial side of the proximal phalanx of the thumb explains its reported role as an abductor of the MCP joint of the thumb. In some individuals the MCP joint functions more as a hinge joint, allowing only flexion and extension [1,12]. Therefore, the role of the abductor pollicis brevis at the MCP joint is probably variable. The muscle is located so that it can produce abduction of the MCP joint, but only in individuals who possess the available motion.

The abductor pollicis brevis also is described as a flexor of the MCP joint of the thumb [19]. EMG studies of the thumb do not offer selective analysis of this role for the abductor pollicis brevis and therefore can neither confirm nor refute this action. Additional research is needed to determine any contribution to MCP flexion [8,9,11].

Although anatomy books typically describe an attachment to the extensor hood of the thumb, there is little or no mention of IP extension in the list of actions by the abductor pollicis brevis [18,30]. Classic studies repeatedly demonstrate EMG activity of the abductor pollicis brevis during extension of the thumb [2,8,11,36]. A study of 11 subjects whose extensor pollicis longus was temporarily paralyzed reveals continued ability to extend the IP joint of the thumb, although through less than the full range of motion (ROM) [36]. This study demonstrates moderate activity in both the abductor pollicis brevis and the flexor pollicis brevis during IP extension without activity in the extensor pollicis longus, suggesting that one or both of these muscles contributes to the motion by way of the thumb's extensor expansion. Disruption of the attachment of the abductor pollicis brevis at the extensor hood also produces an extension impairment [24]. These studies demonstrate the abductor pollicis brevis muscle's participation in IP extension. Under normal circumstances this activity may be important in stabilizing the tendon of the extensor pollicis longus. In the absence of the extensor pollicis longus, however, the thenar muscles, including the abductor pollicis brevis, may provide functionally useful IP extension.

EFFECTS OF WEAKNESS OF THE ABDUCTOR POLLICIS BREVIS

Weakness of the muscle is a common manifestation of a median nerve palsy and often, but not always, occurs with simultaneous weakness of the other thenar muscles. Weakness of the abductor pollicis brevis usually is quite apparent upon inspection. The muscle is superficial, so atrophy of its muscle belly results in a flattening of the thenar eminence (*Fig. 18.2*). Weakness of the abductor pollicis brevis weakens abduction of the CMC joint of the thumb.

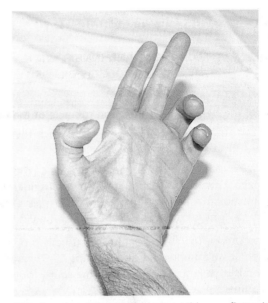

Figure 18.2: Atrophy of the APB is easily visible as a flattening of the thenar eminence. Seen here is an individual with wasting of the thenar eminence resulting from denervation.

Active abduction of the thumb is necessary to position the thumb for grasp or pinch.

The antagonist to the abductor pollicis brevis is the extensor pollicis longus, which lies ulnarly on the dorsum of the thumb and is positioned ideally to adduct the CMC joint of the thumb. Consequently, weakness of the abductor pollicis brevis upsets the delicate balance of strengths within the thumb. The unbalanced pull of the extensor pollicis longus interferes with the ability to position the thumb for pinch or grip and contributes to the characteristic thumb deformity ape thumb. Details of the common hand deformities resulting from muscle imbalances are presented at the end of this chapter. Weakness of the abductor pollicis brevis also leads to decreased strength of pinch and grasp.

Flexor Pollicis Brevis

The flexor pollicis brevis lies on the medial aspect of the abductor pollicis brevis and is approximately the same size as the abductor pollicis brevis [5,15] (*Muscle Attachment Box 18.2*).

ACTIONS

MUSCLE ACTION: FLEXOR POLLICIS BREVIS

Action	Evidence
Flexion of the thumb's CMC joint	Supporting
Abduction and medial rotation of the thumb's CMC joint	Inadequate
Flexion of the thumb's MCP joint	Supporting
Extension of the thumb's IP joint	Supporting

The primary actions of the flexor pollicis brevis are flexion of the thumb's CMC and MCP joints. The medial alignment

MUSCLE ATTACHMENT BOX 18.2

ATTACHMENTS AND INNERVATION OF THE FLEXOR POLLICIS BREVIS

Proximal attachment: The superficial portion comes from the flexor retinaculum and tubercle of the trapezium. The deep portion arises from the capitate and trapezoid bones.

Distal attachment: Radial side of the base of the proximal phalanx of the thumb. There is frequently a sesamoid bone within the tendon. The muscle may also contribute to the extensor hood of the EPL.

Innervation: The superficial head is usually supplied by the median nerve, T1 and perhaps C8. The deep head is usually supplied by the same spinal roots of the ulnar nerve.

Palpation: The flexor pollicis brevis is palpated on the ulnar aspect of the thenar eminence during flexion of the thumb's CMC joint while the MCP joint is extended.

MUSCLE ATTACHMENT BOX 18.3

ATTACHMENTS AND INNERVATION OF THE OPPONENS POLLICIS

Proximal attachment: Flexor retinaculum and the tubercle of the trapezium

Distal attachment: The lateral half of the entire length of the metacarpal of the thumb

Innervation: Median nerve, T1 and perhaps C8. It may also receive innervation from the ulnar nerve.

Palpation: The opponens pollicis can be palpated along the radial aspect of the palmar surface of the thumb's metacarpal during gentle opposition of the thumb. The palpating digit must be slipped between the radial border of the abductor pollicis brevis and the metacarpal. Vigorous opposition will generate contraction of the abductor pollicis brevis, making palpation of the opponens pollicis impossible.

of the flexor pollicis brevis positions it to flex the CMC and MCP joints of the thumb [2,11]. Its attachment into the extensor hood also suggests a role in IP extension like that of the abductor pollicis brevis. EMG data reveal activity of the flexor pollicis brevis during IP extension in the absence of extensor pollicis longus activity [36]. The action of the flexor pollicis brevis also is linked with the action of the opponens pollicis and the adductor pollicis [2,9]. The superficial portion of the flexor pollicis brevis, innervated by the median nerve, is sometimes attached directly to the opponens pollicis. This portion is best suited to position the CMC joint of the thumb [5]. The deeper portion, innervated by the ulnar nerve, is aligned more closely with the adductor pollicis and may function with that muscle at the thumb's MCP joint during pinch.

EFFECTS OF WEAKNESS

Weakness of the flexor pollicis brevis weakens the actions of flexion at the CMC and MCP joints of the thumb, which may have profound functional ramifications, particularly in pinch. This effect is examined more closely in Chapter 19.

Opponens Pollicis

The opponens pollicis is the second largest intrinsic muscle of the thumb and thus offers considerable strength to the base of the thumb [5,25] (*Muscle Attachment Box. 18.3*).

ACTIONS

MUSCLE ACTION: OPPONENS POLLICIS

Action	Evidence
Opposition of the thumb's CMC joint	Supporting

Opposition is the combination of abduction, flexion, and medial rotation of the CMC joint of the thumb. Some references report that the opponens pollicis performs these individual actions, but it is important to recognize that contraction of the opponens pollicis produces abduction, flexion, and medial rotation simultaneously, that is, opposition. Thus the opponens pollicis contributes to the actions of both the abductor pollicis brevis and the flexor pollicis brevis and adds important strength for both muscles [2,5,8]. In a study by Cooney et al. in which the flexor pollicis brevis was studied as part of the opponens pollicis, the opponens pollicis acted as a secondary flexor of the thumb, with increased activity as the force of pinch increased [9]. In this same study the opponens pollicis and abductor pollicis brevis were the primary abductors of the thumb. These data indicate that the opponens pollicis duplicates and reinforces the actions of the other thenar muscles.

EFFECTS OF WEAKNESS

Weakness of the opponens pollicis is usually accompanied by weakness of either or both the abductor pollicis brevis and flexor pollicis brevis. Weakness of the opponens pollicis leads to difficulty in positioning and stabilizing the CMC joint of the thumb during pinch and grasp.

Adductor Pollicis

The adductor pollicis is the largest of the intrinsic muscles of the hand with a physiological cross-sectional area similar to that of the extensor carpi radialis longus and the flexor carpi radialis [5,15,25] (*Muscle Attachment Box 18.4*). This remarkable size reveals that the muscle is specialized for force production.

MUSCLE ATTACHMENT BOX 18.4

ATTACHMENTS AND INNERVATION OF THE ADDUCTOR POLLICIS

Proximal attachment: The oblique head attaches to the anterior surfaces of the bases of the second, third, and perhaps fourth metacarpals; the capitate; the palmar carpal ligaments; and the synovial sheath of the flexor carpi radialis. The transverse head attaches to the distal two thirds of the anterior surface of the long finger's metacarpal bone.

Distal attachment: The base of the thumb's proximal phalanx and the extensor hood of the EPL. There is usually a sesamoid bone within the tendon of the oblique head.

Innervation: Ulnar nerve, C8, and T1

Palpation: The adductor pollicis cannot be palpated.

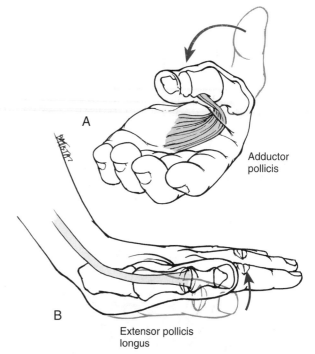

Figure 18.3: The primary adductors of the thumb are the adductor pollicis and the extensor pollicis longus. **A.** The adductor pollicis adducts the thumb to the palm. **B.** The extensor pollicis longus adducts the thumb past the palm (retropulsion).

ACTIONS

MUSCLE ACTION: ADDUCTOR POLLICIS

Action	Evidence
Adduction of the thumb's CMC joint	Supporting
Flexion of the thumb's CMC joint	Supporting
Flexion of the thumb's MCP joint	Supporting
Adduction of the thumb's MCP joint	Inadequate
Extension of the thumb's IP joint	Supporting

The primary actions of the adductor pollicis are flexion and adduction of the CMC joint and flexion of the MCP joint of the thumb. Adduction of the CMC joint of the thumb is defined as movement of the thumb toward (or beyond) the palm of the thumb in a plane perpendicular to the plane of the palm. The adductor pollicis can adduct the thumb only as far as the palm (*Fig. 18.3*). It is the extensor pollicis longus that is aligned to adduct the thumb through its full excursion. EMG data reveal that the adductor pollicis and the extensor pollicis longus are the primary muscles of adduction of the CMC joint [5,9]. Active adduction is most functional in pinch when the thumb is positioned in abduction but must be pulled toward the fingers to maintain pinch (*Fig. 18.4*).

EMG data also support the role of the adductor pollicis as a flexor of both the CMC and MCP joints of the thumb [9]. The transverse head of the adductor pollicis crosses both the CMC and the MCP joints at almost a 90° angle of application at both [5] (*Fig. 18.5*). Its moment arm at the CMC joint is greater than the length of the metacarpal bone. Thus the length of its moment arm and the size of its physiological cross-sectional area make the adductor pollicis an extraordinarily powerful muscle for flexion at the CMC and MCP joints.

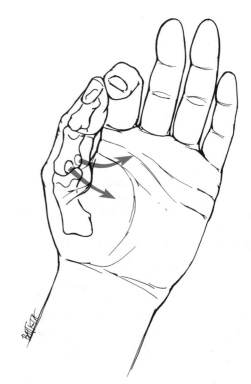

Figure 18.4: The adductor pollicis muscle supplies much of the force of pinch.

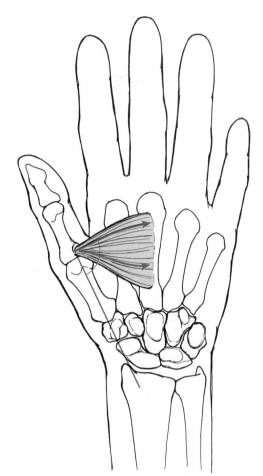

Figure 18.5: The angle of application of the larger, transverse head of the adductor pollicis is almost 90° at both the CMC and MCP joints of the thumb.

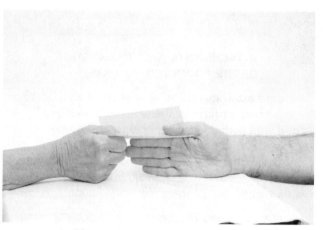

Figure 18.6: Froment's sign. Ability to hold a piece of paper between thumb and palm tests the strength of the adductor pollicis.

Weakness of the adductor pollicis produces weakness in flexion and adduction of the CMC joint and flexion of the MCP joint of the thumb. These impairments can produce severe functional deficits in pinch and grasp [9,20].

Clinical Relevance

FROMENT'S SIGN: *As noted, the adductor pollicis is the largest of the intrinsic muscles of the hand. Weakness in thumb adduction may be the most reliable means of identifying an ulnar nerve palsy [21]. Froment's sign is a classic method to assess adductor pollicis strength. A patient is asked to hold a piece of paper between the thumb and palm while the examiner tries to pull the paper away (Fig. 18.6). An individual with normal strength will be able to hold the paper without difficulty, but an individual with weakness of the adductor pollicis will have difficulty maintaining a hold on the paper.*

Like the abductor pollicis brevis, the adductor pollicis is reported to move the MCP joint of the thumb in the plane of abduction and adduction. The muscle's contribution to actual adduction excursion depends on the joint's shape, although it appears to provide important medial stability regardless of the joint's potential for adduction excursion. The muscle also has an attachment in the extensor hood of the thumb and may participate in IP extension with the abductor and flexor pollicis brevis muscles [9,18,36,40].

EFFECTS OF TIGHTNESS AND WEAKNESS

Tightness of the adductor pollicis may occur in the presence of weakness of the thenar muscles, with a resulting loss of muscle balance. Tightness of the adductor pollicis limits abduction and extension flexibility of the CMC and extension ROM of the MCP joint. These restrictions prevent movement of the thumb away from the palm, which has profound negative effects on the mechanics of pinch and grasp. Severe tightness of the adductor pollicis and flexor pollicis longus contributes to the thumb-in-palm deformity, rendering the thumb useless and compromising the hygiene of the involved hand [29].

PRIMARY INTRINSIC MOVERS OF THE LITTLE FINGER

The hypothenar muscles provide the primary intrinsic control of the little finger (*Fig. 18.7*). The palmar interosseus muscle to the little finger supplies some additional movement and is discussed with the other interossei. The hypothenar muscles are innervated by the ulnar nerve. Their attachments and actions are similar to those of their thenar counterparts. All of the joints of the little finger are influenced by these three muscles.

The CMC articulation of the little finger usually is described as a gliding joint, but Chapter 14 demonstrates that this articulation is more mobile than any other CMC articulation except the thumb. Its surfaces resemble a saddle that allows forward glide and opposition of the little finger [17].

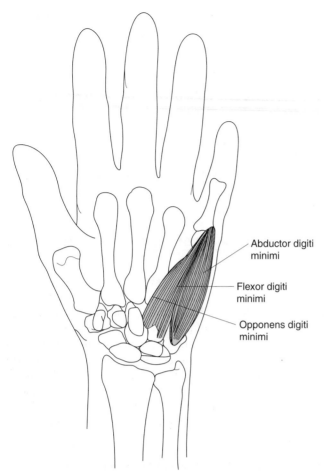

Figure 18.7: The primary intrinsic movers of the little finger include the abductor digiti minimi, flexor digiti minimi, and opponens digiti minimi.

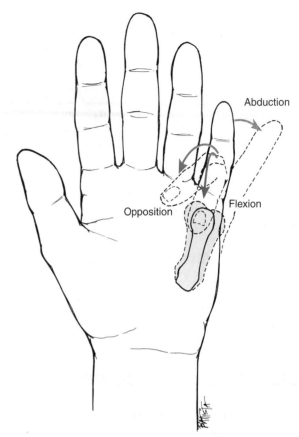

Figure 18.8: Motion at the CMC articulation of the little finger often is described as flexion, rotation, and opposition.

The hypothenar muscles have important effects on this joint. The actions of the hypothenar muscles at the CMC joint are described differently by various authors. Some sources report that the muscular actions of these muscles produce the typical motions of a saddle joint, including flexion, rotation, and opposition (*Fig. 18.8*). Other sources describe the actions according to the direction of movement of the metacarpal, including volar glide and rotation. In this chapter, the actions of the hypothenar muscles at the CMC joint are reported as the actions at a saddle joint, but it is recognized that the joint is only a very mobile gliding joint. Isolated weakness of any of the hypothenar muscles is difficult to identify. The effects of weakness are presented together following the presentation of all three muscles. The effects of intrinsic muscle tightness in the fingers are similar in all of the fingers and are presented later in this chapter.

Abductor Digiti Minimi (Also Known As the Abductor Digiti Quinti)

The abductor digiti minimi is larger than the abductor pollicis brevis and is capable of considerable force production [5,15,25] (*Muscle Attachment Box 18.5*).

ACTIONS

MUSCLE ACTION: ABDUCTOR DIGITI MINIMI

Action	Evidence
Abduction of the little finger's MCP joint	Supporting
Flexion of the little finger's MCP joint	Supporting
Flexion of the little finger's CMC joint	Supporting
Extension of the little finger's IP joints	Supporting

MUSCLE ATTACHMENT BOX 18.5

ATTACHMENTS AND INNERVATION OF THE ABDUCTOR DIGITI MINIMI

Proximal attachment: Pisiform bone, pisohamate ligament, and the tendon of the flexor carpi ulnaris

Distal attachment: Ulnar aspect of the base of the little finger's proximal phalanx and into the extensor hood

Innervation: Ulnar nerve, T1, and perhaps C8

Palpation: The abductor digiti minimi is palpated on the ulnar aspect of the hypothenar eminence during abduction of the little finger's MCP joint.

The primary actions of the abductor digiti minimi occur at the MCP and CMC joints of the little finger. Abduction of the MCP joint of the little finger is the well-recognized role of the abductor digiti minimi [5,19,30,40]. The action of the abductor digiti minimi at the CMC joint is often ignored, even though its attachment on the pisiform produces a large moment arm for flexion at this joint. EMG and clinical studies indicate a clear role for the abductor digiti minimi in stabilizing and flexing the CMC joint. Despite noting an attachment to the extensor hood of the little finger, few anatomy sources report any participation in extension of the IP joints [30,31,40]. Clinical studies and EMG data support the role of the abductor digiti minimi in both MCP flexion and IP extension [2,5].

Flexor Digiti Minimi (Also Known As Flexor Digiti Quinti)

The flexor digiti minimi is the smallest and weakest of the hypothenar muscles [5,15,25] (*Muscle Attachment Box 18.6*).

ACTIONS

MUSCLE ACTION: FLEXOR DIGITI MINIMI

Action	Evidence
Flexion of the little finger's MCP joint	Supporting
Abduction of the little finger's MCP joint	Supporting
Flexion of the little finger's CMC joint	Supporting
Extension of the little finger's IP joints	Supporting

The flexor digiti minimi is functionally important at all of the joints of the little finger. The accepted action of the flexor digiti minimi is flexion of the MCP joint, but its attachment into the extensor hood suggests a role in IP extension. This role is supported by EMG and clinical observations [2,5,11]. These same studies report participation in abduction of the MCP joint along with the abductor digiti minimi. Observation of

the muscle's attachment to the hook of the hamate reveals that the flexor digiti minimi acts with the abductor digiti minimi to flex the CMC articulation of the little finger, and EMG studies support this role [3,11].

Opponens Digiti Minimi (Also Known As Opponens Digiti Quinti)

The opponens digiti minimi is the largest and strongest of the hypothenar muscles [5,15,25] (*Muscle Attachment Box 18.7*). Like the opponens pollicis, the opponens digiti minimi affects only the CMC joint.

ACTIONS

MUSCLE ACTION: OPPONENS DIGITI MINIMI

Action	Evidence
Opposition of the little finger's CMC joint	Supporting

Opposition of the CMC joint of the little finger is the acknowledged action of the opponens digiti minimi [40] and is supported by EMG data [2,5,9,19,30]. Opposition of the little finger is defined as flexion of the CMC joint with rotation so that the pulp of the finger turns toward the thumb. Consequently, some sources also note that the opponens digiti minimi flexes the CMC joint. Opposition of the little finger contributes to the volar arch that is formed by cupping the hand (*Fig. 18.9*).

EFFECTS OF WEAKNESS OF THE HYPOTHENAR MUSCLES

A review of the actions of the hypothenar muscles listed above reveals that the three muscles have very similar actions.

MUSCLE ATTACHMENT BOX 18.7

ATTACHMENTS AND INNERVATION OF THE OPPONENS DIGITI MINIMI

Proximal attachment: Flexor retinaculum and the hook of the hamate

Distal attachment: The ulnar half of the palmar surface of the little finger's metacarpal bone

Innervation: Ulnar nerve, T1, and perhaps C8

Palpation: The opponens digiti minimi can be palpated along the ulnar aspect of the palmar surface of the little finger's metacarpal during gentle opposition of the little finger. As with palpation of the opponens pollicis, the palpating digit must be slipped between the abductor digiti minimi and the metacarpal. Vigorous opposition will generate contraction of the abductor digiti minimi, making palpation of the opponens digiti minimi impossible.

MUSCLE ATTACHMENT BOX 18.6

ATTACHMENTS AND INNERVATION OF THE FLEXOR DIGITI MINIMI

Proximal attachment: Flexor retinaculum and the hook of the hamate

Distal attachment: Ulnar aspect of the base of the little finger's proximal phalanx and into the extensor hood. Its tendon may contain a sesamoid bone.

Innervation: Ulnar nerve, T1, and perhaps C8

Palpation: The flexor digiti minimi is palpated on the radial aspect of the hypothenar eminence.

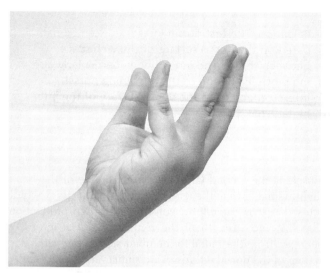

Figure 18.9: Opposition of the little finger moves the little finger toward the thumb and creates the volar arch.

The abductor digiti minimi and flexor digiti minimi flex the CMC joint, and the opponens digiti minimi flexes and rotates the CMC of the little finger toward the thumb. Thus the three muscles all contribute to opposition of the CMC joint of the little finger. The opponens digiti minimi is the largest and strongest of the three. Weakness of the opponens digiti minimi has the greatest effect on opposition strength; however, weakness of any of the three diminishes opposition strength somewhat. Similarly, both the abductor digiti minimi and the flexor digiti minimi are abductors of the MCP joint of the little finger. Because the abductor digiti minimi is larger than the flexor digiti minimi and has a larger abduction moment arm, weakness of the abductor digiti minimi is manifested most clearly by weakness of abduction of the MCP joint, but weakness of the flexor digiti minimi may reduce abduction strength as well. Consequently, it is difficult to ascertain the exact level of weakness of any of these muscles. Despite these difficulties, the clinician can use the following guide to assess hypothenar strength:

- Opposition remains the best indicator of opponens digiti minimi strength.
- MCP abduction strength best indicates abductor digiti minimi strength.
- MCP flexion with IP extension best reflects the strength of the flexor digiti minimi.

Clinical Relevance

WEAKNESS OF THE HYPOTHENAR MUSCLES: *Weakness of the hypothenar muscles impairs the intricate movements of the little finger, especially abduction. This may result in a serious disability in individuals whose occupations depend upon discrete finger movements, such as computer operators or musicians (Fig. 18.10). At least as important and used by*

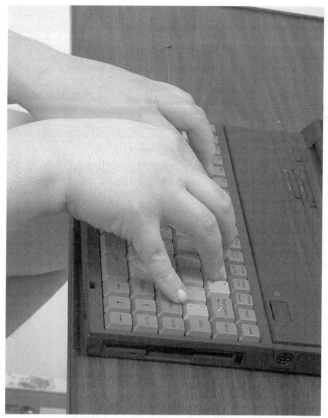

Figure 18.10: Functional activity requiring activity of the intrinsic muscles of the little finger. Abduction or MCP flexion with IP extension of the little finger is a common position required while typing.

almost all humans is the ability to create the volar arch. The volar arch is essential to produce a tight fist (see Fig. 14.45). Because the hypothenar muscles provide the active control of the volar arch, weakness of the hypothenar muscles may impair the ability to make the volar arch, leading to a significant loss in grip strength [3,19].

Weakness of the hypothenar muscles also creates a muscle imbalance in the little finger. In most cases, weakness of the hypothenar muscles is accompanied by weakness of the other muscles of the hand innervated by the ulnar nerve. Consequently, the extrinsic muscles overpower the intrinsic muscles, resulting in a characteristic hand deformity known as a claw hand. A more complete discussion of this deformity is presented later in this chapter.

INTEROSSEI AND LUMBRICALS

Dorsal Interossei

There are four dorsal interosseous muscles in the hand (*Muscle Attachment Box 18.8*)(*Fig. 18.11*). They are bipennate muscles of varying sizes. The first dorsal interosseous

MUSCLE ATTACHMENT BOX 18.8

ATTACHMENTS AND INNERVATION OF THE DORSAL INTEROSSEI

Proximal attachment: Each interosseous muscle arises from the adjacent sides of two metacarpal bones

Distal attachment: The radial two dorsal interossei insert on the radial sides of the bases of the proximal phalanges of the index and long fingers; the ulnar two dorsal interossei insert on the ulnar side of the bases of the proximal phalanges of the ring and long fingers. Each of the dorsal interossei also inserts on the extensor hood of its respective finger.

Innervation: Ulnar nerve, T1, and perhaps C8

Palpation: The first dorsal interosseus can be palpated on the dorsal surface of the web space between thumb and index finger, particularly during pinch. Palpation of the remaining dorsal interossei occurs on the dorsal surface of the intermetacarpal spaces.

muscle is the second largest intrinsic muscle of the hand, slightly smaller than the adductor pollicis [15]. Its size indicates that it is capable of considerable force production. The size and strength of the remaining dorsal interossei decrease from the radial to the ulnar side of the hand. The actions of the dorsal interossei are similar and are presented as a group.

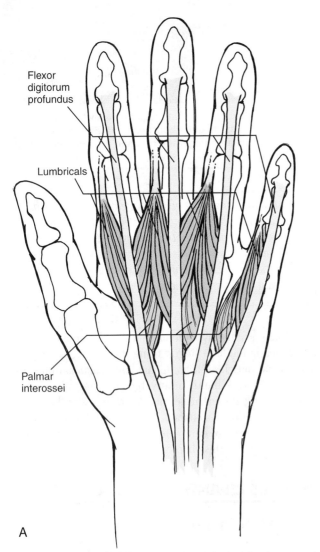

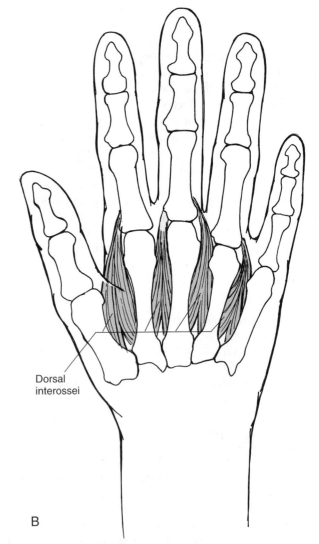

Figure 18.11: Interossei and lumbrical muscles. **A.** The lumbricals and palmar interossei lie in the palm of the hand, with distal attachments to the fingers. **B.** The dorsal interossei are on the dorsum of the hand.

ACTIONS

MUSCLE ACTION: DORSAL INTEROSSEI

Action	Evidence
Abduction of the index, long, and ring fingers' MCP joints	Supporting
Flexion of the index, long, and ring fingers' MCP joints	Supporting
Extension of the index, long, and ring fingers' IP joints	Supporting
Adduction of the thumb's CMC joint by the first dorsal interosseus	Inadequate

To understand the attachments of the dorsal interossei on only the index, ring, and long fingers, it is useful to recognize that the abductor digiti minimi fulfills the role of a dorsal interosseous muscle to the little finger, providing abduction and flexion of the MCP and extension of the IP joints. The little finger has no dorsal interosseous muscle. In addition, because the long finger is the reference for abduction and adduction, it participates in abduction in both the radial and ulnar directions. Thus the long finger has both a radial and an ulnar dorsal interosseous muscle. The role of the dorsal interosseous muscles in abduction and flexion of the MCP joints and in IP extension is well accepted [2,5,19,30,40]. EMG and in vivo muscle stimulation studies confirm their activity in these motions [16,26].

Although the first dorsal interosseous muscle is said to adduct the CMC joint of the thumb and to stabilize the thumb [5,19], an EMG study of isometric abduction and adduction of the thumb reveals minimal activity of the first dorsal interosseous in both directions [9]. EMG data consistently reveal that the muscle is active during pinch, stabilizing either the thumb or index finger or perhaps both [5,9].

EFFECTS OF WEAKNESS

Weakness of the dorsal interossei is manifested most clearly as weakness in abduction of the index, long, and ring fingers. Weakness also contributes to a loss of muscle balance in the hand and thus to the formation of the claw hand. In addition, weakness of the dorsal interossei results in a loss of both pinch and grasp strength [20].

Palmar Interossei

Sources describe either three [5,15,31] or four [19,30,40] palmar interossei (*Muscle Attachment Box 18.9*). The source of variation is the first, or most radial, palmar interosseous muscle, which is described as part of the flexor pollicis brevis or adductor pollicis by those who list only three palmar interossei [37]. Only three palmar interossei are described in this book. The role of the radial muscle belly is included in the description of the actions of the flexor pollicis brevis. The palmar interossei muscles are unipennate, and the three possess similar physiological cross-sectional areas that are generally smaller than those of the dorsal interossei [5,15].

MUSCLE ATTACHMENT BOX 18.9

ATTACHMENTS AND INNERVATION OF THE PALMAR INTEROSSEI

Proximal attachment: The palmar interosseous to the index finger arises from the ulnar surface of the index finger's metacarpal bone. The palmar interossei to the ring and little fingers arise from the radial surface of the ring and little fingers' metacarpal bones, respectively.

Distal attachment: Each of the palmar interossei attaches to the extensor hood of the same finger. The palmar interosseus to the little finger may also insert on the radial side of the proximal phalanx of the little finger.

Innervation: Ulnar nerve, T1, and perhaps C8

Palpation: The palmar interossei cannot be palpated.

ACTIONS

MUSCLE ACTION: PALMAR INTEROSSEI

Action	Evidence
Adduction of the index, ring, and little fingers' MCP joints	Inadequate
Flexion of the index, ring, and little fingers' MCP joints	Inadequate
Extension of the index, long, and ring fingers' IP joints	Inadequate

The absence of a palmar interosseous muscle to the long finger is consistent with the presence of two dorsal interossei to that finger. The actions of the palmar interossei are broadly accepted, although there are few EMG data available assessing their function directly.

EFFECTS OF WEAKNESS

Weakness of the palmar interossei is manifested by weakness in adduction of the fingers. Individuals with palmar interossei weakness are unable to hold their fingers close together with the MCP joints of the fingers extended (*Fig. 18.12*). Weakness also contributes to weakness of MCP flexion with IP extension. Thus, as with the dorsal interossei, weakness of the palmar interossei contributes to weakness in grasp and pinch [6].

 Similarly, weakness of the palmar interossei also contributes to the muscular imbalances leading to the claw hand deformity.

Lumbrical Muscles

The lumbrical muscles are the smallest muscles of the hand and possess the longest muscle fibers of the intrinsic muscles [5,15,25]. They also are among the most unusual muscles in

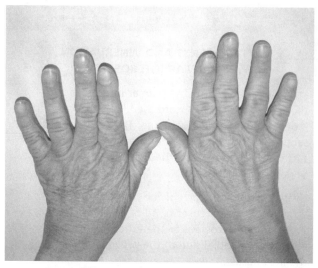

Figure 18.12: Weakness of the palmar interossei. An individual with weakness of the palmar interossei has difficulty holding the fingers together while the MCP joints are extended.

MUSCLE ATTACHMENT BOX 18.10

ATTACHMENTS AND INNERVATION OF THE LUMBRICAL MUSCLES

Proximal attachment: The tendons of the flexor digitorum profundus. The lumbricals to the index and long fingers arise from the radial and palmar surfaces of the tendons to the index and long fingers, respectively. The lumbrical to the ring finger arises from the tendons to the long and ring fingers and the lumbrical to the little finger from the tendons to the ring and little fingers.

Distal attachment: The radial side of the extensor expansion to each finger

Innervation: The lumbricals to the index and long fingers are innervated by the median nerve, T1, and perhaps C8. The lumbricals to the ring and little finger are innervated by the ulnar nerve, T1, and perhaps C8.

Palpation: The lumbricals cannot be palpated.

the body, possessing no bony attachment, instead attaching proximally and distally to tendons that are antagonists to one another [30,40] (*Muscle Attachment Box 18.10*).

ACTIONS

MUSCLE ACTION: LUMBRICALS

Action	Evidence
Flexion of the MCP joints of the fingers	Supporting
Extension of IP joints of the fingers	Supporting
Radial deviation of the MCP joints of the fingers	Inadequate

EMG studies verify the activity of the lumbrical muscles during MCP flexion and IP extension [2,26]. Since these actions are the same as those of the interossei, there has been considerable debate regarding the relative contribution of each muscle group to these motions. The moment arms of the lumbrical muscles are greater than those of the interossei at the MCP joints [5] (*Fig. 18.13*). The moment arms of the dorsal interossei are the smallest. However, the dorsal interossei are the largest of these muscles, and the lumbrical muscles have less than one tenth the physiological

cross-sectional area of the dorsal interossei [5,15]. Therefore, the interossei are considered the primary flexors of the MCP joints when the IP joints are extended, although biomechanical models, cadaver studies, and studies in human subjects consistently demonstrate the lumbricals' ability to flex the MCP joints [23,28,35]. In a study of 80 fingers with interosseus paralysis but intact lumbrical muscles, Srinivasan demonstrated a reduced, but real, capacity to flex the MCP joint while maintaining IP extension [35].

The lumbrical muscles' effects on radial deviation are unclear. Examination of their structure reveals consistent moment arms for radial deviation, but their moment arms are smaller than the moment arms of the corresponding interossei. Since the physiological cross-sectional areas of the interossei are much larger than those of the lumbrical muscles, it is likely that the lumbricals are, at best, accessory muscles for radial deviation. There is no known research that demonstrates that lumbrical contraction produces any functional radial deviation in the absence of the interossei.

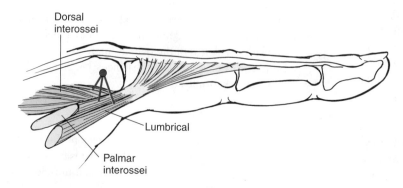

Dorsal interossei
Lumbrical
Palmar interossei

Figure 18.13: The lumbricals have the longest flexion moment arms of the intrinsic muscles at the MCP joints; the dorsal interossei have the shortest.

TABLE 18.1: Muscles Active during Combined Movements and Postures of the MCP and IP Joints of the Fingers

	Concentric MCP Extension	Static Position in MCP Extension	Concentric MCP Flexion	Static Position in MCP Flexion
Static position in IP extension	ED Lumbricals	ED Lumbricals	Interossei Lumbricals	Interossei Lumbricals
Concentric IP extension	NR	ED Lumbricals	NR	Interossei Lumbricals
Static position in IP flexion	ED FDP	ED FDP	FDP	FDP FDS
Concentric IP flexion	NR	ED FDP	NR	FDP

Data from Long C, Brown ME: Electromyographic kinesiology of the hand: muscles moving the long finger. J Bone Joint Surg 1964; 46A: 1683–1706.
FDS, flexor digitorum superficialis; ED, extensor digitorum; NR, not reported; FDP, flexor digitorum profundus.

In contrast, the role of the lumbrical muscles in IP extension is uncontested. The importance of the lumbricals' contribution to IP extension is best understood by analyzing the EMG activity of the intrinsic and extrinsic muscles of the fingers. The results of the classic study of the intrinsic and extrinsic finger muscles by Long and Brown [26] are presented in *Table 18.1*. This study examined muscle activity during various combinations of unresisted isometric or concentric contractions producing flexion or extension of the MCP and IP joints of the long finger. The following conclusions can be drawn from these data:

- The flexor digitorum profundus is active whenever the IP joints are flexed or flexing.
- The flexor digitorum profundus is active with MCP flexion only when the IP joints are flexed or flexing.
- The extensor digitorum is active whenever the MCP joints are extended or extending.
- The extensor digitorum is active in IP extension only when the MCP joints are extended or extending.
- The interossei are active in any combination of isometric or concentric MCP flexion with IP extension.
- The lumbrical muscles are active whenever the IP joints are extended or extending, regardless of MCP position or motion.
- The lumbricals are active during MCP flexion when the IP joints are extended or extending.

The data reported by Long and Brown help explain the critical role played by the lumbrical muscles. Extension by the extensor digitorum is resisted by the passive tension of the tendons of the flexor digitorum profundus. As noted, the lumbricals have unique attachments to tendons. As a lumbrical contracts, it pulls on the flexor digitorum profundus. This pull puts the portion of the flexor digitorum profundus tendon that is distal to the lumbrical attachment on slack, reducing the passive resistance to extension that could be applied by the flexor tendon at the level of the IP joints (*Fig. 18.14*). The primary role of the lumbrical muscles is to reduce the resistance to extension offered by the flexor digitorum profundus, even when extension of the MCP joints stretches

the flexor digitorum profundus. The lumbricals also assist the extensor digitorum in extending the IP joints through the full ROM [26,38].

The data from Long and Brown [26] apply to unresisted motions of the fingers moving in space (open chain motions). More recent studies of finger motion against a resistance or as the fingers press against a load (closed chain activities) suggest a more complex interaction between the intrinsic and extrinsic muscles of the fingers in which precise joint positions influence the relative activity of the muscles [16].

EFFECTS OF WEAKNESS

Isolated weakness of the lumbrical muscles is unusual and difficult to identify. The classic manual muscle test of the lumbrical muscles is resisted flexion of the MCP joints while the IP joints maintain extension [19] (*Fig. 18.15*). However, EMG data convincingly demonstrate that this motion uses the combined activity of the lumbricals and interossei [6,19,26]. Together with weakness of the interossei, weakness of the lumbricals contributes to the classic deformity, the claw hand.

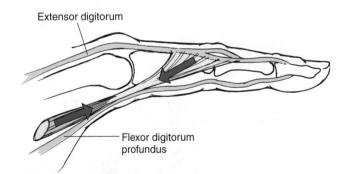

Figure 18.14: Function of the lumbricals. Contraction of the lumbricals pulls the flexor digitorum profundus tendon distally, putting the portion of the tendon that is distal to the lumbrical muscle on slack while increasing the tension in the distal portion of the extensor digitorum (ED). This decreases the passive flexion moment on the IP joints and assists the ED in extending the IP joints.

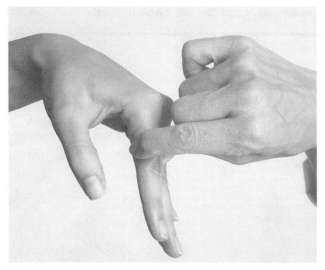

Figure 18.15: The standard manual muscle test procedure for the lumbricals is resisted flexion of the MCP joints with the IP joints extended. EMG data show that the interossei participate in this activity as well.

EFFECTS OF TIGHTNESS OF THE LUMBRICAL, INTEROSSEOUS, AND HYPOTHENAR MUSCLES

The EMG data reported in Table 18.1 reveal that both the interossei and lumbrical muscle groups are active in combined MCP flexion and IP extension of the fingers. The hypothenar muscles participate in the same actions at the little finger. This position is known as the **intrinsic positive,** or **intrinsic plus hand,** since it results from a purely intrinsic contraction (*Fig. 18.16*). Tightness of the intrinsic muscles leads to a static posture in a similar position. Patients frequently demonstrate tightness of the intrinsic muscles after immobilization of the hand, since immobilization must occur with the MCP joints flexed to preserve MCP flexion ROM.

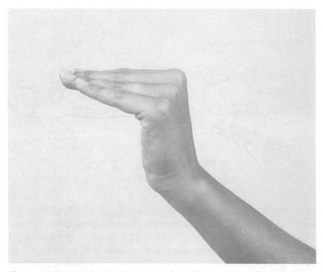

Figure 18.16: An intrinsic positive hand is positioned with the fingers' MCP joints flexed and the IP joints extended.

CLASSIC DEFORMITIES RESULTING FROM MUSCLE IMBALANCES IN THE HAND

To appreciate the deformities resulting from muscle imbalances, it is essential to recognize that the extrinsic muscles of the hand are multijoint muscles, typically crossing three or four joints. The effects of muscles traversing so many joints are similar to the effect of the cords supporting a window blind. The cords lie on both sides of the blind, and are firmly attached to the bottom of the blind. As the cords are pulled together, the blind folds on itself (*Fig. 18.17*). Similarly, when only the extrinsic flexor and extensor muscles pull together on the most distal phalanx, the finger begins to fold on itself, collapsing into a zigzag pattern of joint hyperextension and flexion [33].

Shorter muscles, namely the intrinsic muscles, attaching to the more proximal bones are needed to stabilize the multijointed finger. The loss of balance occurs when the intrinsic muscles are weak or absent and is manifested in the deformities that result from peripheral nerve injuries. The impairments, deformities, and associated functional deficits from specific nerve injuries are presented below.

Ulnar Nerve Injury

The ulnar nerve is susceptible to injury as it wraps around the medial epicondyle of the humerus and as it travels across the wrist into the hand. Injuries at the hand affect the innervation

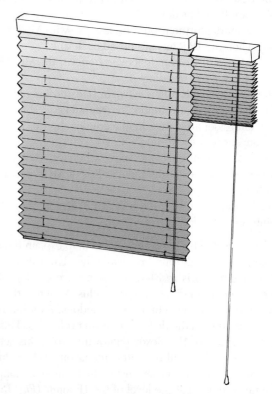

Figure 18.17: Mechanism of a claw hand deformity. When the cords that are attached to the bottom of a window blind are pulled, the blind folds on itself in a zigzag pattern.

of the intrinsic muscles, while injuries at the elbow may affect the muscles receiving innervation from the ulnar nerve in the forearm as well as in the hand.

ULNAR NERVE INJURIES AT THE WRIST

The muscles that may be affected by an ulnar nerve injury at the wrist are listed below:

- Hypothenar muscles: abductor digiti minimi, flexor digiti minimi, opponens digiti minimi
- Dorsal interossei
- Palmar interossei
- Ulnar two lumbrical muscles
- Adductor pollicis
- Deep head of the flexor pollicis brevis

If these muscles are paralyzed, the ulnar two fingers have no intrinsic muscle support, and the long and index fingers have only the remaining lumbrical muscles. The extrinsic muscles pull directly against each other. The extensor digitorum has a larger moment arm at the MCP joint and, consequently, pulls that joint into hyperextension. The extrinsic finger flexors stretch as a result and pull on the phalanges, causing flexion at the PIP and DIP joints. The resulting deformity is the **claw hand** (*Fig. 18.18*). The deformity demonstrates the classic zigzag pattern of joint hyperextension and flexion that follows when the extrinsic flexor and extensor tendons function without the balance of the intrinsic muscles. Because the lumbrical muscles to the index and long fingers remain intact, the clawing is less obvious in these fingers [35]. The claw hand deformity also is characterized by flattening of the hypothenar eminence.

A claw hand deformity produces significant functional deficits. An individual with a claw hand loses grip strength as a result of the loss of intrinsic muscle strength that contributes directly to powerful grasp [4,20]. Loss of the hypothenar muscles results in the inability to form the volar arch actively, resulting in further loss of grip strength. The ability to grasp

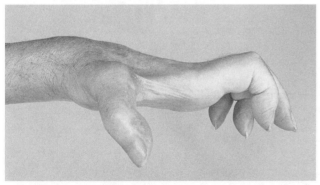

Figure 18.18: In a claw hand deformity, the extrinsic flexor digitorum profundus and the extensor digitorum pull on the distal phalanx. Lacking the control of the intrinsic muscles attached more proximally, the fingers collapse into the zigzag pattern of hyperextension at the MCP joints and flexion at the PIP and DIP joints.

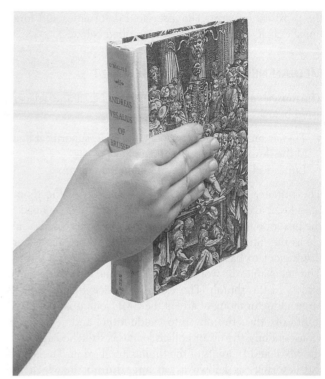

Figure 18.19: Position of the hand to hold a large object. Holding a large object requires MCP flexion of the fingers, with little or no flexion of the IP joints.

large objects also is impaired, since it requires MCP flexion with IP extension (*Fig. 18.19*). The other important loss is the adductor pollicis, resulting in significant impairment to powerful pinch but without an associated deformity.

ULNAR NERVE INJURY AT THE ELBOW

The muscles that may be affected by an ulnar nerve injury at the elbow are listed below:

- Flexor carpi ulnaris
- Flexor digitorum profundus to the ring and little fingers
- The intrinsic muscles listed with ulnar nerve injuries at the wrist

Paralysis of the flexor digitorum profundus to the ulnar two fingers alters the claw deformity slightly in these two fingers. In the absence of the flexor digitorum profundus, the pull from the extrinsic muscles is exerted by the extensor digitorum and the flexor digitorum superficialis. The MCP joints and PIP joints are hyperextended and flexed, respectively, as in a typical claw hand, but the DIP joints in the ring and little fingers remain extended. Paralysis of the flexor carpi ulnaris may result in deviation of the wrist toward extension and radial deviation.

Median Nerve Injury

Median nerve injuries within the carpal tunnel are common, but the nerve also is susceptible to injuries at the elbow or in the proximal forearm. The associated deformities and functional deficits in each lesion are described below.

MEDIAN NERVE INJURY AT THE WRIST

The muscles affected by a median nerve injury at the wrist are listed below:

- Thenar muscles: abductor pollicis brevis, superficial head of the flexor pollicis brevis, opponens pollicis
- Lumbrical muscles to the index and long fingers

The primary loss with this lesion is the loss of the thenar muscles, leaving only the adductor pollicis, the deep head of the flexor pollicis brevis, and the first dorsal interosseus muscle as the intrinsic supply to the thumb. These muscles are insufficient to balance the extrinsic muscles of the thumb. The mechanics at work in the claw hand produce similar effects in the thumb. The extensor pollicis longus with its large adductor moment arm at the CMC joint pulls the CMC joint of the thumb into adduction and extension. Consequently, the flexor pollicis longus is stretched and pulls the MCP and IP joints of the thumb into flexion. The resulting deformity is known as an **ape thumb,** in which the thumb is pulled onto the radial side of the hand, with the CMC joint extended and adducted and the MCP and IP joints flexed (*Fig. 18.20*). This deformity can be very debilitating, since the adducted position precludes normal tip-to-tip or pulp-to-pulp pinch [4].

Clinical Relevance

MEDIAN NERVE INJURY AT THE WRIST:
Orthopaedic surgery to transfer intact muscles to the thumb may be useful in providing some active control of pinch, but a simple splint to position the thumb in opposition also is successful in improving function by placing the thumb in a functional position and allowing the fingers to provide the active pinch against a stable thumb (Fig. 18.21).

MEDIAN NERVE INJURY AT THE ELBOW

The muscles affected when the median nerve is injured at the elbow are listed below:

- Pronator teres
- Flexor carpi radialis
- Palmaris longus
- Flexor digitorum superficialis
- Flexor pollicis longus
- Flexor digitorum profundus to the index and long fingers
- Pronator quadratus
- The intrinsic muscles affected by a median nerve lesion at the wrist

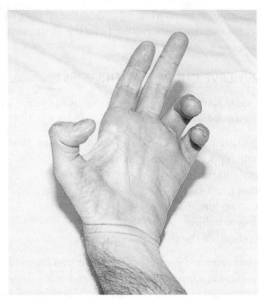

Figure 18.20: An ape thumb deformity in an individual with a peripheral neuropathy is positioned in extension and retropulsion at the CMC joint and flexion at the MCP and IP joints.

These include all of the superficial flexors of the forearm except the flexor carpi ulnaris, the primary pronators of the forearm, the flexor digitorum profundus to the index and long fingers, and the flexor pollicis longus. The ape thumb deformity is altered, since the IP joint remains extended. Similarly the DIP joints of the index and long fingers remain extended. The wrist may be positioned in extension and perhaps ulnar deviation.

Radial Nerve Injury

No intrinsic muscles of the hand are innervated by the radial nerve. Muscular effects are seen in more-proximal radial

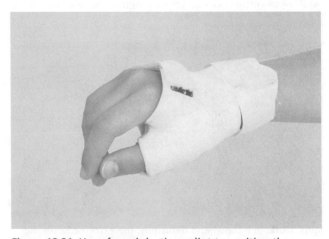

Figure 18.21: Use of an abduction splint to position the thumb in slight opposition can increase an individual's function, even in the presence of significant weakness of the thenar muscles.

nerve injuries. As noted in Chapter 8, the radial nerve is particularly susceptible to injury, as it lies against the humeral shaft in the radial groove. The muscles of the forearm and wrist that are affected in such a lesion are listed below:

- Extensor carpi radialis longus (and perhaps the brachioradialis)
- Extensor carpi radialis brevis
- Extensor digitorum
- Extensor digiti minimi
- Extensor carpi ulnaris
- Supinator
- Abductor pollicis longus
- Extensor pollicis brevis
- Extensor pollicis longus
- Extensor indicis

This list includes all of the wrist extensors and extrinsic extensors to the fingers and thumb. This lesion results in a **drop wrist** deformity. The greatest functional deficit caused by a radial nerve injury is difficulty in positioning the wrist for powerful grasp or pinch. The essential synergy between the wrist extensors and the finger flexors combines the contraction of the extensor carpi radialis longus and brevis and the extensor carpi ulnaris with the flexor digitorum profundus and superficialis. This synergy is necessary to avoid passive insufficiency of the extensor digitorum and active insufficiency of the finger flexors. If the wrist is allowed to remain in flexion in the absence of the wrist extensors, the patient is unable to develop a powerful grasp or pinch (*Fig. 18.22*). A study of 10 healthy individuals with radial nerve blocks reported more than a 75% decrease in grip strength and a 33% loss in pinch strength [22].

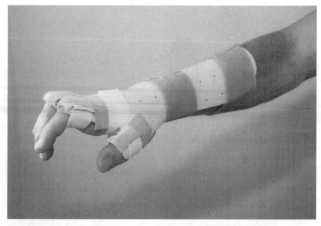

Figure 18.23: An individual with a radial nerve injury can use a splint to position the wrist and fingers in a functional position so that the fingers can develop a powerful grasp.

Clinical Relevance

DROP WRIST DEFORMITY: *The functional need for wrist extension leads surgeons to perform a variety of tendon transfers to restore active control. As in the ape thumb deformity, a splint that helps position the wrist in extension can succeed in providing stability to the wrist in a functional position, allowing the intact finger muscles to perform their roles in grasp and pinch (Fig. 18.23).*

Sensory Deficits Associated with Nerve Injuries to the Hand

Although this book focuses on the mechanics and pathomechanics of the musculoskeletal system, the functional implications of sensory loss to the hand demand at least brief consideration. Sensory distribution to the hand is depicted in *Figure 18.24*. Sensory loss secondary to a median nerve injury presents the greatest functional challenge. Useful pinch requires the integrated control of the intrinsic and extrinsic muscles of the thumb, index, and long finger. However, it also depends on the acute sensory feedback provided by the pulps and nail beds of these digits. Anyone whose hand has "fallen asleep" can appreciate the frustration of lack of sensation in the finger tips.

Sensory loss from a radial or ulnar nerve injury also is a potentially serious lesion. Although feedback from the dorsum or ulnar surface of the hand is less important during pinch and grasp, it is an important warning of injury to the hand. These surfaces are easily bumped on furniture or a hot coil of a stove. Lack of sensation prevents spontaneous recognition of such

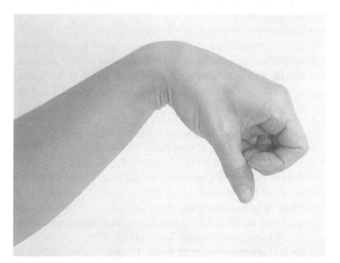

Figure 18.22: An individual with a drop wrist is unable to make a strong fist.

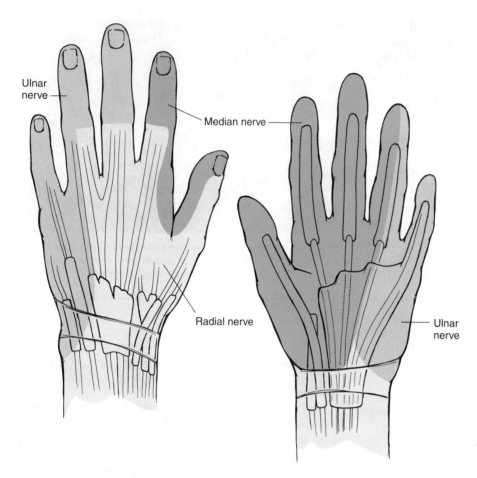

Ulnar nerve

Median nerve

Radial nerve

Ulnar nerve

Figure 18.24: Sensory distribution of the nerves to the hand. Sensory loss in the hand resulting from a peripheral nerve injury can produce severe disability. Fine motor tasks demand sensory input from the pulps of the digits, and the dorsal surface of the hand and fingers is subjected to trauma that, if undetected, can lead to infection and serious impairment.

injuries. If these injuries remain undetected, infection can set in. The clinician must teach the individual to carefully inspect the insensitive skin regularly.

SUMMARY

This chapter presents the intrinsic muscles of the hand, which are integral to the normal function of the hand. The normal interplay of the intrinsic and extrinsic muscles is presented. The primary intrinsic muscles of the thumb are the thenar muscles, innervated by the median nerve, and the adductor pollicis, innervated by the ulnar nerve. Weakness of the thenar muscles leads to an ape thumb deformity, while weakness of the adductor pollicis weakens pinch and grasp. An ulnar nerve injury also leads to reduced grip strength by impairing production of the volar arch and the strength of the intrinsic muscles to the fingers. The following chapter discusses the mechanics and pathomechanics of pinch and grasp. These functions demonstrate the coordinated activity of the intrinsic and extrinsic muscles.

References

1. Barmakian JT: Anatomy of the joints of the thumb. Hand Clin 1992; 8: 683–691.
2. Basmajian JV, DeLuca CJ: Muscles Alive. Their Function Revealed by Electromyography. Baltimore: Williams & Wilkins, 1985.
3. Bendz P: The functional significance of the fifth metacarpus and hypothenar in two useful grips of the hand. Am J Phys Med Rehabil 1993; 72: 210–213.
4. Bowden RE: Peripheral Nerve Injuries. London: HK Lewis & Co, 1958.
5. Brand PW, Hollister A: Clinical Mechanics of the Hand. St. Louis, MO: Mosby-Year Book, 1999.
6. Brandsma JW: Manual muscle strength testing and dynamometry for bilateral ulnar neuropraxia in a surgeon. J Hand Ther 1995; 8: 191–194.
7. Brandsma JW, Oudenaarde EV, Oostendorp R: The abductores pollicis muscles: clinical considerations based on electromyographical and anatomical studies. J Hand Ther 1996; 9: 218–222.
8. Close JR, Kidd CC: The functions of the muscles of the thumb, the index, and the long fingers. J Bone Joint Surg 1969; 51A: 1601–1620.
9. Cooney WP III, An KN, Daube JR, Askew LJ: Electromyographic analysis of the thumb: a study of isometric forces in pinch and grasp. J Hand Surg [Am] 1985; 10A: 202–210.
10. Cooney WP III, Lucca MJ, Chao EYS, Inscheid RL: The kinesiology of the thumb trapeziometacarpal joint. J Bone Joint Surg 1981; 63A: 1371–1381.
11. Forrest WJ, Basmajian JV: Functions of human thenar and hypothenar muscles. An electromyographic study of twenty-five hands. J Bone Joint Surg 1965; 47A: 1585–1594.
12. Hirsch D, Page D, Miller D, et al.: A biomechanical analysis of the metacarpophalangeal joint of the thumb. J Biomech 1974; 7: 343–348.
13. Hollister A, Giurintano DJ: Thumb movements, motions, and moments. J Hand Ther 1995; 8: 106–114.

14. Imaeda T, An KN, Cooney WP III: Functional anatomy and biomechanics of the thumb. Hand Clin 1992; 8: 9–15.

15. Jacobson MD, Raab R, Fazeli BM, et al.: Architectural design of the human intrinsic hand muscles. J Hand Surg [Am] 1992; 17A: 804–809.

16. Kamper DG, Fischer HC, Cruz EG: Impact of finger posture on mapping from muscle activation to joint torque. Clin Biomech 2006; 21: 361–369.

17. Kapandji IA: The Physiology of the Joints. Vol 1, The Upper Limb. Edinburgh: Churchill Livingstone, 1982.

18. Kaplan EB: Anatomy and kinesiology of the hand. In: Flynn JE, ed. Hand Surgery. Baltimore: Williams & Wilkins, 1982; 14–24.

19. Kendall FP, McCreary EK, Provance PG: Muscle Testing and Function. Baltimore: Williams & Wilkins, 1993.

20. Kozin SH, Porter S, Clark P, Thoder JJ: The contribution of the intrinsic muscles to grip and pinch strength. J Hand Surg [Am] 1999; 24A: 64–72.

21. Kuxhaus L, Roach SS, Valero-Cuevas FJ: Quantifying deficits in the 3D force capabilities of a digit caused by selective paralysis: application to the thumb with simulated low ulnar nerve palsy. J Biomech 2005; 38: 725–736.

22. Labosky DA, Waggy CA: Apparent weakness of median and ulnar motors in radial nerve palsy. J Hand Surg [Am] 1986; 11A: 528–533.

23. Leijnes J, Kalker J: A two-dimensional kinematic model of the lumbrical in the human finger. J Biomech 1995; 28: 237–249.

24. Le Viet D, Lantieri L: Ulnar luxation of the extensor pollicis longus. Anatomic and clinical study. Ann Chir Main Membr Super 1993; 12: 173–181.

25. Linscheid RL, An KN, Gross RM: Quantitative analysis of the intrinsic muscles of the hand. Clin Anat 1991; 4: 265–284.

26. Long C, Brown ME: Electromyographic kinesiology of the hand: muscles moving the long finger. J Bone Joint Surg 1964; 46A: 1683–1706.

27. Omokawa S, Ryu J, Tang JB, et al.: Trapeziometacarpal joint instability affects the moment arms of thumb motor tendons. Clin Orthop 2000; 372: 262–271.

28. Ranney DA, Wells RP, Dowling J: Lumbrical function: interaction of lumbrical contraction with the elasticity of the extrinsic finger muscles and its effect on metacarpophalangeal equilibrium. J Hand Surg [Am] 1987; 12A: 566–575.

29. Rayan GM, Saccone PG: Treatment of spastic thumb-in-palm deformity: a modified extensor pollicis longus tendon rerouting. J Hand Surg [Am]. 1996; 21: 834–839.

30. Romanes GJE: Cunningham's Textbook of Anatomy. Oxford: Oxford University Press, 1981.

31. Rosse C, Gaddum-Rosse P: Hollinshead's Textbook of Anatomy. Philadelphia: Lippincott-Raven, 1997.

32. Skoff HD: The role of the abductor pollicis brevis in opposition. Am J Orthop 1998; 27: 369–370.

33. Smith RJ: Balance and kinetics of the fingers under normal and pathological conditions. Clin Orthop 1974; 104: 92–111.

34. Smutz WP, Kongsayreepong A, Hughes RE, et al.: Mechanical advantage of the thumb muscles. J Biomech 2000; 31: 565–570.

35. Srinivasan H: Movement patterns of interosseous-minimus fingers. J Bone Joint Surg 1979; 61A: 557–561.

36. Strong CL, Perry J: Function of the extensor pollicis longus and intrinsic muscles of the thumb: an electromyographic study during interphalangeal joint extension. J Am Phys Ther Assoc 1966; 46: 939–945.

37. Tubiana R, Thomine JM, Mackin E: Examination of the Hand and Wrist. Philadelphia: WB Saunders, 1996.

38. Wang AW, Gupta A: Early motion after flexor tendon surgery. Hand Clin 1996; 12: 43–55.

39. Weathersby HT, Sutton LR, Krusen UL: The kinesiology of muscles of the thumb: an electromyographic study. Arch Phys Med Rehabil 1963; 321–326.

40. Williams P, Bannister L, Berry M, et al: Gray's Anatomy, The Anatomical Basis of Medicine and Surgery, Br. ed. London: Churchill Livingstone, 1995.

Mechanics and Pathomechanics of Pinch and Grasp

T he previous five chapters present the structure and function of the wrist and hand. The bones and joints are discussed to understand the motions available throughout the region. The function of the muscles of the forearm and hand are presented with discussions of the dysfunction resulting from weakness or tightness. One of the primary functions of the hand is to hold onto objects. Therefore a thorough understanding of the wrist and hand requires examination of the roles of the joints and muscles during grasp and pinch.

The purposes of this final chapter on the hand are to detail the requirements of normal pinch and grasp and to discuss the factors contributing to abnormal prehension. Specifically, the goals of this chapter are to

- Discuss the classification schemes describing prehension
- Examine the positions of the joints of the wrist and hand during normal pinch and grasp
- Investigate the muscles needed for powerful pinch and grasp
- Explore the forces to which the digits are subjected during pinch and grasp
- Consider how the forces generated during pinch and grasp can contribute to deformities in the hand

PREHENSION

Prehension pattern is an important defining characteristic of humans. Humans with the ability to oppose the thumb to the fingers exhibit a wide variety of grasping patterns that are typically classified by the position of the fingers and the area of contact between the fingers, thumb, and object grasped. Napier offers the classic description of prehensile patterns [48]. Prehension is classified generally as either pinch or grasp. Pinch is a prehensile pattern that involves the thumb and the distal aspects of the index and/or long finger (*Fig. 19.1*). It is used primarily for precision and fine manipulation. In contrast, grasp typically involves all of the hand, including the digits and the palm [31] (*Fig. 19.2*). Although this classification oversimplifies the enormous variety of prehensile patterns used in daily life, it is a useful means of investigating the basic requirements of each pattern.

The factors distinguishing pinch from grasp are

- Area of contact within the hand
- Number of fingers involved in the activity
- Amount of finger flexion
- Position of the thumb
- Position of the wrist

The following presents the essential elements of pinch and grasp and examines some of the variations available in each pattern.

Necessary Elements of Pinch

Pinch is used for precise manipulation of relatively small objects such as a needle or pen. It may be used in delicate handling of a fragile wing of a butterfly or the powerful twisting of a key in a stubborn lock. Despite the wide variety of

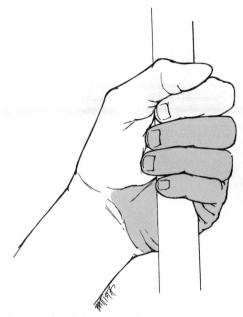

Figure 19.2: Grasp uses all of the digits and the palm.

applications of the pinch, certain characteristics exist. Pinch typically uses the radial side of the hand, primarily the thumb, index, and long fingers. The thumb moves away from the fingers but turns toward them in opposition. The thumb then can hold an object securely against the stable post of the index and long fingers. The thumb's position depends largely on the mobility of its carpometacarpal (CMC) joint, while the relative immobility of the CMC articulation of the index and long fingers provides them the necessary stability to resist the forces from the thumb. It is important to recall that the CMC articulations of the index and long fingers are the least mobile in the hand. This lack of mobility allows these fingers to remain relatively fixed as the thumb pushes against them during pinch.

During pinch, the thumb and fingers assume rather stereotypical positions that are described below. The muscles used to achieve and maintain these positions are then presented. Finally, the effects on the mechanics of pinch when any of the digits is unable to achieve the appropriate position are discussed.

REQUIREMENTS OF NORMAL PINCH

Humans use a wide variety of pinch types (*Fig. 19.3*). Inspection of the basic positions used in the tip-to-tip pinch helps identify the requirements of normal pinch. Tip-to-tip pinch is described as the pinch that forms an "O" between the thumb and a finger, usually the index or long finger (*Fig. 19.4*). It brings the very tips of the digits together and is used to pick up a pin or tiny seed from a table. *Table 19.1* lists the position of the joints of the finger and thumb during tip-to-tip pinch. The wrist maintains a position of extension in most pinch activities.

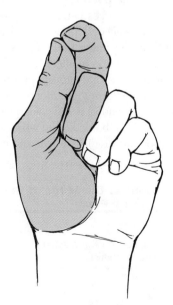

Figure 19.1: Pinch uses the digits on the radial side of the hand.

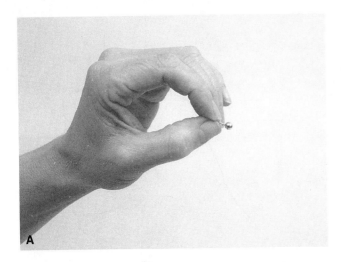

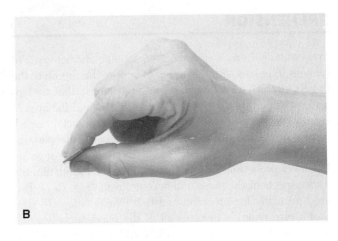

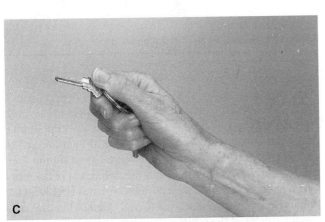

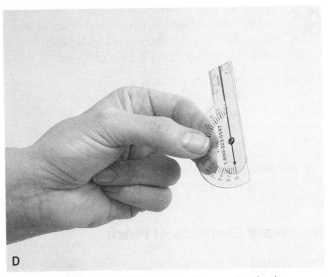

Figure 19.3: Pinch patterns include **(A)** tip-to-tip, **(B)** pulp-to-pulp, **(C)** lateral, or key, pinch, and **(D)** chuck, or three-point chuck.

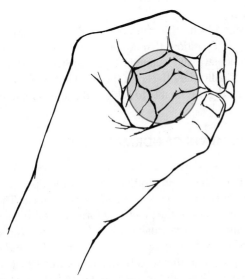

Figure 19.4: Tip-to-tip pinch forms an "O" between the thumb and index finger.

An examination of the positions used in tip-to-tip pinch and consideration of the forces between the opposing digits help explain the muscles needed for normal pinch (*Fig. 19.5*). The DIP joint of the index finger flexes against the thumb as the thumb applies an extension moment to the DIP joint. The index finger requires the flexor digitorum profundus to maintain this position, and the flexor digitorum profundus requires that the wrist remain extended to have adequate contractile length (Chapter 15). Thus the dedicated wrist extensors, particularly the extensor carpi radialis brevis and extensor carpi

TABLE 19.1: Positions of the Joints of the Thumb and Finger in Tip-to-Tip Pinch

	Thumb	Finger
CMC joint	Opposition and extension (radial abduction)	—
MCP joint	Flexion	Flexion
IP (PIP) joint	Flexion	Flexion
DIP joint	—	Flexion

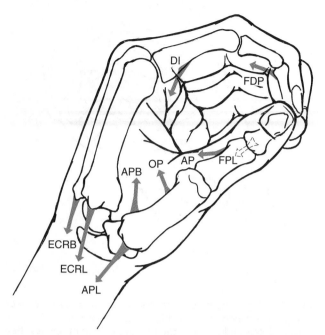

Figure 19.5: Muscles required for tip-to-tip pinch include the dedicated wrist extensors, extensor carpi radialis longus (*ECRL*) and brevis (*ECRB*), the flexor digitorum profundus (*FDP*), the flexor pollicis longus (*FPL*), the abductor pollicis longus (*APL*), the abductor pollicis brevis (*APB*), the opponens pollicis (*OP*), the adductor pollicis (*AP*), and the first dorsal interosseous muscle (*DI*).

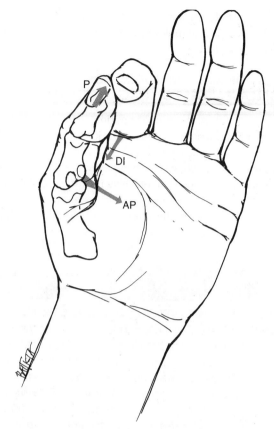

Figure 19.6: The adductor pollicis (*AP*) applies an ulnarly directed force on the index finger, tending to adduct the finger. This adduction is counteracted by the abduction pull of the first dorsal interosseous muscle (*DI*).

ulnaris, are active during pinch [12,38,41]. Similarly, flexion of the interphalangeal (IP) joint of the thumb demands the activity of the flexor pollicis longus [15]. The CMC joint of the thumb then must be stabilized in extension by the abductor pollicis longus against the pull of the flexor pollicis longus as described in Chapter 15 [9,14,58].

Additional intrinsic muscles are essential to normal pinch. The abductor pollicis brevis, the primary abductor of the thumb, is active to position the thumb in abduction (palmar abduction) and medial rotation. The opponens pollicis also helps to position the thumb during pinch [15,19]. Careful observation of the thumb's position relative to the index finger helps to explain the roles of the remaining two intrinsic muscles. Even in tip-to-tip pinch the thumb lies slightly radial to the index finger, exerting an ulnarly directed force on the index finger. The adductor pollicis muscle is perfectly situated to pull the thumb toward the index finger, particularly by flexing the metacarpophalangeal (MCP) joint of the thumb (*Fig. 19.6*). Its size and large moment arm makes the adductor pollicis the most important flexor of the MCP joint. Hence the adductor pollicis is an essential muscle of pinch, particularly in forceful pinch [15,29].

As the thumb exerts a force on the index finger in the ulnar direction, the index finger is pushed ulnarly at the MCP joint. Consequently, the remaining essential muscle in pinch is the first dorsal interosseous muscle. This muscle stabilizes the index finger, preventing ulnar deviation at the MCP joint [15].

To summarize, the thumb muscles essential to a normal tip-to-tip pinch are the flexor pollicis longus, abductor pollicis longus, abductor pollicis brevis, opponens pollicis, and adductor pollicis. At the index finger, the flexor digitorum profundus and first dorsal interosseous muscles are critical to a normal pinch.

The other types of pinch present only minor variations of the requirements of the tip-to-tip pinch. Pulp-to-pulp pinch uses less DIP joint flexion. Consequently, the role of the flexor digitorum profundus may decrease if the individual uses the volar plate to prevent hyperextension. The flexor digitorum superficialis may assume the role of flexor of the PIP and MCP joints. The key, or lateral, pinch and the chuck, or three-jaw chuck, pinches use at least three digits, the thumb, and the index and long fingers. Therefore, these types of pinch are stronger and are used when power is more important than precision [25]. The joint positions and muscle requirements in these forms of pinch are similar to those of tip-to-tip and pulp-to-pulp pinch. Simulations of nerve injuries in cadaver models and in healthy volunteers with temporary, sequential nerve blocks of the median and ulnar nerves at the wrist reveal a 60–77% loss in pinch strength with an ulnar nerve palsy and a 60% loss with a median nerve palsy [36,57]. These data demonstrate the critical contribution to pinch strength made by the intrinsic muscles, even in the presence of intact extrinsic musculature.

EFFECTS OF ABNORMAL JOINT POSITIONS AND MUSCLE WEAKNESS ON PINCH MECHANICS

Inability to achieve the proper position at the thumb or fingers has a chain reaction on the other joints of the digits during pinch because the central goal of pinch remains to hold or manipulate a small object. During pinch, the thumb and fingers function in a closed kinetic chain, with the distal end of each digit fixed. The joints and muscles accommodate in a variety of ways to keep the thumb in contact with the finger and support the object.

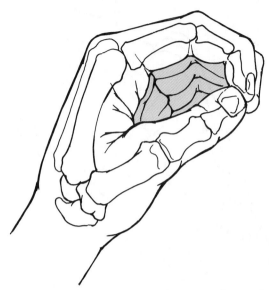

Figure 19.7: Tip-to-tip pinch with inadequate web space between the thumb and index finger exhibits altered positions of both digits, with less abduction of the thumb's CMC joint and less flexion at the finger's MCP joint.

Clinical Relevance

INSUFFICIENT WEB SPACE BETWEEN THE THUMB AND INDEX FINGER: A CASE REPORT: *A student found a growing lump in the web space between the thumb and index finger. The lump was diagnosed as a cyst and was removed surgically. The surgery was more extensive than expected because the cyst had an extensive blood supply. Following the surgery and 3 weeks of immobilization, the patient exhibited a significant scar and limited abduction and extension range of motion (ROM) of the CMC joint of the thumb. The joint end-feel during passive ROM was consistent with soft tissue stretch with no apparent joint capsular restriction, although the joint ROM was limited. The patient reported a pulling discomfort in the scar. The conclusion was that the patient's limited ROM was due to scar formation and inadequate extensibility of the skin in the web space between the thumb and index finger.*

The patient's inability to abduct the CMC joint of the thumb resulted in an abnormal pinch pattern. The pinch was characterized by slight thumb CMC extension and abduction, slight hyperextension of the MCP joint of the thumb, and excessive flexion of the IP joint of the thumb (Fig. 19.7). The index finger exhibited increased flexion of the proximal interphalangeal (PIP) and distal interphalangeal (DIP) joints, with less flexion at the MCP joint. The space bounded by the thumb and index finger was an oval rather than the typical "O" of tip-to-tip pinch. The patient was treated with stretching, gentle soft tissue massage, and splinting. Full ROM and normal function were restored after approximately 3 months.

lead to inability to position the CMC joint properly. Even the presence of long fingernails can alter the relative positions of the fingers and thumb during pinch (*Fig. 19.8*). In any of these cases the thumb lacks the ability to move into sufficient abduction and extension to bring the tip of the thumb to the tip of the index finger. Consequently, to accomplish pinch, the individual alters the position of the other joints of the thumb. In the case report, the individual responded with hyperextension of the MCP joint of the thumb. Other individuals may respond with flexion of the

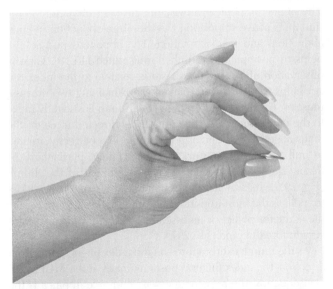

Figure 19.8: Long fingernails alter the positions of the thumb and index finger in pinch.

There are many reasons for abnormal positioning of the CMC joint of the thumb during pinch. These can include weakness of the abductor pollicis longus so that the individual is unable to stabilize the CMC joint of the thumb against the pull of the flexor pollicis longus. Intrinsic weakness with a resulting ape thumb deformity also affects CMC joint position. Instability secondary to arthritic changes can also

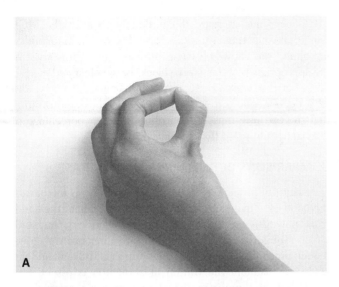

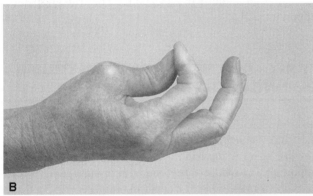

Figure 19.9: Compensation in pinch pattern resulting from limited ROM in the thumb. Different pinch patterns can result from inadequate abduction and extension at the thumb's CMC joint. Both photos reveal limited abduction at the thumb's CMC joint; however, the positions of the MCP and IP joints differ. **A.** Pinch is characterized by hyperextension of the thumb's MCP joint and excessive flexion of the IP joint. **B.** Pinch is characterized by hyperextension of the thumb's IP joint with flexion of the MCP joint.

MCP joint and hyperextension of the IP joint (*Fig. 19.9*). The compensation depends on the available ROMs at the remaining joints. The important element for the clinician to recognize is that the position of the thumb's CMC joint is critical to normal pinch mechanics. Abnormalities at this joint are reflected in the rest of the joints of the participating digits.

Necessary Elements of Powerful Grasp

Powerful grasp is distinguished from pinch by several factors. Grasp uses more of the volar surface of the palm and fingers. It generally uses all of the digits of the hand and, consequently, produces more-forceful prehension. As in pinch, the positions of the digits are somewhat predictable but vary slightly with the type of grasp used.

REQUIREMENTS OF NORMAL POWERFUL GRASP

Like patterns of pinch, patterns of grasp are diverse and serve a variety of purposes (*Fig. 19.10*). The size of the object grasped also affects the grasp pattern. However, certain basic characteristics of grasp exist. The finger joints generally are more flexed than in pinch, and the ulnar fingers exhibit more flexion than the radial fingers. This increased finger flexion on the ulnar side along with the volar arch formed by the movement of the CMC articulations of the little and ring fingers draws the grasped object toward the thumb and clamps it firmly in the palm of the hand (*Fig. 19.11*).

Another distinguishing characteristic of powerful grasp is the position of the thumb. The thumb tends to flex over the fingers and is pulled toward the palm. The CMC joint may remain in a position of slight abduction but less than in pinch. The adductor pollicis forcefully contracts to pull the thumb onto the fingers and object.

The force of the grasp has a significant effect on the characteristics of the grasp. In general, an increase in the force of grasp is accompanied by an increase in the following:

- Flexion of the fingers, particularly at the MCP joints
- Participation of the ulnar side of the hand and the use of the volar arch
- Contact area between the object and the fingers and palm

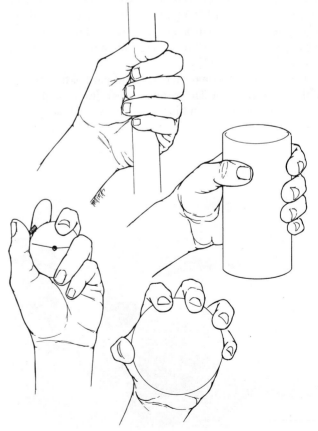

Figure 19.10: Different patterns of grasp demonstrate varied amounts of finger flexion and contact with the palm, leading to varied amounts of grasp force.

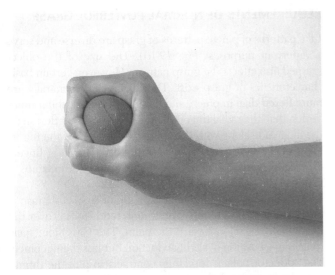

Figure 19.11: Powerful grasp compresses the object into the thenar eminence where the object is covered by the thumb.

Wrist position is more variable in powerful grasp. When making a tight fist, the wrist is extended using the synergy between the dedicated wrist extensor muscles and the finger flexors described in Chapter 15. However, in many forceful activities, the wrist functions in neutral or even slight flexion with ulnar deviation [44,52]. This position aligns the radial side of the hand with the long axis of the forearm. Such positioning is found in activities such as cutting meat or turning a screwdriver (*Fig. 19.12*).

Powerful grasp requires the efforts of most of the muscles of the wrist and hand. The extrinsic finger flexors produce IP flexion. The interossei and lumbricals assist in flexion of the

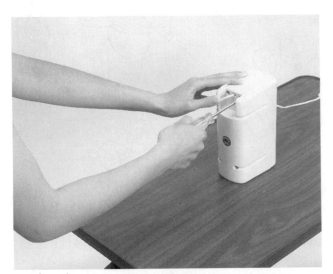

Figure 19.12: Powerful grasp without wrist extension. In some powerful grasps the wrist is in ulnar deviation and neutral flexion, thus aligning the hand with the long axis of the forearm.

MCP joints and increase the flexion moment at the MCP joints. The hypothenar muscles form the volar arch for added force, and the dedicated wrist muscles stabilize the wrist in the appropriate position. Nerve blocks of the ulnar and median nerves at the wrist in healthy individuals produce 38% and 32% decreases in grip strength, respectively, demonstrating that the extrinsic muscles contribute a larger percentage of the strength in grasp than in pinch [36].

COMPARISONS BETWEEN PINCH AND GRASP

The major difference between pinch and grasp is the part of the hand used in each. Pinch uses the radial side of the hand, while powerful grasp depends on the ulnar side of the hand. Greater finger flexion ROM is required in powerful grasp than in pinch. The integrity of the thumb's CMC joint and the ability to maintain the thumb in abduction is essential to pinch, but the thumb's participation in powerful grasp also is important [10].

FORCES ON THE FINGERS AND THUMB DURING ACTIVITIES

An understanding of the forces applied to the structures of the hand is essential to understanding many of the deformities that occur in the hand. An appreciation of these loads is important to avoid loads that can undermine a patient's rehabilitation. For example, the clinician must recognize activities that can disrupt a tendon repair or contribute to joint instability and deformity. This section reviews the analysis used to derive the muscle and joint reaction forces in the digits. The available data reported in the literature regarding these forces are also presented. Finally, the application of these data to typical clinical problems is demonstrated.

Analysis of the Forces in the Fingers

Several investigators have analyzed the forces on the joints and in the muscles of the fingers and thumb during pinch and grasp [2,3,7,8,11,13,20–22,27,40,50,55,57,60]. With the exception of the DIP joint of the fingers and the IP joint of the thumb, several muscles contract simultaneously at each joint during pinch and grasp (*Fig. 19.13*). Consideration of the moments created during pinch helps explain the need for activity of so many muscles. *Examining the Forces Box 19.1* demonstrates the moment applied to the DIP, PIP, and MCP joints of the index finger during tip-to-tip pinch. The pinch force creates an extension moment at each finger joint that increases from distal to proximal. Therefore, the flexion moments needed to stabilize the joints also must increase from distal to proximal [13,18,30,50], which helps explain why there are more muscles available to flex the MCP joint than at the other joints of the fingers [40]. Electromyographic (EMG) data reveal activity in all of these flexors during forceful pinch and grasp [14,19,53].

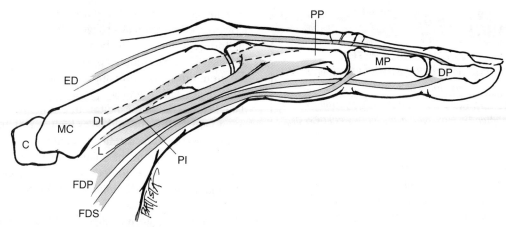

Figure 19.13: The muscles available to flex and extend the joints of the fingers include flexor digitorum profundus (*FDP*), flexor digitorum superficialis (*FDS*), extensor digitorum (*ED*), palmar interossei (*PI*), dorsal interossei (*DI*), and lumbricals (*L*).

EXAMINING THE FORCES BOX 19.1

THE GENERAL MOMENT EQUATION AT EACH FINGER IS:

$$\Sigma M = 0$$

$$M_{internal} + M_{external} = 0$$

where $M_{internal}$ is the moment created by the muscles and ligaments at each joint and $M_{external}$ is the moment generated by the pinch force.

$$M_{internal} = F_m \times x_i$$

where x_i is the perpendicular distance between each muscle force (F_m) and each joint.

$$M_{external} = F_p \times d_i$$

where d_i is the perpendicular distance between the pinch force (P) and the joint (i).

At the DIP the equation becomes

$$(P \times d_1) + (F_{FDP} \times x_{FDP}) = 0$$

At the PIP the equation becomes

$$(P \times d_2) + (F_{FDP} \times x_{FDP}) + (F_{FDS} \times x_{FDS}) = 0$$

At the MCP the equation becomes

$$(P \times d_3) + (F_{FDP} \times x_{FDP}) + (F_{FDS} \times x_{FDS}) + (F_I \times x_I) = 0$$

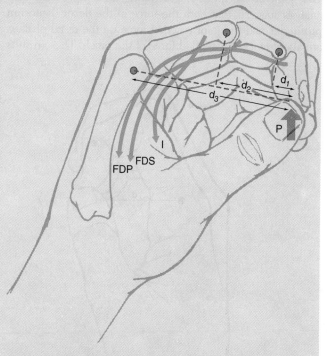

The extension moments from the applied load (*P*) on the joints of the fingers during pinch increase from distal to proximal. The moment arms of the applied load at the DIP, PIP, and MCP joints are d_1, d_2, and d_3, respectively. *FDP*, flexor digitorum profundus; *FDS*, flexor digitorum superficialis; *I*, intrinsic muscles.

Clinical Relevance

PINCH PATTERNS IN INDIVIDUALS WITH WEAKNESS OF THE INTRINSIC MUSCLES: *Patients with significant weakness of the intrinsic muscles of the hand demonstrate the claw hand and ape thumb deformities described in Chapter 18. However, even slight weakness of these muscles impairs the individual's ability to generate a forceful pinch. Because a forceful pinch produces a large extension moment at the MCP joint of the finger, both the intrinsic and extrinsic muscles are needed to create sufficient flexion moment to balance this external moment at the MCP joint. Decreasing the flexion angle at the MCP joint reduces the moment arm of the pinch force and the extension moment applied at the MCP joint (Fig. 19.14). Individuals with even slight-to-moderate weakness of the intrinsic muscles typically pinch with the MCP joint of the finger in extension, effectively reducing the flexion moment needed at the MCP joint.*

Examining the Forces Box 19.2 presents the free-body diagram and the two-dimensional analysis of the forces at the DIP joint of the index finger during tip-to-tip pinch. This analysis suggests that both the force in the flexor digitorum profundus and the joint reaction force on the distal phalanx are about twice the applied force of the pinch. These results

are consistent with results reported in the literature [2,21,60]. However, other estimates suggest that the force in the flexor digitorum profundus may be more than four times the force of pinch [13]. Maximum tip-to-tip pinch forces reported in the literature range from approximately 60 to 120 N (13–27 lb) in males, less in females [17,25,39,45,61]. Based on these data, loads in the flexor digitorum profundus and on the joint are at least 25 lb but could be as high as 200 lb.

Because the force within a tendon is constant along its full length, the data from the solution in Examining the Forces Box 19.2 can be used to determine the muscle forces at the PIP and MCP joints. *Examining the Forces Box 19.3* presents the free-body diagrams and simplified solutions for the forces in the flexor digitorum superficialis and intrinsic muscle group at these joints. The moment arms for the muscles at each joint are based on data found in the literature [1,34]. This example demonstrates the need for additional flexor muscles at each succeeding proximal joint because of the increasing moment exerted by the pinch force.

Review of the Forces Generated during Pinch and Grasp

More complex models than those presented in Examining the Forces Boxes 19.2 and 19.3 allow approximations of the loads in the muscles and ligaments and on the joints of the fingers and thumb. Estimates of the compressive forces on the finger joints vary but increase in magnitude from distal to proximal, since the moment from the external force is increasing [2,13,50]. The types of grasp and the force of the grasp also influence the muscle and joint forces. Lateral, or key, pinch reportedly generates larger muscle and joint reaction forces in the index finger than other forms of pinch [2]. Estimates of compressive loads at the DIP joint during key pinch are as high as 12 times the pinch force [2]. Estimates of the maximum axial loads at the PIP joint during pinch range from 3 to almost 20 times the pinch force [2,7,13,50]. Estimates of the maximal compressive loads at the MCP joint are even greater, ranging from 4 to 27 times the force of pinch.

Generally, evidence suggests that the joint reaction forces on the fingers in grasp exceed those of pinch [2,8,13]. However, the type of grasp and the resulting joint position significantly affects the loads on the joints. For example, a hook grasp in which the MCP joints remain extended and the DIP joints bear no load appears to produce smaller compressive forces on all of the joints of the fingers than any other pinch or grasp pattern studied [2] (*Fig. 19.15*). These findings are consistent with the analysis presented in Examining the Forces Box 19.3, in which the moment arm of the applied load has a dramatic effect on the moments required by the muscles and, ultimately, on the joint reaction forces. Estimates of the loads in the fingers reported by An et al. [2] and by Purves and Berme [50] during a simulation of opening a jar lid are reported in *Table 19.2*.

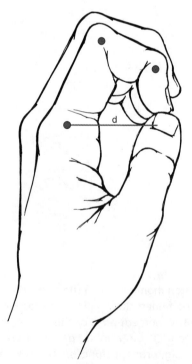

Figure 19.14: Less flexion of the MCP joint reduces the extension moment exerted on the MCP joint by the pinch force by decreasing its moment arm (*d*).

EXAMINING THE FORCES BOX 19.2

CALCULATION OF THE FORCES AT THE DIP JOINT DURING PINCH

M_P moment due to the FDP

F   force applied by the flexor digitorum profundus (FDP)

x   moment arm of the FDP (0.65 cm)

P   pinch force (6 kg)

1.2 cm   moment arm of the pinch force at the DIP

10°   FDP angle of pull

$\Sigma M = 0$

$M_P - (P \times 1.2 \text{ cm}) = 0$

$(F \times x) - (P \times 1.2 \text{ cm}) = 0$

$F = (6 \text{ kg} \times 1.2 \text{ cm}) / 0.65 \text{ cm}$

$F = 11 \text{ kg}$

$\Sigma F_X: \quad J_X + F_X = 0$

$\quad\quad J_X - F \times (\cos 10°) = 0$

$\quad\quad J_X = F \times (\cos 10°)$

$\quad\quad J_X = 10.8 \text{ kg}$

$\Sigma F_Y: \quad J_Y + 6.0 \text{ kg} - F \times (\sin 10°) = 0$

$\quad\quad J_Y = F \times (\sin 10°) - 6.0 \text{ kg}$

$\quad\quad J_Y = -4.1 \text{ kg}$

Using the Pythagorean theorem:

$J^2 = J_X^2 + J_Y^2$

$J \approx 11.5 \text{ kg}$ (approximately 2 times the applied load)

$\sin \alpha = -4.1/11.5$

$\alpha \cong 20°$ from x axis

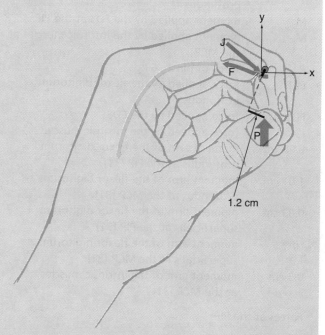

The free-body diagram to calculate the forces at the DIP joint during tip-to-tip pinch identifies the pinch force (*P*), the force in the flexor digitorum profundus (*F*), and the joint reaction force (*J*).

Clinical Relevance

OCCUPATIONAL HAZARDS: *The piano is played by striking the piano keys with the fingertips. Contact with the key is sometimes very soft (pianissimo) but also can be crashing (fortissimo). Professional pianists can develop severe hand problems including tendinitis and joint pain. Studies using models similar to those noted earlier report tendon forces of about three times the force on the keys and joint reaction forces up to seven times the key force [26]. Investigators offer suggestions of wrist and finger positions to minimize the forces on the soft tissue and joints. Musicians are artists, and the physical demands of their profession are rarely appreciated. Recognition of the mechanical stresses of*

playing some instruments may help the clinician direct treatment toward reducing joint stresses and identifying joint protection strategies. Similar approaches are beneficial in assessing the demands of any manual activity, including computer operation, molding pottery, or cutting meat.

Although the data reported in the literature are varied and are only estimates based on mathematical models, they consistently demonstrate that the fingers sustain significant loads during daily activities such as turning a key, playing the piano, turning a water faucet, and opening a jar [2,26,50]. The magnitude of the load on a joint is important, but how that load is distributed across the joint surface also is important. The data

EXAMINING THE FORCES BOX 19.3

CALCULATIONS OF THE FORCES AT THE PIP AND MCP JOINTS DURING PINCH

d_3	the lengths of the moment arms of the pinch force
M_P	moment applied by the flexor digitorum profundus
M_S	moment applied by the FDS at the PIP
M_I	moment applied by the intrinsic muscles at the MCP
P	force of pinch, 6 kg
FDP	force applied by the flexor digitorum profundus
FDS	force applied by the FDS
I	force applied by the intrinsic muscles
0.98 cm	moment arm of the flexor digitorum profundus at the PIP [31]
1.01 cm	moment arm of the flexor digitorum profundus at the MCP [31]
0.83 cm	moment arm of the flexor digitorum superficialis at the PIP [31]
cm	moment arm of the flexor digitorum superficialis at the MCP [31]
0.3 cm	moment arm of the intrinsic muscles at the MCP [31]

Forces at the PIP:

$$\Sigma M = 0$$

$$M_P + M_S - (P \times d_3) = 0$$
$$(11.0 \text{ kg} \times 0.98 \text{ cm}) + M_S - (P \times d_3) = 0$$

where 11.0 kg is the force in the FDP calculated in Examining the Forces Box 19.2

$$d_3 = 2.5 \text{ cm}$$
$$10.8 \text{ kg-cm} + M_S - (6.0 \text{ kg} \times 2.5 \text{ cm}) = 0$$
$$M_S = 15.0 \text{ kg-cm} - 10.8 \text{ kg-cm}$$
$$M_S = 4.2 \text{ kg-cm}$$
$$FDS \times 0.83 \text{ cm} = 4.2 \text{ kg-cm}$$
$$FDS = 5.1 \text{ kg}$$

Forces at the MCP:

$$\Sigma M = 0$$
$$M_P + M_S + M_I - (P \times d_3) = 0$$

Using the force of the flexor digitorum superficialis (FDS) calculated above:

$$(11.0 \text{ kg} \times 1.01 \text{ cm}) + (5.1 \text{ kg} \times 1.21 \text{ cm}) + M_I - (P \times d_3) = 0$$
$$d_3 = 4.1 \text{ cm}$$
$$\text{kg-cm} + 6.2 \text{ kg-cm} + M_I - (6.0 \text{ kg} \times 4.1 \text{ cm}) = 0$$
$$M_I = 7.6 \text{ kg-cm}$$
$$I \times 0.3 \text{ cm} = 7.6 \text{ kg-cm}$$
$$I = 25.3 \text{ kg}$$

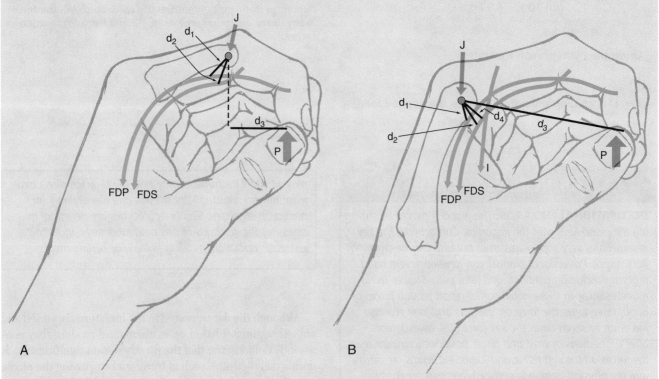

The free-body diagram identifies the forces at the **(A)** PIP joint and at the **(B)** MCP joint during pinch. The lengths of the distal, middle, and proximal phalanges are 1.2 cm, 1.6 cm, and 2.4 cm, respectively.

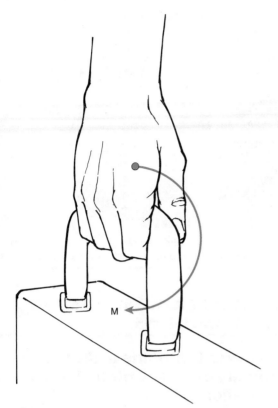

Figure 19.15: A hook grasp produces smaller joint reaction forces at the finger joints because smaller muscle forces are needed to balance the decreased extension moment (M) applied by the briefcase at the MCP joint.

thus far demonstrate that the compressive loads increase from the distal to the proximal joints of the fingers. Analysis of contact areas reveals that the area of contact at the three joints of the index finger decreases from proximal to distal so that the joint reaction forces are distributed over a smaller area at the distal joints than at the proximal joints [38]. Since **stress** is the amount of force applied to an area (force/area), this finding suggests that the stress on the joint increases from proximal to distal. Thus although the joint reaction forces are greatest in the MCP joints, the stresses on the joint appear to be greatest in the DIP joints.

TABLE 19.2: Reported Joint Reaction Forces Generated at the PIP and MCP Joints when Twisting a Jar Lid

	Direction	An et al. [2][a]	Purves and Berme [50][b]
PIP joint	Compressive	7.2–14.2	18.0 ± 13.6
	Dorsal	2.4–4.9	41.6 ± 27.6
	Radial	0.2–0.8	15.5 ± 16.0
MCP joint	Compressive	14.8–24.3	45.2 ± 27.1
	Dorsal	6.5–9.9	15.8 ± 15.5
	Radial	0.2–0.3	12.5 ± 11.4

[a]Reported in units of applied force.
[b]Reported in newtons, mean ± standard deviation, from 10 male and 10 female subjects.

DEGENERATIVE JOINT DISEASE IN THE HAND:
Degenerative joint disease (DJD) of the fingers is most common in the DIP joints and relatively rare in the MCP joints [28,46,47]. Although the link between joint stress and DJD is not clearly identified, data suggest a positive connection between the magnitude of stress to which a joint is subjected and the incidence of DJD [4,5]. The data reported on joint stresses in the fingers support this connection. The joints with the highest stress are the joints that have the greatest incidence of DJD in the hand. Additional research is needed to verify these findings, but the clinician should use these data to implement joint protection strategies with individuals at risk for DJD in the hands.

Models applied to the joints of the thumb also demonstrate large muscle forces and increasing joint reaction forces from distal to proximal. Results are also variable, with joint reaction forces ranging from 2 to 24 times the applied load [7,16,22,27,55]. One study reports that the average maximum external load exerted by the thumb in 70 male subjects (average age, 27 years old) is 20 lb (89 N). This suggests that the thumb joints could sustain reaction forces of almost 500 lb (more than 2000 N). The clinician must keep these values in mind and help to identify individuals at risk of hand pathology. In addition, the clinician can use the perspective gained from such studies to assist individuals in modifying activities to reduce the loads on the thumb and fingers.

Studies of the contact areas at the thumb's CMC joint suggest that contact during pinch occurs over a very small area, leading to very large stresses. The areas of large stress coincide with the sites of significant degenerative change. Thus as in the fingers, stress on the thumb may be associated with degenerative joint diseases [4,5].

Many activities have evolved using unusual finger and thumb positions that while commonly accepted are likely to generate large stresses on the small joints of the hands. For example, flautists often assume positions of extreme hyperextension of the index finger's MCP joint or hyperextension of the thumb's IP joint [35] (*Fig. 19.16*). Individuals performing manual deep tissue massage often use end range hyperextension in finger and thumb joints as their finger flexors fatigue or are too weak to generate adequate force for the massage (*Fig. 19.17*). Such positions alter the contact area of the articulating joint surfaces and typically decrease the total area of contact. Consequently, the joint loads are applied over smaller surfaces and produce increased joint stress. Although the user may feel that such joint positions are the most efficient positions, perhaps even the "proper" position, prolonged use of such extreme positions may lead to overuse syndromes and ultimately to degenerative changes within the joint surfaces. The clinician can play an important role in prevention of joint injuries by helping the individual to understand the

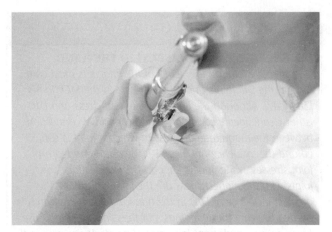

Figure 19.16: Playing the flute often requires extreme positions of the thumb and/or index finger.

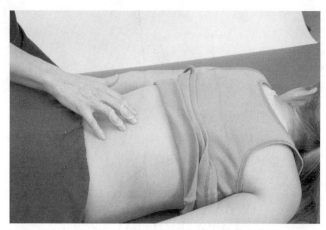

Figure 19.18: A finger splint can protect the fingers from hyperextension during strong pressure such as while giving a massage.

relationship among joint position, joint stress, and joint degeneration, and then assisting the individual to adapt the activity to utilize joint positions that maximize contact area.

Clinical Relevance

FINGER SPLINTS TO OPTIMIZE JOINT ALIGNMENT:
Sometimes an individual is incapable of maintaining good joint alignment throughout an activity. Perhaps maintaining good alignment requires such concentration that the individual is too distracted from the primary activity. Perhaps the individual lacks the muscle strength or endurance to maintain the good alignment for the length of the activity. In such cases, the individual may be best protected by using external supports to maintain the desired position. Simple finger splints are often used by manual therapists themselves to support their fingers while applying deep tissue massages (Fig. 19.18). Such devices can prevent joint pain and fatigue and ultimately may help protect the joint from degenerative joint disease by decreasing prolonged episodes of high joint stress.

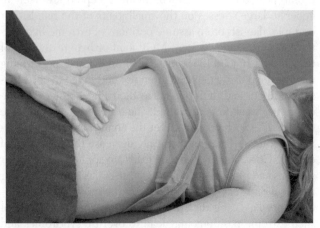

Figure 19.17: Extreme finger positions during massage. Deep tissue massage requires strong pressure through the fingers and often results in hyperextension in finger or thumb joints.

USING FORCE ANALYSIS TO MAKE CLINICAL DECISIONS

How Forces Contribute to the Finger Deformity of Ulnar Drift with Volar Subluxation

The data from the literature thus far focuses primarily on the compressive forces on the joint surfaces. Studies also demonstrate significant forces during both pinch and grasp that pull the fingers in a volar and ulnar direction. These forces are particularly apparent at the MCP joints and contribute to the MCP deformity common in individuals with rheumatoid arthritis. There are many more flexor muscles of the MCP joint than extensor muscles, and these muscles, particularly the extrinsic finger flexors, sustain large forces during pinch and grasp. The normal angle of pull of the flexor tendons is small [34]. Therefore under normal conditions, most of the pull of the flexor tendons is directed parallel to the adjacent phalanx, and only a small component exerts a volar force (*Fig. 19.19*). If the tendon bowstrings, however, its angle of pull increases, and the tendon exerts a larger volar force.

In rheumatoid arthritis affecting the MCP joint, the inflammatory process can lead to laxity in the joint capsule and surrounding ligaments [23]. Even the A1 pulley supporting the tendons at the MCP joint may weaken [53]. Once the pulley is weakened, the pull of the tendons within the pulley contributes to the stretch of the pulley. As the pulley stretches, the tendons begin to bowstring, increasing the volar pull on the proximal phalanx. Because the joint is unstable as a result of the changes in the capsule and ligaments, the proximal phalanx begins to migrate volarly. At the same time, as the pulley loosens, the flexor tendons are able to slip sideways, typically in the ulnar direction [53]. Once the tendons have displaced in the ulnar direction, active contraction of the flexors produces an ulnar pull across the MCP joint (*Fig. 19.20*). Because the joint is unstable, the proximal phalanx migrates in an ulnar direction as it migrates volarly, and the deformity of **ulnar drift** with volar subluxation begins

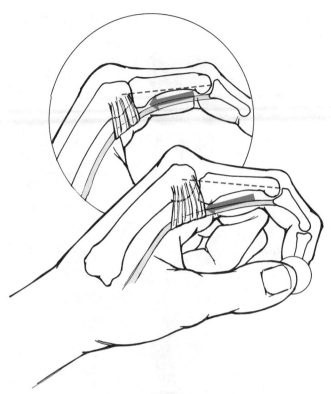

Figure 19.19: Under normal conditions, the pull of the flexor tendons is almost parallel to the long axis of the finger (*inset*). When a tendon bowstrings, its pull exerts a pull that has a component parallel to the phalanx and another significant component aimed in a volar direction.

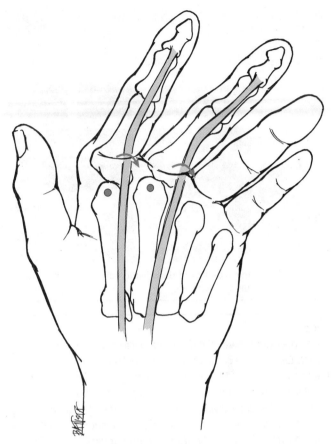

Figure 19.20: Ulnar pull of a subluxed flexor tendon. Once the flexor tendons are displaced, their pull increases the forces pulling the fingers into ulnar deviation.

(*Fig. 19.21*). The tendons of the extensor digitorum also can slide ulnarly and contribute additional deforming forces.

There are additional predisposing factors that contribute to this classic deformity:

- The heads of the metacarpals are normally sloped, so that there is naturally more ROM in ulnar deviation than radial deviation [56,59].
- In many normal activities the fingers are pushed in an ulnar direction by external forces (*Fig. 19.22*).

These predisposing factors combined with the presence of joint instability resulting from the inflammatory process of rheumatoid arthritis and the deforming influence of the flexor tendons create a cascade of factors that can result in a disabling deformity.

Clinical Relevance

JOINT PROTECTION PRINCIPLES: *While some of the elements contributing to an ulnar drift deformity are immutable, others respond to intervention. First, control of the disease process itself is important. Disease-modifying medications and other treatments to decrease the inflammatory process in rheumatoid arthritis are increasingly successful, but*

(continued)

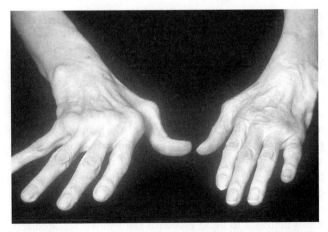

Figure 19.21: Ulnar deviation with volar subluxation of the MCP joints of the fingers in an individual with rheumatoid arthritis occurs when swelling destabilizes the joints and the tendons of the fingers migrate and exert a deforming force. (Reprinted from the AHPA Teaching Slide Collection Second Edition now known as the ARHP Assessment and Management of the Rheumatic Diseases: The Teaching Slide Collection for Clinicians and Educators. Copyright 1997. Used by permission of the American College of Rheumatology.)

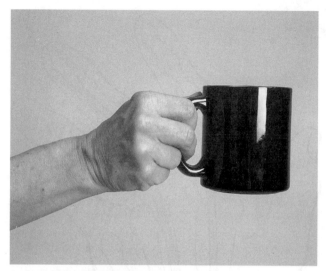

Figure 19.22: Many activities of daily living exert forces that push the fingers into ulnar deviation.

(Continued)

approaches to lessen the deforming factors also are important. Clinicians must be active in instructing patients to modify their activities to reduce the deforming forces of the external load. For example, the throttle-shaped handles on water faucets allow an individual to turn the water on and off using the palm of the hand rather than the fingers, which are pushed ulnarly by the standard tap handle (Fig. 19.23). Similarly, individuals can be instructed to carry items in the palm of the hand rather than in the fingers. Finally, clinicians should recognize the danger in exercises to strengthen the finger flexors, such as squeezing a ball. Such exercises are contraindicated for individuals with unstable MCP joints.

Protecting a Surgically Repaired Tendon in the Finger

The analysis of forces in the fingers during pinch and grasp indicates that the flexor tendons to the fingers can sustain large forces. Awareness of the forces sustained by tendons under various circumstances is critical as a patient resumes motion following a tendon repair. Early motion of the repaired tendon appears essential to enhance lubrication and avoid adhesions and scars that prevent normal excursion of the tendon. However, early motion of the tendon also risks disruption of the repair. The clinician must understand the strength of normal and healing tendons and must be able to adjust activities to avoid excessive loads in the repaired tendon. A detailed discussion of the strength of connective tissues including tendons is presented in Chapter 6.

The strength of different tendon repair techniques is extremely variable. Reported loads at which the repair begins to separate, or gap, range from approximately 5 to 50 N (1 to 10 lb), depending on suture technique [18,54]. Loads that produce complete disruption also depend on repair technique and range from less than 10 N to more than 100 N (2 to 20 lb).

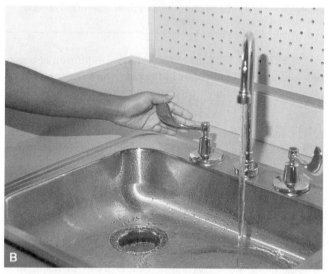

Figure 19.23: Simple changes in activities of daily living help to reduce ulnar forces on the fingers. **A.** Carrying objects in the palm instead of in the fingers reduces the ulnar forces. **B.** Use of push-pull controls on water faucets exerts smaller deforming forces than twist controls.

The goal of rehabilitation is to restore full tendon and joint function, which requires mobilizing the repaired tendon before it has regained its preinjury strength. The therapist responsible for rehabilitation must know how to move the joint and apply loads to the repairing tendon that will not disrupt the repair. In general, this requires that the clinician use active motion only in positions in which the repaired tendon remains on slack and recognize that most functional activities require tendon loads that far exceed the strength of the healing tendon.

Clinical Relevance

RECOMMENDATIONS FOR EARLY ACTIVE MOTION OF TENDON REPAIRS: *Most surgeons and therapists recommend early active motion of a tendon repair in the hand to facilitate tendon lubrication and excursion and limit the effects of scarring and adhesions. Mechanical analysis and review of clinical results suggest that active finger flexion with the wrist extended to 20° or active finger extension with the wrist flexed to 20° can be accomplished safely for flexor and extensor repairs, respectively [18]. Direct measurement of tendon forces reveals loads ranging from about 1 to 5 N (0.2 to 1.1 lb) in the flexor digitorum profundus and from 1 to 10 N (0.2 to 2.25 lb) in the flexor digitorum superficialis during active finger flexion with the wrist at neutral or in 30° of flexion [37]. The higher loads in the flexor digitorum superficialis occurred with the wrist flexed to 30°. Avoidance of extreme finger or wrist positions is necessary to prevent overloading of the repair site. Early mobilization of tendon repairs in the hand appears essential for a favorable outcome of the surgery. However, mobilization of a newly repaired tendon risks disruption of the repair. By appreciating the strength of the repair procedure as well as the loads generated during activity, the therapist can safely guide the patient in activities to enhance the healing process without endangering the integrity of the repair. Therefore, close consultation with the surgeon is essential during the planning and implementation of rehabilitation.*

Relationship between the Forces in the Finger Flexor Muscles and Carpal Tunnel Syndrome

Carpal tunnel syndrome (CTS) is a compression of the median nerve within the carpal tunnel. Symptoms include pain and paresthesia in the hand, particularly in the area of sensory distribution of the median nerve (see Fig. 18.24). Symptoms may also include weakness of the intrinsic muscles innervated by the median nerve. Although there is no clear understanding of the pathomechanics causing CTS, individuals in whom CTS is frequently observed include those whose jobs are characterized by repetitive, high-load manual tasks [42]. Elevated pressure within the carpal tunnel is a commonly proposed explanation for CTS. Pinch loads and finger press activities similar to typing correlate with elevated pressures within the carpal tunnel. These activities require activation of the extrinsic finger flexors, and increased recruitment of these muscles corresponds to increased symptoms in individuals

with CTS [32,51]. One theory to explain this relationship suggests that the tension on the flexor tendons produced by muscle contraction straightens the tendons in the carpal tunnel, causing increased compression of the median nerve [33]. Clinicians may help relieve symptoms by helping patients find ways to decrease the force of contraction in the finger flexor muscles. Prolonged positioning in wrist flexion also appears to pose greater risks of CTS than wrist extension [24]. Wrist flexion puts the finger flexors in a shortened position, which may require increased contraction force, leading to increased carpal tunnel pressures.

Clinical Relevance

CONSERVATIVE MANAGEMENT OF CTS: *Conservative management of CTS typically includes the use of splinting devices to support the wrist to allow muscle relaxation, and patient education to help the patient avoid activities that aggravate the symptoms. Data suggest that resting splints for the wrist should be positioned in slight flexion, but the patient should be taught to perform manual tasks with the wrist in slight extension. The clinician must remain aware of the possible connections between muscle force and pathology. This awareness will enable the clinician to analyze a patient's manual activities when there are complaints of CTS. Even a qualitative analysis of the mechanical requirements of a task may provide insight enabling the clinician to minimize the forces in the finger flexor muscles and thus reduce the compression on the median nerve.*

Forces Are Key in Ergonomic Assessments of Work-Related Musculoskeletal Disorders (WMSDs)

Work-related musculoskeletal disorders are injuries or disorders of the muscles, nerves, joints, and joint tissues that are related to the exposure to risk at work [6]. Many physically demanding jobs can put the worker at high risk for work-related musculoskeletal disorders (WMSDs). In order to decrease the incidence of WMSDs, biomechanists and ergonomists attempt to measure the forces required to perform a task and the number of times an individual can sustain that force safely. Then they create evaluations to identify individuals who can perform the task. For example, individuals who maintain the power lines in the electrical utility industry often must cut aluminum cable, typically 2 cm in diameter. Investigators have demonstrated that using long-handled manual cable cutters to cut a 2-cm cable requires a force on the handles of approximately 500 N (112 lb) [43]. These investigators suggest that less than 50% of the male population and less than 1% of the female population is strong enough to perform this task. Such demands help explain the high incidence of upper extremity WMSDs, including wrist sprains and carpal tunnel syndrome among these workers. Investigations such as these can help establish standards and guidelines for safe and efficient working conditions [49].

Clinical Relevance

FUNCTIONAL CAPACITY EVALUATIONS: *Occupational and physical therapists frequently perform functional capacity evaluations (FCEs) to determine if an individual has the physical capability to begin or return to a certain job. FCEs attempt to replicate or mimic the specific demands of the job in order to determine if the individual can perform the task safely. Being aware of the forces required of the job allows the therapist to specifically assess the individual's ability to perform the task the requisite number of times for successful employment. In the case of rehabilitation, it also allows the therapist to set clear targets for performance and construct a rehabilitation program to achieve those targets.*

SUMMARY

This chapter examines the joint and muscular requirements of pinch and grasp. Normal pinch uses the radial side of the hand and requires activity of intrinsic and extrinsic muscles of the thumb and index finger. Powerful grasp uses the ulnar side of the hand as well as the thumb and also requires intrinsic and extrinsic muscle activity.

A simple analysis of the forces sustained by the muscles and joints during pinch is described. Data from more-complex biomechanical models found in the literature are presented. These data, although varied, demonstrate that during grasp and pinch, the structures of the hand bear loads several times the prehensile load. Generally, loads are greater in grasp than in pinch. Areas of high stress in the fingers and thumb correspond to areas subject to osteoarthritis, suggesting a relationship between the loads sustained in the hand and degenerative changes within the hand. Clinical applications demonstrate how an awareness of the forces present in the structures of the hand during function can affect the integrity of the hand as well as influence the treatment approach.

References

1. An KN, Chao EY, Cooney WP III, Linscheid RL: Normative model of human hand for biomechanical analysis. J Biomech 1979; 12: 775–788.
2. An KN, Chao EY, Cooney WP III, Linscheid RL: Forces in the normal and abnormal hand. J Orthop Res 1985; 3: 202–211.
3. Andrews JG, Youm Y: A biomechanical investigation of wrist kinematics. J Biomech 1979; 12: 83–93.
4. Ateshian GA, Ark JW, Rosenwasser MP, et al.: Contact areas in the thumb carpometacarpal joint. J Orthop Res 1995; 13: 450–458.
5. Ateshian GA, Rosenwasser MP, Mow VC: Curvature characteristics and congruence of the thumb carpometacarpal joint: differences between female and male joints. J Biomech 1992; 25: 591–607.
6. Barr AE, Barbe MF, Clark BD: Work-related musculoskeletal disorders of the hand and wrist: epidemiology, pathophysiology, and sensorimotor changes. J Orthop Sports Phys Ther 2004; 34: 610–627.
7. Berme N: Forces transmitted by the finger and thumb joints. Acta Orthop Belg 1980; 46: 669–677.
8. Berme N, Paul JP, Purves WK: A biomechanical analysis of the metacarpophalangeal joint. J Biomech 1977; 10: 409–412.
9. Brand PW, Hollister A: Clinical Mechanics of the Hand. St. Louis, MO: Mosby-Year Book, 1999.
10. Brandsma JW: Manual muscle strength testing and dynamometry for bilateral ulnar neuropraxia in a surgeon. J Hand Ther 1995; 8: 191–194.
11. Brook N, Mizrahi J, Shoham M, Dayan J: A biomechanical model of index finger dynamics. Med Eng Phys 1995; 17: 54–63.
12. Buchanan TS, Moniz MJ, Dewald JPA, Rymer WZ: Estimation of muscle forces about the wrist joint during isometric tasks using an EMG coefficient method. J Biomech 1993; 26: 547–560.
13. Chao EY, Orpgrande JD, Axmear FE: Three-dimensional force analysis of finger joints in selected isometric hand functions. J Biomech 1976; 9: 387–396.
14. Close JR, Kidd CC: The functions of the muscles of the thumb, the index, and the long fingers. J Bone Joint Surg 1969; 51A: 1601–1620.
15. Cooney WP III, An KN, Daube JR, Askew LJ: Electromyographic analysis of the thumb: a study of isometric forces in pinch and grasp. J Hand Surg [Am] 1985; 10A: 202–210.
16. Cooney WP III, Chao EYS: Biomechanical analysis of static forces in the thumb during hand function. J Bone Joint Surg 1977; 59A: 27–36.
17. Crosby CA, Wehbe MA: Hand strength: normative values. J Hand Surg [Am] 1994; 19A: 665–670.
18. Evans RB, Thompson DE: The application of force to the healing tendon. J Hand Ther 1993; 6: 266–284.
19. Forrest WJ, Basmajian JV: Functions of human thenar and hypothenar muscles. An electromyographic study of twenty-five hands. J Bone Joint Surg 1965; 47A: 1585–1594.
20. Fowler NK, Nicol AC: Measurement of external three-dimensional interphalangeal loads applied during activities of daily living. Clin Biomech 1999; 14: 646–652.
21. Fowler NK, Nicol AC: Interphalangeal joint and tendon forces: normal model and biomechanical consequences of surgical reconstruction. J Biomech 2000; 33: 1055–1062.
22. Giurintano DJ, Hollister AM, Buford WL, et al.: A virtual five-link model of the thumb. Med Eng Phys 1995; 17: 297–303.
23. Hagert CG: Anatomical aspects on the design of metacarpophalangeal implants. Reconstr Surg Traumatol 1981; 18: 92–110.
24. Hagg GM, Oster J, Bystrom S: Forearm muscular load and wrist angle among automobile assembly line workers in relation to symptoms. Appl Ergonomics 1997; 28: 41–47.
25. Halpern CA, Fernandez JE: The effect of wrist and arm postures on peak pinch strength. J Hum Ergol 1996; 25: 115–130.
26. Harding DC, Brandt KD, Hillberry BM: Finger joint force minimization in pianists using optimization techniques. J Biomech 1993; 26: 1403–1412.
27. Hirsch D, Page D, Miller D, et al.: A biomechanical analysis of the metacarpophalangeal joint of the thumb. J Biomech 1974; 7: 343–348.

28. Hochberg MC: Osteoarthritis. B. Clinical features. In: Klippel JH, ed. Primer of the Rheumatic Diseases. Atlanta: Arthritis Foundation, 2001; 289–293.

29. Imaeda T, An KN, Cooney WP III: Functional anatomy and biomechanics of the thumb. Hand Clin 1992; 8: 9–15.

30. Jindrich DL, Balakrishnan AD, Dennerlein JT: Finger joint impedance during tapping on a computer keyswitch. J Biomech 2004; 37: 1589–1596.

31. Kamakura N, Matsuo M, Ishii H, et al.: Patterns of static prehension in normal hands. Am J Occup Ther 1980; 34: 437–445.

32. Keir PJ, Bach JM, Rempel DM: Fingertip loading and carpal tunnel pressure: differences between a pinching and a pressing task. J Orthop Res 1998; 16: 112–115.

33. Keir PJ, Wells RP: Changes in geometry of the finger flexor tendons in the carpal tunnel with wrist posture and tendon load: an MRI study on normal wrists. Clin Biomech 1999; 14: 635–645.

34. Ketchum LD, Thompson D, Pocock G, Wallingford D: A clinical study of forces generated by the intrinsic muscles of the index finger and the extrinsic flexor and extensor muscles of the hand. J Hand Surg [Am] 1978; 3: 571–578.

35. Koppejan S, Snijders CJ, Kooiman T, Van Bemmel B: Hand and arm problems in flautists and a design for prevention. Ergonomics 2006; 49: 316–322.

36. Kozin SH, Porter S, Clark P, Thoder JJ: The contribution of the intrinsic muscles to grip and pinch strength. J Hand Surg [Am] 1999; 24A: 64–72.

37. Kursa K, Lattanza L, Diao E, Rempel D: In vivo flexor tendon forces increase with finger and wrist flexion during active finger flexion and extension. J Orthop Res 2006; 24: 763–769.

38. Labosky DA, Waggy CA: Apparent weakness of median and ulnar motors in radial nerve palsy. J Hand Surg 1986; 11A: 528–533.

39. Lamoreaux L, Hoffer MM: The effect of wrist deviation on grip and pinch strength. Clin Orthop 1995; 314: 152–155.

40. Lee JW, Rim K: Maximum finger force prediction using a planar simulation of the middle finger. Proc Inst Mech Eng [H.] 1990; 204: 169–178.

41. Loren GJ, Shoemaker SD, Burkholder TJ, et al.: Human wrist motors: biomechanical design and application to tendon transfers. J Biomech 1996; 29: 331–342.

42. Loslever P, Ranaivosoa A: Biomechanical and epidemiological investigation of carpal tunnel syndrome at workplaces with high risk factors. Ergonomics 1993; 36: 537–555.

43. Marklin RW, Lazuardi L, Wilzbacher JR: Measurement of handle forces for crimping connectors and cutting cable in the electric power industry. Int J Ind Ergon 2004; 34: 497–506.

44. Marklin RW, Monroe JF: Quantitative biomechanical analysis of wrist motion in bone-trimming jobs in the meat packing industry. Ergonomics 1998; 41: 227–237.

45. Mathiowetz V, Kasperczyk WJ, Volland G, et al.: Grip and pinch strength: normative data for adults. Arch Phys Med Rehabil 1985; 66: 69–72.

46. McFarland GB: Acquired deformities. In: Burton RI, Bayne LG, Becton JL, et al., eds. The Hand. Examination and Diagnosis. Aurora, CO: American Society for Surgery of the Hand, 1978; 64.

47. Moran JM, Hemann JH, Greenwald AS: Finger joint contact areas and pressures. J Orthop Res 1985; 3: 49–55.

48. Napier JR: The prehensile movements of the human hand. J Bone Joint Surg 1956; 38B: 902–913.

49. Potvin JR, Calder IC, Cort JA, et al.: Maximum acceptable forces for manual insertions using a pulp pinch, oblique grasp and finger press. Int J Ind Ergonom 2006; 36: 779–787.

50. Purves WK, Berme N: Resultant finger joint loads in selected activities. J Biomed Eng 1980; 2: 285–289.

51. Rempel D, Keir PJ, Smutz WP, Hargens A: Effects of static fingertip loading on carpal tunnel pressure. J Orthop Res 1997; 15: 422–426.

52. Ryu JR, Cooney WP III, Askew LJ, et al.: Functional ranges of motion of the wrist joint. J Hand Surg 1991; 16A: 409–419.

53. Smith EM, Juvinall RC, Bender LF, Pearson JR: Role of the finger flexors in rheumatoid deformities of the metacarpophalangeal joints. Arthritis Rheum 1964; 7: 467–480.

54. Thurman RT, Trumble TE, Hanel DP, et al.: Two-, four-, and six-strand zone II flexor tendon repairs: an in situ biomechanical comparison using a cadaver model. J Hand Surg [Am] 1998; 23A: 261–265.

55. Toft R, Berme N: A biomechanical analysis of the joints of the thumb. J Biomech 1980; 13: 353–360.

56. Tubiana R, Thomine JM, Mackin E: Examination of the Hand and Wrist. Philadelphia: WB Saunders, 1996.

57. Valero-Cuevas FJ, Towles JD, Hentz VR: Quantification of fingertip force reduction in the forefinger following simulated paralysis of extensor and intrinsic muscles. J Biomech 2000; 33: 1601–1609.

58. Weathersby HT, Sutton LR, Krusen UL: The kinesiology of muscles of the thumb: an electromyographic study. Arch Phys Med Rehabil 1963; 321–326.

59. Weeks PM, Gilula LA, Manske PR, et al.: Acute Bone and Joint Injuries of the Hand and Wrist; A Clinical Guide to Management. St. Louis, MO: CV Mosby, 1981.

60. Weightman B, Amis AA: Finger joint force predictions related to design of joint replacements. J Biomed Eng 1982; 4: 197–205.

61. Young VL, Pin P, Kraemer BA, et al.: Fluctuation in pinch and grip strength in normal subjects. J Hand Surg 1989; 14A: 125–129.

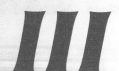
Kinesiology of the Head and Spine

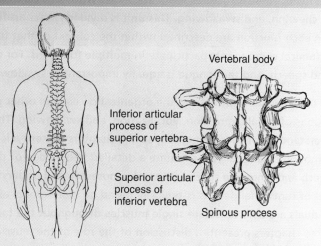

Vertebral body

Inferior articular process of superior vertebra

Superior articular process of inferior vertebra

Spinous process

UNIT 4: MUSCULOSKELETAL FUNCTIONS WITHIN THE HEAD

UNIT 5: SPINE UNIT

The preceding three units examine the structure, function, and dysfunction of the upper extremity, which is part of the appendicular skeleton. Since the function of the remaining appendicular skeleton, the lower extremities, is so intimately related to the spine, it is necessary first to investigate the spine, which is part of the axioskeleton. The axioskeleton includes the head and spine, and this text begins its examination of the axioskeleton at the head and proceeds in a caudal direction. The current unit examines the function and dysfunction of the musculoskeletal components of the head. These structures work in concert with each other in diverse functions including facial expression, vocalization, chewing, and swallowing. This unit is divided rather artificially by function, and the structures most associated with each function are described within the context of that function. However, the reader must recognize that many anatomical components participate in multiple functions. For example, the lips participate in facial expressions, chewing, and speech, and the tongue is equally important in swallowing and speech.

The first three chapters of this unit deviate slightly from the organization used in other parts of this textbook because they focus on the overall functions of facial expression, vocalization, and swallowing. The structure of bones and joints plays a smaller role in the understanding of these functions, so the chapters present a less detailed review of the relevant anatomical structures. Although plastic surgeons require a detailed knowledge of the structures within the face, and otolaryngologists and speech and language specialists need a more detailed understanding of the larynx and pharynx, conservative management of functional deficits is typically based on more-global assessments of impairments in these activities, and few individuals are able to isolate single muscles throughout the face, mouth, and throat. Therefore, each of the next three chapters presents a discussion of the role of the muscles participating in the specified function. The purposes of the first three chapters are to

- Examine the muscles that move the face and eyes (Chapter 20)
- Describe the intrinsic muscles of the larynx and discuss the mechanics of voice production (Chapter 21)
- Review the muscles of the mouth and pharynx and discuss the sequence of movements that constitute the swallow (Chapter 22)

Chapters 23 through 25 in this unit focus on the temporomandibular joint, in which a more detailed understanding of the skeletal, articular, and muscular components is necessary to understand the function and dysfunction of the joint. Consequently, these chapters return to the organization used in most of this text. The purposes of the last three chapters of this unit are to

- Present the bony and articular structures of the temporomandibular joint and describe the motions that occur (Chapter 23)
- Review the muscles of mastication and their contribution to chewing (Chapter 24)
- Review the forces sustained by the temporomandibular joints under various conditions (Chapter 25)

Mechanics and Pathomechanics of the Muscles of the Face and Eyes

The muscles of the face are small and superficial, attaching at least in part to the skin of the face. The resulting skin movement is an essential part of human communication, allowing a face to express love, rage, sadness, fear, and a multitude of other human emotions [14,20,23].

Human expression is enhanced by movements of the eyes, such as when an individual rolls the eyes in disgust. Appropriate and coordinated eye movement also is critical to clear and accurate vision. This chapter presents the muscles that produce facial and ocular movements and discusses the dysfunctions resulting from pathology affecting these muscles. The specific purposes of this chapter are to

- Present the muscles of facial expression
- Discuss the movement dysfunctions that result from weakness in these muscles
- Describe the muscles that move the eyes
- Discuss the coordination of the eye muscles that produces smooth eye movements essential for proper vision

DISTRIBUTION OF THE FACIAL NERVE

The muscles of facial expression are innervated by the motor branch of the seventh cranial nerve, known as the facial nerve (*Fig. 20.1*). As it emerges from the stylomastoid foramen of the temporal bone, the facial nerve gives off a branch, the posterior auricular nerve, to the occipitalis and the posterior auricularis muscle. The terminal portion of the facial nerve, lying within the parotid gland, divides into several branches that go on to supply the rest of the muscles of facial expression:

- The temporal branch supplies the anterior and superior auricular muscles and the frontalis, orbicularis oculi, and corrugator muscles.
- The zygomatic branch supplies the lateral portions of the orbicularis oculi.

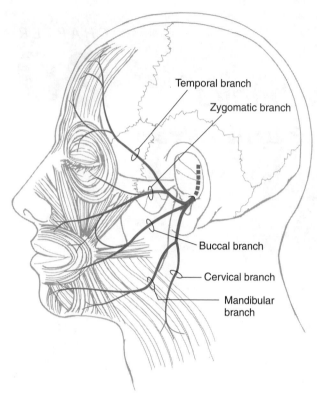

Figure 20.1: The facial nerve gives off the posterior auricular nerve, and then its terminal portion divides into several branches: temporal, zygomatic, buccal, mandibular, and cervical.

of motor control or may be the manifestation of muscle weakness. The clinician requires additional evidence before determining that a muscle is weak. Such corroborating evidence includes the function of surrounding muscles, the resting posture of the face, and the condition of the facial skin.

Clinical Relevance

FACIAL CREASES: *As noted in Chapter 17, most normal skin creases are formed by the pull of underlying muscles that lie perpendicular to the creases. Most facial creases are the consequence of activity of the facial muscles that lie just underneath the skin. Because facial creases are the superficial manifestations of muscle activity under the skin, the absence of facial creases in an adult may indicate weakness in underlying facial muscles. The clinician must be cautious to avoid interpreting the smooth, unlined skin of an elder patient as the consequence of a lifetime of good skin care when it may actually indicate muscular weakness. Careful observation of the wrinkles of both sides of the face allows the clinician to recognize asymmetrical wrinkle patterns that may indicate asymmetrical muscle performance and possible pathology. Since individual palpation of single muscles is impossible, inspection of these facial wrinkles is an important component of an assessment of the facial muscles.*

- The buccal branch innervates the muscles of the nose and the zygomaticus, levator labii superioris, levator anguli oris, orbicularis oris, and buccinator.
- The mandibular branch supplies the muscles of the lower lip and the mentalis.
- The cervical branch supplies the platysma.

 An understanding of the organization of the facial nerve helps the clinician recognize and evaluate the clinical manifestations of facial nerve palsies.

MUSCLES INNERVATED BY THE FACIAL NERVE

Most of the muscles innervated by the facial nerve are **muscles of facial expression,** unique because they cross no joints and attach to aponeuroses and, directly or indirectly, to the skin of the face, producing movement of the facial skin [39,50,51]. There are approximately 21 pairs of muscles in the face. However, asymmetry in movements produced by individual muscles within a pair is common among healthy individuals [13,30,36,44]. Consequently, clinicians must be cautious when determining the clinical significance of asymmetrical facial excursion. For example, many individuals can raise one eyebrow but not the other [13]. The inability to raise an eyebrow may reflect a common lack

The muscles of facial expression surround the **orifices** of the face, regulating their **apertures,** and pull on the skin, thereby modifying facial expressions. The functions of the muscles of facial expression are less well studied than that of the muscles in the limbs and spine. The classic understanding of these muscle actions is reported in standard anatomy texts, which are cited in the discussions that follow [39,51]. However, there is a growing body of literature describing the activity of facial muscles by using electromyography (EMG) to examine the participation of these muscles in facial movements, and these studies also are cited in the following discussions [22,55].

Many of the muscles of the face attach to each other and, therefore, participate together in facial movements. Other muscles, although anatomically separated, appear to function together routinely in certain expressions [40]. The remarkably coordinated contractions of the zygomaticus major, a muscle of the mouth, and the orbicularis oculi, the muscle surrounding the eye, during a smile suggests that these two muscles may even share a common innervation. Other muscles also appear to function in synergies to produce facial expressions that involve most of the face.

Few people can voluntarily contract all of the muscles of the face individually [4]. Unlike most of the muscles of the upper and lower extremities, the muscles of facial expression cannot be assessed individually through palpation or manual muscle testing. Not only do they rarely contract in isolation, they are too small and close together to be palpated. Neely and Pomerantz report the use of a force transducer to assess the strength of facial movements but individual muscles cannot be isolated [34]. The load transducer measurements indicate that movements about the eye and lips can withstand less than one pound of force applied through the transducer.

Since individual muscles cannot be palpated or tested separately, the clinician must assess the muscle's performance during function, that is, by examining the individual's facial function. Therefore, this text groups the muscles together according to the region of the face affected by their contractions. The discussion includes the actions performed by the muscles and the emotional expressions typically associated with the muscle activity. Weakness of these muscles affects facial expressions and facial wrinkles and also has an impact on functional activities such as chewing and speech. The clinical manifestations of weakness are discussed with each muscle.

Muscles of the Scalp and Ears

The muscles of the scalp and ears include the frontalis, occipitalis, and the auricularis anterior, posterior and superior (*Fig. 20.2*). Only the frontalis has a visible and reliable contribution to emotional expression, yet all four muscles may be activated during looks of surprise [3].

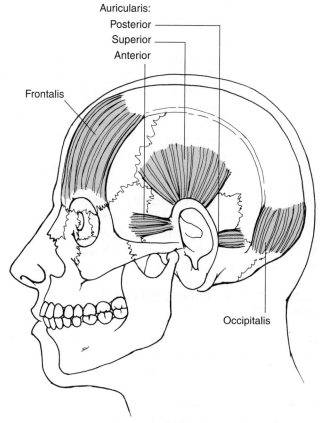

Figure 20.2: The muscles of the scalp and ears include the occipitofrontalis and the auriculares superior, posterior, and anterior.

MUSCLE ATTACHMENT BOX 20.1

ATTACHMENTS AND INNERVATION OF THE OCCIPITOFRONTALIS

Bony/fascial attachment:

Occipitalis: Lateral two thirds of superior nuchal line on the occiput, the mastoid process of the temporal bone, and the epicranial (galea) aponeurosis

Frontalis: Epicranial (galea) aponeurosis

Soft tissue attachment: Skin of the occipital and frontal regions

Innervation:

Occipitalis: Posterior auricular branch of facial nerve

Frontalis: Temporal branches of facial nerve (7th cranial nerve)

FRONTALIS AND OCCIPITALIS

The frontalis and occipitalis actually are the anterior and posterior muscle bellies of a single muscle, the occipitofrontalis, although they are frequently listed separately and can function independently of one another [3,26] (*Muscle Attachment Box 20.1*). They are separated by the galea aponeurotica, which is a large fibrous sheet covering the cranium. The action of the frontalis portion of the muscle is more observable and is the portion typically evaluated clinically.

Actions

MUSCLE ACTION: FRONTALIS

Action	Evidence
Lift eyebrows	Supporting

MUSCLE ACTION: OCCIPITALIS

Action	Evidence
Pull the scalp posteriorly	Supporting

The reported action of the frontalis is to lift the eyebrows. By lifting the eyebrows, the frontalis contributes to a look of surprise [3,36,50]. It also pulls the galea aponeurotica forward, creating the horizontal wrinkles in the forehead. The occipitalis pulls the gala aponeurotica posteriorly, thereby stabilizing it against the pull of the frontalis. The occipitalis also is active in smiling and yawning, although its functional significance is unclear [3].

Weakness

Weakness of the occipitofrontalis is manifested in weakness of the frontalis portion, which limits or prevents the ability to raise the eyebrows. Consequently, the eyebrows are somewhat drooped, stretching the skin of the forehead and reducing or

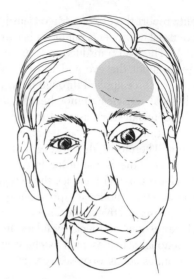

Figure 20.4: A facial nerve palsy produces weakness of the frontalis because the nerve, albeit with input from both hemispheres, does not carry the stimulus to the muscle.

eliminating the forehead wrinkles. When weakness of the frontalis is suspected, careful inspection of the forehead for the presence or absence of wrinkles helps the clinician determine the muscle's integrity.

Weakness of the frontalis is an important clinical finding that helps clinicians distinguish between **upper** and **lower motor neuron lesions** [5]. Most muscles are innervated by nerves that are supplied by the contralateral motor cortex of the brain [31]. The frontalis and part of the orbicularis oculi, however, receive input from the motor cortex of both the contralateral and ipsilateral hemispheres via the temporal branch of the facial nerve through synapses in the facial motor nucleus (FMN) [5,51,52] (*Fig. 20.3*). As a result, a central nervous system disorder such as a cerebral vascular accident (CVA) that affects the motor cortex of one hemisphere may produce weakness of all of the muscles of facial expression except the frontalis, which is only mildly affected since it still receives input from the ipsilateral hemisphere. In contrast, a lower motor neuron lesion to the facial nerve produces weakness in all of the facial muscles including the frontalis, since the facial nerve is the final common pathway to the muscles of facial expression (*Fig. 20.4*). Facial weakness with sparing of the frontalis suggests an upper motor neuron lesion, while facial weakness including the frontalis suggests a lower motor neuron lesion.

AURICULARES ANTERIOR, SUPERIOR, AND POSTERIOR

The auriculares muscles are much less developed in humans than in animals who rotate their ears to localize the sounds of prey or predators (*Muscle Attachment Box 20.2*).

Action

MUSCLE ACTION: AURICULARES

Action	Evidence
Wiggle the ears	Inadequate

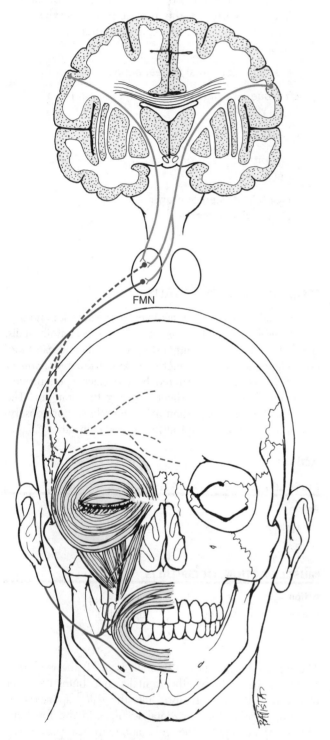

Figure 20.3: The frontalis and part of the orbicularis oculi receive contributions from both hemispheres of the motor cortex, unlike the rest of the facial muscles and most muscles of the body, which receive contributions only from the contralateral hemisphere.

FMN

MUSCLE ATTACHMENT BOX 20.2

ATTACHMENTS AND INNERVATION OF THE AURICULARES

Bony/fascial attachment:

Anterior: Temporal fascia and epicranial aponeurosis

Superior: Epicranial aponeurosis and temporal fascia

Posterior: Surface of the mastoid process of the temporal bone

Soft tissue attachment:

Anterior: Cartilage of the ear

Superior: Cartilage of the ear

Posterior: Cartilage of the ear

Innervation: Posterior auricular and temporal branches of facial nerve (7th cranial nerve)

The theoretical action of the auriculares muscles is to wiggle the ears. In a study of 442 university students, approximately 20% exhibited the ability to move either ear, and slightly less than 20% could move both ears simultaneously [13]. Evaluation of the auriculares muscles is not clinically relevant.

Facial Muscles Surrounding the Eyes

The facial muscles affecting the eyes are the orbicularis oculi, levator palpebrae superioris, and corrugator (*Fig. 20.5*). Contraction of these three muscles manifests a variety of emotions such as anger, confusion, and worry. In addition, the orbicularis oculi plays a critical role in maintaining the health of the eye.

ORBICULARIS OCULI

The orbicularis oculi is a complex muscle that is arranged circumferentially around the eye and is attached to the medial and lateral borders of the orbit (*Muscle Attachment Box 20.3*). Its fibers vary in size and length and are primarily type II fibers with rapid contraction velocities [18,27].

Action

MUSCLE ACTION: ORBICULARIS OCULI

Action	Evidence
Close the eye	Supporting
Pull eyebrows medially	Supporting

The orbicularis oculi is one of the most important muscles of facial expression [17]. By closing the eye in spontaneous blinks, the orbicularis oculi lubricates the eye, spreading the

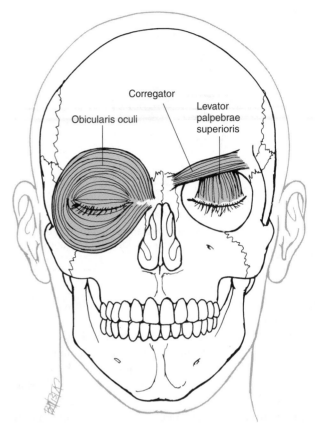

Figure 20.5: The muscles of the face affecting the eye include the orbicularis oculi, the levator palpebrae superioris, and the corrugator.

MUSCLE ATTACHMENT BOX 20.3

ATTACHMENTS AND INNERVATION OF THE ORBICULARIS OCULI

Bony attachment:

Orbital part: Nasal part of frontal bone, frontal process of maxilla, medial palpebral ligament

Palpebral part: Medial palpebral ligament and adjacent bone above and below

Lacrimal part: Crest of the lacrimal bone and fascia

Soft tissue attachment:

Orbital part: Palpebral ligament after arching around the upper and lower eyelid

Palpebral part: Palpebral raphe formed by the interlacing of the fibers at the lateral angle of the eye

Lacrimal part: Medial portion of the upper and lower eyelids with the lateral palpebral raphe

Innervation: Temporal and zygomatic branches of facial nerve (7th cranial nerve)

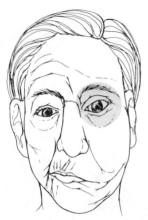

Figure 20.6: Weakness of the orbicularis oculi prevents eye closure and can cause the patient to look surprised because the eye is opened wide.

MUSCLE ATTACHMENT BOX 20.4

ATTACHMENTS AND INNERVATION OF THE LEVATOR PALPEBRAE SUPERIORIS

Bony attachment: Roof of the orbit just in front of the optic canal

Soft tissue attachment: Skin of the upper lid and triangular aponeurosis, which attaches to the midpoint of the medial and lateral orbital margins

Innervation:

Somatic portion: Superior division of the oculomotor nerve (3rd cranial nerve)

Visceral portion: Sympathetic nervous system

tears excreted by the lacrimal gland. **Spontaneous blinks** occur at a rate of approximately 12 or 13 blinks per minute (up to 750 blinks per hour) [18,25]. **Reflex blinks** are critical to protecting the eye from foreign objects. The muscle's high density of type II muscle fibers is consistent with the need to perform rapid, fleeting contractions. In contrast, the orbicularis oculi, like other muscles of facial expression, is unable to tolerate sustained contractions of several seconds duration without fatigue [6,18].

The medial and superior muscle fibers of the orbicularis oculi assist in drawing the eyebrows medially, and the muscle is active during the expression of emotions such as anger and contentment [20,50,51]. The wrinkles formed by the contraction of the orbicularis oculi lie perpendicular to the muscle's fibers and radiate from the corners of the eye in the characteristic "crow's feet" pattern [51].

Weakness

Weakness of the orbicularis oculi results in the inability to close the eye (*Fig. 20.6*). A patient with weakness of the orbicularis oculi often exhibits a perpetual look of surprise because the affected eye is maintained in a wide-open position.

Clinical Relevance

WEAKNESS OF THE ORBICULARIS OCULI: *Weakness of the orbicularis oculi is the most serious consequence of facial weakness because it impairs the lubricating mechanism of the eye. If the eye is unable to close at regular and frequent intervals to spread tears over the surface of the eye, the cornea dries, which can lead to ulceration and impaired vision [17]. In addition, foreign objects may enter the eye without the protection of the reflex blink. Consequently, the patient with facial weakness must obtain immediate consultation with an ophthalmology specialist who can prescribe the appropriate intervention to maintain the necessary lubrication and protection of the eye. The patient may wear a protective eye patch to prevent drying of or trauma to the eye.*

LEVATOR PALPEBRAE SUPERIORIS

The levator palpebrae superioris is technically an **extrinsic muscle of the eye** and, unlike the muscles of facial expression, is innervated by the third cranial nerve, the oculomotor nerve (*Muscle Attachment Box 20.4*). It is discussed here because the levator palpebrae superioris is the antagonist to the orbicularis oculi.

Action

MUSCLE ACTION: LEVATOR PALPEBRAE SUPERIORIS

Action	Evidence
Opens the eye	Supporting

It is because the levator palpebrae is not innervated by the facial nerve that a patient with a facial nerve palsy affecting the orbicularis oculi maintains a wide-eyed expression. In the patient with facial weakness, the levator palpebrae pulls without the normal balance of its antagonist, the orbicularis oculi, and the eye remains wide open. In a healthy awake individual, the levator palpebrae superioris maintains a low level of activity to keep the eye open, but activity decreases as the orbicularis oculi closes the eye. Increased activity occurs when the eye opens wide in a look of surprise or excitement [51].

Weakness

Weakness of the levator palpebrae superioris leads to drooping of the upper eyelid, known as **ptosis.** Ptosis interferes with vision, since the eyelid droops over the eye, obscuring the view. Surgical intervention can be useful in mechanically lifting the eyelid to improve vision.

CORRUGATOR

The corrugator lies deep to the frontalis (*Muscle Attachment Box 20.5*). Unlike the orbicularis oculi, it is composed of approximately equal proportions of type I and type II muscle fibers and, consequently, is more fatigue resistant [18].

MUSCLE ATTACHMENT BOX 20.5

ATTACHMENTS AND INNERVATION OF THE CORRUGATOR SUPERCILII

Bony attachment: Medial bone of the supraciliary arch

Soft tissue attachment: Skin of the medial half of the eyebrow, above the middle of the supraorbital margin, blending with the orbicularis oculi

Innervation: Temporal branch of facial nerve (7th cranial nerve)

Action

MUSCLE ACTION: 6 CORRUGATOR

Action	Evidence
Pull eyebrows medially and down	Supporting

The corrugator contracts with the orbicularis oculi to pull the eyebrows down (*Fig. 20.7*). It is active when an individual squints to protect the eyes from bright lights. Its activity also is a characteristic part of a frown and is associated with emotions such as anger and confusion [15,20,50,51]. Contraction of the corrugator produces vertical creases at the superior aspect of the nose.

Weakness

There is no known functional deficit associated with weakness of the corrugator muscle, but weakness leads to flattening of the skin at the medial aspect of the eyebrow.

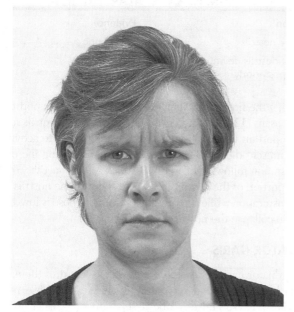

Figure 20.7: Contraction of the corrugator with the medial portion of the orbicularis oculi draws the eyebrows together.

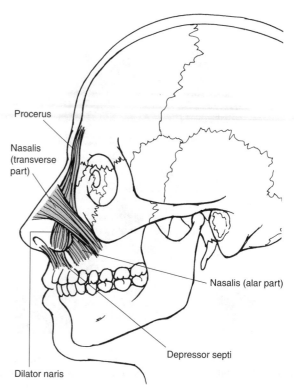

Figure 20.8: Muscles of the nose include the procerus, the transverse and alar portions of the nasalis, the dilator naris, and the depressor septi.

Muscles of the Nose

There are four primary facial muscles of the nose: the procerus, the nasalis with its transverse and alar portions, the dilator naris, and the depressor septi [9,10,12] (*Fig. 20.8*). The procerus appears to function primarily in facial expressions [9,10]. The other muscles of this group also move or stabilize the nose and are active during respiration [9,10,12]. The functional importance of these muscles is not well studied and, consequently, the functional significance of weakness in these muscles is unknown, although weakness does contribute to facial asymmetry. Only the actions of these muscles are discussed below.

PROCERUS

The procerus lies close to the orbicularis oculi and the corrugator (*Muscle Attachment Box 20.6*).

MUSCLE ATTACHMENT BOX 20.6

ATTACHMENTS AND INNERVATION OF THE PROCERUS

Bony attachment: Fascia covering the lower parts of the nasal bone and upper part of the lateral nasal cartilage

Soft tissue attachment: Skin over the lower part of the forehead and between the eyebrows

Innervation: Superior buccal branches of facial nerve (7th cranial nerve)

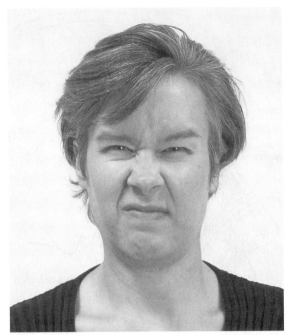

Figure 20.9: Contraction of the procerus produces wrinkles across the bridge of the nose. Contraction often occurs with contraction of the levator labii superioris and the levator anguli oris in a look of distaste.

MUSCLE ATTACHMENT BOX 20.7

ATTACHMENTS AND INNERVATION OF THE NASALIS

Bony attachment:

Transverse part: Upper end of the canine eminence and lateral to the nasal notch of the maxilla

Alar part: Maxilla above the lateral incisor tooth

Soft tissue attachment:

Transverse part: Aponeurosis of the nasal cartilages

Alar part: Cartilaginous ala of the nose and skin of the lateral part of the lower margin of the ala of the nose

Innervation: Superior buccal branches of facial nerve (7th cranial nerve)

Action

MUSCLE ACTION: PROCERUS

Action	Evidence
Pull the nose cranially	Supporting
Pull eyebrows down	Supporting

Contraction of the procerus contributes to the characteristic look of distaste, as an individual wrinkles the nose at an unpleasant smell, flavor, or idea [2,51] (*Fig. 20.9*). The muscle participates with the orbicularis oculi and corrugator in a frown [50,51].

NASALIS

The nasalis consists of two components, the transverse and alar segments [9,10,12,39] (*Muscle Attachment Box 20.7*).

Actions

MUSCLE ACTION: NASALIS, TRANSVERSE SEGMENT

Action	Evidence
Compress and stabilize lateral wall of nose	Supporting

EMG data support the role of the transverse portion of the nasalis muscle in compressing or flattening the nose [12]. Such movement is associated with a look of haughtiness. The movement also is important functionally in closing off the nasal airway during speech when making vocal sounds such as "b" and "p."

Studies report activity in the transverse portion of the nasalis during inspiration [9,10]. These studies suggest that this activity stiffens the outer walls of the nose to prevent collapse as the pressure within the nose decreases during inspiration. Additional studies are needed to verify or refute this explanation.

MUSCLE ACTION: NASALIS, ALAR SEGMENT

Action	Evidence
Dilate nostrils	Supporting
Draw nostrils down and posteriorly	Inadequate

Flaring the nostrils elicits EMG activity in the alar portion of the nasalis [12]. Although the ability to flare the nostrils seems unimportant to most humans, studies demonstrate activity in this muscle during inspiration, particularly during increased respiration following exercise [9,10,12,49]. The activity of the alar portion of the nasalis appears to stabilize the nostrils during inspiration while the pressure within the nose is low, tending to collapse the nostrils.

DILATOR NARIS

The dilator naris is described by some as a part of the nasalis [51] but is described separately in this text because recent studies analyze and describe it separately [9,10,12] (*Muscle Attachment Box 20.8*).

Actions

MUSCLE ACTION: DILATOR NARIS

Action	Evidence
Dilate nostrils	Supporting

The dilator naris appears to function with the alar portion of the nasalis to maintain the shape of the nose during inspiration [9,10,12].

DEPRESSOR SEPTI

The depressor septi is a small muscle lying at the base of the nose (*Muscle Attachment Box 20.9*).

Action

MUSCLE ACTION: DEPRESSOR SEPTI

Action	Evidence
Pull nose down	Supporting
Elevate upper lip	Inadequate

EMG activity is reported in the depressor septi when subjects attempt to flatten the nose or to "look down the nose" in a snobbish manner [9,12]. The muscle also is active during inspiration with the other muscles of the nose, presumably to stabilize the nose.

Muscles of the Mouth

The muscles of the mouth serve several purposes:

- Control the aperture of the mouth
- Stabilize the oral chamber and alter its volume
- Change the position of the mouth and surrounding skin to produce varied verbal sounds and convey a wide spectrum of emotions from elation to abject sorrow

The muscles that attach to the lips and act as **constrictors of the mouth** consist of the orbicularis oris and the mentalis (*Fig. 20.10*). The **dilators of the mouth** are the zygomaticus, risorius, levator labii superioris, levator labii superioris alaeque nasi, levator anguli oris, depressor labii inferioris, depressor anguli oris, and platysma (*Fig. 20.11*). Control of the oral aperture maintains food and liquid within the oral cavity. The size and shape of the mouth also are critical in speech, contributing to the variety of vowel and consonant sounds in oral speech [2,29]. The **volume regulators** are the buccinator muscles.

Although each muscle applies a unique pull on the lips or cheeks, studies consistently demonstrate that muscles of the mouth participate together during eating and speech [2,4,11, 29,53]. It is virtually impossible to activate these muscles

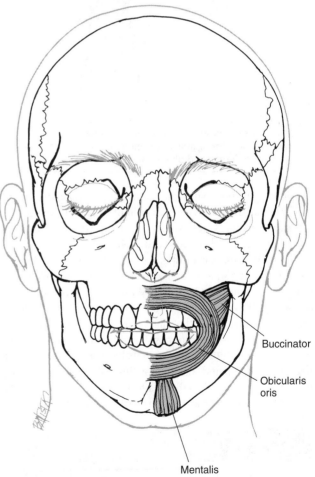

Figure 20.10: Constrictor muscles of the mouth are the orbicularis oris and the mentalis muscles. The buccinator controls the volume of the mouth.

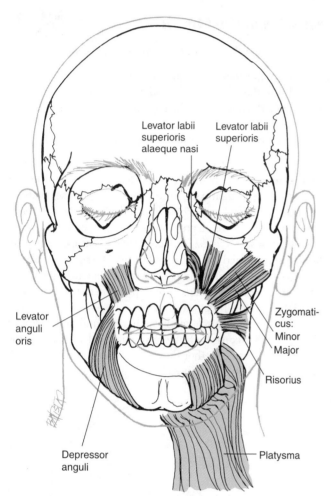

Figure 20.11: Dilator muscles of the mouth are the zygomaticus, risorius, levator labii superioris and levator labii superioris alaeque nasi, levator anguli oris, depressor labii inferioris, depressor anguli oris, and platysma.

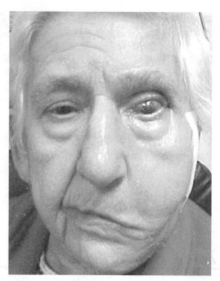

Figure 20.12: A facial nerve palsy on the left produces weakness of the muscles innervated by the facial nerve on the left. This individual displays classic signs of facial weakness, including absence of forehead wrinkles on the left. The left eye is abnormally wide open, and the mouth is pulled to the strong side.

individually through voluntary contraction and almost as difficult to isolate them with electrical stimulation [4]. Consequently, evaluation requires the assessment of the coordinated movements of the mouth in activities such as smiling, eating, and speaking. Weakness is most apparent in the asymmetrical and sometimes grotesque facial movements that result from a loss of balance among these muscles. With weakness of the muscles of the mouth on one side of the face, the unaffected muscles pull the mouth toward the intact side, since there is no counteracting force from the opposite side. It is important for the clinician to recognize that this imbalance produces a mouth that looks smooth and "normal" on the weakened side but contracted and contorted on the unaffected side. Care is needed to correctly distinguish the weak from the unaffected side.

Clinical Relevance

BELL'S PALSY: *Acute idiopathic facial nerve palsy is known as **Bell's palsy** and is characterized by weakness of the muscles innervated by the facial nerve (7th cranial nerve)*

(Fig. 20.12). *It typically is unilateral and usually temporary, although the time course of recovery varies from days to years [8,37]. Exercise and biofeedback have been shown to enhance recovery in patients with facial nerve palsies [7,8]. Clinicians must be able to evaluate the integrity of the muscles of facial expression to establish goals, implement treatment, and monitor progress. It is essential that clinicians be able to identify weakness even when unable to apply a specific muscle assessment to each individual muscle.*

ORBICULARIS ORIS

The orbicularis oris is one of the most important muscles of facial expression because it is the primary constrictor muscle of the mouth (*Muscle Attachment Box 20.10*). Although it usually is described as a single muscle [39], its superior and inferior portions found in the upper and lower lips, respectively, can function independently [2,43,51,54].

MUSCLE ATTACHMENT BOX 20.10

ATTACHMENTS AND INNERVATION OF THE ORBICULARIS ORIS

Soft tissue attachments: To the fibrous intersection of many muscles, known as the modulus, located lateral to the corners of the mouth and into the soft tissue of the lips. It is a sphincter muscle formed by various muscles converging on the mouth.

Innervation: Lower buccal and mandibular branches of facial nerve (7th cranial nerve)

Actions

MUSCLE ACTION: ORBICULARIS ORIS

Action	Evidence
Close lips	Supporting

The orbicularis oris is the **sphincter** for the mouth and is active whenever mouth closure is needed. It is active in chewing, to retain the food within the mouth [45,46,53]. It is used to help slide food from a utensil such as a fork or spoon, and it is essential during sucking through a straw or blowing on a clarinet [33,35,39,51]. It participates in speech to make sounds such as "p" and "b" and assists in the expression of love or friendship, since it is the muscle used to kiss [41,53].

The orbicularis oris has a relatively large cross-sectional area and, consequently, is capable of forceful contractions. Studies report compression forces between the two lips up to 2–4 N (approximately 0.5–1.0 lb) [16,45].

Weakness

Weakness of the orbicularis oris diminishes the ability to close the mouth firmly, producing **oral incontinence.** A patient with weakness of the orbicularis oris muscle reports a tendency to drool or an inability to hold liquid in the mouth. Attempts to whistle are futile, with the air leaking out through the weakened side of the mouth. The patient may also exhibit altered speech, with particular difficulty in pronouncing words that include the sounds of letters such as "p," "b," and "w."

A patient with weakness of the orbicularis oris exhibits flattening of the lips on the affected side. When the muscle contracts, the lips are pulled toward the unaffected side, producing a distorted posture of the mouth, particularly pronounced on the sound side (*Fig. 20.13*).

MUSCLE ATTACHMENT BOX 20.11

ATTACHMENTS AND INNERVATION OF THE MENTALIS

Bony attachment: Incisive fossa of the mandible

Soft tissue attachment: Skin of the chin

Innervation: Mandibular branch of facial nerve (7th cranial nerve)

MENTALIS

Although the mentalis has no direct connection to the lips, it is the only other muscle that can assist the orbicularis oris in closing the mouth (*Muscle Attachment Box 20.11*).

Actions

MUSCLE ACTION: MENTALIS

Action	Evidence
Raise and protrude lower lip	Supporting
Raise and wrinkle skin of chin	Supporting

The mentalis helps the orbicularis oris in sucking actions by pulling the lower lip up and forward, and the muscle is active in such actions as sucking on or blowing through a straw [1,2,43,47,51]. Protrusion of the lower lip also is characteristic of a pouting expression (*Fig. 20.14*).

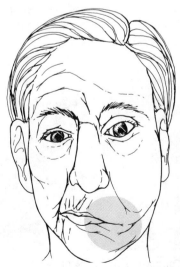

Figure 20.13: Contraction of the orbicularis oris with unilateral weakness pulls the mouth to the strong side and causes the weak side to appear smooth and without wrinkles.

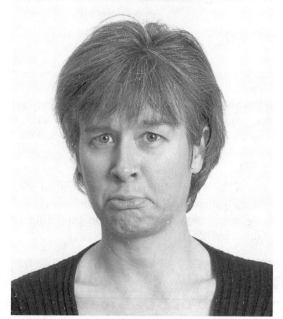

Figure 20.14: Contraction of the mentalis pulls the lower lip anteriorly and superiorly, the characteristic position in a pout.

MUSCLE ATTACHMENT BOX 20.12

ATTACHMENTS AND INNERVATION OF THE ZYGOMATICUS

Bony attachment:

  Major: Zygomatic portion of zygomatic arch

  Minor: Anterior and lateral zygomatic bone

Soft tissue attachment:

  Major: Skin and orbicularis oris at the angle of the mouth

  Minor: Skin and muscle of the upper lip

Innervation: Buccal branches of facial nerve (7th cranial nerve)

Weakness

Weakness of the mentalis limits the ability to protrude the lower lip. The weakness contributes to the asymmetrical posture of the mouth during sucking actions, with the lower lip on the affected side appearing flat while the lip on the unaffected side appears distorted as it protrudes alone.

ZYGOMATICUS

The zygomaticus is one of the muscles that dilate the orifice of the mouth, although its primary functional significance is to express emotion (*Muscle Attachment Box 20.12*).

Actions

MUSCLE ACTION: ZYGOMATICUS

Action	Evidence
Pull edges of mouth superiorly and laterally	Supporting

The zygomaticus is the **smile muscle**, contributing to the characteristic broad full smile that brings the corners of the mouth toward the eyes [2,32,42] (*Fig. 20.15*). It is important, however, to recognize that several muscles are active in this sort of smile. The zygomaticus does not contract alone [24].

Weakness

Weakness of the zygomaticus alters the form of an attempted smile. As the patient smiles, the unaffected muscle pulls the mouth vigorously toward the sound side, producing a rather grotesque image [24] (*Fig. 20.16*).

Clinical Relevance

PSYCHOLOGICAL CHALLENGES FOR A PATIENT WITH FACIAL PALSY: *Weakness of the facial muscles, particularly around the mouth, produces significant social challenges to*

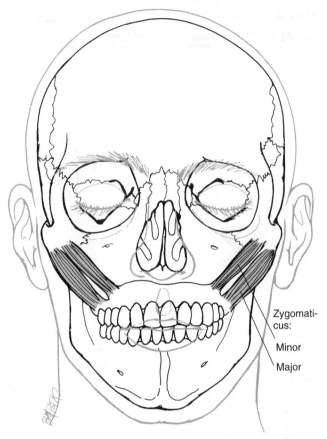

Figure 20.15: The primary muscle of a broad smile is the zygomaticus, but most of the other dilators of the mouth also participate, pulling the lips away from the teeth.

the patient. Weakness of the orbicularis oris may make eating difficult and embarrassing, as the patient is unable to avoid leakage of the food or liquid from the mouth. In addition, facial expressions that are the natural manifestations of emotions such as joy or sorrow are no longer the familiar smiles or frowns but rather grotesque caricatures of such expressions. As a result, many patients are reluctant to leave the privacy of their own homes [48].

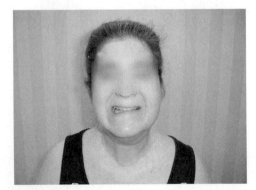

Figure 20.16: Contraction of the dilator muscles with unilateral weakness pulls the mouth to the strong side, leaving the weak side smooth and without wrinkles. (Photo courtesy of Martin Kelley MSPT, University of Pennsylvania Health Systems, Philadelphia, PA.)

MUSCLE ATTACHMENT BOX 20.13

ATTACHMENTS AND INNERVATION OF THE RISORIUS

Bony attachment: Zygomatic bone

Soft tissue attachment: Fascia of the parotid gland, fascia over the masseter muscle, fascia of the platysma, fascia over the mastoid process, and the skin at the angle of the mouth

Innervation: Buccal branches of facial nerve (7th cranial nerve)

MUSCLE ATTACHMENT BOX 20.14

ATTACHMENTS AND INNERVATION OF THE LEVATOR LABII SUPERIORIS AND LEVATOR LABII SUPERIORIS ALAEQUE NASI

Bony attachment: Maxilla and zygomatic bone superior to the infraorbital foramen

Soft tissue attachment: Orbicularis oris of the upper lip and the cartilaginous ala of the nose

Innervation: Buccal branches of facial nerve (7th cranial nerve)

RISORIUS

The risorius is another dilator of the mouth and functions with the zygomaticus (*Muscle Attachment Box 20.13*).

Actions

MUSCLE ACTION: RISORIUS

Action	Evidence
Pull edges of mouth laterally	Supporting

Although the risorius typically contracts with the zygomaticus, when its activity is primary, the risorius produces a grimace that can convey feelings of disgust, dislike, frustration, or other emotions (*Fig. 20.17*).

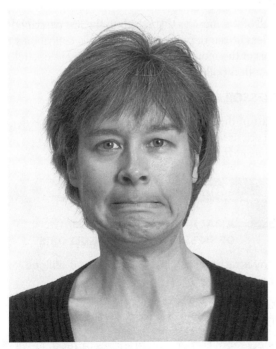

Figure 20.17: When the risorius is the primary muscle active at the mouth, the lips are pulled laterally in a grimace.

Weakness

Weakness of the risorius, like the zygomaticus, results in a distorted smile with the mouth pulled toward the unaffected side.

LEVATOR LABII SUPERIORIS AND LEVATOR LABII SUPERIORIS ALAEQUE NASI

The two levator labii superioris muscles lie between the nose and the mouth, contributing to the characteristic furrow between the side of the nose and the corners of the mouth (*Muscle Attachment Box 20.14*).

Actions

MUSCLE ACTION: LEVATOR LABII SUPERIORIS AND LEVATOR LABII SUPERIORIS ALAEQUE NASI

Action	Evidence
Lift the upper lip and turn it outward	Supporting

The action of the two levator labii superioris muscles produces the common look of disgust or revulsion and typically coincides with contraction of the procerus [10]. These muscles also contribute to retraction of the lips during a large smile [2,42]. The levator labii superioris alaeque nasi also contributes to the dilation of the nostrils with the alar portion of the nasalis and the dilator naris [51].

Weakness

Weakness of the two levator labii superioris muscles contributes to a flattening of the lips in a smile. The patient also may report a tendency to bite the upper lip, particularly while eating. Weakness of these muscles tends to flatten the furrow between nose and mouth. Since this furrow deepens with age normally, weakness of the levator labii superioris muscles tends to make an older individual appear younger.

LEVATOR ANGULI ORIS (ALSO KNOWN AS CANINUS)

The levator anguli oris also contributes to the furrow between the nose and upper lip (*Muscle Attachment Box 20.15*).

MUSCLE ATTACHMENT BOX 20.15

ATTACHMENTS AND INNERVATION OF THE LEVATOR ANGULI ORIS (CANINUS)

Bony attachment: Canine fossa of the maxilla immediately below infraorbital foramen

Soft tissue attachment: Fibers intermingle with the skin and orbicularis oris at the lateral angle of mouth

Innervation: Buccal branches of facial nerve (7th cranial nerve)

Actions

MUSCLE ACTION: LEVATOR ANGULI ORIS

Action	Evidence
Lift lateral aspect of upper lip	Supporting

By lifting the lateral aspect of the lip, the levator anguli oris exposes the canine tooth, which gives the muscle its other name, caninus. Although many individuals are unable to isolate this muscle, its action is associated with a sneering expression (*Fig. 20.18*). Like the other dilator muscles, the levator anguli oris participates in a broad smile [42].

Weakness

Weakness of the levator anguli oris contributes to a distorted smile.

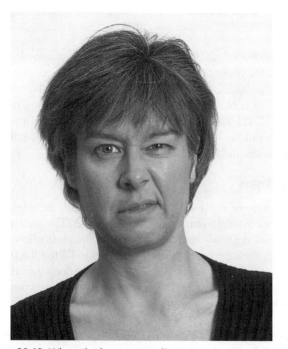

Figure 20.18: When the levator anguli oris is active primarily, the lip is pulled up and laterally in a sneer.

MUSCLE ATTACHMENT BOX 20.16

ATTACHMENTS AND INNERVATION OF THE DEPRESSOR LABII INFERIORIS

Bony attachment: Oblique line of the outer surface of the mandible between the symphysis and mental foramen deep to the depressor anguli oris

Soft tissue attachment: Skin and mucosa of the lower lip, mingling with the orbicularis oris

Innervation: Mandibular branches of facial nerve (7th cranial nerve

DEPRESSOR LABII INFERIORIS

Depressor labii inferioris is a dilator of the mouth, affecting the lower lip (*Muscle Attachment Box 20.16*).

Actions

MUSCLE ACTION: DEPRESSOR LABII INFERIORIS

Action	Evidence
Pull lower lip down and turn it outward	Supporting

Contraction of the depressor labii inferioris exposes the lower teeth. The action of the depressor labii inferioris is generally associated with the emotions of sadness or anger manifested by a frown. However, the muscle also appears to be active in large smiles in which the lips are pulled back from both rows of teeth [38,42].

Weakness

Like all of the muscles that attach to the lips described so far, weakness of the depressor labii inferioris contributes to distortions of the mouth when the patient frowns or smiles, and the mouth is pulled toward the stronger side.

DEPRESSOR ANGULI ORIS

The last of the primary depressors of the lips, the depressor anguli oris, is active with the depressor labii inferioris (*Muscle Attachment Box 20.17*).

MUSCLE ATTACHMENT BOX 20.17

ATTACHMENTS AND INNERVATION OF THE DEPRESSOR ANGULI ORIS

Bony attachment: Mental tubercle and oblique line of mandible

Soft tissue attachment: Orbicularis oris and skin at angle of mouth

Innervation: Mandibular branches of facial nerve (7th cranial nerve)

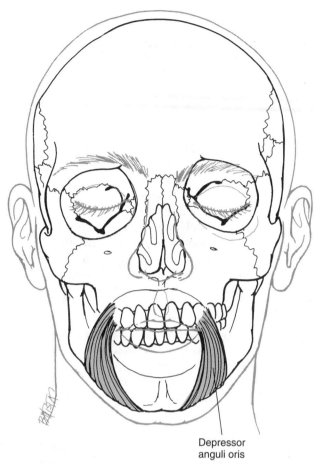

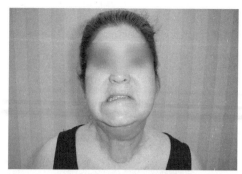

Figure 20.20: Contraction of the depressors of the lip with unilateral weakness pulls the mouth to the strong side, leaving the weak side smooth and without wrinkles. (Photo courtesy of Martin Kelley, MSPT, University of Pennsylvania Health Systems, Philadelphia, PA.)

PLATYSMA

The platysma is a broad, thin sheet of muscle extending from the mouth to the upper thoracic region (*Muscle Attachment Box 20.18*). It is superficial, lying just below the skin in the cervical region.

Actions

MUSCLE ACTION: PLATYSMA

Action	Evidence
Pull corners of mouth and lower lip down	Supporting
Assist in inspiration	Inadequate
Support skin in cervical region	Inadequate

Depressor anguli oris

Figure 20.19: The depressor anguli oris is primarily responsible for the classic frown, although the other depressors of the lips are active as well.

Actions

MUSCLE ACTION: DEPRESSOR ANGULI ORIS

Action	Evidence
Pull angles of mouth down and laterally	Supporting

The action of the depressor anguli oris is associated with the emotion of sadness, since contraction contributes to the classic frown (*Fig. 20.19*).

Weakness

Weakness of the depressor anguli oris contributes, with the other muscles of the mouth, to the distortions of the mouth as it is pulled toward the unaffected side. Loss of the depressor anguli oris is particularly apparent when a patient, depressed or saddened by the effects of the facial weakness, begins to cry. The mouth is pulled down and laterally by the unaffected depressor anguli oris, causing the whole mouth to deviate toward the strong side (*Fig. 20.20*).

MUSCLE ATTACHMENT BOX 20.18

ATTACHMENTS AND INNERVATION OF THE PLATYSMA

Bony attachment: Skin and superficial fascia of the upper pectoral and deltoid regions. Fibers cross the clavicle and pass obliquely upward and medially along the sides of the neck.

Soft tissue attachment: Anterior fibers of either side interlace with each other below the chin, at the symphysis menti. Intermediate fibers attach at the lateral half of the lower lip and lower border of the body of the mandible. Posterior fibers connect with depressor labii inferioris and depressor anguli oris and pass the angle of the jaw to insert into the skin and subcutaneous tissue of the lower part of the face.

Innervation: Cervical branch of the facial nerve (7th cranial nerve)

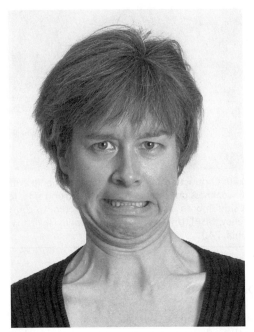

Figure 20.21: Contraction of the platysma contributes to a look of horror.

The actions of the platysma are not well studied. The attachments of the platysma are consistent with the actions listed above [2,51]. Contraction of the platysma often contributes to a look of horror (*Fig. 20.21*). Observation of an individual in respiratory distress typically reveals contraction of the platysma during inspiration, but the significance of such a contraction is unknown.

Weakness

The significance of platysma weakness is unknown.

BUCCINATOR

The buccinator is the muscle of the cheek, with only an indirect attachment to the lips by way of the orbicularis oris (*Muscle Attachment Box 20.19*).

MUSCLE ATTACHMENT BOX 20.19

ATTACHMENTS AND INNERVATION OF THE BUCCINATOR

Bony attachment: Outer surface of alveolar process of maxilla and mandible opposite the sockets of the molar teeth and the anterior border of the pterygomandibular raphe posteriorly

Soft tissue attachment: The orbicularis oris and the lips and submucosa of the mouth

Innervation: Lower buccal branches of facial nerve (7th cranial nerve)

Actions

MUSCLE ACTION: BUCCINATOR

Action	Evidence
Compress the cheek	Supporting

The buccinator muscle is an essential muscle in chewing. By compressing the cheeks, the buccinator keeps the bolus of food from getting caught in the **buccal space,** the space between the mandible and the cheek. The buccinator also controls the volume of the oral cavity and thereby controls the pressure within the cavity. This role is particularly important to musicians who play brass or woodwind instruments but is used by anyone who has blown out the candles on a birthday cake. The buccinator stiffens the cheeks so that the air can be expelled under pressure while contraction of the orbicularis oris muscles directs the air stream toward the target [35].

Weakness

Weakness of the buccinator produces several serious difficulties in chewing. Weakness of the muscle allows the food to become sequestered in the buccal space, so the patient cannot grind the food effectively between the teeth. Prolonged sequestering also can lead to skin breakdown and tooth decay. In addition, with little control of the cheek, a patient is prone to biting the inner wall of the cheek while chewing. Weakness of the buccinator also produces difficulty in blowing air out forcefully through pursed lips, so a patient has difficulty playing a brass or wind instrument.

MUSCLES THAT MOVE THE EYES

There are seven **extrinsic muscles of the eye,** including the levator palpebrae superioris, which is discussed earlier in this chapter. The remaining six muscles are responsible for moving the eye within the orbit and include the superior, inferior, medial, and lateral rectus muscles and the superior and inferior oblique muscles (*Fig. 20.22*). Evaluation and treatment of these muscles are the primary responsibility of ophthalmologists and neurologists. Rehabilitation specialists participate in the conservative management of patients with impairments of these muscles and require an understanding of the basic mechanisms that produce normal eye movements described in this text.

To understand the movements produced by these muscles, it is necessary to appreciate the axes of motion that form the reference frame for eye movement (*Fig. 20.23*). Movements of the eye are described with respect to the axes through the eye itself. **Elevation** and **depression** occur about the medial lateral axis; **medial** and **lateral rotation,** also known as **adduction** and **abduction,** occur about a vertical axis; and **intorsion** and **extorsion** occur about the anterior–posterior axis. Intorsion is defined as the motion that rotates the superior surface of the eye medially toward the nose. Extorsion is motion of the same point laterally toward the ear.

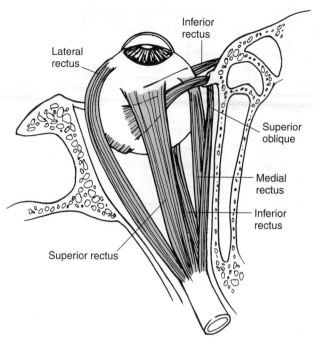

Figure 20.22: The extrinsic muscles that move the eye are the medial and lateral rectus, the superior and inferior rectus, and the superior and inferior oblique muscles.

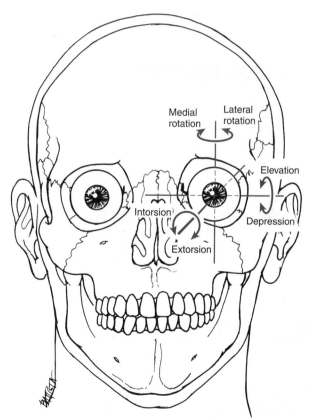

Figure 20.23: Motion about the vertical axis is medial and lateral rotation (adduction and abduction, respectively). Motion about a medial lateral axis is elevation and depression, and motion about an anterior posterior axis is intorsion and extorsion. Intorsion is the movement that moves the superior aspect of the eye medially, and extorsion moves the superior surface of the eye laterally.

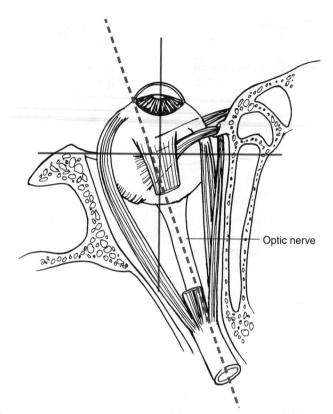

Figure 20.24: Axes of the eye compared with the alignment of the orbit. The axes of the eye are aligned in the cardinal planes of the body; however, the orbits of the eyes project anteriorly and laterally.

The orbit of the eye projects anteriorly and laterally within the skull, but the anterior–posterior axis of each eye lies in the sagittal plane during normal forward vision (*Fig. 20.24*). The differences between the axes of the eye and the axes of the orbit contribute to the complexity of the motions produced by the extrinsic muscles of the eye. Additionally, the extrinsic muscles cannot be observed or assessed by palpation; EMG analysis also is rarely possible. Consequently, these muscles are not well studied. The following provides a basic description of the current understanding of the muscles that move the eye. Effects of weakness are discussed together following the descriptions of all the muscles.

MEDIAL AND LATERAL RECTUS MUSCLES

Both the medial and lateral rectus muscles lie close to the transverse plane when vision is focused on the horizon, so their activity produces movement about a vertical axis through the eye [51] (*Muscle Attachment Box 20.20*).

Actions

MUSCLE ACTION: MEDIAL RECTUS

Action	Evidence
Rotate eye medially (adduct)	Supporting

MUSCLE ATTACHMENT BOX 20.20

ATTACHMENTS AND INNERVATION OF THE MEDIAL AND LATERAL RECTUS MUSCLES

Bony attachment: The optic canal by a common annular ligament

Soft tissue attachment: The medial and lateral scleral surfaces of the eye respectively, posterior to the cornea

Innervation: Medial rectus by the oculomotor nerve (3rd cranial nerve). Lateral rectus by the abducens nerve (6th cranial nerve).

MUSCLE ACTION: LATERAL RECTUS

Action	Evidence
Rotate eye laterally (abduct)	Supporting

The medial and lateral rectus muscles work together to turn the gaze to the right or left [28,51]. As the head faces anteriorly, gaze to the left requires contraction of the left lateral rectus and the right medial rectus (*Fig. 20.25*).

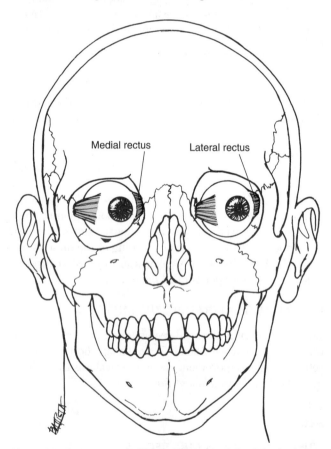

Medial rectus   Lateral rectus

Figure 20.25: Movement of both eyes to the left while the head faces forward requires the medial rectus on the right and the lateral rectus on the left.

MUSCLE ATTACHMENT BOX 20.21

ATTACHMENTS AND INNERVATION OF THE SUPERIOR AND INFERIOR RECTUS MUSCLES

Bony attachment: Optic canal, by a common annular ligament

Soft tissue attachment: Superior and inferior scleral surfaces of the eye, respectively, posterior to the cornea

Innervation: Oculomotor nerve (3rd cranial nerve)

SUPERIOR AND INFERIOR RECTUS MUSCLES

The actions of the superior and inferior rectus muscles are more complex than those of the medial and lateral recti because the superior and inferior recti are more or less aligned along the walls of the orbit and, therefore, pull obliquely with respect to the axes of the eye (*Muscle Attachment Box 20.21*).

Actions

MUSCLE ACTION: SUPERIOR RECTUS

Action	Evidence
Eye elevation	Supporting
Eye medial rotation	Supporting
Eye intorsion	Supporting

The superior rectus clearly contributes to elevation of the eye, but its contribution to the other motions is less obvious. Careful observation of the attachment of the superior rectus reveals that it lies medial to the anterior–posterior and vertical axes, which explains the muscle's contributions to intorsion and medial rotation respectively [28,51] (*Fig. 20.26*).

Actions

MUSCLE ACTION: INFERIOR RECTUS

Action	Evidence
Eye depression	Supporting
Eye medial rotation	Supporting
Eye extorsion	Supporting

The attachment of the inferior rectus muscle on the inferior surface of the eye explains its role as a depressor of the eye. It passes medial to the vertical axis to participate in medial rotation and attaches lateral to the anterior–posterior axis to contribute to extorsion [28,51] (*Fig. 20.25*).

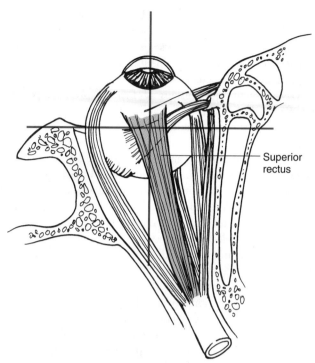

Figure 20.26: The superior rectus is aligned with the orbit of the eye, but its position medial to the vertical and the anterior–posterior axes explains its contributions to medial rotation and intorsion.

SUPERIOR OBLIQUE

The superior oblique muscle travels a circuitous route to the eye, wrapping around a pulley-like structure and traveling posteriorly and laterally to attach posterior to the medial-lateral and vertical axes and lateral to the anterior-posterior axis [28,51,52] (*Muscle Attachment Box 20.22*) (*Fig. 20.22*).

MUSCLE ATTACHMENT BOX 20.22

ATTACHMENTS AND INNERVATION OF THE SUPERIOR OBLIQUE MUSCLE

Bony attachment: Sphenoid bone superior and medial to the optic canal

Soft tissue attachment: Sclera of the eye, posterior to the eye's equator and on the superior lateral surface, between the attachments of the superior rectus and the lateral rectus muscles. As the muscle progresses anteriorly through the orbit toward its attachment on the eye, it passes through a fibrous loop, or pulley, to redirect its fibers posteriorly and laterally.

Innervation: Trochlear nerve (4th cranial nerve)

MUSCLE ATTACHMENT BOX 20.23

ATTACHMENTS AND INNERVATION OF THE INFERIOR OBLIQUE MUSCLE

Bony attachment: the maxilla on the floor of the orbit

Soft tissue attachment: the sclera of the eye, on its inferior, posterior, and lateral surfaces, between the rectus inferior and lateralis muscles

Innervation: Oculomotor nerve (3rd cranial nerve)

Actions

MUSCLE ACTION: SUPERIOR OBLIQUE

Action	Evidence
Eye depression	Inadequate
Eye lateral rotation	Inadequate
Eye intorsion	Inadequate

INFERIOR OBLIQUE

The inferior oblique muscle travels posteriorly and laterally to its attachment posterior and lateral to the axes of the eye [28,51,52] (*Muscle Attachment Box 20.23*).

Actions

MUSCLE ACTION: INFERIOR OBLIQUE

Action	Evidence
Eye elevation	Inadequate
Eye lateral rotation	Inadequate
Eye extorsion	Inadequate

WEAKNESS OF THE MUSCLES THAT MOVE THE EYE

Movements of the eyes appear to be the result of a complex and rhythmic coordination of the muscles of the eye. The eye is moving continuously in individuals with normal motor control of the eyes, and it is likely that all of the muscles of the eyes contract together, producing a steady gaze even when the body or the target moves in space. An imbalance among the extrinsic muscles of the eye produces **strabismus,** the inability to direct the gaze of both eyes toward an object [52]. Strabismus in adults may produce double vision, or **diplopia,** although young children are often able to accommodate by ignoring the input from the misaligned eye. Weakness of either medial or lateral rectus may impair the ability to scan from side to side, creating difficulties in such activities as reading. For example, a lesion of the abducens (sixth cranial nerve) produces weakness of the lateral rectus muscle. The antagonistic medial rectus pulls the eye into medial rotation, producing a "crossed eye." Peripheral vision also is challenged if the lateral rectus is impaired, although compensations by head movements may be available.

Clinical Relevance

RESTORING MUSCLE BALANCE SURGICALLY: *Imbalance in muscle strength of the extrinsic muscles of the eye may produce significant vision disturbances, including double vision, or diplopia. Muscle balance can sometimes be restored by increasing the strength of the weaker muscle through exercise. But sometimes the intervention aims to decrease the effect of the stronger muscle. This can be accomplished surgically by changing the moment that the stronger muscle can generate. Haslwanter and colleagues suggest a procedure to relocate the attachment of the stronger muscle closer to the axis of rotation, thereby reducing the moment generated during muscle contraction [19,21]. The reader may be surprised to recognize that the basic principles of biomechanics learned in Chapter 1 are relevant even in ophthalmic surgery!*

Weakness of the superior oblique deserves special note, since it alone is innervated by the trochlear nerve (fourth cranial nerve). Although both the inferior rectus and superior oblique muscles depress the eye, only the superior oblique can depress the eye when the eye is medially rotated. An individual with weakness of the superior oblique muscle has difficulty looking down and in, a requirement of many activities of daily living such as descending stairs or examining the keyboard of a computer [52].

Clinical Relevance

TROCHLEAR NERVE INJURY: *A patient may be seen for complaints of frequent tripping when descending stairs. Such complaints commonly result from weakness in the lower extremities. However, visual disturbances specifically associated with weakness of the superior oblique muscle of the eye also may produce complaints of difficulty descending stairs. Trochlear nerve lesions may need to be considered in the absence of direct associations between impairments in the lower extremities and the functional complaints.*

SUMMARY

This chapter presents the function of the muscles of facial expression and the muscles that move the eye. The muscles of facial expression are organized around the orifices of the head, ears, eyes, nose, and mouth. The muscles surrounding the eyes and mouth play a vital role in opening and closing their respective orifices. The muscles of utmost importance are the orbicularis oculi, which closes the eye, protecting

it from foreign matter and helping to lubricate it, and the orbicularis oris, which closes the mouth, essential for normal chewing and speech. The muscles surrounding the nose help control the size of the nasal opening and passageways during respiration and speech.

Weakness in the muscles of facial expression poses a significant threat to the eye and produces impairments in chewing and speech. In addition, weakness of the muscles of facial expression alters the normal facial responses and often results in asymmetrical and grotesque facial postures. In many cases the facial skin is pulled toward the strong muscles, producing smooth unwrinkled skin on the weakened side and excessively wrinkled and puckered skin on the strong side.

The extrinsic muscles of the eye work in concert to produce smooth, well-coordinated eye movements, allowing an individual to maintain a steady gaze even as the individual or target moves. Weakness in any of these muscles impairs the coordinated movements of both eyes and may lead to double vision or reduced vision in a specific field.

The muscles of the face and eyes work together in complex combinations to produce finely controlled facial expressions and discrete eye movements. Impairments of single muscles are uncommon, and isolated examination of individual muscles is unrealistic. Therefore, the clinician needs to appreciate the types of disturbances in movement patterns that can occur with weakness of these muscles.

References

1. Ahlgren J: EMG studies of lip and cheek activity in sucking habits. Swed Dent J 1995; 19: 95–101.
2. Basmajian JV, DeLuca CJ: Muscles Alive. Their Function Revealed by Electromyography. Baltimore: Williams & Wilkins, 1985.
3. Berzin F: Occipitofrontalis muscle: functional analysis revealed by electromyography. Electromyogr Clin Neurophysiol 1989; 29: 355–358.
4. Blair C, Smith A: EMG recording in human lip muscles: can single muscles be isolated? J Speech Hear Res 1986; 29: 256–266.
5. Blaustein BH, Gurwood A: Differential diagnosis in facial nerve palsy: a clinical review. J Am Optom Assoc 1997; 68: 715–724.
6. Brach JS, VanSwearingen JM: Measuring fatigue related to facial muscle function. Arch Phys Med Rehabil 1995; 76: 905–908.
7. Brach JS, VanSwearingen JM: Physical therapy for facial paralysis: a tailored treatment approach. Phys Ther 1999; 79: 397–404.
8. Brach JS, VanSwearingen JM, Lenert J, Johnson PC: Facial neuromuscular retraining for oral synkinesis. Plast Reconstr Surg 1997; 99: 1922–1931.
9. Bruintjes TD, van Olphen AF, Hillen B, Huizing EH: A functional anatomic study of the relationship of the nasal cartilages and muscles to the nasal valve area. Laryngoscope 1998; 108: 1025–1032.
10. Bruintjes TD, van Olphen AF, Hillen B, Weijs WA: Electromyography of the human nasal muscles. Eur Arch Otorhinolaryngol 1996; 253: 464–469.
11. Cacou C, Greenfield BE, McGrouther DA: Patterns of coordinated lower facial muscle function and their importance in facial reanimation. Br J Plastic Surg 1996; 49: 274–280.

12. Clark MP, Hunt N, Hall-Craggs M, McGrouther DA: Function of the nasal muscles in normal subjects assessed by dynamic MRI and EMG: its relevance to rhinoplasty surgery. Plast Reconstr Surg 1998; 101: 1945–1955.

13. Code C: Asymmetries in ear movements and eyebrow raising in men and women and right- and left-handers. Percept Mot Skills 1995; 80: 1147–1154.

14. Dimberg U, Thunberg M: Rapid facial reactions to emotional facial expressions. Scand J Psychol 1998; 39: 39–45.

15. Ellis DA: Anatomy of the motor innervation of the corrugator supercilii muscle: clinical significance and development of a new surgical technique for frowning. J Otolaryngol 1998; Aug. 27: 222–227.

16. Gentil M, Tournier CL: Differences in fine control of forces generated by the tongue, lips and fingers in humans. Arch Oral Biol 1998; 43: 517–523.

17. Gittins J, Martin K, Sheldrick J, et al.: Electrical stimulation as a therapeutic option to improve eyelid function in chronic facial nerve disorders. Invest Ophthalmol Vis Sci 1999; 40: 547–554.

18. Goodmurphy CW, Ovalle WK: Morphological study of two human facial muscles: orbicularis oculi and corrugator supercilii. Clin Anat 1999; 12: 1–11.

19. Haslwanter T, Hoerantner R, Priglinger S: Reduction of ocular muscle power by splitting of the rectus muscle I: biomechanics. Br J Ophthalmol 2004; 88: 1403–1408.

20. Hietanen JK, Surakka V, Linnankoski I: Facial electromyographic responses to vocal affect expressions. Psychophysiology 1998; 35: 530–536.

21. Hoerantner R, Priglinger S, Haslwanter T: Reduction of ocular muscle torque by splitting of the rectus muscle II: technique and results. Br J Ophthalmol 2004; 88: 1409–1413.

22. Hu S, Wan H: Imagined events with specific emotional valence produce specific patterns of facial EMG activity. Percept Mot Skills 2003; 97: 1091–1099.

23. Jancke L: Facial EMG in an anger-provoking situation: individual differences in directing anger outwards or inwards. Int J Psychophysiol. 1996; 23: 207–214.

24. Johnson PJ, Bajaj-Luthra A, Llull R, Johnson PC: Quantitative facial motion analysis after functional free muscle reanimation procedures. Plast Reconstr Surg 1997; 100: 1710–1719.

25. Kaneko K, Sakamoto K: Evaluation of three types of blinks with the use of electrooculogram and electromyogram. Percept Mot Skills 1999; 88: 1037–1052.

26. Kendall FP, McCreary EK, Provance PG: Muscle Testing and Function. Baltimore: Williams & Wilkins, 1993.

27. Lander T, Wirtschafter JD, Kirschen McLoon L: Orbicularis oculi muscle fibers are relatively short and heterogeneous in length. Invest Ophthalmol Vis Sci 1996; 37: 1732–1739.

28. Last RJ: Eugene Wolff's Anatomy of the Eye and Orbit. Philadelphia: WB Saunders, 1961.

29. Leanderson R, Persson A, Ohman S: Electromyographic studies of facial muscle activity in speech. Acta Otolaryngol 1971; 361–369.

30. Linstrom CJ: Objective facial motion analysis in patients with facial nerve dysfunction. Laryngoscope 2002; 112: 1129–1147.

31. Liscic RM, Zidar J: Functional organisation of the facial motor system in man. Coll Antropol 1998; 22: 545–550.

32. Messinger DS, Dickson KL, Fogel A: What's in a smile? Dev Psychol 1999; 35: 701–708.

33. Murray KA, Larson CR, Logemann JA: Electromyographic response of the labial muscles during normal liquid swallows using a spoon, a straw, and a cup. Dysphagia 1998; 13: 160–166.

34. Neely JG, Pomerantz RG: Measurement of facial muscle strength in normal subjects. Laryngoscope 2002; 112: 1562–1568.

35. Papsin BC, Maaske LA, McGrail S: Orbicularis oris muscle injury in brass players. Laryngoscope 1996; 106: 757–760.

36. Pennock JD, Johnson PC, Manders EK, VanSwearingen JM: Relationship between muscle activity of the frontalis and the associated brow displacement. Plast Reconstr Surg 1999; 104: 1789–1797.

37. Qiu WW, Yin SS, Stucker FJ, et al.: Time course of Bell palsy. Arch Otolaryngol Head Neck Surg 1996; 122: 967–972.

38. Roedel R, Christen HJ, Laskawi R: Aplasia of the depressor anguli oris muscle: a rare cause of congenital lower lip palsy? Neuropediatrics 1998; 29: 215–219.

39. Romanes GJE: Cunningham's Textbook of Anatomy. Oxford: Oxford University Press, 1981.

40. Root AA, Stephens JA: Organization of the central control of muscles of facial expression in man. J Physiol 2003; 549: 289–298.

41. Ruark JL, Moore CA: Coordination of lip muscle activity by 2-year-old children during speech and nonspeech tasks. J Speech Lang Hear Res 1997; 40: 1373–1385.

42. Rubin LR: The anatomy of the nasolabial fold: the keystone of the smiling mechanism. Plast Reconstr Surg 1999; 103: 687–691.

43. Schievano D, Rontani RM, Berzin F: Influence of myofunctional therapy on the perioral muscles. Clinical and electromyographic evaluations. J Oral Rehabil 1999; 26: 564–569.

44. Schmidt KL, VanSwearingen JM, Levenstein RM: Speed, amplitude, and asymmetry of lip movement in voluntary puckering and blowing expressions: implications for facial assessment. Motor Control 2005; 9: 270–280.

45. Stranc MF, Fogel ML: Lip function: a study of oral continence. Br J Plast Surg 1984; 37: 550–557.

46. Takada K, Yashiro K, Sorihashi Y, et al.: Tongue, jaw, and lip muscle activity and jaw movement during experimental chewing efforts in man. J Dent Res 1996; 75: 1598–1606.

47. Tosello DO, Vitti M, Berzin F: EMG activity of the orbicularis oris and mentalis muscles in children with malocclusion, incompetent lips and atypical swallowing—pt II. J Oral Rehabil 1999; 26: 644–649.

48. VanSwearingen JM, Brach JS: Validation of a treatment-based classification system for individuals with facial neuromotor disorders. Phys Ther 1998; 78: 678–689.

49. Wheatley JR, Brancatisano A, Engel LA: Respiratory-related activity of cricothyroid muscle in awake normal humans. J Appl Physiol 1991; 70: 2226–2232.

50. Wieder JM, Moy RL: Understanding botulinum toxin. Surgical anatomy of the frown, forehead, and periocular region. Dermatol Surg 1998; 24: 1172–1174.

51. Williams P, Bannister L, Berry M, et al.: Gray's Anatomy, The Anatomical Basis of Medicine and Surgery, Br. ed. London: Churchill Livingstone, 1995.

52. Wilson-Pauwels L, Akesson EJ, Stewart PA: Cranial Nerves: Anatomy and Clinical Comments. BC Decker, 1988.

53. Wohlert AB: Perioral muscle activity in young and older adults during speech and nonspeech tasks. J Speech Hear Res 1996; 39: 761–770.

54. Wohlert AB, Goffman L: Human perioral muscle activation patterns. J Speech Hear Res 1994; 37: 1032–1040.

55. Wolf K, Mass R, Kiefer F, et al.: Characterization of the facial expression of emotions in schizophrenia patients: preliminary findings with a new electromyography method. Can J Psychiatry 2006; 51: 335–341.

Mechanics and Pathomechanics of Vocalization

O ral communication is central to the function of most human beings. It is a function that involves several regions of the body including the mouth, the larynx, and even the abdomen and several systems including the musculoskeletal, respiratory, and nervous systems. The diagnosis and treatment of speech problems is outside the purview of most clinicians who specialize in neuromusculoskeletal disorders. However, voice production involves the voluntary and involuntary activity of many structures that are part of the musculoskeletal system. A basic understanding of the structures and mechanisms used to produce voice allows rehabilitation specialists to collaborate constructively with the specialists responsible for treating patients with speech and language impairments. In addition, recent changes in the health care delivery system in the United States have caused patients to receive a large proportion of their health care in the home, where a neuromusculoskeletal expert may be the first, or only, practitioner to see the patient. Therefore, clinicians must be able to recognize signs of speech and swallowing dysfunction. Many muscles that participate in speech also contribute to facial expressions and function in swallowing. Even a basic understanding of the mechanics of speech provides the clinician with additional tools to screen for impairments affecting any of these functions. If impairments are suspected, clinicians are reminded to seek appropriate referrals to qualified health professionals who treat patients with speech disorders.

The purpose of this chapter is to introduce the clinician to the structures of the musculoskeletal system that participate in the production of speech sounds and to provide an overview of the mechanics of voice production. The specific goals of this chapter are to

■ Describe the structures of, and movements in, the larynx that result in voice

■ Present the intrinsic muscles of the larynx and explain their function

■ Explain the musculoskeletal contributions to the production of sounds and words

LARYNX

The larynx, or voice box, consists of a cartilaginous framework composed of three single cartilages and three pairs of cartilages (*Fig. 21.1*). It lies approximately at the level of the third through sixth cervical vertebrae in adult males and slightly more superiorly in females and children [22,25] (*Fig. 21.2*). After puberty the larynx is larger in males than in females, which contributes to the differences in pitch between male and female voices. The larynx performs important functions in swallowing, respiration, and phonation, and the movements that occur in these functions are similar, varying primarily in the amount of movement that is used. The cartilages and their movements are described below.

Laryngeal Cartilages

The three single cartilages of the larynx are the cricoid cartilage, the thyroid cartilage, and the epiglottis. The paired

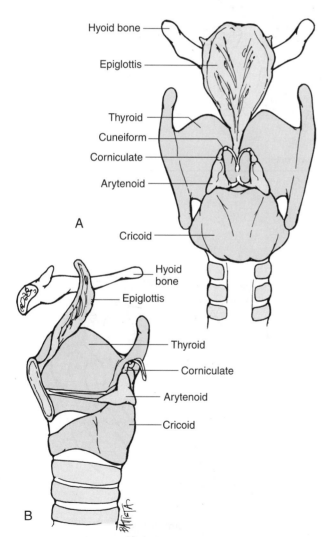

Figure 21.1: The larynx comprises three single cartilages—the thyroid, cricoid, and epiglottis—and three pairs of cartilages—the arytenoid, the corniculate, and the cuneiform cartilages. **A.** Posterior view. **B.** Lateral view.

cartilages are the arytenoid, the corniculate, and the cuneiform cartilages.

CRICOID CARTILAGE

The cricoid cartilage is the base of the larynx, articulating with the trachea inferiorly and attached superiorly to the thyroid cartilage and arytenoid cartilages by synovial joints. The cricoid cartilage forms a complete ring of cartilage with a broad posterior surface, the lamina, and a thin anterior arch so that the ring is shaped like a signet ring (*Fig. 21.3*). Laterally, at the junctions of the lamina and arch, two articular facets face posterolaterally for articulation with the thyroid cartilage. The inferior surface of the cricoid cartilage lies in the transverse plane and attaches to the first tracheal cartilage, while its superior surface slopes posteriorly and superiorly.

THYROID CARTILAGE

The thyroid cartilage is a larger cartilaginous structure than the cricoid cartilage and lies superior to the cricoid. It is composed of two large cartilage wings, or alae, that join together anteriorly, forming the familiar prominence in the throat, the Adam's apple, or laryngeal prominence. Viewed from above the thyroid cartilage is V-shaped, with the opening facing posteriorly (*Fig. 21.4*). The angle of the thyroid cartilage is narrower in males, making the Adam's apple more prominent and the vocal cords longer, thereby contributing to the deeper pitch of male voices. Extending superiorly and inferiorly from the posterior aspect of each wing are projections that articulate superiorly with the hyoid bone, a U-shaped bone at the angle of the mandible, and inferiorly with the cricoid cartilage (*Fig. 21.5*). The inferior projections form a mortise around the cricoid cartilage similar to the mortise for the talus formed by the distal tibia and fibula.

The attachment between the hyoid bone and the thyroid cartilage causes the thyroid cartilage to move with the hyoid bone; when the hyoid bone elevates, the thyroid cartilage elevates, and when the hyoid bone is depressed, the thyroid cartilage is depressed. In contrast, movement between the thyroid cartilage and the cricoid cartilage can be independent or in unison. Elevation of the hyoid bone elevates the cricoid cartilage with the thyroid cartilage. Consequently, elevation of the hyoid bone produces elevation of the larynx. The mortis joint between the cricoid and thyroid cartilages allows the cricoid cartilage to tilt upward or downward with respect to the thyroid cartilage, much as the talus tilts up or down in dorsiflexion or plantarflexion at the ankle joint (*Fig. 21.6*).

EPIGLOTTIS

The epiglottis is a leaf-shaped fibrocartilaginous structure that projects by its stem from the posterior surface of the laryngeal prominence of the thyroid cartilage. The broad, flat portion extends superiorly toward the posterior aspect of the tongue and hyoid bone but remains free of any additional attachment. As the larynx is elevated in swallowing, the epiglottis folds posteriorly, forming a protective lid over the

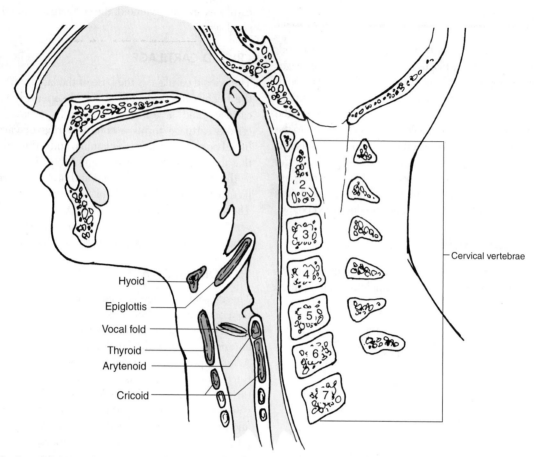

Hyoid

Epiglottis

Vocal fold

Thyroid

Arytenoid

Cricoid

Cervical vertebrae

Figure 21.2: The larynx is located between about the third and sixth cervical vertebrae.

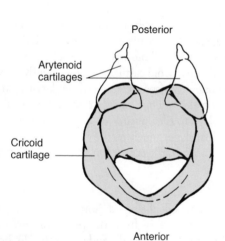

Posterior

Arytenoid
cartilages

Cricoid
cartilage

Anterior

Figure 21.3: The cricoid cartilage is a ring of cartilage with a thin anterior arch and a large posterior lamina, so that the cricoid cartilage looks like a signet ring.

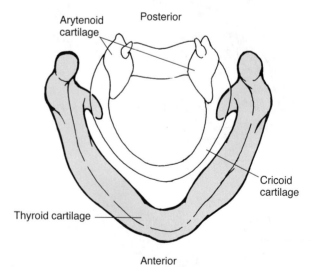

Arytenoid
cartilage

Posterior

Cricoid
cartilage

Thyroid cartilage

Anterior

Figure 21.4: The thyroid cartilage from the superior view forms an angle that opens posteriorly. The anterior aspect of the angle is the laryngeal prominence, or Adam's apple.

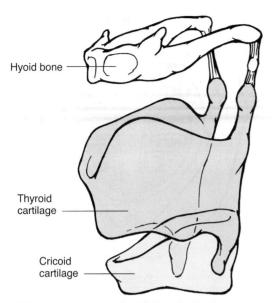

Figure 21.5: The thyroid cartilage articulates with the hyoid bone superiorly and with the cricoid cartilage inferiorly by way of its superior and inferior horns, respectively.

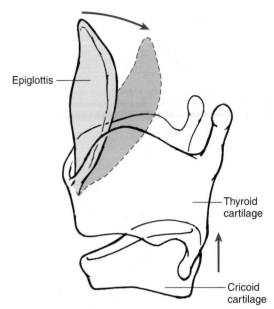

Figure 21.7: Motion of the epiglottis. As the larynx elevates, the epiglottis passively folds over the larynx.

larynx so that the swallowed bolus slides over the epiglottis into the esophagus (*Fig. 21.7*).

ARYTENOID CARTILAGES

The paired arytenoid cartilages rest posteriorly on the superior surfaces of the cricoid cartilage. They are roughly pyramidal, with their bases resting on the cricoid cartilage and the pyramids projecting superiorly toward the posterior aspect of the thyroid cartilage (*Fig. 21.8*). When viewed from above, the base of each arytenoid cartilage exhibits a slight boomerang shape with an anterior vocal process and a posterior and lateral muscular process.

The arytenoid cartilages articulate with the cricoid cartilage by a gliding type of synovial joint supported by a joint capsule and posterior cricoarytenoid ligament. The joints allow rotation of the arytenoid cartilages on the cricoid cartilage in the transverse plane and gliding toward and away from each other. The slope of the cricoid cartilage produces a simultaneous superior translation as the arytenoid cartilages move toward each other, or adduct. Similarly, the arytenoid cartilages glide inferiorly as they move away from each other, or abduct (*Fig. 21.9*).

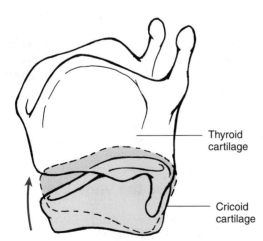

Figure 21.6: Motion of the cricoid cartilage with respect to the thyroid cartilage. The cricoid cartilage rotates about a medial lateral axis within the mortis formed by the inferior horns of the thyroid cartilage.

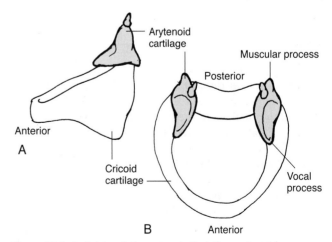

Figure 21.8: A. A lateral view reveals that the arytenoid cartilages are pyramidal, with the apex extending superiorly. **B.** A superior view reveals that the base of the arytenoid cartilages is shaped like a boomerang, with a vocal process anteriorly and a muscular process posteriorly and laterally.

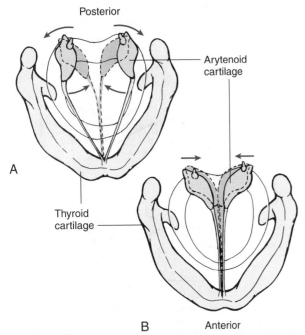

Figure 21.9: Movement of the arytenoid cartilages. **A.** The arytenoid cartilages rotate medially and laterally on the cricoid cartilage. **B.** The arytenoid cartilages translate and produce adduction and abduction of the vocal folds.

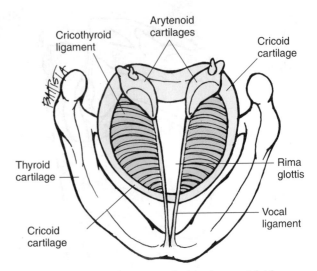

Figure 21.10: A superior view reveals that the vocal folds are formed by the medial borders of the cricothyroid ligaments and are covered by mucous membrane. The opening between the vocal folds is known as the rima glottis.

CORNICULATE AND CUNEIFORM CARTILAGES

The corniculate and cuneiform cartilages are tiny, paired cartilages, the former resting on the superior aspect of the arytenoid cartilages and the latter imbedded in the soft tissue folds that encase the epiglottis and extend to the arytenoid cartilages, the aryepiglottic folds. They provide structural support to the mucous membrane that lines the larynx and thus help to protect the airway [22].

Vocal Folds

The function of the vocal folds is to produce sound by vibrating in much the same way the vibrating string of a violin or guitar produces sound (*Fig. 21.10*). The vocal folds are the thickened, medial borders of two broad ligaments that connect the cricoid, thyroid, and arytenoid cartilages, known as the cricothyroid ligaments. The medial border of each cricothyroid ligament is thickened elastic tissue, the **vocal cord,** which is important during vibration of the folds. The paired vocal folds form a sort of curtain that opens and closes across the larynx and is imbedded in a mucosal lining. The opening between the two vocal folds is known as the **rima glottis,** through which air passes during respiration and vocalization and which closes during swallowing to protect the airway. Control of this aperture between the vocal folds is provided by the intrinsic muscles of the larynx and is the basis for all of the functions of the larynx.

INTRINSIC MUSCLES OF THE LARYNX

The extrinsic muscles of the larynx are those that raise and lower it and include the supra- and infrahyoid muscles, respectively. These muscles are discussed in greater detail in Chapter 22. The **intrinsic muscles of the larynx** lie within the laryngeal cartilage framework and cannot be palpated. These muscles produce discrete motions of the cartilages of the larynx and contribute to the unique functions of the larynx by regulating the size of the rima glottis and the tension of the vocal cords. The intrinsic muscles of the larynx are the cricothyroid muscle, the lateral and posterior cricoarytenoid muscles, the transverse and oblique interarytenoid muscles, and the thyroarytenoid muscle. All but the transverse interarytenoid muscle are paired. Much of the knowledge of the function of the intrinsic muscles of the larynx is based on anatomical studies. More recently, the use of endoscopic imaging and electromyography has advanced the understanding of the role these muscles play during swallowing and vocalization [18,24]. However, the technical difficulty of these measurements and the challenges in controlling for the normal variability of the human voice explain why the number of studies available and the total number of subjects studied remain a fraction of the investigations available for the rest of the musculoskeletal system [13].

Muscles That Close the Vocal Cords

The muscles that close, or adduct, the vocal cords are the transverse and oblique interarytenoid muscles and the lateral cricoarytenoid muscle (*Muscle Attachment Boxes 21.1–21.3*) (*Fig. 21.11*). Adduction of the vocal cords is important in altering pitch during phonation (described later in this chapter). Adduction also assists in protecting the airway during a swallow by contributing to the closure of the larynx.

MUSCLE ATTACHMENT BOX 21.1

ATTACHMENTS AND INNERVATION OF THE OBLIQUE INTERARYTENOID MUSCLE

Attachments: Posterior surface of the muscular process of one arytenoid cartilage to the apex of the opposite arytenoid cartilage

Innervation: Recurrent laryngeal nerve, a branch of the vagus nerve (10th cranial nerve)

ACTIONS OF THE TRANSVERSE AND OBLIQUE INTERARYTENOID MUSCLES

MUSCLE ACTION: OBLIQUE AND TRANSVERSE INTERARYTENOID MUSCLES

Action	Evidence
Adduct the vocal cords	Supporting

Both the transverse and oblique interarytenoid muscles pull the arytenoid cartilages together, producing adduction of the vocal cords [4]. The interarytenoid muscles are active during both phonation and swallowing [15]. An elevation in voice pitch correlates with increased activity of the interarytenoid muscles. These muscles also serve as sphincters to protect the airway during a swallow [17].

ACTION OF THE LATERAL CRICOARYTENOID MUSCLES

MUSCLE ACTION: LATERAL CRICOARYTENOID MUSCLES

Action	Evidence
Adduct the vocal cords	Supporting

The lateral cricothyroid muscles pull the muscular process of the arytenoid cartilage anteriorly, causing the arytenoid cartilages to rotate, moving the vocal processes medially [2,21,22]. Thus the reported action of the lateral cricoarytenoid muscles is adduction of the vocal cords. Studies show that the lateral cricoarytenoid muscles participate in speech, contributing to increases in pitch and helping to regulate the resonance of the voice [4,11,18].

MUSCLE ATTACHMENT BOX 21.2

ATTACHMENTS AND INNERVATION OF THE TRANSVERSE INTERARYTENOID MUSCLE

Attachments: Posterior surface of the muscular processes of both arytenoid cartilages; this is the only unpaired intrinsic muscle of the larynx

Innervation: Recurrent laryngeal nerve, a branch of the vagus nerve (10th cranial nerve)

MUSCLE ATTACHMENT BOX 21.3

ATTACHMENTS AND INNERVATION OF THE LATERAL CRICOARYTENOID MUSCLE

Attachments: Superior border of the cricoid arch anteriorly to the anterior surface of the muscular process of the arytenoid cartilage on the same side

Innervation: Recurrent laryngeal nerve, a branch of the vagus nerve (10th cranial nerve)

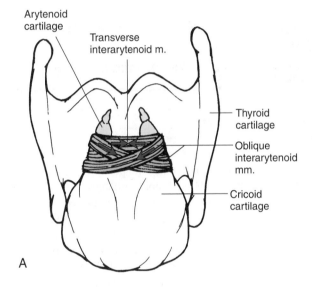

A

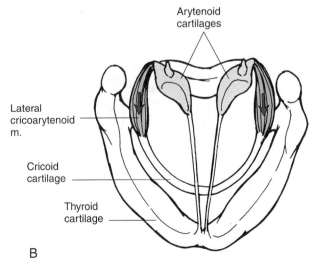

B

Figure 21.11: The muscles that adduct the vocal folds include **(A)** the transverse interarytenoid, the oblique interarytenoid (posterior view), and **(B)** the lateral cricoarytenoid muscles (superior view).

MUSCLE ATTACHMENT BOX 21.4

ATTACHMENTS AND INNERVATION OF THE POSTERIOR CRICOARYTENOID MUSCLE

Attachments: Posterior surface of the cricoid lamina to the muscular process of the arytenoid cartilage on the same side

Innervation: Recurrent laryngeal branch of the vagus nerve (10th cranial nerve)

MUSCLE ATTACHMENT BOX 21.5

ATTACHMENTS AND INNERVATION OF THE CRICOTHYROID MUSCLE

Attachments: Anterior and lateral aspects of the outer surface of the cricoid cartilage passing posteriorly, superiorly and laterally to the anterior border of the thyroid cartilage's inferior horn and to the posterior surface of the lower border of the thyroid lamina

Innervation: External laryngeal branch of the superior laryngeal nerve from the vagus nerve (10th cranial nerve)

Muscles That Open the Vocal Cords

Only the posterior cricoarytenoid muscles widen the rima glottis (*Muscle Attachment Box 21.4*).

ACTION OF THE POSTERIOR CRICOARYTENOID MUSCLES

MUSCLE ACTION: POSTERIOR CRICOARYTENOID MUSCLES

Action	Evidence
Abduct the vocal cords	Supporting

Like the lateral cricoarytenoids, the posterior cricoarytenoids function by rotating the arytenoid cartilages (*Fig. 21.12*). The posterior cricoarytenoid muscles pull the muscular processes posteriorly, thus moving the vocal processes laterally and producing abduction of the vocal cords. Studies demonstrate that the posterior cricoarytenoid muscles actively contract during forced inspiration, apparently to open the airway as much as possible [4–6,18,22]. It also appears that the posterior cricoarytenoid muscles maintain a low level of activity during exhalation, suggesting that a patent airway is maintained through the delicate balance between the adduction and abduction pulls of the surrounding muscles.

Muscles That Alter the Tension in the Vocal Cords

Alteration in the tension of the vocal cords is an important mechanism to alter the pitch of the voice [3]. The muscles that alter the tension of the vocal cords are the cricoarytenoid and thyroarytenoid muscles [2,3,8,23,24] (*Muscle Attachment Boxes 21.5 and 21.6*).

ACTION OF THE CRICOTHYROID MUSCLE

MUSCLE ACTION: CRICOTHYROID MUSCLE

Action	Evidence
Tense the vocal cords	Supporting
Adduct the vocal cords	Conflicting

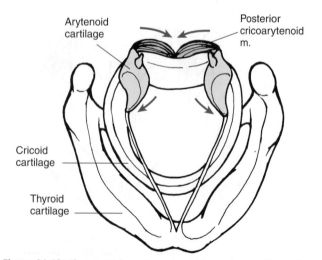

Figure 21.12: The posterior cricoarytenoid muscles are the only muscles that abduct the vocal folds.

MUSCLE ATTACHMENT BOX 21.6

ATTACHMENTS AND INNERVATION OF THE THYROARYTENOID MUSCLE

Attachments: The posterior surface of the angle of the thyroid cartilage to the anterolateral surface of the arytenoid cartilage along the vocal process; the most medial fibers, which attach to the tip of the vocal process and to the vocal ligament, are known as the vocalis muscle

Innervation: Recurrent laryngeal nerve, a branch of the vagus nerve (10th cranial nerve)

The cricothyroid muscle produces motion between the cricoid and thyroid cartilages by lifting the anterior arch of the cricoid cartilage, causing the posterior aspect of the cartilage to tilt inferiorly on the thyroid cartilage [25] (*Fig. 21.13*). This posterior tilt moves the arytenoid cartilages that rest on the cricoid cartilage posteriorly and inferiorly, putting the vocal cords on stretch and elevating pitch [3,9,19,23,26]. There is no clear agreement regarding the cricothyroid muscle's role in opening or closing of the vocal cords. Some investigators report activity during inspiration, suggesting that the muscle participates in abduction of the vocal cords [24]. Others suggest that the muscle adducts the cords because tension in the vocal cords would tend to pull the arytenoids cartilages toward each other (adduction) [22]. Rhythmic activity is also reported in respiration although the significance of that activity is unclear [24]. Poletta et al. report cricothyroid activity during both opening and closing of the vocal cords in respiratory functions such as coughing and sniffing [18]. These authors and others suggest the function of the cricothyroid muscle may be more to stiffen the vocal cords than to adduct or abduct them [4].

ACTION OF THE THYROARYTENOID MUSCLE

MUSCLE ACTION: THYROARYTENOID MUSCLE

Action	Evidence
Tense the vocal cords (vocalis)	Supporting
Adduct the vocal cords (muscularis)	Supporting

The thyroarytenoid muscle is a complex and poorly studied muscle that lies within the vocal fold (*Fig. 21.14*). It consists of a lateral and medial segment [4,20]. The medial segment, also known as the vocalis muscle, attaches directly to the vocal cord, and it is this portion that directly affects the tension

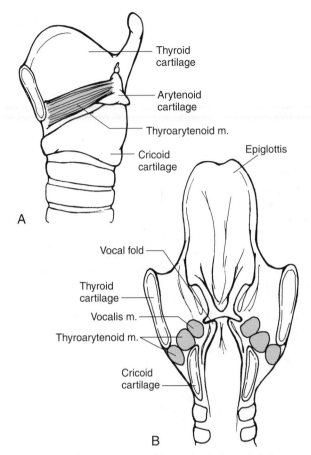

Figure 21.14: The thyroarytenoid muscle. **A.** A medial view reveals that the thyroarytenoid muscle is imbedded within the vocal fold. **B.** A posterior view of the vocal fold reveals that the medial-most portion of the thyroarytenoid muscle is the vocalis muscle, which tenses the vocal fold.

within the vocal cord. The reported action of the vocalis portion of the thyroarytenoid muscle is to increase the tension of the vocal cord. As with the cricothyroid muscle, increased activity in the thyroarytenoid muscle parallels an increase in pitch [9,11,15,23]. The vocalis also may contribute slightly to abduction of the vocal cords [4].

The lateral portion of the thyroarytenoid muscle is known as the muscularis. Studies suggest that this portion contributes significantly to adduction of the vocal cords [4]. This analysis helps explain the finding that the thyroarytenoid muscle also contracts during a swallow, apparently assisting in the closure of the larynx to protect the airway [15,17].

MECHANISM OF VOICE PRODUCTION

Human voice production, or **phonation,** occurs as a result of vibration of the vocal folds by air that is forced past them from the respiratory system. The formation of words from voice sounds is the summated outcome of contributions from the mouth, the larynx, and the pharynx. The intensity and volume of the sound are influenced by the velocity and pressure of the air passing across the folds, which are affected by the

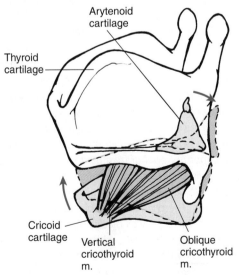

Figure 21.13: Contraction of the cricothyroid muscle lifts the arch of the cricoid cartilage, tipping the lamina posteriorly and stretching the vocal folds.

activity of the abdominal muscles. Thus oral communication requires the coordinated activity of several components of the musculoskeletal system.

Phonation

Phonation is the act of producing sound by vibrating the vocal folds, which is similar to, albeit more complex than, the production of tones by vibrating the string of a guitar [14,22,23]. The basic mechanisms that alter the human sound can be understood by comparing them with the methods used to alter the pitch of any string instrument. The primary mechanisms to alter the tone of a guitar note are alterations in the tension, length, and thickness of a string. Increasing the tension of a string raises the pitch, while increasing the length and thickness of the string decreases pitch. Thus the longer, thicker vocal folds in males produce a voice with a lower pitch. Hoarseness that accompanies a bout with laryngitis demonstrates the effects of thickness of the vocal cords, since it is the swelling of the cords that produces the lower pitch characteristic of a hoarse voice. The instantaneous pitch changes that occur during normal speech are produced by changes in vocal cord tension and in the size of the rima glottis as a result of intrinsic muscle activity.

Increased tension in the vocal cords raises the pitch of a voice just as in a guitar string. Thus contraction of the vocalis and cricothyroid muscles helps raise the pitch [3,8]. Vibration of the surrounding folds also contributes to subtle variations in pitch. Alterations in the width of the rima glottis also affect pitch; adduction of the vocal cords narrows the rima glottis and raises the pitch. The pressure of the expiring air that passes over the vocal folds also affects pitch by producing changes in the vibration pattern of the vocal folds. This helps explains why singers must learn to use the abdominal muscles to control the air pressure while singing [16,23].

All of the vowel sounds and many consonant sounds require vocal cord vibration. However, not all sounds in speech involve the use of the vocal cords. Voiceless consonants are consonants whose sounds do not require vocal fold vibration. These sounds are produced typically with the vocal cords abducted by the posterior cricoarytenoid muscle [10]. The sound of the letter "l" or "b" requires vibration, and consequently, these letters are described as **voiced consonants.** Voiceless consonants include "p," "t," and "s."

Resonance and Pronunciation

Phonation is only one component of normal speech. Anyone who has watched a movie with the sound muted knows that lip motion is frequently sufficient to communicate. Similarly, the verbal speech of an individual who has been deaf from early life often lacks the varied **resonance** and precise **pronunciation** that characterize most verbal communication. Resonance of a voice is produced by the movement of the air within the laryngeal, pharyngeal, nasal, and oral spaces. The muscles that alter the rima glottis help modulate the resonance of the voice by modifying the size of the laryngeal

chambers [11]. Singers know that altering the size and shape of the mouth and pharynx also has a large effect on the resulting sound. Anyone who has ever had a cold with a stuffy nose understands that the nose makes an important contribution to the voice. The lack of resonance within the nasal cavity produces the characteristic "cold in the nose" voice in which the voice exhibits little or no nasal resonance.

Contraction of the muscles of the mouth and nose (described in Chapter 20) and muscles of the tongue and soft palate (described in Chapter 22) produces subtle changes in resonance by altering the contributions of the nose and the volume of the oral cavity. Similarly, the suprahyoid and infrahyoid muscles produce changes in the size and shape of the laryngeal and pharyngeal spaces, producing further changes in resonance [12,22].

Another important influence on resonance is the pressure of the airflow past the vocal cords. The quality of the airflow depends on the status of the respiratory system and on the abdominal musculature. Contraction of the abdominal muscles, particularly the transversus abdominis and the internal and external oblique abdominal muscles, increases abdominal pressure, which increases the force of expiration. Increased airflow pressure raises the volume of the voice and allows the speaker to project the voice, a skill essential to singers and public speakers.

Clinical Relevance

THE ROLE OF BREATH CONTROL IN SPEECH–CASE REPORTS: *The first case involved a 35-year-old woman who was being followed by a multidisciplinary team for rehabilitation following a closed head injury. The patient exhibited several functional problems including speech problems and decreased balance with walking. Her speech problems included vocalization impairment with difficulty in projecting her voice, producing a "breathy" voice quality. The therapist whose primary treatment focus was on the locomotor impairments collaborated with the speech therapist to implement an exercise program for the abdominal muscles to improve voice volume and projection. A common understanding of the mechanics of voice projection allowed the therapists to develop a coordinated treatment regimen directed toward a common goal of improved volume and projection of the voice.*

The second case involved a 5-year-old child with spastic tetraplegia who was being treated by a multidisciplinary team. One important goal of treatment was improved communication skills, including oral communication. At the time of evaluation the patient could verbalize only three syllables between breaths. The child also exhibited impaired trunk control, and the therapist was modifying the child's wheelchair to improve trunk stability, which would also facilitate improved breath control. Improved breath control could improve oral communication, and the therapist collaborated with the speech and language specialist to measure the improvements in breath control and oral communication.

Like resonance, articulation and enunciation use structures beyond the larynx itself. Muscles of facial expression, especially the muscles of the lips and nose, are important in producing the varied sounds of the language [7]. Patients with a facial nerve palsy such as Bell's palsy (described in Chapter 20) frequently exhibit abnormalities in speech, resulting from inadequate control of the lips and cheeks. The intrinsic and extrinsic muscles of the tongue also are essential for precise enunciation of sounds and syllables [1]. Tongue position produces the distinction between the sounds of "d" and "g," and the shape of the tongue contributes to the different sounds of "d" and "l." Thus successful vocalization requires precise coordination of the muscles of the larynx, pharynx, soft palate, nose, and mouth as well as the abdominal muscles.

Common Abnormalities in Voice Production

Diagnosis and treatment of voice problems are the purview of speech and language specialists, but it is useful for all neuromusculoskeletal experts to appreciate the general form of typical voice problems. Voice problems that are based on dysfunctions within the voice production apparatus can be categorized as **hyperfunctional** or **hypofunctional** voices. A hyperfunctional voice results from overuse and is found in individuals who participate in prolonged and violent use of their vocal folds, such as cheerleaders. The prolonged yelling results in repeated and forceful contact between the vocal folds and can lead to the appearance of nodules on the folds themselves. Individuals who frequently clear their throat sustain similar trauma to the vocal folds. During the U.S. presidential campaign, prior to the 1992 election, then-candidate William Clinton sustained trauma to the vocal folds after a period of sustained campaigning and little sleep. As a result, his voice became hoarse and finally required a few days respite from speeches.

Hypofunctional voices are characterized by a lower pitch, an inability to sustain a constant pitch, and hoarseness. Weakness of the laryngeal muscles produces a hypofunctional voice and is a common finding in individuals who have sustained a cerebrovascular accident or head trauma. The speech production in such an individual can be compromised still further by weakness of the tongue and muscles of facial expression.

SUMMARY

This chapter presents a brief review of the structure of the larynx and the intrinsic muscles that control it and provides an overview of the mechanics of voice production. Vibration of the vocal folds produces voice in much the same way that vibration of a guitar string produces a musical note, The intrinsic muscles of the larynx alter the voice's pitch by modifying the aperture between the vocal folds and the rima glottis and also altering the tension within the folds. Narrowing the rima glottis and increasing the tension in the vocal folds increase pitch, while a wider rima glottis and decreased tension in the vocal folds lower the pitch.

The muscles of facial expression, the tongue, the pharynx, and the muscles of respiration also make important contributions to the quality of speech, particularly by modifying resonance and pronunciation. The actions of the lips and tongue allow pronunciation of specific language sounds. Resonance of the voice is modified by changes in the air pressure passing over the vocal folds, controlled by the abdominal muscles and by the volume of the chambers through which the air passes, including the mouth and nose. Muscles of facial expression and the soft palate help control the volume of these chambers and contribute to changes in resonance.

Thus speech results from a complex interaction of muscles throughout the head, neck, and trunk. Rehabilitation specialists possess expertise that can assist speech and language specialists in improving an individual's verbal communication by facilitating the function of the contributing musculoskeletal components, including trunk musculature, muscles of facial expression, and muscles of the tongue, soft palate, and larynx.

References

1. Dworkin JP, Aronson AE: Tongue strength and alternate motion rates in normal and dysarthric subjects. J Commun Disord 1986; 115–132.
2. Farley GR: A biomechanical laryngeal model of voice F0 and glottal width control. J Acoust Soc Am 1996; 100: 3794–3812.
3. Hsiao TY, Solomon NP, Luschei ES, Titze IR: Modulation of fundamental frequency by laryngeal muscles during vibrato. J Voice 1994; 8: 224–229.
4. Hunter EJ, Titze IR, Alipour F: A three-dimensional model of vocal fold abduction/adduction. J Acoust Soc Am 2004; 115: 1747–1759.
5. Kuna ST, Smickley JS, Insalaco G: Posterior cricoarytenoid muscle activity during wakefulness and sleep in normal adults. J Appl Physiol 1990; 68: 1746–1754.
6. Kuna ST, Smickley JS, Insalaco G, Woodsen GE: Intramuscular and esophageal electrode recordings of posterior cricoarytenoid activity in normal subjects. J Appl Physiol 1990; 68: 1739–1745.
7. Leanderson R, Persson A, Ohman S: Electromyographic studies of facial muscle activity in speech. Acta Otolaryngol 1971; 72: 361–369.
8. Lindestad PA, Fritzell B, Persson A: Evaluation of laryngeal muscle function by quantitative analysis of the EMG interference pattern. Acta Otolaryngol 1990; 109: 467–472.
9. Lindestad PA, Fritzell B, Persson A: Quantitative analysis of laryngeal EMG in normal subjects. Acta Otolaryngol 1991; 111: 1146–1152.
10. Lofqvist A, Baer T, McGarr NS, Story RS: The cricothyroid muscle in voicing control. J Acoust Soc Am 1989; 85: 1314–1321.
11. Lofqvist A, McGarr NS, Honda K: Laryngeal muscles and articulatory control. J Acoust Soc Am 1984; 76: 951–954.
12. Lovetri J, Lesh S, Woo P: Preliminary study on the ability of trained singers to control the intrinsic and extrinsic laryngeal musculature. J Voice 1999; 13: 219–226.

13. Ludlow CL, Yeh J, Cohen LG, et al.: Limitations of electromyography and magnetic stimulation for assessing laryngeal muscle control. Ann Otol Rhinol Laryngol 1994; 103: 16–27.

14. Maurer D, Hess M, Gross M: High-speed imaging of vocal fold vibrations and larynx movements within vocalizations of different vowels. Ann Otol Rhinol Laryngol 1996; 105: 975–981.

15. McCulloch TM, Perlman AL, Palmer PM, Van Daele DJ: Laryngeal activity during swallow, phonation, and the Valsalva maneuver: an electromyographic analysis. Laryngoscope 1996; 106: 1351–1358.

16. Perkins WH, Yanagihara N: Parameters of voice production. I. Some mechanisms for the regulation of pitch. J Speech Hear Res 1968; 11: 246–267.

17. Perlman AL, Palmer PM, McCulloch TM, Van Daele DJ: Electromyographic activity from human laryngeal, pharyngeal, and submental muscles during swallowing. J Appl Physiol 1999; 86: 1663–1669.

18. Poletto CJ, Verdun LP, Strominger R, Ludlow CL: Correspondence between laryngeal vocal fold movement and muscle activity during speech and nonspeech gestures. J Appl Physiol 2004; 97: 858–866.

19. Roubeau B, Chevrie-Muller C, Lacau Saint Guily J: Electromyographic activity of strap and cricothyroid muscles in pitch change. Acta Otolaryngol 1997; 117: 459–464.

20. Sanders I, Han Y, Rai S, Biller HF: Human vocalis contains distinct superior and inferior subcompartments: possible candidates for the two masses of vocal fold vibration. Ann Otol Rhinol Laryngol 1998; 107: 826–833.

21. Sanders I, Mu L, Wu BL, Biller HF: The intramuscular nerve supply of the human lateral cricoarytenoid muscle. Acta Otolaryngol 1993; 113: 679–682.

22. Sasaki CT, Isaacson G: Functional anatomy of the larynx. Otolaryngol Clin North Am 1998; 21: 595–612.

23. Titze IR: Current topics in voice production mechanisms. Acta Otolaryngol 1993; 113: 421–427.

24. Wheatley JR, Brancatisano A, Engel LA: Respiratory-related activity of cricothyroid muscle in awake normal humans. J Appl Physiol 1991; 70: 2226–2232.

25. Williams P, Bannister L, Berry M, et al.: Gray's Anatomy, The Anatomical Basis of Medicine and Surgery, Br. Ed. London: Churchill Livingstone, 1995.

26. Yanagihara N, Von Leden H: The cricothyroid muscle during phonation. Ann Otol Rhinol Laryngol 1966; 75: 987–1006.

Mechanics and Pathomechanics of Swallowing

Swallowing dysfunction, known as **dysphagia,** is potentially a life-threatening disorder. The danger associated with swallowing disorders is the possibility of **asphyxia** or **aspiration,** which is the introduction of a solid or liquid, including saliva, into the airway. Aspiration introduces foreign substances including bacteria into the lungs and often leads to **aspiration pneumonia,** one of the leading causes of death in elders [17,19,21]. A basic understanding of the mechanics of swallowing prepares clinicians to identify individuals who may be experiencing difficulty in swallowing and to refer these patients to professionals qualified to evaluate and implement treatment if necessary.

In the United States several different types of health care professionals may participate in the evaluation and treatment of individuals with dysphagia, including otorhinolaryngologists, gastroenterologists, speech and language specialists, occupational therapists, and, less frequently, physical therapists. Because of the potential threat associated with dysphagia, however, any rehabilitation specialists who come in contact with patients who may have swallowing problems require at least rudimentary information regarding the mechanisms of swallowing, even though these clinicians may not treat the dysphagia directly. The clinician's need for a basic understanding of the functional and dysfunctional swallow is made even more acute as the trends in health care continue to cause sicker patients to be followed in a home-care setting, often by a single clinician. The treating clinician must be able to recognize the signs of swallowing impairment to make the appropriate referrals for the patient to obtain the necessary care.

Clinical Relevance

A CASE REPORT: *A family requested a special consultation for a patient who was experiencing increasing difficulties walking and who had fallen several times. A therapist who specialized in locomotion disorders went to see the patient, arriving as he was eating lunch. The therapist waited as the patient ate and noticed that he coughed after every swallow. The therapist questioned the family who reported that the coughing was common when he ate but seemed to subside shortly after the meal. After the patient finished lunch, the therapist proceeded to evaluate his locomotion and instructed the patient and family in a home program of exercises. After leaving the patient, the therapist called the case manager who had requested the consultation and reported the coughing incident and requested that he receive a thorough evaluation of his swallowing function. Follow-up contact revealed that the patient had been hospitalized for dysphagia where further tests and interventions were occurring.*

This case report demonstrates that knowledge of swallowing allowed the therapist to recognize an important sign of swallowing difficulty, coughing specifically related to eating. The therapist was able to inform the case manager, who helped the family access the appropriate services. The swallowing difficulties presented a greater threat to the patient's health than the gait problems and took priority in the patient's treatment regimen.

The focus of this chapter is on presenting the basic mechanics of swallowing, also known as **deglutition,** so that the clinician can appreciate the whole process and the structures that participate in the swallowing event. Specifically, the purposes of this chapter are to

- Briefly describe the parts of the alimentary canal that participate in the swallow
- Present the muscles that are active in the swallowing process
- Describe the series of events that comprise the swallow
- Describe common clinical signs of swallowing problems

FOOD PATHWAY FROM MOUTH TO STOMACH

The **alimentary canal**—the path through which food is ingested, processed, and eliminated—consists of the mouth, pharynx, esophagus, stomach, and intestines and the associated glands. The superior end of the alimentary tract shares many of its structures with the superior end of the **respiratory tract** (*Fig. 22.1*). The two tracts deviate from one another at the level of the larynx. The challenge of the swallow is to transmit the contents of the mouth to the esophagus and stomach without allowing any to enter the areas unique to respiration, including the nose and the trachea. Skeletal muscles move the food from the mouth to the esophagus where further propulsion through the alimentary canal occurs by smooth muscle until the process of elimination of any waste products begins.

Food enters the mouth, where it is prepared for transmission through the alimentary tract. It is then propelled into the oropharynx, but muscle activity is required to prevent any progression into the nasopharynx. From the oropharynx the contents are passed through the laryngopharynx to the esophagus. Skeletal muscles protect the larynx and the primary structures of the respiratory system, and a sphincter guards the entrance into the esophagus. The muscles that assist in the transport of the oral contents to the stomach are discussed in this chapter. The muscles that are specific to the larynx are discussed in the preceding chapter. It is important to note that most of the muscles that prepare the food for swallow and then propel it into the alimentary canal also participate in speech. The muscles of facial expression discussed in Chapter 20 and the muscles of the larynx described in Chapter 21 also participate in swallowing, and the muscles of the tongue and pharynx described in this chapter also participate in oral speech.

MUSCLES OF THE MOUTH

The functions performed in the mouth are

- Preparation of the ingested food into a manageable, rounded mass, or **bolus,** from the contents of the mouth, or **ingestate**

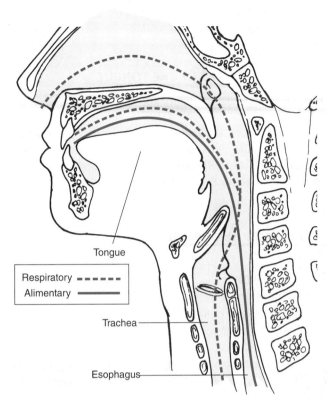

Figure 22.1: The superior end of the alimentary tract is composed of the mouth, pharynx, and esophagus. The respiratory tract shares the mouth and pharynx with the alimentary tract.

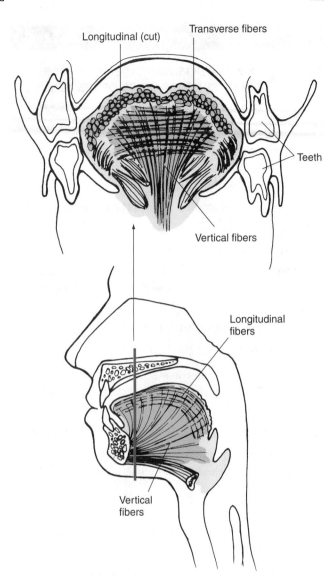

Figure 22.2: The intrinsic muscles of the tongue consist of medial lateral bundles, longitudinal bundles, and bundles that run from the inferior (ventral) to superior (dorsal) surface.

- Location of the bolus in a position that allows efficient transmission into the oropharynx while preventing the contents from leaking into the nose
- Articulation, enunciation, and modulation of vocal resonance creating the unique sounds of voice and language (Chapter 21 describes these functions more fully).

Liquids are localized on the tongue, forming a liquid bolus prior to transmission into the oropharynx. Solid food is formed into a bolus by chewing, or mastication, by the muscles of mastication (discussed in detail in Chapter 24). These muscles elevate the mandible to grind and soften the food. Muscles of the lips and the buccinator also participate in preparation of the bolus, keeping it within the oral cavity by closing the mouth and by compressing the cheeks to keep the food between the teeth. The muscles of the tongue assist the buccinator in positioning the bolus of food during mastication and then propel it into the oropharynx while the muscles of the soft palate close off the nasopharynx. The muscles of the tongue and soft palate are described below.

Muscles of the Tongue

The tongue is a muscular organ that attaches to the mandible and to the hyoid bone, a U-shaped sesamoid bone that lies

posterior to the angle of the mandible. The tongue consists of **intrinsic muscles** that shape the tongue and **extrinsic muscles** that move the tongue (*Fig. 22.2*). The tongue manipulates the contents of the mouth so that the muscles of mastication can process the food. It kneads the food and forms it into a manageable bolus. Then the tongue forms itself into a chute through which the food slides to the oropharynx.

INTRINSIC MUSCLES OF THE TONGUE

The intrinsic muscles of the tongue lie in bundles that run transversely, longitudinally, and vertically from the ventral (underneath) surface to the dorsal (superior) surface [38] (*Muscle Attachment Box 22.1*).

MUSCLE ATTACHMENT BOX 22.1

ATTACHMENTS AND INNERVATION OF THE INTRINSIC MUSCLES OF THE TONGUE

Longitudinal fibers

Attachments: From the hyoid bone and the fibrous tissue at the root of the tongue to the mucosal covering of the tongue anteriorly to the sides and tip of the tongue

Innervation: Hypoglossal nerve (12th cranial nerve)

Transverse fibers

Attachments: From the fibrous septum that runs through the center of the length of the tongue to the mucosal covering of the tongue along the sides of the tongue

Innervation: Hypoglossal nerve (12th cranial nerve)

Vertical fibers

Attachments: From the mucosal covering of the tongue dorsally to the mucosal covering on the ventral surface of the tongue

Innervation: Hypoglossal nerve (12th cranial nerve)

Palpation: Although the tongue is readily palpated, the intrinsic muscles cannot be palpated individually.

Actions

The intrinsic muscles of the tongue change the shape of the tongue.

MUSCLE ACTION: LONGITUDINAL FIBERS

Action	Evidence
Shorten the tongue	Supporting
Curl the tongue up or down	Supporting

MUSCLE ACTION: TRANSVERSE FIBERS

Action	Evidence
Lengthen the tongue	Supporting
Narrow the tongue	Supporting

MUSCLE ACTION: VERTICAL FIBERS

Action	Evidence
Flatten the tongue	Supporting
Widen the tongue	Supporting

These muscles together allow the tongue a broad range of shapes that are essential to the progression of the food into the oropharynx. The diversity in shape also contributes to

word articulation by assisting in creating the differences in sounds between the letters "d" and "l" or between "e" and "i" [9,10,36].

EXTRINSIC MUSCLES OF THE TONGUE

The extrinsic muscles of the tongue move the tongue but also influence its shape [36,38] (*Muscle Attachment Box 22.2*) (*Fig. 22.3*). The extrinsic muscles of the tongue are essential for propelling the bolus into the orophaynx. They also participate in speech by positioning the tongue to create the distinct sounds of vowels and consonants [27].

Actions

MUSCLE ACTION: GENIOGLOSSUS

Action	Evidence
Protrude the tongue	Supporting
Depress the center of the tongue	Supporting
Deviate the tongue to the opposite side	Supporting

MUSCLE ATTACHMENT BOX 22.2

ATTACHMENTS AND INNERVATION OF THE EXTRINSIC MUSCLES OF THE TONGUE

Genioglossus

Attachments: The dorsal surface of the midline of the mandible to the hyoid bone and middle pharyngeal constrictor muscle and to the entire ventral surface of the tongue

Innervation: Hypoglossal nerve (12th cranial nerve)

Hyoglossus

Attachments: The hyoid bone to the lateral aspects of the tongue

Innervation: Hypoglossal nerve (12th cranial nerve)

Styloglossus

Attachments: The styloid process of the temporal bone to the dorsolateral aspect of the tongue

Innervation: Hypoglossal nerve (12th cranial nerve)

Palatoglossus

Attachments: The tendons of the tensor veli palatini muscles in the soft palate to the sides of the tongue

Innervation: Pharyngeal plexus of the vagus nerve (10th cranial nerve)

Palpation: The genioglossus can be palpated intra-orally in the floor of the mouth under the tongue.

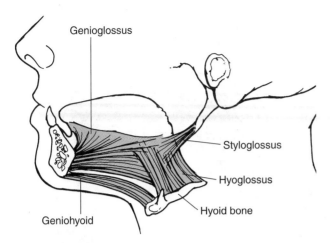

Figure 22.3: The extrinsic muscles of the tongue include the genioglossus, hyoglossus, styloglossus, and palatoglossus (not shown).

MUSCLE ACTION: HYOGLOSSUS

Action	Evidence
Depress the tongue	Supporting
Retract the tongue	Inadequate

MUSCLE ACTION: STYLOGLOSSUS

Action	Evidence
Lifts and retracts tongue	Supporting

MUSCLE ACTION: PALATOGLOSSUS

Action	Evidence
Elevate the back of the tongue	Supporting

By lifting the back of the tongue the palatoglossus separates the oral cavity from the oropharynx. The muscles of the tongue generate large forces to move the bolus in the mouth during mastication and then help to propel the bolus into the oropharynx. Forces of up to 15 N (approximately 3.4 lb) are reported in the tongue during hard swallows [28]. Although it is impossible to test the tongue muscles in isolation, the strength of tongue movements is readily measured. Peak protrusion forces of over 3.0 kg (6.6 lb) are reported, greater in males than in females [10]. Reported peak forces of lateral deviation to the left and right are approximately equal to each other but slightly less than those of protrusion.

Muscles of the Soft Palate

The soft palate is a soft wall of tissue that drapes from the posterior border of the hard palate and is covered by mucosal tissue. Its inferior border contains a central projection, the uvula, which hangs down toward the tongue. Enclosed within the soft palate are two pairs of muscles found in the lateral expanses of the soft palate, the levator and tensor veli

MUSCLE ATTACHMENT BOX 22.3

ATTACHMENTS AND INNERVATION OF THE MUSCLES OF THE SOFT PALATE

Levator veli palatini

Attachments: The temporal bone, the carotid sheath, and the auditory tube to the contralateral levator veli palatini muscle by way of the palatine aponeurosis in the soft palate

Innervation: Pharyngeal plexus of the vagus nerve (10th cranial nerve)

Tensor veli palatini

Attachments: The sphenoid bone and auditory tube to the palatine aponeurosis of the soft palate

Innervation: Mandibular branch of the trigeminal nerve (5th cranial nerve)

Musculus uvulae

Attachments: The palatine bone of the hard palate and the palatine aponeurosis of the soft palate to the mucosal covering of the uvula

Innervation: Pharyngeal plexus of the vagus nerve (10th cranial nerve)

Palatopharyngeus

Attachments: The palatine aponeurosis and mucosal covering of the soft palate to the posterior surface of the thyroid cartilage and the walls of the pharynx

Innervation: Pharyngeal plexus of the vagus nerve (10th cranial nerve)

Palpation: The motion of the soft palate can be observed easily, but direct palpation is not possible.

palatini (*Muscle Attachment Box 22.3*) (*Fig. 22.4*). The musculus uvulae lies in the central portion of the soft palate, projecting into the uvula itself.

LEVATOR VELI PALATINI

MUSCLE ACTION: LEVATOR VELI PALATINI

Action	Evidence
Elevate the soft palate	Supporting
Pull the soft palate posteriorly	Supporting

The levator veli palatini is important for closing off the nasopharynx during a swallow (*Figs. 22.5 and 22.6*). The muscle also closes the nasopharynx to varying degrees during speech.

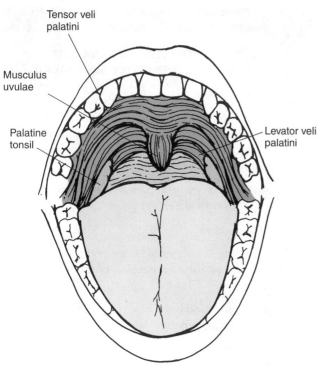

Figure 22.4: The muscles of the soft palate are the levator veli palatini, tensor veli palatini, musculus uvulae, and palatopharyngeus (not shown).

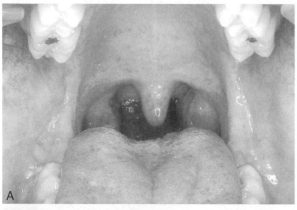

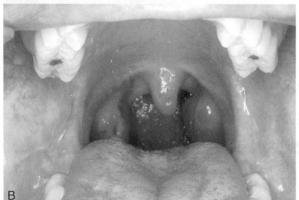

Figure 22.5: Contraction of the muscles of the soft palate elevates the soft palate and closes off the nasopharynx. Contraction occurs when saying "Ah." **A.** Relaxed. **B.** Contracting. (Photo courtesy of Arnold J. Malerman, DDS, PC, Dresher, PA.)

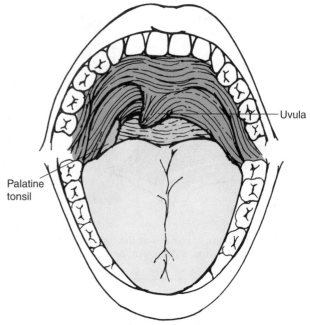

Figure 22.6: With unilateral weakness of the muscles of the soft palate, the soft palate is elevated and pulled toward the strong side.

TENSOR VELI PALATINI

MUSCLE ACTION: TENSOR VELI PALATINI

Action	Evidence
Pull the soft palate taut	Supporting

When both tensor veli palatini muscles contract together, they tighten the soft palate and may help close off the nasopharynx.

MUSCULUS UVULAE

MUSCLE ACTION: MUSCULUS UVULAE

Action	Evidence
Retract the uvula	Supporting

By retracting the uvula the musculus uvulae assists in the closure of the nasopharynx.

PALATOPHARYNGEUS

MUSCLE ACTION: PALATOPHARYNGEUS

Action	Evidence
Elevate the pharynx	Supporting

Elevation of the pharynx helps to shorten the pharynx, thereby facilitating the swallow.

Muscles of the Pharynx

The pharynx is the space posterior to the nasal, oral, and laryngeal spaces. The muscles of the pharynx are found in the walls of the pharynx, where their primary function is to shorten the pharynx, thereby preventing access to the larynx, and to clear any residue of the bolus from the pharynx [16]. Muscles of the pharynx also help to elevate the pharynx during a swallow (*Muscle Attachment Box 22.4*) (*Fig. 22.7*).

MUSCLE ATTACHMENT BOX 22.4

ATTACHMENTS AND INNERVATION OF THE MUSCLES OF THE PHARYNX

Superior constrictor

Attachments: The sphenoid bone, the mandible, and the posterior portion of the lateral aspects of the tongue and indirectly to the base of the occiput to join the fibers of the superior constrictor muscle of the other side

Innervation: Pharyngeal plexus of the vagus nerve (10th cranial nerve)

Middle constrictor

Attachments: The hyoid bone and the stylohyoid ligament to the middle constrictor muscle on the other side by way of the posterior fibrous band known as the median pharyngeal raphe

Innervation: Pharyngeal plexus of the vagus nerve (10th cranial nerve)

Inferior constrictor

Attachments: The cricoid and thyroid cartilages to the inferior constrictor muscle on the other side by way of the posteriorly positioned median pharyngeal raphe

Innervation: Pharyngeal plexus of the vagus nerve (10th cranial nerve)

Stylopharyngeus

Attachments: The styloid process of the temporal bone to the pharyngeal constrictor muscles and the mucosal lining of the pharynx and to the thyroid cartilage

Innervation: Glossopharyngeal nerve (9th cranial nerve)

Salpingopharyngeus

Attachments: The cartilage of the auditory tube to blend with the palatopharyngeus muscle

Innervation: Pharyngeal plexus of the vagus nerve (10th cranial nerve)

Palpation: Not possible.

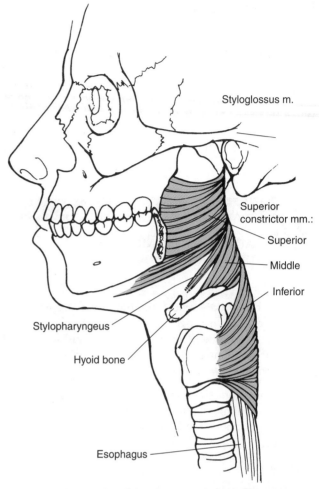

Figure 22.7: The muscles of the pharynx include the superior, middle, and inferior constrictor muscles and the stylopharyngeus and salpingopharyngeus muscles that lie deep to the constrictors (not shown).

These muscles contribute to speech by closing or opening the nasopharynx and thus altering the resonance of the voice.

SUPERIOR, MIDDLE, AND INFERIOR CONSTRICTOR MUSCLES

The constrictor muscles of the pharynx lie in the posterior and lateral walls of the pharynx. Constriction of the pharynx facilitates pharyngeal clearance.

MUSCLE ACTION: CONSTRICTOR MUSCLES

Action	Evidence
Constrict the pharynx	Supporting

MUSCLE ACTION: STYLOPHARYNGEUS AND SALPINGOPHARYNGEUS

Action	Evidence
Elevate the pharynx	Supporting

Suprahyoid Muscles

The suprahyoid and infrahyoid muscles are also known as the **extrinsic muscles of the larynx.** The suprahyoid muscles attach to the hyoid bone and to either the mandible or the temporal bone and play important roles in both swallowing and mastication (*Muscle Attachment Box 22.5*) (*Fig. 22.8*). When the mandible is held fixed by the mandibular elevators, the suprahyoid muscles elevate the hyoid bone, which is how they function in swallowing [35] (*Fig. 22.9*).

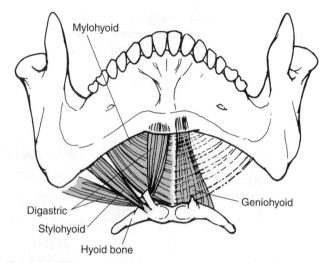

Figure 22.8: The suprahyoid muscles consist of the digastric, stylohyoid, mylohyoid, and geniohyoid muscles.

MUSCLE ATTACHMENT BOX 22.5

ATTACHMENTS AND INNERVATION OF THE SUPRAHYOID MUSCLES

Digastric

Attachments: The posterior belly arises from the mastoid process of the temporal bone, and the anterior belly from the posterior surface of the midline of the mandible. The bellies join at the hyoid bone.

Innervation: The posterior belly is innervated by the facial nerve (7th cranial nerve). The anterior belly is innervated by a branch of the trigeminal nerve (5th cranial nerve).

Stylohyoid

Attachments: The styloid process of the temporal bone to the hyoid bone

Innervation: Facial nerve (7th cranial nerve)

Mylohyoid

Attachments: The posterior surface of the mandible to the hyoid bone. It forms the floor of the mouth.

Innervation: A branch of the trigeminal nerve (5th cranial nerve)

Geniohyoid

Attachments: From the posterior surface of the symphysis of the mandible to the anterior surface of the hyoid bone. It lies superior to the mylohyoid muscle.

Innervation: Fibers from the first cervical nerve carried by the hypoglossal nerve (12th cranial nerve)

Palpation: The mylohyoid and anterior digastric muscles are palpable in the submental space, which is the inferior surface of the chin. The geniohyoid and stylohyoid muscles are not palpable.

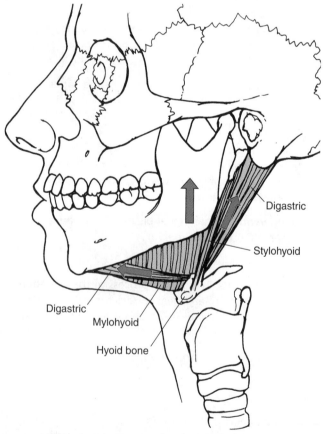

Figure 22.9: Fixation of the mandible during suprahyoid activity. For the suprahyoid muscles to elevate the hyoid bone, their superior attachments on the mandible must be fixed. This fixation occurs by contraction of the mandibular elevators keeping the jaw stabilized so the suprahyoid muscles can pull from their inferior attachments.

Conversely, when the hyoid bone is fixed, the suprahyoid muscles depress the mandible, producing movement at the temporomandibular joints. In this role they participate in chewing, which is discussed in greater detail in Chapter 24 [36]. The suprahyoid and infrahyoid muscles have received little study individually, in part, because they are difficult to isolate. More studies report their group actions during swallowing.

DIGASTRIC

The anterior belly of the digastric muscle has been studied by electromyography (EMG) more extensively than the posterior belly, since it is accessible by surface EMG electrodes in the submandibular space.

Actions

MUSCLE ACTION: DIGASTRIC

Action	Evidence
Elevate the hyoid bone	Supporting
Pull hyoid bone anteriorly	Supporting
Depress the mandible	Supporting

The function of the digastric muscle on the hyoid bone is important during swallowing [35]. With the hyoid bone fixed, the reported action of the digastric muscle is depression of the mandible. The digastric muscle's role in depressing the mandible is relevant in opening the mouth [1,36].

STYLOHYOID

The stylohyoid is not well studied.

Actions

MUSCLE ACTION: STYLOHYOID

Action	Evidence
Elevate the hyoid bone	Supporting
Pull hyoid bone posteriorly	Supporting

This muscle is likely active in swallowing and perhaps in speech, although additional research is needed to describe its function in detail.

MYLOHYOID

The mylohyoid muscle forms the floor of the mouth and is palpable with the anterior belly of the digastric in the submandibular space.

Actions

MUSCLE ACTION: MYLOHYOID

Action	Evidence
Elevate the floor of the mouth	Supporting
Elevate the hyoid bone	Supporting
Depress the mandible	Supporting

The mylohyoid muscle is active in the early phases of the swallow to elevate the hyoid bone [35]. With the hyoid bone fixed, the mylohyoid muscle acts with other suprahyoid muscles in depression of the mandible. The mylohyoid is active with the other mandibular depressors in chewing and opening the mouth wide, as in a yawn.

GENIOHYOID

The geniohyoid is deep to the mylohyoid and cannot be palpated directly.

Actions

MUSCLE ACTION: GENIOHYOID

Action	Evidence
Elevate the hyoid bone	Supporting
Pull hyoid bone anteriorly	Supporting
Depress the mandible	Supporting

Like the other suprahyoid muscles, the geniohyoid muscle is active in swallowing, as it contributes to the elevation of the hyoid bone [35]. With the hyoid bone fixed, the action of the geniohyoid muscle is mandibular depression.

Infrahyoid Muscles

The infrahyoid muscles are strap muscles that extend from the hyoid bone to the thyroid cartilage, also known as the Adam's apple, and to the sternum and scapula (*Fig. 22.10*). They include the sternohyoid, sternothyroid, thyrohyoid, and omohyoid (*Muscle Attachment Box 22.6*).

ACTIONS

MUSCLE ACTION: INFRAHYOID MUSCLES

Action	Evidence
Depress the hyoid bone	Supporting
Fix the hyoid bone	Supporting

The infrahyoid muscles depress the hyoid bone at the end of the swallow and stabilize the hyoid bone when the suprahyoid muscles contract to depress the mandible [1] (*Fig. 22.11*). They also are active during speech, helping to stabilize the larynx, particularly at lower pitches [30]. The sternothyroid and thyrohyoid muscles attach to the thyroid cartilage, which is a component of the larynx. Thus these two muscles can depress and elevate the larynx, respectively, motions that occur during speech. When the infrahyoid and suprahyoid muscles contract together, with the mandible and hyoid bones fixed, they contribute to cervical flexion [14] (*Fig. 22.12*).

Intrinsic Muscles of the Larynx

The larynx is the "voice box" and the entry into the trachea. The intrinsic muscles of the larynx alter the size of the

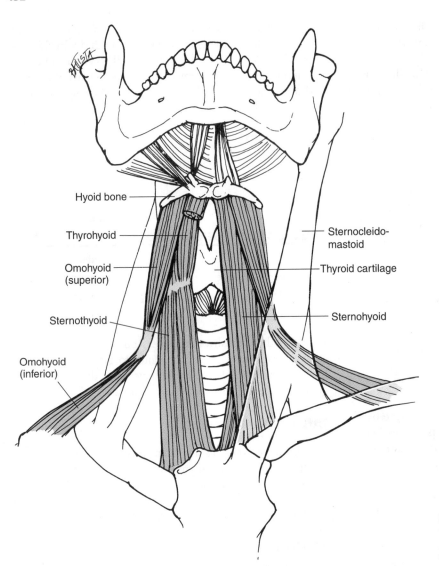

Hyoid bone

Thyrohyoid

Omohyoid
(superior)

Sternothyoid

Omohyoid
(inferior)

Sternocleido-
mastoid

Thyroid cartilage

Sternohyoid

Figure 22.10: The infrahyoid muscles consist of the sternohyoid, sternothyroid, thyrohyoid, and omohyoid muscles.

MUSCLE ATTACHMENT BOX 22.6

ATTACHMENTS AND INNERVATION OF THE INFRAHYOID MUSCLES

Sternohyoid

Attachments: The posterior surface of the medial clavicle and manubrium of the sternum to the inferior aspect of the hyoid bone

Innervation: Ventral rami of C1-C3 via fibers of the ansa cervicalis, which is a loop of nerves from the ventral rami of C2 and C3 and the hypoglossal nerve

Sternothyroid

Attachments: The posterior surface of the sternum and cartilage of the first rib to the laminae of the thyroid cartilage

Innervation: Ansa cervicalis, which is a loop of nerves from the ventral rami of C2 and C3 and the hypoglossal nerve

Thyrohyoid

Attachments: The laminae of the thyroid cartilage to the hyoid bone. It is essentially the continuation of the sternothyroid muscle.

Innervation: Ventral rami of C1 carried by the hypoglossal nerve (12th cranial nerve)

Omohyoid

Attachments: The inferior belly attaches to the superior border of the scapula. The superior belly attaches to the hyoid bone. The two bellies join by an intermediate tendon at the base of the neck, posterior to the sternocleidomastoid muscle.

Innervation: Ansa cervicalis, which is a loop of nerves from the ventral rami of C2 and C3 and the hypoglossal nerve

Palpation: Not palpable.

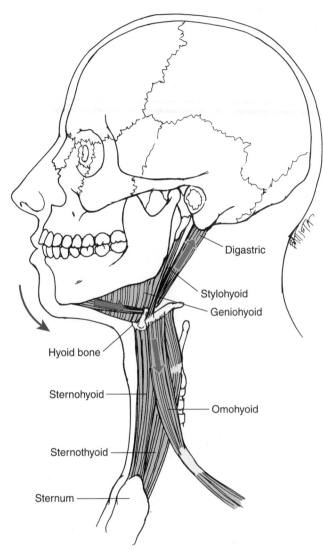

Figure 22.11: Fixation of the hyoid bone by the infrahyoid muscles. Contraction of the infrahyoid muscles holds the hyoid bone inferiorly so that the suprahyoid muscles can contract and depress the mandible.

opening to the trachea and modulate the tension in the vocal folds. The intrinsic laryngeal muscles that function in swallowing are those that close the entrance to the trachea. They include the interarytenoid, the lateral cricoarytenoid, and the thyroarytenoid muscles [22,26,32].

NORMAL SEQUENCE OF SWALLOWING

Swallowing is a complex series of coordinated events that transmit the contents of the oral cavity to the stomach through a region that includes parts of the respiratory tract. The challenge of the swallow is to propel the oral contents past the entries to the dedicated respiratory components, including the nose and trachea.

The swallow consists of four phases, the **oral preparatory, oral, pharyngeal,** and **esophageal phases** [8]. The oral preparatory phase technically precedes the actual swallow and is the period in which the ingested material is chewed and formed into a bolus. This process demands rhythmic coordination among the muscles of facial expression, the tongue, the muscles of mastication, and the suprahyoid and infrahyoid muscles [36]. During the oral preparatory phase the posterior aspect of the tongue elevates to the soft palate, closing off the pharynx and maintaining the food in the mouth. The common admonition "Don't speak with your mouth full" is wise advice, since speaking alters the position of the tongue and can open the passages to the nose and airway. The mechanisms and the muscles that participate in chewing are described in Chapters 23 and 24.

The remaining three phases—oral, pharyngeal, and esophageal—are described below. Although the sequence of events described below is generally accepted, it is important to recognize that individuals exhibit considerable variability in their own swallow patterns, affected by the size and consistency of the bolus, and there is even more variability across individuals [7,20,29]. Swallowing problems are common among the elderly, but aging itself does not appear to alter the normal sequence in a swallow, although the sequence is slowed with age [4,18,29,33].

Oral Phase

The **oral phase** is under voluntary control, while the pharyngeal and esophageal phases are reflexive. However, there is evidence that some reflexive movements within the larynx occur during the oral phase [23,32]. Once the ingestate is adequately prepared for swallowing, during the oral preparatory phase, the process of propelling it to the stomach begins. The oral phase is composed of the tongue movements that thrust the bolus into the pharynx and movements of the pharynx toward the bolus. At the initiation of the swallow, the tip of the tongue lifts the contents of the mouth up against the hard palate [3,39]. Motion of the tongue propagates through the rest of the tongue by contraction of the genioglossus and then the intrinsic muscles of the tongue, creating a peristaltic motion of the tongue that propels the contents posteriorly [8,15]. The back of the tongue then lowers, opening the pharynx, and forms a **chute** that empties into the pharynx. Contact by the bolus on the anterior arch, or **faucial fold,** of the soft palate descending from the uvula triggers the swallow reflex, beginning the pharyngeal phase of the swallow.

Concurrent with the tongue's actions in the oral phase, the suprahyoid muscles begin to pull the pharynx superiorly, which shortens the distance that must be traveled by the bolus, facilitating transmission of the bolus and closure of the vocal cords [3,5,8,23,31,35]. For the suprahyoid muscles to pull the hyoid bone superiorly, their superior attachment on the mandible must be fixed by the mandibular elevators, the masseter, temporalis, and medial pterygoid muscles discussed in Chapter 24 [37]. Thus it is impossible to swallow with the jaw relaxed. The oral phase of a swallow lasts 0.5 to 1.0 second [3,8]. The airway is open during the oral phase of swallowing,

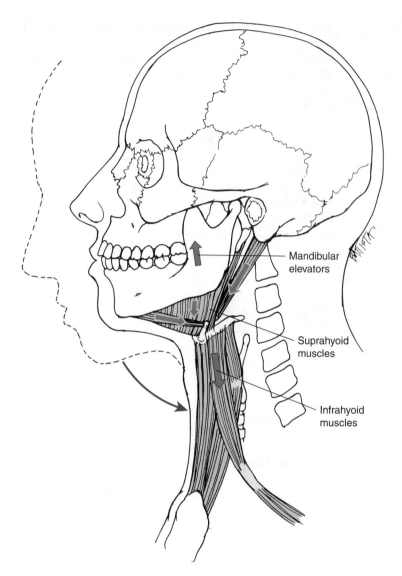

Figure 22.12: Cervical flexion by the suprahyoid and infrahyoid muscles. Simultaneous contraction of the suprahyoid and infrahyoid muscles along with the mandibular elevators contributes to cervical flexion.

and precise muscle control and coordination are required to avoid aspiration.

Pharyngeal Phase

The **pharyngeal phase** of the swallow is under reflex control and consists of several distinct tasks:

- Transmission of the bolus past the nasopharynx and larynx, requiring activity of muscles that close off these spaces
- Continued elevation of the larynx by the suprahyoid muscles assisted by the palatopharyngeus, stylopharyngeus, and salpingopharyngeus
- Action of the pharyngeal constrictor muscles to clear the bolus from the pharynx
- Relaxation of the esophageal sphincter

As the bolus passes the walls of the soft palate, initiating the swallow reflex, the muscles of the soft palate, the levator and tensor veli palatini, and the musculus uvulae contract, pulling the soft palate superiorly and posteriorly, sealing off the nasal cavity from the bolus [24,38,39]. Data from endoscopic videos and from EMG studies reveal continued adduction of the vocal folds and progressive closure of the laryngeal inlet [23,32,35].

Elevation of the hyoid bone and consequently the pharynx, which begins in the oral phase, continues in the pharyngeal phase. This elevation provides additional protection for the airway, because as elevation proceeds, the epiglottis, the leaflike cartilage of the larynx, folds posteriorly, creating a lid over the larynx and entry to the trachea. Maximum elevation of the hyoid bone during a swallow is approximately 1.0 to 1.5 cm [7]. At the same time, the constrictor muscles create a wave of muscle contraction that pushes the bolus inferiorly through the pharynx. The bolus slides over the epiglottis, past the larynx, and into the esophagus [25,26]. The pharyngeal phase of the swallow lasts less than 1 second [3,8].

Esophageal Phase

The bolus enters the esophagus through the esophageal sphincter, also known as the cricopharyngeus muscle. Except during the swallow, this sphincter maintains a low constant level of activity to prevent regurgitation [12,13,24,26,34]. However, contact of the bolus on the sphincter relaxes the muscle reflexively [2]. In addition, elevation of the hyoid bone by the suprahyoid muscles during the oral and pharyngeal phases applies traction to the sphincter, facilitating its opening [8].

The bolus is transmitted through the esophagus via peristaltic contractions of the smooth muscle of the esophagus. The esophagus is a muscular tube that is about 25 cm long, and transport through it can take several seconds [6,38]. After the bolus is entirely within the esophagus and the upper esophageal sphincter closes again, the infrahyoid muscles contract to pull the hyoid bone inferiorly to its resting position.

COMMON ABNORMALITIES IN SWALLOWING

Abnormalities in swallowing may involve any of the phases, including the oral preparatory phase, and can lead to aspiration at any time, before, during, or even after the swallow. Common impairments in the swallow mechanism for each phase are described below.

Impairments of the Oral Preparatory Phase

Impairments during the oral preparatory phase impede the ability to chew the contents of the food and form it into a bolus. Weakness of the facial muscles of the lips and cheeks can allow the contents to leak from the mouth or become sequestered between the cheeks and teeth. Abnormal control of the muscles of mastication impairs the ability to grind the food, and inadequate tongue control makes it difficult to locate the food between the teeth for successful chewing. These impairments may lead to an inability to form a bolus or the production of a bolus that is too large to be propelled easily to the stomach.

Impairments of the Oral Phase

The oral phase requires coordinated movement of the tongue, so impaired tongue movement can result in slowed movement of the bolus toward the pharynx. Conversely, inadequate tongue control also can allow the oral contents to slip too rapidly into the pharynx. Since the airway is open during the oral preparatory and oral phases of swallowing, premature movement of the bolus into the pharynx can lead to aspiration.

Impairments of the Pharyngeal Phase

Impairments of swallowing during the pharyngeal phase result from decreased muscle function and can include inadequate closure of the nasopharynx or larynx and inadequate propulsion of the bolus through the pharynx. Weakness of the muscles of the soft palate can allow the contents of the mouth to enter the nose by way of the nasopharynx. Impaired laryngeal protection may result directly from weakness of the intrinsic muscles of the larynx or from inadequate elevation of the pharynx, so that the protection provided by the tilting of the epiglottis is absent. Inadequate relaxation of the upper esophageal sphincter also may allow the contents to collect at the base of the laryngeal pharynx and slip into the larynx. Weakness of the pharyngeal constrictor muscles may impede the progress of the bolus and again allow it to enter the airway after the laryngeal muscles have relaxed.

Impairments of the Esophageal Phase

Inadequate peristalsis can delay the progression of the bolus through the esophagus. Failure of the cricopharyngeus muscle to close the esophagus at the end of the swallow may allow regurgitation, and aspiration of the regurgitated contents can result.

Signs of Swallowing Impairment

As noted at the beginning of this chapter, the goal of this discussion is to assist a clinician in identifying individuals who may have difficulty in swallowing, to refer the individual to the health care providers best suited to evaluate and treat the condition. Clinicians should suspect swallowing difficulties when an individual coughs regularly or clears the throat regularly before, during, or after a swallow. The material ingested may slip past the mouth before the individual has initiated the swallow, producing a cough before the swallow has even begun. The material may be transmitted appropriately but may slip into an inadequately closed larynx, producing a cough just as the individual swallows. The material may not be transported completely through the pharynx and may become sequestered within the pharynx only to slip later onto the larynx, producing a cough several minutes following the swallow. Since in each of these instances some of the ingested material arrives at the larynx, alterations in voice quality while eating may also suggest inadequate swallow. The voice may sound "wet" or "gurgly," as though the individual needs to clear his or her throat. **Quiet aspiration** also occurs in which there is no coughing or throat clearing to indicate the presence of a liquid or solid at the larynx. Signs of silent aspiration include loss of voice, face reddening, and eye watering.

Examination of the oral cavity to determine if food is sequestered in the cheeks or on the hard palate is useful. Observation of voluntary tongue movements, lip musculature, and muscles of the soft palate is also possible. The muscles of the soft palate contract to close off the nasopharynx when an individual says "ah," and elevation of the soft palate is easily observed for excursion and symmetry. The hyoid bone and the thyroid cartilage of the larynx are palpable during the swallow to assess the motion of the hyoid bone and thus the participation of the supra- and infrahyoid muscles. The clinician must realize that these examination procedures are screening tools to identify patients who may exhibit swallowing disorders. Because swallowing disorders have the potential to lead to lethal sequelae including aspiration pneumonia and asphyxia, the clinician must refer the patient for further, more detailed evaluations by specially trained health care providers who can diagnose and implement treatment for dysphagia.

SUMMARY

This chapter provides an overview of the muscles that participate in swallowing, specifically the muscles of the tongue and soft palate, and the extrinsic muscles of the larynx, the suprahyoid and infrahyoid muscles. The intrinsic muscles of the tongue alter the tongue's shape, while its extrinsic muscles move the tongue, helping to form the bolus and propel it into the oropharynx. The muscles of the soft palate help close off the nasopharynx as the bolus passes into the oropharynx. The suprahyoid muscles elevate the larynx, and the infrahyoid muscles assist in lowering the larynx. Elevation of the larynx along with contraction of the intrinsic muscles of the larynx closes the larynx during the swallow, preventing aspiration.

The swallow is a complex series of coordinated events and consists of four phases—the oral preparatory, oral, pharyngeal, and esophageal phases. Impairments and ensuing dysfunctions can occur in any of the phases, and the chapter lists signs that an individual with swallowing impairments may exhibit, including coughing, a "gurgly" voice, or loss of voice. Because aspiration and aspiration pneumonia are common among the elderly, clinicians who deal with elders must be able to recognize signs of impaired swallowing and refer the

patient to specially trained professionals qualified to diagnose and treat individuals with swallowing disorders.

References

1. Castro HA, Resende LA, Berzin F, Konig B: Electromyographic analysis of the superior belly of the omohyoid muscle and anterior belly of the digastric muscle in tongue and head movements. J Electromyogr Kinesiol 1999; 9: 229–232.
2. Cook IJ: Cricopharyngeal function and dysfunction. Dysphagia 1993; 8: 244–251.
3. Cook IJ, Dodds WJ, Dantas RO, et al.: Timing of videofluoroscopic, manometric events, and bolus transit during the oral and pharyngeal phases of swallowing. Dysphagia 1989; 4: 8–15.
4. Cook IJ, Weltman MD, Wallace K, et al.: Influence of aging on oral-pharyngeal bolus transit and clearance during swallowing: scintigraphic study. Am J Physiol 1994; 266: G972–G977.
5. Curtis DJ, Sepulveda GU: Epiglottic motion: video recording of muscular dysfunction. Radiology 1983; 148: 473–477.
6. Dodds WJ: The physiology of swallowing. Dysphagia 1989; 3: 171–178.
7. Dodds WJ, Man KM, Cook IJ, et al.: Influence of bolus volume on swallow-induced hyoid movement in normal subjects. AJR 1988; 150: 1307–1309.
8. Dodds WJ, Stewart ET, Logemann JA: Physiology and radiology of the normal oral and pharyngeal phases of swallowing. AJR 1990; 154: 953–963.
9. Dworkin JP, Aronson AE: Tongue strength and alternate motion rates in normal and dysarthric subjects. J Commun Disord 1986; 19: 115–132.
10. Dworkin JP, Aronson AE, Mulder DW: Tongue force in normals and in dysarthric patients with amyotrophic lateral sclerosis. J Speech Hear Res 1980; 23: 828–837.
11. Ekberg O: Posture of the head and pharyngeal swallowing. Acta Radiol 1986; 27: 691–696.
12. Elidan J, Gonen B: Electromyography of the inferior constrictor and cricopharyngeal muscles during swallowing. Ann Otol Rhinol Laryngol 1990; 99: 466–469.
13. Elidan J, Shochina M, Gonen B, Gay I: Manometry and electromyography of the pharyngeal muscles in patients with dysphagia. Arch Otolaryngol Head Neck Surg 1990; 116: 910–913.
14. Ferdjallah M, Wertsch JJ, Shaker R: Spectral analysis of surface electromyography (EMG) of upper esophageal sphincter-opening muscles during head lift exercise. J Rehabil Res Dev 2000; 37: 335–340.
15. Kahrilas PJ, Lin S, Jerilyn A, et al.: Deglutitive tongue action: volume accommodation and bolus propulsion. Gastroenterology 1993; 104: 152–162.
16. Kahrilas P, Logemann J, Lin S, Ergun G: Pharyngeal clearance during swallowing: a combined manometric and videofluoroscopic study. Gastroenterology 1992; 103: 128–136.
17. Kikuchi R, Watabe N, Konno T, et al.: High incidence of silent aspiration in elderly patients with community-acquired pneumonia. Am J Respir Crit Care Med 1994; 150: 251–253.
18. Kim Y, McCullough GH, Asp CW: Temporal measurements of pharyngeal swallowing in normal populations. Dysphagia 2005; 20: 290–296.
19. Langmore S, Terpenning M, Schork A, et al.: Predictors of aspiration pneumonia: how important is dysphagia? Dysphagia 1998; 13: 69–81.

20. Lof GL, Robbins J: Test-retest variability in normal swallowing. Dysphagia 1990; 4: 236–242.

21. Lundy D, Smith C, Colangelo L, et al.: Aspiration: cause and implications. Otolaryngol Head Neck Surg 1999; 120: 474–478.

22. McCulloch TM, Perlman AL, Palmer PM, Van Daele DJ: Laryngeal activity during swallow, phonation, and the Valsalva maneuver: an electromyographic analysis. Laryngoscope 1996; 106: 1351–1358.

23. Ohmae Y, Logemann JA, Kaiser P, et al.: Timing of glottic closure during normal swallow. Head Neck 1995; 17: 394–402.

24. Palmer JB: Electromyography of the muscles of oropharyngeal swallowing: basic concepts. Dysphagia 1989; 3: 192–198.

25. Perlman AL, Luschei ES, Du Mond CE: Electrical activity from the superior pharyngeal constrictor during reflexive and nonreflexive tasks. J Speech Hear Res 1989; 32: 749–754.

26. Perlman AL, Palmer PM, McCulloch TM, Van Daele DJ: Electromyographic activity from human laryngeal, pharyngeal, and submental muscles during swallowing. J Appl Physiol 1999; 86: 1663–1669.

27. Perrier P, Payan Y, Zandipour M, Perkell J: Influences of tongue biomechanics on speech movements during the production of velar stop consonants: a modeling study. J Acoust Soc Am 2003; 114: 1582–1599.

28. Pouderoux P, Kahrilas PJ: Deglutitive tongue force modulation by volition, volume, and viscosity in humans. Gastroenterology 1995; 108: 1418–1426.

29. Robbins J, Hamilton JW, Lof GL, Kempster GB: Oropharyngeal swallowing in normal adults of different ages. Gastroenterology 1992; 103: 823–829.

30. Roubeau B, Chevrie-Muller C, Lacau Saint Guily J: Electromyographic activity of strap and cricothyroid muscles in pitch change. Acta Otolaryngol 1997; 117: 459–464.

31. Schultz JL, Perlman AL, VanDaele DJ: Laryngeal movement, oropharyngeal pressure, and submental muscle contraction during swallowing. Arch Phys Med Rehabil 1994; 75: 183–188.

32. Shaker R, Dodds WJ, Dantas RO, et al.: Coordination of deglutitive glottic closure with oropharyngeal swallowing. Gastroenterology 1990; 98: 1478–1484.

33. Shaw DW, Cook IJ, Gabb M, et al.: Influence of normal aging on oral-pharyngeal and upper esophageal sphincter function during swallowing. Am J Physiol 1995; 268: G386–G396.

34. Sivarao DV, Goyal RK: Functional anatomy and physiology of the upper esophageal sphincter. Am J Med 2000; 108: 27S–37S.

35. Spiro J, Rendell JK, Gay T: Activation and coordination patterns of the suprahyoid muscles during swallowing. Laryngoscope 1994; 104: 1376–1382.

36. Takada K, Yashiro K, Sorihashi Y, et al.: Tongue, jaw, and lip muscle activity and jaw movement during experimental chewing efforts in man. J Dent Res 1996; 75: 1598–1606.

37. Tallgren A: Longitudinal electromyographic study of swallowing patterns in complete denture wearers. Int J Prosthodont 1995; 8: 467–478.

38. Williams P, Bannister L, Berry M, et al.: Gray's Anatomy, The Anatomical Basis of Medicine and Surgery, Br. ed. London: Churchill Livingstone, 1995.

39. Zimmerman JE, Oder LA: Swallowing dysfunction in acutely ill patients. Phys Ther 1981; 61: 51–59.

Structure and Function of the Articular Structures of the TMJ

Z. ANNETTE IGLARSH, P.T., PH.D., M.B.A.
CAROL A. OATIS, P.T., PH.D.

CHAPTER CONTENTS

The temporomandibular joint (TMJ) is a potential source of acute and chronic pain in the head and neck regions, and countless types of painful syndromes have been attributed to dysfunction of this joint and its surrounding muscles [24]. Complaints associated with TMJ dysfunction include headaches, **tinnitus** (ringing in the ears), and altered taste. An understanding of the pathomechanics of an impaired TMJ requires a thorough grasp of the structures and function of the TMJ and surrounding tissue [30].

The joint participates in the essential functions of chewing, or **mastication,** and speech [15]. As a consequence, the evaluation and treatment of the joint falls within the scope of practice of dentists and speech and hearing specialists. As a joint of the neuromusculoskeletal system that refers pain to the upper quadrant, it also is studied and treated by therapists and physicians. Consequently, an understanding of the structure and function of the joint can contribute to interdisciplinary collaborations leading to more effective treatments and improved patient outcomes. The purposes of this chapter are to

- Review the structure and function of the articular components of the TMJ
- Describe the motions that occur in the TMJ
- Review the normal ranges of motion of the TMJ
- Describe how TMJ structures and dysfunction may contribute to patient complaint
- Briefly discuss the relationship between the TMJ and posture of the head and cervical spine

BONY STRUCTURES THAT CONSTITUTE AND INFLUENCE THE TMJ

The TMJ, also known as the **craniomandibular joint,** is the articulation between the mandible and the temporal bone of the skull [18] (*Fig. 23.1*). The structural relationship of the mandible to the head contributes to the impact of the TMJ on the muscles of the upper quadrant and the cervical spine. The postures of the mandible with respect to the head and of the head with respect to the neck are so interdependent that it is almost impossible to alter the position of one structure without influencing the other structures [39].

Cranium

The bones of the cranium provide an articular surface for the TMJ and attachments for the muscles of mastication, which are described in Chapter 24. The cranial bones that provide articular surfaces for the TMJ are the temporal and mandibular bones (*Fig. 23.2*). Other bones participate in the function of the joint by providing muscle attachments and articulation for the teeth. The sphenoid and zygomatic bones provide large attachments for the muscles of mastication. The upper teeth articulate with the maxilla, and the palatine bones attach posteriorly to the maxilla, providing additional attachments for the muscles of mastication.

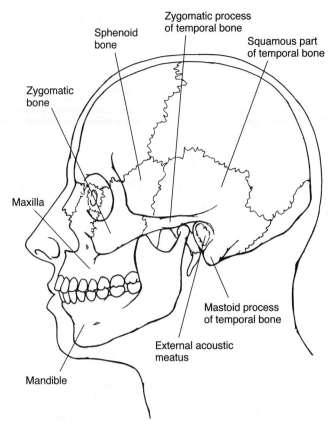

Figure 23.2: Cranial bones particularly relevant to the TMJ are the mandible and the temporal, sphenoid, zygomatic, maxilla, and palatine bones. The palatine bones are not visible in this figure.

TEMPORAL BONE

The temporal bone is a large bone forming part of the lateral wall of the cranium [40,47]. Its inferior surface provides the rostral articular surfaces of the TMJ, including the concave mandibular fossa, or glenoid fossa, and the articular eminence (*Fig. 23.3*). The articular eminence forms the anterior limit of the mandibular fossa and contributes the anteriormost portion of the articular surface of the temporal bone. A styloid process lies slightly posterior to the mandibular fossa, projecting inferiorly from the inferior surface of the temporal bone and providing attachment for muscles of the tongue and pharynx.

Laterally, the temporal bone provides a large relatively flat surface, which together with the lateral aspect of the sphenoid constitutes the temporal fossa that provides attachment for the temporalis muscle. The large, prominent mastoid process lies posterior and lateral to the styloid process. The facial nerve exits the skull at the stylomastoid foramen that lies between the mastoid and styloid processes. The mastoid process is readily palpated and helps orient the clinician to the other structures during a clinical examination.

The external acoustic meatus also is located laterally, superior to the styloid process and slightly posterior to the mandibular fossa. The external auditory meatus leads to the

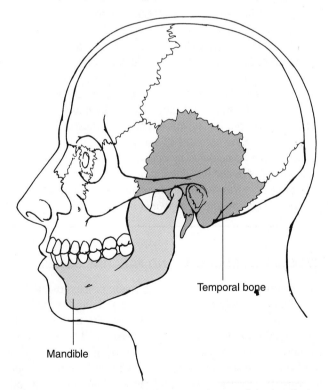

Figure 23.1: The TMJ consists of the articulation of the head of the mandible with the mandibular fossa and articular eminence on the inferior surface of the temporal bone

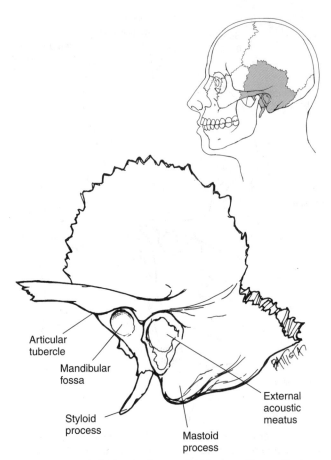

Figure 23.3: Articulating surface on the temporal bone. The mandibular fossa and articular eminence, which form the articular surface for the head of the mandible, lie on the inferior surface of the temporal bone. The styloid and mastoid processes lie posterior to the mandibular fossa.

middle and inner ears, lying within the temporal bone. The proximity of the external, middle, and inner ears to the TMJ may help explain why some individuals with TMJ dysfunction also report impaired hearing [3,9,19].

Clinical Relevance

EAR SYMPTOMATOLOGY WITH TMJ DYSFUNCTION: *Patients with TMJ dysfunction can present in the clinic with complaints of ear pain, ringing in the ears (tinnitus), or even impaired hearing. Such complaints may result from swelling in the area of the TMJ or from direct pressure from the head of the mandible on the inner ear, increasing the pressure around the structures of the ear canal.*

The zygomatic process of the temporal bone projects anteriorly from the lateral aspect of the temporal bone, superior to the external acoustic meatus. The inferior aspect of the root of the zygomatic process and the lateral aspect of

the articular eminence give rise to the articular tubercle that provides attachment for the temporomandibular ligament. The zygomatic process of the temporal bone joins the zygomatic bone anteriorly.

SPHENOID BONE

The sphenoid articulates with the anterior aspect of the temporal bone, contributing to the temporal fossa laterally [20,47]. Along with the palatine bones, the sphenoid bone also contributes to the hard palate of the mouth. The inferior surface of the sphenoid bone contributes to the anterior aspect of the base of the skull, and it is this surface that contains structures that are important to the TMJ (*Fig. 23.4*). The lateral aspect of the inferior surface of the sphenoid bone contributes to the infratemporal fossa and provides the proximal attachment for two of the four primary muscles of mastication, the medial and lateral pterygoid muscles. The medial border of the infratemporal fossa is the lateral pterygoid plate, which projects inferiorly from the inferior surface of the sphenoid bone and contributes an additional attachment for the medial and lateral pterygoid muscles. The medial pterygoid plate also projects inferiorly from the inferior surface of the sphenoid bone and lies medial to the lateral pterygoid plate; it ends anteriorly as the hamulus, which can be palpated intraorally on the hard palate.

Clinical Relevance

PALPATION OF THE HAMULUS: *The hamulus of the sphenoid bone is palpated on the hard palate by placing the palpating finger posterior and medial to the third molar (Fig. 23.5). The pterygomandibular raphe, which is a fibrous band that runs from the hamulus to the mandible, also helps identify the hamulus intraorally, where it too is readily palpated, covered by a layer of mucous membrane. The lateral pterygoid muscle passes just lateral to the hamulus of the sphenoid, and its contraction can be palpated by palpating the lateral aspect of the hamulus as the individual protracts the mandible. Tenderness in this region during contraction may indicate tenderness in the lateral pterygoid muscle.*

ZYGOMATIC, MAXILLA, AND PALATINE BONES

The zygomatic bone joins the zygomatic process of the temporal bone, completing the zygomatic arch, and is known as the cheekbone. The zygomatic arch gives rise to the masseter muscle, an important muscle of mastication. The arch serves to increase the mechanical advantage of the masseter while reinforcing the strength of the zygomatic and temporal bones to resist the forces of powerful jaw closing. The zygomatic bone also contributes to the lateral wall of the eye socket, or orbit, and to the infraorbital fossa. Anteriorly, the zygomatic bones articulate with the maxillae, the largest bones of the

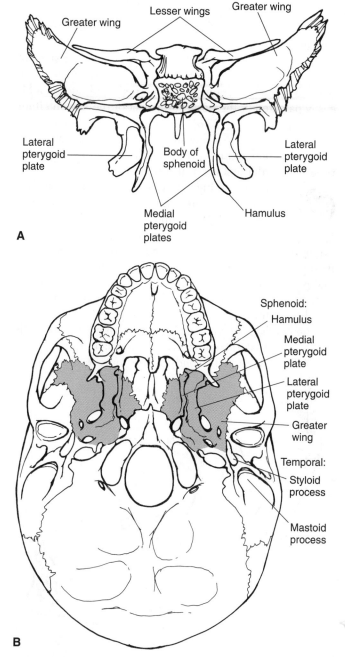

A

B

Figure 23.4: Sphenoid bone. **A.** Posterior view reveals that the inferior surface of the sphenoid bone is marked by the medial and lateral pterygoid plates. The lateral pterygoid plate provides attachment for the medial and lateral pterygoid muscles. **B.** Inferior view reveals only the greater wings of the sphenoid bone and their projections, since the body of the sphenoid is covered by nasal bones. Inferiorly, the medial pterygoid plate contains the projection, the hamulus, palpable inside the oral cavity.

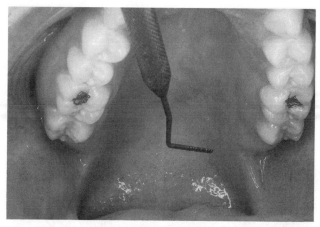

Figure 23.5: The hamulus of the medial pterygoid plate of the sphenoid bone can be palpated intraorally posterior and medial to the third molar. Pterygomandibular raphe attaches to the hamulus and is an easily identified fibrous band, covered by mucous membrane. (Photo courtesy of Arnold J Malerman, DDS, PC, Dresher, PA)

anterior to the TMJ, but its proximity to the joint may explain why some individuals with TMJ symptoms also report chronic sinus pain or irritation. The palatine bones attach between the maxillae and the sphenoid to contribute to the hard palate and floor of the nasal cavity [47].

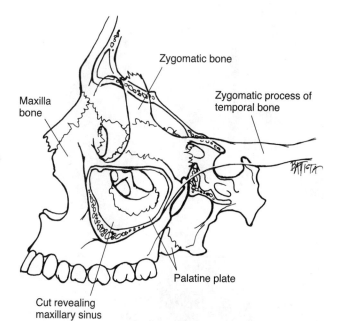

Figure 23.6: Zygomatic bone attaches to the temporal bone and to the maxilla, which contains the upper row of teeth. Palatine bones articulate with the maxilla anteriorly and the sphenoid posteriorly, and together they form the hard palate. The large maxillary sinus found within the maxilla lies anterior to the TMJ. Its proximity to the joint may explain patients' complaints of sinus irritation along with TMJ pain.

face. The maxillae contain the upper row of teeth and form the upper jaw (*Fig. 23.6*). They also compose most of the roof of the mouth and the floor and lateral walls of the nasal cavity and contribute to the infratemporal fossae [20,47]. The large maxillary sinus, a cavity that lies within the maxilla, is

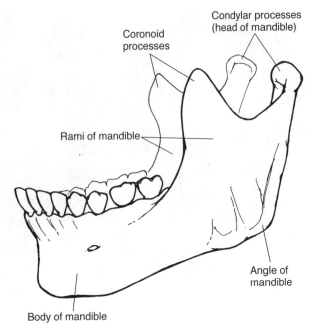

Figure 23.7: The mandible consists of a body and two rami, each ending in coronoid and condylar processes.

MANDIBLE

The mandible, or jaw bone, consists of a U-shaped body containing the lower row of teeth, and two rami projecting posteriorly and superiorly from the right and left sides of the body of the mandible [8,10] (*Fig 23.7*). The angle of the mandible marks the junction of the body and ramus and is easily palpated at the posterior aspect of the jaw on either side of the face (*Fig. 23.8*). The angles of the mandible are important landmarks, lying superior to the posterior tips of the hyoid bone and inferior and anterior to the transverse processes of the first cervical vertebra.

Each mandibular ramus ends superiorly in two processes. The anterior, coronoid process provides attachment for the temporalis muscle. The anterior border of the coronoid process is palpable inferior to the zygomatic arch. The posterior condylar process thickens at its superior end to form the head of the mandible that articulates with the temporal bone in the TMJ. The head narrows inferiorly, forming the neck of the ramus that provides attachment for a portion of the lateral pterygoid muscle.

The condyles of the mandible are shaped like footballs cut in half that tilt anteriorly and medially toward each other (*Fig. 23.9*). The condyles are more curved in the

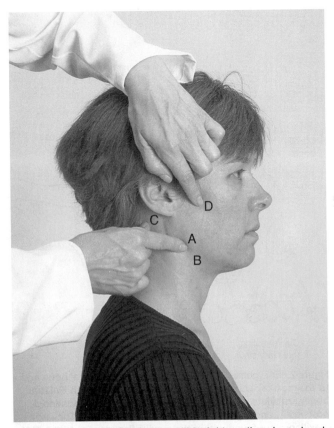

Figure 23.8: The angle of the mandible (*A*) is easily palpated and helps locate the hyoid bone (*B*) inferiorly and the transverse process (*C*) of C1 posteriorly. The coronoid process (*D*) of the mandible is palpable inferior to the zygomatic arch.

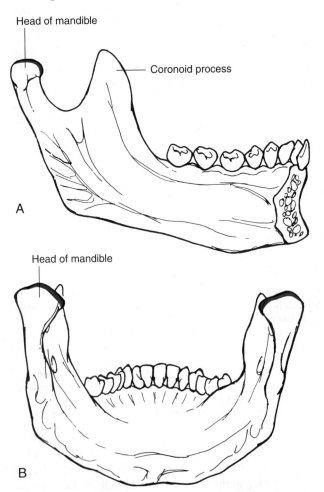

Figure 23.9: **A.** Medial view of the mandible reveals that the articular surfaces of the mandibular condyles face anteriorly. **B.** Posterior view reveals that the articular condyles also face medially.

anterior—posterior direction and slightly flatter in the medial–lateral direction, but show considerable interindividual variability [35,47].

ARTICULAR STRUCTURES OF THE TMJ

The mandible is suspended from the temporal bones at the TMJs, which together form a **compound joint** in which both TMJs must move simultaneously whenever the mandible moves. Although each TMJ often is described as a hinge joint, each joint exhibits more complex motion that occurs in the sagittal, transverse, and frontal planes [7] (*Fig. 23.10*). Opening and closing of the mouth occur primarily in the sagittal plane. Protrusion and retrusion consist primarily of forward and backward translation of the mandible, primarily in the transverse plane, although the shape of the articular eminence requires that the mandible descend as it glides anteriorly and rise as it glides posteriorly. The TMJ allows rotation of the mandible in the transverse plane motion about an axis that projects vertically through a mandibular head. The mandible also can swing from left to right in the frontal plane about an anterior posterior axis. The teeth and the shapes of the articular surfaces guide and limit the motion of the jaw.

The articular surfaces of the mandibular condyle and the articular eminence of the temporal bone are both covered by articular cartilage. Unlike most synovial joints, however, the articular cartilage consists of fibrocartilage rather than hyaline cartilage. As in other synovial joints, the articular cartilage lacks a vascular supply and is nourished and lubricated by the synovial fluid supplied by the surrounding synovial tissue.

Clinical Relevance

WITHSTANDING LARGE FORCES AT THE TMJ: *Most synovial joint surfaces are covered with hyaline cartilage. In contrast, fibrocartilage is found in joints that sustain large forces such as the intervertebral joints of the spine. The presence of fibrocartilage in the TMJ suggests that the TMJ incurs large forces during mastication. Hu et al. suggest that the fibrocartilage is a more important shock absorber at the TMJ than the articular disc [22]. Arthritis and degeneration of the articular cartilage can lead to severe problems in mastication.*

The articular surface of the mandible consists of the superior and anterior surfaces of the mandibular head. The anterior portion of the articular surface on the temporal bone consists of the posterior, convex portion of the articular eminence (*Fig. 23.11*). The remainder of the temporal articular surface is the mandibular fossa that ends posteriorly as the posterior articular ridge, immediately anterior to the external auditory meatus. The shape of the articulating surface of the temporal bone explains the complex motion that occurs during opening and closing the mouth, combining rotation about a medial lateral axis and translation along the curved surface of the articular eminence.

The roof of the mandibular fossa is typically thin and non-weight-bearing. Loads are borne between the mandibular condyle and intraarticular disc and between the disc and articular eminence of the temporal bone. The layer of fibrocartilage covering the entire articulating surface of the temporal bone is thickest on the articular surface of the articular eminence where the stress is the greatest, and thinnest at the roof of the mandibular fossa where little load bearing occurs [38].

Articular Disc

Like the knee, the TMJ contains an intraarticular disc, or meniscus, that separates the joint into a superior joint space, between the disc and the articular eminence, and an inferior joint space, between the disc and the mandibular head [17,18,28,31,34] (*Fig. 23.12*). The disc increases the congruency between the joint surfaces, but also can be a source of pain and dysfunction. The articular disc is concave superiorly to conform to the articular eminence of the temporal bone and concave inferiorly to mold to the convex mandibular head [47].

The disc consists of dense fibrous connective tissue that adheres more firmly to the mandible than to the temporal bone. The stronger inferior connection includes medial and lateral bands from the disc to the articular condyle, a strong anterior connection with the fibers of the lateral pterygoid and a loose fibrous connection posteriorly. The disc is thickest peripherally and thinnest at its center. If the normal anatomical alignment of the joint surfaces is altered, the disc can be torn or perforated as forces compress the thin center of the disc [2,6,17,28,41,49].

The disc continues posteriorly as two layers of loose fibrous tissue, a fibroelastic layer that attaches to the posterior aspect of the mandibular fossa of the temporal bone, and an inferior inelastic layer that attaches to the condyle of the mandible. This **bilaminar region** is highly vascular and rich in nerve endings and fuses with the articular capsule posteriorly as the **retrodiscal pad.** The central portion of the disc is avascular, an indication of its stress-bearing role in TMJ function.

Clinical Relevance

DISC PATHOLOGY: *Many temporomandibular joint dysfunctions involve problems with the disc. The disc can degenerate or tear just as the menisci within the knees do. The bilaminar region and retrodiscal pad can become inflamed and painful from repeated or prolonged compressive forces. Such forces can occur from teeth clenching or grinding. The disc itself can be subluxed (partially dislocated) or dislocated*

(continued)

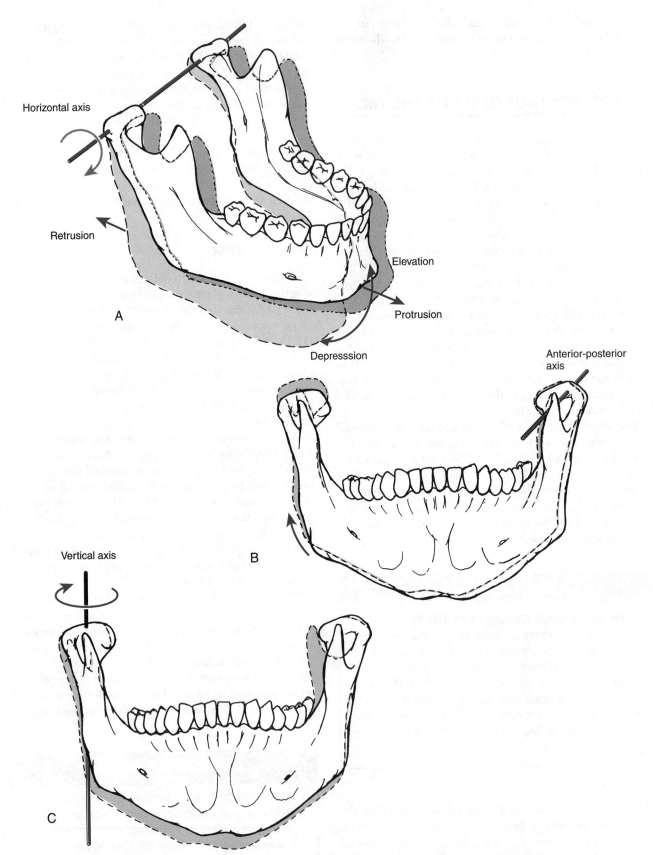

Figure 23.10: The TMJ exhibits three-dimensional motion that includes rotations about medial–lateral **(A)**, anterior–posterior **(B)**, and vertical **(C)** axes. It also allows translation in the sagittal and transverse planes.

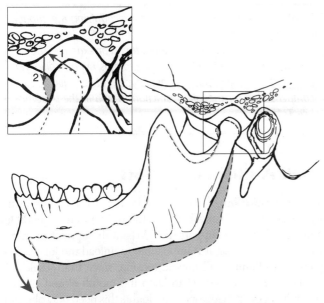

Figure 23.11: The articulating surface of the temporal bone consists of the mandibular fossa and the articular eminence. Opening and closing require rotation of the mandible about a medial lateral axis and translation of the mandibular head along the articular eminence, producing anterior and inferior translation of the mandible.

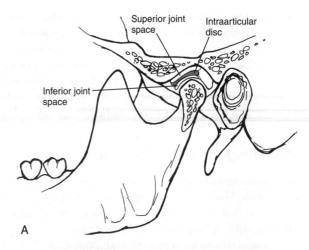

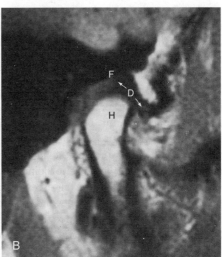

Figure 23.12: The intraarticular disc divides the TMJ into a superior space between the temporal bone and the disc and an inferior space between the disc and the mandibular head. **A.** Sagittal plane view of left disc with the mouth closed. **B.** Sagittal plane MRI of right disc with the mouth closed.

(Continued)
anteriorly (internal derangement of the TMJ), producing abnormal opening and closing patterns of movement and even an inability to fully close the mouth. Just as a complete assessment of the knee includes assessment of the menisci, a thorough assessment of the TMJ includes consideration of the articular disc.

Ligaments

The primary ligamentous supporting structures of the TMJ are the joint capsule and the temporomandibular ligament [17,20,23,28,42,44] (*Fig. 23.13*). Additional ligaments include the sphenomandibular and stylomandibular ligaments. It is important to recognize that stability of the TMJ comes not just from ligamentous support but also from the muscles of mastication that are discussed in detail in Chapter 24 [25].

JOINT CAPSULE

The joint capsule encloses the articular surfaces of the temporal bone and mandibular head, as well as the disc. The capsule can be traced superiorly along the rim of the mandibular fossa, anteriorly around the articular surface of the articular eminence, and inferiorly around the mandibular head.

The horizontal fibers of the joint capsule connect directly to the lateral and medial parts of the disc. The capsule fuses

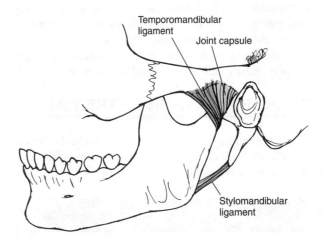

Figure 23.13: Primary ligaments of the TMJ are the joint capsule and the temporomandibular ligament. The stylomandibular and sphenomandibular (not seen in this view) ligaments are accessory ligaments.

with the anterior disc, while posteriorly, the disc connects with the capsule via the retrodiscal pad. Consequently, the disc translates anteriorly easily as its posterior attachments to the retrodiscal pad stretch, but glides little in a posterior direction because of its firm inelastic anterior attachment to the joint capsule. The capsular ligament allows joint motion in the sagittal plane but restricts motion in the frontal and transverse planes [20,25,27].

TEMPOROMANDIBULAR LIGAMENT

The temporomandibular ligament, also known as the lateral temporomandibular ligament, reinforces the joint capsule laterally and consists of two layers, the wide, superficial layer and the medial, deep portion [47]. The superficial portion of the ligament courses downward and posteriorly from the articular tubercle to the posterior surface of the mandibular head, while the deep, or medial, part runs from the articular tubercle and the temporal squama in an anterior and medial direction. These fibers, running horizontally, join the fibers of the joint capsule and disc.

The lateral fibers of the joint capsule limit inferior translations of the mandible. The medial fibers, assisted by the lateral pterygoid muscle, limit posterior translation of the mandible during retrusion or from a direct blow to the jaw. Consequently, these fibers protect the highly vascular and sensitive retrodiscal pad in the posterior joint. Thus the temperomandibular ligament helps prevent excessive jaw opening by checking the mandible's descent beyond the articular eminence [25,27]. It also prevents damage to the retrodiscal pad by preventing excessive posterior translation of the mandible [20].

THE STYLOMANDIBULAR AND SPHENOMANDIBULAR LIGAMENTS

These two ligaments are accessory ligaments and appear to have minor effects on movement of the mandible. Their names reflect their sites of attachment: the stylomandibular ligament starts at the apex of the styloid process and ends on the ramus of the mandible and the sphenomandibular ligament courses from the spine of the sphenoid bone to the mandibular foramen. The stylomandibular ligament may limit forward glide of the mandible during protrusion, but the sphenomandibular ligament appears to have little effect on TMJ motion or stability [47].

ARTICULAR FUNCTIONS OF THE TMJ

The TMJs are unique because they are mechanically linked by the mandible and must work synchronously for the mandible to move normally [17,21,36,39,46].

Clinical Relevance

IMPACT OF SYNCHRONOUS MOVEMENT AND DYNAMIC EVALUATION OF THE TMJ: *When a patient complains of TMJ pain or dysfunction, it is not possible to isolate the cause in one joint without recognizing the impact on the opposite joint. The impairment identified in each joint can be opposite from one another. For example, the practitioner may determine that one joint is hypomobile and then find that the opposite joint is hypermobile, a likely compensation for the joint restrictions found in the hypomobile TMJ.*

Static Positions of the TMJ

The **rest position** of the mandible is a natural position in which there is a balance between the weight of the mandible and the forces that support the TMJs in the upright posture. In the erect position it is impossible to unload the joint completely or eliminate all muscle tension, since the muscles of mastication must contract to keep the mouth closed against the pull of gravity. (Anyone who doubts this need only observe the open-mouthed posture of a student who has fallen asleep in class.) In the normal rest position the tongue is maintained against the hard palate by negative air pressure within the mouth, forming an area referred to as **Donder's space.** The negative air pressure decreases the amount of muscle force needed to support the jaw. The two rows of teeth do not touch in the rest position, but the lips are in gentle contact with each other. In this position, the mandibular head faces the articular eminence of the temporal bone and the disc is seated anteriorly on the mandibular head, between the two articulating surfaces. This combination of disc position and limited muscle activity mechanically unloads the soft tissue of the TMJ. In contrast, the **occlusal position** is defined as the posture in which the two rows of teeth are in gentle contact.

Functional Motions of the TMJ

As noted earlier, the TMJs allow complex three-dimensional motion. The functional movements that allow the jaw to move during mastication and speech are opening and closing the mouth, as well as protrusion, retrusion, and lateral deviation of the jaw.

OPENING AND CLOSING THE MOUTH

Mouth opening, also known as **mandibular depression,** combines rotation about a medial–lateral axis with protrusion in the transverse and sagittal planes. Closing, or mandibular elevation, consists of upward rotation of the mandible and retrusion. Most of the rotation and translation occur simultaneously throughout the range of motion, although the relative contribution of rotation and translation at initial opening is controversial [5,11]. Some investigators suggest that opening begins with rotation, others suggest it begins with translation, and still others report that the contribution is equally distributed [5,11,29]. These differences very well may represent normal individual variation and require additional research to resolve. The rotary motion of the joint occurs mostly in the inferior joint space between the disc and mandibular head. The translation occurs predominantly in the superior joint space as the disc moves to seat itself in the mandibular fossa.

Anterior translation of the disc is necessary to keep the disc in contact with the mandibular head. Forward translation stretches the retrodiscal tissue that contains collagen and elastin fibers. The loose tissue of the retrodiscal pad permits movement of the disc in the mandibular fossa of the temporal bone, and its recoil helps relocate the disc posteriorly. This movement occurs in the superior portion of the joint capsule.

Mouth opening occurs by the following combination of events [32,47]:

- The opening motion, as the mandible descends and the chin lowers, begins with mandibular rotation in the inferior joint space, the space between the disc and the mandibular head. (Slight anterior translation, or protrusion, which occurs in the superior joint space between the disc and temporal fossa may accompany or even precede the mandibular rotation.)
- As the mandible rotates downward, the disc moves posteriorly, relative to the mandibular head, to become seated on top of the mandibular head.
- Ligaments attached to the disc become taut, and the disc is held firmly against the mandibular head.
- Thus this motion is rotation between the disc and the mandibular condyle.
- The disc and mandibular head complex move as a single unit, translating anteriorly and inferiorly along the surface of the articular eminence, producing protrusion and additional depression.

Closing the mouth involves a reversal of the movements of opening, the mandible rotates upward and retrudes, although the mandible's path during closing differs slightly from its opening path [11,43,47,48]. Thus the simple motion of mouth opening or mandibular depression is not a simple hinge action in which the muscles of mastication relax and allow the mandible to rotate downward by gravity. The actions of mouth opening and closing are a complex series of controlled rotations and translations. The role of muscles in depressing and elevating the mandible is presented in Chapter 24.

PROTRUSION, RETRUSION, AND LATERAL MOTION

Protrusion, the motion of "jutting" the jaw forward, is accomplished as the mandibular condyles and the articular disc glide anteriorly and inferiorly along the articular eminence. **Retrusion** occurs in the opposite direction and is limited by taut anterior ligamentous and muscle fibers and the mass of the retrodiscal pad of the disc. Because the retrodiscal tissue is very vascular and well innervated, compression or irritation of the retrodiscal pad by excessive or sustained retrusion may produce TMJ pain.

Lateral deviation of the mandible also involves complex motions of both TMJs. It occurs by protrusion of the mandible on one side while the opposite side rotates about a vertical axis (*Fig. 23.14*). Consequently, one condyle and its disc move anteriorly, inferiorly, and medially along the articular eminence, causing deviation of the mandible toward the opposite side as the opposite condyle rotates laterally around a vertical axis. As in opening and closing, protrusion and lateral motions of the mandible occur by delicately coordinated muscle activity at both TMJs. Mastication is a complex series of motions that includes all the directions of motion discussed above and the corresponding synchronized contraction of the muscles of mastication. This activity is discussed in Chapter 24.

As noted earlier in the chapter, the TMJs are capable of complex three-dimensional motion. Although not specifically measured, the tilting motion of the mandible in the frontal plane, about the anterior–posterior axis, is also an essential movement of the TMJ. This motion allows chewing of a bolus of food on one side of the mouth, critical for controlling the bolus and preparing it for swallow. The tilt increases the joint reaction force on the side to which the mandible tilts.

Disc Movement

Normal movement of the TMJ requires precise synchronization between the movement of the mandible and the movement of the intraarticular disc. Abnormal movements of either can alter the mechanics of the whole TMJ complex

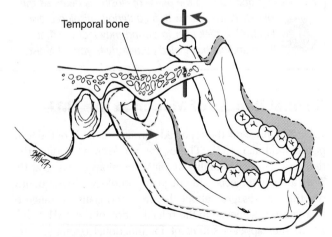

Temporal bone

Figure 23.14: Lateral deviation of the mandible to the left requires protrusion of the right TMJ and rotation of the left TMJ about a vertical axis.

and contribute to patients' signs and symptoms. As the muscles of mastication contract or relax and the mouth closes or opens, the disc remains in contact with the mandibular head and the disc–mandibular head complex moves together in translation [7].

When the mouth is fully open, the intermediate zone of the articular disc is between the articular tubercle of the temporal bone and the dorsal convexity of the condylar process of the mandible, increasing the congruency between the bony surfaces. The posterior retrodiscal cushion is stretched, and the anterior connective tissue is compressed in this position. When the mouth is closed, the retrodiscal cushion is moderately enlarged and the anterior cushion is smaller than when the teeth are in full contact. During protrusion of the mandible, the intermediate zone of the articular disc is between the convexities of the condylar process and the articular eminence. The disc is compressed between the mandible and the temporal bone on the lateral side of the joint. In lateral deviation, the disc is stabilized between the bony joint elements on the side toward which the mandible is deviating. On the opposite side, the articular disc protrudes, with the retrodiscal tissue filling the posterior, lateral half of the mandibular fossa.

Clinical Relevance

SOUNDS ELICITED DURING OPENING AND CLOSING: *The TMJ may emit a variety of sounds during movements, including popping, clicking, or grinding. Some sounds are consistent with normal function such as the popping sound associated with bubbles forming in the synovial fluid. In contrast, clicking and grinding sounds are often associated with joint pathology or impairment and serve as clues to the examining clinician [37]. Grinding, or **crepitus,** suggests increased friction between the articular surfaces and may reflect damage to the articular cartilage. Clicking sounds are often associated with abnormal movement of the intraarticular disc. Some clinicians contend that a clicking sound during opening and early in the phase of closing is heard as the condyle catches up with an anteriorly displaced disc [4,13,16]. A click later in closing may indicate that the mandible has glided posteriorly beyond the disc.*

Normal Ranges of Motion at the TMJ

Table 23.1 presents the reported normal excursion of the temporomandibular [32]. There are no known studies that demonstrate the variability of joint excursions available at the TMJ among subjects without joint pathology. Consequently, practitioners disagree about the preferred goals for range of motion to be achieved in the rehabilitation of the TMJ. While 20–25 mm appears sufficient for functional opening, some practitioners suggest that a patient should achieve a range of motion in excess of 45 mm. Total opening is greater in men than women [11,12]. This difference seems to be primarily the effect of the size of the mandible.

TABLE 23.1: Normal Range of Motion of the Mandible

Depression of the mandible/opening of the mouth:	
Functional active motion	35–55 mm
Minimal opening for functional activity	25–35 mm
Elevation of the mandible/closing of the mouth	
The mandible returns from depression until the teeth of the mandible and maxilla come into contact	
Protrusion of the mandible	
Functional active motion	3–6 mm
Retrusion of the mandible	
Functional active motion	3–4 mm
Lateral deviation of the mandible	
Functional active motion	10–15 mm

Clinical Relevance

MEASURING OPENING: *Because mouth opening is dependent upon the size of the mandible, clinicians may have difficulty judging whether a patient's opening ROM is "normal." Opening can be measured linearly using a ruler, or specialized insert. It can also be assessed functionally by determining the number of knuckles that the patient can comfortably insert into the open mouth (Fig. 23.15). This technique helps adjust for size since the patient's finger size should be proportional to his or her mandible size.*

RELATIONSHIP BETWEEN HEAD AND NECK POSTURE AND THE TMJ

The position of the mandible on the head is inseparably related to the position of the head on the neck [1,7,14,33]. Head position alters the direction of pull of many of the muscles that open the jaw [26]. In the occlusal position, anterior and posterior changes in head and neck postures move the point of contact between the teeth and also alter the joint space of the TMJ [45]. Side bending in the cervical spine reduces the joint space in the ipsilateral TMJ. Reduced joint space may increase the joint reaction forces on the TMJ, contributing to increased joint pain.

Clinical Relevance

HEAD AND NECK POSTURE IN INDIVIDUALS WITH TMJ PAIN: *Head and neck posture may contribute significantly to the pathomechanics of the TMJ, and patients with TMJ pain must undergo a thorough postural evaluation. A forward head posture tends to stretch the soft tissue on the anterior aspect of the cervical spine, including the suprahyoid muscles. Tension in these structures tends to pull the mandible posteriorly, retruding the mandible (Fig. 23.16). A chronically retruded mandible may produce inflammation of the retrodiscal pad, resulting from sustained compression, and also may apply pressure on the middle and inner ears. Thus a forward head posture may produce or contribute to TMJ pain.*

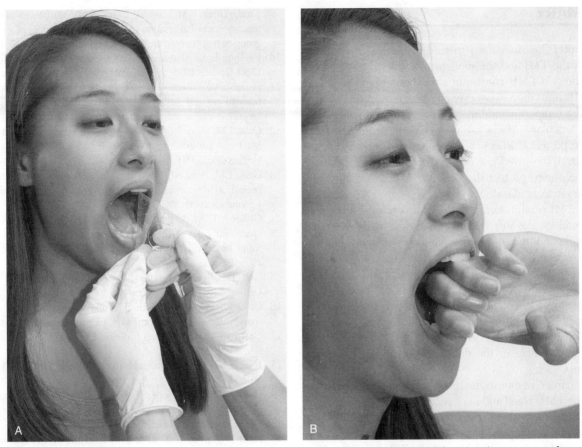

Figure 23.15: Measurement of mouth opening by **(A)** linear measurement of TMJ opening and **(B)** functional assessment of opening by inserting knuckles into the open mouth.

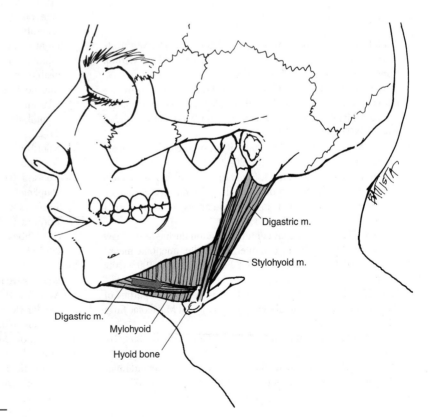

Figure 23.16: A forward head posture stretches the suprahyoid muscles, some of which attach to the mandible. The stretch on these muscles pulls the mandible posteriorly into retrusion, which may lead to compression and irritation of the retrodiscal pad and, consequently, to temporomandibular pain.

SUMMARY

This chapter describes the structure of the bones and ligaments of the TMJ and the motions available to these structures. The two TMJs constitute a compound joint in which both TMJs must move whenever one joint moves. A joint capsule and a temporomandibular ligament support each TMJ, and the articular surfaces are protected by an intraarticular disc. The posterior aspect of the joint space contains highly vascularized, sensitive loose connective tissue, the retrodiscal pad, which helps protect the posterior joint space and supports the intraarticular disc.

Each TMJ exhibits complex three-dimensional motion as the mandible elevates, depresses, or deviates laterally. Opening the mouth requires mandibular depression and protrusion; closing consists of elevation and retrusion. Lateral deviation consists of asymmetrical movement of both TMJs, in which one side protrudes and the opposite side rotates. The disc moves to maintain a cushion between the head of the mandible and the articulating surface of the temporal bone. Impairments of the joint can alter the movement of either the mandible or the disc, contributing to a patient's complaints.

The chapter demonstrates how head and neck posture affects the TMJ. Head and neck posture can alter the area of contact between the teeth as well as the orientation of the mandible on the temporal bone. A careful postural evaluation is an essential component of a thorough TMJ evaluation. The following chapter presents the muscles that provide the coordinated movement of both TMJs essential to mastication and speech.

References

1. Ayub E, Glasheen-Wray M, Kraus S: Head posture: a case study of the effects on the rest position of the mandible. J Orthop Sports Phys Ther 1984; 5: 179–182.
2. Bernasconi G, Marchetti C, Reguzzoni M, et al.: Synovia hyperplasia and calcification in the human TMJ disk: a clinical, surgical, and histologic study. Oral Surg Oral Med Pathol Radiol Endod 1997; 84: 245–252.
3. Bubon MS: Documented instance of restored conductive hearing loss. Funct Orthod 1995; 12: 26–29.
4. Buranastidporn B, Hisano M, Soma K: Effect of biomechanical disturbance of the temporomandibular joint on the prevalence of internal derangement in mandibular asymmetry. Eur J Orthod 2006; 28: 199–205.
5. Chen X: The instantaneous center of rotation during human jaw opening and its significance in interpreting the functional meaning of condylar translation. Am J Phys Anthropol 1998; 106: 35–46.
6. Chin LP, Aker FD, Zarrinnia K: The viscoelastic properties of the human temporomandibular joint disc. J Oral Maxillofac Surg 1996; 54: 315–318.
7. Dale R: TMD: it's our responsibility! J Gen Orthod 1999; 10: 15–20.
8. DelBalso AM: Anatomy of the mandible, temporomandibular joint, and dentition. Neuroimaging Clin N Am 1998; 8: 157–169.
9. Ettala-Ylitalo UM, Laine T: Functional disturbances of the masticatory system in relation to articulatory disorders of speech in a group of 6–8 year old children. Arch Oral Biol 1991; 36: 189–194.
10. Fanibunda K: Anatomical basis for clinical skills: the mandible. Dent Update 1995; 22: 387–391.
11. Ferrario VF, Sforza C, Lovecchio N, Mian F: Quantification of translational and gliding components in human temporomandibular joint during mouth opening. Arch Oral Biol 2005; 50: 507–515.
12. Gallo LM: Modeling of temporomandibular joint function using MRI and jaw-tracking technologies—mechanics. Cells Tissues Organs 2005; 180: 54–68.
13. Gallo LM, Brasi M, Ernst B, Palla S: Relevance of mandibular helical axis analysis in functional and dysfunctional TMJs. J Biomech 2006; 39: 1716–1725.
14. Gillies GT, Broaddus WC, Stenger JM, Taylor AG: A biomechanical model of the craniomandibular complex and cervical spine based on the inverted pendulum. J Med Eng Technol 1998; 22: 263–269.
15. Gole DR: Teeth do more than chew food. J Am Acad Gnathol Orthop 1995; 12: 4–7, 10.
16. Gossi DB, Gallo LM, Bahr E, Palla S: Dynamic intra-articular space variation in clicking TMJs. J Dent Res 2004; 83: 480–484.
17. Guttman GD: Animating functional anatomy for the web. Anat Rec 2000; 261: 57–63.
18. Hanthorne G: Craniomandibular dysfunctions. ASHA 1998; 30: 69–69.
19. Henderson DH, Cooper JC Jr, Bryan GW, et al.: Otologic complaints in temporomandibular joint syndrome (see comments). Arch Otolaryngol Head Neck Surgery 1992; 118: 1208–1213.
20. Hiatt J, Gartner L: Textbook of Head and Neck Anatomy. New York: Appleton-Century-Crofts, 1982.
21. Howard RP, Bowles AP, Guzman HM, Krenrich SW: Head, neck, and mandible dynamics generated by 'whiplash.' Accid Anal Prev 1998; 30: 525–534.
22. Hu K, Qiguo R, Fang J, Mao JJ: Effects of condylar fibrocartilage on the biomechanical loading of the human temporomandibular joint in a three-dimensional, nonlinear finite element model. Med Eng Phys 2003; 25: 107–113.
23. Ishimaru T, Lew D, Haller J, et al.: Virtual arthroscopy of the visible human female temporomandibular joint. J Oral Maxillofac Surg 1999; 57: 807–811.
24. Klausner JJ: Epidemiologic studies reveal trends in temporomandibular pain and dysfunction. J Mass Dent Soc 1995; 44: 21–25.
25. Koolstra JH: Dynamics of the human masticatory system. Crit Rev Oral Biol Med 2002; 13: 366–376.
26. Koolstra JH, van Eijden TMGJ: Functional significance of the coupling between head and jaw movements. J Biomech 2004; 37: 1387–1392.
27. Koolstra JH, van Eijden TMGJ: Three-dimensional dynamical capabilities of the human masticatory muscles. J Biomech 1999; 32: 145–152.
28. Kordass B: The temporomandibular joint in video motion—noninvasive image techniques to present the functional anatomy. Anat Anz 1999; 181: 33–36.
29. Leader JK, Boston JR, Rudy TE, et al.: Relation of jaw sounds and kinematics visualized and quantified using 3-D computer animation. Med Eng Phys 2003; 25: 191–200.
30. LeResche L: Epidemiology of temporomandibular disorders: implications for the investigation of etiologic factors. Crit Rev Oral Biol Med 1997; 8: 291–305.

31. Loughner BA, Gremillion HA, Mahan PE, et al.: The medial capsule of the human temporomandibular joint. J Oral Maxillofac Surg 1997; 55: 363–369.

32. Magee DA: Orthopedic Physical Assessment. Philadelphia: WB Saunders, 1998.

33. McKay DCCLV: Electrognathographic and electromyographic observations on jaw depression during neck extension. J Oral Rehabil 1999; 26: 865–876.

34. Merida-Velasco JR, Rodriguez-Vazquez JR, Merida-Velasco JA, et al.: Development of the human temporomandibular joint. Anat Rec 1999; 255: 20–33.

35. Osborn J, Baragar F: Predicted and observed shapes of human mandibular condyles. J Biomech 1992; 25: 967–974.

36. Packard RC: Epidemiology and pathogenesis of posttraumatic headache. J Head Trauma Rehabil 1999; 14: 9–21.

37. Prinz JF: Physical mechanisms involved in the genesis of temporomandibular joint sounds. J Oral Rehabil 1998; 25: 706–714.

38. Rainer B, Mall G, Landgraf J, Scheck R: Biomechanical analysis of stress distribution in the human temporomandibular-joint. Ann Anat 1999; 181: 55–60.

39. Rocabado M: Physical therapy for the postsurgical TMJ patient. J Craniomandib Disord 1989; 3: 75–82.

40. Romanes GJE: Cunningham's Textbook of Anatomy. Oxford: Oxford University Press, 1981.

41. Rosse C, Gaddum-Rosse P: Hollinshead's Textbook of Anatomy. Philadelphia: Lippincott-Raven, 1997.

42. Sicher H, DuBrul E: Oral Anatomy. St. Louis: CV Mosby, 1975.

43. Slater JJ, Visscher CM, Lobbezoo F, Naeije M: The intra-articular distance within the TMJ during free and loaded closing movements. J Dent Res 1999; 78: 1815–1820.

44. Talebzadeh N, Rosenstein TP, Pogrel MA: Anatomy of the structures medial to the temporomandibular joint. Oral Surg Oral Med Pathol Radiol Endod 1999; 88: 674–678.

45. Visscher CM, Huddleston Slater JJ, Lobbezoo F, Naeije M: Kinematics of the human mandible for different head postures. J Oral Rehabil 2000; 27: 299–305.

46. Weinberg S, Lapointe H: Cervical extension-flexion injury (whiplash) and internal derangement of the temporomandibular joint. J Oral Maxillofac Surg 1987; 45: 653–656.

47. Williams P, Bannister L, Berry M, et al.: Gray's Anatomy, The Anatomical Basis of Medicine and Surgery, Br. ed. London: Churchill Livingstone, 1995.

48. Yatabe M, Zwijnenburg AJ, Megens CC, Naeije M: Movements of the mandibular condyle kinematic center during jaw opening and closing. J Dent Res 1997; 76: 714–719.

49. Zhou D, Hu M, Liang D, et al.: Relationship between fossa-condylar position, meniscus position, and morphologic change in patients with class II and III malocclusion. Chin J Dent Res 1999; 2: 45–49.

Mechanics and Pathomechanics of the Muscles of the TMJ

NEAL PRATT, P.T., PH.D. AND CAROL A. OATIS, P.T., PH.D.

CHAPTER CONTENTS

The preceding chapter presents the bones and connective tissue structures of the temporomandibular joint (TMJ). It also describes the mechanics of movement occurring at the joint. The purpose of this chapter is to review the anatomy of the muscles of mastication and to describe their individual actions and their roles in mastication. As noted in Chapter 23, the two TMJ joints function together, creating a compound joint that permits motion of the mandible. Consequently, the muscles of mastication produce different motions of the mandible, depending on whether they contract unilaterally or bilaterally. The specific purposes of this chapter are to

- Review the structure of the primary muscles of mastication
- Discuss the motions produced by each muscle when contracting unilaterally and bilaterally
- Present the current understanding of the muscles' roles in mastication
- Demonstrate the relationships between the behavior of muscles of mastication and some of the signs and symptoms of patients with TMJ dysfunction

MUSCLES OF MASTICATION

The primary muscles of the TMJ are the masseter and temporalis, which are superficially positioned, and the medial and lateral pterygoids, which occupy the infratemporal fossa (*Fig. 24.1*). Accessory muscles include the buccinator, a muscle of facial expression; the muscles of the tongue; and the suprahyoid muscles, which are the muscles that form the floor of the mouth. These accessory muscles are discussed in detail in Chapters 20 and 21. Their role in chewing, or **mastication,** is presented later in this chapter.

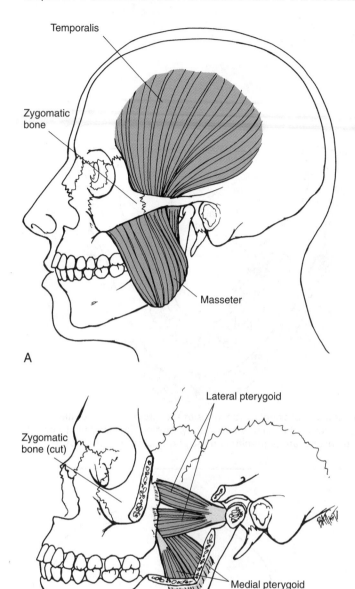

Temporalis

Zygomatic bone

Masseter

A

Lateral pterygoid

Zygomatic bone (cut)

Medial pterygoid

B

Figure 24.1: The primary muscles of mastication are the masseter, temporalis, and medial and lateral pterygoid muscles. **A.** The masseter and temporalis lie on the lateral surface of the joint. **B.** The medial and lateral pterygoid lie on the medial surface of the joint.

The four primary muscles of mastication share several anatomical and functional characteristics. The mandibular elevators, the masseter, temporalis, and medial pterygoid muscles, have large cross-sectional areas indicating their specialization for force production, a necessity for grinding hard, tough foods. The muscles of the TMJ appear to provide the primary stabilizing support to the TMJs [15,17]. Only in extreme mediolateral movements do the ligamentous structures play a primary role.

Sagittal plane or midline motion of the mandible occurs only when both the left and right muscles of a pair contract.

Albeit to different degrees, all of these muscles are oriented obliquely with respect to the axes of the TMJs, so when contracting unilaterally, each produces combinations of motions simultaneously. For example, the lateral pterygoid causes protrusion and deviation of the mandible to the opposite side; the left lateral pterygoid causes deviation of the mandible to the right, and the right lateral pterygoid causes deviation to the left (*Fig. 24.2*). Each lateral pterygoid also produces protrusion of the mandible along with the lateral deviation. Consequently, protrusion in the sagittal plane results only when both right and left lateral pterygoid muscles contract together, counteracting the lateral deviation pull of each muscle individually.

Most skeletal muscles, particularly those in the extremities, can produce motion of either the bone serving as the origin or the bone serving as the insertion. The muscles of mastication arise from the skull and insert on the mandible. Since the skull is fixed relative to the mandible, only the mandible moves with activity of these muscles.

All of the muscles of mastication are innervated by the mandibular division of the trigeminal (5th cranial) nerve (*Fig. 24.3*). The mandibular division branches from the main trunk of the trigeminal nerve in the middle cranial fossa and passes through the foramen ovale into the infratemporal fossa. It branches high in the fossa and, in addition to the muscles, supplies general sensation (not taste) to the mandibular dentition, the mucosa of the cheek, the anterior two thirds of the tongue and the skin superficial to the mandible and posterior temporal region.

Clinical Relevance

TRIGEMINAL NEURALGIA: *Trigeminal neuralgia (tic douloureux) is a syndrome characterized by brief but severe episodes of pain in regions of the head corresponding to the distribution of one or more of the divisions of the trigeminal nerve, most commonly the mandibular nerve. Because the mandibular division supplies the muscles of mastication as well as cutaneous areas, chewing can trigger the onset of pain.*

Masseter

The masseter is positioned superficial to the mandibular ramus, extends from the zygomatic arch to the angle of the mandible, is readily palpable, and is composed of superficial and deep parts (*Fig. 24.4*; Muscle Attachment *Box 24.1*). The superficial part lies more anteriorly than the deep part and is composed of fibers that pass slightly posteriorly from above downward. The deep part is positioned more posteriorly, and consists of more vertically oriented fibers.

ACTIONS

The actions of the masseter are considered unilaterally and bilaterally [1,32,33].

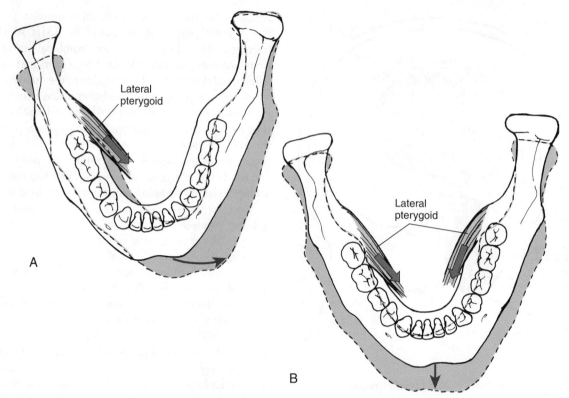

Figure 24.2: Superior view of the motion of the mandible with unilateral and bilateral contractions of the lateral pterygoid muscle. **A.** Unilateral contraction of the lateral pterygoid pulls the ipsilateral ramus of the mandible anteriorly, causing the mandible to deviate toward the contralateral side. **B.** Bilateral and symmetrical contraction of the lateral pterygoid muscles produces protrusion of the mandible, with no lateral deviation.

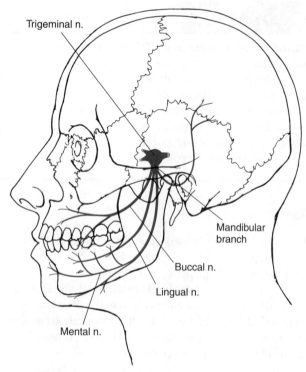

Figure 24.3: The mandibular branch of the trigeminal nerve (5th cranial) innervates the muscles of mastication and provides sensation to the mandibular teeth, the mucosal lining of the cheek, the anterior two thirds of the tongue, and the skin overlying the masseter and posterior temporal region.

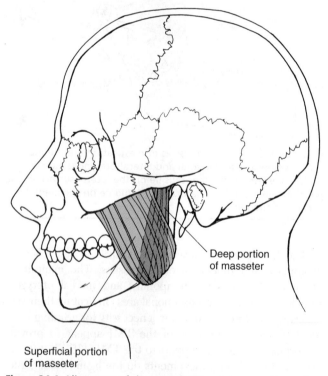

Figure 24.4: Alignment of the superficial and deep portions of the masseter muscle. The fibers of the superficial portion of the masseter run inferiorly and posteriorly, while the fibers of the deep portion are more vertically oriented.

MUSCLE ATTACHMENT BOX 24.1

ATTACHMENTS AND INNERVATION OF THE MASSETER MUSCLE

Cranial attachment:

Superficial part: Lower border of the anterior aspect of the zygomatic arch

Deep part: Deep and lower aspects of the zygomatic arch

Mandibular attachments:

Superficial part: Lateral inferior aspect of the ramus of the mandible

Deep part: Lateral superior aspect of the ramus of the mandible

Innervation: Mandibular division of the trigeminal nerve (5th cranial nerve)

Palpation: The superficial portion of the masseter is easily palpated at the angle of the mandible as the subject gently clenches the teeth.

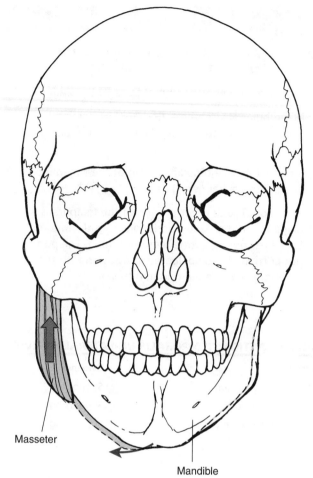

Masseter

Mandible

Figure 24.5: Lateral deviation of the mandible with contraction of the masseter muscle. Unilateral contraction of the masseter produces ipsilateral deviation of the mandible.

MUSCLE ACTION: MASSETER UNILATERAL ACTIVITY

Action	Evidence
Mandibular elevation	Supporting
Ipsilateral deviation of the mandible	Supporting

MUSCLE ACTION: MASSETER BILATERAL ACTIVITY

Action	Evidence
Mandibular elevation	Supporting
Forceful occlusion	Supporting

In the upright posture the weight of the mandible tends to depress it, producing an open mouth. Full opening is prevented in the relaxed upright posture by a low level of activity in the mandibular elevators. However, electromyographic (EMG) studies suggest that the masseter muscles are only minimally active in maintaining resting mandibular posture in the upright position [38,39]. In contrast, the masseter muscles are responsible for producing a powerful bite [26,33]. EMG data reveal that activity in the masseter muscles increases with bite force [3,11,27,29]. The role of the masseter in providing forceful bite is consistent with its large cross-sectional area. In addition, it has the largest moment arm of the mandibular elevators, allowing it to generate the large elevation moments at the TMJ necessary for chewing uncooked carrots or a tough piece of meat [29].

The masseter attaches to the lateral surface of the ramus of the mandible, so contraction pulls the mandible laterally, producing ipsilateral deviation (*Fig. 24.5*) [17,18]. Direct electrical stimulation of the masseter produces elevation, ipsilateral deviation, and slight protrusion [44]. Biomechanical analysis of the masseter's action supports its role in only elevation and ipsilateral deviation [17].

Temporalis

The temporalis muscle is the largest of the masticatory muscles. It is fan-shaped and positioned superficially on the lateral aspect of the skull so it is readily palpable. (Muscle Attachment *Box 24.2*) Since the size of its origin greatly exceeds that of its insertion, the orientation of its fibers varies widely across the whole muscle, so that individual segments of the muscle are capable of distinctly different actions (*Fig. 24.6*). Even though it is commonly divided into anterior, middle and posterior parts, the anterior and middle parts (vertical fibers) and the posterior part (horizontal fibers) form two functional units [3,17,35,40].

ACTIONS

The actions of the temporalis as a whole are considered unilaterally and bilaterally.

MUSCLE ATTACHMENT BOX 24.2

ATTACHMENTS AND INNERVATION OF THE TEMPORALIS MUSCLE

Cranial attachment: Temporal fossa of the skull

Mandibular attachments: Coronoid process and deep surface of the anterior aspect of the ramus of the mandible

Innervation: Mandibular division of the trigeminal nerve (5th cranial nerve)

Palpation: The anterior portion of the temporalis is palpated on the skull superior and slightly anterior to the ear during gentle teeth clenching. The posterior portion may be palpated just posterior to the superior tip of the ear during retrusion.

MUSCLE ACTION: TEMPORALIS BILATERAL ACTIVITY

Action	Evidence
Mandibular elevation	Supporting
Mandibular retrusion	Supporting

The temporalis is considered the primary postural muscle of the mandible in that it maintains mandibular posture in the upright resting position, and it has been described as the most important muscle during both incisor bite and molar occlusion [38,39]. During maximal mandibular depression, as in opening the mouth very wide, it may help to counteract or prevent dislocation of the TMJ by limiting anterior translation of the mandibular condyle [29,37]. Like the masseter, the temporalis pulls the mandible laterally, producing ipsilateral deviation (*Fig. 24.7*) [17,18].

Separate actions of the vertical and horizontal fibers also are reported [3,17,35,40,43]. The horizontal fibers contribute to retrusion, elevation, and lateral deviation of the mandible, while the vertical fibers elevate and deviate the mandible laterally and may provide slight protrusion [40,43]. EMG

MUSCLE ACTION: TEMPORALIS UNILATERAL ACTIVITY

Action	Evidence
Mandibular elevation	Supporting
Mandibular retrusion	Supporting
Ipsilateral deviation of the mandible	Supporting

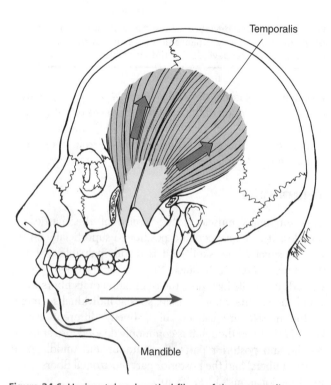

Figure 24.6: Horizontal and vertical fibers of the temporalis muscle. The temporalis is divided functionally into a group of vertical fibers that produce elevation of the mandible and more horizontal fibers that produce elevation and retrusion of the mandible.

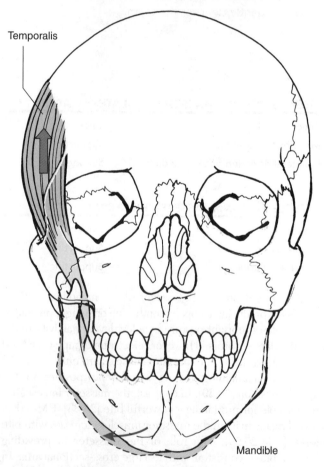

Figure 24.7: Lateral deviation of the mandible with contraction of the temporalis muscle. The attachment of the temporalis on the cranium is lateral to its attachment on the mandible, which is why unilateral contraction of the temporalis muscle produces ipsilateral deviation of the mandible.

studies demonstrate that both portions of the temporalis are active during bite, regardless of whether the bite occurs between the incisor teeth or between the molars [3,24,35]. However, the anterior fibers appear to contribute more than the posterior fibers during an incisal bite [24].

Medial Pterygoid

The medial pterygoid is the deepest of the muscles of mastication and is oriented obliquely in both the sagittal and frontal (coronal) planes. (Muscle Attachment *Box 24.3*) Its sagittal orientation is similar to that of the superficial part of the masseter, so that it inclines posteriorly from superior to inferior. It is more oblique in the frontal plane and inclines considerably laterally as it projects from the skull to the mandible (*Fig. 24.8*).

ACTIONS

The actions of the medial pterygoid muscle are considered unilaterally and bilaterally.

MUSCLE ACTION: MEDIAL PTERYGOID UNILATERAL ACTIVITY

Action	Evidence
Mandibular elevation	Supporting
Contralateral deviation of the mandible	Supporting

MUSCLE ACTION: MEDIAL PTERYGOID BILATERAL ACTIVITY

Action	Evidence
Mandibular elevation	Supporting
Slight mandibular protrusion	Supporting

MUSCLE ATTACHMENT BOX 24.3

ATTACHMENTS AND INNERVATION OF THE MEDIAL PTERYGOID MUSCLE

Cranial attachment: Deep surface of the lateral pterygoid plate of the sphenoid bone

Mandibular attachments: posterior aspect of the medial surface of the mandibular ramus

Innervation: Mandibular division of the trigeminal nerve (5th cranial nerve)

Palpation: The medial pterygoid can be palpated intraorally with care between the medial surface of the ramus of the mandible and the lateral side of the molars.

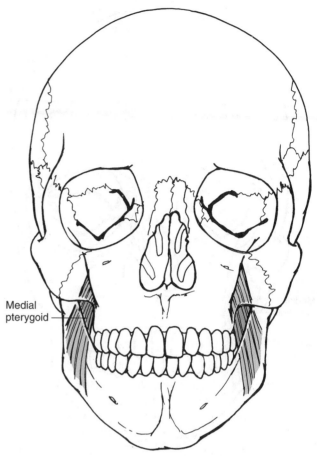

Figure 24.8: Alignment of the medial pterygoid muscle in the frontal plane. The fibers of the medial pterygoid muscle run inferiorly and laterally to attach on the medial side of the mandible.

The location of the medial pterygoid on the deep surface of the mandible explains why it, like the lateral pterygoid, produces contralateral deviation. It pulls the ramus of the mandible medially, shifting the whole mandible toward the contralateral side (*Fig. 24.9*) [17,18]. EMG and biomechanical evidence suggests that the medial pterygoid also is capable of slight protrusion, which is consistent with the sagittal orientation of its fibers [8,17].

Clinical Relevance

BRUXING: *Grinding one's teeth is known as* **bruxing** *and is produced by overactivity of the mandibular elevators. It often occurs while an individual sleeps (*nocturnal bruxing*). Tenderness in the mandibular elevators and even chronic headaches are associated with greater intensity, frequency, and duration of activity of these muscles than in those of nonbruxing healthy control subjects [7,13]. Muscle tenderness may be the direct result of overuse of these muscles [2]. Compression of the retrodiscal tissue of the joint, resulting from retrusion produced by overactivity of the posterior*

(continued)

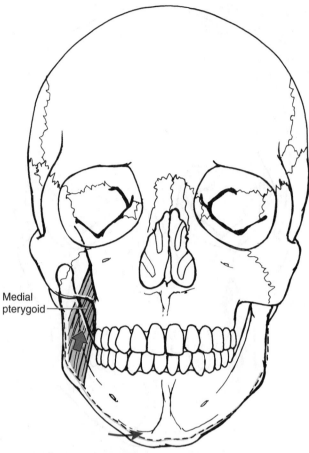

Figure 24.9: Lateral deviation of the mandible with contraction of the medial pterygoid muscle. The alignment of the medial pterygoid produces a medial pull on the mandible during unilateral contraction, producing contralateral deviation of the mandible.

(Continued)

portion of the temporalis muscle, may also contribute to the patient's complaints. The retrodiscal tissue is highly vascular, and compression may produce inflammation and even ischemic pain.

Treatment of the symptoms associated with bruxing includes relaxation exercises, stress management strategies, and oral splints that increase the space between the teeth, preventing contact between the upper and lower teeth [32]. The splints may also position the TMJs to reduce the pressure on the retrodiscal tissue.

Lateral Pterygoid

The lateral pterygoid muscle is oriented horizontally and has distinct superior and inferior parts. (Muscle Attachment *Box 24.4*) From the cranium, the fibers of the two parts converge and pass more obliquely laterally than the medial pterygoid. As a result, balanced bilateral activity of the two lateral pterygoids is necessary if the mandibular and maxillary teeth are to be aligned normally.

MUSCLE ATTACHMENT BOX 24.4

ATTACHMENTS AND INNERVATION OF THE LATERAL PTERYGOID MUSCLE

Cranial attachment: The superior head attaches to the infratemporal surface of the greater wing of the sphenoid bone. The inferior head attaches to the lateral aspect of the lateral pterygoid plate.

Mandibular attachments: The superior head attaches to the articular capsule and intraarticular disc of the TMJ. The inferior head attaches to the pterygoid fovea on the neck of the mandible.

Innervation: Mandibular division of the trigeminal nerve (5th cranial nerve)

Palpation: The lateral pterygoid can be palpated intraorally along the lateral aspect of the hamulus during protrusion (see Fig. 23.5).

ACTIONS

The actions of the lateral pterygoid muscle are considered unilaterally and bilaterally.

MUSCLE ACTION: LATERAL PTERYGOID UNILATERAL ACTIVITY

Action	Evidence
Mandibular protrusion	Supporting
Contralateral deviation of the mandible	Supporting

MUSCLE ACTION: PTERYGOID BILATERAL ACTIVITY

Action	Evidence
Mandibular protrusion	Supporting

EMG and biomechanical studies provide evidence for the lateral pterygoid's role in protrusion and contralateral deviation [17,22] (Fig. 24.2). It is the primary force in protrusion and deviation to the contralateral side [22]. This muscle is particularly important in maintaining continuity between the intraarticular disc and the mandible as the mandible depresses during opening of the mouth. The superior head attaches directly on the intraarticular disc and produces the anterior translation of the disc that occurs in the early stages of mandibular depression. Both heads of the lateral pterygoid muscle also pull the mandibular condyle anteriorly during opening [14,42]. The lateral pterygoid muscle and the posterior fibers of the temporalis, together, control the anterior and posterior translation of the mandible.

Clinical Relevance

HYPERACTIVITY OF THE LATERAL PTERYGOID
MUSCLE: *Excessive activity, or spasm, of the superior head of the lateral pterygoid has been associated with anterior subluxation of the intraarticular disc with respect to the head of the mandible. Conversely, overactivity of the inferior head has been associated with anterior subluxation of the mandible with respect to the disc or even subluxation of the head of the mandible on the articular eminence of the temporal bone [42]. Asynchronous movement of the intraarticular disc and head of the mandible can produce audible clicks with opening or closing of the mouth as the disc and mandible suddenly and forcefully separate or reunite [30].*

Protrusion of the mandible combines anterior and inferior translation of the mandible as the head of the mandible glides along the surface of the glenoid fossa of the temporal bone, which slopes anteriorly and inferiorly (*Fig. 24.10*). Because the lateral pterygoid is the most oblique of the masticatory muscles, it is thought to be responsible for the deviation of the mandible that results from a mandibular nerve injury. With such an injury the mandible is deviated to the side opposite the nerve injury. This deviation may be apparent at rest but is accentuated when the mouth is opened against resistance.

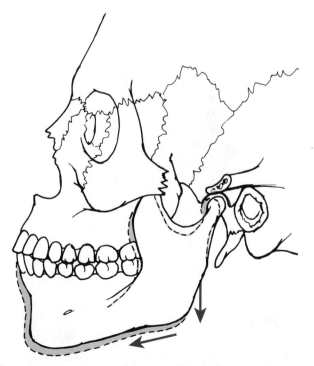

Figure 24.10: Movement of the mandible during protrusion. As the mandible glides anteriorly in protrusion it also glides inferiorly as it follows the surface of the glenoid fossa of the temporal bone.

Accessory Muscles

The accessory muscles of the TMJ include the suprahyoid muscles and the tongue muscles. Although their individual attachments and functions are discussed in Chapter 22, it is useful to review their effects on the TMJ. The suprahyoid muscles form the floor of the mouth and play an important role in mouth opening and during chewing. They function as mandibular depressors when the hyoid bone is fixed by the infrahyoid muscles (*Fig. 24.11*) [17–19]. Thus while the suprahyoid muscles are considered muscles of the TMJ, their effect on the joint requires that they contract in unison with the infrahyoid muscles.

The muscles of the floor of the mouth and the tongue muscles also participate in lateral movement of the mandible. EMG and biomechanical data reveal that the mylohyoid muscle, contracting unilaterally, produces significant lateral deviation of the mandible to the contralateral side [17,18] (*Fig. 24.12*). Bilateral contraction of the tongue muscles helps establish a symmetrical alignment of both TMJs.

Clinical Relevance

TONGUE POSITION DURING ACTIVE EXERCISE OF
THE TMJs: *Lateral deviation of the TMJ frequently occurs during mouth opening in the presence of asymmetrical muscle control. A typical goal of intervention in patients with TMJ dysfunction is to reestablish symmetrical mouth opening. Careful control of tongue position during opening can facilitate symmetrical motion. One useful strategy is to instruct the patient to maintain the tip of the tongue on the highest point of the hard palate whenever performing opening and closing exercises of the mouth (Fig. 24.13). Maintenance of this position requires the contraction of the* *intrinsic and extrinsic muscles of the tongue, which stabilizes the mandible in the transverse plane and limits the unwanted lateral deviation.*

MASTICATION

Chewing is a complex rhythm of mandibular movement, powered by coordinated activity of the muscles of mastication, facial expression, and tongue. The following describes the sequence of mandibular movements that constitute chewing, or mastication, and then discusses the role of the muscles that participate in the function.

Mandibular Motion during Chewing

A single **chewing stroke** consists of one loop of mandibular depression, lateral deviation, and elevation [5,28]. A frontal plane view reveals that the mandible typically follows a path along the midline of the body during depression (*Fig. 24.14*).

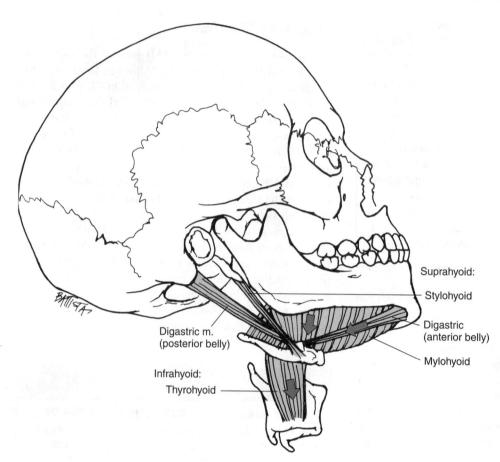

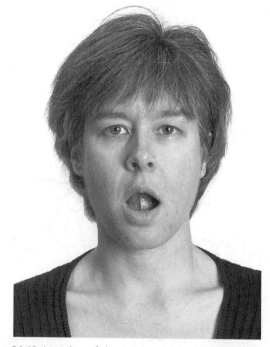

Figure 24.11: Depression of the mandible by the suprahyoid muscles. Contraction of the suprahyoid muscles with simultaneous contraction of the infrahyoid muscles fixes the hyoid bone and allows the suprahyoid muscles to depress the mandible.

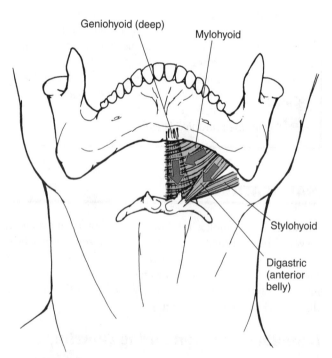

Figure 24.12: Lateral deviation of the mandible with contraction of the muscles of the tongue and floor of the mouth. Ipsilateral contraction of the muscles of the tongue and floor of the mouth assist contralateral deviation of the mandible.

Figure 24.13: Location of the tongue on the hard palate during mouth opening or closing. By locating the tip of the tongue on the hard palate, the individual exhibits symmetrical activity of the tongue muscles and helps maintain symmetrical alignment of the mandible during opening and closing of the mouth.

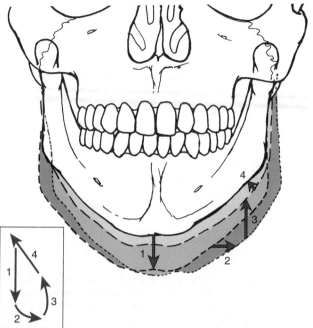

Figure 24.14: Frontal plane view of the path taken by the mandible during a single chewing stroke. Observation of the mandible during chewing reveals that the mandible moves in the sagittal plane as it depresses in the opening phase. As closing begins, the mandible elevates and deviates laterally during the crushing phase. When the two rows of teeth contact each other, mandibular elevation ceases, and the mandible returns to the midline during the grinding phase.

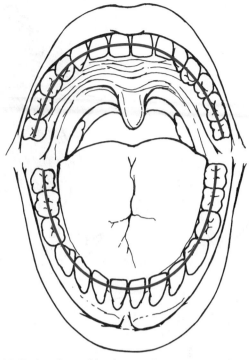

Figure 24.15: Arcs formed by the maxillary and mandibular teeth. The bottom row of teeth (mandibular teeth) forms a smaller arc than the row of teeth on the maxilla. Maximum contact between mandibular and maxillary molars requires lateral deviation of the mandible to one side.

As elevation begins, the path of the mandible deviates laterally and returns to midline as mandibular depression begins again.

In the **rest position,** the upper row of teeth typically does not contact the lower teeth. When the mandible is elevated in the sagittal plane from this position, the teeth of the lower row make only slight contact with the upper row because the mandibular teeth are arranged in a narrower arc than the maxillary teeth (*Fig. 24.15*). To maximize contact between upper and lower teeth, a necessity to grind food, the mandible deviates laterally as it elevates to the maxillary teeth. This explains the small loop that the mandible makes in the frontal plane as it depresses then laterally deviates and elevates to crush the oral contents.

Within the chewing stroke, there are two distinct phases of food preparation by the teeth. The **crushing phase** occurs as the food is compressed between the maxillary teeth and the teeth on the elevating mandible. This phase ends with maximum mandibular elevation. When elevation is complete, contact between the rows of teeth persists as the teeth slide on each other to achieve the **intercuspal position** in which contact between the molars on one side of the mouth is maximal. The gliding between the rows of teeth constitutes the **grinding phase** of mastication. This phase is characterized by transverse plane motion of the mandible, with little or no additional elevation.

Muscle Activity during Mastication

The act of chewing typically occurs on one side of the mouth at a time. The side on which the actual chewing occurs is known as the **working side,** while the opposite side is known as the **balancing side.** EMG studies consistently demonstrate considerable muscle activity on both the working and balancing sides [4,23,31,33].

Several discrete roles of muscle activity during mastication can be described. These functions are to

- Move the mandible in the masticatory path
- Stabilize the balancing side of the mandible
- Maintain appropriate alignment between the disc and the mandibular condyle
- Control the location of the food to optimize mastication

The muscles' participation in these functions is described below.

MUSCLES THAT MOVE THE MANDIBLE DURING MASTICATION

Chapter 23 describes in more detail the movement of the mandible during elevation and depression. Depression of the mandible, or mouth opening, includes rotation about a medial lateral axis and protrusion of the mandible in the transverse plane. As the mandible depresses during the chewing stroke, the suprahyoid muscles contract [18,20,21,34,36,41]. At the

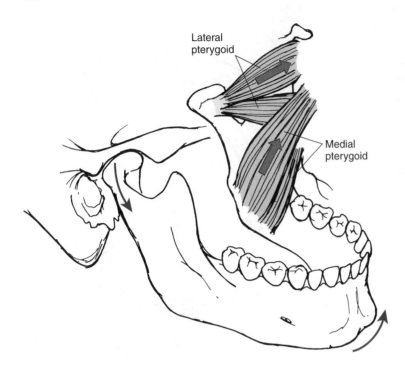

Figure 24.16: Motion on the balancing side of the mandible during bite. As the mandible deviates and rotates to the working (chewing) side, the TMJ on the balancing side undergoes distraction.

same time, the infrahyoid muscles contract, fixing the hyoid bone. As a result, the suprahyoid muscles contribute to mouth opening. Also during the opening phase of mastication, the lateral pterygoid muscle contracts, particularly the inferior head, producing the anterior translation of the mandible that accompanies mandibular depression [6,14,18,21,36].

Mandibular depression and protrusion are followed by lateral deviation, elevation, and retrusion of the mandible for crushing and grinding. These motions occur with the mandibular elevators, the masseter, medial pterygoid, and temporalis muscles as well as the lateral pterygoid [10,18]. Lateral deviation occurs with contraction of the ipsilateral masseter and temporalis and the contralateral medial and lateral pterygoid [5,12]. The temporalis also produces retrusion [4,23,33]. The crushing phase consists of active mandibular elevation and, therefore, the muscle contractions within this phase are primarily concentric. Grinding occurs with little or no additional elevation, so contraction of the mandibular elevators during this phase is primarily isometric. The moment arms for the mandibular elevators increase as the mouth moves from the open toward the closed position [10,16]. The moment arms are maximum at approximately the point at which the mandible is positioned to grind the food, thus optimizing the moments the muscles can generate to chew the food.

The following summarizes the motions of the TMJs during mastication and the muscles primarily responsible for these motions:

- Depression: digastric, mylohyoid, and geniohyoid muscles
- Protrusion: lateral pterygoid muscle
- Elevation: masseter, temporalis, and medial pterygoid muscles

- Lateral deviation: masseter and temporalis on the ipsilateral side and medial and lateral pterygoid on the contralateral side
- Retrusion: temporalis muscle

STABILIZATION OF THE BALANCING SIDE OF THE MANDIBLE

Forceful contraction of the mandibular elevators on the working side produces lateral deviation toward the working side and tends to produce a rotation of the mandible toward the chewing side about an anterior posterior axis [25] (*Fig. 24.16*). This rotation tends to distract the TMJ on the balancing side and to compress the TMJ on the working side. The mandibular elevators on the balancing side of the mandible contract with the contralateral elevators to stabilize the mandible during the crushing and grinding phases [17]. The activity of the muscles on the balancing side adds to the bite force and also stabilizes the mandible to maintain the bite location on the teeth [35]. At the same time the bolus on the teeth of the chewing side tends to distract the TMJ on the chewing (working) side and narrows the joint space on the opposite (balancing) side [9]. This tilt of the mandible helps to explain the large compressive forces that occur on the balancing side. The harder the food is to chew, the more compression occurs on the balancing side [10].

MAINTAIN APPROPRIATE ALIGNMENT BETWEEN THE DISC AND MANDIBULAR CONDYLE

In chewing, the mandible is cyclically opening and closing, requiring repeated anterior and posterior gliding of the mandibular condyle. The intraarticular disc also translates to stay with the head of the mandible and maximize congruency

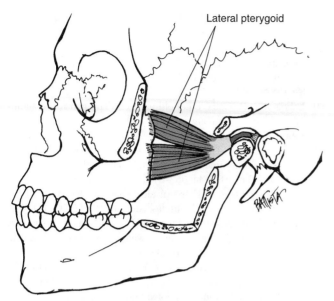

Lateral pterygoid

Figure 24.17: Anterior rotation of the intraarticular disc during bite. During the crushing and grinding phase of the chewing stroke, contraction of the superior head of the lateral pterygoid muscle rotates the intraarticular disc anteriorly, so that it provides cushioning to the anterior surface of the head of the mandible.

between mandible and temporal bone. The lateral pterygoid plays a critical role in stabilizing the disc and maintaining its alignment on the mandible as well as in protruding the mandible. The inferior head of the lateral pterygoid muscle is active during jaw opening, apparently assisting the anterior translation of the mandible. In contrast, EMG studies reveal that the superior head of the lateral pterygoid muscle is active in the mandibular elevation phase of bite [5,14]. This activity appears to stabilize the disc and mandible against the retrusive pull of the mandibular elevators, particularly the temporalis. It also rotates the disc anteriorly to provide cushioning between the mandible and articular eminence of the temporal bone (*Fig. 24.17*).

CONTROL FOOD LOCATION

Regardless of the integrity of the primary muscles of mastication, effective chewing requires that the food be located appropriately between the teeth during the crushing and grinding phases. In addition, the food, moistened by saliva, requires kneading to form a bolus that can be swallowed safely. The buccinator and the intrinsic and extrinsic muscles of the tongue perform this function in mastication. The buccinator is the only muscle that can regulate the lateral part of the cheek between the mandible and maxilla (Chapter 20). This muscle, along with the tongue, is responsible for maintaining the position of a bolus of food between the maxillary and mandibular teeth. The buccinator is essential in preventing food from becoming trapped in the buccal space, between the cheek and the teeth. It must be remembered that the buccinator is paralyzed with an injury of the facial nerve,

making the mucosa of the cheek vulnerable to laceration between the teeth and producing difficulty in chewing.

The tongue muscles also manipulate the food, keeping it between the teeth even while the working side of the mandible is alternated from side to side. As noted in Chapter 22, once the food is prepared thoroughly, the tongue forms a chute and propels the food as the swallow is initiated. Thus mastication is a complex, cyclical movement requiring precise coordination of several muscle groups using concentric, eccentric, and isometric contractions. Mastication is the beginning of the normal digestive process, and pain or incoordination that limits an individual's ability to chew can have profound effects on the person's diet and nutritional status. Restoration of normal muscle balance in patients with temporomandibular dysfunction can provide substantial relief of pain.

Clinical Relevance

MUSCLE DYSFUNCTION IN TMJ DISORDERS: *Just like the muscles of the upper or lower extremity, muscles of mastication and the TMJ's accessory muscles, including the buccinator and tongue muscles, can undergo disuse atrophy and loss of coordination resulting from inactivity. Individuals with severe pain in a TMJ often resort to soft diets because chewing food of typical consistency is too painful. Consequently the individual may lose strength not only in the mandibular elevators, but in the tongue muscles as well. Atrophy and incoordination of the tongue are common impairments seen in individuals with TMJ dysfunction. Happily, the muscles of the tongue appear to be as amenable to exercise and rehabilitation as the muscles of the knee or elbow. Patients with TMJ pain are likely to benefit from tongue exercises as well as from direct intervention at the TMJ.*

SUMMARY

This chapter presents the structure and actions of the four primary muscles of mastication. The three elevators of the mandible—temporalis, masseter, and medial pterygoid muscles—work together to raise and deviate the mandible to produce forceful grinding of food. The lateral pterygoid protrudes the mandible and participates in opening the mouth. It also helps maintain continuity between the intraarticular disc and the mandible. The accessory muscles of mastication include the suprahyoid muscles as well as muscles of the tongue and face. They play an important part in chewing by helping to manipulate the food during chewing and to mold the food into a manageable bolus. These muscles are reviewed briefly since they are covered in greater detail in preceding chapters.

Chewing requires coordinated activity of several muscles to produce the rhythmic opening and closing, protrusion and retrusion, and side-to-side translation that produces the chewing stroke. The following chapter discusses the loads that the TMJ sustains during normal function as well as how those loads may contribute to a patient's complaints.

References

1. Ahlgren J: Kinesiology of the mandible: an EMG study. Acta Odontol Scand 1967; 25: 593–611.

2. Arima T, Svensson P, Arendt-Nielsen L: Experimental grinding in healthy subjects: a model for postexercise jaw muscle soreness? J Orofac Pain 1999; 13: 104–114.

3. Bakke M, Michler L, Han K, Moller E: Clinical significance of isometric bite force versus electrical activity in temporal and masseter muscles. Scand J Dent Res 1989; 97: 539–551.

4. Bishop B, Plesh O, McCall WD: Effects of chewing frequency and bolus hardness on human incisor trajectory and masseter muscle activity. Arch Oral Biol 1990; 35: 311–318.

5. Bourbon B: Craniomandibular examination and treatment. In: Sgarlat Myers R, ed. Saunders Manual of Physical Therapy Practice. Philadelphia: WB Saunders, 1995; 669–725.

6. Chen X: The instantaneous center of rotation during human jaw opening and its significance in interpreting the functional meaning of condylar translation. Am J Phys Anthropol 1998; 106: 35–46.

7. Dahlstrom L: Electromyographic studies of craniomandibular disorders: a review of the literature. J Oral Rehabil 1989; 16: 1–20.

8. Fortinguerra CRH, Vitti M: Estudo eletromiografico d acao do m. pterigoideu medial em movimentos mandibulares. Fev Assoc Paul Cir Dent 1979; 33: 501–508.

9. Fushima K, Gallo LM, Krebs M, Palla S: Analysis of the TMJ intraarticular space variation: a non-invasive insight during mastication. Med Eng Phys 2003; 25: 181–190.

10. Gallo LM: Modeling of temporomandibular joint function using MRI and jaw-tracking technologies—mechanics. Cells Tissues Organs 2005; 180: 54–68.

11. Gervais RO, Fitzsimmons GW, Thomas NR: Masseter and temporalis electromyographic activity in asymptomatic, subclinical, and temporomandibular joint dysfunction patients. J Craniomandib Pract 1989; 7: 52–57.

12. Hiatt J, Gartner L: Textbook of Head and Neck Anatomy. New York: Appleton-Century-Crofts, 1982.

13. Hidaka O, Iwasaki M, Saito M, Morimoto T: Influence of clenching intensity on bite force balance, occlusal contact area, and average bite pressure. J Dent Res 1999; 78: 1336–1344.

14. Hiraba K, Hibino K, Hiranuma K, Negoro T: EMG activities of two heads of the human lateral pterygoid muscle in relation to mandibular condyle movement and biting force. J Neurophysiol 2000; 83: 2120–2137.

15. Koolstra JH: Dynamics of the human masticatory system. Crit Rev Oral Biol Med 2002; 13: 366–376.

16. Koolstra JH, van Eijden TMGJ: The jaw open-close movements predicted by biomechanical modeling. J Biomech 1997; 30: 943–950.

17. Koolstra JH, van Eijden TMGJ: Three-dimensional dynamical capabilities of the human masticatory muscles. J Biomech 1999; 32: 145–152.

18. Koolstra JH, van Eijden TMGJ: A method to predict muscle control in the kinematically and mechanically indeterminate human masticatory system. J Biomech 2001; 34: 1179–1188.

19. Koolstra JH, van Eijden TMGJ: Functional significance of the coupling between head and jaw movements. J Biomech 2004; 37: 1387–1392.

20. Laboissiere R, Ostry DJ, Feldman AG: The control of multimuscle systems: human jaw and hyoid movements. Biol Cybern 1996; 74: 373–384.

21. Langenbach GE, Hannam AG: The role of passive muscle tensions in a three-dimensional dynamic model of the human jaw. Arch Oral Biol 1999; 44: 557–573.

22. Lehr RP Jr, Owens SE Jr: An electromyographic study of the human lateral pterygoid muscles. Anat Rec 1980; 196: 441–448.

23. McCarroll RS, Naeije M, Hansson TL: Balance on masticatory muscle activity during natural chewing and submaximal clenching. J Oral Rehabil 1989; 16: 441–446.

24. Meyer C, Kahn JL, Boutemy P, Wilk A: Determination of the external forces applied to the mandible during various static chewing tasks. J Craniomaxillofac Surg 1998; 26: 331–341.

25. Minagi S: Effect of eccentric clenching on mandibular deviation in the vicinity of mandibular rest position. J Oral Rehabil 2000; 27: 175–179.

26. Mioche L, Bourdiol P, Martin JF, Noel Y: Variations in human masseter and temporalis muscle activity related to food texture during free and side-imposed mastication. Arch Oral Biol 1999; 44: 1005–1012.

27. Naeije M, McCarroll RS, Weijs WA: Electromyographic activity of the human masticatory muscle during submaximal clenching in the inter-cuspal position. J Oral Rehabil 1989; 16: 63–70.

28. Neeman H, McCall W, Plesh O, Bishop B: Analysis of jaw movements and masticatory muscle activity. Comput Meth Programs Biomed 1990; 31: 19–32.

29. Osborn J, Baragar F: Predicted pattern of human muscle activity during clenching derived from a computer assisted model; symmetric vertical bite forces. J Biomech 1985; 18: 599–612.

30. Prinz JF: Physical mechanisms involved in the genesis of temporomandibular joint sounds. J Oral Rehabil 1998; 25: 706–714.

31. Rilo B, da Silva JL, Gude F, Santana U: Myoelectric activity during unilateral chewing in healthy subjects: cycle duration and order of muscle activation. J Prosthet Dent 1998; 80: 462–466.

32. Sessle BJ, Woodside DG, Bourque P, et al.: Effect of functional appliance on jaw muscle activity. Am J Orthod Dentofac Orthop 1990; 98: 222–230.

33. Spencer MA: Force production in the primate masticatory system: electromyographic tests of biomechanical hypotheses. J Hum Evol 1998; 34: 25–54.

34. Takada K, Yashiro K, Sorihashi Y, et al.: Tongue, jaw, and lip muscle activity and jaw movement during experimental chewing efforts in man. J Dent Res. 1996; 75: 1598–1606.

35. Throckmorton G, Groshan GJ, Boyd SB: Muscle activity patterns and control of temporomandibular joint loads. J Prosthet Dent 1990; 63: 685–695.

36. Uchida S, Inoue H, Maeda T: Electromyographic study of the activity of jaw depressor muscles before initiation of opening movements. J Oral Rehabil 1999; 26: 503–510.

37. Vitti M: Estudo electromiografico do musculos mastigadores no cao. Folia Clin Biol 1965; 34: 101–114.

38. Vitti M, Basmajian JV: Muscles of mastication in small children: and electromyographic analysis. Am J Orthod 1975; 68: 412–419.

39. Vitti M, Basmajian JV: Integrated actions of masticatory muscles: simultaneous EMG from eight intramuscular electrodes. Anat Rec 1977; 187: 173–189.

40. Williams P, Bannister L, Berry M, et al.: Gray's Anatomy, The Anatomical Basis of Medicine and Surgery, Br. ed. London: Churchill Livingstone, 1995.

41. Yoshida K: Masticatory muscle responses associated with unloading of biting force during food crushing. J Oral Rehabil 1998; 24: 830–837.

42. Zijun L, Huiyun W, Weiya P: A comparative electromyographic study of the lateral pterygoid muscle and arthrography in patients with temporomandibular joint disturbance syndrome sounds. J Prosthet Dent 1989; 62: 229–233.

43. Zwijnenburg AJ, Kroon GW, Verbeeten B Jr, Naeije M: Jaw movement responses to electrical stimulation of different parts of the human temporalis muscle. J Dent Res 1996; 75: 1798–1803.

44. Zwijnenburg AJ, Lobbezoo F, Kroon GW, Naeije M: Mandibular movements in response to electrical stimulation of superficial and deep parts of the human masseter muscle at different jaw positions. Arch Oral Biol 1999; 44: 395–401.

Analysis of the Forces on the TMJ during Activity

CHAPTER CONTENTS

The temporomandibular joints (TMJs) are the articulation sites for the mandible, a rather small bone of the face with no other additional appendage. The joints serve no function in normal weight bearing and would seem to bear small loads. However, the joints are equipped with intraarticular discs, usually a sign that the joint sustains large stresses. In addition, the muscles that move the TMJs are large and powerful, generating large chewing forces to grind food into a manageable bolus. It is useful for the clinician to investigate the loads sustained by the joint and to consider their contributions to the relatively common complaint of TMJ pain.

The purpose of this chapter is to examine the loads sustained by the TMJs and to review simple analytical tools useful in calculating the loads on the TMJs. Specifically, the objectives of this chapter are to

- Demonstrate a two-dimensional analysis of the forces on the TMJ
- Examine the loads on the structures of the TMJ
- Consider the role that loading may have on the etiology of TMJ dysfunction

TWO-DIMENSIONAL ANALYSIS OF THE FORCES IN THE TMJ COMPLEX

Although the TMJ exhibits motion through three planes, most of the motion of the mandible occurs in the sagittal plane. Thus a two-dimensional model of the joint is an acceptable first approximation of the joint's performance. The free-body diagram of a simplified model is presented in *Examining the Forces Box 25.1* along with an analysis of the forces in the mandibular elevators and the joint reaction force during forceful bite. This example uses a peak bite force on the molars of 500 N (112 lb) [20], although peak bite forces up to 1,000 N (225 lb) are reported in adults [24,27]. Calculations in this example reveal a load of 1013 N (228 lb) in the muscle that elevates the mandible and a joint reaction force on the head of the mandible of 877 N (197 lb) at an angle of 60° from the horizontal.

The example presented in Examining the Forces Box 25.1 uses dimensions reported in the literature but also makes use of an important simplifying assumption [9,21]. The mandibular elevators are represented by a single vertically aligned muscle, the temporalis, despite abundant evidence demonstrating co-contraction of the masseter, medial pterygoid,

EXAMINING THE FORCES BOX 25.1

TWO-DIMENSIONAL ANALYSIS OF THE FORCES IN THE TEMPOROMANDIBULAR JOINT DURING MAXIMAL BITE BETWEEN THE MOLARS

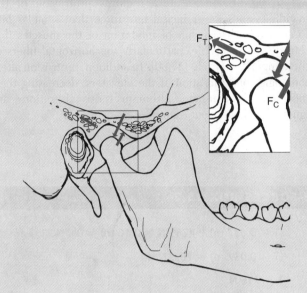

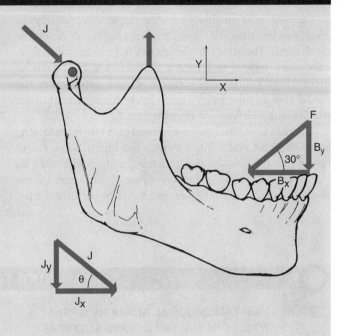

The following data are taken from the literature [9,20,21].

Moment arm of the temporalis (T): 0.037 m
Angle of application of the temporalis:
90° Bite force (F): 500 N
Distance along the x axis from the point of application of the bite force to the joint: 0.063 m
Angle of application of the bite force: 30° from the occlusal plane, which lies on the horizontal

Solve for the temporalis force (T):

$\Sigma M = 0$
$(T \times 0.037 \text{ m}) - (500 \text{ N} \times \sin 30° \times 0.063 \text{ m})$
$- (500 \text{ N} \times \cos 30° \times 0.05 \text{ m}) = 0$
$(T \times 0.037 \text{ m}) = 37.5 \text{ Nm}$
T = 1013 N

Calculate the joint reaction forces (J) on the head of the mandible.

ΣF_X

$J_X + B_X = 0$ where B_X = the bite force $\times$ (cos 30°) in the −x direction

$J_X - 433 \text{ N} = 0$
$J_X = 433 \text{ N}$

ΣF_Y

$J_Y + B_Y + T = 0$ B_Y = the bite force $\times$ (sin 30°) in the −y direction

$J_Y - 250 \text{ N} + 1013 \text{ N} = 0$
$J_Y = -763 \text{ N}$

Using the Pythagorean theorem:

$J^2 = J_X{}^2 + J_Y{}^2$
J ≈ 877 N

Using trigonometry, the direction of J can be determined:

$\sin \theta = J_Y/J$
θ ≈ 60° from the horizontal

both parts of the temporalis, and even the superior head of the lateral pterygoid muscle during bite [4,13,19,25]. This simplification is necessary to solve for the muscle force directly, since inclusion of all of these muscles produces a state of static indeterminacy that allows an infinite number of solutions and requires more sophisticated analysis for a final solution. (See Chapter 1 for more details on static indeterminacy.)

The assumption that only one vertical muscle provides all of the force of mandibular elevation produces an artificially small muscle force and, consequently, underestimates the

joint reaction force. The mandibular elevators and superior head of the lateral pterygoid muscle pull either anteriorly or posteriorly, producing a force couple that rotates the mandible in elevation, while the anterior and posterior pulls counteract each other, producing only slight translation. However, the co-contractions produce large compressive forces on the joint itself. The model also assumes that the mandibular elevator pulls vertically with an optimal 90° angle of application, although analyses reveal that the actual direction of pull of the muscles varies widely, from approximately

30° to 150° [9,24,26]. Angles of application less or greater than 90° require larger muscle forces, since the moment arm of the muscle is smaller when the angle of application is greater or less than 90°. (See Chapter 4 for details of muscle mechanics.) Thus this simplification also produces unrealistically small muscle and joint reaction forces [26]. Despite these simplifications and consequent underestimations, the model reveals substantial muscle loads during forceful bite, which result in large joint reaction forces.

The data presented above are based on a bite force located on the second molar. Anyone who has bitten a raw carrot knows that the jaw also can generate large forces during an incisor bite. *Examining the Forces Box 25.2* examines some of the mechanical alterations produced by an incisal bite.

The free-body diagram in Examining the Forces Box 25.2 demonstrates that an important effect of an incisal bite is an increase in the moment arm of the bite force. The model also uses a smaller peak bite force on the incisors than on the molars. Measurements of peak bite forces between the incisors reveal loads ranging from 150 to almost 400 N (34 to 90 lb). Incisal bite requires protrusion of the mandible, so a lower incisal bite force than a molar bite force may be the result of inhibition of the muscles that retrude the mandible, particularly the horizontal fibers of the temporalis muscle [27,30]. In addition, protrusion alters the angles of application of the elevators, decreasing their mechanical advantage, although these alterations are ignored in the current example.

EXAMINING THE FORCES BOX 25.2

TWO-DIMENSIONAL ANALYSIS OF THE FORCES IN THE TMJ DURING MAXIMAL BITE BETWEEN THE INCISORS

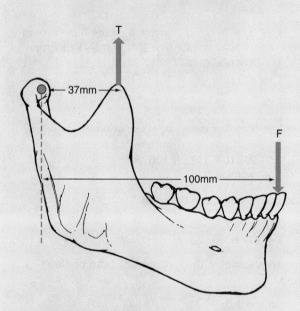

The following data are taken from the literature [9,20,21].

Moment arm of the temporalis (T): 0.037 m
Angle of application of the temporalis: 90°
Bite force (F): 265 N
Distance along the x axis from the point of application of the bite force to the joint: 10 m
Angle of application of the bite force: 90° from the occlusal plane, which lies on the horizontal

Solve for the temporalis force (T):

$\Sigma M = 0$

$(T \times 0.037 \text{ m}) - (265 \text{ N} \times 0.10 \text{ m}) = 0$

$(T \times 0.037 \text{ m}) = 26.5 \text{ Nm}$

T = 716 N

Calculate the joint reaction forces (J) on the head of the mandible.

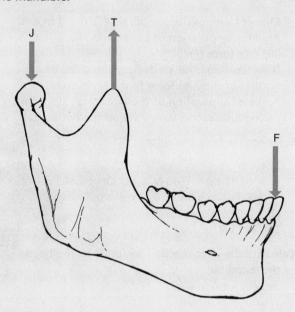

Note that there are no forces in the x direction; therefore $J = J_Y$.

ΣF

$J + T - B = 0$ where B = the bite force

$J + 716 \text{ N} - 265 \text{ N} = 0$

$J = -451 \text{ N}$

J is vertical and pointing down.

The analysis in Examining the Forces Box 25.2 demonstrates that the elevators generate large forces during incisal bite, even though the bite force is smaller than that in the molar bite. The large muscle force is needed because the bite force acts farther from the point of rotation and produces a larger moment. Despite the smaller bite force and large muscle force, the joint reaction force during incisal bite is large although smaller than the joint reaction force during bite on the molars.

The analyses in Examining the Forces Boxes 25.1 and 25.2, albeit oversimplified, reveal substantial loads in the masticatory muscles and on the TMJ. More-accurate calculations require more-sophisticated analyses, and such approaches are less commonly applied to the TMJ than to joints of the upper and lower limbs.

RESULTS FROM SOPHISTICATED MODELING OF THE TMJ

Although the TMJ appears to be a relatively simple mechanical system, it has eluded definitive biomechanical characterization. Several factors help explain the lack of consensus on the forces sustained by the joint's components. Although most of the motion at both joints occurs in the sagittal plane, each joint does exhibit three-dimensional motion. The four primary muscles of each TMJ are large with complex architectures, so the direction of pull and physiological cross-sectional areas are difficult to determine. Consequently, their effects on the joint also are disputed.

The compound nature of the two TMJs also increases the difficulty of analysis. The muscles on one side of the mandible affect both ipsilateral and contralateral joints, although the relative effect on each joint is impossible to measure. As noted in Chapters 23 and 24, in chewing, the side where the bolus is located is known as the **working** side and the opposite side is referred to as the **balancing** side. During mastication muscles at both TMJs contract simultaneously to move and stabilize the joints as they alternate between working and balancing. Consequently, both joints are loaded substantially regardless of which side is actually grinding the food. Finally, the location of the bite force has a significant influence on the muscle forces, as indicated in Examining the Forces Box 25.2. As a result of these challenges to a biomechanical analysis of the TMJ, the literature offers widely varying estimates of the loads applied to the TMJs. The results presented here offer clinicians a perspective on the forces sustained by the joint complex and a framework by which to consider the signs and symptoms reported by patients. Additional research is required to obtain more-precise estimates of the forces to which the structures of the TMJ are subjected.

Bite Force

Peak bite force and forces generated during functional bite are both reported [5,12,21–24,28]. The bite force is greatly influenced by the location of the bite. It is generally agreed that bite forces are greatest when the bite occurs close to the

first molar and are least when it occurs at the incisors [23,24,28]. The decrease in bite force during an incisal bite appears to result from a decrease in the muscles' mechanical advantage and probable inhibition of the temporalis muscle needed to maintain the protruded position [23,28].

The magnitude of reported peak bite forces varies widely because the location and positioning of the measurement device differ substantially among the studies. The position of the mouth during measurement also affects the results and contributes to the diversity in reported bite forces [23]. Reported peak bite forces on the molars range from approximately 500 N to almost 1,000 N (112–225 lb) [1,20,23,24]. Using a load transducer implanted in the crown of a maxillary molar, Kawaguchi et al. report a load of approximately 173 N (39 lb) on a single molar during a maximum contraction of the mandibular elevators [14].

Unlike maximum strengths in the appendicular skeleton, maximum bite force appears less affected by gender and more by physical maturity and by the shape of the cranium and the angles of applications of the muscles [5,21]. Maximum bite strength is less than 100 N (22.5 lb) in children aged 6 to 8 years and appears to increase steadily during maturation.

Despite the variety in reported peak bite forces, there is agreement that peak bite forces are quite large, well over 100 lb in adults. Such loads would seem to have the potential to injure the teeth. However, the arrangement and structure of the teeth appears to provide a protective mechanism [12]. The area of tooth contact, **occlusal contact area,** increases with increasing bite force. As a result, as the bite force increases, so does the area over which the bite force is applied. As the bite force increases, the stress (force/area) decreases, thus decreasing the risk of injury to any tooth.

Although most functional chewing requires submaximal bite forces, the magnitude of a functional bite force is still significant. Measures of the bite forces during mastication of various types of food range from approximately 54 to 88 N (12–20 lb) [22]. However, investigators disagree as to whether there is an actual increase in muscle force with harder foods or whether there is a change in chewing rhythm [4,22].

Clinical Relevance

CHANGES IN DIET IN PATIENTS WITH TMJ DYSFUNCTION: *Because mastication requires large muscle forces, many individuals with chronic TMJ dysfunction find that only a diet of soft foods can be eaten without an increase in symptoms. Instructing an individual to avoid hard, tough food may help control the person's symptoms while normal joint function is being restored.*

Joint Reaction Forces

Although there are several studies that consider the joint reaction forces of the TMJ, most emphasize the factors that influence the validity of the calculations, including the location, magnitude, and direction of the bite force as well as the assumptions made regarding the moment arm and cross-sectional diameters of the active muscles [2,23,27,29]. Actual calculations of peak joint reaction forces on a mandibular condyle are available from only a few studies and range from approximately 400 N to approximately 1,100 N (90–250 lb) [16,18,24]. Although it is generally accepted that the balancing side of the mandible sustains significant loads during bite, only one known study compares the loads on the balancing and working sides, suggesting that the balancing side of the temporomandibular complex sustains approximately twice the load sustained by the working or chewing side [9]. Additional studies report that the joint space is narrower on the balancing side during mastication, supporting the view that the balancing side sustains more compression during chewing than the working side [10,11].

Clinical Relevance

"I CAN'T EVEN CHEW ON THE OPPOSITE SIDE!": *Individuals with acute TMJ pain often assume that chewing on the opposite side of the mouth will help reduce their symptoms. So they continue to bite large tough rolls or chew tough meat. A clinician can help convince a patient to avoid hard, tough foods through the acute phase of a TMJ disorder by helping the patient to understand that the opposite, or balancing, side sustains even larger loads than the chewing, or working, side.*

Some studies examine the stress (force/area) applied to the mandible and intraarticular disc and report that during bite the anterior aspect of the mandibular condyle and neck sustain compressive loads while the posterior aspect and the articular surface of the temporal bone sustain both compressive and tensile loads [7,8] (*Fig. 25.1*). The intraarticular disc

reportedly sustains large stresses in the lateral aspect of the intermediate zone [3]. The chin-cup apparatus used in orthodontic appliances also apparently applies significant stresses to the mandible and joint [8]. Although additional research is needed to evaluate the loads within the TMJ, the available studies consistently demonstrate that the articular structures sustain substantial loads. The magnitude and repetitive nature of these loads may help explain why the TMJ is a frequent site of pain and degeneration.

Clinical Relevance

TRACTION OF THE CERVICAL SPINE: *Traction of the cervical spine is a useful diagnostic procedure as well as a common intervention for pain in the head, neck, or shoulder [17]. Many cervical traction procedures apply a tensile force to the cervical spine through the occiput and mandible (Fig. 25.2). The clinician must exercise considerable care to avoid applying too much force on the mandible, which could produce excessive compression of the TMJ.*

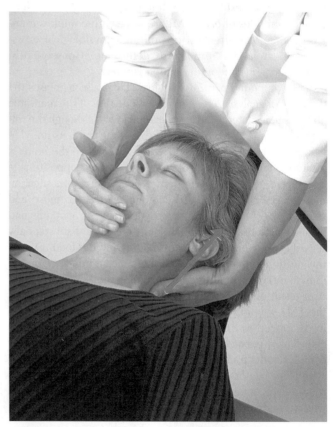

Figure 25.2: Loads on the TMJ during traction of the cervical spine. To apply manual traction to the cervical spine, the therapist must be careful to minimize the load on the mandible, applying most of the force through the occiput, to avoid applying excessive compressive loads to the TMJs.

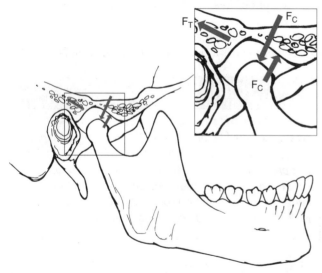

Figure 25.1: Stresses in the TMJ. During bite, the head of the mandible sustains compressive loads (F_C) while the articular surface on the temporal bone sustains both compressive and tensile loads (F_T).

SUMMARY

This chapter provides an overview of the loads sustained by the TMJ during forceful bite and during chewing. While there is no consensus regarding the magnitude and direction of the loads on the TMJ, the joint sustains loads of over 100 lb. Such high loads may help explain why pain in the TMJ is a common complaint.

A simple two-dimensional model was used to examine the mechanics of loading and the effect of bite position on the muscles of mastication and the joint reaction forces. Biting with the incisors differs from chewing with the molars by altering the moment arm of the bite force as well as changing the participation of the muscles of mastication. Instructing an individual to avoid hard foods may help to reduce the muscle and joint reaction forces exerted at the TMJ. Even interventions to treat cervical spine pain may inadvertently produce large forces on the TMJ, and clinicians are cautioned to consider how their treatments may have unintended consequences on the TMJ and to identify ways to protect the joint from excessive loads.

References

1. Bakke M, Michler L, Han K, Moller E: Clinical significance of isometric bite force versus electrical activity in temporal and masseter muscles. Scand J Dent Res 1989; 97: 539–551.
2. Barbenel J: The biomechanics of the temporomandibular joint: a theoretical study. J Biomech 1972; 5: 251–256.
3. Beek M: Three-dimensional finite element analysis of the human temporomandibular joint disc. J Biomech 2000; 33: 307–316.
4. Bishop B, Plesh O, McCall WD: Effects of chewing frequency and bolus hardness on human incisor trajectory and masseter muscle activity. Arch Oral Biol. 1990; 35: 311–318.
5. Braun S: A study of maximum bite force during growth and development. Angle Orthod 1996; 66: 261–264.
6. Chadwick EKJ, Nicol AC: Elbow and wrist joint contact forces during occupational pick and place activities. J Biomech 2000; 33: 591–600.
7. Chen J, Akyuz U, Xu L, Pidaparti RM: Stress analysis of the human temporomandibular joint. Med Eng Phys 1998; 20: 565–572.
8. Deguchi T: Force distribution of the temporomandibular joint and temporal bone surface subjected to the head-chin-up force. Am J Orthod Dentofac Orthop 1998; 114: 277–282.
9. Faulkner MG, Hatcher DC, Hay A: A three-dimensional investigation of temporomandibular joint loading. J Biomech 1987; 20: 997–1002.
10. Fushima K, Gallo LM, Krebs M, Palla S: Analysis of the TMJ intraarticular space variation: a non-invasive insight during mastication. Med Eng Phys 2003; 25: 181–190.
11. Gallo LM: Modeling of temporomandibular joint function using MRI and jaw-tracking technologies—mechanics. Cells Tissues Organs 2005; 180: 54–68.
12. Hidaka O, Iwasaki M, Saito M, Morimoto T: Influence of clenching intensity on bite force balance, occlusal contact area, and average bite pressure. J Dent Res 1999; 78: 1336–1344.
13. Hiraba K, Hibino K, Hiranuma K, Negoro T: EMG activities of two heads of the human lateral pterygoid muscle in relation to mandibular condyle movement and biting force. J Neurophysiol 2000; 83: 2120–2137.
14. Kawaguchi T, Kawata T, Kuriyagawa T, Sasaki K: In vivo 3-dimensional measurement of the force exerted on a tooth during clenching. J Biomech 2007; 40: 244–251.
15. Koh TJ, Herzog W: Increasing the moment arm of the tibialis anterior induces structural and functional adaptation: implications for tendon transfer. J Biomech 1998; 31: 593–599.
16. Koolstra JH, van Eijden TMGJ, Weijs WA, Naeije M: A three-dimensional mathematical model of the human masticatory system predicting maximum possible bite forces. J Biomech 1988; 21: 563–576.
17. Magee DA: Orthopedic Physical Assessment. Philadelphia: WB Saunders, 1998.
18. May B, Saha S, Saltzman M: A three-dimensional mathematical model of temporomandibular joint loading. Clin Biomech 2001; 16: 489–495.
19. McCarroll RS, Naeije M, Hansson TL: Balance on masticatory muscle activity during natural chewing and submaximal clenching. J Oral Rehabil 1989; 16: 441–446.
20. Meyer C, Kahn JL, Boutemy P, Wilk A: Determination of the external forces applied to the mandible during various static chewing tasks. J Craniomaxillofac Surg 1998; 26: 331–341.
21. Moriya Y, Tuchida K, Sawada T, et al: The influence of craniofacial form on bite force and EMG activity of masticatory muscles. VIII-1. Bite force of complete denture wearers. J Oral Sci 1999; 41: 19–27.
22. Neill DJ, Kydd WL, Nairn RI, Wilson J: Functional loading of the dentition during mastication. J Prosthet Dent 1989; 62: 218–228.
23. Osborn J: Features of human jaw design which maximize the bite force. J Biomech 1996; 29: 589–595.
24. Pruim GJ, de Jongh HJ, ten Bosch JJ: Forces acting on the mandible during bilateral static bite at different bite force levels. J Biomechan 1980; 13: 755–763.
25. Spencer MA: Force production in the primate masticatory system: electromyographic tests of biomechanical hypotheses. J Hum Evol 1998; 34: 25–54.
26. Throckmorton G: Quantitative calculations of temporomandibular joint reaction forces-II. The importance of the direction of the jaw muscle forces. J Biomech 1985; 18: 453–461.
27. Throckmorton G: Sensitivity of temporomandibular joint force calculations to errors in muscle force measurements. J Biomech 1989; 22: 455–468.
28. Throckmorton G, Groshan GJ, Boyd SB: Muscle activity patterns and control of temporomandibular joint loads. J Prosthet Dent 1990; 63: 685–695.
29. Throckmorton GS, Throckmorton LS: Quantitative calculations of temporomandibular joint reaction forces- I. The importance of the magnitude of the jaw muscle forces. J Biomech 1985; 18: 445–452.
30. Zwijnenburg AJ, Kroon GW, Verbeeten B Jr, Naeije M: Jaw movement responses to electrical stimulation of different parts of the human temporalis muscle. J Dent Res 1996; 75: 1798–1803.

The spine unit consists of 12 chapters examining the structure and function of the four regions of the spine: cervical, thoracic, lumbar, and pelvic. Each region is described in three chapters, the first discussing the structure of the bones and joints and the factors that influence mobility and stability in each region. The second chapter on each region presents the muscles that support and move the spine as well as those that perform special functions such as the muscles of respiration in the thoracic region. The third chapter of each spinal region examines the forces sustained by the region during daily activities or as a result of trauma commonly associated with the region. By the end of this unit the reader will have an understanding of the features common to the whole spine as well as the unique features that distinguish one region from another.

The purposes of this unit are to

- Relate the structure of the bones and joints of each spinal region to the mobility and stability available in that region
- Discuss the role of the muscles of a spinal region in moving and supporting the region as well as their contributions to special functions
- Consider the effects of joint or muscle impairments on the function of the spinal region
- Examine the loads normally applied to the spinal region and discuss the mechanical factors that contribute to injuries in the spinal regions

Structure and Function of the Bones and Joints of the Cervical Spine

SUSAN R. MERCER, PH.D., B.PHTY., F.N.Z.C.P.

CHAPTER CONTENTS

The cervical spine supports the head, provides attachment for muscles of the neck and upper extremity, and, along with the rest of the spine, protects the spinal cord. It must meet the demand of providing a large range of motion (ROM) to ensure optimal functioning of the special senses such as vision, smell, and hearing that are housed in the head. Yet, it must also serve the contradictory demands of balancing and supporting the head, protecting neural and vascular structures, and providing muscle and ligament attachment. The mechanism of meeting these disparate needs is reflected in the morphology of the bones and joints of the cervical spine. The specific purposes of this chapter are to

- Describe the structure of the individual vertebrae that compose the cervical vertebral column
- Describe the articulations joining the bony elements
- Describe the factors contributing to stability and instability in the cervical spine
- Review the normal ROM of the head and neck

STRUCTURE OF THE BONES OF THE CERVICAL SPINE

The morphology of the cervical spine is complex, yet, compared with the lumbar spine, has been sparsely studied. Consequently, much of what appears as definitive descriptions of the structure and function of the bones and joints of the cervical spine is extrapolation from other areas of the spine.

Throughout this chapter attention is drawn to these problems in the literature. Finally, fundamental to developing an understanding of the cervical spine is an appreciation that each cervical vertebra contributes to the complexities of neck function neither equally nor regularly.

The cervical vertebral column consists of seven vertebrae, of which the first two are morphologically distinct, while the third through seventh vertebrae follow a typical morphology with minor variations. For ease of study, two distinct units

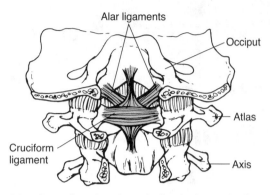

Figure 26.1: Coronal section through the craniovertebral region reveals articulations of the atlas with the occiput and axis. The posterior portions of the bone are removed, leaving a posterior view of the anterior ligaments.

within the cervical vertebral column may be described. These are the craniovertebral, or suboccipital, region, comprising the atlas and axis, and the lower cervical vertebral column, comprising vertebrae C3 through C7. Together they contribute to the function of the neck.

Craniovertebral Vertebrae

ATLAS

The atlas sits like a washer between the skull and the lower cervical spine (*Fig. 26.1*). It functions to cradle the occiput and to transmit forces from the head to the cervical spine. Secondarily, it is adapted for attachment of ligaments and muscles. Its distinctive morphology of two large lateral masses vertically aligned below the occipital condyles reflects these functions. Slender arches join the lateral masses anteriorly and posteriorly, transforming the atlas into a ring and allowing the lateral masses to act in parallel [59] (*Fig. 26.2*).

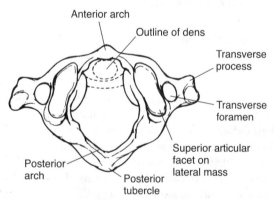

Figure 26.2: Superior view of the lateral masses of the atlas. The superior surface of the lateral masses contain kidney-shaped articular facets for the occiput and form a ring by anterior and posterior arches.

The superior aspect of each lateral mass exhibits a deep socket that is concave anteroposteriorly and mediolaterally, consistent with the curvature of the occipital condyles so that the skull rests securely on the atlas. The size and shape of the sockets vary greatly, but in general, the articular surfaces of these superior facets are directed upward and medially, with their outer margins projecting more superiorly [93]. In long, deeply concave sockets the anterior wall may face backward, and the posterior wall forward. In most C1 vertebrae, each socket is completely or incompletely divided into two facets or into a dumbbell-shaped facet having a nonarticular waist. The atlantal sockets typically exhibit right–left asymmetry [37,86].

Clinical Relevance

ATLANTO-OCCIPITAL RANGE OF MOTION: *The large variation in normal morphology of the atlantal sockets means that the apparent differences in motion between right and left atlanto-occipital joints or among individuals may be due to normal differences in the joint structure and may not indicate joint impairment. Clinicians must identify relationships between ROM measures and other signs and symptoms to suspect that differences in motion reflect true impairments.*

The occipital condyles transmit the weight of the head to the axis (C2) via the large lateral masses of the atlas (C1). This is achieved by an articulation between the apparently flat, broad inferior articular surfaces of the lateral masses, which are directed inferiorly and medially to the wide shoulders of the superior articular facets of the axis below (*Fig. 26.1*).

The robust transverse processes of the atlas are the primary site of muscle attachment for this vertebra. The size of each transverse process accommodates the loading associated with suspension of the scapula through the attachment of the levator scapulae muscle. Consequently, any movement of the upper limb exerts compressive forces on the entire cervical spine. The length of each transverse process increases the moment arms of the muscles attached to it, but also allows the vertebral artery to clear the large lateral masses of the axis below (*Fig. 26.2*).

The anterior arch that joins the lateral masses of the atlas is short and slender, since it is uninvolved in transmitting large forces. A small, smooth facet lies centrally on the posterior aspect of the anterior arch for articulation with the odontoid process of the axis. The position of the anterior arch against the odontoid process ensures that there is a bony block to posterior translation of the atlas. Enclosed by the anterior and posterior arches and lateral masses, the central foramen of the atlas has two distinct parts. The smaller anterior part partially encircles the odontoid process, or dens, while the larger posterior portion is the vertebral foramen proper (Fig. 26.2).

AXIS

The axis accepts the load of the head and atlas and transmits that load to the remainder of the cervical spine. It also provides axial rotation of the head and atlas. The broad, laterally placed, superior articular facets of the axis accept and transmit loads from the head and atlas, while the centrally placed odontoid process, or dens, acts as a pivot around which the anterior arch of the atlas spins and glides to produce axial rotation (*Fig. 26.3*).

The superior articular facets of the axis are lateral to the dens and face upward and laterally and slope inferiorly and laterally. They support the lateral masses of the atlas and transmit the load of the head and atlas inferiorly and anteriorly to the C2-3 intervertebral disc and inferiorly and posteriorly to the C2-3 zygapophysial, or facet, joints. The inferior articular facet is located posterior to the superior facet in a position similar to the articular processes of the lower cervical vertebrae (*Fig. 26.3B*).

The laminae of the axis are broad and robust, meeting at a broad, roughened spinous process. The size and strength of the spinous process reflect the number, size, and direction of pull of the attaching muscles. Like the transverse processes of the lower cervical vertebrae, each transverse process of the atlas and axis contains a transverse foramen that, with the other foramina on the same side, form a canal through which the vertebral artery travels on its way to the foramen magnum. Each transverse process of the axis is short, ending in a single tubercle, while each transverse process of the atlas is long. Consequently, as the canal for the vertebral artery approaches the inferior surface of the superior articular mass, it turns sharply laterally to exit beneath the lateral margin of the superior articular facet.

Lower Column C3–C7 Vertebrae

The lower five cervical vertebrae must support the axial load of the head and vertebrae above, keep the head upright, support the reactive forces of muscles, yet provide for mobility of the head. The vertebrae, therefore, exhibit features that reflect these load-bearing, stability, and mobility functions. Together, the lower five vertebrae may be considered as a triangular column consisting of an anterior pillar composed of the vertebral bodies and two posterior columns composed of the right and left articular pillars of the articulating superior and inferior articular processes (*Fig. 26.4*).

The vertebral bodies exhibit a modified blocklike quality reflecting their ability to bear and transmit axial loads (*Fig. 26.5*). Due to the presence of the uncinate processes along the posterolateral margins, the superior surface of the body of a lower cervical vertebra is concave transversely, while in the sagittal plane, the superior surface slopes forward

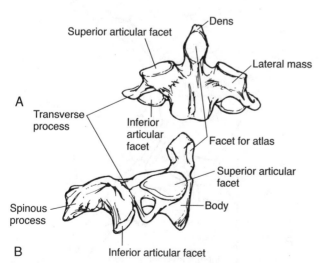

Figure 26.3: Axis viewed anteriorly **(A)** and laterally **(B)**. The axis includes the dens, short transverse processes, and a long spinous process. The superior articular processes slope inferiorly and laterally and face upwardly and posteriorly. The inferior facets lie posterior to the superior facets.

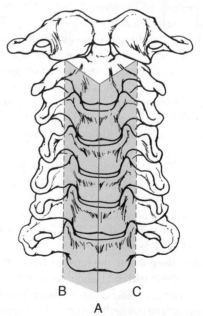

Figure 26.4: Anterior view of the cervical vertebral column. The cervical vertebral column consists of a central anterior pillar *(A)* and the right *(B)* and left *(C)* articular pillars, forming a triangular column.

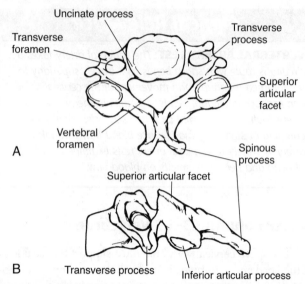

A

B

Figure 26.5: Typical cervical vertebra viewed superiorly **(A)** and laterally **(B)**. The superior surface of the body of a typical cervical vertebra is concave from side to side and slopes inferiorly and anteriorly. The superior facets face posteriorly and superiorly; the inferior facets face anteriorly and inferiorly.

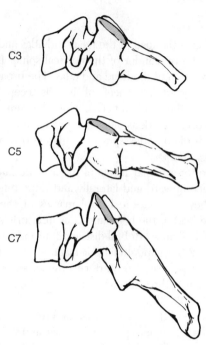

Figure 26.6: The superior facets of C3 face slightly medially as well as superiorly and posteriorly. The superior facets of C3 and C7 are more steeply oriented than those of C5.

and downward. Inferiorly, the surface of the body is concave anteroposteriorly, with an anterior lip that projects anteroinferiorly toward the anterior superior edge of the vertebra below [10]. Appreciation of such detail regarding the geometry of the articular surfaces is vital to understanding the patterns of segmental motion.

Posteriorly, the articular processes bear the superior and inferior articular facets. Generally, the superior facets are directed superiorly and posteriorly, while the inferior facets are directed anteriorly and inferiorly (Fig. 26.5). The orientation of the facets contributes to the function of each vertebra. In the upright posture, the superior facet lies between the transverse and frontal planes, and as a consequence, it helps support the weight of the head and stabilizes the vertebra above against forward translation. However, at each level there are subtle differences in orientation of the facets [56, 70,94] (*Fig. 26.6*). In addition to facing superiorly and posteriorly, the superior facet of C3 also faces medially by about 40° [61,94]. Consequently, the superior articular processes of C3 form a socket into which the inferior articular processes of C2 nestle [10]. The superior articular facets change from a posteromedial orientation at the C2/C3 level to posterolateral orientation at C7/T1. The transition typically occurs at the C5/C6 level [71].

Descending the column, the superior facets sit higher relative to the superior vertebral endplate, and the C3 and C7 facets are steeper [66]. Knowledge of the height of the articular processes is important, as it has been demonstrated that the height of the articular processes is perfectly related to the location of the instantaneous axes of rotation. It is articular height, not slope, that is the major determinant of the patterns of motion of the cervical vertebrae [66].

The unique morphology exhibited by the seventh cervical vertebra reflects its load-bearing function (*Fig. 26.7*). It is the point where the neck is cantilevered off the more

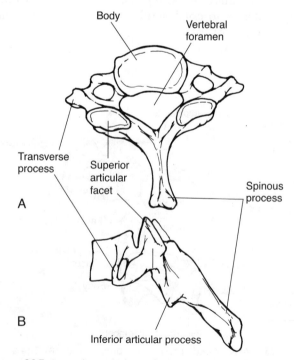

A

B

Figure 26.7: Seventh cervical vertebra: superior view **(A)** and lateral view **(B)**. The spinous process of C7 is long and robust. The superior articular facets sit high relative to the superior surface of the vertebral body and are steeply inclined in the coronal plane.

rigid thoracic spine [14,43,44]. It also is the site of attachment of several structures, including the raphe of the ligamentum nuchae, the large, middle portion of the trapezius, the rhomboid minor, and the muscles of respiration, scalenus medius, scalenus posterior, and levator costae. Consequently, the spinous process and posterior tubercles are long and robust. The superior articular facets sit high relative to the superior surface of the vertebral body and are steeply inclined in the coronal plane. Such geometry appears to provide optimal stability, guarding against forward translation at this transition from the cervical to the thoracic spine [66].

JOINTS OF THE CERVICAL SPINE

Just as the bones of the cervical region are organized into two distinct regions, the joints of the cervical spine also are described in two regions. The craniovertebral joints exhibit specialized characteristics that dictate the mobility and stability of the upper cervical region. The joints of the lower cervical segments exhibit modified interbody and facet joints, reflecting the stability, mobility, and load-bearing roles of the lower neck.

Craniovertebral Joints

The two atlanto-occipital joints are found between the superior concave sockets of the atlas and the occipital condyles of the skull (Fig. 26.1). Being typical synovial joints, they are enclosed by a joint capsule and contain intra-articular inclusions. These are fat pads that sit in the nonarticular waist of the bean-shaped articular surface of the atlas and act as deformable space fillers [57].

The atlantoaxial joints consist of three synovial joints: the left and right lateral atlantoaxial joints and the median atlantoaxial joint. Together these joints allow axial rotation of the head and atlas where the centrally placed odontoid process acts as a pivot around which the anterior arch of the atlas spins. This movement is accommodated anteriorly by the median atlantoaxial joint and inferiorly by the lateral atlantoaxial joints. The median atlantoaxial joint lies between the odontoid process and osseoligamentous ring made by the anterior arch of the atlas and the transverse ligament (*Fig. 26.8*).

At the lateral atlantoaxial joints, the superior articular surfaces of the axis and the corresponding inferior articular surfaces of the atlas appear flat (Fig. 26.3). In vivo, however, they are covered by articular cartilage that is convex in the sagittal plane [48] (*Fig. 26.9*). The apex of this convexity lies along a ridge passing downward and laterally across the articular facet so that each cartilaginous facet presents a curved posterior and anterior slope. In the neutral position, the apex of the cartilage of the inferior articular facet sits on the apex of the superior articular cartilage of the axis. Large intraarticular **meniscoids** fill the spaces between the articular spaces

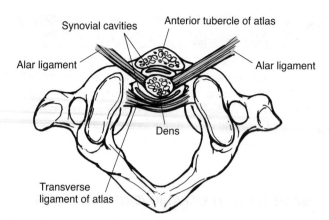

Figure 26.8: Superior view of a transverse section through the atlas and dens reveals the median atlantoaxial joint and supporting ligaments.

anteriorly and posteriorly [57]. These meniscoids act not only as moveable space fillers, but also protect those articular surfaces that are not in contact with one another by ensuring that a film of synovial fluid coats them.

Little research has been undertaken regarding the structure of the joint capsule of the lateral atlantoaxial joints, although it is described as loose and thin [96]. The capsule must be lax to allow approximately 45° of axial rotation in each direction, yet it contributes to stability of the joint at the end range of these movements [20].

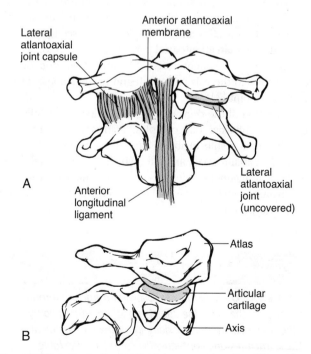

Figure 26.9: Lateral atlantoaxial joints: anterior view **(A)** and lateral view **(B)**. Covered by articular cartilage, the articular surfaces of the lateral atlantoaxial joints are convex.

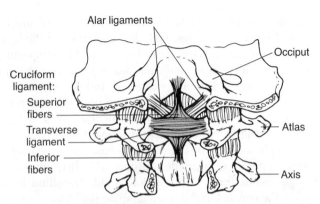

Figure 26.10: Coronal section of the occiput, atlas, and axis, with the posterior section removed, reveals the transverse and alar ligaments. The transverse ligament combines with the longitudinally oriented superior and inferior fibers to form the cruciform ligament.

LIGAMENTS OF THE CRANIOVERTEBRAL JOINTS

Many supposedly definitive descriptions of the structure and function of the ligaments of the cervical spine are extrapolations from other areas of the spine or are impressions, rather than results of systematic anatomical studies. In particular, many structures have been described as ligaments that are in fact only fascial membranes. True or **proper ligaments** are composed predominately of strong collagen fibers oriented in the direction of the movement that they are designed to resist, and they attach bone to bone. This chapter distinguishes between such proper ligaments and fascial membranes, or **false ligaments,** which differ by consisting of collagen that is loosely arranged and therefore not strong.

Transverse Ligament

The transverse ligament is classified as a proper ligament, being a well-defined and strong structure consisting almost exclusively of collagen fibers. It spans the anterior portion of the central foramen, attaching on the inner surface of each lateral mass of the atlas, and so completes the osseoligamentous ring of the median atlantoaxial joint (Figs. 26.1, 26.8, 26.10). The transverse ligament resists forward translation of the atlas relative to the axis and is integral to the stability of the atlantoaxial joint [31,34].

Disruption of the transverse ligament does not totally disable the atlantoaxial joint complex. Transection of the transverse ligament results in about 4 mm of forward translation of the median atlantoaxial joint, after which the joint is stabilized by the alar ligaments (described later), which prevent the head from moving relative to the axis and restrict the motion of the interposed atlas [27].

The cruciform or cruciate ligament is formed by the transverse ligament, with associated superior and variably present inferior bands that together make a cross-shaped structure (*Fig. 26.10*). The functional significance of these longitudinally directed median bands, which cannot be classed as proper ligaments because of their attachment sites, has not been determined.

Alar Ligaments

The anatomy of the two alar ligaments appears to differ from the descriptions provided in the traditional textbooks of anatomy. The morphology of these proper ligaments has been reexamined by Dvorak and Panjabi [29]. Textbooks tend to depict each alar ligament as passing steeply upward and laterally from the odontoid process to the margins of the foramen magnum. In fact, the orientation of the alar ligaments is closer to being horizontal, running from the lateral aspect of the odontoid process to the margins of the foramen magnum (Figs. 26.1, 26.8, 26.10). In some specimens, a small portion of the alar ligament has been observed to run between the dens and the lateral masses of the atlas. However, the functional significance of this small portion has not been described further than reinforcing the intimate relationship of the atlas interposed between the occiput and axis [29].

The absence of elastic fibers and the strictly parallel orientation of the collagen fibers in the alar ligaments mean that elongation of these ligaments is almost impossible [83]. Apart from stabilizing the atlantoaxial joint with respect to anterior translation, flexion, and lateral bending, the alar ligaments are of critical importance in limiting rotation of the head and atlas on the axis. Because the odontoid attachment of the alar ligament lies posteriorly on the dens, as the neck rotates, the contralateral alar ligament wraps around the circumference of the dens, thereby increasing tension in the ligament. The length between the origin and insertion of the ligament is not a straight line during rotation but a curve around the perimeter of the odontoid process, and therefore, tension develops quickly. Following this model, Dvorak et al. report that axial rotation slackens the ipsilateral ligament [31].

Disagreement exists regarding the role of both alar ligaments in limiting rotation. Some authors report that both alar ligaments are involved in the control of axial rotation to one side. A model of upper cervical axial rotation predicts that both alar ligaments must be intact for axial rotation to be checked [20]. Transecting cadaver alar ligaments reveals that axial rotation increases in both directions when a single alar ligament is cut [72]. Using computed tomography (CT) scanning, Dvorak et al. show that axial rotation increases by about 11° (30%) following transection of a contralateral alar ligament [30]. While agreement exists that these paired ligaments play a vital role in stabilizing and limiting the motion in the craniovertebral region, the precise role played by each ligament remains debatable.

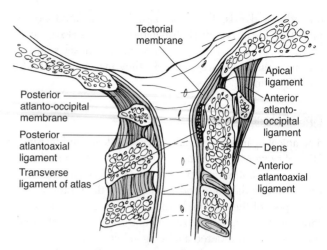

Figure 26.12: Median sagittal section through the craniovertebral region. Ligaments and membranes associated with the craniovertebral region include the transverse ligament, the apical ligament, the anterior and posterior atlanto-occipital membranes, the anterior and posterior atlantoaxial membranes, and the tectorial membrane.

Clinical Relevance

REAR-END MOTOR VEHICLE ACCIDENTS: *In an unexpected rear-end collision, the neck may be slightly rotated when undergoing a flexion–extension injury [30]. In this position the alar ligament is particularly susceptible to strain or rupture. It has been suggested that subluxation or dislocation of the atlantoaxial joint implies destruction of both transverse and alar ligaments [34].*

Membrana Tectoria

The membrana tectoria, or tectorial membrane, is a wide sheet of collagen fibers that covers the atlantoaxial ligament complex (*Fig. 26.11*). It extends from the posterior surface of

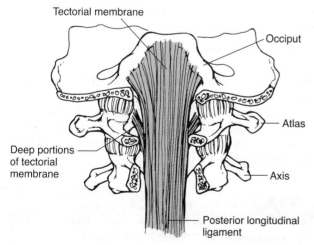

Figure 26.11: Tectorial membrane, posterior view. The tectorial membrane is the superior extension of the posterior longitudinal ligament onto the anterior and lateral margins of the foramen magnum. It lies posterior to the transverse and alar ligaments.

the vertebral body of the axis up to the margins of the foramen magnum and is the direct proximal continuation of the posterior longitudinal ligament (*Fig. 26.12*). It may, therefore, be classified as a proper ligament. Little research has been undertaken to determine the role of the membrana tectoria in craniovertebral stability [67,95]. However, following transection studies on cadavers, Oda et al. state that the membrana tectoria plays a role in multidirectional stability of the upper spine, particularly in upper cervical flexion and axial rotation [67].

Atlanto-Occipital and Atlantoaxial Membranes

The anterior and posterior atlanto-occipital membranes and anterior and posterior atlantoaxial membranes are often described as ligaments associated with the craniovertebral joints. Interestingly, although the atlanto-occipital membranes are consistently described in anatomical textbooks, the atlantoaxial membranes are often not mentioned [82,96], or a picture may be presented but a description of the structure not supplied [64]. Such variability in presentation raises questions regarding their structural and functional significance. The anterior and posterior atlanto-occipital membranes are found spanning the space between the upper border of the anterior arch of the atlas and the basiocciput and the posterior arch and posterior margin of the foramen magnum (Fig. 26.12). They appear to consist of dense areolar tissue that is not particularly organized.

Ramsey sectioned these posterior membranes and found some elastic fibers, although fewer than typically seen in the ligamentum flavum [79]. He feels that these structures should be considered being "in series" with the ligamentum flavum. As these membranes are found in the anterior and posterior spaces between the occiput and atlas and between the atlas and axis, they may also be considered nothing more than fascial curtains between the external space occupied by the posterior vertebral or prevertebral muscles and the internal epidural space. As such, they may be classified as false ligaments.

Apical Ligament

The apical ligament is trivial in size, very thin, and missing in 20% of persons. The ligament has no known biomechanical importance. Rather, it represents the vestigial remains of the cranial end of the notochord passing from the posterior superior aspect of the odontoid process to the anterior rim of the foramen magnum (Fig. 26.12) [74,89]. This ligament should, therefore, be considered a false ligament.

Joints of the Lower Cervical Spine

INTERBODY JOINTS

As elsewhere in the vertebral column, the vertebral bodies below C2 are joined via intervertebral discs. These discs provide separation of adjacent vertebral bodies, thereby allowing the superior vertebra to move on the lower vertebra. The interposed disc must be able to accommodate the motion occurring between vertebrae, be strong enough to transfer loads, and not be injured during movement [11]. The form and function of the cervical intervertebral disc is, however, distinctly different from those of the lumbar intervertebral disc [58]. In the adult, the anulus fibrosus in the cervical region is a discontinuous structure surrounding a fibrocartilaginous core, instead of being a fibrous ring enclosing a gelatinous nucleus pulposus like the anulus fibrosus in the lumbar region. Anteriorly, the anulus fibrosus in the cervical spine is a thick crescent of oblique fibers joining the vertebral bodies to constitute a strong interosseous ligament located at the pivot point of axial rotation [59]. Posteriorly, the anulus is a thin, narrow, vertically oriented band of fibers joining the vertebral bodies. Laterally, there is no distinct anulus, only flimsy fascial tissue that is continuous with the periosteum (*Fig. 26.13*).

Penetrating the fibrocartilaginous core to a greater or lesser extent are uncovertebral clefts, which are considered normal features of cervical intervertebral discs. Found opposite the uncinate processes, they have been shown to develop following the maturation of the uncinate processes at approximately 9 years of age. With age, the clefts progress medially into the disc to form transverse clefts, which may completely transect the posterior two thirds of the disc [58,68,76,88]. It is these normally developing clefts or fissures that effectively form a joint cavity between the vertebral bodies and allow the swinging movement of the posterior inferior surface of the upper vertebral body within the concavity of the uncinate processes. The clefts, therefore, enable the interbody joint to accommodate the coupling of lateral flexion and axial rotation that is determined by the geometry of the zygapophysial joints [77].

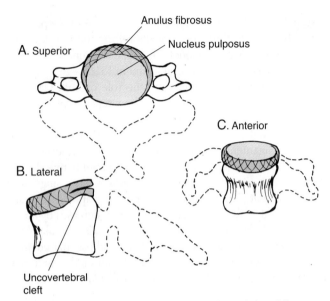

Figure 26.13: Cervical disc: superior view **(A)**, lateral view **(B)**, anterior view **(C)**. A typical cervical disc contains a distinct, strong anulus fibrosus anteriorly, which is discontinuous with the thin vertically oriented fibers of the posterior anulus fibrosus. Uncovertebral clefts form opposite the unciform processes and may eventually form clefts that transect the posterior two thirds of the disc.

Clinical Relevance

DISCOGENIC PAIN: *The recently described morphology of the adult cervical intervertebral disc must raise questions for clinicians concerning the etiology and mechanism of cervical discogenic pain. This pain cannot arise from posterolateral fissures in the anulus fibrosus, as occurs in the lumbar disc, since there is no posterolateral anulus fibrosus in a cervical disc [63]. Given the morphology of the cervical intervertebral disc, possible sources of disc-related pain in the cervical spine are strain or tears of the anterior anulus fibrosus, especially following hyperextension trauma, and strain of the lateral (alar) portions of the posterior longitudinal ligament by a bulging disc [58].*

The nucleus pulposus of the cervical intervertebral disc is also distinctly different from the lumbar nucleus. At birth, the nucleus comprises less than 25% of the discs, whereas in the lumbar disc, it comprises at least 50% [87]. The adult cervical nucleus is characterized by fibrocartilage, with no gelatinous component [10,58,68,88].

Clinical Relevance

CERVICAL DISC STRUCTURE: *The absence of a gelatinous nucleus pulposus has implications for assessment and treatment techniques that assume that a cervical intervertebral*
(continued)

(Continued)
disc is composed of a gelatinous nucleus pulposus encircled by an anulus fibrosus [60]. Although the validity and effectiveness of such techniques require direct assessment, the biological explanations for these techniques appear implausible.

ZYGAPOPHYSEAL JOINTS

The cervical zygapophyseal, or facet, joints are formed by the articulation of the inferior articular cervical vertebra with the ipsilateral superior articular process of the vertebra below. As typical synovial joints, the articular surfaces are lined by articular cartilage and enclosed by a joint capsule. A variety of intraarticular inclusions are found within the joint, with fibroadipose meniscoids always present along the ventral aspect of the joint and frequently also present along the dorsal aspect [57]. The articular facets may be round or oval, and there is often right–left asymmetry [71].

Clinical Relevance

WHIPLASH INJURIES: *Rear-impact motor vehicle collisions produce hyperextension movements of the head and neck. It has been postulated that these movements cause impingement of the meniscoids, which could become inflamed and so be a source of undiagnosed neck pain following whiplash injuries [47].*

The capsules of the zygapophysial joints consist of well-orientated collagen and elastic fibers. The medial, anterior, and lateral parts of the joint capsule have been described as thicker than the thinner posterior part [35,74,90], although Johnson et al. state that the posterior portion is thick [45]. The elastic fibers of the medial aspect are oriented like those of the ligamentum flavum, projecting vertically from one articular process to the other, and may join with the ligamentum flavum. Anterolaterally, the elastic fibers are less concentrated, are oriented obliquely in the transverse and sagittal planes, and appear to provide an important barrier to anteroposterior shear [90].

In the neutral position, the capsules of the zygapophysial joints are lax. This laxity is the large range of gliding that occurs between the articular facets during the normal movements of flexion–extension and rotation of the cervical motion segments. However, at the extremes of these motions, the capsules are taut and hence function as stabilizing or resisting ligaments. It is for this reason that some persons refer to these structures as the **capsular ligaments.**

LIGAMENTS OF THE LOWER CERVICAL SPINE

Longitudinal Ligaments

A variety of descriptions of the structure and function of the anterior longitudinal ligament exists, but few studies have specifically examined the cervical ligaments. Most descriptions extrapolate structure and function from the lumbar portion of the ligament. Being arranged essentially in a uniaxial manner, these ligaments resist tension [98].

Traditionally, descriptions of the anterior longitudinal ligament suggest that it is a multilayered ligament firmly adherent to the intervertebral discs and to the margins of adjacent vertebral margins and, therefore, may be considered a proper ligament [96]. The posterior longitudinal ligament is a broad, thick ligament that blends with the posterior surface of the intervertebral discs and attaches to the vertebral bodies near their upper and lower margins and somewhat over their posterior surfaces [96]. It, too, may be considered a proper ligament. Cranially, the ligament expands to form the membrana tectoria, which attaches to the anterior and lateral margins of the foramen magnum (Fig. 26.11).

More-recent descriptions of the morphology of the cervical longitudinal ligaments reveal that the anterior longitudinal ligament is a centrally placed, thin structure composed of four distinct layers of fibers. This ligament, therefore, provides a thin covering to the front of the disc. The thicker posterior longitudinal ligament covers the entire floor of the cervical vertebral canal and is also distinctly multilayered. It reinforces the deficient posterior anulus fibrosus with **longitudinal** and **alar** fibers. This geometry also allows the ligament to resist tensile forces in a range of directions [58]. The morphology of the longitudinal ligaments and anulus fibrosus of the adult cervical disc suggests that the posterior longitudinal ligament and anterior anulus fibrosus are the important stabilizers of each interbody segment.

Ligamentum Flavum

The ligamentum flavum lacks studies that examine the form and function of its cervical portion. The ligamentum flavum in the neck is considered to be considerably thinner than in the lumbar region, but it maintains similar attachments and so may be classed as a proper ligament. This elastic ligament passes from the border of the lamina of one vertebra to the anterior surface of the lower edge of the vertebra above, leaving a space between the dorsal surface of ligamentum flavum and the inferior margin of the lamina of the upper vertebra (*Fig. 26.14*). The space is filled with fascia and some fat. As in the lumbar region, the ligamentum flavum seems to serve to provide a smooth, somewhat elastic posterior wall to the vertebral canal, thereby protecting the spinal cord against any buckling of the ligament that might occur if the ligament were fibrous.

Ligamentum Nuchae

The literature offers three opposing descriptions of the ligamentum nuchae. The most common description is that the ligamentum nuchae is a median fibrous septum, triangular

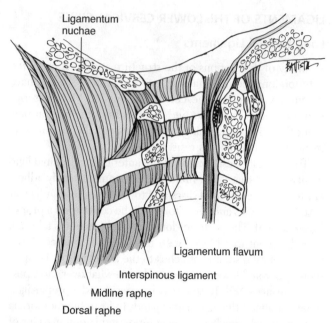

Figure 26.14: The ligamentum nuchae in the cervical region can be described with two distant parts, a dorsal raphe and a ventral midline septum.

tissue is continuous between the spinous processes, so no definite interspinous ligaments are found. In the suboccipital region, the fascia is confluent with the posterior atlanto-occipital and atlantoaxial membranes [33,40]. Consequently, in the cervical spine, there is no classically defined supraspinous ligament, nor is the ligamentum nuchae a proper ligament.

Clinical Relevance

LIGAMENTUM NUCHAE: *The absence of firm tendinous attachments of the ligamentum nuchae to the cervical spine raises questions regarding the importance of this structure in stabilizing the head or as the source of pain from tendinitis of the ligament's insertion at the tips of the cervical spinous processes.*

in shape, which divides the muscles of the posterior neck into right and left compartments and provides attachment for the upper fibers of trapezius, rhomboid minor, splenius capitis, and serratus posterior superior. It is composed of a free posterior border that extends between the external occipital protuberance and the spinous process of the seventh cervical vertebrae, an anterior border that is firmly attached to the cervical spinous processes, and a short superior border that extends along the external occipital crest [64,96]. The clinical literature portrays this ligament as a substantial midline structure that is important in control of head posture [7,78].

A second description found in a small number of texts characterizes the nuchal ligament as being no more than a thin fibrous intermuscular septum [1,38,80,101]. The third description of the ligamentum nuchae, favored by this author, presents the ligament with two distinct parts: a dorsal raphe and a ventral, midline septum (Fig. 26.14). The dorsal raphe is firmly attached to the external occipital protuberance and spans the cervical spine to attach to the spinous process of C7 and C6. It is formed by the interlacing of the tendons of the cervical portion of trapezius, splenius capitis, and rhomboid minor muscles. The midline septum, which consists of unoriented fascia embedded with fat and blood vessels, extends from the ventral aspect of the dorsal raphe attaching to the external occipital protuberance, to the external occipital crest, and to the tips of the cervical spinous processes. This fascial

NORMAL RANGE OF MOTION

Total Motion of the Cervical Spine

Because the American Medical Association (AMA) *Guides for the Assessment of Impairment* stipulate that ROM of the head be used to determine impairment of the neck, the clinician must appreciate the limitations in the current knowledge of ROM measures for the neck [4]. Total motion of the cervical spine is typically determined by describing head motion relative to the thorax or shoulder girdle. The wide variety of instruments and lack of standardized procedures that have been used in both reliability and descriptive studies have contributed to the wide range of published norms for active (*Table 26.1*) and passive neck ROM [3,8,36,50,51,55,69, 85,99] (*Table 26.2*). In addition, age and sex have been associated with variations in neck ROM [17,18,26,51,53,65,91,99]. Normal variation in ROM in subjects suggests that when measuring individual patients, a clinician should allow for natural variation of 12–20° [19].

Clinical Relevance

CERVICAL RANGE OF MOTION: *Clinicians must recognize the wide range of reported values for normal neck motion in addition to the normal variation reported for individual subjects when using neck motion to determine response to treatment or making disability ratings. Small changes in cervical motion may be attributable to normal variability and may have little to do with the impairment or intervention.*

TABLE 26.1: Reported Extremes of Active Range of Motion

ROM	R Axial Rotation	L Axial Rotation	R Lateral Flexion	L Lateral Flexion	Flexion	Extension
Minimum	70	66	38	38	35	50
Maximum	93	93	49	53	70	93

TABLE 26.2: Reported Extremes of Passive Range of Motion

ROM	R Axial Rotation	L Axial Rotation	R Lateral Flexion	L Lateral Flexion	Flexion	Extension
Minimum	79	81	39	46	59	53
Maximum	97	95	61	65	76	77

Because of the complex anatomy of the cervical spine, global ranges of neck motion are unable to differentiate movement occurring within the functional units of the upper and lower cervical spine and, therefore, do not reflect motion occurring at the segmental level. It has been demonstrated that in full extension, the entire cervical spine is in lordosis. However, during flexion the degree of kyphosis achieved in the upper and lower regions of the cervical spine varies, depending upon the posture adopted by the upper cervical spine. During head and neck flexion and extension, motion occurring in both the upper and lower regions of the cervical spine must be observed if the full potential of cervical flexion is to be assessed [97]. To establish full range of flexion of both the upper and lower cervical spine, upper cervical flexion should be examined with the lower cervical region in neutral, and then lower cervical flexion should be examined with the upper cervical region in slight extension [24]. This method ensures that total ROM in both functional units is assessed.

The traditional descriptions of neck ROM have been of total ROM. Yet the total ROM of the neck is not the arithmetic sum of the segmental ROMs. Total ROM appears to be as much as 10–30° less than the sum of the maximum segmental ROMs [92]. Segmental ROM in normals varies from day to day and depends on whether the motion is measured from an initial starting position of flexion or extension [92]. Further, in individuals reporting neck pain, dysfunctional segments have been demonstrated at levels other than those responsible for the pain [5]. These findings challenge the clinical relevance of considering the neck as a single entity and determining impairment on the basis of the ROM of the head and neck as a whole. Because global ROMs do not fully describe what is occurring in the neck, attempts to determine segmental mobility in both cadavers and in vivo are important.

Segmental Motion of the Craniovertebral Joints

ATLANTO-OCCIPITAL JOINTS

The functional challenge for the atlanto-occipital joints is to provide stability for the balance of the head on the cervical spine yet allow mobility. The geometry of the atlantal sockets, designed primarily for stability, determines the pattern of motion. The deep walls of each atlantal socket prevent translation of the occipital condyle laterally, anteriorly, or posteriorly, but the concave shape permits nodding movements of the head [13].

The nodding motion that occurs during flexion of the head is the result of rolling and sliding of the occipital condyles in their sockets. As the head nods forward, the occipital condyles roll forward in the atlantal sockets, tending to roll up the anterior wall of the socket. Because of the compression loading exerted by the mass of the head, the flexor musculature, or tension in the joint capsules, the occipital condyles concomitantly translate downward and backward [13]. As a result, anterior rotation is coupled with downward and posterior sliding, and the condyles effectively stay nestled in the floor of the atlantal sockets, ensuring maximum stability of the head on the neck. The converse occurs during extension of the head on the atlas.

The results of studies that have described range of flexion and extension at the atlanto-occipital joints are reported in *Table 26.3*. Examination of this table reveals the large variation in reported normal range for this joint. The total range of flexion–extension observed in vivo varies between a mean value of 14 and 35°. Brocher observes a range from 0 to 25° (mean, 14.3°), while Lind et al. find a mean value of 14°, but with a standard deviation of 15° [15,53].

TABLE 26.3: Range of Flexion–Extension at the Atlanto-Occipital Joint

Source	Subject	Mean ROM (°)	Range	SD
Brocher [15]	In vivo	14.3	0–25	
Lewit & Krausova [52]	In vivo	15		
Markuske [54]	In vivo	14.5		
Fielding [34]	In vivo	35		
Kottke & Mundale [49]	In vivo		0–22	
Lind et al. [53]	In vivo	14		15
Werne [95]	Cadaver		13	
Worth & Selvik [97]	Cadaver	18.6		0.6

Clinical Relevance

DISTINGUISHING NORMAL AND ABNORMAL RANGE OF MOTION: *The wide variation in reported ROM has important implications for clinicians who are attempting to differentiate normal from abnormal ROMs at the atlanto-occipital joint. In view of normal variation in morphology and ROM, the clinician must use additional information, including the patient's symptoms, to identify real impairments in ROM in the cervical region.*

Although commonly described, axial rotation (about a vertical axis) is not a true physiological movement of the atlanto-occipital joint. For true axial rotation to occur, the contralateral occipital condyle must translate posteriorly while the ipsilateral condyle translates anteriorly. As these translations are prevented by the steep walls of the atlantal sockets, axial rotation can only occur if sufficient torque is applied to the head. This would force the occipital condyles to rise up the walls of the sockets, which are wider at their mouths than at their depths. Axial rotation may, therefore, occur only if accompanied by upward vertical motion of the occiput. The alar ligaments and tension within the capsules of the atlanto-occipital joints resist this vertical displacement. As depicted in *Table 26.4*, the ROM that has been reported is small (–2-7°), and only one study has measured ROM in vivo.

Clinical Relevance

ATLANTO-OCCIPITAL ROTATION: *Although clinicians often report restrictions in atlanto-occipital rotation, the small values reported in the literature cast doubt on the validity of such clinical observations.*

Atlanto-occipital lateral flexion in vivo has not been systematically studied, although it has been examined in cadavers, with a reported ROM from 2.3 to 11° [73,97] (*Table 26.4*). Because of the geometry of the atlantal socket, either the contralateral occipital condyle must slide up and out of its deep atlantal socket while pivoting on the ipsilateral condyle, or both condyles must slide in parallel up the contralateral walls of their respective sockets. These articular surface

movements are not physiological but may be induced during manual examination. When induced, lateral flexion is coupled with flexion, extension, or axial rotation [97]. Since the pattern of coupling depends on the shape of the joint surfaces, and asymmetry of these joint surfaces has been extensively documented, no single rule for a pattern of coupling can be applied [93].

ATLANTOAXIAL JOINTS

Few studies are available that have fully investigated the available range and patterns of motion of the atlantoaxial joints. Most studies have used plain radiography and have only reported ranges of flexion and extension. Axial rotation has been either inferred from these plain films or biplanar radiography, although more recently, functional CT scanning has been undertaken. The clinician should note the methodology used when interpreting each study, because the measurement methodology may affect the results.

Axial rotation at the atlantoaxial level is extremely important functionally, for movement at this level accounts for 50% of the total range of axial rotation of the neck. Indeed, the first 45° of rotation of the head to either side occurs at the C1–C2 level before any lower cervical segments move in this plane.

Axial rotation of the atlas to the left requires anterior displacement of the right lateral mass and a reciprocal posterior displacement of the left lateral mass. The inferior articular cartilages of the atlas must therefore slide down the respective slopes of the convex superior articular cartilages of the axis (*Fig. 26.15*). The atlas, accordingly, screws down on the axis as it rotates [48]. Any asymmetry between the articular cartilages results in coupling of ipsilateral or contralateral side-bending with the axial rotation, the side of coupling depending upon the direction of the asymmetry [75]. Here, as at the atlanto-occipital joint, normal asymmetry of the articular surfaces has been documented [81]. At the limits of axial rotation, the lateral joints are almost subluxed. The alar ligaments are ideally located to act as the principal structures to restrain axial rotation, with the lateral atlantoaxial joint capsules playing a secondary role [20,30]. Limitation of axial rotation is essential, as the spinal cord and vertebral arteries cross this joint [20]. The reported normal range of axial rotation to one side in living subjects is between 39 and 49° (*Table 26.5*).

The shape of the odontoid process allows the anterior arch of the atlas to slide upward and slightly backward, thereby

TABLE 26.4: Range of Motion for Lateral Flexion and Axial Rotation at the Atlanto-Occipital Joint

Source	Subjects	Total Lateral Flexion	Axial Rotation
Panjabi et al. [73]	Cadaver	3.9 ± 1.6	7
Penning [75]	Cadaver		0
Penning & Wilmink [77]	In vivo		1 (–2–5)
Werne [95]	Cadaver		0
Worth & Selvik [97]	Cadaver	11.0	

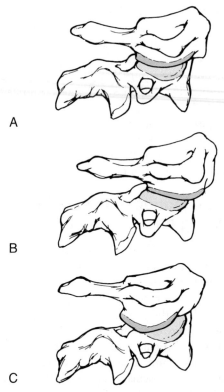

Figure 26.15: In axial rotation of the atlantoaxial joint from the neutral position **(A)**, the inferior articular facet of the atlas slides down the anterior slope of the convex superior facet of the axis during contralateral rotation **(B)** or down the posterior slope of the convex superior facet of the axis during ipsilateral rotation **(C)**.

producing extension of the atlas on the axis [95]. Flexion takes place by a downward and forward glide, with an additional slight anterior translation of the anterior arch on the odontoid process. The total range of flexion–extension reported in vivo varies between 11 and 21° (*Table 26.5*). Panjabi et al. report 11.5° of flexion and 10.9° of extension in cadavers [73].

The reported ROM for side-bending at the atlantoaxial joint in cadavers ranges between 5° and 10° [22,75]. Side-bending does not result from pure lateral translation. As the superior articular facets of the axis slope down and laterally, lateral translation would produce impaction of the contralateral lateral mass of the atlas on the superior lateral mass of the axis (*Fig. 26.16*). Consequently, the inferior facet must ride down the superior facet while the contralateral inferior facet must ride up the contralateral superior facet, thereby imparting a lateral tilt to the atlas. The contralateral alar ligament offers primary resistance to this motion, but ultimately, the motion is resisted by impaction of the contralateral lateral mass onto the lateral aspect of the odontoid process [12,72].

SEGMENTAL CRANIOVERTEBRAL MOTION

The characteristic movements of the atlanto-occipital and atlantoaxial joints that have been described do not occur in isolation. Rather, these joints of the head, atlas, and axis normally function as a composite unit. As noted previously, the atlas acts essentially as a passive washer, structurally tied to the occipital condyles by joint geometry and soft tissues.

Consequently, when the head moves during axial rotation, the head and atlas move in concert on the axis. During flexion and extension of the head and neck, the atlas exhibits what is known as paradoxical motion. For example, during flexion, the atlas may flex or it may extend, and during extension of the neck, the atlas may also flex or it may extend [75,92]. This incongruity occurs because the convexities of the inferior facets of the atlas rest on the convexities of the superior facets of the axis (*Fig. 26.9*). The equilibrium of the resting position is thus susceptible to small variations in the position of compression forces passing through the lateral masses. If the compression load is exerted anterior to the fulcrum of the articular surfaces of the lateral atlantoaxial joint, the atlas tilts into flexion. If the compression load is exerted posterior to the fulcrum, the atlas tilts into extension [59].

TABLE 26.5: Average Motion at the Atlantoaxial Joint Complex

Source	Subjects	Axial Rotation One-Sided ROM	Axial Rotation Total ROM	Flexion–Extension
Brocher [15]	In vivo			18 (2–16)
Dvorak et al. [30]	Cadaver	32		
Dvorak et al. [28]	In vivo	43.3 ± (5.5)		
Fielding [32]	In vivo		90	15
Hohl & Baker [39]	Cadaver	30		
Kottke & Mundale [49]	In vivo			11
Lewit & Krausova [52]	In vivo			16
Lind et al. [53]	In vivo			13 ± 5
Markuske [54]	In vivo			21
Panjabi et al. [73]	Cadaver	38.9		
Penning & Wilmink [77]	In vivo	40.5 (29–46)		
Werne [95]	Cadaver		47 (22–58)	10

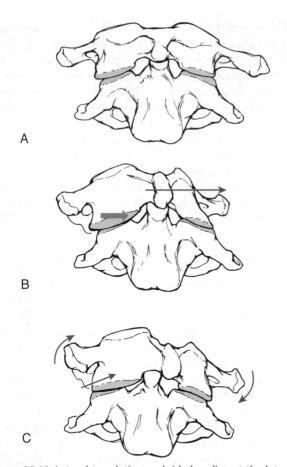

A

B

C

Figure 26.16: Lateral translation and side-bending at the lateral atlantoaxial joints. **A.** The superior articulating facets of the axis slope laterally and inferiorly. **B.** As the atlas translates laterally, its inferior facet impacts on the superior facet on the axis. **C.** As the atlas translates, one inferior facet slides up on the underlying superior facet as the other rides down, imparting a lateral tilt to the atlas.

Clinical Relevance

HEAD POSTURE AFFECTS CERVICAL RANGE OF MOTION: *Posture of the head and neck influences whether flexion or extension of the atlas occurs during cervical spine motion. If the chin is protruded as the neck flexes, the atlas flexes in accord with the other cervical vertebrae as the compression force on the atlas is displaced anteriorly. If the chin is tucked, the atlas extends when the other cervical vertebrae flex as the compression load moves posteriorly within the lateral atlantoaxial joint. Initial head posture may, therefore, influence craniovertebral movement patterns.*

During side-bending of the head to the left, the atlas rotates to the right while the axis rotates to the left [41,42]. This combination of movements occurs because side-bending exerts a downward load on the ipsilateral articular pillar. The compressive load of the head passes from the ipsilateral lateral mass of the atlas down to the C2/3 zygapophysial joint and

zygapophysial joints below. Due to the slope of the articular facets, the inferior process of C2 moves down and backward along the superior articular facet of C3. This backward motion causes the axis to rotate toward the direction of side-bending. However, to ensure that the face is directed forward during side-bending, the atlas undergoes contralateral axial rotation. If, however, the patient is not asked to look forward or the therapist does not maintain the forward head position, the patient's head naturally rotates to the same side as the side-bend of the neck because of the coupled motion in the lower cervical region.

Segmental Motion of the Lower Cervical Region

Because of the technical difficulties involved in studying segmental motion, studies of the lower cervical spine have concentrated on flexion–extension movements. The nature and range of segmental motion in the lower cervical spine are influenced by both the geometry of the zygapophysial joints and the morphology of the interbody joints. The orientation and height of the articular processes oblige coupling of certain movements. Pure anterior translation cannot occur because the inferior articular processes of the upper vertebra impact against the superior articular processes of the lower vertebra. Further, translation occurs if the upper vertebra tilts forward, drawing its inferior articular processes up the superior articular processes below. Flexion in the lower cervical spine, therefore, is always a combination of anterior translation and anterior rotation in the sagittal plane. The reverse occurs in extension, with coupling of posterior sagittal rotation and posterior translation (*Fig. 26.17*).

It is the height, not the slope, of the caudal adjacent superior articular processes that dictates the relative amounts of sagittal translation and sagittal rotation that occur at any level [66]. In the cervical spine, the superior articular processes become progressively taller from C3 down to C7. At more cranial levels, therefore, a greater amount of sagittal translation can be achieved with less sagittal rotation, because of the smaller height of the superior articular processes.

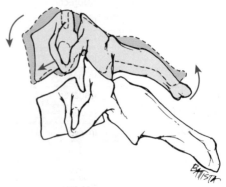

Figure 26.17: Flexion in the lower cervical spine combines anterior translation and sagittal plane rotation of the superior vertebra.

TABLE 26.6: Normal Ranges of Segmental Motion during Cervical Spine Flexion and Extension

Source	Number	C2–3	C3–4	C4–5	C5–6	C6–7
Aho et al. [2]	15	12 ± 5	15 ± 7	22 ± 4	28 ± 4	15 ± 4
Bakke [6]	15	13 (3–22)	16 (8–23)	17 (11–24)	20 (12–29)	18 (11–26)
Bhalla & Simmons [9]	20	9 ± 1	15 ± 2	23 ± 1	19 ± 1	18 ± 3
de Seze [23]	9	13	16	19	28	18
Dvorak et al. [26]	28	10 ± 3	15 ± 3	19 ± 4	20 ± 4	19 ± 4
Buetti-Bauml [16]	30	11 (5–18)	17 (13–23)	21 (16–28)	23 (18–28)	17 (13–15)
Kottke & Mundale [49]	78	11	16	18	21	18
Lind et al. [53]	70	10 ± 4	14 ± 6	16 ± 6	15 ± 8	11 ± 7
Zietler & Markuske [100]	48	16 (4–23)	23 (13–38)	26 (10–39)	25 (10–43)	22 (13–29)
Mestdagh [61]	33	11	12	18	20	16
Johnson et al. [46]	44	12	18	20	22	21
Dunsker et al. [25]	25	10 (7–16)	13 (8–18)	13 (10–16)	20 (10–30)	12 (6–15)

A wide range of measurements is reported for normal ranges of segmental motion during cervical spine flexion and extension (*Table 26.6*). Despite the variability in reported ROMs, the data consistently show progressively larger contributions to flexion and extension from the C2–C3 segment to the C5–C6 segment, followed by a decrease in motion occurring at C6–C7. However, those studies report mean values and standard deviations that highlight the huge variation seen in normal data [2,9,26,53].

Using CT scanning, Penning and Wilmink estimate the range of axial rotation for each segment of the lower cervical spine (*Table 26.7*) [77]. The only other study examining segmental motion in detail was undertaken by Mimura et al., who used trigonometric reconstructions of motion recorded via biplanar radiography (*Table 26.8*) [62]. These authors also report ranges of coupled motions, and it is interesting to note that axial rotation is coupled with side-bending of essentially the same magnitude [13].

Traditionally it has been taught that side-bending of a segment is coupled with axial rotation and axial rotation is coupled with side-bending, the basis for this coupling lying in the morphology of the articular processes. During axial rotation the contralateral inferior articular process impacts the superior articular process of the vertebra below, and axial rotation only continues if the inferior articular process glides up the superior facet, resulting in an ipsilateral side-bend of the

TABLE 26.7: Mean Values and Ranges of Segmental Axial Rotation

Segment	Mean (°)	Range (°)
C2/C3	3.0	0–10
C3/C4	6.5	3–10
C4/C5	6.8	1–12
C5/C6	6.9	2–12
C6/C7	2.1	2–10
C7/T1	2.1	–2–7

moving vertebra above. Therefore axial rotation is always coupled with ipsilateral side-bending (*Fig. 26.18*).

Reciprocally, during side-bending, as the ipsilateral inferior articular process moves down the slope of the superior articular process of the vertebra below, the inferior process is driven into the superior process. The inferior articular process must, therefore, move backward, and it is this backward movement that results in the vertebra rotating toward the side of the side-bending. Side-bending is, therefore, always coupled with ipsilateral axial rotation (*Fig. 26.19*).

Examination of the structure of the cervical joints reveals that the movements of side-bending and horizontal rotation

TABLE 26.8: Normal Range of Axial Rotation with Coupled Flexion–Extension and Side-Bending

Segment	Axial Rotation	Flexion/Extension	Side-Bending
C2/C3	7 ± 6	0 ± 3	–2 ± 8
C3/C4	6 ± 5	–3 ± 5	6 ± 7
C4/C5	4 ± 6	–2 ± 4	6 ± 7
C5/C6	5 ± 4	2 ± 3	4 ± 8
C6/C7	6 ± 3	3 ± 3	3 ± 7

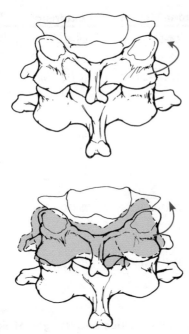

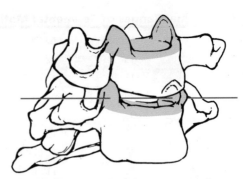

Figure 26.20: The interbody joint of the lower cervical region can be described as a saddle joint, with the convex inferior surface of the superior vertebra cradled in the concave superior surface of the inferior vertebra.

Figure 26.18: Coupling of motion during rotation in the lower cervical spine. Traditionally, axial rotation to the left is described as coupled with ipsilateral side-bending resulting from the right inferior facet gliding superiorly on the underlying superior facet.

are an artificial construct, and motion should be considered as occurring in the plane of the zygapophysial joints [13,76]. Since side-bending and rotation cannot occur independently, they can never be considered separate movements. In fact, each is only a partial manifestation of a single gliding motion

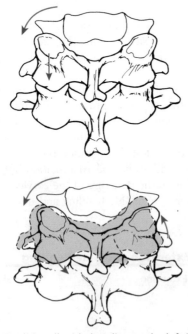

Figure 26.19: Traditionally side-bending to the left in the lower cervical spine is described as coupled with ipsilateral rotation resulting from the posterior glide of the left inferior facet on the underlying superior facet.

in the plane of the zygapophysial joint. When viewed in this plane, the interbody joint emerges as a saddle joint, and the functional implications of the specialized morphology of the cervical intervertebral disc become apparent (*Fig. 26.20*).

The substantial anterior anulus fibrosus and the gentle curving of the vertebral bodies in the sagittal plane make flexion and extension the predominant motion in the lower cervical spine. If the profile of the vertebral bodies is considered parallel to the plane of the facet joints, the posterior aspect of the superior vertebra is convex and the reciprocal posterior aspect of the inferior vertebra is concave. This structure suggests that the superior vertebral body can rock side to side within the concavity of the uncinate processes, pivoting about the anterior anulus fibrosus while the facets slide freely upon one another (*Fig. 26.21*) [13]. This second form of pure motion available is, therefore, rotation about an axis perpendicular to the facets. Since the facets are oriented at about 45° to the transverse plane of the vertebrae, the axis of rotation is 45° from the conventional axes of both horizontal rotation and side-bending [13,66]. Therefore, as

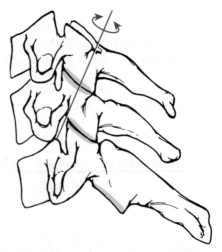

Figure 26.21: The motion of the saddle joint between adjacent lower cervical vertebrae occurs in the plane of the facet joints, about an axis perpendicular to the plane.

horizontal rotation and side-bending are always coupled, the rules commonly learned for coupled motion are unnecessary if motion is considered in the plane of the facet rather than in the coronal or transverse plane.

SUMMARY

The morphology of each of the cervical vertebrae reflects the function of the neck. The deep atlantal sockets of the atlas cradle the occipital condyles of the skull. The pivot joint of the median atlantoaxial joint and broad facets of the lateral atlantoaxial joints ensure stability of the atlas and head while allowing for a large range of axial rotation. The lower cervical vertebrae must continue the transmission of the axial load of the head and vertebrae above but also provide for mobility yet stability of the neck. This is achieved through a saddlelike joint between the vertebral bodies, and zygapophysial joints that permit predominately flexion and extension and rotation in the plane of the facet yet ensure stability. Research describing the functional morphology and kinematics of the cervical spine is sparse, yet the studies available indicate that the cervical spine cannot be considered similar to the lumbar spine. It has a complex structure reflecting its role in orienting the head in three-dimensional space. The following chapter examines the muscles that move the head and neck and contribute to the region's stability.

References

1. Agur AMR: Grant's Atlas of Anatomy. Baltimore: Williams & Wilkins, 1991.
2. Aho A, Vartianen O, Salo O: Segmentary antero-posterior mobility of the cervical spine. Ann Med Intern Fenn 1955; 44: 287–299.
3. Alaranta H, Hurri H, Heliovaara M, et al.: Flexibility of the spine: normative values of goniometric and tape measurements. Scand J Rehabil Med 1994; 26: 147–154.
4. American Medical Association. Guides to the Evaluation of Permanent Impairment. Chicago: American Medical Association; 1988.
5. Amevo B, Aprill C, Bogduk N: Abnormal instantaneous axes of rotation in patients with neck pain. Spine 1992; 17: 748–756.
6. Bakke SN: Rontgenologische Beobachtungen uber die Bewegengen der Wirbelsaule. Acta Radiol Suppl 1931; 13: 1–76.
7. Bateman JE: The Shoulder and Neck. London: WB Saunders, 1978.
8. Bennett JG, Bergmanis LE, Carpenter JK, Skowlund HV: Range of motion of the neck. J Am Phys Ther Assoc 1963; 43: 45–47.
9. Bhalla SK, Simmons EH: Normal ranges of intervertebral joint motion of the cervical spine. Can J Surg 1969; 12: 181–187.
10. Bland J, Boushey DR: Anatomy and physiology of the cervical spine. Semin Arthritis Rheum 1990; 20: 1–20.
11. Bogduk N: Clinical Anatomy of the Lumbar Spine and Sacrum. Edinburgh; Churchill Livingstone, 1987.
12. Bogduk N, Major GA, Carter J: Lateral subluxation of the atlas in rheumatoid arthritis: a case report and post-mortem study. Ann Rheum Dis 1984; 43: 341–346.
13. Bogduk N, Mercer SR: Biomechanics of the cervical spine. Part 1. Normal kinematics. Clin Biomech 2000; 15: 633–648.
14. Breathnach AS: Frazer's Anatomy of the Human Skeleton. London: J & A Churchill Ltd, 1965.
15. Brocher JEW: Die occipito-cervical-gegend. Eine diagnostiche pathogenetische studie. Stuttgart: Georg Thieme Verlag, 1955.
16. Buetti-Bauml C: Funcktionelle Rontgendiagnsotik der Halswirbelsaule. Stuttgart: Georg Thieme Verlag, 1954.
17. Castro WHM, Sautmann A, Schilgen M, Sautmann M. Noninvasive three-dimensional analysis of cervical spine motion in normal subjects in relation to age and sex. Spine 2000; 25: 443–449.
18. Chen J, Solinger AB, Poncet JF, Lantz CA: Meta-analysis of normative cervical motion. Spine 1999; 24: 1571–1578.
19. Christensen HW, Nilsson N: Natural variation of cervical range of motion: a one-way repeated-measures design. J Manip Physiol Ther 1998; 21: 383.
20. Crisco JJ, Oda T, Panjabi MM, et al.: Transections of the C1-C2 joint capsular ligaments in the cadaveric spine. Spine. 1991; 16: S474–S479.
21. Croft AC: Biomechanics. In: Foreman SM, Croft AC, eds. Whiplash Injuries. The Cervical Acceleration/Deceleration Syndrome. Baltimore; Williams & Wilkins, 1995; 1–92.
22. Dankmeijer J, Rethmeier BJ: The lateral movement in the atlanto-axial joints and its clinical significance. Acta Radiol 1943; 24: 55–66.
23. De Seze S: Etude radiologique de la dynamique cervicale dans la plan sagittale. Rev Rhum Mal Osteoartic 1951; 3: 111–116.
24. Dirheimer Y: The craniovertebral region in chronic inflammatory rheumatic diseases. Berlin: Springer-Verlag, 1977.
25. Dunsker SB, Coley DP, Mayfield FH: Kinematics of the cervical spine. Clin Neurosurg 1978; 25: 174–183.
26. Dvorak J, Antinnes J, Panjabi M, et al.: Age and gender related normal motion of the cervical spine. Spine 1992; 17: 393–398.
27. Dvorak J, Froehlich D, Penning L, et al.: Functional radiographic diagnosis of the cervical spine: flexion/extension. Spine 1988; 13: 748–755.
28. Dvorak J, Hayek F, Zehnder R: CT functional diagnostics of the rotatory instability of the upper cervical spine. Part 2. An evaluation on healthy adults and patients with suspected instability. Spine 1987; 12: 726–731.
29. Dvorak J, Panjabi MM: Functional anatomy of the alar ligaments. Spine. 1987; 12: 183–189.
30. Dvorak J, Panjabi MM, Gerber M, Wichmann W: CT functional diagnostics of the rotatory instability of the upper cervical spine. Part 1. An experimental study on cadavers. Spine 1987; 12: 197–205.
31. Dvorak J, Schneider E, Saldinger P, Rahn B: Biomechanics of the craniocervical region: the alar and transverse ligaments. J Orthop Res 1988; 6: 452–461.
32. Fielding JW: Cineroentgenography of the normal cervical spine. J Bone Joint Surg 1957; 39: 1280–1288.
33. Fielding JW, Burstein AH, Frankel VH: The nuchal ligament. Spine 1975; 1: 3–14.
34. Fielding JW, Cochran GVB, Lawsing JF, Hohl M: Tears of the transverse ligament of the atlas. J Bone Joint Surg 1974; 56A: 1683–1691.
35. Giles LG, Taylor JR: Human zygapophyseal joint capsule and synovial fold innervation. Br J Rheumatol 1987; 26: 93–98.
36. Glanville AD, Kreezer G: The maximum amplitude and velocity of joint movements in normal male human adults. Hum Biol 1937; 9: 197–211.

37. Gottlieb MS: Absence of symmetry in superior articular facets on the first cervical vertebra in humans: implications for diagnosis and treatment. J Manip Physiol Ther 1994; 17: 314–320.

38. Halliday D, Sullivan C, Hollinshead W, Bahn R: Torn cervical ligaments: necropsy examination of the normal cervical region of the spinal column. J Trauma 1964; 4: 219–232.

39. Hohl M, Baker HR: The atlanto-axial joint. J Bone Joint Surg 1964; 64A: 1739–1752.

40. Hollinshead WH: Anatomy for Surgeons. Vol 3. The Back and Limbs. London: Harper & Row, 1969.

41. Jirout J: Synkinetic contralateral tilting of atlas and head on lateral inclination. Part I. Manuelle Med 1985; 1: 116–120.

42. Jirout J: Synkinetic contralateral tilting of atlas and head on lateral inclination. Part II. Manuelle Med 1985; 1: 121–125.

43. Johnson G, Bogduk N, Nowitzke A, House D: Anatomy and actions of the trapezius. Clin Biomech 1994; 9: 44–50.

44. Johnson G, Spalding D, Nowitzke A, Bogduk N: Modelling the muscles of the scapula. Morphometric and coordinate data and functional implications. J Biomech 1996; 29: 1039–1051.

45. Johnson RM, Crelin ES, White AA, et al.: Some new observations of the functional anatomy of the lower cervical spine. Clin Orthop 1975; 111: 192–200.

46. Johnson RM, Hart DL, Simmons EH, et al.: Cervical orthoses. A study comparing their effectiveness in restricting cervical motion. J Bone Joint Surg 1977; 59A: 332–339.

47. Kaneoka K, Ono K, Inami S, Hayashi K: Motion analysis of cervical vertebrae during whiplash loading. Spine 1999; 24: 763–770.

48. Koebke J, Brade H: Morphological and functional studies on the lateral joints of the first and second cervical vertebrae in man. Anat Embryol 1982; 164: 265–275.

49. Kottke FJ, Mundale MO: Range of mobility of the cervical spine. Arch Phys Med Rehabil 1959; 40: 379–382.

50. Kuhlman KA: Cervical range of motion in the elderly. Arch Phys Med Rehabil 1959; 40: 379–383.

51. Lantz CA, Chen J, Buch D: Clinical validity and stability of active and passive cervical range of motion with regard to total and unilateral uniplanar motion. Spine 1999; 24: 1082–1089.

52. Lewit K, Krausova L: Messungen von vor-und ruckbeuge in den kopfgelenken. Fortschr Roentgenst. 1963; 99: 538–549.

53. Lind B, Sihlbom H, Nordwall A, Malchau H: Normal range of motion of the cervical spine. Arch Phys Med Rehabil 1989; 70: 692–695.

54. Markuske H: Untersuchungen zur Statik und Dynamik der kindlichen Halswirbelsaule: der Aussagewert seitlicher Rontgenaufnahmen. Die Wirbelsaule in Forschung und Praxis. Stuttgart: Hippokrates, 1971.

55. McClure P, Siegler S, Nobilini R: Three-dimensional flexibility characteristics of the human cervical spine in vivo. Spine 1998; 23: 216–223.

56. Med M: Articulations of the cervical vertebrae and their variability. Folia Morphol 1973; 21: 324–327.

57. Mercer SR, Bogduk N: Intraarticular inclusions of the cervical synovial joints. Br J Rheumatol 1993; 32: 705–710.

58. Mercer SR, Bogduk N: The ligaments and anulus fibrosus of human adult cervical intervertebral discs. Spine 1999; 24: 619–626.

59. Mercer SR Bogduk N: The joints of the cervical vertebral column. J Orthop Sports Phys Ther 2001; 31: 174–182.

60. Mercer SR, Jull GA: Morphology of the cervical intervertebral disc: implications for McKenzie's model of the disc derangement syndrome. Manual Ther 1996; 2: 76–81.

61. Mestdagh H: Morphological aspects and biomechanical properties of the vertebro-axial joint (C2-C3). Acta Morphol Neerl Scand 1976; 14: 19–30.

62. Mimura M, Moriya H, Watanabe T, et al.: Three-dimensional motion analysis of the cervical spine with special reference to the axial rotation. Spine 1989; 14: 1135–1139.

63. Moneta GB, Videman T, Kaivanto K, et al.: Reported pain during lumbar discography as a function of anular ruptures and disc degeneration. A re-analysis of 833 discograms. Spine 1994; 17: 1968–1974.

64. Moore KL, Dalley AF: Clinically Oriented Anatomy. 4th ed. London: Williams & Wilkins, 1999.

65. Netzer O, Payne VG: Effects of age and gender on functional rotation and lateral movements of the neck and back. Gerontology 1993; 39: 320–326.

66. Nowitze A, Westaway M, Bogduk N: Cervical zygapophysial joints: geometrical parameters and relationship to cervical kinematics. Clin Biomech 1994; 9: 342–347.

67. Oda T, Panjabi MM, Crisco JJ: Role of the tectorial membrane in the stability of the upper cervical spine. Clin Biomech 1992; 7: 201–207.

68. Oda J, Tanaka H, Tsuzuki N: Intervertebral disc changes associated with aging of human cervical vertebra. From the neonate to the eighties. Spine 1988; 13: 1205–1211.

69. Ordway NR, Seymour R, Donelson RG: Cervical sagittal range-of-motion analysis using three methods: cervical range-of-motion device, 3 space, radiography. Spine 1997; 22: 501–508.

70. Pal GP, Routal RV: A study of weight transmission through the cervical and upper thoracic regions of the vertebral column in man. J Anat 1986; 148: 245–261.

71. Pal GP, Routal RV, Saggu SK: The orientation of the articular facets of the zygapophyseal joints at the cervical and upper thoracic region. J Anat 2001; 198: 431–441.

72. Panjabi M, Dvorak J, Crisco J, et al.: Flexion, extension and lateral bending of the upper cervical spine in response to alar ligament transections. J Spinal Dis 1991; 4: 157–167.

73. Panjabi M, Dvorak J, Duranceau J, et al.: Three dimensional movement of the upper cervical spine. Spine 1988; 13: 726–730.

74. Panjabi MM, Oxland TR, Parks EH: Quantitative anatomy of cervical spine ligaments. Part 1. Upper cervical spine. J Spinal Dis 1991; 4: 270–276.

75. Penning L: Normal movements of the cervical spine. Am J Roentgenol 1978; 130: 317–326.

76. Penning L: Differences in anatomy, motion, development and aging of the upper and lower cervical disk segments. Clin Biomech 1988; 3: 37–47.

77. Penning L, Wilmink JT: Rotation of the cervical spine. A CT study in normal subjects. Spine 1987; 12: 732–738.

78. Porterfield JA, DeRosa C: Mechanical Neck Pain. Perspectives in Functional Anatomy. London: WB Saunders, 1992.

79. Ramsey RH: The anatomy of the ligamenta flava. Clin Orthop 1966; 44: 129–140.

80. Romanes GJ: Cunningham's Textbook of Anatomy. London: Oxford University Press, 1964.

81. Ross JK, Bereznick DE, McGill SM: Atlas-axis facet asymmetry. Spine 1999; 24: 1203–1209.

82. Rosse C, Gaddum-Rosse P: Hollinhead's Textbook of Anatomy. New York: Lippincott Raven, 1997.

83. Saldinger P, Dvorak J, Rahn BA, Perren SM: Histology of the alar and transverse ligaments. Spine 1990; 15: 257–261.

84. Schonstrom N, Twomey L, Taylor J: The lateral atlanto-axial joints and their synovial folds: an in vitro study of soft tissue injuries and fractures. J Trauma 1993; 35: 886–892.

85. Sharpe KP, Rao S, Ziogas A: Evaluation of the effectiveness of the Minerva cervicothoracic orthosis. Spine 1995; 20: 1475–1479.

86. Singh S: Variations of the superior articular facets of the atlas vertebrae. J Anat 1965; 99: 565–571.

87. Taylor JR. Regional variation in the development and position of the notochordal segments of the human nucleus pulposus. J Anat 1971; 110: 131–132.

88. Tondury G: The Behaviour of Discs during Life. In: Hirsch C, Zotterman Y, eds. Cervical Pain. Oxford: Pergamon Press, 1972; 59–66.

89. Tubbs RS, Grabb P, Spooner A, et al.: The apical ligament: anatomy and functional significance. J Neurosurg (Spine 2) 2000; 92: 197–200.

90. Tonnetti J, Peoc'h M, Merloz P, et al.: Elastic reinforcement and thickness of the joint capsules of the lower cervical spine. Surg Radiol Anat 1999; 21: 35–39.

91. Trott PH, Pearcy MJ, Ruston SA, et al.: Three-dimensional analysis of active cervical motion: the effect of age and gender. Clin Biomech 1996; 11: 201–206.

92. Van Mameren H, Drukker J, Sanches H, Beursgens J: Cervical spine motion in the sagittal plane (I) Range of motion of actually performed movements, an x-ray cinematographic study. Eur J Morphol 1990; 28: 47–68.

93. Van Roy P, Caboor D, de Boelpaep S, et al.: Left-right asymmetries and other common anatomical variants of the first cervical vertebra. Part 1: left–right asymmetries in C1 vertebrae. Manual Ther 1997; 2: 24–36.

94. Velaneau C: Vertebral structural peculiarities with a role in the cervical spine mechanics. Folia Morphol 1971; 14: 388–393.

95. Werne S: The possibilities of movement in the craniovertebral joints. Acta Orthop Scand 1959; 28: 165–173.

96. Williams PL, Bannister LH, Berry MM, et al.: Gray's Anatomy. The Anatomical Basis of Medicine and Surgery. 38th ed. Edinburgh: Churchill Livingstone, 1995.

97. Worth DR, Selvik G: Movements of the craniovertebral joints. In: Grieve G, ed. Modern Manual Therapy of the Vertebral Column, Edinburgh: Churchill Livingstone, 1994: 53–68.

98. Yoganandan N, Kumaresan S, Pintar FA. Biomechanics of the cervical spine. Part 2. Cervical spine soft tissue responses and biomechanical modelling. Clin Biomech 2001; 16: 1–27.

99. Youdas JW, Garrett TR, Suman VJ, et al.: Normal range of motion of the cervical spine: an initial goniometric study. Phys Ther 1992; 72: 770–780.

100. Zietler E, Markuske H: Rontegenologische Bewengungsanalyse der Halswirbelsaule bei gesunden Kinden. Forstschr Roentgestr 1962; 96: 87–93.

101. Zuckerman S: A New System of Anatomy. London: Oxford University Press, 1961.

Mechanics and Pathomechanics of the Cervical Musculature

PETER PIDCOE P.T., D.P.T., PH.D. AND THOMAS MAYHEW P.T., PH.D.

CHAPTER CONTENTS

The musculature of the human cervical region has developed in response to two major functional demands. With the development of bipedal gait and upright posture, the position of the skull has moved more directly over the cervical spine. Large posterior muscles that support the weight of the head in animals in the quadruped position have become much smaller in humans, because the skull is balanced on the atlas with a larger bony brain case and smaller facial skeleton. In the standing position, however, the center of gravity of the human skull does fall in front of the articular condyles of the occiput and, therefore, creates a flexion moment on the neck; the mass of the cervical posterior/extensor muscles continues to be larger than that of the anterior/flexor muscles to offset this tendency for the skull to fall forward. A study comparing the relative force-generating capability of the neck flexors and extensors found an extension–flexion ratio of 1.7 to 1.0 in both men and women [8].

Another major function of the cervical vertebrae and surrounding musculature, in addition to supporting the weight of the skull, is to position the special sense organs located in the skull optimally to respond to stimuli. The need to move the skull in response to auditory or visual stimuli to place the ears or eyes in a favorable position may be very rapid, requires precision, and is often mediated reflexively. Patients' chief complaints are often related to the pain associated with these rapid movements, or the inability to move the head and neck appropriately. The proximity of the small and large muscles located in the cervical region to the head and associated sense organs can lead to a number of debilitating conditions when there are movement problems.

There are many muscles located in the neck region, and it would seem logical to organize them according to movements produced at the head and/or neck. Many of these muscles, however, have several actions on both the head and neck and have very different actions when considered ipsilaterally or in combination with their counterparts on the contralateral side. Another problem related to categorizing muscle function in the cervical region is the depth at which many of the muscles lie and the vital structures located in the area. Because many of the deeper muscles are covered with three or four layers of muscle and fascia, surface electromyographic (EMG) evidence is lacking, and palpation is difficult. Use of fine wire electrodes is risky because of the number of important vessels and nerves located so close to these muscles. Anything more than general movement categorizations are therefore artificial. Commonly, however, the muscles can be categorized according to their bilateral function and region with accompanying descriptions of secondary actions. This is the categorization scheme used in this chapter.

The purposes of this chapter are to

- Present the structure and function of the muscles of the cervical spine
- Discuss the literature concerning the activity patterns of these muscles
- Discuss the contributions of these muscles to complaints of head and neck pain in individuals

EXTENSORS OF THE HEAD AND NECK

This group includes muscles that extend the head on the neck (atlanto-occipital joint) and muscles that extend the cervical spine. Kapandji provides a useful description of this region by dividing it into four planes [10]. The deep plane consists of the suboccipital and segmentally located transversospinal muscles. The semispinalis plane contains the semispinalis capitis and semispinalis cervicis. The plane of the splenius and levator scapulae includes the splenius capitis, splenius cervicis, levator scapulae, and longissimus capitis. The superficial plane is composed of the trapezius (Kapandji includes the posterior part of the sternocleidomastoid, but this muscle is discussed with the anterolateral group).

Deep Plane

SUBOCCIPITAL MUSCLES

The suboccipital muscles are deeply situated in the posterior cervical area below the occipital region of the head (*Fig. 27.1*). These muscles are a group of four deeply placed muscles spanning the distance from the axis (C2) to either the atlas (C1) or the skull. Consequently, based upon their attachments and direction of muscle fibers, their combined actions are to extend the head on the upper cervical spine while ipsilaterally they produce rotation and lateral flexion of the head [20]. These muscles include the rectus capitis posterior major, obliquus capitis inferior (inferior oblique), obliquus capitis superior (superior oblique), and rectus capitis posterior minor. The first three of the above participate in a significant anatomical landmark, the suboccipital triangle. Located within this triangle are two important structures: the vertebral artery and the suboccipital nerve (dorsal ramus of C1).

Actions

MUSCLE ACTION: RECTUS CAPITIS POSTERIOR MAJOR UNILATERAL ACTIVITY

Action	Evidence
Ipsilateral rotation	Supporting
Lateral bending	Supporting

MUSCLE ACTION: RECTUS CAPITIS POSTERIOR MAJOR BILATERAL ACTIVITY

Action	Evidence
Extension of the head on the atlas	Supporting

MUSCLE ACTION: RECTUS CAPITIS POSTERIOR MINOR UNILATERAL ACTIVITY

Action	Evidence
Ipsilateral rotation	Supporting

MUSCLE ACTION: RECTUS CAPITIS POSTERIOR MINOR BILATERAL ACTIVITY

Action	Evidence
Extension of the head on the atlas	Supporting

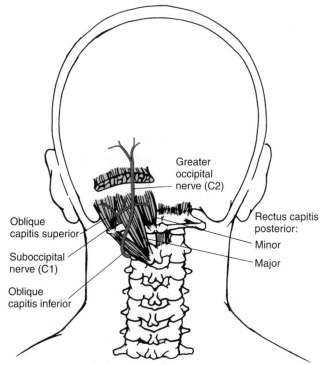

Figure 27.1: Suboccipital muscles include the rectus capitis posterior major and minor and the obliquus capitis superior and inferior.

MUSCLE ACTION: SUPERIOR OBLIQUE UNILATERAL ACTIVITY

Action	Evidence
Ipsilateral rotation	Supporting

MUSCLE ACTION: SUPERIOR OBLIQUE BILATERAL ACTIVITY

Action	Evidence
Extension of the head on the atlas	Supporting

MUSCLE ACTION: INFERIOR OBLIQUE UNILATERAL ACTIVITY

Action	Evidence
Ipsilateral rotation	Supporting

Two of the four suboccipital muscles, the rectus capitis posterior minor (*Muscle Attachment Box 27.1*) and the superior oblique (*Muscle Attachment Box 27.2*), only extend from the atlas to the skull, and their line of action produces atlanto-occipital extension or lateral flexion, respectively. The rectus capitis posterior major (*Muscle Attachment Box 27.3*) extends from the spinous process of the axis to the occiput, and the inferior oblique (*Muscle Attachment Box 27.4*) from the spine of the axis to the transverse process of the atlas. The transverse process of the atlas and the spine of the axis are prominent and, therefore, the moment arms for these two muscles are good for the production of atlanto-occipital extension (rectus capitis posterior major) and rotation of the atlas on the axis (inferior oblique).

The size of these muscles must be taken into consideration when evaluating their ability to produce force and contribute in movements of the head and neck. They are quite small compared with the large posterior muscles superficial to them. It has been suggested that the suboccipital muscles may be active in "fine-tuning" head and neck movements in response to the needs of the special sense organs, while the larger muscles are the prime movers and postural stabilizers over these joints. The finding that there is a large concentration of muscle spindles located in small muscles such as the suboccipital muscles supports this theory [2].

Clinical Relevance

CERVICAL HEADACHES: *All of these muscles are innervated by the dorsal ramus of C1 (suboccipital nerve), which exits within the suboccipital triangle, superior to the arch of the atlas. It is primarily a motor nerve but can have cutaneous branches [33] that may result in pain if stretched or trapped. More often, headaches of cervical origin have*

MUSCLE ATTACHMENT BOX 27.1

ATTACHMENTS AND INNERVATION OF THE RECTUS CAPITIS POSTERIOR MINOR

Proximal attachment: Posterior tubercle on the posterior arch of C1 (atlas)

Distal attachment: Occipital bone inferior to the inferior nuchal line

Innervation: Dorsal ramus of C1 (suboccipital nerve)

Palpation: Not palpable.

MUSCLE ATTACHMENT BOX 27.2

ATTACHMENTS AND INNERVATION OF THE SUPERIOR OBLIQUE

Proximal attachment: Superior surface of the transverse process of C1 (atlas)

Distal attachment: Smaller lateral impression between the superior and inferior nuchal lines on the posterior aspect of the occipital bone

Innervation: Dorsal ramus of C1 (suboccipital nerve)

Palpation: Not palpable.

MUSCLE ATTACHMENT BOX 27.3

ATTACHMENTS AND INNERVATION OF THE RECTUS CAPITIS POSTERIOR MAJOR

Proximal attachment: Posterior edge of the spinous process of C2 (axis)

Distal attachment: Occipital bone inferior to the inferior nuchal line

Innervation: Dorsal ramus of C1 (suboccipital nerve)

Palpation: Not palpable.

MUSCLE ATTACHMENT BOX 27.4

ATTACHMENTS AND INNERVATION OF THE INFERIOR OBLIQUE

Proximal attachment: Lateral surface of the spinous process of the C2 vertebra (axis)

Distal attachment: Inferior surface of the transverse process of the C1 vertebra (atlas)

Innervation: Dorsal ramus of C1 (suboccipital nerve)

Palpation: Not palpable.

been attributed to the greater occipital nerve (dorsal ramus of C2), which innervates much of the posterior aspect of the head up to the vertex. This nerve exits below the inferior oblique (external to the suboccipital triangle) and curves superiorly to pierce the semispinalis capitis (Fig. 27.1). It has been suggested that entrapment or stretching of the nerve as it passes between the lamina of the axis and the inferior oblique muscle may result in headaches or posterior neck pain [3].

The suboccipital muscles are deep and difficult to palpate. Several layers of large muscles and dense fascia are interposed between the skin and this muscle group. Empirically, then, it would be difficult to isolate pain resulting from muscular tightness or trigger points as coming from these muscles. Kendall describes pain associated with muscle tightness in this area as a result of postural problems [11]. She observes that patients with a marked forward head and kyphotic upper thoracic region have a compensatory hyperextension of the cervical spine and head (Fig. 27.2). This position may lead to shortening of the suboccipital muscles and "stretch weakness" of the anterior neck muscles. The mechanism of pain would be an abnormally large compression force on the articular facets due to the altered and sustained pull of the shortened muscles. However, the specific association between impairments of the suboccipital muscles and patient symptoms remains theoretical.

TRANSVERSOSPINAL MUSCLES

This group of muscles occupies the space between the transverse and spinous processes of the very short fibers (extending a few segments) and a relatively small moment arm for joint movement. Anatomy texts describe two layers of muscle located in this gutter area. The deeper of the two layers is

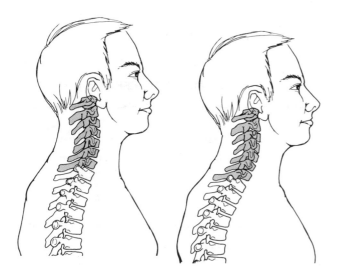

Figure 27.2: Forward head position shows that the hyperextension at the cervical spine could result in shortening of the neck extensor musculature.

MUSCLE ATTACHMENT BOX 27.5

ATTACHMENTS AND INNERVATION OF THE MULTIFIDUS

Proximal attachment: Spinous processes and laminae of C2–C7 vertebrae, spanning one to three vertebrae

Distal attachment: Transverse processes of upper thoracic vertebrae and articular processes of C7–T2

Innervation: Dorsal rami of cervical spinal nerves

Palpation: Not palpable.

made up of the rotatores muscle, but this layer is only well developed in the thoracic region and is not relevant to the cervical region [17,26]. The multifidus muscle makes up the more superficial layer (*Muscle Attachment Box 27.5*). Anatomy texts describe this muscle quite simply as fibers that arise from transverse processes and extend two to four segments to attach on the spinous processes above.

Actions

MUSCLE ACTION: MULTIFIDUS UNILATERAL ACTIVITY

Action	Evidence
Lateral flexion	Insufficient
Contralateral rotation	Insufficient

MUSCLE ACTION: MULTIFIDUS BILATERAL ACTIVITY

Action	Evidence
Extension of the spine	Insufficient

Further examination of this muscle group demonstrates a much more complicated picture of fiber arrangement and innervation pattern [13] (*Fig. 27.3*). Macintosh demonstrates, based on innervation, that the multifidus runs in a spinotransverse direction rather than a transversospinal orientation and has many important functions in spinal stabilization. The multifidus, however, is much more developed in the lumbar region, and studies describing its function usually are confined to effects on the lumbar spine. On the basis of its small size, deep location, and relatively poor moment arm, it can be hypothesized that it may act more as an organ of proprioception than as a prime mover in the cervical region.

Semispinalis Plane

SEMISPINALIS CAPITIS AND CERVICIS

The semispinalis capitis and cervicis constitute a large group of muscle fibers that originate from the transverse processes of the upper thoracic vertebrae. The capitis

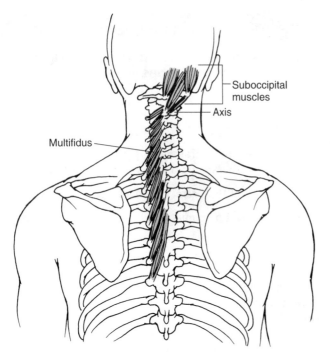

Figure 27.3: Fibers in the multifidus run obliquely superiorly and medially.

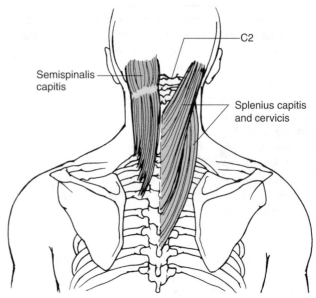

Figure 27.4: This figure demonstrates the excellent line of pull of the semispinalis capitis for neck extension. The convergence of semispinalis cervicis on the spinous process of C2 is also evident.

(*Muscle Attachment Box 27.6*) inserts centrally on the occipital bone between the superior and inferior nuchal lines (*Fig. 27.4*). The cervicis fibers converge on the spinous processes of C2 through C5 with the largest concentration on C2 (*Muscle Attachment Box 27.7*). This muscle is bulky and easily palpable just lateral to the ligamentum nuchae in the upper cervical region.

Actions

The arrangement of fibers in these muscles makes them important extensors of the head and neck, but EMG studies report conflicting evidence of action during functional activities [4,12,23,27].

MUSCLE ATTACHMENT BOX 27.6

ATTACHMENTS AND INNERVATION OF THE SEMISPINALIS CAPITIS

Proximal attachment: Transverse processes of C7 and T1–T6 vertebrae

Distal attachment: Medial half of the area between the superior and inferior nuchal lines on the occipital bone

Innervation: Dorsal rami of cervical spinal nerves

Palpation: Deep to the upper trapezius and levator scapulae and not palpable.

MUSCLE ACTION: SEMISPINALIS CAPITIS UNILATERAL ACTIVITY

Action	Evidence
Extension with slight lateral flexion	Supporting

MUSCLE ACTION: SEMISPINALIS CAPITIS BILATERAL ACTIVITY

Action	Evidence
Extension of the head	Supporting
Extends the cervical spine	Supporting
Accentuation of cervical lordosis	Supporting

MUSCLE ACTION: SEMISPINALIS CERVICIS UNILATERAL ACTIVITY

Action	Evidence
Extension of cervical spine	Supporting
Lateral flexion of lower cervical spine	Supporting

MUSCLE ACTION: SEMISPINALIS CERVICIS BILATERAL ACTIVITY

Action	Evidence
Extension of the lower cervical spine	Supporting

MUSCLE ATTACHMENT BOX 27.7

ATTACHMENTS AND INNERVATION OF THE SEMISPINALIS CERVICIS

Proximal attachment: Transverse processes of T1–T6

Distal attachment: Cervical spinous processes of C2–C5

Innervation: Dorsal rami of cervical spinal nerves

Palpation: Deep to the upper trapezius and levator scapulae and not palpable.

No known studies directly address weakness in these muscles, but it can be hypothesized that maintenance of upright head posture would be compromised by weakness of the semispinalis muscles. Because the semispinalis cervicis may stabilize the axis and potentiate the function of two of the suboccipital muscles, weakness in the semispinalis cervicis could affect the ability of these suboccipital muscles to fine-tune head movements in response to stimuli.

These two muscles are perhaps the prime movers for cervical spine and head extension. Their line of pull, from the upper thoracic area to the occiput, is well positioned to produce pure extension and maintenance of the cervical lordosis [18]. In the cadaver, the semispinalis cervicis is striking for its large convergence of fibers on the spinous process of C2. Indeed, this is a landmark for locating this structure (C2) and the associated suboccipital muscles arising from it. This convergence suggests that the semispinalis cervicis has an important stabilizing function on the axis that improves the ability of the rectus capitis posterior major and the inferior oblique to carry out their functions.

As straightforward as the actions of these two muscles appear to be from their anatomical positions, controversy exists in the literature regarding their activity during various activities. The location of the semispinalis group is superficial enough to allow investigators to record activity using fine wire EMG electrodes. Pauley reports that the semispinalis capitis and cervicis are continually active during upright posture to help support the head [21]. A later study verifies that the major function of this muscle group is extension of the head on the neck but notes that the semispinalis muscles are silent during quiet standing when the head is balanced over the cervical spine [27]. In contrast to the usual description in anatomy texts, EMG data suggest that the semispinalis group does not participate in rotation of the head or cervical spine [27].

Clinical Relevance

IMPAIRMENTS OF THE SEMISPINALIS CAPITIS MUSCLE: *The previously described course of the greater occipital nerve included the fact that it pierces the semispinalis capitis on its way to the vertex of the head (Fig. 27.1). Entrapment or tension on the nerve can occur within the semispinalis capitis. Travell describes a condition in which pain and burning occur in the distribution of the greater occipital nerve in response to spasms in the semispinalis capitis [28]. As this muscle group is often activated during normal upright activities, continued irritation might occur during ordinary activities of daily living.*

Splenius and Levator Scapulae Plane

SPLENIUS CAPITIS AND CERVICIS

The splenius muscles are a large flat group that covers the superior–medial aspect of the posterior neck (*Fig. 27.5*) (*Muscle Attachment Box 27.8*). This muscle group is considered a spinotransverse muscle group because it originates medially on spinous processes and passes laterally and superiorly to attach to cervical transverse processes and the skull. The lower fibers insert into the posterior tubercles of the upper two or three cervical vertebrae posterior to the attachment of the levator scapulae and are, therefore, named splenius cervicis. The remainder of the muscle fibers course superolaterally to the lateral half of the superior nuchal line and the mastoid process. This part is called the splenius capitis.

Actions

This muscle group exerts force over both the cervical spine and the atlanto-occipital joint (head on neck).

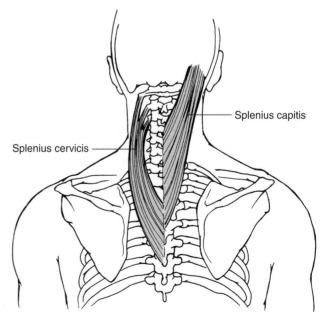

Figure 27.5: Splenius capitis and cervicis run in a spinotransverse direction to attach to the skull and transverse processes of cervical vertebrae, respectively.

MUSCLE ATTACHMENT BOX 27.8

ATTACHMENTS AND INNERVATION OF THE SPLENIUS CAPITIS AND CERVICIS

Proximal attachment: Inferior one half of mastoid process of the temporal bone, the ligamentum nuchae and the spinous processes of T1–T6 vertebrae

Distal attachment: Capitis—lateral aspect of the mastoid process and the lateral one third of the superior nuchal line of the occipital bone (deep to the sternocleidomastoid m.); cervicis—posterior tubercles of the transverse processes of C1–C4 vertebrae (posterior to the levator scapulae m.)

Innervation: Dorsal rami of cervical spinal nerves

Palpation: Deep to the upper trapezius and levator scapulae and not palpable.

MUSCLE ACTION: SPLENIUS CAPITIS AND CERVICIS UNILATERAL ACTIVITY

Action	Evidence
Extension of the head and cervical spine	Supporting
Lateral flexion of the head and cervical spine	Supporting
Ipsilateral rotation	Supporting

MUSCLE ACTION: SPLENIUS CAPITIS AND CERVICIS BILATERAL ACTIVITY

Action	Evidence
Extension of the head and cervical spine	Supporting
Accentuation of cervical lordosis	Supporting

According to Basmajian [1], the splenius capitis is extremely active in ipsilateral neck rotation and may be as important as the sternocleidomastoid in this function. The splenius group is intermediate in depth in this region and thus has an excellent moment arm for extension and rotation of the head and neck. EMG studies show that the splenius group is very active during extension of the head and cervical spine [1] but relatively silent during normal standing posture without head movement [27].

Clinical Relevance

IMPAIRMENTS OF THE SPLENIUS CERVICIS: *Little information is found concerning clinical syndromes and the splenius group. Kendall names it as one of the muscles*

affected by the posture of forward head with slumped, round upper back and hyperextension of the cervical spine (Fig. 27.2) [11]. In this condition, the splenius capitis is theoretically shortened, which contributes to an overall increase in compression on the posterior elements of the articular processes and vertebral bodies. This evidence is largely anecdotal, and further research is necessary to verify these relationships.

Calliet suggests that during car accidents in which the vehicle is stopped abruptly (front end collision), the neck is forcefully flexed, which quickly stretches posterior tissues [3]. Posterior extensor muscles are "overwhelmed" and are torn before the neuromuscular system can prevent it. Pain afterward is felt in the neck locally and referred in the distribution of the myotomes and dermatomes. The splenius group is likely involved in this type of injury.

LEVATOR SCAPULAE

Actions

Functionally this muscle is usually considered with the muscles that rotate or fix the scapula (see Chapter 9). Its proximal attachments, however, are from the transverse processes of the upper four cervical vertebrae and it can move the cervical spine when the scapula is *fixed* through synergistic muscle action (*Muscle Attachment Box 27.9*).

MUSCLE ATTACHMENT BOX 27.9

ATTACHMENTS AND INNERVATION OF THE LEVATOR SCAPULAE

Proximal attachment: Posterior tubercles of transverse processes of C1–C4 vertebrae

Distal attachment: Superior part of medial border of scapula

Innervation: Dorsal scapular nerve (C5), ventral rami of cervical nerves (C3 and C4)

Palpation: Deep to the upper trapezius, the levator scapulae can be palpated between the upper trapezius and sternocleidomastoid muscles. To promote levator scapulae muscle action with a minimum of upper trapezius activity, ask the patient to place the forearm in the small of the back to downwardly rotate the scapula and then shrug the shoulder.

MUSCLE ACTION: LEVATOR SCAPULAE UNILATERAL ACTIVITY

Action	Evidence
Extension of the cervical spine with scapula fixed	Supporting
Lateral flexion of the cervical spine with scapula fixed	Supporting
Ipsilateral rotation of the cervical spine with scapula fixed	Supporting
Scapular elevation, downward rotation and adduction with cervical spine fixed	Supporting

MUSCLE ACTION: LEVATOR SCAPULAE-BILATERAL ACTIVITY

Action	Evidence
Extension of the cervical spine with scapula fixed	Supporting
Accentuation of cervical lordosis	Supporting

From the superior angle of the scapula, this muscle passes medially and anteriorly to reach the transverse processes of the upper four cervical vertebrae (*Fig. 27.6*). The location of this relatively large neck muscle is significant both functionally and clinically. As the muscle passes superiorly and anteriorly, it twists from a frontal plane to a sagittal plane and separates into distinctive fleshy slips that attach to the individual transverse processes. Considered bilaterally, the levator scapulae appear to be posterior "guy wires" that stabilize the cervical spine with co-contraction from antagonistic anterior muscles (*Fig. 27.7*). This mechanism helps keep the head balanced over the cervical spine more efficiently and helps maintain the cervical lordosis.

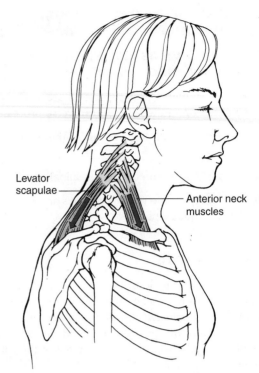

Figure 27.7: The "guy wire" arrangement of the levator scapulae and antagonistic anterior neck muscles. The levator scapulae and anterior cervical muscles provide opposing forces that help stabilize the cervical spine.

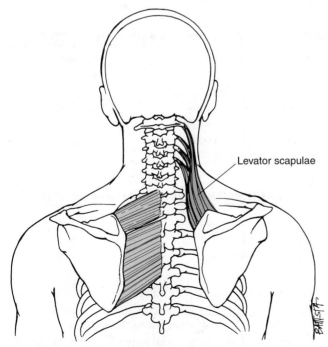

Figure 27.6: Levator scapulae runs superiorly and medially to attach to transverse processes of cervical vertebrae.

Clinical Relevance

NECK AND SHOULDER PAIN ASSOCIATED WITH THE LEVATOR SCAPULAE: *The levator scapulae muscles probably play an important role, as previously mentioned, in maintenance of optimal head and neck alignment. In this role the muscle may be continuously active to counterbalance the tendency for forward flexion. Jull characterizes the levator scapulae as one of the muscles in the neck–shoulder girdle region that becomes overactive with poor posture such as forward-head [9]. Over time, length-associated changes in this muscle would occur as a result of this position, however, in the short term, the overuse of the muscles could result in pain and discomfort. Patients with neck pain and postural problems often complain of pain in the region of the upper medial scapula, and point tenderness is frequently found at the superior–medial border of the scapula, site of attachment of the levator scapulae. Articular structures in this region may already be experiencing altered loads as a result of suboptimal postural changes. Pain and spasm of this muscle may further compromise these articular structures, as they will not receive the adequate support usually provided by the "guy wire" mechanism.*

MUSCLE ATTACHMENT BOX 27.10

ATTACHMENTS AND INNERVATION OF THE LONGISSIMUS CAPITIS

Proximal attachment: From superior thoracic transverse processes and the cervical transverse processes

Distal attachment: Mastoid process of the temporal bone

Innervation: Dorsal rami of cervical spinal nerves

Palpation: Deep to the upper trapezius and levator scapulae, it is not palpable.

LONGISSIMUS CAPITIS

This relatively small muscle is the most superior part of the long, intermediately placed longissimus erector spinae muscle (*Muscle Attachment Box 27.10*). It lies lateral to the semispinalis capitis and proceeds to insert on the mastoid process of the skull, deep to the attachment of the splenius capitis and sternocleidomastoid (*Fig. 27.8*).

Actions

MUSCLE ACTION: LONGISSIMUS CAPITIS UNILATERAL ACTIVITY

Action	Evidence
Extension of the head	Supporting
Lateral flexion of the head	Supporting
Ipsilateral rotation of the head and cervical spine	Supporting

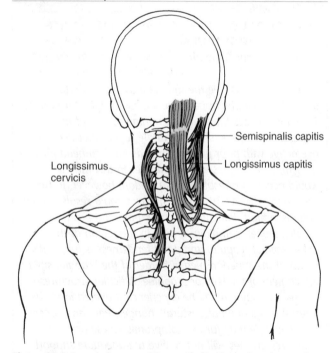

Figure 27.8: Longissimus capitis muscle lies lateral to the semispinalis capitis.

MUSCLE ACTION: LONGISSIMUS CAPITIS BILATERAL ACTIVITY

Action	Evidence
Extension of the head	Supporting

This muscle is far smaller than the semispinalis capitis, closer to the joints (reduced mechanical advantage), and more laterally placed, so its lateral flexion moment arm enhances the muscle's role in frontal plane stabilization as one of the "guy wires" arranged around the skull. The longissimus capitis appears to provide little stabilization in the sagittal plane, probably because of its lateral position [10].

Superficial Plane

TRAPEZIUS

This muscle is immediately deep to the superficial fascia and skin of the posterior neck region (*Fig. 27.9*). It is a very large flat muscle extending from the superior nuchal line of the skull to the spine of the twelfth thoracic vertebra (*Muscle Attachment Box 27.11*). Its upper fibers course inferolaterally to the clavicle and acromion, its middle fibers pass to the scapular spine, and its lower fibers pass to the tubercle on the base of the spine of the scapula. It is apparent from a posterior view of the trapezius that this muscle anchors the shoulder girdle to the axial skeleton. The primary function of the trapezius is movement of the shoulder girdle and associated movements of the upper extremity (Chapter 9); however, when the scapulae are fixed, it may act on the head and cervical spine. The trapezius is easily palpable and is responsible for the contour of the lateral neck area.

Actions

MUSCLE ACTION: TRAPEZIUS UNILATERAL ACTIVITY

Action	Evidence
Lateral flexion of the cervical spine with scapula fixed	Supporting
Contralateral rotation of the cervical spine with scapula fixed	Supporting
Scapular elevation, depression, upward rotation, and adduction	Supporting

MUSCLE ACTION: TRAPEZIUS BILATERAL ACTIVITY

Action	Evidence
Extension of the head	Supporting
Increase cervical lordosis	Supporting

Owing to the expanse of this muscle and the variety of fiber directions, the trapezius needs to be separated into three parts. The lower fibers depress the scapula. The middle fibers adduct the scapula. The upper fibers elevate the tip of the shoulder; acting with the lower fibers they rotate the scapula so that the glenoid fossa faces superiorly (to facilitate

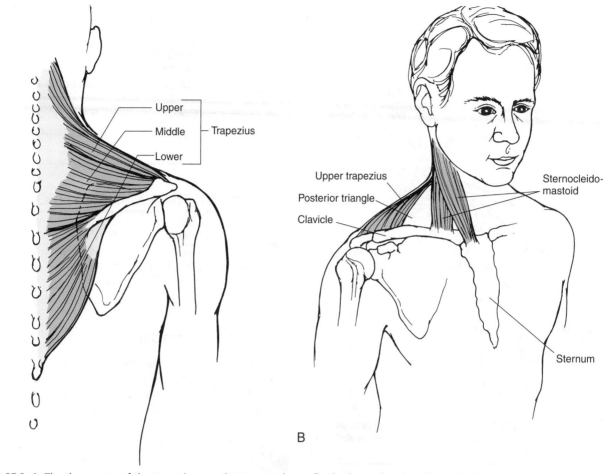

Figure 27.9: **A.** The three parts of the trapezius constitute a very large, flat back muscle primarily involved in upper extremity movements. **B.** The sternocleidomastoid forms the anterior border of the posterior triangle whose posterior border is the upper trapezius.

MUSCLE ATTACHMENT BOX 27.11

ATTACHMENTS AND INNERVATION OF THE TRAPEZIUS

Proximal attachment: Medial one third of superior nuchal line, external occipital protuberance, ligamentum nuchae, spinous processes of C7–T12

Distal attachment: Lateral one third of clavicle, acromion, and spine of scapula

Innervation: Spinal root of accessory nerve (CN XI), cervical nerves (C3 and C4)

Palpation: Palpate the entire trapezius by asking the patient to abduct the shoulder and adduct the scapula. To activate upper trapezius only, ask the patient to elevate the scapula (shrug the shoulder) and palpate between the spine of the scapula or acromion and the medial one third of the superior nuchal line.

glenohumeral motions). Acting on a fixed scapula, the upper fibers flex the neck laterally and rotate it to the contralateral side as a synergist to the ipsilateral sternocleidomastoid. Contracting bilaterally and acting on a fixed scapula, these fibers reportedly extend the head and increase the cervical lordosis.

Clinical Relevance

WEAKNESS AND STRAINS OF THE TRAPEZIUS MUSCLE: *The trapezius is commonly evaluated during a neurological examination because it is innervated by a cranial nerve. Paralysis of the trapezius results in an inferiorly sagging shoulder tip. In addition, the inferior angle of the scapula protrudes dorsally and creates a ridge in the skin of the back that disappears with flexion of the upper extremity and becomes more pronounced during glenohumeral abduction [26] (Fig. 27.10). This is in contrast to the "winging" observed with paralysis of the serratus anterior, which is*

(continued)

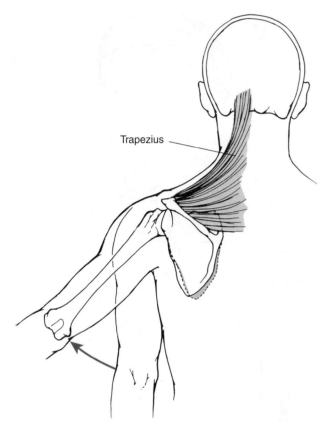

Trapezius

Figure 27.10: With a weak trapezius there is a dorsal protrusion of the inferior angle of the scapula while attempting to abduct the glenohumeral joint.

(Continued)

made worse during glenohumeral flexion and helps in the differential diagnosis between injuries to the respective nerves (Chapter 9).

Usually, the cardinal sign of trapezius paralysis (and possible injury to the accessory nerve) is drooping and inability to elevate the tip of the ipsilateral shoulder. For the superior fibers of the trapezius to elevate the shoulder, however, antagonistic muscles must stabilize the cervical spine and skull. Injury to these antagonistic muscles would result in an inability of the trapezius to elevate the scapula, appearing to be a problem with the trapezius or accessory nerve. Porterfield and DeRosa have identified these supporting muscles as the longus colli and longus capitis, which stabilize the head and neck and prevent extension moments [23]. These authors also describe the pathomechanics of shoulder limitations after acceleration injuries such as whiplash. With this type of injury, there is an uncontrolled extension movement that can injure the anterior muscles (longus colli and capitis). These muscles are no longer able to stabilize the head and neck and provide a stable base for the trapezius to act [23].

The mechanics of acceleration injuries such as whiplash are complex and beyond the scope of this chapter. The

above description of the injury indicates that there is an uncontrolled extension motion that can damage the anterior musculature. Usually, following this extension movement, there is rapid forward translation of the head and, subsequently, flexion movement that can damage the posterior elements including musculature such as the superior fibers of the trapezius. Calliet finds that following this type of injury the upper trapezius becomes tender and nodular [3].

FLEXORS OF THE HEAD AND NECK

This group includes muscles that are located antero-laterally around the neck and defy anything global organization. The muscles that are discussed in this region include the sternocleidomastoid, longus colli, longus capitis, scalenes, and the two anterior rectus muscles.

STERNOCLEIDOMASTOID

This large muscle passes from the medial clavicle and manubrium of the sternum to the mastoid process and lateral half of the superior nuchal line (*Muscle Attachment Box 27.12*). It is superficial, is easily palpated, and, because of its extensive course, has many functions (*Fig. 27.9*). Anatomically, it forms the anterior border of the posterior triangle and the lateral border of the anterior triangle. Asymmetries in these triangles may be observable in clinical conditions such as forward head posture, primarily because of the prominence of the sternocleidomastoid.

MUSCLE ATTACHMENT BOX 27.12

ATTACHMENTS AND INNERVATION OF THE STERNOCLEIDOMASTOID

Proximal attachment: Superior attachment—lateral surface of the mastoid process of the temporal bone and the lateral one half of the superior nuchal line of the occipital bone

Distal attachment: Sternal head—anterior surface of the manubrium of the sternum, lateral to the jugular notch; clavicular head—superior surface of the medial one third of the clavicle

Innervation: Spinal root of the accessory nerve (CN XI) and branches of the 2nd and 3rd cervical nerves (C2 and C3)

Palpation: With the subject seated, palpate along a line between the mastoid process and the sternoclavicular joint. Ask the subject to turn the his or her head to the opposite side you are palpating.

Actions

MUSCLE ACTION: STERNOCLEIDOMASTOID UNILATERAL ACTIVITY

Action	Evidence
Extension of the head	Supporting
Lateral flexion	Supporting
Contralateral rotation of the head and neck	Supporting

MUSCLE ACTION: STERNOCLEIDOMASTOID BILATERAL ACTIVITY

Action	Evidence
Extension of the head	Supporting
Flexion of the cervical spine	Supporting

EMG analysis of the superficially located sternocleidomastoid has been provided by two investigators [5,31]. They report that the sternocleidomastoid is quiet in relaxed sitting, breathing, deep expiration, and swallowing. As expected, there is marked activity during resisted neck flexion, side-bending, and rotation to the opposite side. Inspiration, coughing, and resisted backward extension elicit variable activity. This evidence clearly indicates the varied and frequent activity of this important muscle.

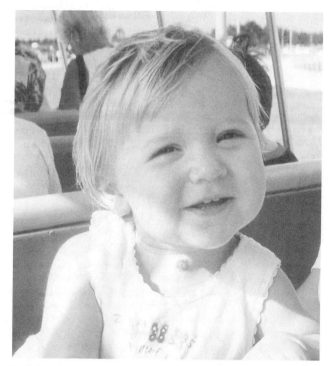

Figure 27.11: Torticollis is the deformity resulting from tightness or spasm of the sternocleidomastoid muscle. It consists of ipsilateral side-bending and contralateral rotation of the head.

Clinical Relevance

TORTICOLLIS: *Probably the most common clinical condition involving the sternocleidomastoid is **torticollis** (Fig. 27.11). There are two general forms of torticollis: congenital and spasmodic. The most common congenital form is the prenatal development of a fibrous tissue tumor in the sternocleidomastoid, turning the infant's head to one side in utero [25]. This may result in a breech delivery and subsequent tearing of sternocleidomastoid fibers or damage to the accessory nerve. Fibrosis and shortening of the fibers may lead to the torticollis.*

Spasmodic torticollis is a condition in which there is involuntary contraction of the sternocleidomastoid, resulting in repeated or sustained lateral flexion, rotation, and extension of the head and neck [6]. It usually occurs in individuals between the ages of 20 and 60 and may involve more than one muscle. It is usually accompanied by neck pain.

The previous discussion of the trapezius noted that acceleration injuries often damage anterior structures including muscles that are active in resisting extension moments [23]. In support of this, McNab finds that the sternocleidomastoid is the most commonly damaged muscle during an acceleration injury in which the impact comes from behind [16]. This follows from the knowledge that the sternocleidomastoid is a strong flexor of the cervical spine and may be stretched or injured during such an impact.

LONGUS CAPITIS AND LONGUS COLLI

These prevertebral muscles are located deep in the anterior neck and cover the cervical vertebrae (*Fig. 27.12*). The longus capitis extends superomedially from cervical transverse processes to the basilar part of the occipital bone (*Muscle Attachment Box 27.13*). The longus colli has a much more complicated arrangement (*Muscle Attachment Box 27.14*). Inferior fibers pass superolaterally, superior fibers pass superomedially, and intermediate fibers travel straight up from lower cervical levels to upper cervical segments. The shape of the muscle is triangular.

Actions

These muscles function to stabilize the head and neck as well as flex them.

MUSCLE ACTION: LONGUS CAPITIS UNILATERAL ACTIVITY

Action	Evidence
Ipsilateral rotation of the head	Insufficient

MUSCLE ACTION: LONGUS CAPITIS BILATERAL ACTIVITY

Action	Evidence
Flexion of the head	Insufficient

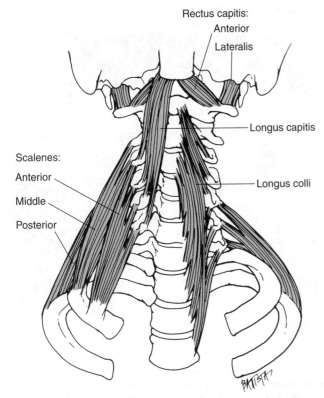

Rectus capitis:
Anterior
Lateralis

Longus capitis

Longus colli

Scalenes:
Anterior
Middle
Posterior

Figure 27.12: Deep flexor muscles include the longus colli and longus capitis, the rectus capitis anterior and lateralis, and the scalenes.

MUSCLE ATTACHMENT BOX 27.13

ATTACHMENTS AND INNERVATION OF THE LONGUS CAPITIS

Proximal attachment: Superior attachment—basilar part of occipital bone

Distal attachment: Inferior attachment—anterior tubercles of C3–C6 transverse processes

Innervation: Ventral rami of C1–C3

Palpation: Not palpable.

MUSCLE ATTACHMENT BOX 27.14

ATTACHMENTS AND INNERVATION OF THE LONGUS COLLI

Proximal attachment: Inferior attachment—bodies of C5–T3 vertebrae, transverse processes of C3–C5 vertebrae

Distal attachment: Lowest fibers insert on transverse processes of C3–C5, superior fibers insert on bodies of C1–C3 and anterior tubercle of the atlas

Innervation: Ventral rami of C2–C6

Palpation: Not palpable.

MUSCLE ACTION: LONGUS COLLI UNILATERAL ACTIVITY

Action	Evidence
Lateral flexion of the cervical spine	Supporting
Ipsilateral rotation of the cervical spine	Insufficient

MUSCLE ACTION: LONGUS COLLI BILATERAL ACTIVITY

Action	Evidence
Cervical flexion	Supporting

These two muscles are especially active in protection of anterior structures during forceful extension motions. EMG recordings of the longus colli show activity patterns similar to those of the sternocleidomastoid muscle: quiet in relaxed sitting and breathing, with marked activity during resisted flexion and side-bending. No known EMG studies investigate the longus capitis.

Clinical Relevance

WHIPLASH INJURIES TO THE LONGUS COLLI AND CAPITIS: *Injury to these muscles is discussed in the trapezius muscle section. Forceful hyperextension movements of the neck (auto accident) may stretch and tear the longus colli and capitis, thereby reducing the ability of these muscles to provide a stable base on which the trapezius muscle can act. Palpation in the region of the longus colli and capitis muscles and/or resisted neck flexion (such as raising the head in the supine position) would be painful. In the short term, the patient may not even be able to lift the head while lying down, although the sternocleidomastoid and scalene muscles may substitute and provide an adequate flexion moment to flex the neck [23].*

RECTUS CAPITIS LATERALIS AND RECTUS CAPITIS ANTERIOR

These two muscles arise from the anterior part of the atlas and insert on the base of the skull (*Muscle Attachment Boxes 27.15 and 27.16*). They are, therefore, very short, have a limited moment arm, and probably do not produce significant force (*Fig. 27.12*). Their lines of action suggest that they flex the head on the atlas when contracting bilaterally and perhaps laterally flex when acting alone. No EMG data are available, as these muscles are quite deep and in a dangerous location for fine wire EMG.

MUSCLE ACTION: RECTUS CAPITIS ANTERIOR AND LATERALIS UNILATERAL ACTIVITY

Action	Evidence
Lateral flexion of the cervical spine	Insufficient

MUSCLE ACTION: RECTUS CAPITIS ANTERIOR AND LATERALIS BILATERAL ACTIVITY

Action	Evidence
Flexion of the head	Insufficient

MUSCLE ATTACHMENT BOX 27.15

ATTACHMENTS AND INNERVATION OF THE RECTUS CAPITIS ANTERIOR

Proximal attachment: Base of the skull just anterior to the occipital condyle

Distal attachment: Anterior surface of the lateral mass of the atlas

Innervation: Branches from loop between C1 and C2 spinal nerves

Palpation: Not palpable.

MUSCLE ATTACHMENT BOX 27.16

ATTACHMENTS AND INNERVATION OF THE RECTUS CAPITIS LATERALIS

Proximal attachment: Jugular process of the occipital bone

Distal attachment: Transverse process of the atlas

Innervation: Branches from loop between C1 and C2 spinal nerves

Palpation: Not palpable.

MUSCLE ATTACHMENT BOX 27.17

ATTACHMENTS AND INNERVATION OF THE ANTERIOR SCALENE

Proximal attachment: Posterior tubercles of transverse processes of C3–C6

Distal attachment: Superior surface of first rib, anterior to groove for subclavian artery

Innervation: Ventral rami of C4–C6

Palpation: Palpated posterior to the inferior portion of the sternocleidomastoid muscle.

MUSCLE ATTACHMENT BOX 27.18

ATTACHMENTS AND INNERVATION OF THE MIDDLE SCALENE

Proximal attachment: Posterior tubercles of transverse processes of C4–C6 vertebrae

Distal attachment: Superior surface of first rib, posterior groove for subclavius artery

Innervation: Ventral rami of cervical spinal nerves

Palpation: Not palpable.

MUSCLE ATTACHMENT BOX 27.19

ATTACHMENTS AND INNERVATION OF THE POSTERIOR SCALENE

Proximal attachment: Posterior tubercles of transverse processes of C4–C6 vertebrae

Distal attachment: External border of second rib

Innervation: Ventral rami of C7 and C8

Palpation: Not palpable.

SCALENE MUSCLES

This is a group of three deeply placed muscles in the lateral region of the neck that arise from the transverse processes of cervical vertebrae (*Muscle Attachment Boxes 27.17, 27.18, and 27.19*). The anterior and middle scalenes attach to the first rib on either side of the neurovascular bundle leaving the root of the neck (*Fig. 27.13*). This bundle includes the subclavian artery and brachial plexus, which create a shallow groove on the first rib. The posterior scalene passes to the second rib, running just anterior to the levator scapulae.

Actions

This group generally functions together to laterally flex the neck, stabilize the neck with the actions of other cervical muscles, and elevate the ribs as accessory muscles of respiration.

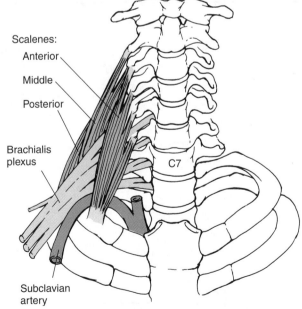

Figure 27.13: The scalenes are intimately related to the brachial plexus and subclavian artery, which pass between the anterior and middle scalenes.

MUSCLE ACTION: SCALENES UNILATERAL ACTIVITY

Action	Evidence
Lateral flexion of the cervical spine	Supporting
Contralateral rotation	Supporting
Elevation of ribs	Supporting

MUSCLE ACTION: SCALENES BILATERAL ACTIVITY

Action	Evidence
Flexion of cervical spine	Supporting

EMG recordings from the anterior scalene confirm its action in neck flexion and rotation [1]. The three muscles appear to be perfectly positioned to help stabilize the vertebral column in synergy with the larger muscles around the head and neck.

Clinical Relevance

SCALENUS ANTICUS SYNDROME: The narrow triangular opening between the anterior scalene, the middle scalene, and their attachments on the first rib transmits the subclavian artery and brachial plexus and is a potential problem site (Fig. 27.13). Compression of these structures in this space can lead to symptoms such as diminished sensation, weakness, "pins and needles" paresthesia, and pain. Patients with this anterior scalene syndrome (scalenus anticus syndrome) complain of numbness and tingling in the arm and fingers [3]. The exact cause of this condition is unknown; however, hypotheses include muscle spasm as a result of exercise, anxiety, tension, trauma, or tightness resulting from postural problems.

MUSCLE FUNCTION IN THE CERVICAL SPINE

Based on previous descriptions and as a review, the muscles of the their respective functions can be found in *Table 27.1*. With the actions of these muscles described and their clinical relevance discussed, their interaction can be explored from both a mechanical and a motor control sense.

As noted in Chapter 26, the cervical spine is composed of seven cervical vertebrae. These are designed to support the head in space while at the same time allowing movement of the head for interaction with the surrounding environment. Two major functions of the neck musculature are (a) to stabilize the head during external perturbations or body movements and (b) to provide orienting or voluntary head movements [22]. Stability implies support and is related to the stiffness of the

TABLE 27.1: Cervical Muscles Grouped According to Their Actions

Group	Muscle Name	Action			
		Extension	Flexion	Lateral Flexion	Rotation
Extensor	Rectus capitis posterior major	Bilateral		Ipsilateral	Ipsilateral
	Rectus capitis posterior minor	Bilateral			Ipsilateral
	Superior oblique	Bilateral			Ipsilateral
	Inferior oblique				Ipsilateral
	Semispinalis capitis	Bi-, unilateral		Ipsilateral	
	Semispinalis cervicis	Bi-, unilateral		Ipsilateral	
	Splenius capitis and cervicis	Bi-, unilateral		Ipsilateral	Ipsilateral
	Levator scapulae	Bi-, unilateral		Ipsilateral	Ipsilateral
	Longissimus capitis	Bi-, unilateral		Ipsilateral	Ipsilateral
	Trapezius	Bilateral		Ipsilateral	Contralateral
Flexor	Sternocleidomastoid		Bilateral	Ipsilateral	Contralateral
	Longus colli		Bilateral	Ipsilateral	Ipsilateral
	Longus capitis		Bilateral	Ipsilateral	Ipsilateral
	Rectus capitis lateralis		Bilateral	Ipsilateral	
	Rectus capitis anterior		Bilateral	Ipsilateral	
	Scalene muscles		Bilateral	Ipsilateral	Contralateral

supporting structure. In the vertebral column, muscular and ligamentous connections provide this stiffness. Cervical mobility is provided, in part, by the discs that separate each vertebral component. Facets that articulate with the facets of adjacent vertebrae guide this movement. Facet orientation promotes motion in certain directions while limiting motion in others. The cervical vertebrae also act to protect neural and vascular structures associated with the region and serve as outriggers for the attachment of muscles and ligaments.

Motion of the cervical spine is described in detail in Chapter 26. A typical cervical motion segment (two adjacent vertebrae and the intervening disc) has six degrees of freedom (DOF), translations in each plane and rotations in each axis (*Fig. 27.14*). These motions are often coupled such that motions around one axis are consistently associated with motions around another axis. The coupling relationships depend on the spinal posture, orientation of the articulating facets, thickness of the intervertebral disc, and extensibility of the muscles surrounding the joint.

In normal posture, the cervical vertebrae form a lordotic curve. This curve is supported and accentuated by the semispinalis capitis, splenius capitis and cervicis, trapezius, and levator scapulae muscles. In a cervical lordotic position, anterior and posterior stresses on the cervical vertebral bodies are nearly uniform and minimal compared with those in other postures [7]. With a kyphotic cervical posture, compression forces on the anterior margins of the vertebrae can be 6 to 10 times larger [7].

The cervical lordosis improves the ability of the spine to absorb axial loads. When a cervical spine is straightened and axially loaded, the time to failure and total displacement at failure are significantly lower than their lordotic counterparts [19]. This implies that a nonlordotic cervical spine has a decreased ability to absorb axial force. The presence of the cervical lordosis provides shock absorption for the head from forces that are transferred from the body and lower extremities. Similar curves in the thoracic and lumbar spine also contribute to shock absorption. Loss of the cervical lordosis can result in a decrease in shock absorption capability of the spine [32]. Cervical lordosis results from the shape of the discs and vertebrae in this region.

For the entire spine, intervertebral discs make up 20–30% of the column length. The discs increase in size from the cervical to lumbar region. The ratio of disc thickness to vertebral body thickness is greatest in the cervical and lumbar regions and least in the thoracic; the higher the ratio, the greater the mobility due to a greater range of motion (ROM) at the symphysis joints between the vertebral bodies.

Muscle Interactions and Activation Patterns

Redundancies in the musculature of the cervical spine allow multiple muscles to perform similar actions. In essence, there are more muscles than there are motions. As a result, there can be a variety of muscle activation patterns that produce or contribute to a single movement. A single muscle can potentially contribute to head movements in multiple directions [12]. For any given cervical muscle, the muscle moment arm, line of action, and muscle force production determine the resulting action of the head.

Activation of multiple muscles to produce a movement is called a **muscle synergy.** This method of control is not exclusive to the cervical region and occurs throughout the human body. An example of a synergy in the cervical region is the activation of the trapezius muscle and sternocleidomastoid

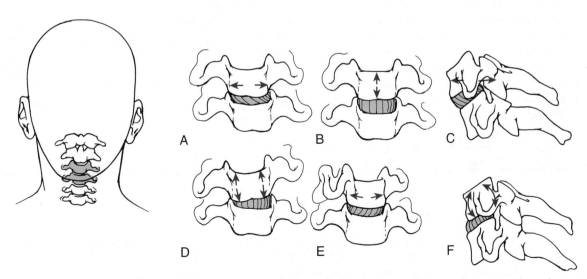

Figure 27.14: A typical cervical vertebral motion segment is able to translate along three axes and rotate about those three axes. Consequently, the motion segment has six degrees of freedom (DOF), three translations and three rotations: A. side-to-side translation in the frontal plane, B. superior–inferior translation, C. anterior–posterior translation in the sagittal plane, D. side-to-side rotation in the frontal plane, E. rotation in the transverse plane around a superior–inferior axis, F. anterior–posterior rotation in the sagittal plane.

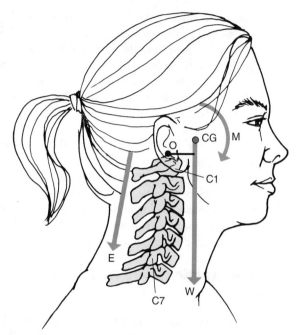

Figure 27.15: Sagittal plane view of the head and neck illustrates a flexion moment *(M)* around the point of rotation, or axis, *(O)* produced by the weight of the head *(W)*. The weight of the head is applied at the head's center of gravity *(CG)*. The extensor musculature must produce an extension moment *(E)* to balance the head.

the neck extensor muscles bilaterally. In this situation, one of three things can happen. (*a*) If the combination of the forces results in no movement, the muscle contraction is defined as **isometric.** The flexion moment created by gravity and the extension moment created by the muscle activation are equal. (*b*) If the combination of the forces results in acceleration of the head in a flexion direction, the flexion moment created by gravity is greater than the extension moment provided by the muscles, and the muscle contraction is an **eccentric,** or lengthening, contraction. (*c*) If the combination of forces results in acceleration of the head in an extension direction, then the extension moment provided by the muscles is greater than the flexion moment created by gravity. The muscle contraction is a **concentric,** or shortening, contraction.

By viewing the movement of the head as resulting from an imbalance in moments, the reader can visualize the contributions of various muscle groups and types of contractions. The moment produced by the weight of the head is a function of body position. As a result, muscle activity differs with body position. Some of these differences are highlighted in *Table 27.2.* The descriptions of active muscles are, for the most part, kept in an extensor/flexor format. The reader can refer to *Table 27.1* for the specific muscles in each of these groups.

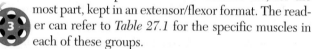

Effects of Posture on Cervical Muscles

Most neck muscles maintain at least 80% of their peak force-generating capacity throughout full cervical ROM (29). The analysis of neck musculature is complex, however, since length–tension relationships affect the force-generation capability of a given muscle. The length–tension relationship, combined with moment arm changes throughout the ROM, alters a muscle's moment or torque-generating capability (Chapter 4). On the basis of their muscle lengths, moment arms, and EMG activation patterns, the posterior neck muscles appear to be most efficient when the head is in a neutral position [14]. Muscle length, which is a function of head position, is probably the main influencing factor in this relationship, suggesting that maintaining a neutral head position is important in reducing the load on the cervical extensor muscles. Cervical muscles with the largest moment arms include the sternocleidomastoid muscles (flexion and lateral flexion),

muscle to create contralateral cervical rotation. These muscles produce opposing force vectors. The interaction of these force vectors produces rotation and is an example of an **anatomical force couple.** Force couples can theoretically produce pure rotational movements by canceling opposing translatory components. They also can produce motion in directions not available from a single muscle's line of action.

When a muscle is active, it produces a moment or torque around the joint on which it is acting. Muscle activation results during the initiation of voluntary activities and in response to direct and indirect forces imposed on the system. External forces produce moments as well. In a normal sitting posture, there is an external flexion moment on the cervical spine due to the weight of the head, which must be countered by an internal extension moment if the head is to remain upright (*Fig. 27.15*). The extension moment in this case is provided by

TABLE 27.2: Types of Contractions of Cervical Muscles: How Position Alters the Muscle Group and Type of Contraction Used during Specific Motions

Movement	Position	Active Muscle
Flexion	Sitting	Eccentric extensors bilaterally
	Supine	Concentric flexors bilaterally
Extension	Sitting	Concentric extensors bilaterally followed by eccentric flexors (once cervical extension reaches the point where gravity produces an extension moment)
	Prone	Concentric extensors bilaterally
Lateral flexion	Sitting	Eccentric contralateral flexors and extensors
	Side-lying	Concentric ipsilateral flexors and extensors
Rotation	Sitting	Ipsilateral splenius capitis, longissimus capitis, and levator scapula (if scapula fixed); contralateral sternocleidomastoid and upper trapezius

semispinalis capitis and splenius capitis muscles (extension), and trapezius muscles (rotation) [29]. These muscles are expected to be the most efficient at producing their respective movements, but the magnitude of the moment produced is not only a function of moment arm, but also a function of muscle force production and the muscle's physiological cross-sectional area. A positive correlation between muscle strength and physiological cross-sectional area is found for muscles in the cervical region just as in muscles throughout the appendicular skeleton [15].

Changes in posture alter the moment produced by the weight of the head by changing the location of the head's center of gravity with respect to the point of rotation in the cervical spine. This relationship influences the way people interact with their environment. The posture assumed while working on a computer, for instance, can affect the muscles used to perform that task. Data show that increased cervical flexion produces increased EMG activation of the trapezius muscles bilaterally in some subjects [30]. Backward leaning (reclining the trunk) decreases the activation of the trapezius muscles bilaterally in some subjects. Higher computer screen heights result in subjects assuming a more erect cervical spine posture and a more backward-leaning position. This example demonstrates that there are a variety of changes in muscle activity that may occur with relatively small modifications to a work environment. The muscle forces required to compensate for different head positions can be modeled biomechanically. *Fig. 27.16* demonstrates that a forward head position can result in a fourfold increase in the requirements of the extensor musculature.

The interaction of cervical musculature has not yet been fully explored, in part, because of the complex nature of the instrumentation required to perform the measurements. Cadaver studies and EMG studies combine to provide rough estimates or ranking of muscle moment production capabilities [5,13,15,21,27]. Biomechanical models provide suggested

ergonomic solutions for posturally related problems [7,14,18,29,33]. This section demonstrates that an understanding of the role of the cervical muscles in functional activities requires attention to postural attitudes, since head alignment affects the external moments on the cervical spine. The following chapter provides additional examples of the loads sustained by the cervical spine.

SUMMARY

This chapter examines the discrete actions of each muscle of the cervical spine as well as the combined actions of muscle groups. Because the muscles of the cervical spine are usually paired, the effects of unilateral and bilateral contractions are also discussed. The extensors of the head and neck are arranged in four planes from deep to superficial. Besides extending the head and neck, many of these muscles contribute to lateral flexion and to either ipsilateral or contralateral rotation of the head and neck. Similarly, the flexors provide side-bending and rotation. Evidence suggests that many muscles contract together as synergists to move the head and neck while stabilizing the region. Available studies of the effects of muscle impairments are reviewed, and clinical examples provided. Finally, this chapter demonstrates that gravity and posture play important roles in determining muscle activation in the cervical spine.

References

1. Basmajian JV, DeLucca C: Muscles Alive: Their Functions Revealed by Electromyography. 5th ed. Baltimore: Williams & Wilkins, 1985.
2. Buxton DF, Peck D: Neuromuscular spindles relative to joint movement complexities. Clin Anat 1989; 2: 211–220.
3. Calliet R: Neck and Arm Pain. 3rd ed. Philadelphia: FA Davis, 1991.
4. Cromwell RL, Aadland-Monahan TK, Nelson AT, et al.: Sagittal plane analysis of the head, neck, and trunk kinematics and electromyographic activity during locomotion. J Orthop Sports Phys Ther 2001; 31: 255–262.
5. deSousa T, Furlani J, Vitti M: Etude electromyographique du m. sternocleidomastoideus. Electromyogr Clin Neurophysiol 1973; 13: 93–106.
6. Fahn S, Bressman SB, Brin MF: Dystonia. In: Rowland LP, ed. Merritt's Textbook of Neurology. Baltimore: Williams & Wilkins, 1995.
7. Harrison DE, Harrison DD, Janik TJ, et al.: Comparison of axial and flexural stresses in lordosis and three buckled configurations of the cervical spine. Clin Biomech 2001; 16: 276–278.
8. Jordan A, Mehlsen J, Bulow PM, et al.: Maximal isometric strength of the cervical musculature in 100 healthy volunteers. Spine 1999; 24: 1343–1348.
9. Jull GA: Headaches of cervical origin. Phys Ther Cerv Thorac Spine 2000: 261–285.
10. Kapandji IA: Physiology of the Joints: Trunk and the Vertebral Column. New York: Churchill Livingstone, 1974.
11. Kendall HO, Kendall FP, Boynton DA: Posture and Pain. Huntington: Robert E. Krieger, 1952.

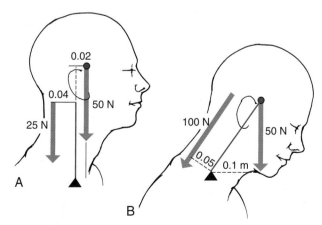

Figure 27.16: Biomechanical model of the force couples required to balance the head in two different head positions. A. Neutral head position requires 25 N of muscle force to balance the system. B. Forward head position requires 100 N of muscle force to balance the system.

12. Keshner EA, Campbell D, Katz RT, Peterson BW: Neck muscle activation patterns in humans during isometric head stabilization. Exp Brain Res 1989; 75: 335–344.

13. Macintosh JE, Valencia F, Bogduk N, Munro RR: The morphology of the lumbar multifidus muscles. Clin Biomech 1986; 1: 196–204.

14. Mayoux-Behamou MA, Revel M: Influence of head position on dorsal neck muscle efficiency. Electromyogr Clin Neurophysiol 1993; 33: 161–166.

15. Mayoux-Behamou MA, Wybier M, Revel M: Strength and cross-sectional area of the dorsal neck muscles. Ergonomics 1989; 32: 513–518.

16. McNab I: Acceleration injuries of the cervical spine. J Bone Joint Surg [Am] 1964; 46: 1797–1799.

17. Moore KL, Dalley AF: Clinically Oriented Anatomy. 4th ed. Baltimore: Lippincott Williams & Wilkins, 1999.

18. Nolan JP, Sherk HH: Biomechanical evaluation of the extensor musculature of the cervical spine. Spine 1988; 13: 9–11.

19. Oktenoglu T, Ozer AF, Ferrara LA, et al.: Effects of cervical spine posture on axial load bearing ability: a biomechanical study. J Neurosurg 2001; 94(1 suppl): 108–114.

20. Palastanga N, Field D, Soames R: Anatomy of Human Movement: Structure and Function. 3rd ed. Oxford: Butterworth-Heinemann, 1998.

21. Pauley JE: An electromyographic analysis of certain movements and exercises. Part I. Some deep muscles of the back. Anat Rec 1966; 155: 223–234.

22. Peterson BW, Keshner EA, Banovitz J: Comparison of neck muscle activation patterns during head stabilization and voluntary movements. Prog Brain Res 1989; 80: 363–371.

23. Porterfield JA, DeRosa C: Musculature of the Cervical Spine. In: Porterfield JA, DeRosa C, eds. Mechanical Neck Pain: Perspectives in Functional Anatomy. Philadelphia: WB Saunders, 1995; 47–81.

24. Queisser F, Bluthner R, Brauer D, Seidel H: The relationship between electromyogram amplitude and isometric extension torques of the neck muscles at different positions of the cervical spine. Eur J Appl Physiol Occup Physiol 1994; 68: 92–101.

25. Raffensperger JG: Congenital cysts and sinuses of the neck. In: Raffensperger JG, ed. Swenson's Pediatric Surgery. Norwalk, CT: Appleton & Lange, 1990.

26. Stern JT: Essentials of Gross Anatomy. 1st ed. Philadelphia: FA Davis, 1988.

27. Takebe K, Vitti M, Basmajian JV: The functions of semispinalis capitis and splenius capitis muscles: an electromyographic study. Anat Rec 1974; 179: 477–480.

28. Travell JG, Simmons DG: Myofascial Pain and Dysfunction. Baltimore: Williams & Wilkins, 1983.

29. Vasavada AN, Li S, Delp SL: Influence of muscle morphometry and moment arms on the moment-generating capacity of human neck muscles. Spine 1998; 23: 412–422.

30. Villanueva MB, Jonai H, Sotoyama M, et al.: Sitting posture and neck and shoulder muscle activities at different screen height settings of the visual display terminal. Ind Health 1997; 35: 330–336.

31. Vitti M, Fujiwara M, Iida M, Basmajian JV: The integrated roles of longus colli and sternocleidomastoid muscles: an electromyographic study. Anat Rec 1973; 177: 471–484.

32. White AA, Panjabi MM: Clinical Biomechanics of the Spine. 2nd ed. Baltimore: Lippincott Williams & Wilkins, 1990.

33. Williams P, Bannister L, Berry M, et al.: Gray's Anatomy: The Anatomical Basis of Medicine and Surgery, Br. ed. London: Churchill Livingstone, 1995.

CHAPTER

28

Analysis of the Forces on the Cervical Spine during Activity

CHAPTER CONTENTS

he cervical spine is a common site for complaints of pain and stiffness, and cervical spine pathology also often produces symptoms in the upper extremity. Although the cause of such complaints often is unclear, mechanical stresses on the spine are frequently implicated [23,24]. Similarly, an appreciation of the nature of the mechanical loads applied to the cervical spine in whiplash injuries is important for understanding the mechanisms of injury [28,29,47]. Impact loads on the cervical spine also can produce catastrophic results including tetraplegia [6]. Thus an appreciation of the loads sustained by the cervical spine may help health care providers optimize treatment and develop more effective prevention strategies.

The purpose of this chapter is to examine the ability of the cervical spine to withstand loads. Specifically, the objectives of this chapter are to

- Use two-dimensional examples to estimate the loads to which the cervical spine is subjected
- Examine the maximum static loads the cervical spine can sustain before it fails
- Discuss the mechanisms of injury in dynamic loading that occur in impact and whiplash injuries

TWO-DIMENSIONAL ANALYSIS OF THE LOADS ON THE CERVICAL SPINE

Normal upright posture is characterized by a lordotic curve in the cervical spine so that the atlanto-occipital (AO) junction lies anterior to the cervicothoracic junction (C7–T1) (*Fig. 28.1*). Because the center of mass of the head lies anterior to the AO joint, the head creates a flexion moment at both the AO and C7–T1 junctions [48]. Many readers know this intuitively, since they have inadvertently fallen asleep while sitting upright, only to have the head fall forward as the extensor muscles relax. *Examining the Forces Box 28.1* details the

two-dimensional analysis to determine the joint reaction force on the occiput during upright posture. The extension moment needed to keep the head upright is produced by the extensor muscles, represented as a single extension force, *E*. The free-body diagram reveals that the moment arm of the weight of the head is approximately one half of the moment arm of the extensor muscles, putting the muscles at a mechanical advantage [42]. The extensor muscle force needed to support the head is approximately 19 N (4.3 lb), or about one half the weight of the head. The joint reaction force on the occiput maintaining the head in an upright position is approximately 46 N (10.3 lb), or 1.2 times the weight of the head.

511

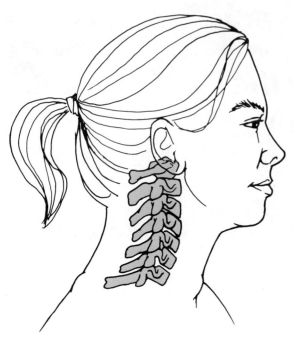

Figure 28.1: The cervical spine is normally aligned in a lordosis in which the middle cervical spine tends to extend and the lower cervical spine tends to flex.

The analysis in Examining the Forces Box 28.2 determines the extensor muscle force at the C7–T1 joint to maintain the head's upright position. The analysis reveals that the extensor muscle force needed is approximately 75 N (17 lb) and the joint reaction force on C7 is 112 N (25 lb). The greater loads in the extensor muscles and on the vertebra are consistent with the C7–T1 joint's position with respect to the center of mass of the head. In contrast to the AO junction, the moment arm of the weight of the head with respect to the point of rotation at C7–T1 is twice the moment arm of the extensor muscles at C7–T1, putting the muscles at a mechanical disadvantage. Therefore, the muscles must exert more force to maintain the position of the head and, consequently, the joint reaction force increases. The results presented in *Examining the Forces Boxes 28.1 and 28.2* are, at best, approximations of the real loads sustained by the structures of the cervical spine in upright posture. The analyses examine loads in only two dimensions and use simplifying assumptions such as activity in only one muscle and the location of the axis of rotation at a single point. Although the results of the calculations are only estimates, they provide a perspective on the loads sustained by the cervical spine and the means to examine the consequence of altered posture on these loads.

EXAMINING THE FORCES BOX 28.1

CALCULATION OF THE MUSCLE AND JOINT REACTION FORCES AT THE ATLANTO-OCCIPITAL JOINT

The following dimensions are based on a 534 N (120 lb) female [38]:

Weight of the head (7% of body weight)	37.4 N
Moment arm of the head weight	0.02 m
Moment arm of the extensor muscle force (E)	0.04 m

Solve for the extensor muscle force (E):

$\Sigma M = 0$

$(E \times 0.04 \text{ m}) - (37.4 \text{ N} \times 0.02 \text{ m}) = 0$

$E = 0.75 \text{ Nm}/0.04 \text{ m}$

E = 18.75 N, or approximately one half the weight of the head

Calculate the joint reaction forces (J) on the occiput. Assume that the extensor muscle force is applied in the *y* direction

ΣF_x: no forces in the *x* direction

ΣF_y: $J - E - W = 0$

where E is the extensor muscle force and is equal to 18.75 N, and W is the head weight, equal to 37.4 N

$J = 37.4 \text{ N} + 18.75 \text{ N}$

J = 46.15 N, or approximately 1.2 times the weight of the head

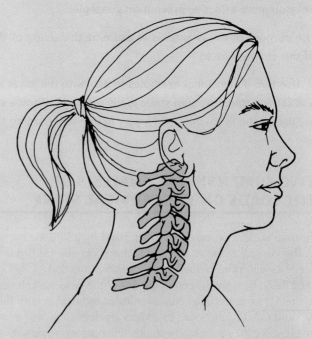

Free-body diagram of atlanto-occipital (AO) joint. The weight of the head *(W)* produces a flexion moment at the AO joint that must be balanced by the extension moment from the force of the extensor muscles *(E)*.

EXAMINING THE FORCES BOX 28.2

CALCULATION OF THE MUSCLE AND JOINT REACTION FORCES AT THE C7–T1 JOINT

The following dimensions are based on a 534 N (120 lb) female [38]:

Weight of the head (7% of body weight)	37.4 N
Moment arm of the head weight	0.04 m
Moment arm of the extensor muscle force (E)	0.02 m

Solve for the extensor muscle force (E):

$\Sigma M = 0$

$(E \times 0.02 \text{ m}) - (37.4 \text{ N} \times 0.04 \text{ m}) = 0$

$E = 1.5 \text{ N m}/0.02 \text{ m}$

$E = 75 \text{ N}$

Calculate the joint reaction forces (J) on the occiput. Assume that the extensor muscle force is applied in the y direction

ΣF_x: no forces in the x direction

ΣF_y: $J - E - W = 0$

where **E** is the extensor muscle force and is equal to 75 N, and W is the head weight equal to 37.4 N

$J = 112.4 \text{ N}$

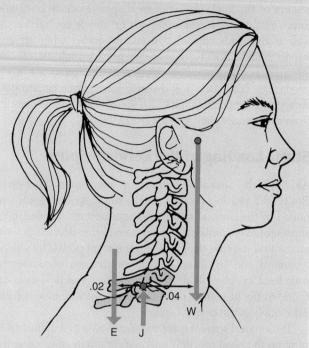

Free-body diagram of the cervicothoracic (C7–T1) joint. The weight of the head *(W)* produces a flexion moment at the C7–T1 joint that must be balanced by the extension moment from the force of the extensor muscles *(E)*.

Clinical Relevance

CERVICAL DISC DEGENERATION: *Cervical disc degeneration is common; one study reports finding degeneration in over 80% of the cervical discs examined in asymptomatic individuals over 60 years of age [18]. Disc degeneration is considerably more common in the lower cervical region than in the upper cervical region. Although several factors contribute to the disparity in incidence between the upper and lower cervical regions, one factor may be the magnitude of the loads to which each region is subjected on a daily basis [12,23,45]. Many activities require flexion of the head and neck and may lead to increased cervical spine loads. Redesigning work sites to decrease the amount of head and neck flexion may help prevent disc degeneration in the cervical spine. The loads on the lower cervical region also are likely to increase in abnormal head alignments such as in* **forward head posture,** *in which the head is positioned even farther anterior to the C7–T1 junction, increasing its flexion moment on the lower cervical spine (Fig. 28.2). Interventions to reduce forward head posture may be important in preventing disc degeneration, as well as in treating the symptoms associated with cervical disc degeneration [7,19].*

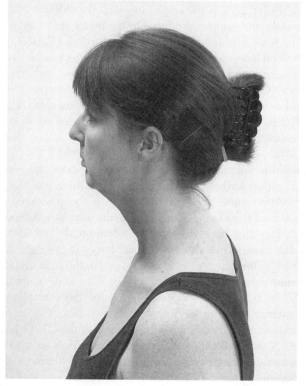

Figure 28.2: Forward head alignment produces an increased flexion moment at the C7–T1 junction because the moment arm of the weight of the head increases as the head translates anteriorly.

LOADS ON THE CERVICAL SPINE

Studies of the loads on the cervical spine examine the static forces attributable to external loads or muscle contraction, as well as the loads applied dynamically during whiplash and impact injuries. Both types of loading provide clinically relevant information. Degenerative changes in the spine are likely affected by both static and dynamic loads, while catastrophic damage to the cervical spine and spinal cord typically results from dynamically applied loads [10,12,48].

Static Loading of the Cervical Spine

Although the analyses described in Examining the Forces Boxes 28.1 and 28.2 provide rough estimates of the loads sustained by the cervical spine in upright posture, the examples represent oversimplifications of the real situation. As in most anatomical regions, the cervical spine is supported by several ligaments and by simultaneous contractions of numerous muscles. Considerably more sophisticated analytical tools are found in the literature, providing more realistic biomechanical models of the cervical spine.

The cervical spine is quite mobile, allowing an individual to position the head precisely and easily, thereby optimizing the function of the special senses of vision, hearing, and smell. Moving the head slightly from the neutral position requires minimal muscle force. The **neutral zone** of the cervical spine describes the arc of motion that is available around the neutral position without passive resistance to the motion (*Fig. 28.3*). The neutral zone is the region in which the stiffness of the cervical spine complex produced by the bones, discs, and soft tissue is minimal [20,32,46]. The neutral zone for flexion and extension is approximately 10°, for side-bending less than 10°, and approximately 35° for rotation [1,46]. The midcervical region (C2–C5) is stiffer and thus less mobile than the upper and lower cervical regions [8,37], and the cervical spine is less stiff than the thoracic and lumbar spines and uses less muscle force to produce motion [9,22,33].

While little muscle force is required to move the head through small arcs of motion in the upright position, as the head moves farther from the neutral zone, the muscle force needed to move the head increases as the resistance to movement from the joints and ligaments increases. A model including the trapezius, sternocleidomastoid, and rectus capitis muscles calculates very small forces in the right and left trapezius muscles (13 N or 3 lb) and in the right and left sternocleidomastoid muscles (34 N or 8 lb) to maintain the head in the upright position [38]. Like the examples in Examining the Forces Boxes 28.1 and 28.2, the model demonstrates a larger joint reaction force at the C7–T1 joint (130 N or 29 lb) than at the AO joint (70 N or 16 lb). Forward-bending from the upright position increases the muscle and joint reaction forces at both locations. At 30° of cervical flexion the model calculates joint reaction forces of approximately 75 N (17 lb) and 250 N (56 lb) at the AO and C7–T1 joints, respectively.

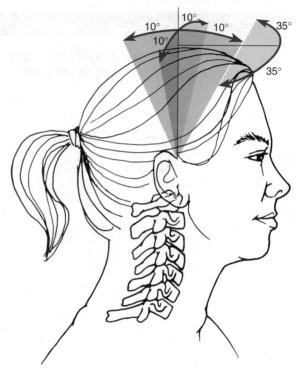

Figure 28.3: The neutral zone is the region through which the head and neck can move with little passive resistance from ligaments, joints, and muscles.

Biomechanical models simulating cervical rotations also report that unresisted axial rotation within the neutral zone generates minimal loading of the vertebrae and requires little muscular force. However, axial rotation to approximately 35° produces compressive forces on the cervical spine of approximately 100 N (22.5 lb) while developing muscle moments of about 2 Nm [1,38]. The muscle forces increase as passive resistance to rotation increases. The relatively large compressive loads result from the increased muscle forces and the co-contractions of muscles on all sides of the neck necessary to maintain an erect position of the head during the movement. Loads on the cervical spine during more-forceful contractions are also reported [23]. Loads on the C4–C5 junction during maximal isometric contraction are reported in a model using 14 pairs of muscles. This model yields average compressive loads of 1160 N (261 lb) during isometric extension and more than 750 N (169 lb) in side-bending and rotation.

Internal pressures within the cervical intervertebral disc also are useful indicators of the loads on the cervical spine. Average intradiscal pressures at C3–C4 and at C5–C6 measured in seven human cadaveric spines range from 0.16 MPa (megapascals) in axial rotation to 0.32 MPa in flexion/extension [35]. These measurements are based on bending moments of no more than 0.5 Nm with a compressive load of 10 N (2.25 lb, less than the weight of the head). Similar intradiscal pressures are reported based on a mathematical model of the cervical spine [8]. Simulated co-contractions of three pairs of muscles produce varied increases in intradiscal pressure, ranging from approximately 10 to 400% increases in pressure [35]. The largest increases are reported during flexion/extension and side-bending. The reported increases in pressure are consistent with the increased compressive loads reported during simulated co-contractions. The intradiscal pressures in the cervical spine can be compared to pressures of 4.0–6.0 MPa found at the hip joint during weight bearing [14] and 2.3–3.6 MPa at the elbow during vigorous elbow extension [21] and reveal substantial loading of the cervical spine, even though it supports only the weight of the head.

STRENGTH OF THE CERVICAL SPINE TO RESIST STATIC LOADS

Failure strength of a tissue is the maximum load the tissue can sustain and still fulfill its function (Chapter 2). Bones fail by fracturing, ligaments and muscles fail by tearing. Although the loads in the cervical spine reported so far are well below the failure strengths of the cervical spine, they may be important in the degenerative changes in cervical discs and in arthritic changes at the facet joints as the result of repetitive or prolonged loading. In the upright posture, most of the load is borne through the intervertebral disc, and flexion of the cervical spine increases the load on the discs [8,15]. Extension of the cervical spine reduces the load on the intervertebral discs while increasing the loads on the facet joints [8].

During small movements of the head from the neutral position only slight loads are generated in the cervical spine. Larger movements of the head produce larger loads on the vertebrae and discs. To put the loads sustained by the cervical spine on a regular basis in perspective, it is useful to compare these values with the reported loads at which the cervical spine fails. Most of the data describing the failure strength of the cervical spine are based on mechanical testing of cadaver specimens and thus do not adequately represent the physiological response of an intact cervical spine. Yet these data are useful in understanding how the loads sustained by the cervical spine during everyday activities compare with the theoretical failure points of the spine.

The failure strength of the cervical spine in static loading typically reflects the ability of the cervical spine to withstand bending in either flexion or extension, with and without the addition of a compressive load [22,34,37,47]. Failure of the cervical spine occurs by vertebral fracture, disc disruption, or tears of the ligaments or muscles so that the cervical spine is no longer able to support or move the head. Available studies are hard to compare because the modes of loading and the specific regions of the cervical spine tested vary. Failure of the cervical spine is reported when it is subjected to flexion moments of approximately 7 Nm in the midcervical region, but a 12-Nm flexion moment with an additional 2000-N compression load (450 lb) is reported before failure occurs in the lower cervical region [37]. Nightingale et al. report an average moment at failure of 24 Nm in the upper cervical region (occiput to C2) during flexion and 43 Nm for extension [26]. Another study also reports failure of the entire head-neck complex with approximately 2000 N when loading with the

cervical spine flexed [34]. Testing the cervical spine when it is held in combined axial rotation and flexion reveals increases in the stiffness of the spine, and the moment at failure is greater than when the cervical spine is flexed alone. However, the damage to the tissue is greater at failure when the spine fails in combined flexion and rotation [13,37,47]. Failure moments reported for the cervical spine are lower than those reported for the lumbar spine [22]. These data demonstrate that the loads sustained by the cervical spine during active motion are well below the static loading limits of the cervical spine. To put these moments in perspective, it is useful to recall that the elbow reportedly sustains moments of approximately 12 Nm during propulsion of a wheelchair [36].

Dynamic Loading of the Cervical Spine

Typically, failures of the cervical spine in healthy individuals result from high-velocity dynamic loading. Loading rate affects the mechanical properties of bones and connective tissues (Chapters 3 and 6). Like the studies examining static loads on the cervical spine, the studies that examine the response of the cervical spine to dynamic loads vary in the rates and modes of loading studied and in the part of the spine analyzed, as well as its position [16,25,28,34,44,47]. Despite these differences, data suggest that the stiffness of the cervical spine and the load that it can sustain before failure increase with increasing loading rates [34,44]. The increased stiffness and load to failure with increased loading rates demonstrate the **viscoelastic behavior** of the cervical spine. Studies of impact loading are useful in understanding the incidents that most often lead to spinal cord injuries. Acceleration, or whiplash, injuries to the cervical spine also occur, frequently as the result of automobile accidents. Although whiplash injuries rarely produce the catastrophic results that occur in impact injuries, they are extremely common and can be very costly, both physically and financially [28,47].

IMPACT LOADING OF THE CERVICAL SPINE

Most catastrophic injuries to the cervical spine result from high-velocity collisions between the head and relatively fixed objects, such as when a football player uses his head to tackle another player or when a swimmer's head hits a rock or pool bottom [2,5].

Several factors contribute to the severity of the injuries that result from impact loading of the head and neck. The force of impact is quite large because the head comes to an abrupt stop after traveling at a high speed. Recalling the relationship between force and acceleration ($\Sigma F = ma$) discussed in Chapter 1, it is clear that the deceleration from a high velocity to zero velocity requires large deceleration forces. Burstein provides an example of a football player moving at a velocity of 5 m per second whose average deceleration at the time of impact with another player is about 415 m/sec^2, compared with the acceleration of gravity, 9.8 m/sec^2 [5]. The average force of impact for the football player is approximately 2000 N (450 lb).

Clinical Relevance

AMERICAN FOOTBALL: *American professional football players may be exposed to compression forces on the cervical spine of more than 5,000 N (approximately 1,125 lb) when involved in helmet-to-helmet impacts in which the striking player lowers his head and hits the other player with the top of his helmet [43]. Such tackling is known as "spearing." While exceptional strength of the cervical muscles appears to help protect most professional players from catastrophic cervical damage, players with less strength are unlikely to sustain such impacts safely. These data emphasize the need for parents, coaches, and officials to enforce the no-spearing (tackling a player by hitting with a lowered head) rules that currently exist in football.*

An impact force on the head may produce axial loading and compressive loads on the cervical spine or a flexion or extension moment on the head and neck, depending on the location of the force with respect to the joints of the cervical spine (*Fig. 28.4*). Studies of the force of impact on the head when it collides with a more rigid structure while traveling at similar, or even slower, speeds than the football player reveal impacts ranging from 2000 to 11,000 N (450–2472 lb) and bending moments on the neck from 40 to 150 Nm [25]. Loads and moments of such magnitudes produce diffuse and catastrophic damage to the bones, ligaments, and discs of the cervical spine and ultimately to the spinal cord housed within it [25].

Another important factor in the morbidity of impact accidents is the continued movement of the body after the head has impacted the object. At the time of impact, the body is traveling at approximately the same speed as the head.

However, after the head comes to a stop, the rest of the body continues to move toward the head, so the entire mass of the body exerts a force on the cervical spine, producing additional deformation of the cervical spine [5,25] (Fig. 28.5). Studies show that if the head is capable of moving out of the way of the oncoming trunk, the cervical spine may survive the impact and avoid significant damage [25]. Studies of the mechanics of such collisions and the resultant injuries have lead to national standards for swimming pool designs and changes in athletic equipment, including football helmets. Clinicians who understand the mechanisms leading to the failure of the cervical spine are better able to participate in public education and equipment design to prevent such accidents [6].

ACCELERATION INJURIES TO THE CERVICAL SPINE

Although impact injuries of the cervical spine are the primary cause of catastrophic injuries of the cervical spine, the most common trauma to the cervical spine is whiplash injuries. Rarely catastrophic, these injuries nevertheless cause substantial cost in human suffering, lost wages, and medical expenditures [28,47]. As in impact injuries, major contributors to the cervical spine injuries in whiplash incidents are the accelerations imparted to the head and neck when the body is suddenly slowed, as well as the continued movement of the trunk toward the head and neck. In an automobile accident in which a car at rest is hit from behind, the car and its contents are accelerated forward. If the driver is secured in the seat by a lap and shoulder belt, the driver accelerates forward with the car [3]. However, the flexible cervical spine allows the head to lag behind the trunk, producing cervical hyperextension, stretching the anterior structures of the neck, and causing compression loading of the posterior structures [3,33] (*Fig. 28.6*). Almost simultaneously, the occupant's trunk rises toward the head, applying a compressive load to the lower cervical region [3]. Conversely, the car that impacts an

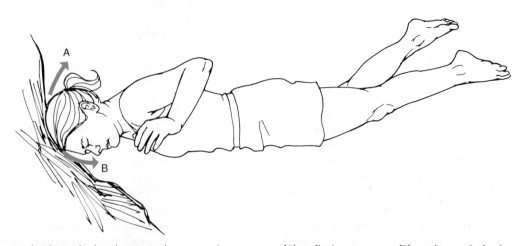

Figure 28.4: Impact loads on the head may produce extension moments **(A)** or flexion moments **(B)** on the cervical spine.

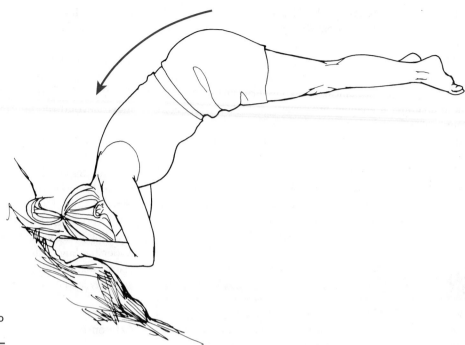

Figure 28.5: The trunk's effect on the cervical spine in impact injuries. After the head comes to a stop during an impact injury, the body continues to move toward the head, contributing to additional deformation of the spine.

immovable object from the front comes to an abrupt halt, but the relatively mobile head and neck accelerate forward. High-velocity impacts may cause a rebound movement of the head and neck before the head finally comes to rest, producing diffuse injury to the cervical spine [25].

Studies of rear impacts at relatively low velocities, 8 kph (approximately 5 mph), suggest that the head and neck complex are subjected to accelerations as high as 13 times the acceleration due to gravity and extension moments of approximately 30 Nm [16,29]. Investigations into the effects of front or rear impacts on the structures of the cervical spine present conflicting conclusions [17,27]. However, the weight of the evidence suggests that even impacts at low velocities can produce increased deformation in ligaments and muscles, increased pressures within the intervertebral discs, and increased loads on the facet joints [3,11,16]. Experiments

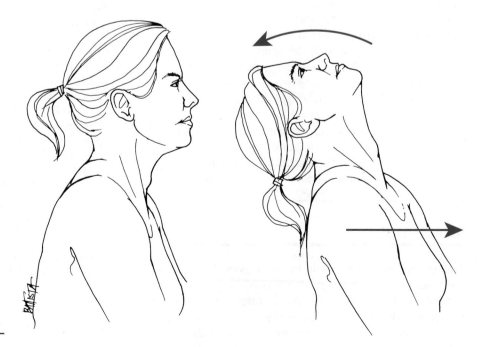

Figure 28.6: When a car is rear-ended, the vehicle and driver accelerate forward, but the head lags behind in hyperextension, putting strain on the anterior structures of the cervical spine.

using cadaver specimens yield evidence of strain (percentage change in length) beyond physiological tolerance within the intervertebral discs and excessive narrowing of the intervertebral foramena following impact [30,31]. Individuals who sustained whiplash injuries with their heads rotated also exhibit evidence of torn alar, apical, and transverse ligaments [13]. These anatomical changes are consistent with the frequent complaints of headaches, neck pain, and radicular pain (pain radiating into the arm) that many individuals report following motor vehicle accidents [4,31]. The combined use of shoulder and lap belt restraint systems and properly positioned head rests in automobiles decreases collisions between the head and rigid objects within the car and limits the excursion of the head and neck on the more stationary body, thereby reducing the soft tissue injuries sustained in whiplash injuries [16].

Clinical Relevance

MOTOR VEHICLE ACCIDENTS: *Health care providers frequently treat the pain and impairments resulting from motor vehicle accidents. The most common of these is whiplash injury. Because not all individuals involved in front or rear-impact collisions report neck pain, there is a tendency among some health professionals to dismiss the complaints. However, the biomechanical data suggest that if the conditions are right, a small "fender bender" can indeed produce a significant injury. Abnormal head posture appears to increase the risk of neck injury in such motor vehicle accidents [39]. Women demonstrate more cervical motion and higher accelerations of the head following low-velocity impacts, which may help to explain why women have an increased incidence of whiplash injuries [40,41].*

Another common cause of acceleration injuries to the cervical region is deployment of the front seat airbag. The injury occurs when the bag deploys with an explosive force into the face and head of the passenger, forcing the neck into hyperextension. Children and small adults are particularly susceptible because of the position of the airbag in relationship to the passenger's head. Unlike whiplash injuries, these injuries typically involve the upper cervical region despite the fact that the upper cervical region appears to be stronger in extension than the lower and middle regions of the cervical spine [26]. These data help reinforce the need to keep children riding in the back seat of the car until they attain the required height.

SUMMARY

This chapter provides simple two-dimensional analyses of the forces on the upper and lower cervical spine that are generated while holding the head upright. The analyses demonstrate the differences in mechanical advantage of the cervical extensor muscles between the upper and lower

regions. These differences lead to differences in the joint reaction forces sustained by the two regions. In upright postures, calculations determine loads of approximately 1.2 times the weight of the head at the AO joints and loads of approximately 3 times head weight at the C7–T1 juncture. Loads on the cervical spine increase as the head and neck move beyond the neutral zone, and loads of over 50 lb on the C7–T1 joint are reported during forward-bending. However, typical loads in the cervical region to move the head and neck are well below those that produce failure.

This chapter also discusses the mechanics of injury to the cervical region produced by dynamic loading. Injuries to the cervical spine typically involve large accelerations that produce very large forces and moments on the cervical spine, resulting in significant soft tissue and bony tissue trauma. An understanding of the mechanics of such injuries allows a clinician to contribute to the development of prevention strategies and may lead to more effective treatment regimens.

References

1. Bernhardt P, Wilke HJ, Jungkunz B, et al.: Multiple muscle force simulation in axial rotation of the cervical spine. Clin Biomech 1999; 14: 32–40.
2. Blanksby BA, Wearne FK, Elliott BC, Blivitch JD: Aetiology and occurrence of diving injuries. A review of diving safety. Sports Med. 1997; 23: 228–246.
3. Bogduk N, Yoganandan N: Biomechanics of the cervical spine part 3: minor injuries. Clin Biomech 2001; 16: 267–275.
4. Brault J, Wheeler JB, Siegmund GP, Brault EJ: Clinical response of human subjects to rear-end automobile collisions. Arch Phys Med Rehabil 1998; 79: 72–80.
5. Burstein AH, Wright TM: Fundamentals of Orthopaedic Biomechanics. Baltimore: Williams & Wilkins, 1994.
6. Carter DR, Frankel VH: Biomechanics of hyperextension injuries to the cervical spine in football. Am J Sports Med 1980; 8: 302–307.
7. Enwemeka C, Bonet IM, Ingle JA, et al.: Postural corrections in persons with neck pain II. Integrated electromyography of the upper trapezius in three simulated neck positions. J Orthop Sports Phy Ther 1986; 8: 240–242.
8. Goel VK, Clark CR, Gallaes K, King Lui Y: Moment-rotation relationships of the ligamentous occipito-atlanto-axial complex. J Biomech 1988; 21: 673–680.
9. Goel VK: Prediction of load sharing among spinal components of a C5-C6 motion segment using the finite element approach. Spine 1998; 23: 684–691.
10. Hendriksen IJ, Holewijn M: Degenerative changes of the spine of fighter pilots of the Royal Netherlands Air Force (RNLAF). Aviat Space Environ Med 1999; 70: 1057–1063.
11. Howard RP, Bowles AP, Guzman HM, Krenrich SW: Head, neck, and mandible dynamics generated by 'whiplash.' Accid Anal Prev 1998; 30: 525–534.
12. Joosab M, Torode M, Rao PV: Preliminary findings on the effect of load-carrying to the structural integrity of the cervical spine. Surg Radiol Anat 1994; 16: 393–398.
13. Kaale BR, Krakenes J, Albrektsen G, Wester K: Head position and impact direction in whiplash injuries: associations with MRI-verified lesions of ligaments and membranes in the upper cervical spine. J Neurotrauma 2005; 22: 1294–1302.

14. Krebs DE, Robbins CE, Lavine L, Mann RW: Hip biomechanics during gait. J Orthop Sports Phys Ther 1998; 28: 51–59.

15. Kumaresan S, Yoganandan N, Pintar FA, Maiman DJ: Finite element modeling of the cervical spine: role of intervertebral disc under axial and eccentric loads. Med Eng Phys 1999; 21: 689–700.

16. Luo ZP, Goldsmith W: Reaction of a human head/neck/torso system to shock. J Biomech 1991; 24: 499–510.

17. Maak TG, Tominaga Y, Panjabi MM, Ivancic PC: Alar, transverse, and apical ligament strain due to head-turned rear impact. Spine 2006; 31: 632–638.

18. Matsumoo M, Fujimura Y, Suzuki N, et al: MRI of cervical intervertebral discs in asymptomatic subjects. J Bone Joint Surg [Br] 1998; 80: 19–24.

19. Mayoux-Benhamou MA, Revel M: Influence of head position on dorsal muscle efficiency. Electromyogr Clin Neurophysiol 1993; 33: 161–166.

20. McClure P, Siegler S, Nobilini R: Three-dimensional flexibility characteristics of the human cervical spine in vivo. Spine 1998; 23: 216–223.

21. Merz B, Eckstein F, Hillebrand S, Putz R: Mechanical implications of humero-ulnar incongruity: finite element analysis and experiment. J Biomech 1997; 30: 713–721.

22. Moroney SP, Schultz AB, Miller AA, Andersson GR: Load-displacement properties of lower cervical spine motion segments. J Biomech 1988; 21: 769–779.

23. Moroney S, Schultz AB, Miller JA: Analysis and measurement of neck loads. J Orthop Res 1988; 6: 713–720.

24. Mundt DJ, Kelsey JL, Golden AL, et al.: An epidemiologic study of sports and weight lifting as possible risk factors for herniated lumbar and cervical discs. Am J Sports Med 1993; 21: 854–860.

25. Nightingale RW, McElhaney JH, Richardson WJ, Myers BS: Dynamic responses of the head and cervical spine to axial impact loading. J Biomech 1996; 29: 307–318.

26. Nightingale RW, Winkelstein BA, Knaub KE, et al.: Comparative strengths and structural properties of the upper and lower cervical spine in flexion and extension. J Biomech 2002; 35: 725–732.

27. Nuckley DJ, Van Nausdle JA, Raynak GC, et al: Examining the relationship between whiplash kinematics and a direct neurologic injury mechanism. Int J Vehicle Design 2003; 32: 68–83.

28. Panjabi MM, Cholewicki J, Nibu K, et al.: Simulation of whiplash trauma using whole cervical spine specimens. Spine 1998; 23: 17–24.

29. Panjabi MM, Cholewicki J, Nibu K, et al.: Capsular ligament stretches during in vitro whiplash simulations. J Spinal Disord 1998; 11: 227–232.

30. Panjabi MM, Ito S, Pearson AM, Ivancic PC: Injury mechanisms of the cervical intervertebral disc during simulated whiplash. Spine 2004; 29: 1217–1225.

31. Panjabi MM, Maak TG, Ivancic PC, Ito S: Dynamic intervertebral foramen narrowing during simulated rear impact. Spine 2006; 31: E128–E134.

32. Panjabi MM, Summers DJ, Pelker RR, et al.: Three-dimensional load-displacement curves due to forces on the cervical spine. J Orthop Res 1986; 4: 152–161.

33. Panjabi MM, White AA: Physical properties and functional biomechanics of the spine. In: White AA, Panjabi MM, eds. Clinical Biomechanics of the Spine. Philadelphia: JB Lippincott, 2001; 3–81.

34. Pintar FA, Yoganandan N, Voo L: Effect of age and loading rate on human cervical spine injury threshold. Spine 1998; 23: 1957–1962.

35. Pospiech J, Stolke D, Wilke HJ, Claes LE: Intradiscal pressure recordings in the cervical spine. Neurosurgery 1999; 44: 379–384 [discussion 384–385].

36. Robertson RN, Boninger ML, Cooper RA, Shimada SD: Pushrim forces and joint kinetics during wheelchair propulsion. Arch Phys Med Rehabil 1996; 77: 856–864.

37. Shea M, Edwards WT, White AA, Hayes WC: Variations of stiffness and strength along the human cervical spine. J Biomech 1991; 24: 95–107.

38. Snijders CJ, Hoek Van Dijke GA, Roosch ER: A biomechanical model for the analysis of the cervical spine in static postures. J Biomech 1991; 24: 783–792.

39. Stemper BD, Yoganandan N, Pintar FA: Effects of abnormal posture on capsular ligament elongations in a computational model subjected to whiplash loading. J Biomech 2005; 38: 1313–1323.

40. Stemper BD, Yoganandan N, Pintar FA: Gender- and region-dependent local facet joint kinematics in rear impact: implications in whiplash injury. Spine 2004; 29: 1764–1771.

41. Tierney RT, Sitler MR, Swanik CB, et al.: Gender differences in head-neck segment dynamic stabilization during head acceleration. Med Sci Sports Exerc 2005; 37: 272–279.

42. Vasavada AN, Li S, Delp SL: Influence of muscle morphometry and moment arms on the moment-generating capacity of human neck muscles. Spine 1998; 23: 412–422.

43. Viano DC, Pellman EJ: Concussion in professional football: biomechanics of the striking player—Part 8. Neurosurgery 2005; 56:266–280.

44. Voo LM, Pintar FA, Yoganandan N: Static and dynamic bending responses of the human cervical spine. J Biomech Eng 1998; 120: 693–696.

45. Wainner RS, Gill H: Diagnosis and nonoperative management of cervical radiculopathy. J Orthop Sports Phys Ther 2000; 30: 728–744.

46. White AA III, Panjabi MM: Kinematics of the Spine. In: Cooke DB, ed. Clinical Biomechanics of the Spine. Philadelphia: JB Lippincott, 1990; 85–126.

47. Winkelstein BA, Nightingale RW, Richardson WJ, Myers BS: The cervical facet capsule and its role in whiplash: a biomechanical investigation. Spine 2000; 25: 1238–1246.

48. Yoganandan N, Kumaresan S, Pintar FA: Biomechanics of the cervical spine part 2: cervical spine soft tissue responses and biomechanical modeling. Clin Biomech 2001; 16: 1–27.

Structure and Function of the Bones and Joints of the Thoracic Spine

CHAPTER CONTENTS

Thoracic vertebrae exhibit the articular attachments typical of much of the vertebral column, including the interbody and facet (zygapophyseal) joints. The thoracic spine differs from the cervical and lumbar spinal segments by virtue of its participation in the thoracic cage that encloses the thoracic viscera (*Fig. 29.1*). Along with intervertebral articulations, the thoracic vertebrae provide attachments for the ribs, and these additional articulations influence the structure of the individual thoracic vertebrae and the mobility and stability of the thoracic spine. The articulations between thoracic vertebrae and the rest of the thorax also affect the mechanics of respiration.

The three chapters on the thoracic spine review its structure and how its structure affects the mechanics and pathomechanics of the region. The first chapter presents the skeletal composition of the thorax and the mobility allowed by the articulations. The second chapter discusses the function of the muscles of the thoracic spine, and the third chapter discusses the forces sustained by the thoracic spine and how those forces contribute to common pathologies.

The current chapter discusses the structure of the thoracic vertebrae and ribs and how their architecture influences the mobility, stability, and function of the thoracic cage. The objectives of this chapter are to

- Describe the unique structural features of the thoracic vertebrae and the functionally relevant features of the ribs
- Discuss the joints of the thorax and their supporting structures
- Compare the mobility and stability of the thoracic, cervical, and lumbar spines
- Discuss the mobility of the costal articulations
- Review the basic mechanics of ventilation

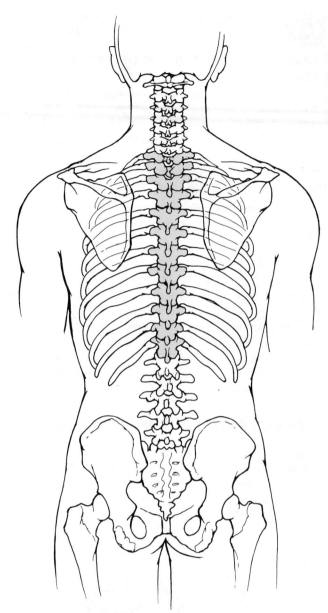

Figure 29.1: The thoracic spine is the transition between cervical and lumbar regions and is an integral part of the thoracic cage.

STRUCTURE OF THE THORACIC VERTEBRAE

The thoracic region of the spine, the longest segment of the vertebral column, consists of 12 separate vertebrae and acts as a transition between the cervical and lumbar spines [47]. The thoracic vertebrae have several features in common with each other and contain the typical elements of a vertebra, the body and the vertebral arch with its sites for muscular attachments, the transverse and spinous processes. However, some individual variations have lead to the identification of three distinct regions within the thoracic spine [34]. The **upper thoracic spine** consists of the first through fourth thoracic vertebrae

(T1–T4), which have many features similar to those of the lower cervical vertebrae. The middle region extends from the fourth through the ninth or tenth thoracic vertebrae and exhibits the classic characteristics of thoracic vertebrae. The **lower region** consists of the lowest two or three thoracic vertebrae, which have features similar to those of the upper lumbar vertebrae [35].

Bodies of Thoracic Vertebrae

The bodies of the vertebrae increase in size from the second cervical vertebra through the lumbar vertebrae. Consequently, the body of the twelfth thoracic vertebra is larger than the body of the first thoracic vertebra [37,54] (*Fig. 29.2*). This progressive increase in size is consistent with the increasing load that is borne by underlying vertebrae. The superior and

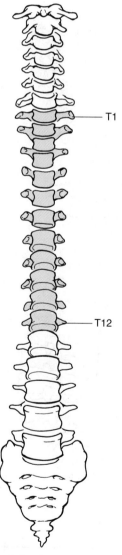

Figure 29.2: The bodies of the thoracic vertebrae increase in size from superior to inferior vertebrae and within each vertebra from superior to inferior surface.

inferior surfaces of the vertebral bodies, known as **endplates,** exhibit similar size progressions, the inferior surface of each vertebra being larger than its superior surface. The diameters of the bodies are slightly larger in an anterior–posterior direction than in a medial–lateral direction [34,37]. The ratio between the anterior–posterior and medial–lateral diameters varies only slightly throughout the thoracic spine.

The bodies of the thoracic vertebrae are wedge shaped, thicker posteriorly than anteriorly (*Fig. 29.3*). Wedging of the vertebral bodies is the primary cause for the normal kyphotic curve of the thoracic spine that is characterized by a posterior convexity [26,34]. The normal kyphosis of the thoracic spine and wedging of its vertebrae result in large loads applied to the thoracic vertebral bodies and may help explain why compression fractures of the vertebral bodies in individuals with osteoporosis are more common in the thoracic spine [2,49].

Clinical Relevance

COMPRESSION FRACTURES OF THE THORACIC VERTEBRAE: *Osteoporosis, common in postmenopausal women, decreases the load-bearing capacity of bone, predisposing an individual to **fragility fractures** and progressive kyphosis, the so-called **widow's hump** deformity. Approximately 25% of postmenopausal women and more than 50% of women 85 years or older are affected by vertebral fractures [20,27]. Fragility fractures are most commonly seen in the lower thoracic spine [27].*

The bodies of the thoracic vertebrae contain facets for articulation with the heads of the ribs. With the exception of the first, tenth, eleventh, and twelfth vertebral bodies, the bodies possess half, or demi, facets at their posterolateral aspects on both the superior and inferior borders [34,39,54] (*Fig. 29.4*). The half facet on the superior aspect of one vertebral body pairs with the inferior half facet of the body above to form the socket for the head of a rib. The first, tenth, eleventh, and twelfth vertebral bodies have full facets and provide the entire attachment for the head of a rib.

Vertebral Arch of a Thoracic Vertebra

The vertebral arch in the thoracic region, as in the rest of the vertebral column, is formed by the posteriorly projecting pedicles and medially projecting laminae (*Fig. 29.5*). As the laminae converge and join together, the vertebral arch is formed. In the thoracic region, the pedicles project less

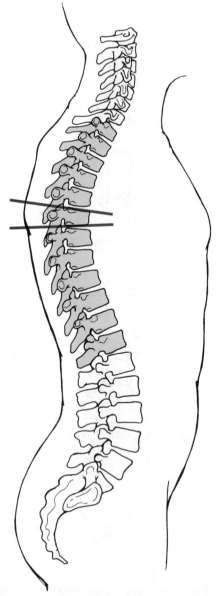

Figure 29.3: The wedge-shaped bodies of the thoracic vertebrae are the primary source of the normal thoracic kyphosis.

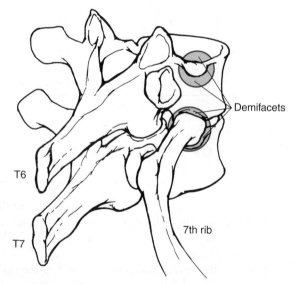

Figure 29.4: Demifacets on the thoracic vertebrae are located at the posterolateral aspect of the superior and inferior surfaces of the vertebral bodies and provide attachment for the heads of articulating ribs. The inferior vertebra attaches to the rib of the same number.

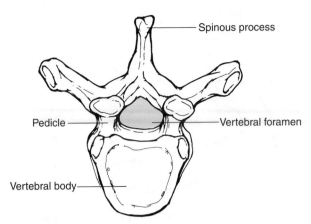

Figure 29.5: The spinal canal within the thoracic region is narrow because the pedicles of the vertebrae project posteriorly with little lateral angulation.

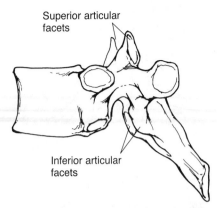

Figure 29.6: The articular processes of the thoracic region are almost vertically aligned. The superior articulating facets in the thoracic region face posteriorly and slightly laterally and superiorly; the inferior articulating facets face anteriorly and slightly medially and inferiorly.

laterally than they do in either the cervical or lumbar regions, contributing to a narrower spinalcanal.

The spinal canal contains the spinal cord, and its size and shape are important factors in avoiding impingement of the spinal cord. In general, the spinal canal is smaller in the thoracic region than in the cervical or lumbar regions where the spinal cord enlarges, providing the large spinal nerves that form the brachial and lumbosacral plexuses of the upper and lower extremities, respectively. The spinal cord occupies approximately 40% of the spinal canal in the thoracic region but only about a quarter of the canal in the cervical region [34,47]. Within the thoracic region, the spinal canal is largest at the level of the first thoracic vertebra and is smallest in the midthoracic region. The area increases again in the lower thoracic region.

Clinical Relevance

SPINAL CORD IMPINGEMENT: *Because the spinal canal is relatively small in the thoracic region, space-occupying lesions such as tumors or disc herniations put the spinal cord at risk [47]. Careful screening for signs of spinal cord compression is an important component of the assessment of an individual with thoracic spine dysfunction. Signs of spinal cord compression include motor or sensory changes in the lower extremities as well as hyperreflexia. Loss of bowel or bladder control also may suggest spinal cord involvement.*

ARTICULAR PROCESSES OF A THORACIC VERTEBRA

The articular processes extend superiorly and inferiorly from the junction of the pedicles and laminae. Each process contains an articular facet that provides articular surfaces for a facet, or zygapophyseal, joint (*Fig. 29.6*). The orientation of the articular processes and facets directly affects the available

spinal motion. In the thorax, the articular processes are more vertically aligned than in the cervical region [33]. The angle between the facets and the transverse plane increases steadily through the cervical and upper thoracic vertebrae. The facets throughout most of the thoracic region lie approximately 70–80° from the transverse plane, with the facets of the lower thoracic vertebrae slightly more vertical than those of the upper thoracic vertebrae [25,33]. In addition, the facets on the superior articular processes face posteriorly and slightly laterally, while the inferior facets face anteriorly and slightly medially. These facets lie at approximately 10° from the frontal plane, which is similar to those of the cervical vertebrae [25,30,33]. In contrast, the lumbar facets lie closer to the sagittal plane [33,37,46].

The alignment of the articular facets helps explain the regional differences in mobility. The vertical alignment of the thoracic facets has a limiting effect on flexion, since the inferior facet of the vertebra above can glide only slightly anteriorly on the superior facet of the vertebra below. Because the thoracic facets lie close to the frontal plane, the articular surfaces provide little limitation to axial rotation. Side-bending also is relatively unobstructed by bony contact at the facet joints. However, as the facets become more medially and laterally aligned in the lower thoracic vertebrae, rotation is more limited, as it is throughout the lumbar region.

MUSCULAR PROCESSES OF A THORACIC VERTEBRA

The transverse and spinous processes of the thoracic vertebrae exhibit unique characteristics. The transverse processes of the thoracic vertebrae vary in length. They are longest in the upper thoracic region and shortest in the lower thoracic region [34]. The lateral aspect of the anterior surface of each transverse process contains a facet for articulation with the tubercle of a rib. The spinous processes are longer in the thoracic region than anywhere else in the vertebral column and project inferiorly, so that throughout most of the thorax the palpable tip of a thoracic spinous process is in line with the

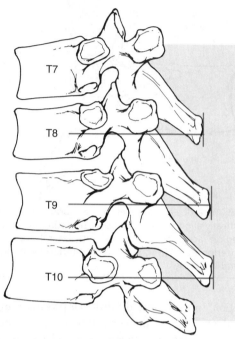

Figure 29.7: The spinous processes of the thoracic region are long and project inferiorly so that the palpable tip of the spinous process is in line with the body of the vertebra below.

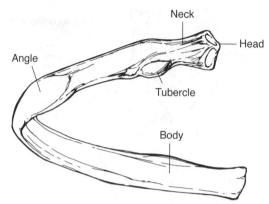

Figure 29.8: A typical rib possesses a head, neck, and body.

body of the inferior thoracic vertebra (*Fig. 29.7*). This relationship is found from approximately the second or third thoracic vertebra to the ninth or tenth vertebra. The upper thoracic vertebrae have more horizontally aligned spinous processes, similar to the cervical vertebrae. The spinous processes of the eleventh and twelfth thoracic vertebrae are somewhat shorter than those of the rest of the thoracic vertebrae and project more posteriorly, becoming more like the spinous processes of the lumbar vertebrae.

Clinical Relevance

PALPATION OF THE THORACIC SPINE: *Clinicians frequently palpate the spinous processes of the vertebral column. A clear understanding of the relationship between a spinous process and neighboring vertebrae allows accurate location of a patient's complaints or the site of impairment.*

BONES OF THE THORACIC CAGE

Ribs

Twelve pairs of ribs and the sternum, along with the thoracic vertebrae, form the thoracic cage. Ribs are long, curved strips of bone composed of head, neck, and body (*Fig. 29.8*). The head and neck form the most dorsal portion of each rib and articulate with the vertebral column. The body, or shaft, constitutes most of each rib and provides attachment to the costal cartilages for all but the last two pairs of ribs [39,54].

The second through ninth pairs of ribs consist of **typical ribs.** The head of a typical rib has a superior and an inferior facet that articulate with the demifacets on the vertebral bodies. The neck of the rib extends laterally and slightly posteriorly from the head, ending with a tubercle on the posterior surface of the rib for articulation with a transverse process. The body of the rib extends laterally from the neck and then curves anteriorly from the angle of the rib. The bodies of the ribs provide attachments for several muscles, including the intercostal muscles, the erector spinae muscles, and the abdominal muscles. The anterior tip of the rib is slightly concave for articulation with a costal cartilage.

The first rib is the shortest and most curved and has a single facet on its head to articulate with the first thoracic vertebra. The tenth, eleventh, and twelfth ribs also typically have only one facet on the heads of the ribs to articulate with their respective vertebrae [39,54].

Sternum

The sternum as a whole is convex anteriorly and concave posteriorly, contributing to the normal contour of the anterior chest wall. It is a flat bone that is composed of three segments, the manubrium, the body, and the most inferior and smallest segment, known as the xiphoid process (*Fig. 29.9*). The manubrium is the proximal and widest segment of the sternum. Its superior border lies at approximately the level of the third thoracic vertebra and contains the palpable sternal, or jugular, notch, which is bordered laterally by the facets for the sternoclavicular joints. The sternal notch is a useful landmark to identify the sternoclavicular joints [39,54].

The body is the longest segment of the sternum, spanning the fifth through ninth thoracic vertebrae [54]. It is notched laterally by facets for the costal cartilages of the second through seventh pairs of ribs. The manubrium and body are joined by a cartilaginous joint that may ossify with age. This joint, the sternomanubrial junction, is readily palpable, since the manubrium and sternal body join at an angle of approximately 160°, known as the sternal angle, or angle of Louis. While mobile, the joint bends a few degrees in the sagittal

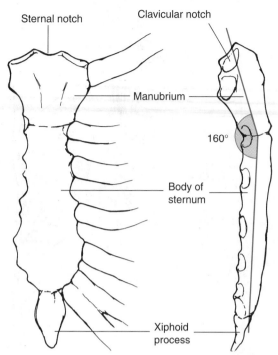

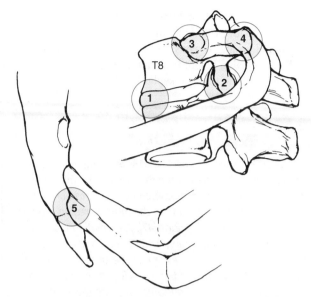

Figure 29.9: The sternum consists of the manubrium, body, and xiphoid process. A lateral view reveals the angle of the sternum, or sternomanubrial junction, formed by the cartilaginous joint between the manubrium and body.

Figure 29.10: The joints of the thoracic region participate in articulations between adjacent vertebral bodies *(1)*, between articulating facets *(2)*, between the ribs and vertebrae at the bodies *(3)* and transverse processes *(4)*, and indirectly with the sternum *(5)*.

plane during respiration, especially during forced respiration [15,40,54]. The xiphoid process is the smallest portion of the sternum and attaches to the inferior aspect of the sternal body. Its shape is more variable than that of the other portions of the sternum, but typically ends in a point inferiorly. The xiphoid process projects inferiorly or inferiorly and posteriorly and may or may not be palpable. The xiphisternal junction is cartilaginous and typically ossifies by 40 years of age.

JOINTS OF THE THORACIC REGION

The thoracic vertebrae are joined at the vertebral bodies by the intervertebral discs and at the spinal arches by the facet joints *(Fig. 29.10)*. In addition, the ribs articulate with the vertebrae and with the sternum by way of the costal cartilages.

Joints between Adjacent Vertebrae

The joints tethering the thoracic vertebrae together consist of the interbody joints, or symphyses, and the synovial facet joints.

INTERBODY JOINTS

The joints between adjacent vertebral bodies are formed by the binding of the intervertebral disc to the adjacent vertebrae. The disc consists of the gelatinous nucleus pulposus and the anulus fibrosus composed of concentric cartilaginous rings that bind the adjacent vertebrae together at their endplates [36].

The structure and mechanical properties of a typical lumbar intervertebral disc are discussed thoroughly in Chapter 32. Thoracic discs differ from discs in the lumbar region in size and shape. Although the discs generally increase in size from superior to inferior, the thinnest discs of the vertebral column are found in the upper thoracic region. The ratio between the disc height and the height of the vertebral body is smaller in the thoracic region than in the cervical and lumbar regions [15,54] *(Fig. 29.11)*. Because deformation of the intervertebral discs contributes to motion of the spine, the decreased ratio

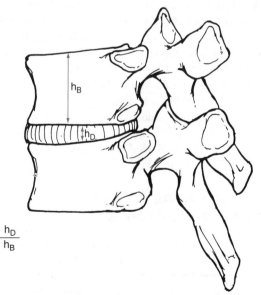

Figure 29.11: The ratio of intervertebral disc height to vertebral body height is smallest in the thoracic region.

between disc and vertebral body height in the thoracic region contributes to lower mobility in the thoracic spine than in the cervical and lumbar regions. The thoracic intervertebral discs are almost equal in height from anterior to posterior and contribute little to the thoracic kyphosis [26,34].

Clinical Relevance

HERNIATION OF THORACIC DISCS: *Herniations of the intervertebral disc occur in the thoracic region, although most apparently remain asymptomatic. Symptomatic disc herniations are less common in the thoracic region than in the cervical or lumbar regions [47]. A herniation may produce nerve root compression with dermatomal or myotomal signs at the level of impingement or, because the spinal canal is relatively small in the thoracic region, spinal cord compression with signs and symptoms into the lower extremities.*

FACET JOINTS

The facet joints of the thoracic region are gliding synovial joints supported by joint capsules like facet joints throughout the vertebral column. The capsules in the thoracic and lumbar regions are tauter than those in the cervical region and help limit flexion and anterior translation of a superior vertebra on an inferior vertebra [32,36].

SUPPORTING STRUCTURES

Besides the capsular ligaments, the thoracic spine is supported by several sets of ligaments common to the rest of the vertebral column: the anterior and posterior longitudinal ligaments, the inter- and supraspinous ligaments, the ligamentum flavum, and the intertransverse ligaments (*Fig. 29.12*). Serial transection of these ligaments in the thoracic region using cadaver specimens reveals that anterior instability of the thoracic spine with intact vertebrae occurs only after transection of all of the posterior ligaments and the posterior portion of the disc [31]. Similarly, posterior instability of the thoracic spine occurs only with transection of the anterior longitudinal ligament and the anterior portion of the disc. Removal of small portions of the disc alone for treatment of disc herniations does not appear to impair spinal stability in the thoracic region [3].

Articulations Joining the Ribs to the Vertebrae and Sternum

The ribs, thoracic vertebrae, and sternum form the thoracic cage, which must be rigid enough to protect the heart and lungs but flexible enough to participate in respiration and to allow spinal motion. The rib cage plays an important role in supporting the entire thoracic spine [8,31,32,35]. With an intact thoracic cage, the thoracic spine can sustain four times

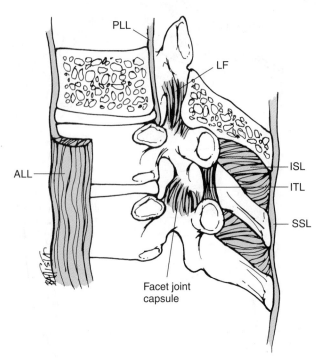

Figure 29.12: Ligaments supporting the thoracic spine consist of the capsular ligaments of the facet joints, the anterior and posterior longitudinal ligaments (*ALL* and *PLL*), the supra- and interspinous ligaments (*SSL* and *ISL*), the ligamentum flavum (*LF*), and the intertransverse ligaments (*ITL*).

the compressive load it can support without the thoracic cage [1,37]. In fact, without the rib cage, the thoracic spine would barely be able to support the weight of the head [35].

ARTICULATIONS BETWEEN THE RIBS AND THE VERTEBRAE

The posterior ends of the ribs articulate with the vertebrae at the bodies and transverse processes, forming the **joints of the costal heads** (also known as the **costovertebral joints**) and the **costotransverse joints,** respectively. Although each articulation is described as a gliding, or plane, joint, together they allow rotational movement of a rib.

The joints of the costal heads typically consist of the junction between the head of a rib and the demifacets of two vertebral bodies [39,54] (*Fig. 29.13*). With the exception of the first, tenth, eleventh, and twelfth pairs of ribs, the head of each rib attaches to the bodies of two adjacent vertebrae, to the vertebra at the same thoracic level as the rib, and to the vertebra above. The rib also attaches to the intervening intervertebral disc. The first pair of ribs attaches only to the lateral surfaces of the first thoracic vertebra. Typically, the tenth through twelfth pairs of ribs articulate with single vertebrae, T10 through T12.

The joints of the costal heads are supported by synovial capsules and by intraarticular ligaments that extend medially from the tips of the heads of the ribs to the intervertebral discs. Each joint capsule is reinforced on its superficial surface by a radiate ligament, so named because it radiates from

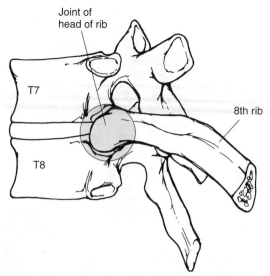

Figure 29.13: Joints of the costal heads consist of the head of a rib, the posterolateral surface of the inferior surface of the superior vertebral body, and the superior surface of the vertebral body of the adjacent vertebra.

Consequently, blows to the chest more frequently produce rib fractures than dislocations of these joints [56].

the rib to the bodies of the superior and inferior vertebrae and to the intervening disc [38,52] (*Fig. 29.14*).

The costotransverse joints are the junctions between the facet on the tubercle of the neck of each rib and the facet on the anterior surface of each transverse process. Each rib articulates with the transverse process of the vertebra of the same number. The costotransverse joint is supported by a joint capsule that is reinforced by a costotransverse ligament, and by posterior and lateral costotransverse ligaments (*Fig. 29.15*). Ligamentous support affords considerable stability to the joints of the costal heads and the costotransverse joints.

ARTICULATIONS BETWEEN THE RIBS AND STERNUM

All but the last two pairs of ribs join the sternum by costal cartilages that are lengths of hyaline cartilage (*Fig. 29.16*). The first pair of ribs attaches to the lateral facets on the manubrium just inferior to the sternoclavicular joints. The second pair articulates with the sternum at the junction of the manubrium and body. The second rib is readily palpated at the sternomanubrial junction (*Fig. 29.17*). The third through seventh pairs attach to the lateral sides of the sternal body. Because of their direct attachment with the sternum, the first seven pairs of ribs are known as **vertebrosternal ribs.** Rib pairs eight through ten join the costal cartilages of the rib above and eventually join the costal cartilages of the seventh ribs. These ribs are referred to as **vertebrochondral ribs.**

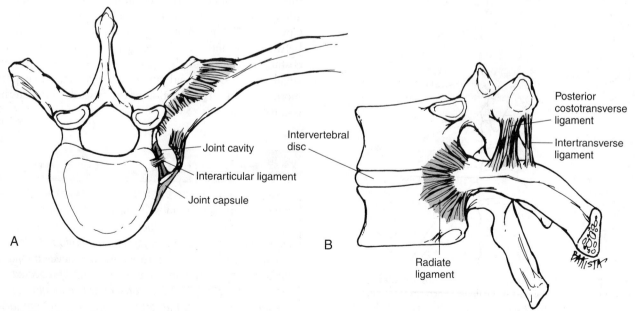

Figure 29.14: A joint of the costal head is supported by a capsule that is reinforced by the radiate ligament (**B**) and by an intraarticular ligament between the head of the rib and the adjacent intervertebral disc (superior view) (**A**).

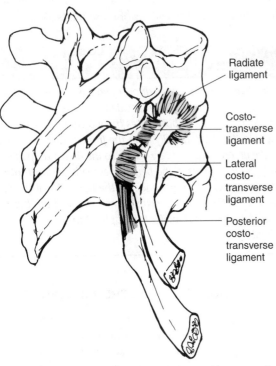

Figure 29.15: A costotransverse joint is supported by a capsule, a costotransverse ligament, and posterior and lateral costotransverse ligaments.

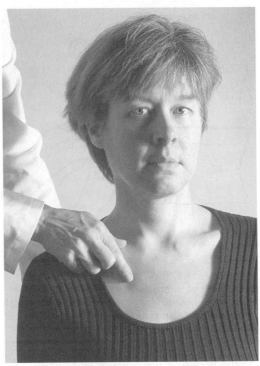

Figure 29.17: The second rib is easily palpated at the sternomanubrial junction.

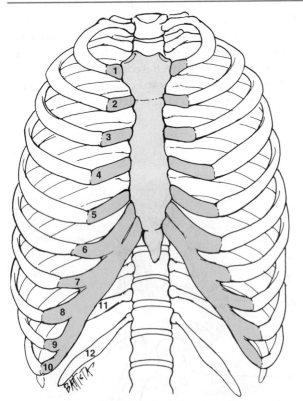

Figure 29.16: The seven superior pairs of ribs articulate with the sternum by individual costal cartilages. Each rib from eight through ten joins the costal cartilage of the rib immediately superior to it. Ribs eleven and twelve have only small cartilaginous tips and do not articulate with the sternum.

The last two pairs of ribs, known as **vertebral ribs,** have no costal cartilage attachments, so their ventral tips, covered by a thin layer of cartilage, have no bony attachment anteriorly and are often palpable. Although often referred to as the **floating ribs,** these last two rib pairs are secured by muscles and ligaments and are not free to "float" in the thorax.

The costal cartilages adhere to the ribs by a blending of the periosteum and perichondrium, as well as by a continuation of the collagen matrix within the bones and cartilages. Consequently, no motion is available at the junctions between ribs and costal cartilages. In contrast, most of the costal cartilages join the sternum by synovial joints with small joint capsules and supporting ligaments that permit motion [38,54]. The junction of the first rib to the sternum is cartilaginous.

Clinical Relevance

PAIN AT THE COSTOSTERNAL JUNCTIONS: *Because the junctions between most of the costal cartilages and the sternum are synovial, they are relatively mobile and capable of subluxation and joint inflammation. An individual with bronchitis or pneumonia may develop inflammation at a costosternal joint as the result of repeated vigorous coughing that generates repetitive loading on the joints by muscles that attach to the ribs and produce the cough.*

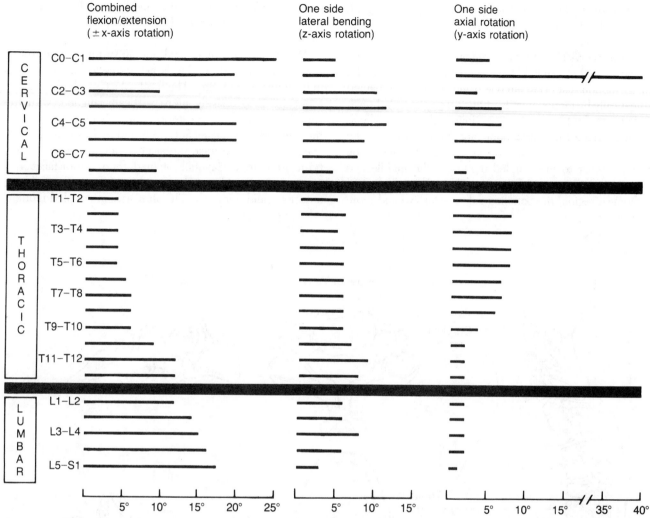

Figure 29.18: Segmental motion varies throughout the vertebral column. (Reprinted with permission from White AA III, Panjabi MM: Kinematics of the spine. In: White AA III, Panjabi MM, eds. Clinical *Biomechanics of the Spine. 2nd ed.* Philadelphia: JB Lippincott, 1990.)

MOVEMENTS OF THE THORACIC SPINE AND THORAX

Thoracic Spine Motion

Motion of the thoracic spine, like that of the cervical and lumbar regions (Chapters 26 and 32), depends on the orientation of the facet joints and on the thickness of the intervertebral discs. In addition, the motion of the thoracic spine is influenced greatly by the presence of the ribs [32,37]. To understand the motion in the thoracic spine, the clinician must appreciate the **segmental mobility** that is available at an individual thoracic motion segment (two adjacent thoracic vertebrae with the intervening disc) as well as the **total motion** from all of the thoracic vertebrae. Thoracic spine motion is less thoroughly studied than the motions in other regions of the spine.

SEGMENTAL MOTION

In general, the thoracic spine exhibits less segmental mobility than the cervical or lumbar regions [24,36,52] (*Fig. 29.18*). The segments in the upper and middle regions of the thoracic spine display approximately 2–6° of combined flexion and extension, with approximately equal flexion and extension excursions [24,32,36,43,52]. The thoracic spine is slightly less stiff in flexion than in extension, requiring less force to flex than to extend [30]. Flexion and extension mobility increases in the lower thoracic spine in the presence of the vertebral ribs.

Segmental side-bending is less in most of the thoracic region than in the cervical region and similar to that available in the lumbar region. The ribs limit side-bending in the thoracic region. Consequently, side-bending increases in the lower thoracic region, where the ribs have no sternal attachment and provide little barrier to side-bending motion. Segmental rotation in the upper and middle thoracic regions is greater than segmental rotation in the lumbar region. Rotation in the lower thoracic region is similar to lumbar segmental rotation.

As in the cervical and lumbar regions, the motions of the thoracic spine are coupled. A **coupled motion** consists of a primary motion that occurs in one plane and is accompanied automatically by motion in at least one other plane. Although coupling appears to occur in all motions of the vertebral column, it is greatest in side-bending and rotation [52]. In the upper thoracic region, side-bending is coupled with ipsilateral rotation, similar to the coupled motion in the middle and lower cervical regions (Chapter 26). Throughout the rest of the thoracic region, the coupling is less extensive and more variable. Side-bending in the middle and lower thoracic regions can be accompanied by either ipsilateral or contralateral rotation.

Differences in segmental mobility among the spinal regions can be attributed in large degree to the differences in facet joint orientation. The facets of a typical thoracic vertebra are progressively more vertically aligned, with the superior facets facing posteriorly and slightly laterally and the inferior facets facing anteriorly and slightly medially [30] (*Fig. 29.19*). In contrast, the facets of a typical cervical vertebra are more horizontally aligned, the superior facets facing posteriorly and superiorly and the inferior facets facing anteriorly and inferiorly. The similarity in coupled motions

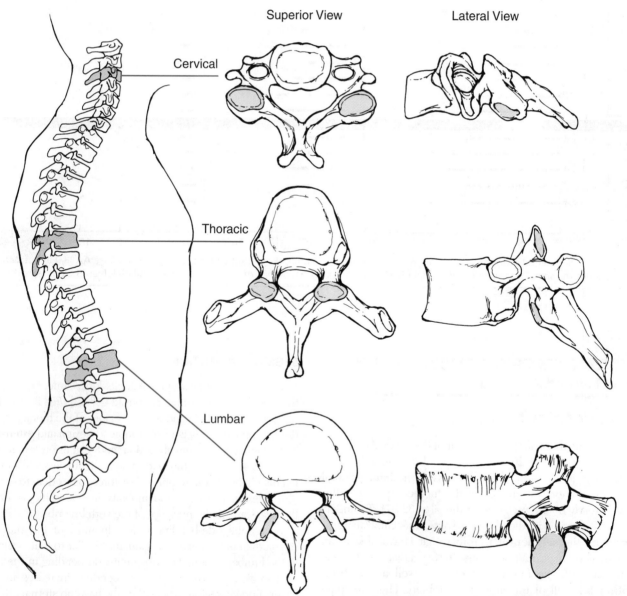

Superior View   Lateral View

Cervical

Thoracic

Lumbar

Figure 29.19: Superior and lateral views reveal that the thoracic and lumbar vertebral facets are more vertically aligned than the cervical facets. The cervical and thoracic facets face more anteriorly and posteriorly; the lumbar facets face more medially and laterally.

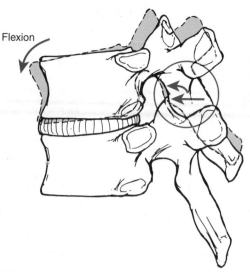

Figure 29.20: Flexion of the thoracic spine requires anterior translation of the inferior facet, limited by the vertical orientation of the facet and by the facet joint capsule.

between the cervical and upper thoracic regions results from the gradual transition from cervical to thoracic facet orientations [30]. Typical lumbar facets are almost vertical but face more medially or laterally than either the cervical or thoracic vertebrae [36].

The facet alignment in the thoracic region allows easy mobility in axial rotation, limited by the posterior ligaments [29,52]. The vertical orientation of the thoracic facets and their position close to the frontal plane require that flexion of one vertebra on another be accompanied by superior translation of the inferior facets on the superior facets (*Fig. 29.20*). The facet alignment and joint capsules help limit the translation [29,47]. Similarly, the facet orientation produces compressive forces between articulating facets during extension, limiting extension range of motion (ROM). The anterior longitudinal ligament and intervertebral disc limit extension excursion that may also be limited by the inferiorly projecting spinous processes of the thoracic region [52]. The ribs contribute to a reduction in segmental mobility in all directions [1,32,35,37].

TOTAL MOBILITY OF THE THORACIC SPINE

Few reports exist describing the total excursion available in the thoracic spine, and only one known report describes the

source of the data [9,10]. *Table 29.1* reveals wide variations in reported total motion in the thoracic spine and demonstrates the lack of accepted norms for the excursions available in the thoracic region in individuals without pathology. Despite the lack of normative data for total excursions, evidence demonstrates that left–right symmetry in rotation and side-bending excursions is a normal finding in individuals without impairments [18]. Research is required to determine the relative flexibility in rotation, side-bending, flexion, and extension as well as to determine the range of mobility available in individuals with no spinal impairments. Establishing normative data describing total excursions of the thoracic spine will assist clinicians in identifying joint impairments in patients with thoracic spine dysfunction.

Motion of the Rib Cage

The ribs attach to the vertebrae by gliding synovial joints, and all but the last two pairs are attached indirectly to the corresponding rib on the opposite side by the costal cartilages and sternum. Thus the rib pair forms a closed loop, or **closed kinetic chain,** fixed at both ends to the thoracic vertebrae. The primary motion of the ribs is the elevation and depression that is a part of respiration. Because the ribs are attached to the thoracic vertebrae, they also move in response to thoracic motion. Motions of the ribs apply forces on the costal cartilages, and the resulting alterations in the shapes of the costal cartilages also play a role in respiration.

TABLE 29.1: ROM of the Thoracic Spine in Individuals without Spinal Impairment

Little information is available on the total motion exhibited by the thoracic spine in individuals with no thoracic impairments.

	Flexion/Extension	Side-Bending to One Side	Rotation to One Side
American Academy of Orthopaedic Surgeons [10]	63°	68°	62°
Gerhardt and Rippstein [9]	85° flexion; 30° extension	30°	45°

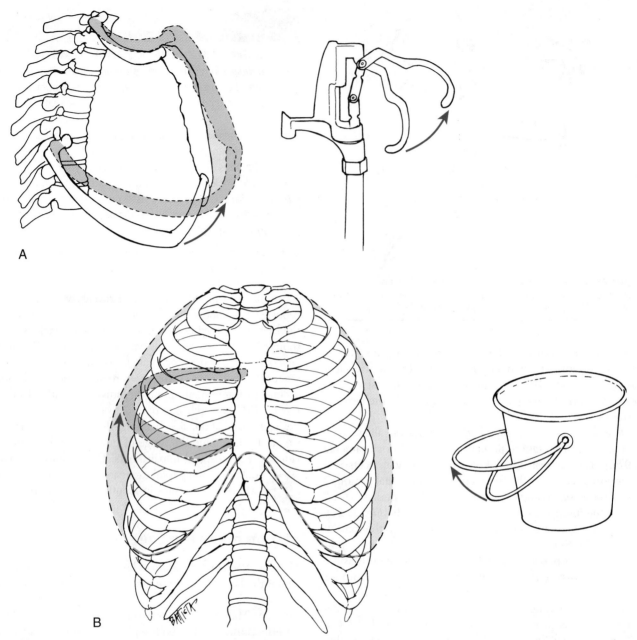

Figure 29.21: A. Pump handle motion occurs in the sagittal plane. **B.** Bucket handle motion occurs in the frontal plane.

ELEVATION AND DEPRESSION OF THE RIBS

Although the ribs exhibit complex three-dimensional motion [39,54], the motions of the ribs in elevation and depression can be described mechanically as hingelike. Rib movements classically are compared to the hinged movements of a pump handle and a bucket handle [12,23,55] (*Fig. 29.21*). The handle represents the closed kinetic chain that consists of a pair of ribs attached by costal cartilage and the sternum. The axis of motion passes approximately through the length of the rib neck, and the costotransverse joint and joint of the head of the rib together constitute a hinge-like unit on each side of the

vertebral column. **Pump-handle motion** of the ribs refers to their motion in the sagittal plane, and **bucket-handle motion** represents frontal plane excursion.

Although each rib moves in both the sagittal and frontal planes, sagittal plane, or pump-handle, movement predominates in the upper thoracic region, where the neck of the ribs, and hence the putative axis of motion, lies closer to the frontal plane. [7,17,22]. The lower thoracic region exhibits more equally distributed motion in both the sagittal and frontal planes, and it is unclear if one motion predominates [7,17,22,55]. Angular measurements of elevation and depression reveal larger total excursions of the upper ribs than of the middle and lower ribs [21,55].

Total chest expansion measurements are more clinically feasible than measurements of discrete rib motion and are standard components of the assessment of pulmonary function [13]. Average chest expansion during forced inspiration and expiration in individuals with normal pulmonary function is presented in *Table 29.2*. Young adults show average chest expansions of approximately 7.0 cm or more; women exhibit slightly less excursion than men [28]. Chest expansion appears to increase from adolescence to adulthood and then begins to decrease in elders [4,28]. Measurements are influenced by the location of the measurement within the chest and by the position of the subject during the measurement. Chest excursion is a common clinical assessment in individuals

 with suspected pulmonary dysfunction, and clinicians must choose consistent measurement techniques to ensure valid assessments.

Clinical Relevance

CHEST EXPANSION IN PATIENTS WITH ANKYLOSING SPONDYLITIS: *Many disorders restrict the motion of the ribs and affect pulmonary function negatively. One such disorder is **ankylosing spondylitis,** which is an inflammatory disease affecting the joints of the spine and thorax. Joints of the lower extremities such as the hips and knees may also be affected [16]. Inflammation and subsequent ankylosis, or fusion, of the joints of the spine and ribs lead to decreased*

chest expansion. Measurements of chest expansion are useful outcome variables to assess a patient's progress or the effectiveness of an intervention [48].

MOTIONS OF THE RIBS WITH THORACIC MOTION

Because ribs are attached to all of the thoracic vertebrae, movement of these vertebrae also produces rib motion [40, 42]. Flexion and extension of the thoracic spine are accompanied by depression and elevation of the ribs, respectively. Flexion of the thoracic spine causes approximation of the ribs, which contributes to the limitation of total thoracic flexion ROM. Similarly, extension of the thoracic spine causes the ribs to separate and consequently tends to expand the chest. Side-bending of the thorax produces approximation of the ribs on the side of the concavity and separation on the side of the convexity, contributing to the limitation in side-bending excursion.

Rotation of a thoracic vertebra in the transverse plane affects the paired ribs attached to it asymmetrically. Rotation of a vertebra is named according to the side to which the vertebral body turns; hence right rotation indicates that the body of the vertebra turns to the right. Because the center of rotation (COR) for a thoracic vertebra rotating in the transverse plane lies somewhere in the vertebral body, rotation to the right is accompanied by anterior movement of the left transverse process and posterior movement of the right transverse process, producing asymmetric movement of the left and right ribs [15,51] (*Fig. 29.22*). Rotation to the right tends to push the left rib anteriorly and to pull the right rib posteriorly. Thus rotation of the thoracic spine alters the contour of the thorax [15,22].

TABLE 29.2: Circumferential Chest Excursions in Subjects with Normal Pulmonary Function

Circumferential chest expansion measurements are similar in men and women but appear to vary with age, subject position, and measurement site.

	Axillary Site (cm)	Xiphoid Process Site (cm)
Carlson [5][a]	8.48 ± 0.64	
Harris et al. [12]	7.6 ± 1.2[b]	7.4 ± 1.7
	7.1 ± 1.3[c]	6.9 ± 1.6
	6.8 ± 1.6[d]	8.2 ± 1.4
	6.8 ± 1.3[e]	7.6 ± 1.5
LaPier et al. [19]	4.75[f]	4.75
Moll and Wright [28]	6.0 ± 2.14[g]	
	4.82 ± 1.29[h]	
Burgos-Vargas et al. [4]		5.6 ± 1.76[i]

[a]13 females and 6 males, aged 20 to 30 years, in supine; mean ± standard error of the mean.
[b]30 males, aged 19 to 34 years, in supine; mean ± standard deviation.
[c]30 females, aged 19 to 34 years, in supine; mean ± standard deviation.
[d]30 males, aged 19 to 34 years, in standing position; mean ± standard deviation.
[e]30 females, aged 19 to 34 years, in standing position; mean ± standard deviation.
[f]20 male and female subjects, aged 20 to 69 years, in standing position; data reported graphically without standard deviations.
[g]16 males, aged 45–54 years, in standing position; mean ± standard deviation.
[h]26 females, aged 45–54 years, in standing position; mean ± standard deviation.
[i]57 adolescents (112 boys and 45 girls, mean age of 13 years ± 1.1), in standing position; mean ± standard deviation.

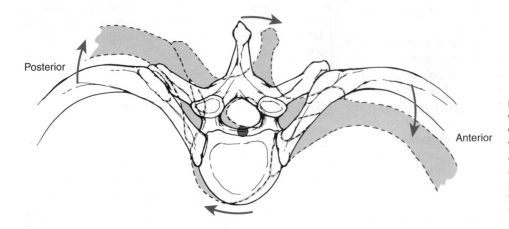

Figure 29.22: Right rotation of the thoracic spine in the transverse plane rotates the right transverse process posteriorly and the left transverse process anteriorly. This rotation tends to pull the right rib posteriorly and to push the left rib anteriorly.

Clinical Relevance

COUPLED MOTIONS AND IDIOPATHIC SCOLIOSIS IN THE THORACIC SPINE:

*Although coupled motions in the thoracic spine are variable in normal motion, side-bending and contralateral rotation appear more systematically coupled in individuals with idiopathic scoliosis. **Idiopathic scoliosis** is the most common form of scoliotic deformity, typically arising in adolescent girls with apparently normal musculoskeletal systems [50]. The deformity is characterized by a frontal plane curve that is accompanied by transverse plane rotation of the involved thoracic vertebrae to the side of the convexity [44,45,51,53]. Rotation applies posteriorly directed stresses to the rib on the convex side and anteriorly directed stresses to the rib on the concave side. The angle of the rib on the convex side becomes more prominent and produces the characteristic **rib hump** (Fig. 29.23). The rib hump,*

always found on the convex side of the curve, is the result of the asymmetrical stress on the attached ribs, contributing to asymmetrical growth of the ribs.

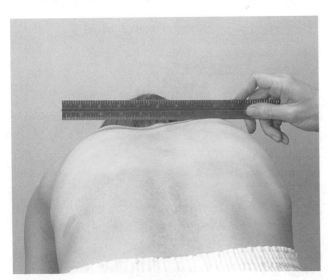

Figure 29.23: An individual with idiopathic scoliosis in the thoracic region exhibits a rib hump.

MOVEMENTS OF THE COSTAL CARTILAGES AND STERNUM

Because most ribs are attached to the vertebral column and to each other by means of the costal cartilages and sternum, movement of the ribs is accompanied by movement of these other structures as well. During elevation of the ribs the sternum rises and moves slightly anteriorly [14,23] (*Fig. 29.24*). The difference in lengths of the superior and inferior ribs produces an unequal anterior movement that induces a slight bending or flexion of the sternum at the sternomanubrial junction [15,40].

Although the sternum rises during rib elevation, its movement is less than the movement of the ribs. The difference in movement between the ribs and sternum twists the costal cartilages [11]. The passive torsion applied to the costal cartilages allows the cartilages to store **elastic energy** that is

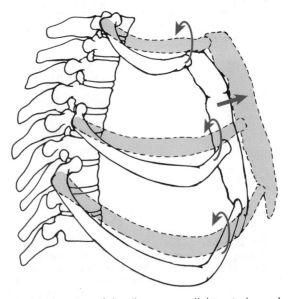

Figure 29.24: Elevation of the ribs causes a slight anterior and superior movement of the sternum and torsion of the costal cartilages.

released as the cartilages recoil [38]. Their passive recoil helps lower the ribs and reduce thoracic volume during exhalation, without the need for muscle contraction.

Clinical Relevance

INCREASED STIFFNESS OF THE COSTAL CARTILAGES WITH AGING: *Aging produces increased stiffness in the costal cartilages as well as in the lung tissue itself. Increased stiffness increases ventilatory resistance, intensifying the work of respiration in elders [6,15].*

MECHANICS OF RESPIRATION

Respiration, the exchange of oxygen and carbon dioxide within the lungs, is largely a mechanical process that pumps air in and out of the lungs. This process, known as **ventilation,** is the function of rib motion and operates on the simple inverse relationship between volume and pressure in a closed space. **Boyle's law** relating pressure and volume of a gas states:

$$P_1V_1 = PV = \text{constant}$$

where P is pressure and V is volume. The respiratory pump moves air by altering the volume of the thoracic cage, thus altering the internal pressure within the thoracic cavity (*Fig. 29.25*). When pressure within the cavity is high, air is expelled, and when pressure is low, air flows in. Specifically, elevation of the ribs or contraction of the diaphragm muscle increases the volume of the thorax, decreasing the internal pressure, and inspiration begins. As the lungs fill with air, internal pressure rises, and the muscles that have increased the thoracic volume gradually relax. The elastic recoil of the chest wall and of the lungs themselves reduces the volume of the thorax, elevating the internal pressure, and air flows out of the lungs [11]. Active contraction of the abdominal muscles can facilitate the descent of the ribs, contributing to a rapid, more forceful retraction of the thorax and volume reduction during forced expiration.

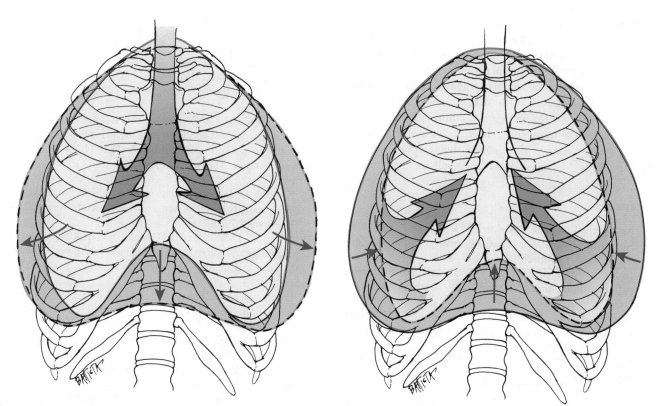

Figure 29.25: An increase in thoracic volume decreases thoracic pressure and air rushes in (*left*); a decrease in thoracic volume increases thoracic pressure and forces air out of the thoracic cage (*right*).

SUMMARY

This chapter reviews the structure and motion of the thoracic spine and rib cage. As in other regions of the vertebral column, the mobility of the thoracic spine depends on the alignment of the articular facets and the ligamentous supports. The superior facets of the thoracic spine face posteriorly and slightly laterally, and the inferior facets face in the opposite direction. The alignment of the facets in the thoracic spine contributes to limits in flexion and extension while providing little restraint to axial rotation. The mobility and stability of the thoracic spine also are influenced by the rib cage, which limits excursion of the thoracic spine while helping to stabilize it. Segmental flexion and extension in the thoracic spine are smaller than that available in the cervical and lumbar regions. Thoracic segmental rotation is greater than lumbar rotation except in the lower thoracic region. Segmental side-bending in the thoracic and lumbar regions is less than that in the cervical regions.

Motions of the ribs are less well studied, but data suggest that normal chest expansion is approximately 7.0 cm (approximately 3 in) in young adults without impairments and decreases in elders. The motion of the ribs and thoracic spine contributes significantly to the mechanics of respiration. Respiration includes the mechanical pumping action of the ribs, known as ventilation, which is governed by Boyle's law. Elevation of the ribs increases thoracic volume and decreases thoracic pressure, allowing air to flow into the thoracic cavity. Depression of the ribs reverses the volume and pressure so that air is expelled.

Motions of the thoracic spine also influence the position of the ribs. In particular, rotation of the thoracic spine distorts the thorax by pushing one rib anteriorly and pulling the opposite rib posteriorly. This normal rib and costal cartilage deformation helps explain the characteristic rib hump in structural scoliosis deformities. Thus the structure and function of the thoracic portion of the vertebral column and the rib cage attached to it are intimately related to each other. The following chapter reviews the muscles that support and move the thoracic region and discusses their role in respiration.

References

1. Andriacchi T, Schultz A, Belytschko T, Galante J: A model for studies of mechanical interactions between the human spine and rib cage. J Biomech 1974; 7: 497–507.
2. Biyani A, Ebraheim NA, Lu J: Thoracic spine fractures in patients older than 50 years. Clin Orthop 1996; 328: 190–193.
3. Broc GG, Crawford NR, Sonntag VK, Dickman CA: Biomechanical effects of transthoracic microdiscectomy. Spine 1997; 22: 605–612.
4. Burgos-Vargas R, Castelazo-Duarte G, Orozco JA, et al.: Chest expansion in healthy adolescents and patients with the seronegative enthesopathy and arthropathy syndrome or juvenile ankylosing spondylitis. J Rheumatol 1993; 20: 1957–1960.
5. Carlson B:. Normal chest excursion. Phys Ther 1973; 53: 10–14.
6. Clough P: Restrictive lung dysfunction. In: Allen A, ed. Essentials of Cardiopulmonary Physical Therapy. Philadelphia: WB Saunders, 2001; 183–256.
7. De Groote A, Wantier M, Cheron G, et al.: Chest wall motion during tidal breathing. J Appl Physiol 1997; 83: 1531–1537.
8. Edmondston SJ, Allison GT, Althorpe BM, et al.: Comparison of ribcage and posteroanterior thoracic spine stiffness: an investigation of the normal response. Manual Ther 1999; 4: 157–162.
9. Gerhardt JJ, Rippstein J: Measuring and Recording of Joint Motion Instrumentation and Techniques. Lewiston, NJ: Hogrefe & Huber, 1990.
10. Greene WB, Heckman JD: The Clinical Measurement of Joint Motion. Rosemont, IL: American Academy of Orthopaedic Surgeons, 1994.
11. Han JN, Gayan-Ramirez G, Dekhuijzen R, Decramer M: Respiratory function of the rib cage muscles. Eur Respir J 1993; 6: 722–728.
12. Harris J, Johansen J, Pederson S, LaPier TK: Site of measurement and subject position affect chest excursion measurements. Cardiopulm Phys Ther 1997; 8: 12–17.
13. Hidding A, van der Linden S, Gielen X, et al.: Continuation of group physical therapy is necessary in ankylosing spondylitis: results of a randomized controlled trial. Arthritis Care Res 1994; 7: 90–96.
14. Jordanoglou J: Rib movement in health, kyphoscoliosis, and ankylosing spondylitis. Thorax 1969; 24: 407–414.
15. Kapandji IA: The Physiology of the Joints. Vol 3, The Trunk and the Vertebral Column. Edinburgh: Churchill Livingstone, 1974.
16. Keat AM: Seronegative spondyloarthropathies C. Ankylosing spondylitis. In: Klippel JH, ed. Primer on Rheumatic Diseases. Atlanta: Arthritis Foundation, 2001; 250–254.
17. Kondo T, Kobayashi I, Taguchi Y, et al.: A dynamic analysis of chest wall motions with MRI in healthy young subjects. Respirology 2000; 5: 19–25.
18. Kumar S, Panjabi MM: In vivo axial rotations and neutral zones of the thoracolumbar spine. J Spinal Disord 1995; 8: 253–263.
19. LaPier TK, Cook A, Droege K, et al.: Intertester and intratester reliability of chest excursion measurements in subjects without impairment. Cardiopulm Phys Ther 2000; 11: 94–98.
20. Lee Y, Yip K: The osteoporotic spine. Clin Orthop 1996; 323: 91–97.
21. Lemosse D, LeRue O, Diop A, et al.: Characterization of the mechanical behaviour parameters of the costo-vertebral joint. Eur Spine J 1998; 7: 16–23.
22. Leong JC, Lu WW, Luk KD, Karlberg EM: Kinematics of the chest cage and spine during breathing in healthy individuals and in patients with adolescent idiopathic scoliosis. Spine 1999; 24: 1310–1315.
23. Loring SH, Woodbridge JA: Intercostal muscle action inferred from finite-element analysis. J Appl Physiol. 1991; 70: 2712–2718.
24. Magee DA: Orthopedic Physical Assessment. Philadelphia: WB Saunders, 1998.
25. Masharawi Y, Rothschild B, Dar G, et al.: Facet orientation in the thoracolumbar spine: three-dimensional anatomic and biomechanical analysis. Spine 2004; 29: 1755–1763.
26. Mcinerney J, Ball PA: The pathophysiology of thoracic disc disease. Neurosurg Focus 2000; 9: 1–8.

27. Melton LJI: Epidemiology of spinal osteoporosis. Spine 1997; 22: 2S–11S.

28. Moll JM, Wright V: An objective clinical study of chest expansion. Ann Rheum Dis 1972; 31: 1–8.

29. Oxland TR, Lin RM, Panjabi MM: Three-dimensional mechanical properties of the thoracolumbar junction. J Orthop Res 1992; 10: 573–580.

30. Pal G, Routal R, Saggu S: The orientation of the articular facets of the zygapophyseal joints at the cervical and upper thoracic region. J Anat 2001; 198(pt 4): 431–441.

31. Panjabi MM, Brand RA, White AA III: Three-dimensional flexibility and stiffness properties of the human thoracic spine. J Biomech 1976; 9: 185–192.

32. Panjabi MM, Hausfeld JN, White AA III: A biomechanical study of the ligamentous stability of the thoracic spine in man. Acta Orthop Scand 1981; 52: 315–326.

33. Panjabi MM, Oxland T, Takata K, et al.: Articular facets of the human spine. Spine 1993; 18: 1298–1310.

34. Panjabi MM, Takata K, Goel V, et al.: Thoracic human vertebrae: Quantitative three-dimensional anatomy. Spine 1991; 16: 888–901.

35. Panjabi MM, White AA: Physical properties and functional biomechanics of the spine. In: White AA, Panjabi MM, eds. Clinical Biomechanics of the Spine. Philadelphia: JB Lippincott, 2001; 3–81.

36. Panjabi MM, White AA III: Basic biomechanics of the spine. Neurosurgery 1980; 7: 76–93.

37. Resnick DK, Weller SJ, Benzel EC: Biomechanics of the thoracolumbar spine. Neurosurg Clin North Am 1997; 8: 455–469.

38. Roberts SB, Chen PH: Elastostatic analysis of the human thoracic skeleton. J Biomech 1970; 3: 527–545.

39. Romanes GJE: Cunningham's Textbook of Anatomy. Oxford: Oxford University Press, 1981.

40. Saumarez RC: An analysis of possible movements of human upper rib cage. J Appl Physiol 1986; 60: 678–689.

41. Shen W, Niu Y, Stuhmiller JH: Biomechanically based criteria for rib fractures induced by high-speed impact. J Trauma 2005; 58: 538–545.

42. Smith JC, Mead J: Three degree of freedom description of movement of the human chest wall. J Appl Physiol. 1986; 60: 928–934.

43. Sran MM, Khan KM, Zhu Q, Oxland TR: Posteroanterior stiffness predicts sagittal plane midthoracic range of motion and three-dimensional flexibility in cadaveric spine segments. Clin Biomech 2005; 20: 806–812.

44. Stokes IAF, Bigalow LC, Moreland MS: Three-dimensional spinal curvature in idiopathic scoliosis. J Orthop Res. 1987; 5: 102–113.

45. Stokes IAF, Laible JP: Three-dimensional osseo-ligamentous model of the thorax representing initiation of scoliosis by asymmetric growth. J Biomech 1990; 23: 589–595.

46. Tulsi RS, Hermanis GM: A study of the angle of inclination and facet curvature of superior lumbar zygapophyseal facets. Spine 2001; 18: 1311–1317.

47. Vanichkachorn JS, Vaccaro AR: Thoracic disk disease: diagnosis and treatment. J Am Acad Orthop Surg 2000; 8: 159–169.

48. Viitanen JV, Suni J, Kautiainen H, et al.: Effect of physiotherapy on spinal mobility in ankylosing spondylitis. Scand J Rheumatol 1992; 21: 38–41.

49. White AA III, et al.: The clinical biomechanics of kyphotic deformities. Clin Orthop 1977; 128: 8–17.

50. White AA III, Panjabi MM: The clinical biomechanics of scoliosis. Clin Orthop 1976; 118: 100–112.

51. White AA III, Panjabi MM: The basic kinematics of the human spine. A review of past and current knowledge. Spine 1978; 3: 12–20.

52. White AA III, Panjabi MM: Kinematics of the Spine. In: Cooke DB, ed. Clinical Biomechanics of the Spine. Philadelphia: JB Lippincott, 1990; 85–126.

53. White AA III, Panjabi MM: Practical biomechanics of scoliosis and kyphosis. In: Cooke DB, ed. Clinical Biomechanics of the Spine. Philadelphia: JB Lippincott, 1990; 127–163.

54. Williams P, Bannister L, Berry M, et al.: Gray's Anatomy, The Anatomical Basis of Medicine and Surgery, Br. ed. London: Churchill Livingstone, 1995.

55. Wilson TA, Rehder K, Krayer S, et al.: Geometry and respiratory displacement of human ribs. J Appl Physiol 1987; 62: 1872–1877.

56. Yoganandan N, Morgan RM, Eppinger RH, et al.: Thoracic deformation and velocity analysis in frontal impact. J Biomech Eng 1995; 117: 48–52.

Mechanics and Pathomechanics of the Muscles of the Thoracic Spine

CHAPTER CONTENTS

The preceding chapter describes the bony architecture of the thoracic region, its supporting structures, and available motion. The current chapter presents the muscles of the thoracic region. These muscles support and move the thoracic spine and also participate in respiration.

The goals of this chapter are to

- Present the reported actions of the muscles found in the thoracic region
- Discuss the muscles' functional significance
- Consider the functional consequences of impairments in these muscles
- Examine the role these muscles play in respiration

Muscles affecting the thoracic region include the muscles of the shoulder, posterior thoracic spine, and abdomen, and those intrinsic to the thoracic cage, which attach the ribs to the sternum, to vertebrae, or to each other (Fig. 30.1). Muscles of the shoulder are discussed in Chapter 9 and are discussed only briefly in the current chapter. Abdominal muscles produce flexion of both the thoracic and lumbar spines and are presented in Chapter 33.

MUSCLES OF THE POSTERIOR THORAX

Muscles of the posterior thorax are grouped in a variety of ways. The current chapter describes two layers, a superficial and deep layer. The superficial layer consists of shoulder muscles, specifically the trapezius, the rhomboids major and minor, and the latissimus dorsi. The deep layer contains the erector spinae, the transversospinales muscles, and the interspinous and intertransverse muscles.

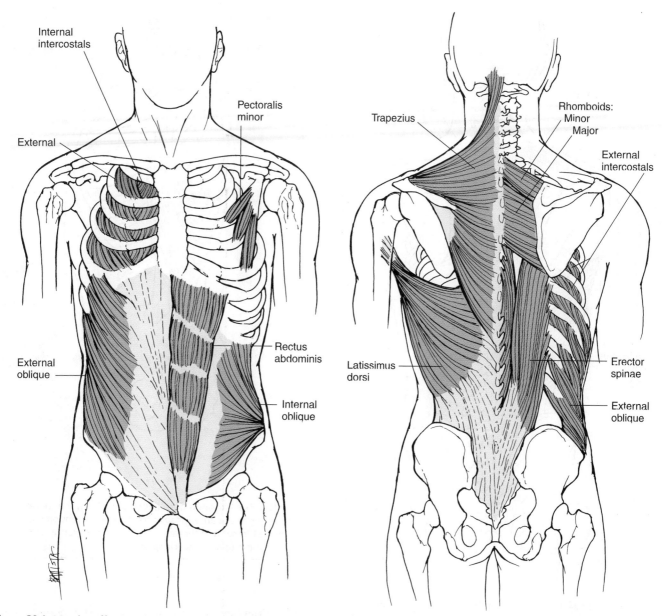

Figure 30.1: Muscles affecting the thorax include shoulder muscles, muscles of the posterior spine, abdominal muscles, and muscles intrinsic to the thorax.

Superficial Layer

MUSCLE ACTION: TRAPEZIUS AND RHOMBOIDS

Action	Evidence
Thoracic spine extension (bilateral contraction)	Inadequate
Thoracic spine side bending (unilateral contraction)	Inadequate
Contralateral rotation of thoracic spine (unilateral contraction)	Inadequate

MUSCLE ACTION: LATISSIMUS DORSI

Action	Evidence
Thoracic spine extension (bilateral contraction)	Conflicting

MUSCLE ACTION: LATISSIMUS DORSI (Continued)

Action	Evidence
Thoracic spine side bending (unilateral contraction)	Supporting
Ipsilateral rotation of thoracic spine (unilateral contraction)	Supporting

The muscles of the superficial layer of the posterior thorax assist in supporting the thorax (*Fig. 30.2*). They attach to spinous processes of thoracic vertebrae. With their distal attachments on the scapula and humerus fixed, these muscles may move the thoracic spine. Just as bilateral contraction of the upper trapezius produces extension of the cervical spine, bilateral contraction of the trapezius and/or

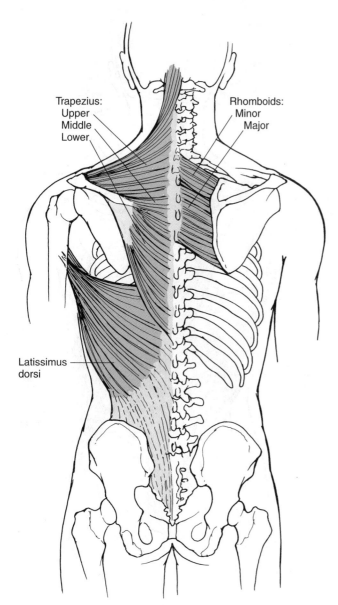

Figure 30.2: Superficial muscles of the posterior thorax are shoulder muscles and include the trapezius, the rhomboids major and minor, and the latissimus dorsi.

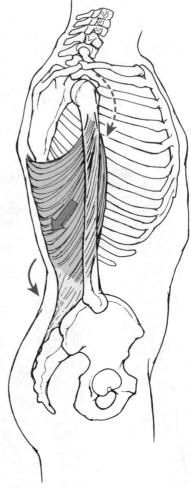

Figure 30.3: The latissimus dorsi lies diagonally on the thorax from the posterior to the anterior surface. It has an extension moment arm on the lumbar and thoracic spines but may exert a flexion moment on the upper thoracic spine.

rhomboids major and minor may help support the thoracic spine in extension, although there are minimal data verifying such a role [43].

The latissimus dorsi exhibits an extension moment arm in the lumbar region and participates in extension of the lumbar spine [35,38]. Its role in flexion and extension in the thoracic spine is controversial, because as the latissimus dorsi projects to its distal attachment on the humerus, it appears to pass from the posterior to the anterior surface of the thorax (*Fig. 30.3*). Measurement of its flexion and extension moment arms using magnetic resonance imaging (MRI) suggests that it continues to have an extension moment arm to at least the fifth thoracic vertebra [35]. Others suggest that it develops a flexion moment arm on the thoracic spine at its humeral end

[12,42]. Tightness of the latissimus dorsi reportedly contributes to excessive thoracic kyphosis, although there are no known studies verifying this association [25].

Unilateral contraction of the trapezius, rhomboids, and latissimus dorsi reportedly produces side-bending and rotation of the thoracic spine, although only the latissimus dorsi has data directly supporting its contributions to these actions [35,38]. In individuals with idiopathic scoliosis, the trapezius on the convex side exhibits a relative increase in type I muscle fibers with a slight atrophy of type II fibers, and the trapezius and rhomboid muscles may contribute to the spinal deformity [41,60,61].

Electromyography (EMG) data reveal activity of the latissimus dorsi during ipsilateral rotation with its inferior attachment fixed [39] (*Fig. 30.4*). With their distal attachments fixed, contraction of the trapezius and rhomboids major and minor could potentially produce contralateral rotation by pulling the spinous processes toward the distal attachment. No known data are available to identify if, or under what conditions, the

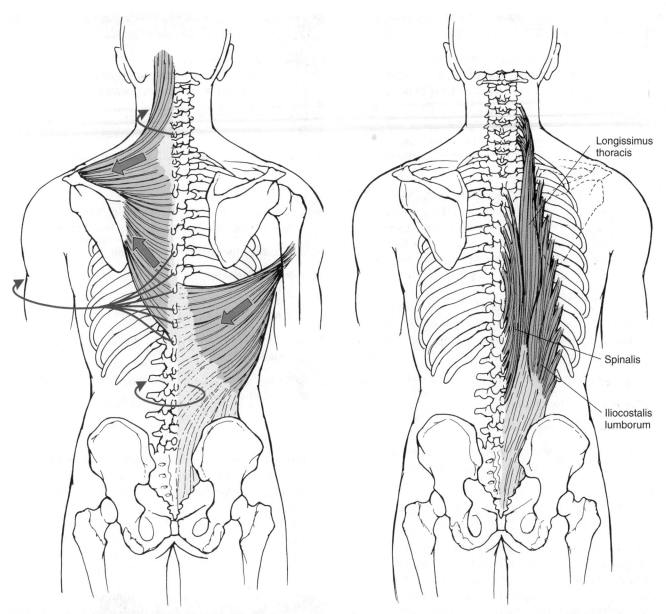

Figure 30.4: The latissimus dorsi pulls the shoulder girdle posteriorly and participates in ipsilateral rotation of the thorax. The trapezius and rhomboids major and minor pull on the spinous processes of the thoracic spines and, consequently, produce contralateral rotation.

Figure 30.5: The three groups of the erector spinae are, from lateral to medial, the iliocostalis, longissimus, and spinales muscle groups.

trapezius and rhomboid muscles contribute to movement of the thoracic spine, and further research is needed to clarify their participation in thoracic spine motion. [25]

Deep Layer of the Posterior Thoracic Region

The deep muscular layer of the back is separated from the superficial layer by the thoracolumbar fascia. The deep layer can be divided into additional muscular subsets: the erector spinae, the transversospinales, and the deepest layer consisting of the interspinales and intertransversarii.

ERECTOR SPINAE

The erector spinae extends from the pelvis to the occiput and consists of three main groups of muscles: the iliocostalis, longissimus, and spinalis muscles (*Fig. 30.5*) (*Muscle Attachment Boxes 30.1–30.3*). The spinales are found in the thoracic, cervical, and occipital regions only. The longissimus consists of longissimus thoracis, cervicis, and capitis. The longissimus thoracis contains both a thoracic portion (the longissimus thoracis pars thoracis) and a lumbar portion (the longissimus thoracis pars lumborum) [28,29]. The iliocostalis consists of cervical, thoracic, and lumbar segments but, like the longissimus thoracis, the iliocostalis lumborum

MUSCLE ATTACHMENT BOX 30.1

ATTACHMENTS AND INNERVATION OF THE ILIOCOSTALIS MUSCLES AFFECTING THE THORACIC AND LUMBAR SPINES

Iliocostalis thoracis:

Inferior attachment: Upper borders of the lower six rib angles medial to the insertion of the iliocostalis lumborum

Superior attachment: Superior borders of the upper six ribs at their angles and the posterior aspect of the transverse processes of the seventh cervical vertebra. The iliocostalis thoracis lies between the iliocostalis lumborum pars thoracis and the longissimus thoracis pars thoracis.

Iliocostalis lumborum pars thoracis:

Inferior attachment: Crest of the ilium from the posterior superior iliac spine laterally approximately 5 cm

Superior attachment: Angles of all 12 ribs

Iliocostalis lumborum pars lumborum:

Inferior attachment: Iliac crest

Superior attachment: Transverse processes of the first four lumbar vertebrae and thoracolumbar fascia

Innervation: Dorsal rami of the thoracic and lumbar spinal nerves.

Palpation: The erector spinae can be palpated as a group through the thoracolumbar fascia as the muscles parallel the vertebral column in the lumbar and thoracic regions. The iliocostalis can not be distinguished from the rest of the erector spinae.

contains a thoracic component (the iliocostalis lumborum pars thoracis) and a lumbar portion (the iliocostalis pars lumborum).

Action

MUSCLE ACTION: ERECTOR SPINAE

Action	Evidence
Trunk extension (bilateral contraction)	Supporting
Trunk side bending (unilateral contraction)	Supporting
Ipsilateral rotation of trunk (unilateral contraction)	Supporting

The spinalis thoracis and iliocostalis thoracis span only the thoracic region and act only to extend the thoracic spine. In

MUSCLE ATTACHMENT BOX 30.2

ATTACHMENTS AND INNERVATION OF THE LONGISSIMUS MUSCLES AFFECTING THE THORACIC AND LUMBAR SPINES

Longissimus thoracis pars thoracis:

Inferior attachment: Fibers contribute to the erector spinae aponeurosis and the spinous processes of the lumbar and sacral vertebrae and onto the ilium.

Superior attachment: Transverse processes of all thoracic vertebrae and the lower eight or nine ribs

Longissimus thoracis pars lumborum:

Inferior attachment: Posterior superior iliac spine

Superior attachment: Transverse and accessory processes of the lumbar vertebrae

Innervation: Dorsal rami of the lumbar and thoracic spinal nerves

Palpation: Cannot be differentiated from the rest of the erector spinae.

contrast, the longissimus thoracis and iliocostalis lumborum with their pars thoracis and pars lumborum components cross the thoracic and lumbar regions, producing combined thoracic and lumbar extension [28,29]. A detailed description of their effects on the lumbar spine is found in Chapter 33.

EMG data verify the role of the erector spinae as a whole in extension of the trunk during bilateral contraction [1,2]. The

MUSCLE ATTACHMENT BOX 30.3

ATTACHMENTS AND INNERVATION OF THE SPINALIS MUSCLES OF THE THORACIC SPINE

Spinalis thoracis:

Inferior attachment: Arises by three to four tendons from the eleventh thoracic to the second lumbar vertebral spines running medial to, and blending with, iliocostalis thoracis

Superior attachment: Spines of the upper four to eight thoracic vertebrae by separate tendons and blending with semispinalis thoracis

Innervation: Dorsal rami of thoracic spinal nerves

Palpation: Cannot be differentiated from the rest of the erector spinae.

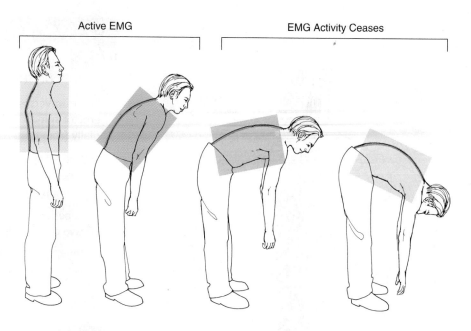

Active EMG   EMG Activity Ceases

Figure 30.6: EMG studies demonstrate that the erector spinae cease electrical activity about halfway through a full forward bend and remain silent until the individual returns about halfway toward the upright position.

muscles contract eccentrically during forward-bending from a standing position and concentrically as the spine returns to an erect position. The erector spinae becomes **electrically silent** during forward flexion when the trunk reaches approximately two thirds of its maximal available excursion, and remains silent as the trunk initiates the return to the erect posture [1,2,10,19,23,26] (*Fig. 30.6*). Only after the trunk reaches approximately 45° do the muscles resume activity. The posterior ligaments of the spine and intervertebral discs provide the primary support to the spine in the maximally flexed position, and the passive recoil of these tissues, combined with the action of the superficial back muscles and hip extensors, helps initiate the return to upright posture [2,19,40].

Unilateral contraction of the iliocostalis and longissimus muscles is associated with side-bending and with ipsilateral rotation of the spine [1,46,58]. The erector spinae as a whole exhibits a side-bending moment arm of 25 to 35 mm in the thoracic region, compared with moment arms of approximately 50 mm for extension [35,38]. The moment arms of muscles within the erector spinae are quite varied, so that substantial moment arms in both extension and side-bending are exhibited by at least some segments of the erector spinae [29,30].

It is important to recognize that from the erect posture, the erector spinae contract eccentrically to control forward-bending of the trunk and contract concentrically briefly to initiate either extension or side-bending (*Fig. 30.7*). Continuation of hyperextension or side-bending is facilitated by the moments exerted by the weight of the head and trunk. The abdominal muscles contract eccentrically to control the extension moment of the head and trunk [2]. Similarly, side-bending of the trunk from the upright posture is controlled by the abdominal muscles and contralateral erector spinae [1,2,36].

The erector spinae in the thoracic region are composed primarily of type I fibers, or slow-twitch fibers (approximately 75%), but the erector spinae in the lumbar region exhibit a more even distribution of type I and type II fibers (approximately 57% type I) [50]. The preponderance of fatigue-resistant muscle fibers in the thoracic spine suggests that the erector spinae in the thoracic region plays a primary role in postural support and in stabilizing the costovertebral joints [47].

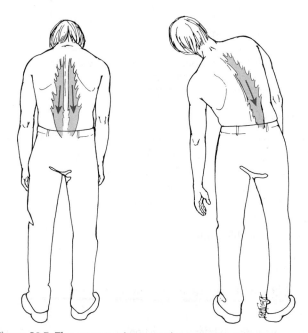

Figure 30.7: The erector spinae muscles typically contract to control forward-bending or side-bending, requiring an eccentric contraction of the whole group during forward-bending and the contralateral group during side-bending.

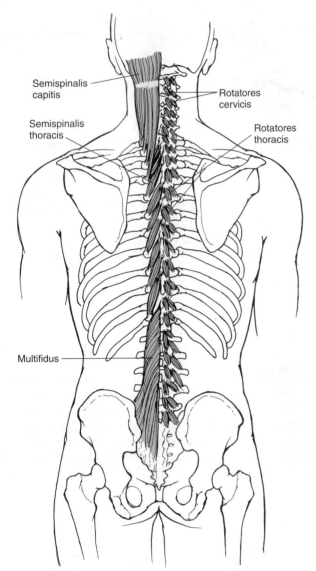

Semispinalis
capitis

Semispinalis
thoracis

Rotatores
cervicis

Rotatores
thoracis

Multifidus

Figure 30.8: Transversospinales muscles include the semispinalis, multifidus, and rotatores muscles.

TRANSVERSOSPINALES

The transversospinalis muscle group consists of the semi-spinales, multifidus, and rotatores muscles (*Fig. 30.8*) (*Muscle Attachment Boxes 30.4–30.6*). The group is so named because of its attachments, which consist of an inferior attachment on a transverse process and a superior attachment on a spinous process [46,58]. Like the erector spinae, these muscles are more thoroughly studied in the lumbar region.

Action

MUSCLE ACTION: TRANSVERSOSPINALES

Action	Evidence
Trunk extension (bilateral contraction)	Supporting
Trunk side bending (unilateral contraction)	Supporting
Contralateral rotation of trunk (unilateral contraction)	Supporting

MUSCLE ATTACHMENT BOX 30.4

ATTACHMENT AND INNERVATION OF THE SEMISPINALIS MUSCLES

The transversospinales muscle group lies deep to the erector spinae with fibers running superiorly and me-dially from transverse processes to spinous processes.

Semispinalis thoracis:

Inferior attachment: Transverse processes of the sixth to the tenth thoracic vertebrae by tendinous slips

Superior attachment: Spinous processes of the lower two cervical and upper four thoracic vertebrae

Innervation: Dorsal rami of the cervical and tho-racic spinal nerves

Palpation: Cannot be palpated directly.

MUSCLE ATTACHMENT BOX 30.5

ATTACHMENT AND INNERVATION OF THE MULTIFIDUS

Inferior attachment: Arises from the transverse processes of thoracic vertebrae

Superior attachment: Fibers run superiorly and medi-ally in the space between the transverse processes to their spinous process insertions along the length of the spine. Fasciculi vary in length, with the most superficial running from one vertebra to the third or fourth above, the next deepest running from one vertebra to the second or third above and the deep-est connecting adjacent vertebrae.

Innervation: Dorsal rami of the thoracic spinal nerves

Palpation: Cannot be palpated.

MUSCLE ATTACHMENT BOX 30.6

ATTACHMENT AND INNERVATION OF THE ROTATORES

Rotatores thoracis:

Superior attachment: Eleven pairs of muscles that take origin from the lower border and lateral surfaces of the lamina from the first to the eleventh vertebra

Inferior attachment: Upper and posterior portions of the transverse processes of the vertebra below

Innervation: Dorsal rami of the thoracic spinal nerves

Palpation: Cannot be palpated.

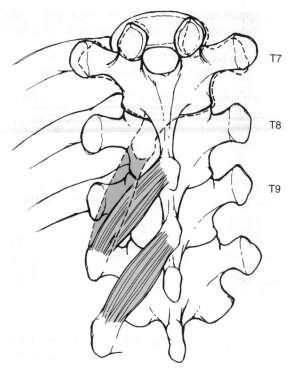

MUSCLE ATTACHMENT BOX 30.7

ATTACHMENT AND INNERVATION OF THE INTERSPINALES

Attachments: The interspinales are most distinct in the cervical and lumbar regions running along either side of the interspinous ligaments to connect the apices of contiguous spinous processes. Occasionally a pair may be found between the last thoracic and first lumbar vertebrae and between the fifth lumbar and the sacrum, and they may be absent in the thoracic region.

Innervation: Dorsal rami of the spinal nerves

Palpation: Cannot be palpated.

Figure 30.9: The transversospinales muscles produce contralateral rotation by pulling the spinous process of the superior vertebrae toward the transverse process of the inferior vertebrae.

IMPAIRMENT OF THE MUSCLES OF THE POSTERIOR THORAX

Discrete impairments of the deep posterior thoracic muscles are difficult to identify. The erector spinae muscles in the thoracic region contribute to the extension moment of the thoracic and lumbar regions. Consequently, weakness of the thoracic erector spinae contributes to a decrease in total trunk extension strength. Individuals with idiopathic scoliosis exhibit atrophy of the muscles of the posterior thorax, particularly on the concave side, and a higher than normal percentage of type I muscle fibers on the convex side of the deformity, but the clinical significance of these differences is unclear [15,60,62].

Like the erector spinae, these muscles contract eccentrically to control flexion and contralateral side-bending from the upright position. They produce contralateral rotation by pulling the spinous processes of the superior vertebrae toward the transverse processes of the inferior vertebrae (*Fig. 30.9*). The thoracic multifidi are longer and thinner, with longer and more obliquely aligned tendons than those in the lumbar region [4]. Thus while the multifidi in the lumbar region may contribute significantly to the compressive loads on the lumbar vertebrae, the multifidi in the thoracic region may contribute more to side-bending and rotation moments. The multifidi in the thoracic region are, like the erector spinae, composed mostly of type I fibers (approximately 75%) and exhibit a slightly smaller concentration of type I fibers (63%) in the lumbar region [50].

The rotatores are more fully developed in the thoracic region than anywhere else, yet they are still very small and hence not very powerful. They may act more as position sensors than as torque producers, but additional research is needed to verify this hypothesis.

INTERSPINALES AND INTERTRANSVERSARII

The interspinales and intertransversarii muscles are found at only a few of the thoracic vertebral levels, primarily at the superior and inferior aspects of the thorax, and may even be absent completely in the thoracic region [46,58] (*Muscle Attachment Boxes 30.7 and 30.8*). Their functional significance is unclear.

INTRINSIC MUSCLES OF THE THORAX

The intrinsic muscles of the thorax consist of those muscles that attach the ribs to the vertebral column, to the sternum, or to other ribs. This group includes the posterior serratus

MUSCLE ATTACHMENT BOX 30.8

ATTACHMENT AND INNERVATION OF THE INTERTRANSVERSARII

Attachments: The intertransversarii are sets of muscles running between vertebrae and are most distinct in the cervical spine. In the thoracic region, down to the first lumbar vertebra, intertransversarii connect transverse processes as a single muscle slip.

Innervation: Dorsal rami of thoracic spinal nerves with ventral rami contribution

Palpation: Cannot be palpated.

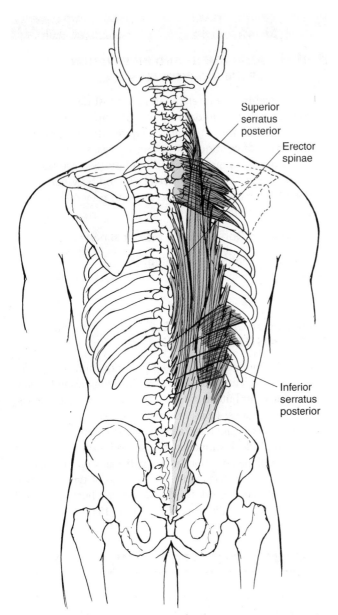

Figure 30.10: The superior and inferior serratus posterior muscles lie deep to the superficial muscles of the posterior thorax and superficial to the erector spinae.

superior and inferior; the external, internal, and innermost intercostals; the transversus thoracis, subcostales, levator costarum, and the diaphragm.

Serratus Posterior Superior and Inferior

MUSCLE ACTION: SERRATUS POSTERIOR SUPERIOR AND INFERIOR

Action	Evidence
Elevate the ribs (superior)	Inadequate
Depress the ribs (inferior)	Inadequate

MUSCLE ATTACHMENT BOX 30.9

ATTACHMENTS AND INNERVATION OF THE SERRATUS POSTERIOR SUPERIOR

Superior attachment: Arises from the inferior part of the ligamentum nuchae and the spines of the upper three or four thoracic vertebrae and seventh cervical vertebrae

Inferior attachment: Four digitations descend inferiorly and laterally to insert just lateral to the angles of the second, third, fourth, and fifth ribs on their superior and superficial surfaces.

Innervation: Second to the fourth intercostal nerves. The fifth intercostal nerve may also contribute.

Palpation: Cannot be palpated.

The serratus posterior superior and inferior muscles attach the ribs to the thoracic vertebrae (*Fig. 30.10*) (*Muscle Attachment Boxes 30.9 and 30.10*). Neither muscle is well studied, and the posterior serratus inferior is absent in some individuals [58]. The serratus posterior superior is aligned to elevate the ribs and thus may be active in inspiration; the serratus posterior inferior may lower the ribs and perhaps participates in exhalation.

Intercostal Muscles

The intercostal muscles include the external, internal, and innermost intercostal muscles (*Fig. 30.11*) (*Muscle Attachment Boxes 30.11–30.13*).

MUSCLE ATTACHMENT BOX 30.10

ATTACHMENTS AND INNERVATION OF THE SERRATUS POSTERIOR INFERIOR

Superior attachment: The outer surface and inferior borders of the lower four ribs just lateral to their angles by four digitations. Fewer digitations may be present, and infrequently the entire muscle may be absent.

Inferior attachment: The spines of the upper two or three lumbar vertebrae and lower two thoracic vertebrae and their supraspinous ligaments. It may also attach to the thoracolumbar fascia.

Innervation: Ninth through eleventh or twelfth intercostal nerves.

Palpation: Cannot be palpated.

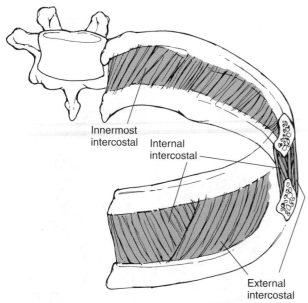

Figure 30.11: The intercostal muscles include the external, internal, and innermost intercostal muscles.

MUSCLE ATTACHMENT BOX 30.12

ATTACHMENT AND INNERVATION OF THE INTERNAL INTERCOSTALS

Superior attachment: Eleven pairs of muscles arise anteriorly at the costal cartilages of the first seven ribs and the cartilaginous ends of the remaining ribs, with continuing attachment along the floor of the costal grooves back to the rib angles. From the rib angles, they continue as an aponeurotic layer called the internal intercostal membrane and blend with the superior costotransverse ligaments.

Inferior attachment: Fibers descend obliquely from the superior rib to the upper border of the rib below in a direction nearly perpendicular to fibers of the external intercostals. Fibers of the lower two rib spaces may blend with the internal oblique muscle.

Innervation: The corresponding intercostal nerves

Palpation: In the spaces between the upper ribs, just lateral to the sternum where the external intercostal muscles are membranous.

MUSCLE ATTACHMENT BOX 30.11

ATTACHMENT AND INNERVATION OF THE EXTERNAL INTERCOSTALS

Superior attachment: Tubercles of the ribs, blending with the posterior fibers of the costotransverse ligaments, continuing along the lower rib borders almost to the costal cartilages, where it then proceeds anteriorly toward the sternum as an aponeurotic layer called the external intercostal membrane.

Inferior attachment: Eleven pairs of muscles run from their superior attachment to the upper border of the rib below. Fibers travel obliquely downward and laterally at the back of the thorax and downward, medially and forward on the anterior thorax. In the lower two rib spaces, fibers attach to the ends of the costal cartilages; in the upper two or three rib spaces, they do not quite reach the rib ends. Fibers from the lower intercostal spaces may blend with the external oblique muscle.

Innervation: The corresponding adjacent intercostal nerves

Palpation: The intercostals are palpated together in the intercostal spaces.

ACTION

MUSCLE ACTION: INTERCOSTALS EXTERNAL AND INTERNAL

Action	Evidence
Contralateral trunk rotation (external)	Supporting
Ipsilateral trunk rotation (internal)	Supporting
Inspiration (external)	Conflicting
Exhalation (internal)	Conflicting

MUSCLE ATTACHMENT BOX 30.13

ATTACHMENT AND INNERVATION OF THE INNERMOST INTERCOSTAL MUSCLES (INTERCOSTALES INTIMI)

Attachments: Pairs of muscles attach to the internal aspect of two adjacent ribs. They lie deep to the internal intercostals, with fibers running in the same direction. The innermost intercostal muscles become more substantial posteriorly and in the middle two quarters of the lower intercostal spaces. They are smaller and may be absent at the higher thoracic levels.

Innervation: The corresponding intercostal nerves

Palpation: Cannot be palpated directly.

Several studies investigated the role of the external and internal intercostal muscles but few studies have investigated the function of the innermost intercostal muscles that lie parallel to the internal intercostals and are smaller, more variable, and sometimes absent. Their actions are inferred from studies of the internal intercostal muscles [58]. Despite efforts to define the functional role of the external and internal intercostal muscles, controversy remains. Intercostal muscles are difficult to study because they are thin and overlie each other through most of their lengths [57]. The external intercostal is the only intercostal muscle belly in an intercostal space between the angle of the rib and tubercle of the rib. Similarly, the only location where the internal intercostal muscles are not covered by external intercostal muscles is in the spaces between the costal cartilages. In this region they are known as the **parasternal intercostal** muscles. Most of the studies of the internal intercostal muscles are investigations of the parasternal muscles [28,48].

EMG data reveal activity of the external intercostal muscles during contralateral rotation and activity in the internal intercostal muscles during ipsilateral rotations [45,56]. These actions parallel the actions of the oblique abdominal muscles, which have similar lines of pull. The intercostal muscles appear to play an important role in trunk rotation; however, their short fiber length suggests that additional muscles are necessary to produce an excursion through the full available range of motion.

Some EMG studies and biomechanical models support the traditional view that the external intercostal muscles participate in inspiration and the internal intercostal muscles in expiration [28,31,44,47,59], although most studies agree that at least the parasternal portion of the internal intercostal muscles are active in inhalation [6,8,11,20,28,55]. Other studies identify activity in both muscle groups during both inspiration and exhalation [11,58]. Simultaneous activity of the intercostal muscles suggests that the muscles may work together to stabilize the rib cage against the changing pressures of the thoracic cavity and the displacement of the diaphragm [6,11,47,58].

The mechanics of ventilation are based on the relationship between pressure and volume of a gas. This relationship dictates that as volume increases, pressure decreases, and as volume decreases, pressure increases. Decreased pressure within the thoracic cavity causes air to enter the lungs. The internal pressure of the thorax tends to have the same effect on the flexible walls of the thorax (*Fig. 30.12*). To prevent the collapse of the rib cage during inhalation and its expansion during exhalation, the intercostal muscles contract simultaneously to support the thorax. The fibers of the internal and external intercostal muscles are approximately perpendicular to each other and thus are well aligned to function together to stiffen the thoracic walls and stabilize the ribs.

IMPAIRMENT OF THE INTERCOSTAL MUSCLES

Weakness of the intercostal muscles may occur in individuals following cervical or thoracic spinal cord injury as well as in other neuromuscular and musculoskeletal disorders [3,7,

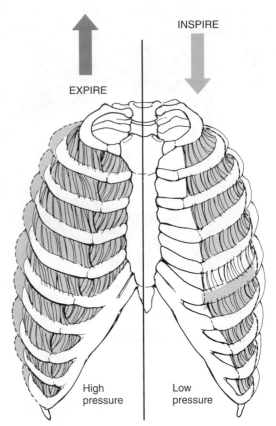

Figure 30.12: During inspiration, the pressure within the thorax is low and tends to collapse the rib cage. During expiration, the pressure within the thorax is high and tends to expand the thorax.

18,51]. Isolated evaluation of these muscles is impossible because of their location and because they function as a group with the diaphragm during respiration. Consequently, assessment is based on clinical observations and pulmonary function tests, including maximum inspiratory and expiratory pressures and vital capacity [3,7,18]. Studies show that muscles of respiration are amenable to exercise and demonstrate improved function following exercise [34,44].

Clinical Relevance

PARADOXICAL BREATHING: *Paradoxical breathing is a breathing pattern in which the change in circumference of either the thorax or abdomen is opposite that expected from the relationship of volume and pressure in normal respiration. A patient with flaccid paralysis of the intercostal muscles following a cervical or high thoracic spinal cord injury demonstrates paradoxical breathing with abnormal movement of the rib cage during respiration. Inspiration occurs by means of contraction of the diaphragm, which increases the volume of the thoracic cage and decreases the pressure. In the absence of intercostal muscle activity to stabilize the ribs, the decrease in thoracic pressure also causes the thorax to collapse toward*

(continued)

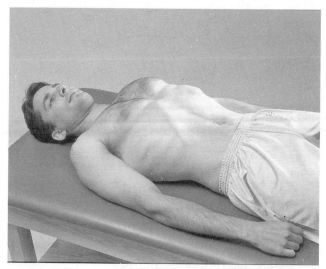

Figure 30.13: Paradoxical breathing is movement of the thorax or abdomen in a direction opposite to the expected direction for the phase of respiration. Pictured is paradoxical breathing in which the circumference of the abdomen decreases during inspiration, when it is expected to expand.

MUSCLE ATTACHMENT BOX 30.14

ATTACHMENT AND INNERVATION OF THE SUBCOSTALES

Superior attachment: Internal surface of the ribs near the angle

Inferior attachment: Internal surface of the second or third rib below, traveling with the innermost intercostal muscles between the intercostal vessels and nerves and the pleura. They usually are most developed in the lower thorax, with the fibers running parallel to those of the internal intercostal muscles.

Innervation: The corresponding intercostal nerves

Palpation: Cannot be palpated.

(Continued)
the lungs. Consequently, the circumference of the thorax decreases during inspiration instead of increasing.

Paradoxical breathing also occurs if the intercostal muscles contract in the absence of diaphragmatic activity; inspiration occurs with chest expansion, but the diameter of the abdomen decreases as the diaphragm is pulled into the thoracic cavity (Fig. 30.13). Paradoxical breathing patterns, identifiable by careful observation, provide valuable clinical information to the clinician regarding the patient's respiratory function.

The transversus thoracis and subcostales lie on the deep surface of the thoracic cage, and the levator costarum muscles lie on the posterior aspect of the thorax. These muscles are not well studied (*Fig. 30.14*) (*Muscle Attachment Boxes 30.14–30.16*). The transversus thoracis (also known as the triangularis sterni) depresses the lower ribs and participates in expiration [13,28,46,58]. The subcostales muscles lie parallel to the internal intercostal muscles and are found primarily in the lower thoracic region [46,58]. They appear to depress the ribs, although no known studies verify that function. The levator costarum, as its name suggests, appears to elevate the ribs [28,46,58].

Tightness of the intrinsic muscles of the thorax may occur following thoracic surgery or be present on the concave side of a thoracic scoliosis. Tightness of the intrinsic muscles restricts the mobility of the rib cage and, in particular, limits chest expansion. Individuals with scoliosis demonstrate decreased pulmonary function attributed to the diminished chest expansion resulting from the deformity [27,53]. Stretching exercises may improve pulmonary function in these patients [49,54].

Transversus Thoracis, Subcostales, and Levator Costarum

MUSCLE ACTION: TRANSVERSUS THORACIS, SUBCOSTALES, LEVATOR COSTARUM

Action	Evidence
Depress the ribs (transversus thoracis)	Supporting
Depress the ribs (subcostales)	Inadequate
Elevate the ribs (levator costarum)	Supporting

MUSCLE ATTACHMENT BOX 30.15

ATTACHMENT AND INNERVATION OF TRANSVERSUS THORACIS

Superior attachment: Fibers diverge into slips passing from their inferior attachment to insert onto the lower borders and inner surfaces of the costal cartilages of the second to the sixth ribs.

Inferior attachment: Lower third of the posterior surface of the sternum, the xiphoid process, and the costal cartilages of the lower three or four true ribs near their sternal ends. Lower slips run horizontally and are contiguous with superior fibers of transversus abdominis; the upper slips run obliquely upward and laterally.

Innervation: The corresponding intercostal nerves

Palpation: Cannot be palpated.

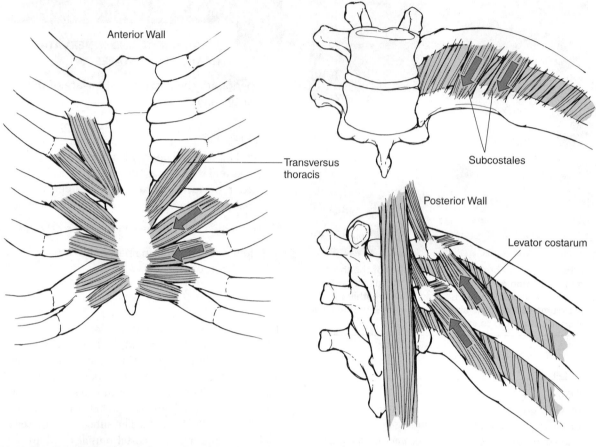

Figure 30.14: The deep layer of intrinsic muscles of the thorax includes the subcostales and transversus thoracis, lying on the deep surface of the thoracic wall, and the levator costarum on the posterior surface of the thorax.

MUSCLE ATTACHMENT BOX 30.16

ATTACHMENT AND INNERVATION OF THE LEVATORES COSTARUM

Superior attachment: Twelve pairs of triangular muscle bundles arise from the tips of the transverse processes of the seventh cervical and the first to the eleventh thoracic vertebrae.

Inferior attachment: Superior and outer edge of the rib immediately below the vertebra of origin between the tubercle and angle. Fibers run laterally and inferiorly, paralleling the posterior borders of the external intercostals. The lower four muscle pairs may have an additional attachment to the second rib below their origin.

Innervation: Lateral branches of the dorsal rami of the corresponding thoracic spinal nerves

Palpation: Cannot be palpated.

Diaphragm

The diaphragm is an unusual muscle because it is a somewhat circular sheet of muscle with a central tendon and bony attachment only along its circumference. During contraction it pulls from its periphery to its central tendon (*Fig. 30.15*) (*Muscle Attachment Box 30.17*).

ACTION

MUSCLE ACTION: DIAPHRAGM

Action	Evidence
Lower floor of thoracic cavity	Supporting
Elevate the lower ribs	Supporting

Because the diaphragm's actions increase thoracic volume, the diaphragm is unquestionably a muscle of inspiration [8,9,11,17,46,58]. The diaphragm contracts from its peripheral attachments on the lower ribs and vertebrae and pulls on the central tendon, thereby pulling the central tendon inferiorly and increasing the vertical length of the thoracic cavity.

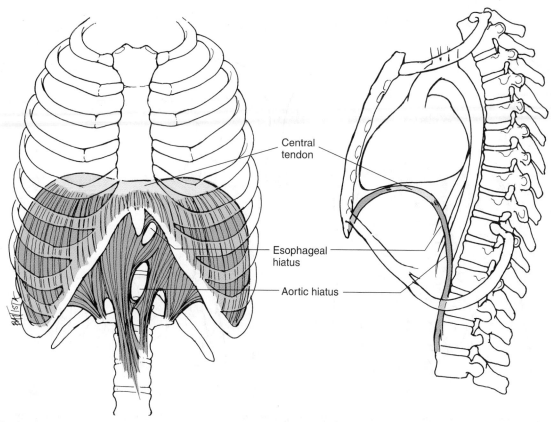

Figure 30.15: The diaphragm forms a movable floor of the thoracic cavity, attached peripherally to the sternum, lower ribs, lumbar vertebrae, and the fibrous arches surrounding the aorta and esophagus.

As the thoracic floor lowers, the volume of the abdominal cavity decreases, and abdominal pressure increases. If the abdominal wall remains relaxed, the abdominal viscera are pushed anteriorly, and the anterior–posterior diameter of the abdominal cavity increases [16]. Although the diaphragm lies deep to the lower ribs and cannot be palpated, its contraction is readily inferred by observing the movements of the abdominal contents.

The abdominal viscera limit the full descent of the diaphragm allowable by the contractile length of the diaphragm's muscle fibers. Continued contraction of the diaphragm after it reaches its maximum descent onto the viscera elevates the lower ribs, continuing to increase thoracic volume [46,58] (*Fig. 30.16*).

MUSCLE ATTACHMENT BOX 30.17

ATTACHMENT AND INNERVATION OF THE DIAPHRAGM

Attachments: The diaphragm attaches peripherally in three parts: sternal, costal, and lumbar or crural. The sternal portion attaches to the posterior surface of the xiphoid process. This attachment may be absent. The costal portion attaches to the deep surfaces of the lower six costal cartilages and ribs. The lumbar portion arises from the lumbar vertebrae and from two aponeurotic arches and the medial and lateral arcuate ligaments. The peripheral attachments converge to attach on a central tendon that has no bony attachments.

Innervation: Phrenic nerve (C3-5)

Palpation: Cannot be palpated.

Clinical Relevance

VALSALVA MANEUVER: The **Valsalva maneuver** is the sustained simultaneous elevation of thoracic and abdominal pressure and is a natural response during vigorous muscle contractions such as lifting a heavy weight or defecating. It is performed at the end of inspiration by holding the breath and contracting the abdominal muscles. At the end of inspiration, the diaphragm is contracted, which increases abdominal pressure. Simultaneous contraction of the muscles of the abdominal wall increases abdominal pressure further. At the same time, thoracic pressure is high because air fills the thoracic cavity, and the airway is closed. High thoracic pressure inhibits venous return to the heart and elevates blood pressure. It also

(continued)

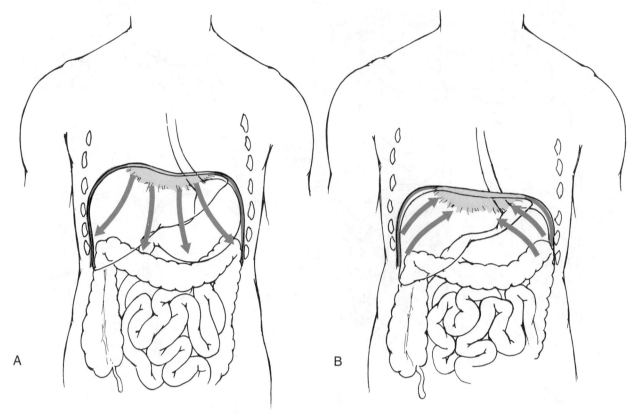

Figure 30.16: Action of the diaphragm. **A.** Contraction of the diaphragm lowers the thoracic floor. **B.** When the descent of the diaphragm is stopped by the viscera, continued contraction elevates the lower ribs.

> *(Continued)*
> *increases the resistance to blood flow to and from the lungs. These changes are dangerous in an individual with hypertension or other forms of cardiopulmonary disorders. Individuals at risk of cardiopulmonary dysfunction must be instructed to avoid the maneuver.*

IMPAIRMENT OF THE DIAPHRAGM

Weakness and or paralysis of the diaphragm can occur in individuals with high cervical spinal cord injuries (C3) who also exhibit weakness or loss of the intercostal muscles and scalenes. Such patients have profound impairment of inspiration and require at least intermittent mechanical ventilation. Weakness of the diaphragm, even with intact rib cage muscles, produces substantial impairment of the inspiratory apparatus. Isolated weakness of the diaphragm produces a paradoxical breathing pattern in which the circumference of the abdominal cavity decreases during inspiration.

MUSCLE ACTIVITY DURING RESPIRATION

The primary role of the muscles of respiration is to regulate volume of the thoracic cavity and hence to control the pressure within the cavity. Muscles of inspiration are those that increase thoracic volume, and muscles of expiration decrease thoracic volume.

Muscles of Inspiration

Although individuals exhibit variability in respiratory muscle activation, the diaphragm is the primary muscle of inspiration [14,58]. It is responsible for approximately 60% of vital capacity (the amount of inspired and expired air during maximal inspiration and expiration) and 70% of tidal volume (the volume of inspired and expired air during relaxed breathing) [14,58]. The diaphragm is not, however, the sole muscle of inspiration [8,11,16]. The intercostal muscles participate either directly to elevate or depress the ribs or indirectly to stabilize the thorax. The parasternal intercostal muscles and the scalene muscles in the cervical region also participate in relaxed inspiration, elevating the ribs in the sagittal plane as the diaphragm increases the vertical and lateral dimensions of the thorax [6,11,14]. Quiet breathing in standing relies more on rib cage movement than on abdominal excursion [11,53]. There are many additional muscles, including the sternocleidomastoid, the suprahyoids, and the pectoralis major and minor, that may be recruited with more-vigorous inspiratory efforts [11,21,22,24,32,52]. Increased respiratory challenge induces greater recruitment of the muscles that attach to the upper rib cage than of the diaphragm [5,11,37].

Muscles of Expiration

The passive recoil of the rib cage and lungs provides most of the volume reduction of the thorax necessary for quiet breathing. Activity of the diaphragm, parasternal intercostal muscles, and the scalenes continues into early expiration, contracting eccentrically to control the recoil of the rib cage [8,24]. As respiratory effort increases, however, as during a cough or sneeze, active muscle contraction facilitates the volume reduction in the thorax. Contraction of the muscles of the abdominal wall compresses the abdominal contents and depresses the ribs, pushing the diaphragm superiorly and decreasing the thoracic cavity (*Fig. 30.17*). The quadratus lumborum and the erector spinae also can depress the ribs. Shoulder muscles appear to function as either inspiratory or expiratory accessory muscles, depending upon the position and stabilization of the shoulder. Both the trapezius and latissimus dorsi are reportedly active during respiration [58].

SUMMARY

This chapter discusses the muscles of the thorax, including the muscles that support and extend the spine and those that move the ribs. The extensors of the thoracic spine include shoulder muscles as well as muscles that span the entire vertebral column. The thoracic erector spinae extend the thoracic spine but also contain segments that extend both the thoracic and lumbar regions together. The extensor muscles of the spine function primarily to control forward-bending through eccentric contractions. The superficial and deep extensor muscles also contribute to side-bending and rotation of the trunk. The deep extensor muscles of the thoracic spine are characterized by an unusually high type I muscle fiber content, consistent with a primary role in postural support.

The intrinsic muscles of the thorax are responsible for ventilation by elevating and depressing the ribs and, in the case of the diaphragm, by lengthening and shortening the vertical dimension of the thoracic cavity. Action of these muscles alters the volume of the thorax and induces inspiration or expiration. The diaphragm is the primary muscle of inspiration, but increased resistance to inspiration yields increased recruitment of intercostals, cervical, and shoulder muscles. Exhalation occurs by the passive recoil of the costal cartilages, although contraction of the abdominal muscles contributes to forced exhalation. Assessment of the muscles of the thorax must include careful observations of a patient's breathing pattern as well as an assessment of the patient's respiratory function.

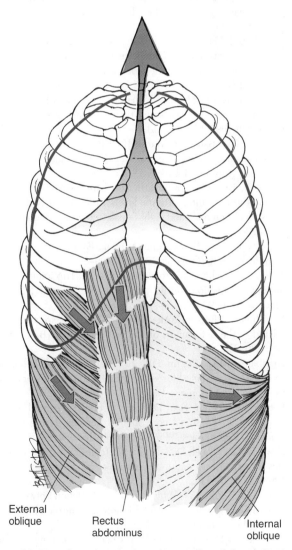

Figure 30.17: In forced expiration, the muscles of the abdominal wall compress the abdominal cavity and depress the ribs, decreasing the volume of the thoracic cavity and forcing air out.

External oblique

Rectus abdominus

Internal oblique

References

1. Bankoff MD, Moraes AC, Salve MG, et al.: Electromyographical study of the iliocostalis lumborum, longissimus thoracis and spinalis thoracis muscles in various positions and movements. Electromyogr Clin Neurophysiol 2000; 40: 345–349.
2. Basmajian JV, DeLuca CJ: Muscles Alive. Their Function Revealed by Electromyography. Baltimore: Williams & Wilkins, 1985.

3. Baydur A: Respiratory muscle strength and control of ventilation in patients with neuromuscular disease. Chest 1991; 99: 330–338.

4. Bojadsen TW, Silva ES, Rodrigues AJ, Amadio AC: Comparative study of mm. multifidi in lumbar and thoracic spine. J Electromyogr Kinesiol 2000; 10: 143–149.

5. Breslin EH, Garoutte BC, Kohlman-Carrieri V, Celli BR: Correlations between dyspnea, diaphragm and sternomastoid recruitment during inspiratory resistance breathing in normal subjects. Chest 1990; 98: 298–302.

6. Cala SJ, Kenyon CM, Lee A, et al.: Respiratory ultrasonography of human parasternal intercostal muscle in vivo. Ultrasound Med Biol 1998; 24: 313–326.

7. Clanton TL, Diaz PT: Clinical assessment of the respiratory muscles. Phys Ther 1995; 75: 983–995.

8. De Troyer A, Estenne M: Coordination between rib cage muscles and diaphragm during quiet breathing in humans. J Appl Physiol Respir Environ Exerc Physiol 1984; 57: 899–906.

9. De Troyer A, Sampson M, Sigrist S, Macklem PT: The diaphragm: two muscles. Science 1981; 213: 237–238.

10. Dolan P, Mannion A, Adams M: Passive tissues help the back muscles to generate extensor moments during lifting. J Biomech 1994; 27: 1077–1085.

11. Druz WS, Sharp JT: Activity of respiratory muscles in upright and recumbent humans. J Appl Physiol 1981; 51: 1552–1561.

12. Dumas GA, Poulin MJ, Roy B, et al.: Orientation and moment arms of some trunk muscles. Spine 1991; 16: 293–303.

13. Estenne M, Zocchi L, Ward M, Macklem PT: Chest wall motion and expiratory muscle use during phonation in normal humans. J Appl Physiol 1990; 68: 2075–2082.

14. Farkas GA, Cerny FJ, Rochester DF: Contractility of the ventilatory pump muscles. Med Sci Sports Exerc 1996; 28: 1106–1114.

15. Ford DM, Bagnall KM, McFadden KD, et al.: Paraspinal muscle imbalance in adolescent idiopathic scoliosis. Spine 1984; 9: 373–376.

16. Gilbert R, Auchincloss JH Jr, Peppi D: Relationship of rib cage and abdomen motion to diaphragm function during quiet breathing. Chest 1981; 80: 607–612.

17. Goldman MD, Mead J: Mechanical interaction between the diaphragm and rib cage. J Appl Physiol 1973; 35: 197–204.

18. Gorini M, Ginanni R, Spinelli A, et al.: Inspiratory muscle strength and respiratory drive in patients with rheumatoid arthritis. Am Rev Respir Dis 1990; 142: 289–294.

19. Gupta A: Analyses of myo-electrical silence of erectors spinae. J Biomech 2001; 34: 491–496.

20. Han JN, Gayan-Ramirez G, Dekhuijzen R, Decramer M: Respiratory function of the rib cage muscles. Eur Respir J 1993; 6: 722–728.

21. Hollowell DE, Suratt PM: Activation of masseter muscles with inspiratory resistance loading. J Appl Physiol 1989; 67: 270–275.

22. Johnson MW, Remmers JE: Accessory muscle activity during sleep in chronic obstructive pulmonary disease. J Appl Physiol Respir Environ Exerc Physiol. 1984; 57: 1011–1017.

23. Jonsson B: Electromyography of the erector spinae muscle. Med Sport 1973; 8: 294–300.

24. Kapandji IA: The Physiology of the Joints. Vol 3, The Trunk and the Vertebral Column. Edinburgh: Churchill Livingstone, 1974.

25. Kendall FP, McCreary EK, Provance PG: Muscle Testing and Function. Baltimore: Williams & Wilkins, 1993.

26. Kippers V, Parker AW: Posture related to myoelectric silence of erectores spinae during trunk flexion. Spine 1984; 9: 740–745.

27. Leong JC, Lu WW, Luk KD, Karlberg EM: Kinematics of the chest cage and spine during breathing in healthy individuals and in patients with adolescent idiopathic scoliosis. Spine 1999; 24: 1310–1315.

28. Loring SH, Woodbridge JA: Intercostal muscle action inferred from finite-element analysis. J Appl Physiol 1991; 70: 2712–2718.

29. Macintosh JE, Bogduk N: The morphology of the lumbar erector spinae. Spine 1987; 12: 658–668.

30. Macintosh JE, Bogduk N: The attachments of the lumbar erector spinae. Spine 1991; 16: 783–792.

31. Macklem PT, Gross D, Grassino A, Roussos C: Partitioning of inspiratory pressure swings between diaphragm and intercostal/accessory muscles. J Appl Physiol Respir Environ Exerc Physiol 1978; 44: 200–208.

32. Martin JG, De Troyer A: The behaviour of the abdominal muscles during inspiratory mechanical loading. Respir Physiol 1982; 50: 63–73.

33. McConnell AK, Romer LM: Respiratory muscle training in healthy humans: resolving the controversy. Int J Sports Med 2004; 25: 284–293.

34. McCool FD, Tzelepis GE: Inspiratory muscle training in the patient with neuromuscular disease. Phys Ther 1995; 75: 1006–1014.

35. McGill SM, Santaguida L, Stevens J: Measurement of the trunk musculature from T6 to L5 using MRI scans of 15 young males corrected for muscle fibre orientation. Clin Biomech 1993; 8: 171.

36. McGill S: A myoelectrically based dynamic 3-D model to predict loads on lumbar spine tissues during lateral bending. J Biomech 1992; 25: 395–414.

37. Mengeot PM, Bates JH, Martin JG: Effect of mechanical loading on displacements of chest wall during quiet breathing in humans. J Appl Physiol 1985; 58: 477–484.

38. Moga PJ, Erig M, Chaffin DB, Nussbaum MA: Torso muscle moment arms at intervertebral levels T10 through L5 from CT scans on eleven male and eight female subjects. Spine 1993; 18: 2305–2309.

39. Mooney V, Pozos R, Vleeming A, et al.: Exercise treatment for sacroiliac pain. Orthopedics 2001; 24: 29–32.

40. Nemeth G, Ekholm J, Arborelius UP, et al.: Hip joint load and muscular activation during rising exercises. Scand J Rehabil Med 1984; 16: 93–102.

41. Nudelman W, Reis ND: Anatomy of the extrinsic spinal muscles related to the deformities of scoliosis. Acta Anat (Basel) 1990; 139: 220–225.

42. Nussbaum MA, Chaffin DB, Rechtien CJ: Muscle lines-of-action affect predicted forces in optimization-based spine muscle modeling. J Biomech 1995; 28: 401–409.

43. Potten YJ, Seelen HA, Drukker J, et al.: Postural muscle responses in the spinal cord injured persons during forward reaching. Ergonomics 1999; 42: 1200–1215.

44. Powers SK, Criswell D: Adaptive strategies of respiratory muscles in response to endurance exercise. Med Sci Sports Exerc 1996; 28: 1115–1122.

45. Rimmer KP, Ford GT, Whitelaw WA: Interaction between postural and respiratory control of human intercostal muscles. J Appl Physiol 1995; 79: 1556–1561.

46. Romanes GJE: Cunningham's Textbook of Anatomy. Oxford: Oxford University Press, 1981.

47. Saumarez RC: An analysis of action of intercostal muscles in human upper rib cage. J Appl Physiol 1986; 60: 690–701.

48. Saumarez RC: An analysis of possible movements of human upper rib cage. J Appl Physiol 1986; 60: 678–689.

49. Sciaky A, Stockford J, Nixon E: Treatment of acute cardiopulmonary conditions. In: Hillegass EA, Sadowsky HS, eds. Essentials of Cardiopulmonary Physical Therapy. Philadelphia: WB Saunders, 2001; 647–676.

50. Sirca A, Kostevc V: The fibre type composition of thoracic and lumbar paravertebral muscles in man. J Anat 1985; 141: 131–137.

51. Tantucci C, Massucci M, Piperno R, et al.: Control of breathing and respiratory muscle strength in patients with multiple sclerosis. Chest 1994; 105: 1163–1170.

52. Van Der Schans CP, De Jongi W, De Vries G, et al.: Respiratory muscle activity and pulmonary function during acutely induced airways obstruction. Physiother Res Int 1997; 2: 167–194.

53. Verschakelen JA, Demedts MG: Normal thoracoabdominal motions: influence of sex, age, posture, and breath size. Am J Respir Crit Care Med 1995; 151: 399–405.

54. Weiss HR: The effect of an exercise program on vital capacity and rib mobility in patients with idiopathic scoliosis. Spine 1991; 16: 88–93.

55. Whitelaw WA, Feroah T: Patterns of intercostal muscle activity in humans. J Appl Physiol 1989; 67: 2087–2094.

56. Whitelaw WA, Ford GT, Rimmer KP, De Troyer A: Intercostal muscles are used during rotation of the thorax in humans. J Appl Physiol 1992; 72: 1940–1944.

57. Whitelaw WA, Markham DR: Electrode for selective recording of electromyograms from intercostal muscles. J Appl Physiol 1989; 67: 2125–2128.

58. Williams P, Bannister L, Berry M, et al: Gray's Anatomy, The Anatomical Basis of Medicine and Surgery, Br. ed. London: Churchill Livingstone, 1995;

59. Wilson TA, Legrand A, Gevenois P, De Troyer A: Respiratory effects of the external and internal intercostal muscles in humans. J Physiol 2001; 530: 319–330.

60. Yarom R, Robin GC: Studies on spinal and peripheral muscles from patients with scoliosis. Spine 1979; 4: 12–21.

61. Yarom R, Wolf E, Robin G: Deltoid pathology in idiopathic scoliosis. Spine. 1982; 7: 463–470.

62. Zetterberg C, Aniansson A, Grimby G: Morphology of the paravertebral muscles in adolescent idiopathic scoliosis. Spine 1983; 8: 457–462.

Loads Sustained by the Thoracic Spine

The preceding two chapters discuss the structure and function of the bones, joints, and muscles of the thoracic spine. It is well supported by ligaments, muscles, and the rib cage. Yet the thoracic spine undergoes mechanical failure when it sustains excessive loads or when the spine is weakened so that it is unable to withstand normal loads. Fractures are a common form of mechanical failure in the thoracic spine and can result from trauma that exerts excessive loads on the vertebrae. More commonly, fractures of the thoracic vertebrae are fragility fractures produced by normal loads applied to bones weakened by osteoporosis [12]. The current chapter describes the mechanical factors that play a role in compression fractures as well as in progressive kyphotic deformities of the thoracic spine. The specific objectives of this chapter are to

■ Use two-dimensional examples to calculate the in vivo forces on the thoracic spine
■ Discuss the mechanical factors that lead to compression fractures or excessive kyphotic deformities in the thoracic spine
■ Examine the strength of thoracic vertebrae

TWO-DIMENSIONAL ANALYSIS OF THE FORCES ON THE THORACIC SPINE

The normal thoracic kyphosis subjects the vertebral bodies to compressive loads. The two-dimensional examples presented in *Examining the Forces Boxes 31.1 and 31.2* demonstrate the relationship between the kyphosis and compressive loads on the vertebral bodies. In the upright posture, the superincumbent weight of the head and neck is distributed between the vertebral bodies and the columns formed by the articular processes, with more load on the bodies than on the articular processes [19] (*Fig. 31.1*). The anterior concavity of the thoracic spine places the center of gravity of the head and cervical spine anterior to much of the thoracic spine, thereby producing a flexion moment on the thoracic spine [24] (*Examining the Forces Box 31.1*) [14, 23]. The farther a thoracic vertebra is from the line of force of the head and neck weight, the greater the flexion moment on the thoracic vertebra. An increase in thoracic flexion or in the thoracic kyphosis lengthens the moment arm of the head and neck weight and increases the flexion moment on the thoracic spine.

In static equilibrium, **external moments** produced by the weight of a body segment or external load must be balanced by **internal moments** produced by muscles and ligaments. An increase in the external flexion moment on the thoracic spine resulting from an increased thoracic kyphosis is balanced by an

EXAMINING THE FORCES BOX 31.1

FLEXION MOMENTS ON THE THORACIC SPINE

External flexion moments (M_{EXT}) are exerted on the thoracic vertebrae by the superincumbent weight of the head, neck, and superior vertebrae (W_S). In normal upright posture, the flexion moment on the first thoracic vertebra (T1) is smaller than the flexion moment on the fourth thoracic vertebra (T4) because the moment arm (x) of the superincumbent weight is shorter for T1 than for T4 and because the superincumbent weight at T1 includes the head and cervical vertebrae, while the force producing a flexion moment on T4 includes the weight of the head, cervical spine, and the first three thoracic vertebrae.

$$M_{EXT} = W_s \times x$$

As the thoracic kyphosis increases, the external flexion moment on the thoracic spine increases because the moment arm (x) of the superincumbent weight increases, even though the weight (W_s) remains the same.

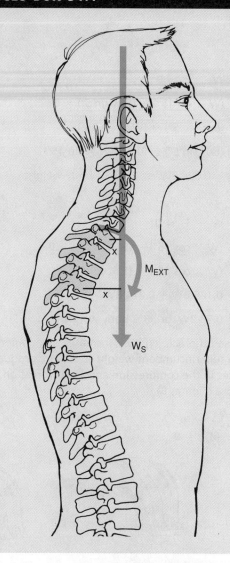

EXAMINING THE FORCES BOX 31.2

COMPRESSIVE LOADS ON A THORACIC VERTEBRA

To determine the reaction force on the fifth thoracic vertebra (T5), the extension force in the muscles and posterior ligaments (E) needed to balance the flexion moment of the weight of the head, neck, and upper thoracic vertebra (W) must first be determined (Figure, A). The following anthropometric data are based on data from the literature [2,14,21,24].

Weight of head, neck and superior vertebrae (W):	11% of body weight (BW)
Moment arm of W:	5 cm
Moment arm of the extensor muscles and ligaments:	2 cm

$\Sigma M = 0$

$M_{EXT} + M_{INT} = 0$

$(W \times 5.0 \text{ cm}) - (E \times 2.0 \text{ cm}) = 0$

$0.11 \text{ BW} \times 5.0 \text{ cm} = E \times 2.0 \text{ cm}$

E = 0.275 BW, or 27.5% of body weight

Calculate the compressive and shear forces $(J_C$ and $J_s)$ on T5. The coordinate system is placed within the vertebra so that the compressive force (J_C) is along the y axis and the shear force (J_s) is along the x axis.

(continued)

EXAMINING THE FORCES BOX 31.2 *(Continued)*

ΣF_X:

$J_S + W_X - E_X = 0$

$J_S + (W \times \sin 15°) - (E \times \sin 5°) = 0$

$J_S = (E \times \sin 5°) - (W \times \sin 15°)$

$J_S = (E \times \sin 5°) - (0.11\ BW \times \sin 15°)$

$J_S = -0.004\ BW$, or 0.4% of body weight

ΣF_Y:

$J_C - W_Y - E_Y = 0$

$J_C - (W \times \cos 15°) - (E \times \cos 5°) = 0$

$J_C = (W \times \cos 15°) + (E \times \cos 5°)$

$J_C = 0.106\ BW + 0.274\ BW$

$J_C = 0.38\ BW$, or 38% body weight

Increased thoracic kyphosis increases the moment arm of the superincumbent weight to 9.5 cm, producing changes in the compression and shear forces on the vertebra (Figure, B).

$\Sigma M = 0$

$M_{EXT} + M_{INT} = 0$

$(W \times 9.5\ cm) - (E \times 2.0\ cm) = 0$

$0.11\ BW \times 9.5\ cm = E \times 2.0\ cm$

$E = 0.5225\ BW$ or 52.25% of body weight

ΣF_X:

$J_S - E_X + W_X = 0$

$J_S - (E \times \sin 5°) + (W \times \sin 30°) = 0$

$J_S = (E \times \sin 5°) - (W \times \sin 30°)$

$J_S = 0.046\ BW - 0.055\ BW$

$J_S = -0.009\ BW$, or almost 1.0% body weight

ΣF_Y:

$J_C - W_Y - E_Y = 0$

$J_C - (W \times \cos 30°) - (E \times \cos 5°) = 0$

$J_C = (W \times \cos 30°) + (E \times \cos 5°)$

$J_C = 0.095\ BW + 0.52\ BW$

$J_C = 0.61\ BW$, or 61% body weight

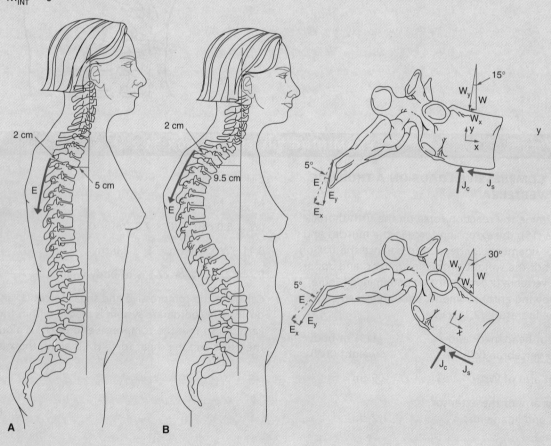

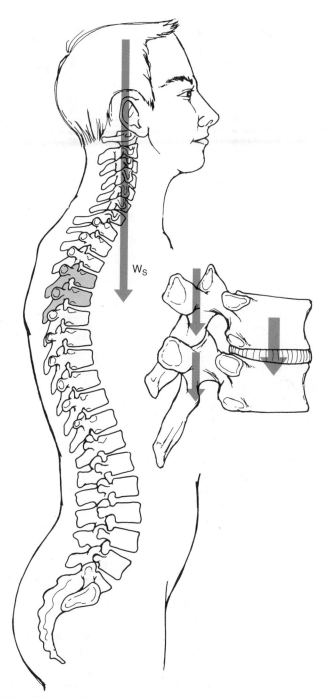

Figure 31.1: The superincumbent weight (W_S) from the head and neck is distributed between the thoracic vertebral bodies and the facet joints, with more load on the vertebral bodies.

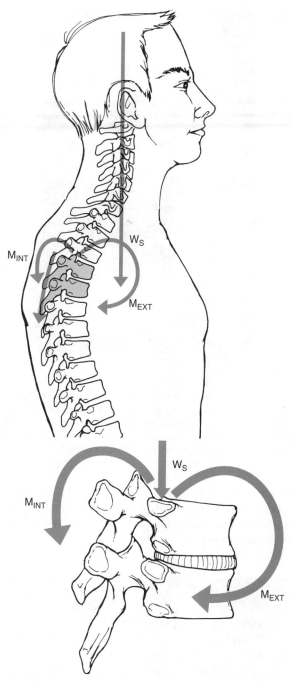

Figure 31.2: The extensor muscles and posterior ligaments apply an internal extension moment (M_{INT}) to balance the external flexion moment (M_{EXT}) applied by the superincumbent weight (W_S).

increased internal extension moment to keep the thoracic spine from flexing more (*Examining the Forces Box 31.2*). The extension moment can be exerted by extensor muscles and also by the posterior ligaments [1,7] (*Fig. 31.2*). The reaction force on the vertebral body is determined from the static equilibrium relationship, $\Sigma F = 0$. As the kyphosis increases, the external flexion moment and resulting internal

extension moment increase, producing an increased reaction force on the vertebral bodies, including the compressive component. Increased compressive forces on the vertebral bodies can lead to compressive failures. A compression failure in the thoracic region commonly occurs in the anterior portion of a vertebral body, creating a **wedge fracture.** The collapse of the anterior portion of the body of a

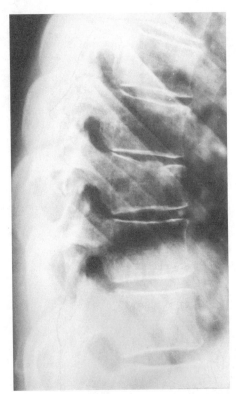

Figure 31.3: Compression fractures in the thoracic region typically occur in the anterior portion of the vertebral body and contribute to an increase in the kyphosis. (Reprinted with permission from RB Salter: Textbook of Disorders and Injuries of the Musculoskeletal System. 3rd ed. Baltimore: Williams & Wilkins, 1999.)

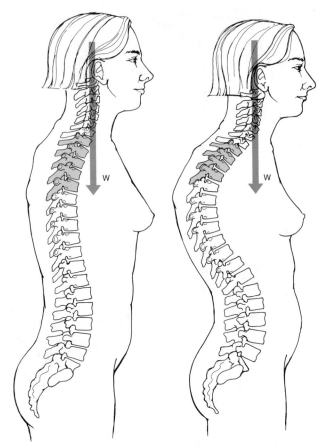

Figure 31.4: Severe thoracic kyphosis secondary to osteoporosis. Osteoporosis can produce a downwardly spiraling set of events in which the osteoporosis leads to a compression fracture that increases the thoracic kyphosis, producing an increased flexion moment and further compression failures.

thoracic vertebra increases the kyphotic deformity (*Fig. 31.3*). A wedge fracture contributes to a downward spiral of excessive kyphosis, compressive failure, increased kyphosis, and further compressive failure [4] (*Fig. 31.4*).

Clinical Relevance

COMPRESSION FRACTURES IN THE THORACIC SPINE, WEDGE AND BURST FRACTURES: *Fractures of the vertebral body in the thoracic spine result from compressive loading. When the loading is accompanied by significant flexion, the anterior portion of the body fractures, producing a* **wedge fracture.** *Large compressive forces applied to a relatively straight spine produce a* **burst fracture** *in which the endplate of the vertebral body fractures, and the nucleus pulposus is forced into the vertebral body [11,17]. Fortunately, vertebral body fractures alone in the midthoracic region rarely produce spinal cord impingement [10].*

Because wedge fractures contribute to an increased kyphosis and an increased risk of additional fractures, these fractures are sometimes treated with **kyphoplasty,** *in which an inflatable balloon is inserted into the fractured vertebral body. The insert is designed to elevate the compressed vertebral body, thereby reducing or controlling the kyphotic deformity [15].*

LOADS ON THE THORACIC SPINE

Loads on the thoracic spine are contributing factors in the failure of the thoracic vertebrae, although they are less well studied than in the cervical and lumbar regions. Knowledge of the strength of healthy thoracic vertebrae may help clinicians and scientists develop strategies to prevent thoracic fractures in the future. Most studies of the mechanical properties of the thoracic spine examine the ultimate strength of the thoracic spine in compression, since most of the failures of the thoracic spine in vivo occur under compressive loading. The **ultimate strength** of bone is the maximum load the bone can support without fracture. Studies of cadaver specimens from adults ranging in age from 26 to 98 years demonstrate increasing load to failure from the superior to inferior thoracic vertebrae [3,5,9,18]. These findings are consistent with the increase in the size of the vertebral bodies from the upper to lower thoracic spine described in Chapter 29 [16,18]. As the size and load to failure increase from the upper to the lower thoracic vertebrae, the load each vertebra bears also increases. Anther important measure of bone strength is ultimate stress, the maximum stress

(stress = load/area) sustained without failure. Ultimate stress remains relatively constant or actually decreases from the upper to the lower thoracic vertebrae [5,18]. This may help explain the increased incidence of vertebral fractures in the middle and lower thoracic regions.

The magnitude of the load to failure in the thoracic spine depends on many factors, including subject characteristics as well as characteristics of the mechanical testing procedures used in the experiments. Subject characteristics that influence the ultimate strength of the thoracic vertebrae in compression include gender, bone mineral density, and bone mineral content [3,9,18]. Although there is no known study that specifically examines the effect of age on the strength of thoracic vertebrae, it follows that since bone mineral content and bone mineral density decrease with age, failure strength of thoracic vertebrae also decreases with age.

Testing procedures have a significant influence on the determination of ultimate strength of thoracic bone. Chapter 2 describes the effect that loading rate can have on the mechanical properties of materials, and this is borne out in the thoracic spine, where tests reported in the literature vary in loading rates from approximately 0.1 mm/sec to almost 1000 mm/sec [3,9,18]. Position of the spine during loading also affects the strength of the spine [13]. Consequently, there is no single value of bone strength for the thoracic spine (or any other biological tissue, for that matter). The clinician can use the literature to obtain a general concept of the range of strength in thoracic vertebrae and to recognize the clinically relevant factors that influence strength.

Reported loads to failure applied at slow loading rates in the upper thoracic region are on the order of approximately 2600 N (approximately 600 lb) [3,9,18]. However, in a study of cadavers of elderly subjects (aged 46–98 years), failure loads as low as 613 N (138 lbs) are reported [3]. At higher loading rates, upper thoracic vertebrae exhibit ultimate loads of 3000–4500 N (675–1000 lb) in the same region [3,9]. Slowly applied loads to failure in the lower thoracic spine range from 4000 to 5000 N (approximately 900–1100 lb) [3,9]. Failure loads of approximately 8500 N (almost 2 tons) are reported in the lower thoracic spine during rapidly applied loading [9]. These data demonstrate the increased strength of the lower thoracic vertebrae. They also reveal that bone strength, as measured by ultimate failure loads, increases with increased loading rates, consistent with the **viscoelastic** nature of bone.

Bone mineral content and bone mineral density are correlated with bone strength [3,18]. These relationships help explain the increase in ultimate strength in the lower thoracic spine where the vertebrae are larger. These correlations also help explain the greater bone strength in men than in women, since men, on average, have larger bones. In fact, research suggests that **ultimate stress** (force/area) in the thoracic spine is similar in men and women [5]. Finally, these relationships are particularly useful in explaining the increase in incidence of vertebral fractures identified in postmenopausal women who undergo accelerated loss of bone mass at menopause [8,10].

Clinical Relevance

SPONTANEOUS VERTEBRAL FRACTURES: *Individuals reach peak bone mass in their mid-20s. After reaching their peak bone mass, premenopausal women begin to lose approximately 0.3% of their bone mass per year.*

Menopausal and postmenopausal women experience accelerated bone loss during menopause and for approximately the next 5 or 10 years, losing approximately 2% of bone mass yearly, although later in life bone loss slows again. Individuals with extremely low body weight and body mass index (BMI) also experience accelerated rates of bone loss [6,25]. The sustained increased rate of bone loss leads to a cumulative loss that drastically alters the ultimate strength of bone [22]. Osteoporosis is defined as bone mass more than 2.5 standard deviations below peak bone mass [10,22]. Postmenopausal women are most likely to be affected by osteoporosis; however, younger women with a very low BMI, such as highly trained athletes or women with eating disorders such as anorexia nervosa, also are at increased risk of osteoporosis [20,25].

Individuals with osteoporosis are at risk for vertebral fractures and may report a sudden sharp pain in the midback, perhaps following a sneeze but often with no precipitating event at all. Some individuals may deny any discomfort but report an increase in a midback hump or a loss of standing height. These clinical findings are consistent with a spontaneous fracture of one or more thoracic vertebrae. A precipitating event such as a sneeze produces a large flexion moment that cannot be sustained by the thoracic vertebrae weakened by loss of bone mass. In the presence of severe osteoporosis, the superincumbent weight in an individual with an excessive kyphosis may be sufficient to produce a fracture with no precipitating event.

SUMMARY

This chapter presents two-dimensional models to demonstrate the mechanical factors that contribute to fractures of the thoracic spine. The bodies of the thoracic vertebrae are predisposed to high loads because of the normally occurring thoracic kyphosis. Although thoracic vertebrae can sustain compressive loads of several hundred pounds or more before failure, fractures of thoracic vertebrae occur as the result of excessive loads or, more commonly, from normal loads applied to weakened thoracic vertebrae. As the thoracic kyphosis increases, the flexion moment applied by the weight of the head and neck increases, producing larger compressive loads on the vertebral bodies, which may result in fracture. The presence of osteoporosis is a primary factor that precipitates a cascade of events producing a downward spiral: kyphotic deformity, increased load, fracture, increased deformity, and increased load.

References

1. Basmajian JV, DeLuca CJ: Muscles Alive. Their Function Revealed by Electromyography. Baltimore: Williams & Wilkins, 1985.

2. Braune W, Fischer O: Center of gravity of the human body. In: Krogman WM, Johnston FE, eds. Human Mechanics; Four Monographs Abridged AMRL-TDR-63-123. Wright-Patterson Air Force Base, Ohio: Behavioral Sciences Laboratory, 6570th Aerospace Medical Research Laboratories, Aerospace Medical Division, Air Force Systems Command, 1963; 1–57.

3. Burklein D, Lochmuller EM, Kuhn V, et al.: Correlation of thoracic and lumbar vertebral failure loads with in situ vs. ex situ dual energy x-ray absorptiometry. J Biomech 2001; 34:579–587.

4. Chew F, Maldjian C, Leffler SG: Musculoskeletal Imaging: A Teaching File. Philadelphia: Lippincott Williams & Wilkins, 1999.

5. Eckstein F, Fischbeck M, Kuhn V, et al.: Determinants and heterogeneity of mechanical competence throughout the thoracolumbar spine of elderly women and men. Bone 2004; 35: 364–374.

6. Grinspoon S, Thomas E, Pitts S, et al.: Prevalence and predictive factors for regional osteopenia in women with anorexia nervosa. Ann Intern Med 2000; 133: 790–794.

7. Gupta A: Analyses of myo-electrical silence of erectors spinae. J Biomech 2001; 34: 491–496.

8. Harma M, Heliovaara M, Aromaa A, Knekt P: Thoracic spine compression fractures in Finland. Clin Orthop 1986; 205: 188-195.

9. Kazarian L, Graves GA Jr: Compressive strength characteristics of the human vertebral centrum. Spine 1977; 2: 1–14.

10. Lane J, Russell L, Khan S: Osteoporosis. Clin Orthop 2000; 372: 139–150.

11. Leventhal MR: Fractures, dislocations, and fracture-dislocations of spine. In: Canale ST, ed. Campbell's Operative Orthopaedics. St. Louis: Mosby, 1998; 2704–2790.

12. Melton LJI: Epidemiology of spinal osteoporosis. Spine 1997; 22: 2S–11S.

13. Panjabi MM, Oxland TR, Kifune M, et al.: Validity of the three-column theory of thoracolumbar fractures. A biomechanic investigation. Spine 1995; 20: 1122–1127.

14. Pearsall DJ, Reid JG, Livingston LA: Segmental inertial parameters of the human trunk as determined from computed tomography. Ann Biomed Eng 1996; 24: 198–210.

15. Pradhan BB, Bae HW, Kropf MA, et al.: Kyphoplasty reduction of osteoporotic vertebral compression fractures: correction of local kyphosis versus overall sagittal alignment. Spine 2006; 31: 435–441.

16. Resnick DK, Weller SJ, Benzel EC: Biomechanics of the thoracolumbar spine. Neurosurg Clin North Am 1997; 8: 455–469.

17. Salter RB: Textbook of Disorders and Injuries of the Musculoskeletal System. 3rd ed. Baltimore: Williams & Wilkins, 1999;

18. Singer K, Edmondston S, Day R, et al.: Prediction of thoracic and lumbar vertebral body compressive strength: correlations with mineral density and vertebral region. Bone 1995; 17: 167–174.

19. Toh E, Yerby SA, Bay BK, et al.: The effect of anterior osteophytes and flexural position on thoracic trabecular strain. Spine 2001; 26: 22–26.

20. Treasure J, Serpell L: Research and treatment in eating disorders. Psychiatr Clin North Am 2001; 24: 359–370.

21. Vasavada AN, Li S, Delp SL: Influence of muscle morphometry and moment arms on the moment-generating capacity of human neck muscles. Spine 1998; 23: 412–422.

22. Watts NB: Osteoporotic vertebral fractures. Neurosurg Focus 2001; 10: 1–6.

23. White AA III, Panjabi MM: Practical biomechanics of scoliosis and kyphosis. In: Cooke DB, ed. Clinical Biomechanics of the Spine. Philadelphia: JB Lippincott, 1990; 127–163.

24. White AA III, Panjabi MM, Thomas CL: The clinical biomechanics of kyphotic deformities. Clin Orthop 1977; 128: 8–17.

25. Zipfel S, Seibel MJ, Löwe B, et al.: Osteoporosis in eating disorders: A follow-up study of patients with anorexia and bulimia nervosa. J Clin Endocrinol Metab 1986; 86: 5227–5233.

Structure and Function of the Bones and Joints of the Lumbar Spine

PAUL F. BEATTIE, P.T., PH.D.

T he lumbar spine functions as a complex interplay of musculoskeletal and neurovascular structures creating a mobile, yet stable, transition between the thorax and pelvis. The lumbar region repetitively sustains enormous loads throughout one's lifetime, while still providing the mobility necessary to allow a person to perform myriad tasks associated with daily living. In addition, the lumbar spine provides the fibro-osseous pathway for the inferior portion of the spinal cord, the cauda equina and lumbosacral spinal nerves traveling to and from the trunk and lower extremities. Considering the magnitude and complexity of these functional demands, it is not surprising that the low back is a common site of dysfunction, with low back pain syndromes representing the most frequent musculoskeletal problem encountered by health care professions [16,17,26]. The high prevalence of this condition and the enormous variability of its clinical manifestations create a challenge when studying spinal motion or when diagnosing sources of low back pain.

The purpose of this chapter is to describe the bony structures of the lumbar spine as well as its joint components and to relate these to the spine's functional demands of stability, mobility, and protection of neurovascular elements. Emphasis is placed upon the clinical significance of various structures as they relate to trauma and degeneration.

The specific objectives of this chapter are to

- Describe and discuss the bony geometry and other unique morphology of the lumbar vertebrae
- Describe the structure and unique biomechanical functions of the lumbar spinal ligaments, facet joints, intervertebral discs (IVDs), and intervertebral joints
- Identify and define spinal gross and segmental motions
- Compare various methods of lumbar motion assessment
- Relate the objectives above to commonly observed clinical conditions

STRUCTURE OF THE BONES AND LIGAMENTS OF THE LUMBAR SPINE

General Overview of the Osteocartilaginous Lumbar Spine

The human spine acts as a multisegmental, flexible rod forming the central axis of the neck and trunk. The normal bony spine consists of 24 presacral vertebrae that combine to form the three major curves on the sagittal plane. Lordotic curves (apex anterior) are present in the lumbar and cervical spines, with a kyphotic curve (apex posterior) present in the thoracic spine. These curves help to enhance the repetitive load-bearing capacity of the spine by providing "flex," or damping function. The junctions between these curves are areas of great force concentration and are called *transitional zones (Fig. 32.1)*. These zones are frequent sites of tissue injury resulting in dysfunction and nociception. For example, in the lumbar spine the junction between L5 and S1 (lumbosacral joint) is a very common site of pain complaint [19]. Vertebrae near and within transitional zones have unique characteristics and are referred to as *atypical vertebrae.*

Interposed between the vertebrae are the fibrocartilaginous IVDs, the principle component of the intervertebral joints. These symphysis-type joints create a flexible interspace to maintain the vertical length of the lumbar spine and permit three-dimensional displacement [23]. Posteriorly, articular processes projecting from adjacent vertebrae join to form the paired facet or apophyseal joints. These synovial joints act to guide and restrict the directions of motion available at different segmental levels [13,19]. Conceptually, the intervertebral joints and the paired facet joints act to form the motion segment, or "articular tripod" [53], in which these three joints function as a closed chain system, i.e., displacement of one joint requires a specific displacement of the other two joints *(Fig. 32.2A)*. Consider the spine, therefore, to be a series of links (segmental levels) of three joint systems helping to fill the lumbar spine's demands of mobility and stability *(Fig. 32.2B)*.

In addition to the mechanical demands of mobility and stability, each motion segment forms three important

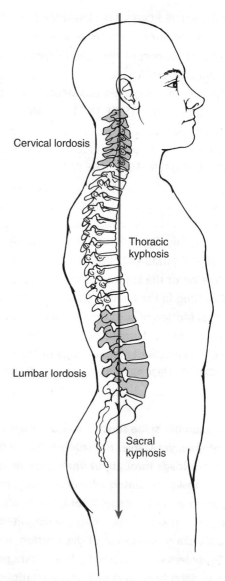

Cervical lordosis

Thoracic kyphosis

Lumbar lordosis

Sacral kyphosis

Figure 32.1: Sagittal view of the entire spine. Note the anteriorly convex lumbar and cervical lordosis and the posteriorly convex thoracic kyphosis. A plumb line dropped through the center of the spine transects the transitional zones.

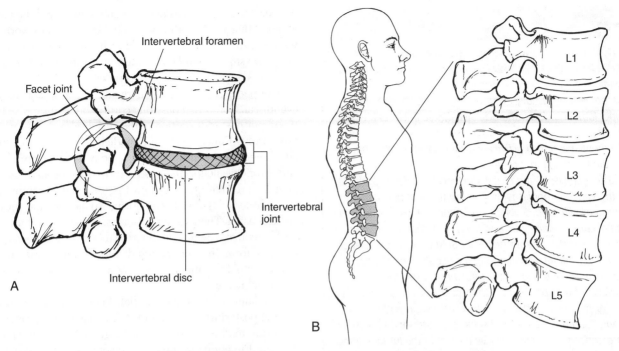

Figure 32.2: A. Lateral view of two adjacent vertebrae and the interposed intervertebral disc. This system, along with associated soft tissues, is referred to as a *lumbar motion segment*. Note the intervertebral joint anteriorly and the paired facet joints posteriorly. **B.** When the motion segments are joined, a complex multijoint system is formed.

fibro-osseous canals to house and protect the important neurovascular elements of the lumbar spine. The vertebral foramen is formed within the center of the vertebrae, and the paired intervertebral foramina are formed laterally between adjacent vertebrae.

The osseous lumbar spine comprises five vertebrae (L1-5). Occasionally, the junction between the first and second sacral vertebrae fails to fuse, creating a condition known as *lumbarization*. This results in six mobile lumbar vertebrae. In some cases, the lumbosacral junction fuses during growth and development, resulting in *sacralization* of L5. This results in only four mobile lumbar vertebrae. While the mechanical influence of these anatomical variations is uncertain, it is important to note that neither lumbarization nor sacralization appears to increase the risk of low back pain [72].

Anatomically, each vertebra consists of a large, cylindrical vertebral body anteriorly, with a bony ring or "neural arch" posteriorly (*Fig. 32.3*). The vertebral bodies, along with the IVDs, provide the vertical dimension (length) of the lumbar spine and sustain most of the compressive loading [13,23,46]. The neural arch forms a protective bony ring around the neural elements of the lumbar region while providing numerous bony projections or processes that serve to form the surfaces of the facet joints or act as sites of attachment for spinal muscles and ligaments. The neural arch, along with the IVDs, sustains most of the torsional load bearing acting on the lumbar spine [13,59].

VERTEBRAL BODIES

The vertebral bodies are primarily composed of well-vascularized cancellous bone. Roughly cylindrical, they narrow slightly in their midsection to create a shape similar to an "hourglass" [13]. This unique biconcave arrangement provides a deep passageway for neurovascular structures along the midportion of the vertebral body and, coupled with the vertical and transverse arrangement of the bony trabeculae, creates a system that is well designed to tolerate compressive loads. For example, in upright postures the vertebral bodies of the lumbar spine assume 80–90% of the compressive load bearing [13,23]. This capacity is further enhanced by an abundance of potential spaces within the cancellous bone that are occupied by blood and hematopoietic tissues helping to reinforce the bony trabeculae by occupying the empty spaces. Interestingly, the "reinforced scaffolding" created by the alignment of the bony trabeculae lacks a substantial number of obliquely orientated trabeculae, which results in a poor capacity of the lumbar vertebrae to tolerate rotational stresses. In situ, this is compensated for by the IVDs and posterior bony structures as well as by muscular support.

At their superior and inferior margins, the lumbar vertebral bodies widen slightly and are covered by the cartilaginous **vertebral endplates.** This widening corresponds to the epiphyseal ring and forms the site of the strong peripheral attachments of the IVD. The vertical dimension of the lumbar vertebral bodies is higher anteriorly, forming a slight wedge shape that results in adjacent vertebrae forming a natural lordotic curve. Consistent with the rest of the spine, the vertebral bodies become progressively larger from superior (L1) to inferior (L5) as a function of progressively increasing load demands from rostral to caudal.

NEURAL ARCH

The neural arch is a bony ring spanning posteriorly from the vertebral bodies. It consists of the paired pedicles that bind the vertebral bodies and neural arch together and the paired laminae that enclose the posterior portion of the vertebral foramen. Arising from the neural arch are seven bony projections: two superior and inferior articular processes, two transverse processes, and one spinous process.

The pedicles in the lumbar region are stout and roughly cylindrical. Composed of strong cortical bone, they arise from the upper posterior portion of the vertebral body and project posteriorly. Functionally, the pedicles are the only bony attachment between the vertebral body and the neural arch and strongly anchor these structures to one another. The pedicles are often called upon to sustain high compressive and tensile loads that occur during spinal rotation, flexion, and extension. Their strong, tubular shape and amount of cortical bone make them well suited to this task. Additionally, the pedicles form the superior and inferior boundaries of the intervertebral foramina, providing a reinforced pathway for the spinal nerves.

The laminae are relatively flat, blade-shaped bones that project posteriorly from lateral to medial, converging at the posterior midline of the trunk to give rise to the spinous process. Functionally, the laminae act primarily as a posterior bony boundary of the neural arch. While having less load-bearing demand than the pedicles, they are responsible for shunting forces between the spinous processes and the articular processes, as may occur with forceful lumbar rotation [13]. Recognizing this, spinal surgeons use great care to

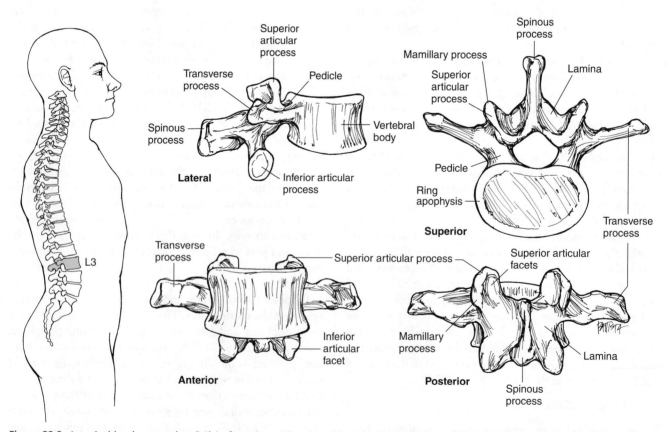

Figure 32.3: A typical lumbar vertebra (L3) in four views. The views identify all of the relevant landmarks of a typical lumbar vertebra.

minimize removal of laminae (laminectomy) during posterior-approach spinal surgery.

Arising from the junction of the posterior pedicles and lateral laminae are the important superior and inferior articular processes. These processes articulate with the opposite articular processes from adjacent vertebrae (i.e., a superior articular process articulates with the inferior articular process of the vertebra above it). The superior articular process is the larger of the two articular processes. It projects upward, providing an articular surface on its medial aspect, thus forming the outer bony component of the facet joint. The thick bone of the superior articular process is critical in resisting lumbar rotation and, by doing so, protecting the IVD from excessive torsional stress [13]. The inferior articular process projects downward and provides an articular surface on its lateral side. As it "nests" into the vertebra below, it forms the inner portion of the facet in a manner similar to two paper cups being placed one into the other.

As noted in the cervical and thoracic regions, the orientation of the articular processes as they form the facet joint is critical to understanding the directions in which a motion segment is able to displace and thus is critical to the understanding of spinal motion [13,19,50,60]. In the lumbar spine, the facet joint planes lie roughly parallel to the sagittal plane; thus movements in this plane (flexion and extension) have larger excursions than movements in the transverse plane (lumbar rotation) or frontal plane (lumbar side-bending) [50,69]. It is important to note, however, that anatomical variation in the facet joint planes is common. For example, the facet joint plane on one side of a vertebra may be orientated more obliquely than the facet joint plane on the opposite side, leading to asymmetrical side-bending or rotation [19,77].

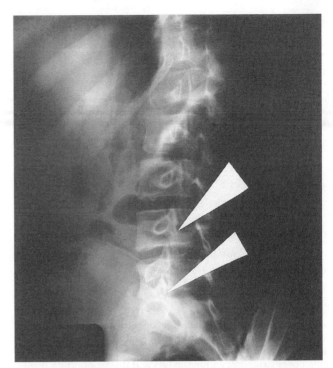

Figure 32.4: An oblique view radiograph of the lumbar spine reveals a normal pars interarticularis *(upper arrow)* and a fractured pars interarticularis (i.e., spondylolysis) *(lower arrow)*.

Clinical Relevance

SPONDYLOLYSIS: *Between the superior and inferior articular processes is a relatively flat isthmus of bone known as the **pars interarticularis**. Clinically, this area is of great importance, as it is often the site of bone failure during excessive or repetitive lumbar extension and/or rotation. Fractures in this area are called spondylolysis and are visible on plane film oblique radiographs (Fig. 32.4). Occasionally, stress fractures can occur in this area that are not easily detectable radiographically. These are extremely common in young gymnasts and springboard divers. In some cases, bilateral spondylolysis can occur. This can result in anterior slippage of the lumbar vertebra known as spondylolisthesis [2,41].*

The spinous and transverse processes have no joint surfaces but serve a very important function as "outriggers" for the attachment of muscles, ligaments, and fascia. The spinous processes in the lumbar spine are relatively thick, with a quadrangular shape. Their posterior tips are easily palpable and are on the same transverse plane as the vertebral body. Along its superior and inferior surface, the spinous process is the point of attachment of the interspinous ligament, and posteriorly it provides an enhanced moment arm for the attachment of the thoracolumbar fascia (TLF) and the multifidus muscle [74,77].

The transverse processes are long and flat. The widest transverse processes (an important radiographic landmark) are found on the third lumbar vertebra and the thickest are part of the fifth lumbar vertebra. Several structures that provide stability in the frontal plane have attachments to the transverse processes, including the quadratus lumborum muscle, fibers from the TLF, and the iliolumbar ligaments (L4-5).

VERTEBRAL FORAMINA

Of critical importance are the three fibro-osseous passageways within the bony lumbar spine. Located centrally is the vertebral foramen, while the paired intervertebral foramina are positioned laterally. The vertebral foramen is typically triangular, bordered anteriorly by the posterior aspects of the vertebral body and IVD, laterally by the pedicle, and posteriorly by the lamina and ligamentum flavum. When considering the lumbar spine as an entire unit, the vertebral foramina and associated soft tissues form the spinal or vertebral canal. In the upper lumbar spine this canal is oval and contains the conus medullaris, the lower portion of the spinal cord. Progressing inferiorly, the canal becomes wider and flatter while containing the cauda equina [15]. The lateral portions

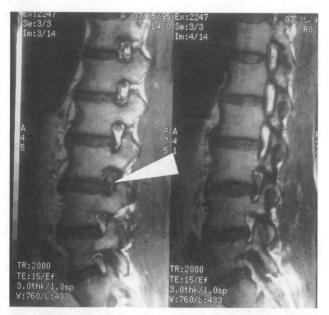

Figure 32.5: Parasagittal lumbar magnetic resonance image of the intervertebral foramen (IVF) of a lumbar motion segment. Note the oblong shape. In situ the spinal nerve roots (seen as small gray structures within the IVF) and their supporting tissues travel through the superior portion of the IVF and thus are a considerable distance from the IVD. At the L3-4 level, a disc herniation encroaches upon the intervertebral foramen but does not compress the spinal nerve (arrow).

of the vertebral foramen just medial to the intervertebral foramen are known as the **lateral recesses** and are a common location for nerve entrapment by disc herniation [9].

The intervertebral foramina are bordered anteriorly by the posterior aspects of the vertebral bodies and anulus fibrosus. The pedicles form the superior and inferior borders, while posteriorly the ligamentum flavum and anterior portion of the facet joint capsule complete the perimeter (*Fig. 32.5*).

In the normal lumbar spine the ratios between the size of the vertebral foramen and the size of the nerves is quite large, providing, in the normal state, ample room for the neural and vascular structures within the vertebral foramina [9,15]. Representative values are reported by Dommisse [15], who describes the anterior–posterior (AP) diameter at L1 level as approximately 16 mm and the transverse diameter as approximately 21 mm, with the neural contents approximately 10 mm. At the L3 level, the canal becomes flatter and wider (AP, 15 mm; transverse, 22 mm), and at the S1 level, it narrows slightly, with an AP diameter of approximately 13 mm and a transverse diameter of approximately 30 mm.

Of great interest is the change in the shape and diameter of the vertebral and intervertebral foramina during spinal motion and how these changes influence the neural structures. The theoretical basis behind many spinal treatments relates to relieving nerve compression by lumbar movement [40,41,73]. In normal subjects, there is an approximately 10%

increase in the area of the vertebral foramen during flexion and a 10% decrease during extension [13].

Clinical Relevance

SPINAL STENOSIS: *Spinal stenosis is a narrowing of the vertebral foramina. Persons with spinal stenosis typically find positions of lumbar flexion more comfortable than positions of extension. This clinical finding is consistent with the data that show an increase in the vertebral foramina with flexion. This increased space reduces compression on the neural structures [2,41].*

Panjabi et al. [49] compare the size and shape of the intervertebral foramina in normal and degenerative motion segments (i.e., two adjacent vertebra). The authors report a 20% decrease in the area during lumbar extension and a 30% increase during lumbar flexion. Hasue [22] and Mayoux-Benhamou [38] describe the intervertebral foramen as pear-shaped in flexion and triangular in extension.

Despite the changes in shape and area, the ratio between the intervertebral foramen and the nerve root remains quite large, so that nerve root compression rarely occurs in the intervertebral foramen of the lumbar spine. In a recent study, only 4 of 408 subjects with presumed nerve compression had evidence of compression in the intervertebral foramen [9]. However, a very large number of these individuals demonstrated compression in the lateral portion of the vertebral foramen, the area known as the lateral recess.

Ligamentous Support of the Lumbar Spine

The lumbar spine contains a very complex ligament system that provides a critical component of its mobility and stability characteristics. On gross inspection, the ligaments are intermeshed with fascia, tendinous attachments of muscle, and, in some cases, the outer portion of the IVD [13,77]. The lumbar ligaments may be classified as extrasegmental (anterior longitudinal, posterior longitudinal, and supraspinous), segmental ligaments (ligamentum flavum, interspinous, and intertransverse) or regional (iliolumbar) (*Fig. 32.6*).

A primary function of the lumbar ligaments is to provide a restraint for motion. Biomechanically, the spinal ligaments, with the exception of the ligamentum flavum, are relatively inelastic and exhibit a **viscoelastic** response, or time-dependent elongation, to loading [13]. (See Chapter 2 for a more detailed discussion of viscoelasticity.) By identifying the location of a ligament and the direction of its fibers, one may hypothesize the motions that a given ligament resists. For example, those ligaments posterior to the axis of rotation of a motion segment: posterior longitudinal, interspinous, ligamentum flavum, and supraspinous ligament are restraints

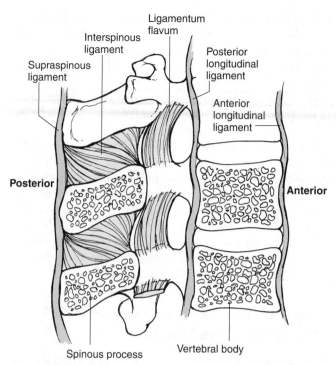

Figure 32.6: Midsagittal view of the lumbar spine demonstrates the spinal ligament system.

against flexion, while the anterior longitudinal ligament restrains extension (*Table 32.1*) [13,77].

The anterior longitudinal ligament is a large, broad band that spans the anterior portion of the vertebral bodies and anulus fibrosus. It is strongly anchored to the anterior sacrum and is a strong reinforcing tissue against anterior displacement of the IVD [13]. The posterior longitudinal ligament spans the posterior aspect of the vertebral bodies. It is characteristically hourglass shaped, with the widest portion covering the posterior, but not posterior lateral, portions of the IVD. The interspinous ligament runs between the spinous process, while the supraspinous ligament travels from the posterior tips of the spinous processes. These two ligaments help to provide posterior stability for the motion segment [20].

TABLE 32.1: Displacements Opposed by Lumbar Ligaments

Ligament	Displacements Resisted
Anterior longitudinal	Vertical separation of anterior vertebral bodies (e.g., lumbar extension, anterior bowing of the lumbar spine)
Posterior longitudinal	Separation of posterior vertebral bodies
Supraspinous	Separation of the spinous process
Ligamentum flavum	Separation of the laminae
Interspinous	Separation of posterior vertebral bodies, i.e. lumbar flexion, posterior translation of superior vertebral bodies
Intertransverse	Separation of transverse processes
Iliolumbar	Flexion, extension, rotation, and lateral bending

Unique among the lumbar ligaments is the ligamentum flavum. This ligament travels between adjacent laminae anteriorly and blends with the anterior portion of the facet joint capsule. In so doing, it forms the posterior aspect of the vertebral foramen. Characterized by its yellow color, this ligament contains large amounts of the elastic protein known as **elastin**. Approximately 80% of its mass is elastin. Unlike other ligaments, the ligamentum flavum can be passively elongated to 40% of its resting length without tissue failure. This elasticity allows the ligamentum flavum to tolerate the large displacements between adjacent laminae during lumbar flexion and yet not buckle and displace into the vertebral foramen during lumbar extension [13].

The iliolumbar ligament is a series of bands that run from the transverse processes of L5 to the ilium. Basadonna et al. [4] describe it as having an anterior band traveling from the anterior–inferior–lateral part of the transverse process and widening to attach on the anterior part of the iliac tuberosity. Additionally, a posterior band arises from the apex of the transverse process and attaches superior to the anterior band. Because of its central location at the lumbosacral joint it acts to resist flexion, extension, rotation, and lateral bending. Sprain of this ligament, especially the weak posterior band, has been hypothesized as a common cause of low back pain.

While traditional beliefs have classified lumbar ligaments as the primary stabilizers of the spine, the actual role of these structures may be more complex. Work by Lucas and Bresler [33] indicates that the spine, without muscular support, buckles under only 2 kg of loading, implying that ligaments provide only a small portion of the stability necessary for the spine. Others confirm that the stress–strain characteristics of the spinal ligaments provide minimal support to spinal stability during normal lumbar motion (see Chapters 33 and 34).

What then is the primary role of the lumbar ligament system? Close inspection reveals that the lumbar ligaments are blended and interconnected with many other structures such as deep and superficial fascia as well as tendon and muscle fibers. Histological studies identify large densities of sensory end-organs, including free nerve endings and mechanoreceptors [12,28,54,78]. This observation has led authors [62] to postulate that the ligament system may be a major part of a reflex arc, with the lumbar muscles providing important information regarding the position of the motion segment, which in turn influences lumbar muscle tension. Examining this hypothesis on animal models and a small sample of patients, Solomonow et al. report that a primary reflex arc exists between the mechanoreceptors in the supraspinous ligament and the multifidus muscle [62]. When the supraspinous ligament is loaded, the multifidus muscle contracts to increase the stiffness in the motion segment. The magnitude of contraction increases as the load increases, implying a protective mechanism. The authors postulate that similar arcs exist from the other spinal ligaments as well as the IVD and the facet joint capsule. This fascinating theory supports the importance of interplay of the fibro-osseous and neuromuscular structures in the normal function of the spine.

Thoracolumbar Fascia

The TLF is a complex array of dense connective tissue covering the lumbar region. It interconnects with an extraordinary number of bony and soft tissue structures while providing critical support to the spine during lumbar flexion and lifting activities [18,74]. Anatomically it consists of three layers (*Fig. 32.7*). The anterior and middle layers arise from the transverse processes of the lumbar vertebrae and join together laterally, encompassing the quadratus lumborum while blending with the fascia of the transversus abdominis and internal oblique abdominis muscles. This creates a direct connection between the bony spine and the deep abdominal muscles and appears to be an important relationship for the dynamic stabilization of the lumbar spine. The large posterior layer of the TLF arises from the spinous processes of the thoracic, lumbar, and sacral vertebrae and covers the erector spinae muscles. Laterally, it blends with the latissimus dorsi muscle, and inferiorly it blends with the gluteus maximus muscle, thus forming a direct connection between the proximal humerus (the distal attachment of the latissimus dorsi) and proximal femur (distal attachment of the gluteus maximus muscle).

To conceptualize one of the important functions of the TLF, imagine being in the position of lumbar forward-bending, with the hips and knees slightly flexed, while pulling an object toward you. This requires activity of the gluteus maximus, lumbar erector spinae, abdominal muscles, and latissimus dorsi, all of which have central attachments to the TLF. The TLF is then strongly tensed, providing stability to the posterior aspect of the lumbar spine as it reinforces the posterior ligaments and muscular system [18,74].

Palpable Bony and Ligamentous Structures of the Lumbar Spine

Palpation of the bony structures of the lumbar spine is a vital component of the physical examination. Palpation can assist in identifying the segmental level of pain [35] and may provide general information about the mobility of a given motion segment [67].

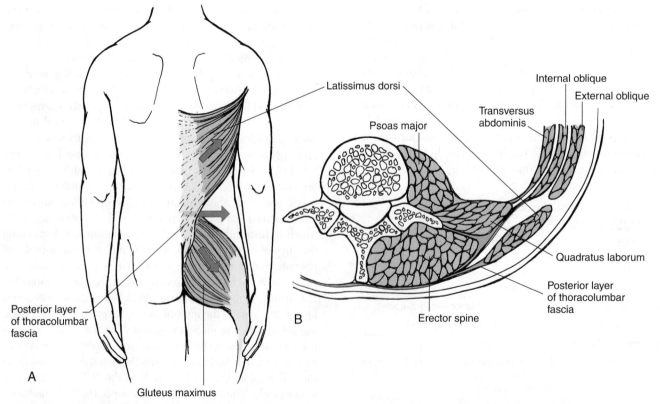

Figure 32.7: A. Posterior view of the TLF. Note how various muscles act to exert tension on this structure, thus providing dynamic stability to the low back. **B.** Axial (transverse) view of the posterior lumbar spine shows the layers and attachments of the TLF.

The only bony structures that can be easily palpated in the lumbar spine are the spinous processes. Clinically, a useful technique for this is to use the radial surface of the index finger to identify the iliac crests in a standing or prone patient. If the examiner brings his or her thumbs directly toward the midline, they intersect roughly at the level of the L4-5 interspace. The spinous process below is that of L5, while that above is L4. A second technique is to palpate the inferior surfaces of the posterior superior iliac spines (PSISs). This corresponds to the S2 level. After identifying the spinous process of L5, the remaining lumbar vertebrae can be determined by counting the spinous processes. The interspace between the spinous processes is occupied by the supraspinous and interspinous ligaments and the TLF.

STRUCTURE OF THE JOINTS OF THE LUMBAR SPINE

The joint system of the lumbar spine comprises the large symphysis joint (the intervertebral joint) anteriorly and the paired synovial joints (the facet or apophyseal joints) posteriorly.

These three joints form an anatomically unique three-joint complex [29], or "articular tripod" [53]. This joint system forms the basis of dynamic stability, allowing the spine to tolerate loads while traveling through an arc of motion.

Facet Joints

The paired facet joints of the lumbar spine are located posteriorly but are intimate with the vertebral and intervertebral foramina. These unique joints are formed by the inferior articular processes of the vertebrae above "nesting" into the superior articular process of the vertebrae below (*Fig. 32.8*). Because of their flat appearance, the facet joints are classed as planar joints. However, upon closer inspection, the articular surfaces are typically J-shaped, with the lower portion or hook of the "J" being most anterior [13]. The facet joints have a unique joint capsule. As with all synovial joints, the capsule is lined with synovium and covered by a layer of dense ordinary connective tissue. The capsule attaches just beyond the periphery of the joint surfaces. Inferiorly and superiorly, the capsule tends to bow outward away from the joint surface, creating a redundancy. This

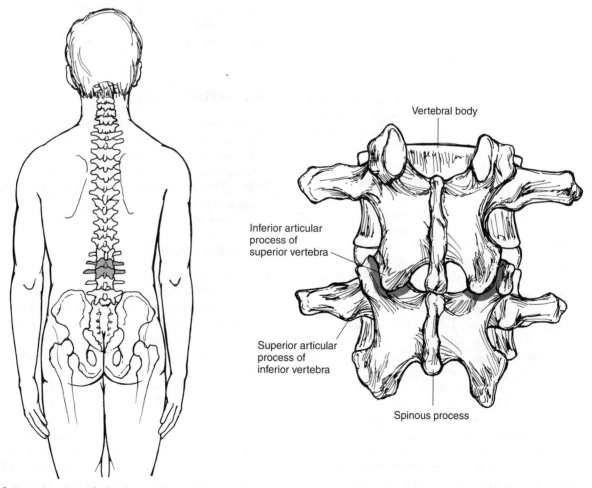

Figure 32.8: Posterior view of a lumbar motion segment illustrates the bony components of the lumbar facet joints. Note how the inferior articular processes of the superior segment "nest" into the superior articular processes of the inferior segment.

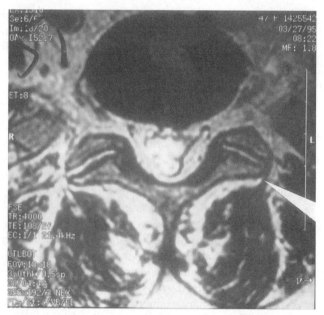

Figure 32.9: An axial view MRI demonstrates the attachment of the lumbar multifidus muscle to the facet joint capsule *(arrow)*.

appears to allow extra "joint play," increasing the magnitude of joint motion [67]. Overall, however, the redundancy is not large, since the capacity for fluid within the facet joint is only approximately 2 mL [24]. Interestingly, the ligamentum flavum attaches to the anterior–superior portion of the capsule and exerts tension during lumbar flexion. The multifidus muscle sends fibers to attach on the superior–posterior portion of the capsule and exerts tension when active concentrically during lumbar extension or eccentrically during lumbar flexion (*Fig. 32.9*).

As previously stated, a primary function of the facet joint is to guide segmental motion. This is a function of the direction of the facet planes. The general direction of the facet planes in the lumbar spine is parallel to the sagittal plane; thus the lumbar spine flexes and extends through a large arc of motion, while rotation and side-bending are much less.

The facet joints also serve other important roles in the load bearing of the lumbar spine. They act to resist anterior shear forces and, along with the IVD, resist torsion [59]. Additionally, the facet joints play a role in resisting compressive forces. During upright posture, approximately 18–20% of the compressive load acting upon the lumbar spine is exerted at the facets [13]. This value, however, varies as a function of the position of the center of gravity of the head, arms, and trunk. With increased lordosis, the center of gravity shifts posteriorly, producing an extension moment on the lumbar spine and increasing the load on the lumbar facets. A decreased lordosis shifts the center of gravity of the head, arms, and trunk anteriorly and shifts the load to the vertebral bodies and intervertebral joints [30,46,58].

Intervertebral Joint

The intervertebral, or interbody, joint is a symphysis-type articulation that joins two adjacent vertebral bodies. Its primary components are the superior and inferior surfaces of the vertebral bodies, the vertebral endplates, and the IVD (*Fig. 32.10*) [23,31]. The intervertebral joint serves the critical function of providing a mechanism for motion and load bearing between the vertebrae.

VERTEBRAL ENDPLATE

The vertebral endplate is a flat structure composed of hyaline and fibrocartilage that is approximately 0.6–1.0 mm thick [13]. Located within the inner margin of the epiphyseal rings on the superior and inferior surfaces of the vertebral bodies, the endplate acts as a boundary between the IVD and vertebra [23]. In certain places, the subchondral bone deep to the endplate is thin or absent, creating a portal for tissue fluid to travel between the bone marrow and the IVD. This is an important consideration in understanding the nutrition of the largely avascular IVD. The endplate is more strongly bound to the disc than to the vertebral body; thus certain types of trauma can tear the endplate away from the bone [1]. Additionally, the vertebral endplate may be fractured following rapidly applied compression loads to the spine such as those sustained when a person slips and falls on the ischial tuberosities. Although usually quite painful, these fractures may not be easily visible on

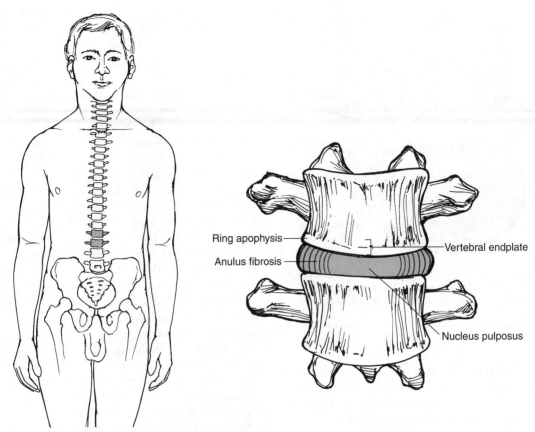

Figure 32.10: The lumbar intervertebral joint consists of the IVD, the vertebral endplate, and the ring apophysis.

radiographs and may require further investigation using magnetic resonance imaging or bone scan procedures.

INTERVERTEBRAL DISC

The IVD is an extraordinary structure that is the central figure in spinal mechanics and pathology [1,6,31,40,42]. It is typically described as consisting of an outer fibrous covering, the anulus fibrosus, and an inner gel-like region known as the nucleus pulposus [13,23,24]. This distinction between the nucleus pulposus and the anulus fibrosus often is used to describe disc biomechanics; however, in vivo these are neither independent nor isolated structures [7,23,24]. The nuclear zone actually develops as a transition from a lesser hydrated area in the periphery to a more highly hydrated central region [7,27]. This distinction becomes less apparent with disc degeneration. For clarity, however, the current discussion describes the anulus fibrosus and the nucleus pulposus as separate structures.

Anulus Fibrosus

The anulus fibrosus is predominately composed of rings of fibrocartilage forming the outer portion of the IVD. Taylor describes the typical lumbar anulus fibrosus as consisting of between 10 and 20 layers of collagen fibers that are obliquely oriented to one another [66]. This plywood-like system forms a strong surrounding band of tissue to protect and isolate the nucleus pulposus while tolerating high-magnitude tensile loads [13,23]. Strong attachments exist between the anulus fibrosus and the outer portion of the vertebral bodies and vertebral endplates as well as with the anterior longitudinal ligament.

When viewed on the transverse plane, the IVD is not circular but rather has a noticeable concavity in its central, posterior portion (*Fig. 32.11*) [13]. This concavity increases the amount of anulus fibrosus material posteriorly to resist the flexion loads common in daily activities. The posterior longitudinal ligament also reinforces the posterior anulus; however, the posterior–lateral portion of the anulus is not as well reinforced. This contributes to the predominance of posterior and posterior–lateral disc herniations [9,41].

In addition to its capacity for load bearing, recent work demonstrates an abundance of mechanoreceptors and free nerve endings in the outer layer of the anulus, suggesting an important role in proprioception as well as in pain production [29,41,62]. A recent surgical development, anuloplasty, thermally denervates the outer anulus in an attempt to control pain. The efficacy of this procedure is not currently known.

Nucleus Pulposus

The nucleus pulposus represents the inner portion of the IVD. Histologically, the nucleus pulposus is a mucopolysaccharide

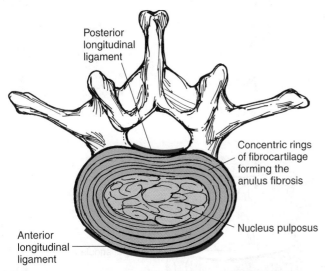

Figure 32.11: Axial view of the lumbar IVD. Note the posterior concavity and the close relationships of the anterior and posterior longitudinal ligaments to the anterior and posterior anulus fibrosus.

gel that is approximately 70–90% water, although this water concentration typically decreases with aging. The dry weight of the nucleus pulposus is composed of 65% proteoglycans, approximately 20% of which is collagen, with the rest being elastic fibers and various proteins [13,23,27]. These structures aggregate to form a relatively soft, gel-like substance that interfaces with the anulus fibrosus to provide a hydraulic load-bearing system [70,76]. Because it is more hydrated than the anulus fibrosus, the nucleus pulposus of the IVD is clearly visible on T2-weighted magnetic resonance images (*Fig. 32.12*) [3,6,9,10].

Its hydrophilic capacity, (i.e., its ability to bind water) is critical to the function of the IVD [13,23,70,71]. Consider that with the exception of the very periphery of the anulus fibrosus, the IVD is avascular [13]. Such avascularity is necessary because if this structure relied upon arterial flow, sustained compression such as occurs during upright activities would impede blood flow and lead to ischemia. Thus the disc maintains its hydration by diffusion of tissue fluid, mediated by mechanical forces and osmotic gradients. To clarify this, Urban et al. [70,71] describe the fluid content of the disc as a balance of the hydrostatic and osmotic pressures. Hydrostatic pressures are created by the external loads acting upon the disc, such as those from muscle and ligamentous tension. Osmotic pressures are generated within the disc by proteoglycan molecules that have water-binding properties. Thus cyclic loading in the presence of a normal concentration of proteoglycans within the IVD creates a series of events that move tissue fluid in and out of the disc. Considering the numerous variations in a person's posture from one moment to the next and, therefore, changing loads over a 24-hour period, one can see that the disc is constantly changing its shape and fluid content. An interesting and clinically relevant application of this process relates to diurnal variations in the fluid content of the disc. During loading, the disc initially adapts by slight movements in the collagen fibers; however with sustained loading, fluid is lost from the disc [70,71], resulting in a loss of vertical dimension. During periods of reduced loading, such as recumbency while sleeping, the osmotic gradient is greater, and fluid travels back into the disc. This explains why persons are taller (sometimes up to 2 cm!) in the early morning than in the evening. This phenomenon is exaggerated by exposure to weightless environments during space travel.

Clinical Relevance

THE FLUID CONTENT OF THE IVD AND ITS RELATIONSHIP TO LOW BACK PAIN: *Because of the great importance of maintaining adequate hydration of the disc, factors that adversely influence this may lead to disc degeneration and spinal dysfunction. For example, the synthesis of proteoglycans may be impaired by smoking or during prolonged immobilization [47]. Exposure to vibration also has been postulated to cause this.*

Considering the diurnal variations in the disc, Snook et al. [61] describe a randomized clinical trial on persons with chronic low back pain. Noting that most lifting injuries to the low back occurred in the morning, the authors postulated that flexion avoidance in the morning might help to reduce pain. In their study, one group of persons with low back pain avoided early morning lumbar flexion and had much better outcomes than a second group that performed stretching exercises in the early morning. The authors suggest that the elevated disc fluid volume early in the morning predisposed the disc to injury during lumbar flexion. This is an intriguing finding and may have implications for instruction to patients performing exercises for low back pain.

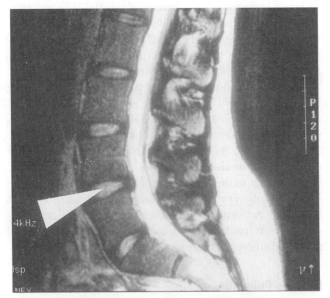

Figure 32.12: Midsagittal T2-weighted lumbar MRI. Note the high (*white*) signal from the region of the nucleus pulposus (*arrow*) and the low (*dark*) signal from the anular region.

MECHANICAL PROPERTIES OF THE IVD

Humzah provides an appropriate description of the IVD, referring to it as a "flexible interspace" between the vertebrae [23]. The IVD's extraordinary ability to absorb and transmit forces is accomplished by developing a hydraulic effect during loading [13,30,70,76]. The IVD allows joint displacement to occur by maintaining a separation between the vertebral bodies (i.e., acting as a "spacer") and by being capable of deformation in all planes of motion. The uniqueness of the mechanics of the IVD, coupled with its central role in the generation of low back pain, make it one of the most highly investigated musculoskeletal tissues. To understand the mechanical properties of the IVD, it is first important to consider the external forces to which it is subjected. The basic external stresses acting upon the IVD can be classified as compression and tension, bending and rotation.

Compression

External forces that tend to approximate the vertebral bodies exert compressive loads on the IVD. In general, the disc tolerates these loads by converting vertically applied compression into circumferentially applied tension by a phenomenon known as **hoop stress** (*Fig. 32.13*) [41,53,76]. **Pascal's law** states that pressure applied to a liquid is distributed equally in all directions. As the compressive load is applied, pressure within the nucleus pulposus increases, but because water is incompressible, the nucleus pulposus in turn exerts pressure against the surrounding anulus fibrosus through a process

known as **radial expansion.** The anulus fibrosus then resists this load through tension developed in its collagen fibers. The nucleus pulposus also exerts pressure against the superior and inferior vertebral endplates, thus serving to transmit part of the load from one vertebra to the next. Enormous loads can be tolerated in this fashion. Because of their association with the vertebral body, the endplates do not deform unless large-magnitude, damaging forces are applied.

Bogduk and Twomey [13] describe a second property of the disc as the ability to store energy during loading and to recoil elastically once the load is released. This mechanism is critical to the load-bearing capacity of the motion segment and the ability of trabecular bone in the vertebral body to function as a shock absorber. This hypothesis is supported by recent work that shows the presence of elastic fibers in the anulus fibrosus and nucleus pulposus, implying a dynamic flexibility to the IVD and the capacity for viscoelastic behavior [24,27].

The normal disc, therefore, functions hydrostatically, with internal pressures increasing in relation to externally applied forces. With dehydration or surgical excision of the nucleus pulposus, the capacity of the IVD to tolerate compressive loads is altered. Short applications of light compressive loads to denucleated discs can be tolerated by the anulus fibrosus alone; however, higher forces or prolonged application of forces are problematic because of the inability of the disc to develop internal fluid pressure and transform the compressive load to radial forces on the anulus fibrosus [76]. This leads to excessive loading on the vertebral bodies, which often results in further degenerative changes.

Bending

The behavior of the IVD during bending motions, such as occur with many of activities of daily living, is of great interest both as a mechanism to understand tissue injury and as a strategy for exercise prescription. Consider that the nucleus pulposus is not a rigid sphere but is capable of deformation in three directions. In 1935, Steindler [63] postulated that the nucleus pulposus deforms in the direction opposite to the motion during sagittal or frontal plane motions, so that during lumbar extension, the nucleus pulposus displaces anteriorly and vice versa. This theory has been confirmed in several studies using cadaveric material and living subjects, supporting the notion of the intact nucleus pulposus functioning as a ball bearing during spinal motion [56,76] (*Fig. 32.14*).

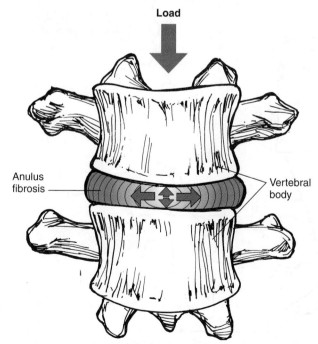

Figure 32.13: An example of the "hoop stress" created within the IVD during compressive load bearing. Compressive loading on the nucleus pulposus causes it to exert radial stresses on the anulus fibrosus.

Load

Anulus fibrosis

Vertebral body

Clinical Relevance

DEFORMATION OF THE NUCLEUS PULPOSUS AS A BASIS FOR BACK EXERCISES: *The deformation of the nucleus pulposus during lumbar motion forms the basis for the repeated prone press-up exercises advocated by McKenzie [40]. McKenzie's hypothesis is that as a patient flexes his or her lumbar spine, the nucleus pulposus*

(continued)

(Continued)

displaces posteriorly, while during lumbar extension, it displaces anteriorly, away from the pain-sensitive structures in the vertebral and intervertebral foramina. Thus exercises and postures are prescribed to influence the position of the IVD. Both discography and magnetic resonance imaging demonstrate this phenomenon in normal discs [7,56]. Thus during lumbar bending, a normal nucleus pulposus deforms in a direction opposite that of the applied load.

It is important to realize, however, that the nucleus pulposus is deforming, not actually displacing or moving across bone, during lumbar motions. As previously stated, the nucleus pulposus is not a discrete structure, but actually represents an area of the disc with greater hydration than the periphery [23]. Dehydration of the discs leads to an even less clear distinction between the nucleus and anulus. Interestingly, in discs with evidence of degeneration or herniation, the nucleus pulposus has been shown to have an inconsistent pattern of deformation [7]. This may explain why certain patients with disc pathology have symptom enhancement with lumbar extension and others do not. White and Panjabi [76] point out that during

bending, the anulus fibrosus is compressed on the side to which the subject bends. For example, the posterior portion of the IVD is compressed during extension but is exposed to tensile loading on the opposite side (Fig. 32.15). Therefore, with lumbar extension, a posterior bulging of the anulus fibrosus and nucleus pulposus may be present, especially in patients with degenerative IVDs. The clinical significance of this is unknown.

Rotation

While well suited to withstand compressive loads, the disc is much less able to tolerate torsional (rotational) forces. During torsional stress on the IVD, the anulus fibrosus is loaded in tension. Recall, however, that the anulus fibrosus is a series of obliquely arranged fibers; thus during rotation of a vertebral body, a portion of these fibers is not under tension [13] (*Fig. 32.16*). Therefore, only a portion of the anulus fibrosus is able to resist a torsional stress. Fortunately for the lumbar spine, the sagittal plane arrangement of the facet joints in this region limits rotation and thus protects against these forces. This protective mechanism is significantly reduced when the spine

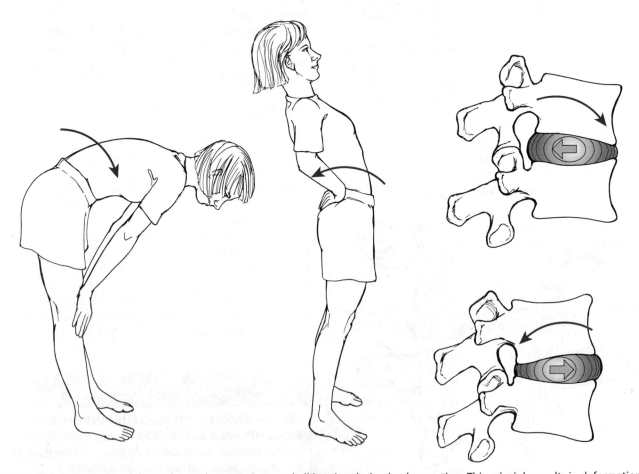

Figure 32.14: The concept of the nucleus pulposus acting as a ball bearing during lumbar motion. This principle results in deformation of the nucleus in the direction opposite the motion. During lumbar flexion, the nucleus pulposus tends to deform posteriorly; in lumbar extension, the nucleus pulposus tends to deform anteriorly.

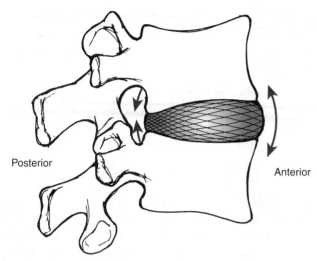

Figure 32.15: As an individual bends backward, the posterior aspect of the IVD sustains compressive forces while the anterior aspect of the disc undergoes tensile loading.

is in flexion [13,19]; thus a common mechanism of disc injury is combined rotational and forward-bending movements [1,40,51,61].

IVD Pressures during Activities of Daily Living

Of great interest clinically is the effect of various activities and postures on the intradiscal pressure. While this mechanism

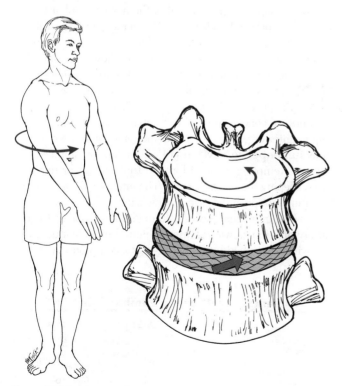

Figure 32.16: Stress on the fibers of the anulus fibrosus during lumbar rotation. The criss-cross arrangement of the collagen fibers results in only a portion of the fibers being loaded.

has been studied extensively [1,2,30,46,58], the classic work was reported by Nachemson et al. [46]. Using a pressure sensor inserted into the nucleus pulposus of the L3 disc, these authors demonstrated a linear relationship between intradiscal pressure and the moment acting upon the disc. The moment is the product of the superincumbent load, including the mass of the head, arms, and trunk plus anything being lifted or carried, and the length of the moment arm of the superincumbent load.

Activities that increase intradiscal pressure often involve lumbar flexion from the upright position and/or increased trunk muscle activity. For example, Nachemson reports that lying supine results in 250 N (56 lb) of intradiscal pressure, which increases to 500 N (112 lb) when standing erect [46]. Forward-bending 40°, which increases the moment arm of the superincumbent weight, raises the pressure to 1000 N (224 lb). Lifting 100 N (22.5 lb), which increases the superincumbent mass, elevates the pressure to 1700 N (382 lb), and holding 50 N (11 lb) at arm's length, increasing both the moment arm and the superincumbent mass, raises the pressure to 1900 N (427 lb). Coughing (which requires contraction of the trunk muscles) increases the pressure to 700 N (157 lb). Clinically, increases in symptoms during forward-bending, lifting, or coughing are common findings in persons with IVD pathology.

When sitting in an unsupported position and thus reducing the normal lumbar lordosis, intradiscal pressure rises to 700 N (200 N, or 45 lb, greater than standing). This decreases to 400 N (90 lb) when the lumbar spine is supported. Considering this, it is not surprising that persons with symptomatic herniated lumbar IVDs have increased symptoms when sitting, which is often considered to be light duty! Use of a lumbar roll to maintain a normal lumbar lordosis and thus reduce intradiscal pressure is often a very useful intervention for persons with discogenic low back pain [40].

Clinical Relevance

THE INTERVERTEBRAL DISC AS A SOURCE OF SYMPTOMS OF LOW BACK PAIN: *Disorders of the IVD are one of the most common sources of low back symptoms and lumbar nerve root compression. Numerous hypotheses have been proposed. The three primary ways in which an abnormal IVD may cause symptoms are (a) direct injury to the pain-sensitive outer portion of the anulus fibrosus, (b) a herniated disc in which nuclear material breaks through its boundaries created by the anulus fibrosus and causes mechanical pressure and chemical irritation of the pain-sensitive structures in the vertebral foramina, and (c) a degenerative disc that loses vertical dimension and causes the vertebrae to approximate one another, leading to a reduction in the stability of the segment.*

(continued)

(Continued)

Interestingly, not all herniated discs cause symptoms, and most degenerative discs do not. Numerous factors such as the ratio of disc abnormality to the size of the vertebral canal [9], the degree of instability at the motion segment [29], and various biochemical issues [41,47] must also be considered. This lack of linearity between pathology and symptoms makes the evaluation and treatment of persons with low back pain extremely challenging [5,9].

TABLE 32.2: Gross Motions of the Lumbar Spine Based upon Cardinal Planes

Motion	Cardinal Plane
Flexion (forward-bending)	Sagittal
Extension (backward-bending)	Sagittal
Side or lateral bending	Frontal
Rotation	Transverse

MOTION OF THE LUMBAR SPINE

Motion occurring at the lumbar spine is critical to a person's ability to perform the numerous tasks of daily living. Lumbar motion can range from very small displacements providing a "damping effect" during loading to very large arcs of motion that occur with bending and reaching tasks. Abnormalities of lumbar motion can manifest themselves as various combinations of reduced, excessive, or poorly timed joint displacements. These abnormalities are a primary source of symptoms and often lead to tissue degeneration through repetitive, abnormal loading. In the clinical environment, accurate assessment of impairment of lumbar motion and its relationship to a person's symptoms and functional limitations is a critical component of the assessment process. In this section, the motion of the lumbar spine is discussed from a variety of perspectives, including gross motions, osteo- and arthrokinematics, and clinical measurement.

Gross Motion of the Lumbar Spine

When considering the lumbar spine as an entire unit, motions traditionally are described using cardinal planes as a reference (*Table 32.2*). This system is quite useful as a classification of joint displacement, as it provides a conceptual framework for lumbar ROM by creating common reference points. It is important to note, however, that under the conditions of loading associated with daily activities, the lumbar spine is nearly always undergoing multidirectional displacement. In fact, at the level of the joint surface, pure single-plane movement may not exist [19].

When determining the nature of gross motions of the lumbar spine, the plane of the facet joints dictates the directions

of displacement possible. For example, the sagittal plane alignment of the lumbar facet joints favors flexion and extension but greatly limits rotation. The height of the IVD acts to maintain the alignment of the joint surfaces as well as tension on the segmental ligaments. The vertical dimension of the IVD space also is related to the available motion at a given motion segment, since the deformation of the disc contributes to the motion between adjacent vertebrae. In the lumbar spine, the normal disc spaces are larger than those of the thoracic spine. This contributes to the relatively large arc of motion that is possible in the lumbar spine. With disc space narrowing such as occurs with disc degeneration, changes in the positional relationships of the vertebrae to one another can adversely affect joint mechanics [7,29,41,76].

LUMBAR FLEXION

Lumbar flexion (forward-bending) is achieved by a "flattening" or perhaps a slight reversal of the normal lumbar lordosis. When a person bends forward from the standing position, segments are recruited from rostral to caudal (i.e., the upper lumbar segments move into flexion first followed by the middle then lower segments) [13]. Lumbar flexion is limited by tension in the posterior anulus fibrosus and the posterior ligament system (*Table 32.3*).

A critical concept related to lumbar flexion is its relationship to anterior pelvic rotation, a phenomenon often referred to as **lumbopelvic rhythm** [14]. This concept applies to a person attempting to bend forward to touch his or her toes while keeping the knees straight. The interplay between lumbar spine motion and pelvic motion is integral to understanding how an individual moves. Although there appears to be a variety of lumbopelvic rhythms exhibited by individuals, the following, described by Calliet [14], is a commonly reported

TABLE 32.3: General Trends for Angular Displacement at the Segmental Levels of the Lumbar Spine (in°)

	L1-2	L2-3	L3-4	L4-5	L5-S1	Total
Flexion	6–8	7–10	7–12	8–13	7–9	35–52
Extension	4–5	3–5	1–6	2–7	5–6	15–29
Side bending	3–6	3–6	5–6	4–5	1–2	16–25
Rotation	1–4	1–3	1–3	1–3	1–3	5–16

Data from Grieve GP: Common Vertebral Joint Problems. New York: Churchill-Livingstone, 1981 and Pearcy M, Portek I, Shepherd J: Three dimensional x-ray analysis of normal movement in the lumbar spine. Spine 1984; 9: 294–297.

sequence of lumbar spine and pelvic movement. Initially the trunk inclines forward as the lumbar lordosis flattens. Once full lumbar flexion is achieved, the additional forward inclination of the trunk occurs from the pelvis rotating anteriorly upon the hip joints. The forward rotation of the trunk is in turn typically limited by tension in the hamstring muscles. Thus a person's ability to touch his or her toes relies upon pelvic rotation and extensible hamstring muscles, as well as the ROM of lumbar flexion.

Clinical Relevance

THE RELATIONSHIP OF INEXTENSIBLE HAMSTRING MUSCLES TO LOW BACK PAIN: *The concept of lumbo-pelvic rhythm illustrates the potential relationship of inextensible hamstring muscles to excessive flexion forces on the lumbar spine during forward-bending. For example, if a patient has inextensible hamstring muscles, forward rotation of the pelvis when standing may be prematurely restricted. In an attempt to reach forward and down, a person may try to compensate for this by increasing the amount of lumbar flexion, often causing injury to the posterior lumbar structures. Stretching the hamstring muscles, therefore, is often a critical portion of treatment for low back pain.*

LUMBAR EXTENSION

Lumbar extension, or backward-bending, occurs in a similar, but opposite manner to lumbar flexion (i.e., it is an increase in the lumbar lordosis). The overall magnitude of lumbar extension is much less than that of lumbar flexion because of the unique bony geometry of the lumbar vertebrae. As the lumbar spine extends from a normal lordosis, the spinous processes approach one another, and tension in the anterior longitudinal ligament restricts motion.

The relationship of pelvic displacement to lumbar extension is also limited. In the standing position, posterior pelvic rotation is limited by the tension in the iliolumbar ligaments and the hip flexor muscles that restrict hip extension and, therefore, pelvic rotation. Clinically, inextensible hip flexor muscles can act to hold the pelvis in anterior rotation, which in turn increases the lumbar lordosis, especially when a person attempts to extend the hip. The resulting excessive lumbar extension places increased loads on the posterior elements of the lumbar spine and may be associated with symptoms and tissue degeneration.

Another commonly observed clinical phenomenon relates to how a person returns to the upright position from a position of forward-bending. Typically, a person initially rotates the pelvis posteriorly, followed by a return to the normal lumbar lordosis. Occasionally, one may initially arch the back to regain the lumbar lordosis while flexing the hip and knees and "walking" the hands up the thighs. This abnormal lumbopelvic rhythm may indicate some lumbar spine segmental instability [41].

LUMBAR ROTATION AND SIDE-BENDING

Lumbar rotation, or twisting, as previously described, is potentially deleterious to the IVDs if it is excessive. Because of the roughly sagittal plane alignment of the facet joints, the transverse plane motion of rotation is quite restricted in the lumbar spine, limited by the approximation of the facet joint surfaces. Anatomically, the facet joints surfaces at L5–S1 tend to have a more oblique arrangement than the other segments of the lumbar spine. Because of this, authors have proposed that more lumbar rotation occurs at this segment than in the other segments of the lumbar spine [19,76]. Recent findings by Pearcy et al. [50] have contested this. The mechanics of the lumbosacral junction are discussed in greater detail in Chapter 35.

Despite the very limited degree of lumbar rotation, most persons are able to compensate by achieving a relatively large arc of total trunk and neck rotation. For example, the amount of total rotation necessary to back up one's car is provided by the contributing motions of the thoracic and cervical spine.

Lumbar side-bending in the lumbar spine, displacement in the frontal plane, has a larger ROM than rotation but substantially less than the sagittal plane motions [50,65,68]. The amplitude of motion appears relatively evenly distributed over all segments except L5–S1, which is quite restricted by bony geometry and tension from the iliolumbar ligament [4]. Side-bending cannot occur without some lumbar rotation (and vice versa) because of the phenomenon known as **joint coupling.** Joint coupling occurs when two motions are linked together so that one cannot occur without the other.

Joint Coupling in the Lumbar Spine

In the discussion above, lumbar motion is described from a "neutral" starting point. This neutral position can be considered a normal lumbar lordosis with no appreciable rotation or side-bending. In most activities of daily living, the spine moves in and out of a neutral position. How does this change the nature of spinal motion? Interestingly, lumbar rotation and side-bending depend upon one another (i.e., their motions are "coupled"). The degree of coupling is determined primarily by two factors: the direction of the articular processes acts to guide specific displacements at the joint surface, and the position of the spine determines the relative tension on various soft tissue structures [19]. For example, in the neutral position, rotation is limited by approximation of the articular processes and by tension in the anulus fibrosus and posterior longitudinal ligaments [19,20]. Lumbar flexion and extension reduce the available range of side-bending and rotation, while the position of side-bending reduces the available range of flexion and extension. When the lumbar spine is in a position of side-bending, rotation is greater to the opposite side (toward the convexity) than to the same side (toward the concavity). Thus, when the lumbar spine is in flexion, side-bending and rotation occur to the same side (e.g., left rotation is accompanied by left side-bending). When the lumbar spine is in a neutral or extended position, side-bending and rotation occur opposite one another (e.g., left rotation is accompanied by right side-bending) [19].

Segmental Motion of the Lumbar Spine

The preceding section describes motions that encompass the entire lumbar spine. Movement between adjacent vertebrae is also described. It is important for the clinician to clarify which motions are being discussed. Movement occurring at a single motion segment is called **segmental motion,** while gross motion of the entire lumbar spine is a multisegmental phenomenon.

To understand the complexity of spinal motion, it is important to recall that the stability and mobility of the lumbar spine result from an interplay of the bony elements and their associated joint structures under the guidance of an elegant neuromuscular control system. As stated in Chapter 7, joint motion is described in terms of **osteokinematics** (displacement of a bone) and **arthrokinematics** (displacement occurring at specific joint surfaces). The combination of these two events allows a joint to move through a given ROM. As opposed to joints of the appendicular skeleton, such as the hip, where a small number of relatively large bones move around a single axis, spinal motion occurs as a result of numerous small bones moving around several axes. Conceptually, the elbow joint can be viewed as a lever pumping up and down, while the lumbar spine moves like an accordion opening and closing.

The multijoint system of the lumbar spine serves beautifully to absorb and attenuate forces and to make the myriad of finely tuned adjustments required of the spine during activities of daily living. It makes, however, the quantification of spinal motion difficult. Each motion segment has the potential to displace through angular (rotary) and linear (translatory) motion in each of the three planes. This produces 6 degrees of freedom. Because each displacement can occur in opposite directions (e.g., anterior and posterior translation in the sagittal plane), a motion segment has a total of 12 possible movements (2 types of motion in 2 directions in 3 planes) (*Table 32.4*).

Segmental motion of the spine occurs at the three-joint complex of the motion segment or vertebral unit, which is composed of two adjacent vertebrae and the tissues included within them. The plane of its facet joints and the height of the IVD influence the movements of a motion segment.

TABLE 32.4: The Twelve Motions of a Lumbar Motion Segment

Axis of Movement	Type of Movement
Sagittal	Anterior and posterior translation Anterior and posterior rotation
Frontal	Left and right translation Left and right side rotation
Transverse	Distraction and compression Left and right rotation

SEGMENTAL MOTION IN THE SAGITTAL PLANE

Because of the roughly sagittal plane alignment of the articular processes in the lumbar spine, segmental motion in the sagittal plane, grossly described as flexion and extension, is the closest to occurring in a single plane of motion. During flexion, each lumbar vertebra displaces by rotating in an anterior direction. This is coupled with a slight anterior translation, so that the facet joint surfaces of the inferior articular processes of the superior vertebra slide superiorly, reducing contact between the joint surfaces and allowing a slight anterior translation to occur [13,59,60]. This anterior displacement is limited by the bony geometry of the facet joints [31], while the tension in the posterior anulus fibrosus and posterior ligament system resist anterior rotation.

At the joint surfaces, extension occurs in a manner similar to lumbar flexion; however, the unique bony geometry of the lumbar vertebrae acts to restrict lumbar extension to a much smaller ROM than lumbar flexion [19,50]. During extension, the lumbar vertebrae rotate posteriorly accompanied by a small posterior translation. As the superior articular processes slide inferiorly during extension, the spinous processes of adjacent vertebrae impact upon one another to restrict extension. Further lumbar extension is limited by the approximation of the articular processes and spinous processes [13].

Clinical Relevance

FLEXION VERSUS EXTENSION EXERCISES: *With increasing flexion, compressive load bearing is shifted anteriorly away from the facet joints and the posterior IVD while increasing the area of the vertebral foramen [49]. With increasing extension, compressive load bearing is shifted posteriorly away from the IVD toward the facet joints while decreasing the area of the vertebral foramen. This principle provides the basis for two major biomechanical treatment approaches for persons with low back pain. For persons with symptoms related to lumbar flexion, reducing pressure on the IVD by limiting lumbar flexion is often a useful approach. Conversely, for persons with symptoms during lumbar extension, a useful treatment approach is to limit extension and thereby reduce pressure on the facets joints as well as prevent narrowing of the vertebral foramina.*

*Abnormal displacement of vertebrae, which occurs during lumbar motion, is thought to be a primary contributor to symptoms of low back pain and, in some cases, to transient nerve compression (dynamic stenosis). If the facet joints are unable to resist anterior translation during flexion or during flexion combined with rotation, excessive movement may occur, creating a condition known as **segmental instability,** or **hypermobility** [29,41]. Conversely, it has been hypothesized that shortening of the facet joint capsule can lead to limited displacement of a motion segment and result in symptoms caused by premature end-range loading, a condition known as segmental **hypomobility** [67].*

SEGMENTAL MOTION IN THE TRANSVERSE AND FRONTAL PLANE

Consistent with the morphology of the motion segment, joint movement in the transverse plane, rotation, is quite restricted throughout the lumbar spine. Because of their oblique alignment, the collagen fibers within the anulus fibrosus are quickly loaded in tension during lumbar rotation. Bogduk and Twomey [13] report that stretching a collagen fiber beyond 4% of its resting length can lead to failure. These authors calculate that lumbar segmental rotation beyond 3° in a given direction can lead to injury of the anulus fibrosus. Fortunately, unilateral rotation rarely exceeds 3° under normal conditions [50]. As previously stated, the mechanism providing the primary restraint is approximation of the plane of the facet joints. For example, if the vertebral body rotates to the left (left rotation of the motion segment), the joint surfaces of the right facet approximate one another while the joint capsule of the left facet is stretched, or loaded in tension. This restraint mechanism is not as effective during lumbar flexion, which may help explain the increased incidence of lumbar IVD injuries that occur during combined flexion–rotation activities.

As noted earlier, segmental motion in the frontal plane, side-bending, is coupled with rotation. There is more displacement in side-bending than in rotation, with the exception of L5–S1, where both motions are limited. Tension in the intertransverse ligament and the capsule of the contralateral facet joint and approximation of the ipsilateral facet joint surfaces all act to restrict side-bending.

Clinical Methods of Lumbar Range of Motion Assessment

Assessment of ROM in the clinical setting is a fundamental component of the physical examination. This section discusses (a) the variables that must be considered to understand the measurement of lumbar motion and (b) the general trends of lumbar ROM on the basis of age and gender.

Numerous techniques have been described to assess lumbar motion in the clinical setting, including observation, palpation of active and passive motion, and the use of instruments such as goniometers, tape measures, inclinometers, and spondylometers [11,21,32,34–37,43,44,50,57,64,65,68,69,75]. Recently, several types of computer-based motion analysis systems have been described in the literature. Because of the cost and lack of general accessibility of these systems, this discussion is limited to those methods commonly used in clinical practice.

Two common procedures to assess lumbar motion are goniometry and the fingertips-to-floor method. Unfortunately, both of these techniques are problematic. A goniometer is a single-axis device typically used to measure ROM in joints of the extremities. However, its use for lumbar motion assessment is not appropriate (with the possible exception of lumbar rotation) because spinal motion is the result of several joints moving around numerous axes [44]. The fingertips-to-floor method attempts to assess lumbar flexion by simply measuring the distance of the fingertips to the floor when a person bends forward from a standing position. This procedure is inexpensive and easy to perform but is of limited use because it does not differentiate between lumbar flexion and forward inclination of the pelvis. The distance to which a person can reach toward the floor is a function of both lumbar flexion and pelvic rotation. For example, as noted earlier in this chapter, a patient might have normal lumbar flexion, but inextensible hamstring muscles, limiting the distance he or she may reach the fingertips to the floor. This can lead an examiner to conclude falsely that the lumbar spine is restricted in forward-bending. Conversely, someone with very extensible hamstring muscles may be able to touch the floor easily, even with limited ROM of the lumbar spine.

Considering that the limitations of the techniques above are caused by the unique multisegmental motion of the lumbar spine, it is not surprising that a common way to obtain reliable and valid measures in the clinical setting is to break down lumbar motion into two primary dimensions: linear displacement of spinous processes and angular displacement of a given point on the trunk relative to the pelvis.

LINEAR DISPLACEMENT OF THE SPINOUS PROCESSES OF THE LUMBAR SPINE

Clinicians can easily perform a gross assessment of the linear displacement of the spinous processes occurring during sagittal motion. In 1937, Schober [57] described the following simple procedure. The examiner places the tip of his or her little finger over the posterior tubercle of S1 and then places the index finger over a spinous process approximately 10 cm superiorly. By having the subject bend forward, the distraction between the spinous process and the posterior tubercle can be appreciated. During lumbar backward-bending (extension), an approximation or attraction of these bony prominences may be felt, providing the examiner with a gross assessment of lumbar motion. To quantify lumbar flexion using this principle, Macrae and Wright [34] and Moll and Wright [43,44] use a tape measure over the lumbar spine with the inferior landmark 5 cm inferior to the lumbosacral joint and the superior landmark 10 cm superior. Beattie et al. [11] use the same landmarks to assess lumbar extension (*Fig. 32.17*). Both of these studies report that the tape measure technique (distraction method for forward-bending and attraction method for backward-bending) yields reliable measures and is a simple, inexpensive technique for clinical use.

ANGULAR DISPLACEMENT OF THE LUMBAR SPINE

Angular measures of lumbar ROM are obtained using a variety of instruments that typically provide a single angle of trunk displacement relative to the ground or to the sacrum. Reliable measures are reported from the use of spondylometers [21,64], flexible rulers [32], and inclinometers, which are fluid-filled instruments measuring the angle in degrees that the trunk makes with the vertical [36,37,75]. Of these, the inclinometer appears to be the most inexpensive and easiest to use.

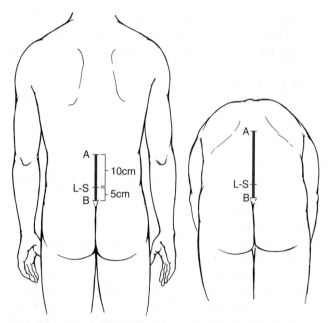

Figure 32.17: Landmarks used to perform measurements of lumbar flexion (distraction method) and lumbar extension (attraction method). This figure demonstrates the method for assessing flexion excursion. The landmarks are located when the subject is standing in a neutral posture. The reference locations are the lumbosacral region (L-S) at 0 cm, a second point (A) at 10 cm superior to L-S, and a third point (B) located 5 cm inferior to L-S that acts as an anchor point for the tape measure. At the end of the subject's available lumbar flexion, the distance between the reference point and the superior point is measured again. Ten centimeters is subtracted from this new value to yield a linear measurement of the subject's flexion. For example, if the second measurement is 15 cm, the subject's flexion excursion is 5 cm (15 cm − 10 cm = 5 cm) [7,43].

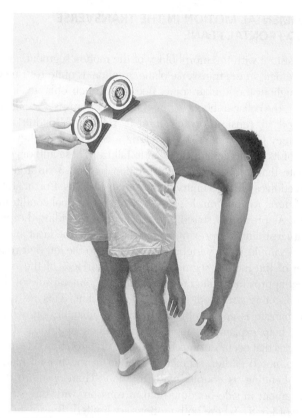

Figure 32.18: Use of an inclinometer to measure angular motion of the lumbar spine. Two inclinometers are placed, one on the sacrum and one at the proximal aspect of the lumbar spine. The difference between the two measurements indicates the lumbar spine angular motion.

Mayer et al. [37] describe the two-inclinometer method. During this procedure, an examiner identifies a point on the sacrum in the standing subject and places one inclinometer over this area. A second inclinometer is placed over the spinous process of L1. The subject then performs forward-bending (*Fig. 32.18*). The upper inclinometer indicates the total anterior displacement of the trunk, while the lower inclinometer indicates pelvic rotation. By subtracting the lower value from the upper value, the degree of angular motion for lumbar flexion is obtained. A similar procedure is used for

backward-bending. Because the pelvis does not typically displace laterally during standing side-bending, a single inclinometer over the upper lumbar spine is adequate. Lumbar rotation is not measured with an inclinometer.

Waddell et al. [75] report acceptable reliability for use of the double inclinometer technique and identify differences between nonpatients and persons with chronic low back pain (*Table 32.5*). Patients with chronic low back pain exhibit significantly less motion for anterior rotation of the pelvis, total flexion, total extension, and lateral flexion.

TABLE 32.5: Normal Values (95% Confidence Intervals) for Adults without LBP and with Chronic LBP (in°)

Motion	Normal Subjects (n = 70)	Patients (n = 120)
Lumbar flexion	42.4 (39.8–44.9)	48.7 (46.0–51.4)
Anterior rotation of pelvis	57.1 (54.1–59)	30.7 (27.4–34)
Total flexion	99.5 (96.2–102.8)	79.3 (74.7–83.9)
Total extension	26.5 (24.4–28.6)	18.4 (17.0–19.8)
Lateral flexion	29.4 (27.9–31.0)	22.7 (21.3–24.1)

Adapted from Waddell G, Somerville D, Henderson I, et al.: Objective clinical evaluation of physical impairment in chronic low back pain. Spine 1992; 17: 617–628.

Normative Values for Lumbar Range of Motion

A fundamental question is, "What is normal lumbar ROM for the lumbar spine?" While general trends of motion are known, *exact values* for normal lumbar ROM are difficult to establish. To understand this, consider the concept of normative data. Normative data can be thought of as a distribution of measures obtained from a large number of persons to determine an "average score" [55]. For these values to be meaningful, several factors must be considered, including the specific way in which the measures are obtained, the specific characteristics of the population sampled, and the variation within the distribution of measures. In other words, establishment of normative values requires an evaluation procedure that yields reliable and valid measures that are obtained from a clearly defined group of persons (consider age, gender, pathology, etc.), and provide a mechanism to determine how much variation from the average score (mean or other description of central tendency) is considered "normal." If one considers the large number of measures used to describe lumbar ROM as well as the numerous factors influencing ROM, it is not surprising that a single set of normative values has not yet been agreed upon. Thus it is very difficult in a clinical setting to identify a threshold for determining the presence of abnormal motion of the lumbar spine.

Twomey and Taylor [68] report age and gender differences in lumbar motion measured by a special instrument known as a spondylometer, which reports an overall angular displacement in a given plane of motion. The results of the study are described in *Table 32.6* and reveal the following general trends: (*a*) considerably more lumbar flexion–extension than rotation is present throughout life; (*b*) teenage females have more flexion, extension, and rotation than teenage males; (*c*) young adult females have slightly more flexion–extension

than young adult males; and (*d*) older adults have less ROM than younger adults or teenagers; however, there is little difference between the genders in this group.

Several factors can influence the measurements obtained over time by the same or different examiners, and these must be considered when reviewing any measurement of lumbar motion. Four primary concerns relative to a measure include (*a*) device error, (*b*) human–device interface or procedural error, (*c*) human performance variability, and (*d*) lack of training among test administrators [36].

MANUAL ASSESSMENT OF PASSIVE INTERVERTEBRAL MOTION

Determining the degree of passive motion available at an individual motion segment is of interest to clinicians. Although several variations have been described, the primary technique for this involves either (*a*) applying varying degrees of pressure to lumbar spinous processes to determine displacement or (*b*) passively moving the spine while palpating changes in the size of the intersegmental spaces. Although these techniques are still widely taught, recent work has demonstrated low agreement between examiners relative to the amount of motion available [35]. Because of the small amounts of displacement and relatively large variability among subjects, the validity of the manual assessment of segmental motion remains unproved.

RELATING THE OSTEOCARTILAGINOUS LUMBAR SPINE TO FUNCTIONAL DEMANDS

Throughout this chapter, the emphasis has been upon the multiple factors that contribute to function (and dysfunction) of the lumbar spine. While it is convenient to describe form and function by considering one tissue and one motion at a time, the lumbar spine, like the transmission in a car, relies upon the proper functioning and interplay of numerous structures. The osteocartilaginous lumbar spine is associated with muscles, ligaments, and fascia arising from the pelvis, thoracic spine, and extremities. The lumbar spine, therefore, provides a series of mobile links within a kinetic chain that includes the sacroiliac joints, pubic symphysis, and lower extremities as well as the cervicothoracic spine and upper extremities (in other words, everything). Mechanical loading of these structures greatly influences the lumbar spine and vice versa. Clinically, it is critical to assess these structures carefully when working with persons who have lumbar spine problems. For example, a limb length discrepancy resulting from tibial shortening following a fracture can dramatically change the loading patterns on the lumbar spine [8]. Conversely, excessive lumbar lordosis associated with anterior pelvic rotation can change loading patterns on the hip joint. Limited ROM of the hip is a frequent finding in persons with chronic low back pain [52].

TABLE 32.6: Approximate Mean Values for Lumbar Range of Motion (in°) as Measured with a Spondylometer

Motion	Age	Male	Female
Flexion	13–19	33	42
	20–35	33	38
	36–59	28	27
	60+	22	22
Extension	13–19	9	13
	20–35	15	18
	36–59	11	13
	60+	10	10
Rotation	13–19	16	20
	20–35	18	19
	36–59	13	13
	60+	12	12

Adapted from Twomey LR: The effects of age on the ranges of motions of the lumbar region. Aust J Physiother 1979; 25: 257–262.

Recall that in addition to protecting neurovascular elements, the primary function of the lumbar spine is to provide stability while allowing adequate mobility for activities of daily living. As with most joint systems this is really an issue of *dynamic stability*. Stability in the presence of motion at any given vertebral level is a function of bony architecture, disc height and mechanics, facet joint orientation, ligamentous support, and motor control in response to the load being applied. When this system is working properly, the lumbar spine is capable of withstanding large loads throughout the ROM. However, when any component of the system becomes impaired (e.g., fracture, disc herniation, soft tissue trauma, or loss of motor control), relatively minor loads can result in further trauma and symptoms (*Box 32.1*).

Finally, when applying the information from this chapter in the clinical environment, the clinician must relate the structure and mechanics of the lumbar spine to the physical and emotional stresses encountered by the patient. The problem of low back pain and associated spinal disorders remains a major public health consideration throughout the world. Considerable suffering and loss of quality of life have resulted from these conditions. Through an understanding of the structure and function of the lumbar spine, the disorders of the lumbar spine, and most importantly the persons who must endure these conditions, clinicians have the opportunity to make great contributions.

SUMMARY

This chapter examines the bones and joints of the lumbar spine and describes how these structures influence the mobility and stability of the region. The structures of the lumbar spine are specialized to perform load-bearing functions, and they sustain large loads during most activities. The ligaments of the lumbar spine contribute to stability but also appear to play a role in the motor control of the region by providing important sensory feedback. The IVDs absorb and transmit forces and work as dynamic spacers that allow more mobility between lumbar vertebrae. The contribution of these structures to common lumbar disorders is introduced.

Total lumbar motion as well as segmental motion is reviewed. The lumbar spine exhibits greatest motion in the sagittal plane as a result of the alignment of the facet joints. Transverse and frontal plane motions are more limited and coupled with each other. Normative data on the mobility of the spine are reviewed. Mobility of the lumbar spine is affected by age and gender.

The lumbar spine is a fascinating system of bones, joints, ligaments, and fascia under the control of a very sophisticated neuromuscular mechanism. Providing a protected pathway for neurovascular structures, this complex interplay of mobility and stability acts as a critical pivot in the center of the human skeleton. The following chapter describes the muscles' participation in the support and movement of the lumbar spine.

EXAMINING THE FORCES BOX 32.1

SUMMARY OF STRUCTURES THAT RESIST LOADING IN THE LUMBAR SPINE AND COMMON INJURIES THAT OCCUR FROM EXCESSIVE LOADING

Compressive (Axial) Loading

Tissues resisting: Vertebral bodies and intervertebral disc, abdominal mechanism

Injury: Vertebral body or endplate fracture

Rotational and Side-Bending Stress

Tissues resisting: Facet joints, pedicles, abdominal mechanism, quadratus lumborum, superficial and deep back muscles

Injury: Fracture of pars interarticularis, pedicle

Flexion Stress

Tissues resisting: Posterior ligament system, posterior anulus fibrosus, thoracodorsal fascia, superficial and deep back muscles

Injury: Anular tear, disc herniation, muscle injury

Extension Stress

Tissues resisting: Anterior ligament system, posterior bony elements, abdominal mechanism

Injury: Pars fracture, traumatic spondylolisthesis

Protection of Neurovascular Elements

Tissues resisting: Fibro-osseous foramina

Injury: Entrapment of cauda equina and/or nerve roots

References

1. Adams MA, Hutton WC: Gradual disc prolapse. Spine 1985; 10: 524–531.
2. Andersson GBJ, McNeill TW: Lumbar Spine Syndromes: Evaluation and Treatment. New York: Springer-Verlag, 1989; 1–28.
3. Aprill C, Bogduk N. High intensity zone: a diagnostic sign of painful lumbar disc on magnetic resonance imaging. Br J Radiol 1992; 65: 361–368.
4. Basadonna P-T, Gasparini D, Rucco V: Iliolumbar ligament insertions. Spine 1996; 21: 2313–2316.
5. Beattie P: The use of an eclectic approach for the treatment of low back pain: a case report. Phys Ther 1992; 72: 923–928.
6. Beattie P: The relationship between symptoms and abnormal magnetic resonance images of lumbar intervertebral discs. Phys Ther 1996; 76: 601–608.

7. Beattie P, Brooks W, Rothstein J, et al.: Effect of lordosis on the position of the nucleus pulposus in supine subjects. Spine 1994; 19: 2096–2102.

8. Beattie P, Issacson K, Riddle D, Rothstein JM: Validity of derived measurements of leg-length differences obtained by the use of a tape measure. Phys Ther 1990; 70: 150–157.

9. Beattie P, Meyers S, Stratford P, et al.: Associations between patient report of symptoms and anatomic impairment visible on lumbar magnetic resonance. Spine 2000; 25: 819–828.

10. Beattie P, Meyers SM: Lumbar magnetic resonance imaging: general principles and diagnostic efficacy. Phys Ther 1998; 78: 738–753.

11. Beattie P, Rothstein JM, Lamb RL: Reliability of the attraction method of measuring lumbar spine backward bending. Phys Ther 1987; 67: 364–369.

12. Bogduk N: The innervation of the lumbar spine. Spine 6: 286–293, 1983.

13. Bogduk N, Twomey LT: Clinical Anatomy of the Lumbar Spine. 2nd ed. New York: Churchill-Livingstone, 1991.

14. Calliet R: Low Back Pain Syndrome. 5th ed. Philadelphia: FA Davis, 1995.

15. Dommisse GF: Morphological aspects of the lumbar spine and lumbosacral region. Orthop Clin North Am 1975; 6: 163–175.

16. Frymoyer JW: Epidemiological studies of low back pain. Spine 1980; 5: 419.

17. Frymoyer JW: An overview of the incidence and costs of low back pain. Orthop Clin North Am 1991; 22: 262–271.

18. Gracovetsky S: The optimum spine. Spine 11: 543–73, 1986.

19. Grieve GP: Common Vertebral Joint Problems. New York: Churchill-Livingstone, 1981.

20. Gunzberg R, Hutton WC, Crane G, et al.: Role of the capsulo-ligamentous structures in rotation and combined flexion-rotation of the lumbar spine. J Spinal Disord 1992; 5: 1–7.

21. Hart FD, Strickland D, Cliffe P: Measurement of spinal mobility. Ann Rheum Dis 1974; 33: 136–139.

22. Hasue M, Kikuchi S, Sakutama Y, et al.: Anatomical study of the interrelation between lumbosacral nerve roots and their surrounding tissues. Spine 1983; 8: 50–58.

23. Humzah MD, Soames RW: The human intervertebral disc. Anat Rec 1988; 220: 337–356.

24. Iatridis JC, Weidenbaum M, Setton LA, et al.: Is the nucleus pulposus a solid or a fluid? Mechanical behaviors of the nucleus pulposus of the human intervertebral disc. Spine 1996; 21: 1174–1184.

25. Jackson RP: The facet syndrome: myth or reality? Clin Orthop 1992; 279: 110–120.

26. Jette AM, Smith K, Haley SM, Davis K: Physical therapy episodes of care for patients with low back pain. Phys Ther 1994; 74: 101–115.

27. Johnson EF, Chetty IM, Moore A, et al.: Distribution and arrangement of elastic fibres in intervertebral discs of adult humans. J Anat 1982; 136: 301–309.

28. Kellgren JH: On the distribution of pain arising from deep somatic structures with charts of segmental pain areas. Clin Sci 1938; 3: 175–190.

29. Kirkaldy-Willis WH: A more precise diagnosis for low back pain. Spine 1979; 4: 102.

30. Langrana NA, Edwards WT, Sharma M: Biomechanical analyses of loads on the lumbar spine. In: The Lumbar Spine, 2nd ed. Eds: Wiesel SW, Weinstein JN, Herkowitz HN, et al. Philadelphia: WB Saunders, 1996; 163–180.

31. Lewin T, Moffet B, Viidik A: The morphology of the lumbar synovial intervertebral joints. Acta Morphol Neerl Scand 1962; 4: 29–319.

32. Loebl WY: Measurement of spinal posture and range of spinal movement. Ann Phys Med 1967; 9: 103–110.

33. Lucas D, Bresler B: Stability of Ligamentous Spine. Report no. 40. University of California, San Francisco/Berkeley: Biomechanics Laboratory, 1961; 1–41.

34. Macrae IF, Wright V: Measurement of back movement. Ann Rheum Dis 1969; 28: 584–589.

35. Maher C, Adams R: Reliability of pain and stiffness assessments in clinical manual lumbar spine examination. Phys Ther 1995; 74: 801–811.

36. Mayer TG, Kondraske G, Beals SB, et al.: Spinal range of motion: accuracy and sources of error with inclinometric measurement. Spine 1997; 22: 1976–1984.

37. Mayer TG, Tencer AF, Kristoferson S, et al.: Use of noninvasive techniques for quantification of spinal range-of-motion in normal subjects and chronic low-back dysfunction patients. Spine 1984; 9: 588–595.

38. Mayoux-Benhamou MA, Revel M, Aaron C, et al.: A morphometric study of the lumbar foramen. Surg Radiol Anat 1989; 11: 97–102.

39. McGill SM: Low back pain exercises: evidence for improving exercise regimens. Phys Ther 1998; 78: 754–765.

40. McKenzie R: The Lumbar Spine: Mechanical Diagnosis and Therapy. Waikanae, New Zealand: Spinal Publications, 1981.

41. McNab I., McCulloch J: Backache. 2nd ed. Baltimore: Williams & Wilkins, 1990.

42. Mixter W, Barr J: Rupture of the intervertebral disc with involvement of the spinal canal. New Engl J Med 1934; 211: 210.

43. Moll JMH, Wright V: Normal range of spinal mobility: an objective clinical study. Ann Rheum Dis 1971; 30: 381–386.

44. Moll JMH, Wright V: Measurement of spinal movement. In: Jason M, ed. The Lumbar Spine and Back Pain. New York: Pittman Medical, 1976; 93–112.

45. Mooney V, Robertson J: The facet syndrome. Clin Orthop 1976; 115: 149–156.

46. Nachemson AL. Intravital dynamic pressure measurements in lumbar discs. Scand J Rehabil Med 1970; 1(suppl): 1–40.

47. Nachemson AL: Advances in low back pain. Clin Orthop 1985; 200: 266–278.

48. O'Sullivan PB, Twomey LT, Allison GT: Evaluation of specific stabilizing exercise in the treatment of chronic low back pain with radiologic diagnosis of spondylolysis or spondylolisthesis. Spine 1997; 22: 2959–2967.

49. Panjabi PM, Takata D, Goel VK: Kinematics of the lumbar intervertebral foramen. Spine 1983; 8: 348–357.

50. Pearcy M, Portek I, Shepherd J: Three dimensional x-ray analysis of normal movement in the lumbar spine. Spine 1984; 9: 294–297.

51. Pope MH, Frymoyer JW, Lehman TR: Structure and Function of the Lumbar Spine. in Occupational Low Back Pain: Assessment, Treatment, and Prevention. Pope MA, Andersson GBJ, Frymoyer JW, Chaffin DB, eds. St. Louis: Mosby Yearbook, 1991; 3–19.

52. Porter JL, Wilkinson A: Lumbar-hip flexion motion: a comparative study between asymptomatic and chronic low back pain in 18- to 36-year-old men. Spine 1997; 22: 1508–1514.

53. Porterfield J, DeRosa C: Mechanical Low Back Pain: Perspectives in Functional Anatomy. Philadelphia: WB Saunders, 1991.

54. Rhalmi W, Yahia H, Newman N, et al.: Immunohistochemical study of nerve in lumbar spine ligaments. Spine 1993; 18: 264–267.

55. Rothstein JM, Echternach JL: Primer on Measurement: An Introductory Guide to Measurement Issues.: American Physical Therapy Association. Alexandria, VA: 1993; 46–54.

56. Schnebel BE, Watkins RG, Dillin W: A digitizing technique for the study of movement of intradiscal dye in response to flexion and extension of the lumbar spine. Spine 1988; 13: 309–312.

57. Schober P. The lumbar vertebral column and backache. Muench Med Wochenschr 1937; 84: 336–338.

58. Schultz AB, Brinckman P, Pope M, et al.: Biomechanical analyses of loads on the lumbar spine. In: Weinstein JN, Wiesel SW, eds. The Lumbar Spine. Philadelphia: WB Saunders, 1990; 160–171.

59. Sharma M, Langrana NA, Rodriquez J: Role of ligaments and facets in lumbar spinal stability. Spine 1995; 20: 887–900.

60. Shiraxi-Adi A: Biomechanics of the lumbar spine in sagittal/lateral moments. Spine 1994; 19: 2407–2414.

61. Snook S, Webster BS, McGorry RW, et al.: The reduction of chronic nonspecific low back pain through the control of early morning lumbar flexion. Spine 1998; 23: 2601–2607.

62. Solomonow M, Bing-He Z, Harris M, et al.: The ligamento-muscular stabilizing system of the spine. Spine 1998; 23: 2552–2562.

63. Steindler A: Mechanics of Normal and Pathological Locomotion in Man. Springfield, IL: Thomas Books, 1935.

64. Sturrock RD, Wojtulewski JA, Hart FD: Spondylometry in a normal population and in ankylosing spondylitis. Rheumatol Rehabil 1973; 12: 135–142.

65. Taylor J, Twomey L: Sagittal and horizontal plane movement of the human lumbar vertebral column in cadavers and in the living. Rheumatol Rehabil 1980; 19: 223–232.

66. Taylor JR: The development and adult structure of lumbar intervertebral discs. J Manual Med 1990; 5: 43–47.

67. Twomey L: A rationale for the treatment of back pain and joint pain by manual therapy. Phys Ther 1992; 72: 885–892.

68. Twomey LR: The effects of age on the ranges of motions of the lumbar region. Aust J Physiother 1979; 25: 257–262.

69. Twomey LR, Taylor JR: Sagittal movements of the human lumbar vertebral column: a quantitative study of the role of the posterior vertebral elements. Arch Phys Med Rehab 1983; 64; 322–325.

70. Urban JPG, Holm SH, Lipson SJ: Biochemistry. In: Weinstein JN, Wiesel SW, eds. The Lumbar Spine. Philadelphia: WB Saunders, 1990; 231–242.

71. Urban JP, McMullin JF: Swelling pressure of the lumbar intervertebral disc: influence of age, spinal level, composition, and degeneration. Spine 1988; 13: 179–187.

72. van Tulder MW, Assendelft WJ, Koes BW, et al.: Spinal radiographic findings and nonspecific low back pain. Spine 1997; 22: 427–434.

73. van Tulder MW, Koes BW, Bouter LM: Conservative treatment of acute and chronic nonspecific low back pain: a systematic review of randomized controlled trials of the most common interventions. Spine 1997; 22: 2128–2156.

74. Vleeming A, Pool-Gooudzwaard AL, Stoeckart R: The posterior layer of the thoracolumbar fascia: its function in load transfer from spine to legs. Spine 1995; 20: 753–758.

75. Waddell G, Somerville D, Henderson I, et al.: Objective clinical evaluation of physical impairment in chronic low back pain. Spine 1992; 17: 617–628.

76. White AA, Panjabi MM. Clinical Biomechanics of the Spine. Philadelphia: JB Lippincott, 1978.

77. Williams PL, Warwick R: Gray's Anatomy. 36th ed. Philadelphia: WB Saunders, 1980.

78. Yahia H, Newman N, Richards C, et al.: Neurohistology of lumbar spine ligaments. Acta Orthop Scand 1988; 59: 508–512.

Mechanics and Pathomechanics of Muscles Acting on the Lumbar Spine

STUART M. McGILL, PH.D.

Traditional description of the spine musculature is from a posterior vantage point, but many of the functionally relevant aspects are better viewed in the sagittal plane. (For a nice synopsis of the sagittal plane lines of action, see Bogduk et al. [3].) This traditional approach has hindered understanding of the many roles that muscles play in lumbar mechanics. Furthermore, understanding of muscle function is typically obtained by simply interpreting the lines of action and region of attachment, which may be misleading. Understanding the function and purpose of each muscle requires knowledge of muscle morphology, together with knowledge of activation of the musculature over a wide variety of movement and loading tasks. Muscles create force, but these forces play roles in moment production for movement and for stabilizing joints for safety and performance. Further, interpreting anatomy, mechanics, and activation profiles is the only way to understand motor control system strategies chosen to support external loads and maintain stability. This chapter enhances the discussion of anatomically based issues of the spine musculature and blends the results of various electromyographic (EMG) studies to help interpret function and the functional aspects of motor control. The purposes of this chapter are to

- Present the current understanding of the functional roles of the muscles of the lumbar spine
- Demonstrate the application of this knowledge in the design of exercises for the lumbar spine

MUSCLE SIZE

As noted in Chapter 4 on the mechanics of muscle, the physiological cross-sectional area (PCSA) of muscle determines the force-producing potential, while the line of action and moment arm determine the effect of the force in moment production, stabilization, etc. It is erroneous to estimate force on the basis of muscle volume without accounting for fiber architecture or by taking transverse scans to measure anatomical cross-sectional areas [13], as has often occurred in interpreting spine mechanics. In such cases, muscle forces are underestimated, as a large number of muscle fibers are not "seen" in a single transverse scan of a pennated muscle. Thus, areas obtained from magnetic resonance imagery (MRI) or computed tomography (CT) scans must be corrected for fiber architecture and scan plane obliquity [14]. In *Figure 33.1,*

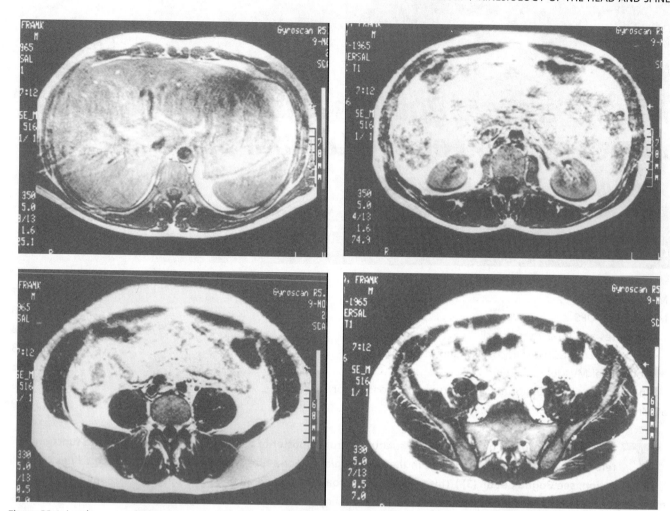

Figure 33.1: Lumbar musculature in cross section. Transverse scan of one subject (supine) at the level of (left to right) T9, L1 (top) and L4, S1 (bottom); anterior is the top of each scan. (Reprinted with permission from McGill SM, Santaguida L, Stevens J: Measurement of the trunk musculature from T6 to L5 using MRI scans of 15 young males corrected for muscle fiber orientation. Clin Biomech 1993; 8: 171–178.)

transverse scans of one subject show the changing shape of the torso muscles over the thoracolumbar region, highlighting the need to combine transverse scan data with data documenting fiber architecture obtained from dissection. In this example, the thoracic extensors seen at T9 provide an extensor moment at L4 even though they are not "seen" in the L4 scan. Only their tendons overlie the L4 extensors.

Raw muscle PCSAs and moment arms [14] are provided in *Tables 33.1–33.3*. Areas corrected for oblique lines of action are shown in *Table 33.4* for some selected muscles at several levels of the thoracolumbar spine. Guidelines for estimating true physiological areas are provided in McGill et al. [13].

Moment arms of the abdominal musculature reported in CT- or MRI-based studies have recently been shown to underestimate true values by 30%, given the supine posture required in the MRI or CT scanner. This posture causes the abdominal contents to collapse posteriorly under gravity [10]. In real life, the abdominals are pushed away from the spine by visceral contents when standing. In summary, muscle areas obtained from various medical imaging techniques need to be corrected to account for fiber architecture and contractile components

that do not appear in the particular scan level (only the tendon passes the level). Further, moment arms for muscle line of action obtained from subjects who are lying down need to be adjusted for application to real life and upright postures.

MUSCLE GROUPS

Rotatores and Intertransversarii

MUSCLE ACTION: ROTATORES

Action	Evidence
Trunk rotation	Inadequate
Proprioception and position sense	Inadequate

MUSCLE ACTION: INTERTRANSVERSARII

Action	Evidence
Trunk lateral flexion	Inadequate
Proprioception and position sense	Inadequate

TABLE 33.1: Raw Cross-Sectional Areas (mm²) (Standard Deviation) Measured Directly from MRI Scans

Muscles	Vertebral Level												
	L5	L4	L3	L2	L1	T12	T11	T10	T9	T8	T7	T6	T5
R. Rectus abdominis	787(250)	750(207)	670(133)	712(239)	576(151)								
L. Rectus abdominis	802(247)	746(181)	693(177)	748(240)	514(99)								
R. External oblique		915(199)	1276(171)	1158(222)									
L. External oblique		992(278)	1335(213)	1351(282)									
R. Internal oblique		903(83)	1515(317)	1055(173)									
L. Internal oblique		900(115)	1424(310)	1027(342)									
R. Trans. abdominis	119(22)	237(82)	356(110)	596(50)									
L. Trans. abdominis	175(57)	224(48)	376(115)	646(183)									
R. Abdominal wall[a]	1104(393)	2412(418)	3269(422)	3051(463)									
L. Abdominal wall[a]	1146(377)	2420(475)	3329(468)	3111(556)									
R. Longissimus thor.			47(162)	1175(370)	1248(228)	1095(222)	938(49)						
L. Longissimus thor.			782(129)	1089(251)	1180(184)	1258(347)	938(21)						
R. Iliocostalis lumb.			1368(341)	1104(181)	1181(316)	921(339)	556(234)						
L. Iliocostalis lumb.			1395(223)	1150(198)	1158(247)	835(400)	551(170)						
R. Multifidus			447(271)	343(178)	290(96)	289(66)	331(89)	351(90)	312(97)				
L. Multifidus			472(269)	366(157)	324(95)	312(76)	327(80)	353(53)	355(73)				
R. Latissimus dorsi			232(192)	429(202)	717(260)	1014(264)	1254(281)	1368(330)	1458(269)	1581(159)	1764(289)	1876(432)	2477(246)
L. Latissimus dorsi			256(217)	372(161)	682(260)	960(310)	1102(316)	1239(257)	1417(293)	1582(281)	1697(189)	2013(422)	2596(721)
R. Erector mass[b]	905(331)	2151(539)	2831(458)	2854(547)	2615(405)	2614(584)	1832(282)	1690(210)	1413(304)	1049(201)	842(165)	777(189)	743(70)
L. Erector mass[b]	986(338)	2234(476)	2933(382)	2833(456)	2723(428)	2601(559)	2041(285)	1722(279)	1471(351)	1129(100)	879(114)	779(95)	675(76)
R. Psoas	1606(198)	1861(347)	1594(369)	1177(285)	513(329)	330(210)							
L. Psoas	1590(244)	1820(272)	1593(291)	1211(298)	488(250)	462(190)							
R. Quadratus lumb.		725(209)	701(212)	552(192)	392(249)	320(197)							
L. Quadratus lumb.		625(249)	746(167)	614(189)	404(220)	326(5)							
Disc area	1360(276)	1459(270)	1415(249)	1332(294)	1334(285)	1241(166)	1133(124)	1015(125)	933(112)	798(91)	797(104)	741(80)	671(82)
Total area	52912(9123)	51813(9845)	54286(8702)	55834(8112)	59091(6899)	63287(9153)	59249(7272)	61051(7570)	61732(6960)	65794(5254)	67782(3982)	66410(2372)	69337(2233)

[a] Abdominal wall includes external and internal oblique and transverse abdominis.
[b] Erector mass includes longissimus thoracis, iliocostalis lumborum, and multifidus.
Reprinted with permission from McGill SM, Santaguida L, Stevens J: Measurement of the trunk musculature from T6 to L5 using MRI scans of 15 young males corrected for muscle fibre orientation. Clin Biomech 1993; 8: 171–178.

TABLE 33.2: Raw Lateral Distances (mm) between Muscle Centroids and Intervertebral Disc Centroid (Standard Deviation)

Muscles	Vertebral Level												
	L5	L4	L3	L2	L1	T12	T11	T10	T9	T8	T7	T6	T5
R. Rectus abdominis	32(5)	38(7)	43(7)	46(8)	37(8)								
L. Rectus abdominis	−33(6)	−36(7)	−38(8)	−43(7)	−35(17)								
R. External oblique		125(13)	130(10)	140(5)									
L. External oblique		−120(9)	−125(9)	−133(7)									
R. Internal oblique		109(11)	116(8)	123(9)									
L. Internal oblique		−103(9)	−112(8)	−121(11)									
R. Transverse abdominis	99(1)	108(11)	112(9)	117(9)									
L. Transverse abdominis	−101(1)	−101(9)	−107(7)	−109(9)									
R. Abdominal wall[a]	102(8)	113(12)	119(8)	123(9)									
L. Abdominal wall[a]	−102(9)	−115(14)	−114(7)	−120(9)									
R. Longissimus thoracis			22(4)	32(2)	32(6)	30(2)	29(1)						
L. Longissimus thoracis			−19(5)	−30(6)	−37(12)	−34(4)	−36(7)						
R. Iliocostalis lumborum			52(4)	58(4)	68(10)	65(7)	61(4)						
L. Iliocostalis lumborum			−48(6)	−60(10)	−65(9)	−67(7)	−67(11)						
R. Multifidus			11(1)	13(4)	13(3)	10(3)	8(2)	11(2)	12(2)				
L. Multifidus			−14(7)	−12(3)	−11(3)	−11(2)	−12(2)	−12(2)	−15(10)				
R. Latissimus dorsi			102(8)	108(8)	122(12)	129(10)	129(9)	140(9)	141(8)	145(7)	146(7)	153(7)	153(4)
L. Latissimus dorsi			−104(15)	−107(9)	−117(11)	−128(7)	−129(10)	−137(9)	−139(8)	−143(6)	−147(10)	−153(5)	−151(5)
R. Erector mass[b]	22(6)	34(7)	40(4)	42(4)	44(5)	42(3)	34(4)	34(4)	32(4)	31(7)	30(4)	25(5)	27(2)
L. Erector mass[b]	−21(5)	−33(6)	−38(5)	−41(6)	−41(7)	−40(4)	−40(3)	−36(3)	−35(4)	−33(6)	−31(2)	−29(3)	−27(6)
R. Psoas	54(4)	50(3)	44(3)	39(2)	32(3)	32(3)							
L. Psoas	−54(5)	−48(4)	−42(3)	−38(3)	−31(3)	−32(2)							
R. Quadratus lumborum		81(5)	75(6)	63(5)	46(6)	46(11)							
L. Quadratus lumborum		−78(12)	−73(4)	−64(5)	−50(6)	−47(5)							
Total area	0(2)	1(3)	−2(4)	−1(3)	−1(4)	0(3)	1(3)	0(2)	0(2)	2(1)	2(1)	1(3)	2(3)

[a]Abdominal wall includes external and internal oblique and transverse abdominis.
[b]Erector mass includes longissimus thoracis, iliocostalis lumborum, and multifidus.
Reprinted with permission from McGill SM, Santaguida L, Stevens J: Measurement of the trunk musculature from T6 to L5 using MRI scans of 15 young males corrected for muscle fibre orientation. Clin Biomech 1993; 8: 171–178.

TABLE 33.3: Raw Anterior–Posterior Distances (mm) between Muscle Centroids and Intervertebral Disc Centroid (Standard Deviation)

Muscles	Vertebral Level												
	L5	L4	L3	L2	L1	T12	T11	T10	T9	T8	T7	T6	T5
R. Rectus abdominis	81(16)	73(14)	79(13)	90(14)	109(8)								
L. Rectus abdominis	80(15)	73(14)	80(14)	92(14)	112(6)								
R. External oblique		35(10)	20(14)	28(12)									
L. External oblique		32(18)	19(11)	28(11)									
R. Internal oblique		41(12)	25(9)	36(17)									
L. Internal oblique		41(17)	26(12)	40(16)									
R. Transverse abdominis	55(0)	28(11)	22(11)	36(6)									
L. Transverse abdominis	50(5)	30(14)	23(10)	44(5)									
R. Abdominal wall[a]	58(16)	31(12)	17(12)	30(15)									
L. Abdominal wall[a]	59(17)	32(13)	20(12)	31(11)									
R. Longissimus thoracis			−61(6)	−62(7)	−60(7)	−60(6)	−56(4)						
L. Longissimus thoracis			−61(5)	−63(6)	−60(7)	−59(8)	−52(4)						
R. Iliocostalis lumborum			−57(7)	−61(7)	−62(5)	−59(7)	−57(1)						
L. Iliocostalis lumborum			−57(7)	−61(6)	−61(4)	−58(6)	−56(2)						
R. Multifidus			−55(7)	−55(6)	−52(6)	−51(3)	−47(5)	−49(4)	−48(2)				
L. Multifidus			−53(7)	−56(5)	−51(5)	−50(3)	−47(5)	−47(3)	−47(2)				
R. Latissimus dorsi			−45(16)	−47(12)	−47(10)	−39(8)	−32(7)	−24(7)	−22(7)	−18(9)	−17(6)	−12(3)	−17(5)
L. Latissimus dorsi			−43(17)	−46(10)	−46(7)	−37(8)	−28(9)	−23(7)	−19(7)	−17(7)	−15(8)	−11(7)	−19(3)
R. Erector mass[b]	−64(6)	−61(5)	−61(5)	−61(5)	−59(5)	−56(5)	−54(4)	−54(4)	−52(4)	−52(3)	−52(4)	−47(4)	−50(3)
L. Erector mass[b]	−63(5)	−61(5)	−61(5)	−62(5)	−60(4)	−57(5)	−52(4)	−52(4)	−51(4)	−51(3)	−51(4)	−46(5)	−50(3)
R. Psoas	18(9)	1(5)	−7(5)	−9(5)	−11(6)	−14(2)							
L. Psoas	19(8)	2(4)	−6(4)	−8(2)	−11(4)	−11(1)							
R. Quadratus lumborum		−36(9)	−37(6)	−37(6)	−35(4)	−31(6)							
L. Quadratus lumborum		−31(5)	−34(6)	−36(5)	−34(4)	−32(8)							
Total area	1(10)	−2(9)	1(8)	9(8)	18(5)	24(7)	29(8)	30(9)	32(7)	36(7)	37(6)	32(10)	34(5)

[a] Abdominal wall includes external and internal oblique and transverse abdominis.
[b] Erector mass includes longissimus thoracis, iliocostalis lumborum, and multifidus.
Reprinted with permission from McGill SM, Santaguida L, Stevens J: Measurement of the trunk musculature from T6 to L5 using MRI scans of 15 young males corrected for muscle fibre orientation. Clin Biomech 1993; 8: 171–178.

TABLE 33.4: Examples of Corrected Cross–Sectional Areas and A–P and Lateral Moment Arms Perpendicular to the Muscle Fiber Line of Action Using the Appropriate Cosines: These Values Should Be Used in Biomechanical Models Rather Than the Uncorrected Values Obtained Directly from Scan Slices

Muscle		Cross-Sectional Area (mm)^2	Anterior–Posterior (mm)	Lateral (mm)
Longissimus pars lumborum[a]	L3-4	644	51	17
Quadratus lumborum	L1-2	358	31	43
	L2-3	507	32	55
	L3-4	582	29	59
	L4-5	328	16	39
External oblique	L3-4	1121	17	110
Internal oblique	L3-4	1154	20	89

[a]Longissimus pars lumborum at the L4-5 level would have been listed here by virtue of their cosines, but were not, as they could not be distinguished on all scan slices.

Many anatomical textbooks describe the function of the small rotator muscles of the spine, which attach to adjacent vertebrae, as creating axial twisting torque, consistent with their nomenclature (*Muscle Attachment Box 33.1*). Similarly, the intertransversarii are often assigned the role of lateral flexion (*Muscle Attachment Box 33.2*). There are several problems with these proposals. First, these small muscles (*Fig. 33.2*) have such small PCSAs that they can only generate a few newtons of force, and second, they work through such a small moment arm that their total contribution to rotational axial twisting and bending torque is minimal. It would appear that they have some other function.

There is evidence to suggest that these muscles are highly rich in muscle spindles, approximately 4.5–7.3 times richer than the multifidus [16]. This evidence suggests that they are involved as length transducers or vertebral position sensors at every thoracic and lumbar joint. In some EMG experiments performed in the author's laboratory a number of years ago, some indwelling electrodes were placed very close to the vertebrae. In one case, there was strong suspicion that the electrode was in a rotator muscle. Isometric twisting efforts with the spine untwisted (or constrained in a neutral posture) were attempted in both directions but produced no EMG activity from the rotator—only the usual activity in the abdominal obliques, etc. However, when twisting was attempted in one direction (with minimal muscular effort), there was no response, while in the other direction, there was major activity. It appeared that this particular rotator was not activated to create axial twisting torque but acted in response to twisted position change. Thus its activity, elicited as a function of twisted position, was not consistent with the role of creating torque to "twist" the spine.

MUSCLE ATTACHMENT BOX 33.1

ATTACHMENTS AND INNERVATION OF THE ROTATORES

Inferior attachment: Superior and posterior portion of the transverse process of one vertebra

Superior attachment: Inferior and lateral border of the lamina of the vertebra immediately above the inferior attachment. The rotatores lie deep to the multifidus. The rotatores are less fully developed in the lumbar than in the thoracic region.

Innervation: Dorsal rami of spinal nerves

Palpation: Not palpable.

MUSCLE ATTACHMENT BOX 33.2

ATTACHMENTS AND INNERVATION OF INTERTRANSVERSARII

Inferior attachment: Transverse process of one vertebra

Superior attachment: Transverse process of the vertebra above. In the lumbar region there are two sets of muscles, medial and lateral, each lying posterior to the ventral ramus. The lateral lumbar portion is further divided into ventral and dorsal sections.

Innervation: The nerve supply for the medial portion of the muscle is the dorsal ramus of the associated spinal nerve, while the lateral lumbar portion is innervated by the ventral ramus of the spinal nerve.

Palpation: Not palpable.

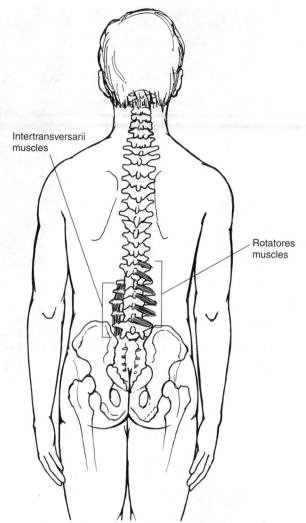

Intertransversarii muscles

Rotatores muscles

Figure 33.2: The small rotator muscles of the lumbar spine, the rotatores and intertransversarii, are seen crossing the joints of the lumbar region.

Clinical Relevance

MANUAL THERAPY AND THE FUNCTION OF THE ROTATORES AND INTERTRANSVERSARII: *It is suspected that these "muscles" are actually length transducers, and thereby position sensors, sensing the positioning of each spinal motion unit. It is very likely that these structures are affected during various types of manual therapy with the joint at end range of motion.*

Extensors: Longissimus, Iliocostalis, and Multifidus Groups

MUSCLE ACTION: EXTENSORS

Action	Evidence
Trunk extension	Supporting
Anterior shear support (longissimus and iliocostails)	Supporting

MUSCLE ATTACHMENT BOX 33.3

ATTACHMENTS AND INNERVATION OF THE LONGISSIMUS THORACIS PARS LUMBORUM

Inferior attachment: Posterior superior iliac spine

Superior attachment: Transverse and accessory processes of the lumbar vertebrae

Innervation: Dorsal rami of the lumbar spinal nerves

Palpation: Cannot be separately identified deep to the thoracolumbar fascia.

The major extensors of the thoracolumbar spine are the longissimus, iliocostalis, and multifidus groups (*Muscle Attachment Boxes 33.3–33.5*). The longissimus and iliocostalis groups are often separated in anatomy books, although it may be more enlightening, in a functional context, to recognize the thoracic portions of both of these muscles as one group and the lumbar portions of these muscles as another group, since the lumbar and thoracic portions are architecturally [3] and functionally different [12]. Bogduk [3] partitions the lumbar and thoracic portions of these muscles into longissimus thoracis pars lumborum and pars thoracis and iliocostalis lumborum pars lumborum and thoracis.

MUSCLE ATTACHMENT BOX 33.4

ATTACHMENTS AND INNERVATION OF THE ILIOCOSTALIS LUMBORUM

Iliocostalis lumborum pars thoracis:

Inferior attachment: Crest of the ilium from the posterior superior iliac spine laterally approximately 5 cm

Superior attachment: Angles of all 12 ribs

Palpation: Palpable with other erector spinae along thoracic vertebrae.

Iliocostalis lumborum pars lumborum:

Inferior attachment: Iliac crest

Superior attachment: Transverse processes of the first four lumbar vertebrae and thoracolumbar fascia

Innervation: Dorsal rami of the thoracic and lumbar spinal nerves

Palpation: Cannot be separately identified deep to the thoracolumbar fascia.

MUSCLE ATTACHMENT BOX 33.5

ATTACHMENTS AND INNERVATION OF THE MULTIFIDUS

Inferior attachment: Posterior surface of the sacrum, aponeurosis of the erector spinae muscles, posterior superior iliac spine (PSIS) and sacroiliac ligaments, and mamillary processes of the lumbar vertebrae

Superior attachment: Superficially to the third or fourth vertebra above, intermediately to the second or third vertebra above, and deeply to the vertebra directly above the inferior attachment. The multifidus muscles lie deep to the semispinalis and erector spinae muscles.

Innervation: Dorsal rami of the spinal nerves

Palpation: Not palpable.

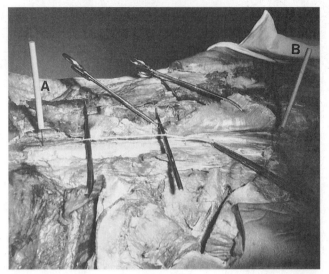

Figure 33.3: A bundle of longissimus thoracis pars thoracis isolated inserting on the ribs at T6 (*probe A*), with their tendons lifted by the probes, course over the full lumbar spine to their sacral origin (*probe B*). They have a very large extensor moment arm. (Reprinted with permission from McGill SM: Biomechanics of the thoracolumbar spine. In: Dvir Z, ed. Clinical Biomechanics. New York: Churchill Livingstone, 2000.)

These two functional groups (pars lumborum, which attach to lumbar vertebrae, and pars thoracis, which attach to thoracic vertebrae) form quite a marvelous architecture for several reasons and are discussed in a functional context with this distinction (i.e., pars lumbar vs. pars thoracic). Fiber-typing studies note differences between the lumbar and thoracic sections, as the thoracic sections contain approximately 75% slow twitch fibers, while lumbar sections are generally evenly mixed [17]. The pars thoracis components of these two muscles attach to the ribs and vertebral components and have relatively short contractile fibers with long tendons that run parallel to the spine to their origins over the posterior surface of the sacrum and medial border of the iliac crests (*Fig. 33.3*). Furthermore, their line of action over the lower thoracic and lumbar region is very superficial, such that forces in these muscles have the greatest possible moment arm and, therefore, produce the greatest amount of extensor moment with a minimum of compressive penalty to the spine (*Fig. 33.4*). When seen on a transverse MRI or CT scan at a lumbar level, their tendons have the greatest extensor moment arm, overlying the lumbar bulk—often over 10 cm [13,14] (see Fig. 33.1).

The lumbar components of these muscles (iliocostalis lumborum pars lumborum and longissimus thoracis pars lumborum) are very different anatomically and functionally from their thoracic namesakes. They connect to the mamillary, accessory, and transverse processes of the lumbar vertebrae and attach distally over the posterior sacrum and medial aspect of the iliac crest. Each vertebra is connected bilaterally with separate laminae of these muscles (*Fig. 33.5*). Their line of action is not parallel to the compressive axis of the spine, but rather has a posterior and caudal direction, which causes them to generate posterior shear forces together with an extensor moment on the superior vertebrae. These posterior shear forces support any anterior reaction shear forces of the

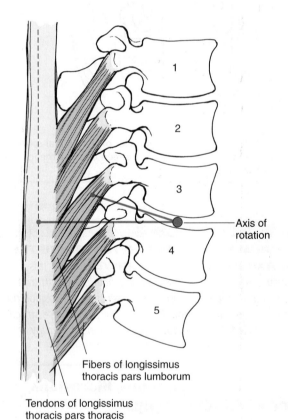

Figure 33.4: Tendons from the longissimus thoracis pars thoracis have a large extensor moment arm as they cross the lumbar joints. (Note that the actual muscle belly is in the thoracic region.) Fibers of longissimus thoracis pars lumborum connect to each lumbar vertebra, and these shorter muscles create extensor moments together with posterior shear forces on the superior vertebrae.

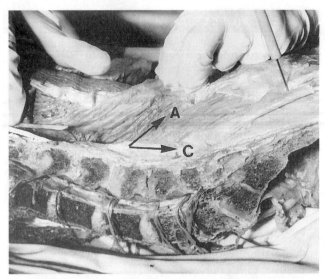

Figure 33.5: The lumbar extensor muscles, the iliocostalis lumborum pars lumborum and longissimus thoracis pars lumborum, originate over the posterior surface of the sacrum, follow a very superficial pathway, and then dive obliquely to their vertebral attachments. Thus, their line of action *(A)* is oblique to the compressive axis *(C)*, and they create posterior shear forces and extensor moments on each successive superior vertebra. (Reprinted with permission from McGill SM: Biomechanics of the thoracolumbar spine. In: Dvir Z, ed. Clinical Biomechanics. New York: Churchill Livingstone, 2000.)

upper vertebrae that are produced as the upper body is flexed forward in a typical lifting type of posture. A discussion of this possible injury mechanism together with activation profiles during clinically relevant activities is addressed in a following section.

The multifidus muscles perform quite a different function, particularly in the lumbar region where they attach posterior spines of adjacent vertebrae or span two or three segments (*Fig. 33.6*). Their line of action tends to be parallel to the compressive axis or, in some cases, runs anteriorly and caudal in an oblique direction. But, the major mechanically relevant feature of the multifidi is that since they span only a few joints, their forces only affect local areas of the spine. Therefore, the multifidus muscles are involved in producing extensor torque (together with very small amounts of twisting and side-bending torque) but only provide the ability for corrections or moment support at specific joints that may be foci of stresses. An injury mechanism involving inappropriate neural activation signals to the multifidus is proposed in the next chapter, using an example of injury observed in the laboratory.

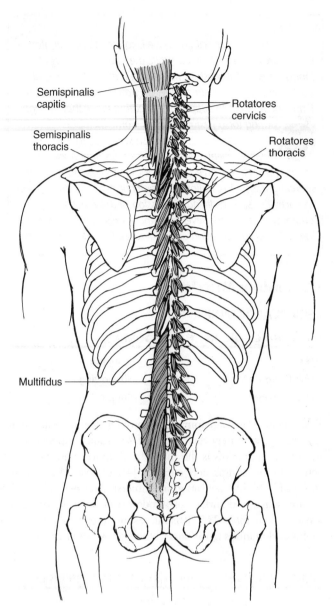

Figure 33.6. The multifidus consists of multiple bundles, or fasciculi, that lie almost parallel to the lumbar spine, each bundle spanning no more than a few lumbar motion segments.

Clinical Relevance

EXERCISE FOR THE EXTENSOR MUSCLES OF THE LOW BACK: *The thoracic extensors (longissimus thoracis pars thoracis and iliocostalis lumborum pars thoracis) that attach in the thoracic region are the most efficient lumbar extensors, since they have the largest moment arms as they*

course over the lumbar region. The clinical practice of "isolating muscle groups," in this case the lumbar extensors for the lumbar spine, needs to be revisited. Specifically, the "lumbar" extensors located in the lumbar region only contribute a portion of the total lumbar extensor moment. Training of the lumbar extensor mechanism must involve the extensors that attach to the thoracic vertebrae, whose bulk of contractile fibers lie in the thoracic region but whose tendons pass over the lumbar region and have the greatest mechanical advantage of all lumbar muscles. Thus, exercises to "isolate" the lumbar muscles cannot be justified from either an anatomical basis or a motor control perspective in which all "players in the orchestra" must be challenged during training.

(continued)

(Continued)

Another important clinical issue is founded upon anatomical features of the extensors. While the lumbar sections of the longissimus and iliocostalis muscles that attach to the lumbar vertebrae create extensor torque, they also produce large posterior shear forces to support the shearing loads that develop during torso flexion postures. Some therapists unknowingly disable these shear force protectors by having patients fully flex their spines during exercises, creating myoelectric quiescence in these muscles, or by recommending the subject maintain a posterior pelvic tilt during flexion activities such as lifting. Discussion of this functional anatomy is critical for developing the strategies for injury prevention and rehabilitation and is described in the next chapter.

Abdominal Muscles

RECTUS ABDOMINIS

MUSCLE ACTION: RECTUS ABDOMINIS

Action	Evidence
Trunk flexion	Supporting
Rib depression	Supporting

While many classic anatomy texts consider the entire abdominal wall to be an important flexor of the trunk, it appears that the rectus abdominis is the major trunk flexor (and the most active during sit-ups and curl-ups [4]) (*Muscle Attachment Box 33.6*). Muscle activation amplitudes obtained from both intramuscular and surface electrodes, over a variety of tasks, are shown in *Table 33.5*. It is interesting to consider why the rectus abdominis is partitioned into sections rather than being

MUSCLE ATTACHMENT BOX 33.6

ATTACHMENTS AND INNERVATION OF THE RECTUS ABDOMINIS

Inferior attachment: Pubic crest and adjacent symphysis

Superior attachment: Fifth, sixth, and seventh costal cartilages and anterior surface of the xiphoid process. The rectus abdominis widens as it ascends and contains three transverse tendinous intersections that adhere to the rectus sheath. One of the intersections is at the umbilicus, one at the end of the xiphoid, and the third one midway in between these two.

Innervation: Ventral rami of lower six or seven thoracic spinal nerves

a single long muscle, given that the sections share a common nerve supply and that a single long muscle would have the advantage of broadening the force–length relationship over a greater range of length change. Perhaps a single muscle would bulk upon shortening, compressing the viscera, or be stiff and resistant to bending. Not only does the "sectioned" rectus abdominis limit bulking upon shortening, but also the sections have a "bead effect" that allows bending at each tendon to facilitate torso flexion–extension or abdominal distension or contraction as the visceral contents change volume [2]).

Another clinical issue surrounds the controversy regarding upper and lower abdominals. It appears that while the obliques are regionally activated (and have functional separation

TABLE 33.5: Subject Averages of EMG Activation Normalized to 100% MVC—Mean and (Standard Deviation)

Abdominal Tasks	Quadratus Lumborum	Psoas 1$_i$	Psoas 2$_i$	EOi	IOi	TAi	RAs	RFs	ESs
Straight leg situps		15(12)	24(7)	44(9)	15(15)	11(9)	48(18)	16(10)	4(3)
Bent knee situps	12(7)	17(10)	28(7)	43(12)	16(14)	10(7)	55(16)	14(7)	6(9)
Press heel situps		28(23)	34(18)	51(14)	22(14)	20(13)	51(20)	15(12)	4(3)
Bent knee curlup	11(6)	7(8)	10(14)	19(14)	14(10)	12(9)	62(22)	8(12)	6(10)
Bent knee leg raise	12(6)	24(15)	25(8)	22(7)	8(9)	7(6)	32(20)	8(5)	6(8)
Straight leg raise	9(2)	35(20)	33(8)	26(9)	9(8)	6(4)	37(24)	23(12)	7(11)
Isom. hand-to-knee LH-RK		16(16)	16(8)	68(14)	30(28)	28(19)	69(18)	8(7)	6(4)
RH-LK		56(28)	58(16)	53(12)	48(23)	44(18)	74(25)	42(29)	5(4)
Cross curlup RS-across	6(4)	5(3)	4(4)	23(20)	24(14)	20(11)	57(22)	10(19)	5(8)
LS-across	6(4)	5(3)	5(5)	24(17)	21(16)	15(13)	58(24)	12(24)	5(8)
Isom. side bridge	54(28)	21(17)	12(8)	43(13)	36(29)	39(24)	22(13)	11(11)	24(15)
Dyn. side bridge		26(18)	13(5)	44(16)	42(24)	44(33)	41(20)	9(7)	29(17)
Pushup from feet	4(1)	24(19)	12(5)	29(12)	10(14)	9(9)	29(10)	10(7)	3(4)
Pushup from knees		14(11)	10(7)	19(10)	7(9)	8(8)	19(11)	5(3)	3(4)

Note: Psoas channels, quadratus lumborum, external oblique, internal oblique, transverse abdominals are intramuscular electrodes; rectus abdominis, rectus femoris, erector spina are surface electrodes. RH-LK, right hand-left knee; LH-RK, left hand-right knee; RS, right shoulder; LS, left shoulder.

between upper and lower regions), all sections of the rectus are activated together at similar levels during flexor torque generation. It appears that there is not a significant functional separation between upper and lower rectus [5] in most persons. Research reporting that there are differences in upper and lower rectus activation sometimes suffer from the absence of normalization of the EMG signal during processing. Briefly, raw amplitudes of myoelectric activity (in millivolts) have been used to conclude that there is more, or less, activity relative to other sections of the muscle, but the magnitudes are affected by local conductivity characteristics. Thus, amplitudes must be normalized to a standardized contraction and expressed as a percentage of this activity (rather than in millivolts). Additional details regarding normalization of EMG are found in Chapter 4.

ABDOMINAL WALL

MUSCLE ACTION: EXTERNAL OBLIQUE ABDOMINAL MUSCLE

Action	Evidence
Trunk flexion	Supporting
Contralateral trunk rotation	Supporting
Increase intraabdominal pressure	Supporting
Rib depression	Supporting
Spinal stabilization	Supporting

MUSCLE ACTION: INTERNAL OBLIQUE

Action	Evidence
Trunk flexion	Supporting
Ipsilateral trunk rotation	Supporting
Increase intraabdominal pressure	Supporting
Rib depression	Supporting
Spinal stabilization	Supporting

MUSCLE ACTION: TRANSVERSUS ABDOMINIS

Action	Evidence
Increase intraabdominal pressure	Supporting
Spinal stabilization	Supporting

The three layers of the abdominal wall (external oblique, internal oblique, transverse abdominis) perform several functions (*Muscle Attachment Boxes 33.7–33.9*). The oblique muscles are involved in flexion and appear to have the ability to flex, enhanced by their attachment to the linea semilunaris (*Fig. 33.7*) [9], which redirects the oblique muscle forces down the rectus sheath to effectively increase their flexor moment arm. Specifically, a large portion of the obliques does not have an anterior bony attachment, but attaches to the rectus abdominis via the linea semilunaris. In this way, the rectus abdominis actually carries some of the oblique muscle forces, enhancing the flexor moment potential of the torso [14]. The obliques are involved in torso twisting [7] and lateral bending [8] and appear to play some role in lumbar stabilization, since the obliques increase their activity, to a small degree,

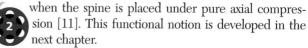

ATTACHMENTS AND INNERVATION OF THE EXTERNAL OBLIQUE

Inferior attachment: Anterior two thirds of the outer lip of the iliac crest and aponeurosis

Superior attachment: Outer surfaces of lower eight ribs, interdigitating with serratus anterior and latissimus dorsi. The external oblique runs in an inferior and anterior direction and is the largest and most superficial of the three muscles of the abdominal wall (external oblique, internal oblique, and transversus abdominis).

Innervation: Ventral rami of lower six thoracic spinal nerves

Palpation: May be palpable in thin individuals with well-developed muscles interdigitated with the serratus anterior on the lateral side of the trunk.

when the spine is placed under pure axial compression [11]. This functional notion is developed in the next chapter.

The fibers of the transversus abdominis run transversely and consequently produce little or no flexion force [15]. Rather the muscle is well aligned to contract with the oblique abdominal muscles to increase intraabdominal pressure for functions such as coughing, defecation, and childbirth. The role of increased intraabdominal pressure in stabilizing the low back is discussed in detail in Chapter 34. Isolated contraction of the transversus abdominis is rare.

MUSCLE ATTACHMENT BOX 33.8

ATTACHMENTS AND INNERVATION OF THE INTERNAL OBLIQUE

Inferior attachment: Thoracolumbar fascia, anterior two thirds of the intermediate line of the iliac crest, lateral two thirds of the inguinal ligament, and the fascia on the iliopsoas muscle

Superior attachment: Inferior borders and tips of the last three or four ribs and cartilage and the aponeurosis. The internal oblique runs superiorly and anteriorly and is thinner and lies beneath the external oblique.

Innervation: Ventral rami of lower six thoracic and first lumbar nerves

Palpation: Not palpable

MUSCLE ATTACHMENT BOX 33.9

ATTACHMENTS AND INNERVATION OF THE TRANSVERSUS ABDOMINIS

Superior attachment: Deep surfaces of the costal cartilages of the lower six ribs, interdigitating with the diaphragm, thoracolumbar fascia between iliac crest and 12th, anterior two thirds of the inner lip of the iliac crest, lateral one third of the inguinal ligament, and fascia over the iliacus muscle

Inferior attachment: The pubic crest and the aponeurosis that fuses with the posterior layers of the aponeurosis of the internal oblique. The transversus abdominis is the innermost of the three muscles of the abdominal wall.

Innervation: Ventral rami of lower six thoracic and first lumbar spinal nerves

Palpation: Not palpable

Clinical Relevance

ABDOMINAL MUSCLE EXERCISES: *The functional divisions of the abdominal muscles justify the need for several exercise techniques to enhance their multiple roles. While the obliques are regionally activated, there appears to be no functional separation of upper and lower rectus abdominis. All parts are activated together at similar amplitudes in most persons. This can be seen in the clinic if care is taken to normalize the channels of EMG as described briefly in Chapter 4. Thus a curl-up exercise activates all of the rectus abdominis. However, upper and lower portions of the oblique abdominal muscles are activated separately, depending upon the demands placed on the torso.*

Special Case of the Quadratus Lumborum and Psoas Major

While the psoas major, a muscle of the hip and lumbar spine, has often been regarded as a good stabilizer of the lumbar spine, it is the opinion of this author that such a role is unlikely (see Chapter 39 for details on the psoas major). This issue is highlighted by a comparison with the quadratus lumborum. Like the lumbar portion of the psoas major, the quadratus lumborum attaches to the lumbar vertebrae, but it also exhibits several structural differences from the psoas major. It has many more fibers cross-linking the vertebrae than does the psoas; it has a larger lateral moment arm via the transverse process attachments; and it traverses the rib cage and iliac crests (*Muscle Attachment Box 33.10*). Thus, while both

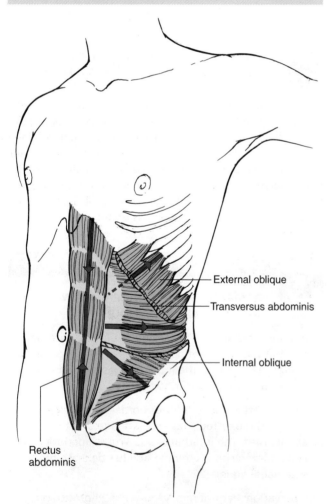

- External oblique
- Transversus abdominis
- Internal oblique
- Rectus abdominis

Figure 33.7: The oblique muscles transmit force along their fiber lengths and then redirect the force along the rectus abdominis, via their attachment to the linea semilunaris, to enhance their effective flexor moment arm. (Reprinted with permission from McGill SM: J Biomech 1996; 29: 973–977.)

MUSCLE ATTACHMENT BOX 33.10

ATTACHMENTS AND INNERVATION OF THE QUADRATUS LUMBORUM

Inferior attachment: Iliolumbar ligament, posterior iliac crest, transverse processes of lower lumbar vertebrae

Superior attachment: Medial one half of the lower border of the 12th rib, transverse processes of upper lumbar vertebrae and 12th thoracic vertebra. The quadratus lumborum lies between the anterior and middle layers of the thoracolumbar fascia, anterior to the erector spinae muscles and posterior to the abdominal organs.

Innervation: Ventral rami of the 12th thoracic and upper three or four lumbar spinal nerves

Palpation: Not palpable.

muscles could buttress shear instability, the quadratus is more effective in all loading modes, by design. In addition, psoas activation profiles are not consistent with that of a spine stabilizer [4] (see Table 33.5). These data indicate that the role of the psoas major is primarily as a hip flexor and to provide hip stiffness. In contrast, activation profiles support the notion of the stabilizing role of the quadratus. It is active during a variety of flexion-dominant, extension-dominant, and lateral-bending tasks of the lower back [1,11]. Further, Andersson et al. [1] find that the quadratus lumborum does not relax with the trunk extensors during the flexion—relaxation phenomenon. The flexion–relaxation phenomenon is an interesting task, since there is no substantial lateral or twisting torque and the extensor torque appears to be supported passively. Continued activity in the quadratus lumborum suggests that the muscle plays a stabilizing role. An experiment in which subjects stand upright but hold buckets in either hand as a load is incrementally added to each bucket reveals that the quadratus lumborum increases its activation level (together with the obliques) as more stability is required [11] (*Fig. 33.8*). This task forms a special situation, since only compressive loading is applied to the spine in the absence of any bending moments.

It is interesting to consider why the psoas major courses over the lumbar spine. Why not just let the iliacus, another hip muscle, perform the role of hip flexion? Without the psoas major, the iliacus would rotate the pelvis upon hip flexion, placing large bending stresses on the lumbosacral junction (in the direction to cause excessive lordosis). The psoas major disperses these stresses over the length of the lumbar region.

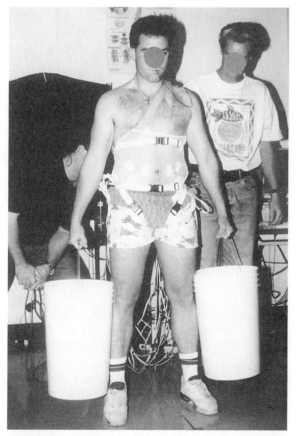

Figure 33.8: Role of active muscle to stabilize the spine. Loading the upright vertebral column (as shown here with the person standing while having weight loaded into baskets in each hand) requires guy wire support from the musculature to prevent buckling. This is an interesting test since muscles, in this posture, are recruited to prevent buckling and not to support moments. In this task, the motor control system appears to choose the abdominal obliques and, to some degree, the quadratus lumborum to provide stability.

Clinical Relevance

QUADRATUS LUMBORUM: *Myoelectric evidence, together with anatomical analysis, suggests that the psoas major acts primarily to flex the hip and that its activation is minimally linked to spine demands. The quadratus lumborum appears to be involved with stabilization of the lumbar spine with other muscles, suggesting clinical focus on the quadratus lumborum may be warranted. Exercises emphasizing activation of the quadratus lumborum are described in the next chapter.*

SUMMARY

This chapter provides an overview of the roles of the muscles of the trunk in moving and stabilizing the lumbar spine. It presents the posterior muscles in four large functional groups. The deepest group appears to act as a position sensor rather than as a generator of torque. The more superficial extensors fall into three categories to (*a*) generate large extension moments, (*b*) generate posterior shear, or (*c*) affect only one or two lumbar segments. The roles of the abdominal muscles in trunk flexion and in trunk stabilization are also discussed, together with the roles of psoas and quadratus lumborum. The abdominal muscles and quadratus lumborum appear to play important roles in stabilizing the spine, but the psoas major appears to be less important for lumbar stabilization. It is clear from this discussion that many muscles play a large role in protecting the low back from injury. Applications of these findings to exercise regimens for individuals with low back pain are presented in the following chapter.

Acknowledgment

The author wishes to acknowledge the contributions of several colleagues who have contributed to the collection of works reported here: Daniel Juker, M.D.; Craig Axler, M.Sc.; Jacek Cholewicki, Ph.D.; Robert Norman, Ph.D.; Michael Sharratt, Ph.D.; John Seguin, M.D.; and Vaughan Kippers, Ph.D. Also the continual financial support from the Natural Science and Engineering Research Council, Canada, has made this series of work possible.

References

1. Andersson EA, Oddsson LIE, Grundstrom H, et al.: EMG activities of the quadratus lumborum and erector spinae muscles during flexion–relaxation and other motor tasks. Clin Biomech 1996; 11: 392–400.
2. Belanger M: Personal communication, University of Quebec at Montreal, 1996.
3. Bogduk N: A reappraisal of the anatomy of the human lumbar erector spinae. J Anat 1980; 131: 525.
4. Juker D, McGill SM, Kropf P, Steffen T: Quantitative intramuscular myoelectric activity of lumbar portions of psoas and the abdominal wall during a wide variety of tasks. Med Sci Sports Exerc 1998; 30: 301–310.
5. Lehman G, McGill SM: Quantification of the differences in EMG magnitude between upper and lower rectus abdominis during selected trunk exercises. Phys Ther 2001; 1096–1101.
6. Macintosh JE, Bogduk N: The morphology of the lumbar erector spinae. Spine 1987; 12: 658.
7. McGill SM: Electromyographic activity of the abdominal and low back musculature during the generation of isometric and dynamic axial trunk torque: implications for lumbar mechanics. J Orthop Res 1991; 9: 91.
8. McGill SM: A myoelectrically based dynamic 3-D model to predict loads on lumbar spine tissues during lateral bending. J Biomech 1992; 25: 395.
9. McGill SM: A revised anatomical model of the abdominal musculature for torso flexion efforts. J Biomech 1996; 29: 973.
10. McGill SM, Juker D, Axler CT: Correcting trunk muscle geometry obtained from MRI and CT scans of supine postures for use in standing postures. J Biomech 1996; 29: 643–646.
11. McGill SM, Juker D, Kropf P: Quantitative intramuscular myoelectric activity of quadratus lumborum during a wide variety of tasks. Clin Biomech 1996; 11: 170.
12. McGill SM, Norman RW: Effects of an anatomically detailed erector spinae model on L4/L5 disc compression and shear. J Biomech 1987; 20: 591.
13. McGill SM, Patt N, Norman RW: Measurement of the trunk musculature of active males using CT scan radiography: duplications for force and moment generating capacity about the L4/L5 joint. J Biomech 1988; 21: 329.
14. McGill SM, Santaguida L, Stevens J: Measurement of the trunk musculature from T6 to L5 using MRI scans of 15 young males corrected for muscle fiber orientation. Clin Biomech 1993; 8: 171.
15. McGill SM: Ultimate back fitness and performance. Backfitpro Inc. www.backfitpro.com 2006.
16. Nitz AJ, Peck D: Comparison of muscle spindle concentrations in large and small human epaxial muscles acting in parallel combinations. Am Surg 1986; 52: 273–277.
17. Sirca A, Kostevc V: The fibre type composition of thoracic and lumbar paravertebral muscles in man. J Anat 1985; 141: 131.

Analysis of the Forces on the Lumbar Spine during Activity

STUART M. McGILL, PH.D.

CHAPTER CONTENTS

This chapter examines the biomechanical evidence regarding the loads and loading mechanisms of the lumbar spine available to date and uses it to assist clinicians in designing and prescribing better rehabilitative exercise on the basis of the best available scientific evidence. While clinicians strive to attain evidence-based practice, too often the prescription of exercise falls short of this laudable objective.

The purpose of this chapter is to lay a scientific foundation upon which the real clinical issues pertaining to optimal rehabilitation may be based. A description of relevant normal biomechanics of the lumbar spine, together with some injury mechanics, is combined with the information from the previous chapter on muscle.

The specific objectives of this chapter are to

- Discuss the forces developed in the low back tissues during selected activities
- Review the biomechanics of the passive tissues (vertebrae, discs, ligaments, fascia)
- Discuss the concepts of spine stability
- Provide guidelines and caveats to assist the development of better rehabilitative exercise programs

The professional challenge for clinicians is to make wise decisions by blending laboratory evidence with clinical experience.

NORMAL BIOMECHANICS AND PATHOMECHANICS OF THE LUMBAR SPINE

Loads on the Low Back during Lifting and Walking

The common activities of lifting and walking generate forces on the low back tissues that are introduced here to "calibrate" the reader for the ensuing discussion. Tissue loads during lifting result from muscle and ligament tension required to support the static posture while holding a load and to facilitate movement. Lifting techniques modulate the distribution of force among the tissues. Given all the possible techniques, it is how these forces are distributed that is so important in

determining the risk of injury from excessive loading. The following example demonstrates this concept.

A man is lifting 27 kg (approximately 60 lb) held in his hands, using a squat lift style. This produces an extensor reaction moment in the low back of 450 Nm (332 ft-lb). The forces in the various tissues that support this moment impose a compressive load on the lumbar spine of over 7,000 N (1,568 lb). Contributions to the total extension moment and to the forces from the muscular components are detailed in *Table 34.1*. These forces and their effects are predicted by a sophisticated modeling approach that uses body segment displacement, spine curvature, and muscle electromyographic (EMG) signals obtained directly from the subject. The interested reader is urged to consult McGill [49] or Cholewicki and McGill [17] for details. It should be noted here that 7,000 N (1,568 lb) of compression begins to cause damage in very

TABLE 34.1: Musculature Forces and Shear and Compressive Contributions to Spine Load during a Squat Lift of 27 kg That Required a Lumbar Extensor Moment of 450 Nm

Muscle[a]	Force (N)	Moment (Nm)	Compression (N)	Shear (N)
Rectus abdominis	25	–2	24	5
External oblique 1	45	1	39	24
External oblique 2	43	–2	30	31
Internal oblique 1	14	1	14	–2
Internal oblique 2	23	–1	17	–16
Longissimus thoracis pars lumborum L4	862	35	744	–436
Longissimus thoracis pars lumborum L3	1514	93	1422	–518
Longissimus thoracis pars lumborum L2	1342	121	1342	0
Longissimus thoracis pars lumborum L1	1302	110	1302	0
Iliocostalis lumborum pars thoracis	369	31	369	0
Longissimus thoracis pars thoracis	295	25	295	0
Quadratus lumborum	393	16	386	74
Latissimus dorsi L5	112	6	79	–2
Multifidus 1	136	8	134	18
Multifidus 2	226	8	189	124
Psoas L1	26	0	23	12
Psoas L2	28	0	27	8
Psoas L3	28	1	27	6
Psoas L4	28	1	27	5

[a]Muscles include both left and right sides of the body.
Note: Negative moments correspond to flexion; negative shear corresponds to L4 shearing posteriorly on L5.

weak spines, although the tolerance of the lumbar spine in an average healthy young man probably approaches 12–15 kN [1] (2,688–3,360 lb). In extreme cases, compressive loads on the spines of competitive weight lifters have safely exceeded 20 kN (4,480 lb).

The individual muscle forces, their contribution to supporting the low back, and their components of compression and shear force that are imposed on the spine are very useful information. In this particular example, the lifter avoided full spine flexion by flexing at the hip, minimizing ligament and other passive tissue tension, and relegating the moment generation responsibility to the musculature. An example in which the spine is flexed is presented later in this chapter. As can be seen, the pars thoracis extensors described in the preceding chapter are very effective lumbar spine extensors, given their large moment arm. Also, since the lifter's upper body is flexed, large reaction shear forces on the spine are produced (the rib cage is trying to shear forward on the pelvis). These shear forces are supported to a very large degree by the pars lumborum extensor muscles. Furthermore, it is clear that the abdominal muscles are activated but produce a negligible contribution to moment–posture support. Why are they active? These muscles are activated to stabilize the spinal column, although this mild abdominal activity imposes a compression penalty to the spine. A more robust explanation of stabilizing mechanics follows in this chapter.

The preceding example demonstrates to the reader how diffusely the forces are distributed and illustrates how proper clinical interpretation requires anatomically detailed free-body diagrams that represent reality (*Fig. 34.1*). It is the opinion of this author that oversimplified free-body diagrams have overlooked the important mechanical compressive and, especially, shear components of muscular force. This has compromised assessment of injury mechanisms and the formulation of optimal therapeutic exercise.

During walking, thousands of low-level loading cycles are endured by the spine every day. While the small loads in the low back during walking suggest it is a safe and tolerable activity, clinicians have found that walking provides relief to some individuals but is painful to others. Recent work has suggested that walking speed affects spine mechanics and may account for these individual differences. During walking, the compressive loads on the lumbar spine of approximately 2.5 times body weight, together with the very modest shear forces, are well below any known in vitro failure load.

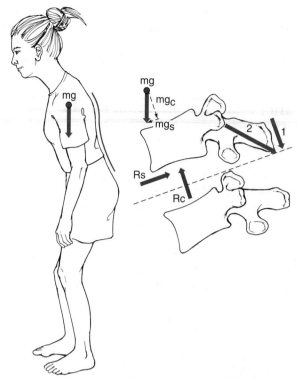

Figure 34.1: Free-body diagram of forward-bending while keeping the lumbar spine erect shows how the lumbar extensors support the reaction shear of the upper body. Specifically, the lumbar fibers of the longissimus and iliocostalis muscles *(2)* create posterior shear to offset the reaction shear *(Rs)* of gravity on the upper body. *1*, the force from the pars thoracis muscles spanning the lumbar segments; *Rc*, the compression reaction force; *mg*, the superincumbent weight.

swinging, with all other factors controlled, results in lower lumbar spine torques, muscle activity, and loading. Swinging the arms may facilitate efficient storage and recovery of elastic energy, reducing the need for concentric muscle contraction together with reduction in upper body accelerations associated with each step. It is interesting to note that fast walking has been shown to be a positive cofactor in prevention of, and more successful recovery from, low back troubles [55].

An appreciation of the magnitude and direction of loads sustained by tissues of the trunk is essential to understanding the mechanisms of low back injury and repair. This brief discussion of the spine and spine tissue forces will assist in building the foundation needed for developing better clinical practice.

BIOMECHANICS OF THE PASSIVE TISSUES OF THE LUMBAR SPINE

Interpretation of the forces described in the previous section is limited to neutral spine postures, therefore only muscle contributions are considered. However, as the spine flexes, bends,

Clinical Relevance

WALKING AND LOW BACK PAIN: *"Strolling" reduces spine motion and produces static loading of tissues, whereas faster walking, with arms swinging, causes cyclic loading of tissues [14]. This change in motion may begin to explain the relief walking provides some people who have low back pain. Arm*

and twists, passive tissues are stressed, and their resultant forces change the interpretation of injury exacerbation and/or the discussion of clinical issues. For this reason, the mechanics of passive tissues is introduced below, followed by some examples illustrating the effects on clinical mechanics.

Functional Consideration for the Interspinous and Supraspinous Ligaments

The interspinous and supraspinous ligaments are important contributors to lumbar flexion mechanics. These ligaments are often described as a single structure in anatomy texts, although functionally they appear to have quite different roles. The interspinous ligaments connect adjacent posterior spines but are not oriented parallel to the compressive axis of the spine. Rather, they have a very large angle of obliquity (Fig. 34.2) [27], which is often shown incorrectly in anatomy texts. Heylings [27] suggests that the interspinous ligaments act like collateral ligaments similar to those in the knee, controlling the vertebral rotation throughout the flexion range.

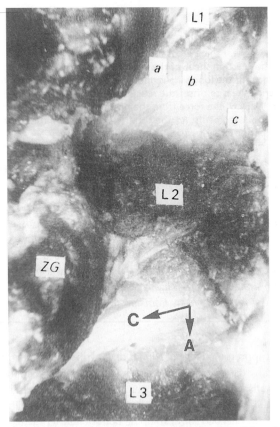

Figure 34.2: The interspinous ligament runs obliquely (C) to the compressive axis (A) and thus has limited capacity to check flexion rotation of the superior vertebral. Rather, the interspinous may act as a collateral ligament, controlling vertebral rotation and imposing anterior shear forces on the superior vertebrae. L1, L2, and L3 indicate the spinous processes of the respective vertebrae. Interspinous ligament between L1 and L2 is indicated by a, b, and c. Anterior is to the left. (Reprinted with permission from Heylings D: J Anat 1978; 123: 127–131.)

This control, in turn, assists the facet joints to remain in contact, gliding with rotation. Furthermore, with their oblique lines of action, these ligaments protect against posterior shearing of the superior vertebrae on its inferior partner. The supraspinous ligament, on the other hand, is aligned parallel to the compressive axis of the spine, connecting the tips of the posterior spines. It appears to provide resistance against excessive forward flexion.

Determining the roles of ligaments has involved qualitative interpretation using their attachments and lines of action together with functional tests in which successive ligaments are destroyed, and the joint motion reassessed. Early studies to determine the relative contribution of each ligament to restricting flexion, in particular, were performed on cadaveric preparations that were not preconditioned prior to testing, resulting in an abnormally large disc space. This suggests that early data that described the relative roles of various ligaments are incorrect. For example, upon death, the discs, being hydrophilic, increase their water content and, consequently, their height. The "swollen" discs in cadaveric specimens result in an artificial preload on the ligaments closest to the disc, causing the earlier studies to suggest that the capsular and longitudinal ligaments are more important in resisting flexion than is actually true in vivo. The work of Sharma et al. [64] shows that the major ligaments for resisting flexion are the supraspinous complex.

MECHANISMS OF INJURY

The lumbar spine is subjected to large compressive and shear forces. However, the margin of safety is much larger in compressive loading than in shear loading since the spine can tolerate well over 10kN in compression, but 1,000 N of shear force causes injury with cyclic loading (one-time loading of 2,000 N [448 lb] is very dangerous.) As noted earlier in this chapter, compressive loads arise from the weight of the head, arms, and trunk and any loads being carried, but also from contractions of the supporting trunk musculature. Although compressive loading can produce injuries, it is likely that more low back injuries result from shear loading.

In a previous section, lifting with the torso flexing about the hips, rather than the spine, is analyzed. Now the exercise is reexamined, but the lifter has elected to flex the spine sufficiently to cause the posterior ligaments to strain (Fig. 34.3). This lifting strategy (spine flexion) has dramatic effects on shear loading of the intervertebral column and the resultant risk of injury. First, the dominant direction of the pars lumborum fibers of the longissimus thoracis and iliocostalis lumborum muscles noted in the previous chapter, causes these muscles to produce a posterior shear force on the superior vertebra. In contrast, with spine flexion, the interspinous ligament complex generates forces with the opposite obliquity and, therefore, imposes an anterior shear force on the superior vertebra (see Figs. 34.2 and 34.3). Thus, the posture, or curvature, of the spine is important in influencing the interplay between passive tissues and muscles that ultimately modulates the risk of several types of injury.

larger in the compressive mode than in the shear mode, since the spine can safely tolerate well over 10 kN in compression, but 1,000 N of shear force causes injury with cyclic loading. This example also illustrates the need for clinicians to consider more loading modes than simple compression. In this example, the real risk is anterior–posterior shear load.

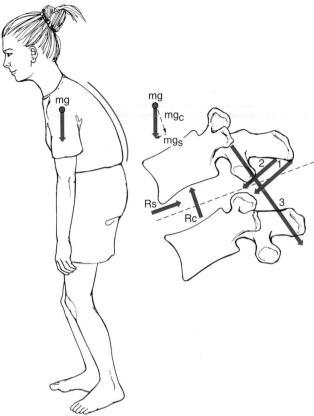

Figure 34.3: Free-body diagram while bending forward with lumbar spine flexion shows that the anterior shear forces can reach dangerous levels from the upper body reaction *(Rs)*, interspinous ligaments *(1 and 2)*, and reorientation of the lumbar extensor fibers of longissimus and iliocostalis muscles *(3)*, which decrease their ability to support shear as they change their orientation during lumbar flexion. *Rc,* compression reaction force; *mg,* superincumbent weight.

> ## Clinical Relevance
>
> **LIFTING POSTURE:** *Most individuals recognize that lifting a load safely requires bending the knees. An understanding of shear forces on the spine leads to the recognition that lifting safety is enhanced when the lifter maintains a neutral spine. This posture allows the trunk extensors to exert a posterior pull to oppose the anterior shear forces from the body weight and the additional shear forces from the load.*

If a subject holds a load in the hands with the spine fully flexed, sufficient to achieve **myoelectric silence** in the extensors (reducing their tension as the result of the flexion–relaxation phenomenon) and with all joints held still so that the low back moment remains the same, then the recruited ligaments appear to contribute to the anterior shear force, so that shear force levels are likely to exceed 1,000 N (224 lb). Such large shear forces are of great concern from an injury risk viewpoint. However, when a more neutral lordotic posture is adopted, the extensor musculature is responsible for creating the extensor moment and at the same time provides a posterior shear force that supports the anterior shearing action of gravity on the upper body and hand-held load. Thus using muscle to support the moment in a more neutral posture, rather than being fully flexed with ligaments supporting the moment, greatly reduces shear loading *(Table 34.2)*.

This example demonstrates that the spine is at a much greater risk of sustaining shear injury (>1,000 N) (224 lb) than compressive injury (3,000 N) (672 lb), simply because the spine is fully flexed, or in a position at the end range of motion (for a more comprehensive discussion see references 37, 42, and 43). As noted earlier the margin of safety is much

Although lifting is a familiar mode of low back injury, falls and other traumatic mechanisms can also produce injury. Such injuries are characterized by their high velocities and the resulting high rates of strain applied to the tissue.

King [29] notes that soft tissue ligamentous injuries are much more common during high-energy traumatic events such as automobile collisions and impact scenarios in athletics. Our own observations on pig and human specimens loaded at slow load rates in bending and shear forces most frequently suggest that excessive tension in the longitudinal ligaments results in avulsion or bony failure as the ligament pulls some bone away from its attachment. Noyes and colleagues [54] noted that slower strain rates (0.66%/sec) produced more ligament avulsion injuries, while faster strain rates (66%/sec) resulted in more ligamentous failure of the fiber bundles in the middle region of the ligament, at least in monkey knee ligaments. (Chapter 6 discusses in detail the effects of loading rate on connective tissue.)

Rissanen [60] reports that approximately 20% of cadaveric spines possessed visibly ruptured lumbar interspinous ligaments in their middle, not at their bony attachment. This report also notes that dorsal and ventral portions of the interspinous ligaments, together with the supraspinous ligament, remained intact.

Given the oblique fiber direction of the interspinous complex, a very likely scenario to damage this ligament would be slipping, falling, and landing on one's behind, driving the pelvis forward on impact and creating a posterior shearing of the lumbar joints when the spine is fully flexed *(Fig. 34.4)*. The interspinous ligament is a major load-bearing tissue in this example of high-energy loading in which anterior shear displacement is combined with full flexion. Given the available data, it is the opinion of this author that damage to the ligaments of the spine during lifting or other normal occupational

TABLE 34.2: Individual Muscle and Passive Tissue Forces and the Lumbar Moments, Compression, and Shear Forces during Full Flexion Together with Just the Forces in a More Neutral Lumbar Posture, Demonstrating the Shift from Muscle to Passive Tissue and the Resultant Effects on Joint Compression and Shear

| Muscle | Fully Flexed Lumbar Spine | | | | | | | Neutral Lumbar Spine |
| | Moment (Nm) | | | Compression (N) | Shear (N) | | Muscle Forces (N) | Muscle Forces (N) |
	Flexion	Lateral	Twist		Anteroposterior	Lateral		
R Rectus abdominis	-2	1	1	15	5	-4	16	39
L Rectus abdominis	-2	-1	-1	15	5	4	16	62
R External oblique 1	-1	1	1	8	7	-3	10	68
L External oblique 1	-1	-1	-1	8	7	3	10	40
R External oblique 2	-1	1	0	6	2	-3	7	62
L External oblique 2	-1	-1	-0	6	2	3	7	31
R Internal oblique 1	0	3	-2	21	-19	20	35	130
L Internal oblique 1	0	-3	2	21	-19	-20	35	102
R Internal oblique 2	-2	2	-3	8	-17	21	29	116
L Internal oblique 2	-2	-2	3	8	-17	-21	29	88
R Pars lumborum (L1)	2	1	0	21	6	2	21	253
L Pars lumborum (L1)	2	-1	-0	21	6	-2	21	285
R Pars lumborum (L2)	2	1	0	26	8	2	27	281
L Pars lumborum (L2)	2	-1	-0	26	8	-2	27	317
R Pars lumborum (L3)	1	1	0	29	-4	6	31	327
L Pars lumborum (L3)	1	-1	-0	29	-4	-6	31	333
R Pars lumborum (L4)	1	1	-0	30	-7	6	32	402
L Pars lumborum (L4)	1	-1	0	30	-7	-6	32	355
R Iliocostalis lumborum	5	4	1	57	14	-1	58	100
L Iliocostalis lumborum	5	-4	-1	57	14	1	58	137
R Longissimus thoracis	7	4	0	91	23	-6	93	135
L Longissimus thoracis	7	-4	-0	91	23	6	93	179
R Quadratus lumborum	1	2	-0	25	-1	1	25	155
L Quadratus lumborum	1	-2	0	25	-1	-1	25	194
R Latissimus dorsi (L5)	1	1	-0	14	-1	-6	15	101
L Latissimus dorsi (L5)	1	-1	0	14	-1	6	15	115
R Multifidus 1	1	1	1	26	6	9	28	80
L Multifidus 1	1	-1	-1	26	6	-9	28	102
R Multifidus 2	1	1	0	28	6	0	28	87

L Multifidus 2	1	−0	28	6	0	28	90
R Psoas (L1)	1	0	24	0	6	25	61
L Psoas (L1)	−1	−0	24	0	−6	25	69
R Psoas (L2)	−1	0	24	0	6	25	62
L Psoas (L2)	−0	−0	24	0	−6	25	69
R Psoas (L3)	−0	0	24	0	7	25	62
L Psoas (L3)	−0	−0	24	0	−7	25	69
R Psoas (L4)	−0	1	24	0	8	25	61
L Psoas (L4)	−0	−1	24	0	−8	25	69
Ligament							
Anterior longitudinal	0	0	0	0	—	0	0
Posterior longitudinal	2	0	261	44	—	86	0
Ligamentum flavum	1	0	21	2	—	21	3
R Intertransverse	0	0	13	3	—	14	0
L Intertransverse	0	−0	13	3	—	14	0
R Articular	2	1	65	40	—	74	0
L Articular	2	−1	65	40	—	74	0
R Articular 2	3	2	84	−3	—	103	0
L Articular 2	3	−2	84	−3	—	103	0
Interspinous 1	18	0	273	142	—	301	0
Interspinous 2	14	0	233	268	—	345	0
Interspinous 3	10	0	194	238	—	298	0
Supraspinous	41	0	591	79	—	592	0
R Lumbodorsal fascia	8	−0	109	−1	—	122	0
L Lumbodorsal fascia	−1	0	109	−1	—	122	0
Passive tissue							
Disc	9	0	—	0	—	—	1
Gut, etc.	11	0	—	0	—	—	2

Note: The extensor moment with full lumbar flexion is 171 Nm, producing 3,145 N of compression and 954 N of anterior shear. In the more neutral posture, an extension moment of 170 Nm produces 3,490 N of compression and 269 N of shear.

607

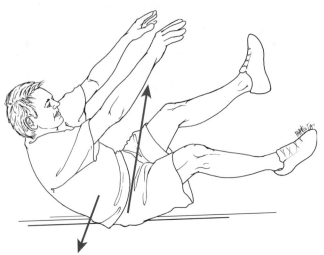

Figure 34.4: Loads during a fall. Landing on the buttocks pushes the pelvis anteriorly and creates a posterior shear on the lumbar spine.

activities, particularly to the interspinous complex, is more uncommon than common. Rather, it appears much more likely that ligament damage occurs during a more traumatic event, particularly landing on one's behind during a fall, and leads to joint laxity and acceleration of subsequent arthritic changes. As has been often said in reference to the knee joint, "ligament damage marks the beginning of the end."

Clinical Relevance

LOW BACK INJURIES FROM FALLS: *As in lifting injuries, shear forces appear to be the culprit in low back injuries from falls. Yet the direction of the damaging shear force is in the opposite direction compared with lifting. Consequently, the motions that reproduce the symptoms as well as those that reduce symptoms are likely to differ from those motions in an individual with a lifting injury. Understanding the mechanism of injury helps the clinician to identify strategies to reduce pain.*

Functional Consideration of the Vertebrae

THE VERTEBRAL BODY

While many consider the vertebrae to be stiff, rigid structures, in fact, they are not. The vertebral bodies themselves may be likened to a barrel in which the round walls are formed with relatively stiff cortical bone. However, the top and bottom of the barrel are formed with a more deformable cartilage plate (endplate), while the inside of the body is filled with cancellous bone. The trabecular arrangement within the cancellous bone is aligned with the trajectories of stress to

which it is exposed, dominated by compression and thus a vertical arrangement. This is a very special architecture in terms of how the vertebral bodies bear compressive load and fail under excessive loading. Two major types of injury appear to occur, endplate fracture and cancellous bone fracture within the body, both of which are discussed below.

While the walls of the vertebra appear to be rigid upon compression, the nucleus of the disc is pressurized, as demonstrated by the classic work by Nachemson [50,53]. This pressure causes the cartilaginous endplates of the vertebra to bulge inward, seemingly to compress the cancellous bone [10]. In fact, under compression, it is the cancellous bone that fails first [10], making it the tissue that determines the compressive strength of the spine (at least when the spine is in a neutral posture and not positioned at the end range of motion). It is difficult to injure the anulus fibrosus under compressive loading. Mechanisms that lead to anular failure are discussed later in this chapter. While this notion of compressibility of the vertebral endplate is contrary to the concept that the vertebral bodies are rigid, the functional interpretation of this anatomy suggests the presence of a very clever shock-absorbing and load-bearing system. Farfan [21] proposes the notion that the vertebral bodies act as shock absorbers of the spine, although this theory is based on vertebral body fluid flow and not endplate bulging. Since the nucleus pulposus is an incompressible fluid, under compressive loading the vertebral endplates bulge inward, suggesting fluid expulsion from the vertebral bodies, specifically blood through the perivertebral sinuses [61]. This suggests protective dissipation of stress during quasi-static and dynamic compressive loading of the spine. The question is, how do the endplates bulge inward into seemingly rigid cancellous bone? The answer appears to be in the architecture of the cancellous bone, which is dominated by the system of columns of bone with much smaller transverse bony ties. Upon axial compression, as the endplates bulge into the vertebral bodies, these columns experience compression and appear to bend in a buckling mode. Fyhrie and Schaffler [22] demonstrate that under excessive load, these columns buckle as the small bony transverse ties fracture (*Fig. 34.5*). In this way, the cancellous bone can rebound back to its original shape (at least 95% of the original unloaded shape) when the load is removed, even after suffering fractures of the transverse ties. This architecture appears to afford superior elastic deformation, even after marked damage, and allows the bone to heal and regain its original structure and function.

Under excessive compressive loading, endplates bulge into the vertebral bodies, causing radial stresses in the endplate sufficient to cause fracture in a "stellate" pattern. These fractures or cracks in the endplate are sometimes large enough to allow the nucleus pulposus to squirt through into the vertebral body [53], forming Schmorl's node. The classic **Schmorl's node** is nuclear material found within the vertebral body and surrounded by bone (*Fig. 34.6*). This type of injury is associated with compression of the spine when the spine is not at the end range of motion (i.e., neither flexed, bent, nor twisted).

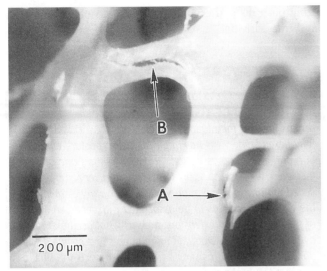

Figure 34.5: Trabecular bone fractures. Under compressive loading, bulging of the endplate can cause buckling fractures in the vertical trabeculae **(A)**. These generate tensile stresses in the transverse trabeculae that can produce tensile cracks **(B)**. (Reprinted with permission from Fyhrie DP, Schaffler MB: Failure mechanisms in human vertebral cancellous bone. Bone 1994; 15: 105–109.)

Clinical Relevance

ENDPLATE FRACTURES: *It is the opinion of this author that endplate fractures, with the loss of nuclear fluid through the crack into the vertebral body (often forming Schmorl's nodes), are very common compressive injuries and perhaps the most misdiagnosed. Loss of the nucleus pulposus results in a flattened interdiscal space that when seen on planar x-rays is usually diagnosed as a herniated disc. However, the anulus of the disc remains intact. It is simply a case of the nucleus squirting through the endplate crack into the cancellous core of the vertebra. True disc herniation requires very special conditions, which are described shortly.*

POSTERIOR ELEMENTS OF THE VERTEBRA

The facet joint complex is described in Chapter 32. However, a relevant biomechanical feature is that the neural arch made up of the pedicles and laminae appears to be somewhat flexible [7,20]. Failure of these elements together with facet damage leads to **spondylolisthesis,** an anterior displacement of the superior vertebra on the inferior vertebra. It is often blamed exclusively on anterior–posterior shear forces. There is no doubt that excessive shear forces also cause injury to these elements. Posterior shear of the superior vertebra can lead to ligamentous damage but also to failure in the vertebra itself as the endplate avulses from the rest of the vertebral body, particularly in adolescent and geriatric spines. Further,

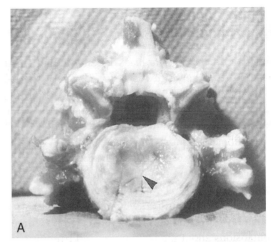

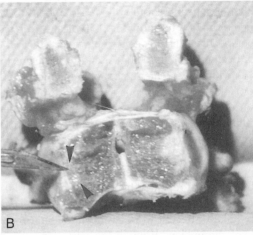

Figure 34.6: **A.** The stellate pattern of an endplate fracture. **B.** Intrusion of nuclear material (shown at the tip of the scalpel) into the vertebral body from compressive loading of a spine in a neutral posture. Both photos are of porcine specimens. (Reprinted with permission from McGill SM: Biomechanics of low back injury: implications on current practice and the clinic. J Biomech 1977; 30: 465–475.)

anterior shear of the superior vertebra has been documented to cause pars and facet fracture leading to spondylolisthesis [68], with a typical tolerance of an adult lumbar spine of approximately 2,000 N (448 lb) [18]. This magnitude of force may be created during a slip and fall, producing a posterior shear, or during lifting with a fully flexed spine, producing an anterior shear as noted in a previous section of this chapter. It appears from both mechanical analysis and epidemiological evidence that damage to these posterior elements may also be associated with repeated, full range of motion, such as that sustained by gymnasts and Australian cricket players [26]. These sorts of activities cause stress reversals in the pars with each cycle of bending (full flexion and extension), causing cracks to form and propagate, eventually fracturing the arch. These fractures are examples of fatigue fractures. Thus, the facet joint complex is susceptible to injury from activities that produce excessive loading as well as from low load, high repetition activities.

Functional Consideration of the Intervertebral Disc

The ability of the disc to bear loads depends upon its anatomical structure together with the posture or curvature of the spine. Twisting of the spine is a good example of this dependance. As noted in Chapter 32, the collagen fibers within the concentric rings of the anulus fibrosus are arranged with one half of the fibers oblique to the other half (*Fig. 34.7*). In this way, the anulus is able to resist twisting. However, only half of the fibers are able to support this mode of loading, while the other half become disabled, resulting in a substantial loss of strength or ability to bear load with increasing twist.

From a review of the literature, one can make three general conclusions about anulus injuries and true disc herniations. First, it appears that the disc must be bent to the full end range of motion to herniate [2]. Typically, from a functional perspective, this means the spine must be at the end range of flexion. Also, herniations tend to occur in younger spines [3], with higher water content [4] and more-hydraulic behavior. Older spines do not appear to exhibit "classic" extrusion of nuclear material, but rather are characterized by delamination of the anulus layers, and radial cracks that progress with repeated loading. A nice review is provided by Goel et al. [23]. Furthermore, disc herniation is associated not only with extreme postures (either fully flexed or side-bent), but also with repeated bending at least 20 or 30 thousand times, highlighting the role of fatigue as a mechanism of injury [24,29]. Recent work has documented progressive tracking of the nucleus through the posterior parts of the anulus with continual full-flexion bending. Finally, epidemiological data link herniation with sedentary occupations and the sitting posture [66]. In fact, Wilder et al. [67] document anular tears in young calf spines from prolonged simulated sitting postures and cyclic compressive loading (i.e., simulated truck driving).

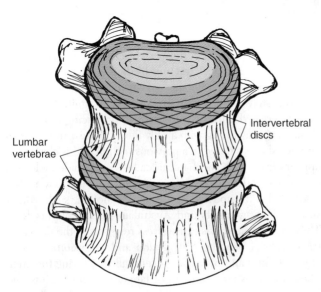

Figure 34.7: Collagen fibers of the anulus are arranged with one half of the fibers being oblique to the other half so that during twisting only half of the fibers bear load.

Lumbar vertebrae

Intervertebral discs

Clinical Relevance

MECHANISMS OF TISSUE FAILURE: *Damage to the anulus fibrosus (herniation) appears to be associated with a fully flexed spine. This has implications on posture correction and exercise prescription. Prolonged sitting and abdominal exercises such as "crunches" are characterized by a fully flexed lumbar spine. Damage to posterior bony elements of the vertebrae appears to be associated with repeated cycles of full flexion to full extension, such as what occurs during gymnastic routines. Damage to ligaments is associated with ballistic insults such as slips and falls or impacts in athletic or other traumatic situations.*

FUNCTIONAL CONSIDERATION FOR THE LUMBODORSAL FASCIA

Recent studies attribute various mechanical roles to the lumbodorsal fascia (LDF). In fact, there have been some attempts to recommend lifting techniques based on these hypotheses. But are they consistent with experimental evidence? Suggestions were originally made [25] that lateral forces generated by the internal oblique and transverse abdominis muscles are transmitted to the LDF via their attachments to the lateral border, with claims that the fascia could support substantial extensor moments. This lateral tension on the LDF was hypothesized to increase longitudinal tension by virtue of the collagen fiber obliquity in the LDF, causing the posterior spinous processes to move together, resulting in lumbar extension. This proposed sequence of events formed an attractive proposition because the LDF has the largest moment arm of all extensor tissues. As a result, any extensor forces within the LDF would impose the smallest compressive penalty to vertebral components of the spine.

However, this hypothesis was examined by three studies, all published about the same time, which collectively challenge its viability: Tesh et al. [65], who performed mechanical tests on cadaveric material; Macintosh et al. [32], who recognized the anatomical inconsistencies with the abdominal activation; and McGill and Norman [48], who tested the viability of LDF involvement with latissimus dorsi as well as with the abdominals. These collective works show that the LDF is not a significant active extensor of the spine. Nonetheless, the LDF is a strong tissue with a well-developed lattice of collagen fibers, suggesting that its function may be that of an extensor muscle retinaculum [8] or nature's abdominal belt. The tendons of longissimus thoracis and iliocostalis lumborum pass under the LDF to their sacral and iliac attachments. It appears that the LDF may provide a form of "strapping" for the low back musculature.

SPINE STABILITY: MUSCLE STIFFNESS AND CO-CONTRACTION, MOTOR CONTROL, AND THE LINK TO THE CLINIC

The concept of stability is being used in the clinic to enhance rehabilitation outcomes and justify better injury prevention strategies. In fact, "stability" is the foundation for the current paradigm shift now occurring in rehabilitation. An earlier section of this chapter documents abdominal wall activity during a lift. Why does the motor control system expend energy in this way?

It is clear that abdominal activity during lifting is counterproductive for producing an extensor moment that is needed to support the lifting posture. Consider that a spine without muscular support fails under compressive loading in a buckling mode, at about 20 N (5 lb) [30]. In other words, a bare spine is unable to bear compressive load! The spine can be likened to a flexible rod that buckles under compressive loading. However, if the rod has guy wires connected to it, like the rigging on a ship's mast, more compression is ultimately experienced by the rod, but the rod is able to bear much more compressive load as it is stiffened and becomes more resistant to buckling (*Fig. 34.8*). The co-contracting musculature of the lumbar spine performs the role of stabilizing guy wires to each lumbar vertebra of the flexible column, bracing the spine against buckling.

Understanding stability from a clinical perspective requires several steps. First, there is a critical link between muscle activation and stiffness. Activating a muscle increases stiffness of both the muscle and the joint(s) [16]. Activating a group of muscle synergists and antagonists in the optimal way now becomes a critical issue. From a motor control point of view, the analogy of an orchestra is useful. The orchestra must play together, or in clinical terms, the full complement of the stabilizing musculature must work together to achieve stability. One instrument out of tune ruins the sound. One muscle with inappropriate activation or force-stiffness can produce instability or at least unstable behavior will result at lower externally applied loads.

It has been claimed for many years that intraabdominal pressure (IAP) plays an important role in support of the lumbar spine, especially during strenuous lifting. Although it was thought that IAP directly reduced compressive loads on the spine, it was found that the abdominal muscle activity needed to create higher IAP actually increased spine compression [47,52]. Despite adding additional compressive force to the lumbar spine, IAP through contraction of the abdominal muscles appears to stabilize the spine. The mechanism of this increased stability remains controversial. Some suggest that IAP produces an extensor moment that assists the erector spinae in supporting the spine [19]. Others suggest that the abdominal muscles with other trunk muscles serve to stiffen the spine, effectively creating a flexible corset or air splint

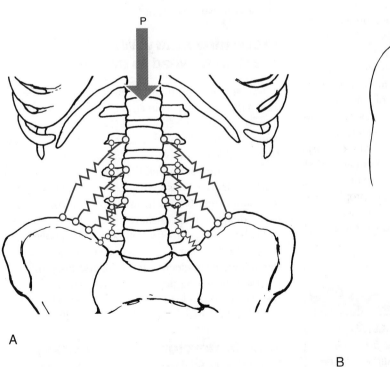

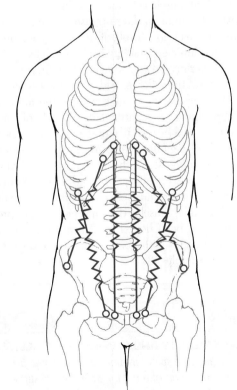

Figure 34.8: Co-contracting muscles stabilize the spine to prevent buckling. **A.** Paraspinal muscles stiffen and stabilize the vertebrae directly (a few are seen). **B.** The abdominal wall stabilizes the spine by its attachment to the rib cage and pelvis. Buckling can occur when one or more muscles have an inappropriate amount of stiffness, determined by the activation level of the muscles.

around the spine [16,47]. Regardless of the mechanism, stability of the spine is the result.

Clinicians are very aware of patients who co-contract their torso muscles to stabilize a joint. This type of behavior makes sense, and in fact, it is the only way to stabilize a joint actively. However, the clinical question then becomes how much stability is necessary? The concept of "sufficient stability" is essential for clinicians to consider.

For a joint to bear larger loads, more stability is required. In most activities only a modest amount of stability is required. Too much stiffness from muscle activation imposes a severe load penalty by increasing joint compression forces on the joint. Excessive stiffness also impedes the joint's motion. In normal joints, with fit motor control systems, appropriate stability is achieved. In addition to muscular sources of joint stiffness, individual joints have passive stiffness. **Stiffness** is defined as the ratio between the force applied to an object and the object's resulting change in shape (Chapter 2). Following injury, passive tissue stiffness is reduced. Also, reports document that the motor system is altered, resulting in inappropriate muscle activation sequences. The biomechanist's contribution is to quantify the loss of passive stiffness and determine how much muscular stiffness is necessary for stability. Once this amount of stability is determined, the clinician will then wish to add a modest amount of extra stability to form a margin of safety. This is known as "sufficient stability."

The stability concept is revolutionizing rehabilitation. The biomechanists are beginning to provide clinicians with specific target levels of muscle activation to achieve sufficient stability. Interestingly enough, large muscular forces are rarely required. Instead, low levels of muscular co-contraction are required for sufficient stability in almost all tasks. This means that a patient must be able to maintain sufficient stability getting on and off the toilet, in and out of the car, up and down stairs, etc. This argument suggests that the margin of safety when performing tasks, particularly the tasks of daily living, is not compromised by insufficient strength but rather by insufficient muscular endurance or muscle coordination. We are beginning to understand the mechanistic pathway of those studies showing the efficacy of endurance training, rather than strength of the muscles that stabilize the spine. Having strong abdominal muscles does not provide the prophylactic effect that had been hoped for. However, recent work suggests that muscles with good endurance reduce the risk of future back troubles [31].

Clinical Relevance

JOINT STABILITY AND CLINICAL PRACTICE: *Stiffness and stability of a spinal motion segment come from both muscle contraction and the inherent passive stiffness of the joint. Clinicians who practice manual therapy attempt to identify spinal segments that are not moving correctly or are "blocked" or "stiff." Recalling that the definition of stiffness*

implies that a "stiff" joint requires increased force to move it, a stiff joint actually is a more stable joint and requires a very large perturbation to become unstable. In contrast, the clinical expression "stiff joint" usually means that the joint lacks range of motion. However, the joint that lacks mobility often is supported by weaker tissue and is more susceptible to injury from high loads. (Chapter 6 describes the effects of immobilization on connective tissue.)

A common goal of therapy is to restore normal motion, but more motion requires more stability. Clinicians should give due consideration to enhancing spinal stability from muscular sources following mobilization therapy. Furthermore, there may be a peril in mobilization producing too much motion, increasing the importance of specific training for muscular endurance and motor control to enhance spine stability [41].

CLINICAL APPLICATION: USING BIOMECHANICS TO BUILD BETTER REHABILITATION PROGRAMS FOR LOW BACK INJURY

Reducing the pain and improving function for patients with low back pain involves two components: removing the stressors that create or exacerbate damage and enhancing activities that build healthy supportive tissues. This section begins with a brief listing of considerations for prophylaxis and then focuses on issues relevant to wise exercise prescription.

Preventing Injury: What Does the Patient Need to Know?

A few universal guidelines can be based on the foundation laid in this and the previous chapters. Perhaps the single most important guideline should be "Don't do too much of any one thing." Either too much loading or too little is detrimental. Other guidelines include (a) avoid repeated or prolonged end-range lumbar motion that puts the disc at risk; (b) design work to vary positions so that loads are rotated among the various supporting tissues to minimize the risk of accumulated tissue deformation; (c) allow time for tissues to restore their unloaded rest geometry following the application of prolonged loads when creep has occurred prior to performing demanding tasks (such as in prolonged stooping); (d) don't sit too long (how long depends on the patient's history and status); (e) keep the loads close to the low back. A much more developed list may be found in McGill [46].

Toward Developing Scientifically Justified Low Back Rehabilitation Exercises

The "art" of rehabilitation is to find the optimal physical challenge—not too much and not too little. The "science" of rehabilitation provides the foundation to find the optimum.

While it is outside the scope of this chapter, the interested reader is urged to consult the literature for a description of the scientific methods used to develop the following program [17,28,36,49].

A lot of the notions that clinicians consider principles for exercise prescription may not be as well supported by data as one might think. For example, most individuals are instructed to perform sit-ups with bent knees. Why? Similarly, many clinicians emphasize performing a pelvic tilt when performing many types of low back exercises. What is the scientific evidence for such recommendations? An examination of the literature reveals that the scientific foundation upon which many exercise notions are based is extremely thin.

Clinical Relevance

BENT-KNEE SIT-UPS: *Several hypotheses to justify bent-knee sit-ups have suggested that this disables the psoas major and/or changes its line of action. Recent magnetic resonance imagery (MRI)-based data [63] demonstrate that the psoas major's line of action does not change because of lumbar or hip posture (except at L5–S1), since the psoas laminae attach to each vertebra and "follow" the changing orientation of the spine. However, there is no doubt that the psoas major is shortened with the flexed hip, which decreases its force production. But the question remains, is there a reduction in spine load with the legs bent? McGill [38] found no major difference in lumbar load as the result of bending the knees with average moments of 65 Nm in both straight and bent knees in 12 young men. The reported compression loads are 3,230 N (723 lb) with straight legs and 3,410 N (763 lb) with bent knees. Reported shear forces are 260 N (58 lb) with straight legs and 300 N (67 lb) with bent knees. Compressive loads in excess of 3,000 N (672 lb) certainly raise questions of safety in both exercises.*

This type of quantitative analysis is necessary to demonstrate that the issue of performing sit-ups using bent knees or straight legs is probably not as important as the issue of whether to prescribe sit-ups at all! There are better ways to challenge the abdominal muscles. Furthermore, certain types of low back injuries are characterized by very specific tissue damage that may require quite different exercise rehabilitation programs for different people. For example, because flexion is a potent way to herniate the anulus the individual with a posterior disc herniation would do well to avoid full-spine flexion maneuvers, particularly with concomitant muscle activity causing significant compressive loading. Yet this spine posture is often unknowingly adopted by patients or consciously advocated by clinicians who demand a full pelvic tilt.

Several exercises are required to train all the muscles of the lumbar torso, and the exercises that best suit the individual depend on a number of variables, such as fitness level, training

goals, history of previous spinal injury, and other factors specific to the individual. However, depending on the purpose of the exercise program, several principles apply. For example, an individual beginning a postinjury program is better advised to avoid loading the spine throughout the range of motion, while a trained athlete may indeed achieve higher performance levels by doing so. Selection of the exercises described in this chapter is biased toward safety, minimizing spine loading during muscle challenge. Therefore, a "neutral" spine (neutral lordosis) is emphasized while the spine is under load; that is, the spine is in neither hyperlordotic nor hypolordotic posture. A general rule of thumb is to preserve the normal low back curve similar to that of standing upright or some variation that minimizes pain. The neutral spine is neither flexed nor extended, but is in a position of elastic equilibrium in which the passive tissues are in the least stressed conformation. Rotating the vertebrae from this neutral posture increases the loading on the spine. Thus, performing a pelvic tilt increases the stress within the spinal tissues and is not in the best interest of minimizing loads during activities such as exercise that places additional loads on the spine. A final caveat for those in pain is to let pain guide small modifications to the initial position of elastic equilibrium, allowing the pain-free position to serve as their neutral spine. In the past, performing a pelvic tilt when exercising has been recommended. However, it should be clear to the reader that this is not justified, because the pelvic tilt increases spine tissue loading, since the spine is no longer in static–elastic equilibrium. It appears to be unwise to recommend the pelvic tilt when challenging the spine.

ISSUES OF FLEXIBILITY

Training to optimize spine flexibility depends on the person's injury history and exercise goal. There are two opposing considerations for the clinicians. First, training for flexibility can lead to exacerbation of troubles, yet having spinal mobility enables spine motion with lower stresses from passive tissues whose role is to define the end-range. However, it is the opinion of this author that training for spine flexibility is overemphasized. Generally, for the injured back, spine flexibility should not be emphasized until the spine has stabilized and has undergone strength and endurance conditioning. Some individuals may never reach this stage! Despite the notion held by some, there are few quantitative data to support a major emphasis on trunk flexibility to improve back health and lessen the risk of injury. In fact, some exercise programs that have included loading of the torso throughout the range of motion (in flexion–extension, lateral bend, or axial twist) have had negative results [33,51]. In addition, greater spine mobility has been, in some cases, associated with low back trouble [11,51]. Further, having spine flexibility has been shown to have little predictive value for future low back trouble [6,51]. The most successful programs appear to emphasize trunk stabilization through exercise with a neutral spine [62] but emphasize mobility at the hips and knees. Bridger et al. [9] demonstrate advantages for hip and knee flexibility in sitting and standing, while McGill and Norman [49] outline advantages for lifting.

For these reasons, specific torso flexibility exercises should be limited to unloaded flexion and extension for those concerned with safety, but perhaps not those interested in specific athletic performance. (Of course spinal flexibility may be of greater desirability in athletes who have never suffered back injury). A very conservative method is to have the patient cycle through full flexion and extension in a slow, smooth motion, while in a hands and knees posture (*Fig. 34.9*).

Issues of Strength and Endurance

The link between previous back injuries resulting in lower muscle strength and endurance performance is well documented. However, does less strength cause injury? The few

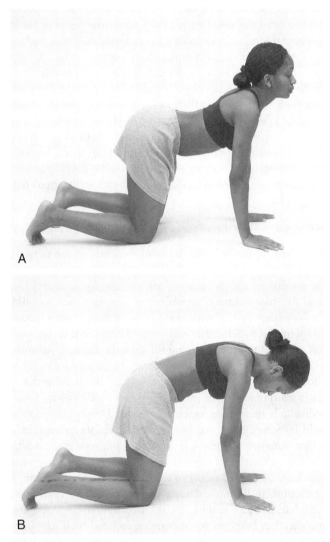

Figure 34.9: The flexion–extension exercise is performed by slowly cycling through full spine flexion **(A)** to full extension **(B)**. Spine mobility is emphasized rather than "pressing" at the end range of motion. This exercise provides motion for the spine with very low loading of the intervertebral joints and reduces viscous stresses for subsequent exercise.

studies available suggest that endurance has a much greater prophylactic value than strength [31]. Furthermore, it appears that emphasis placed on endurance should precede specific strengthening exercise in a graduated progressive exercise program (i.e., longer-duration, lower-effort exercises).

AEROBIC EXERCISE

The mounting evidence supporting the role of aerobic exercise in both reducing the incidence of low back injury [12] and in treating patients with low back pain is compelling [55]. Recent investigation into the loads sustained by the low back tissues during walking [14] confirm very low levels of supporting passive tissue load coupled with mild, but prolonged, and beneficial activation of the supporting musculature.

Exercises for the Abdominal Muscles (Anterior and Lateral) and Quadratus Lumborum

The role of the abdominal muscles in stabilizing the low back is discussed earlier in this chapter. The question remains, what is the best way to train these muscles to perform their stabilizing role? It is important to clarify first that all of the muscles of the abdominal wall participate in stabilization [15,56,57]. Studies of the transversus abdominis demonstrate its participation in stabilization, but clinicians are cautioned from attributing exclusive or unique roles to this muscle. Thus, exercises are needed that elicit activity from each muscle of the abdominal wall to educate individuals to utilize their stabilizing contributions. Unfortunately, there is no single abdominal exercise that challenges all of the abdominal musculature. Consequently, clinicians must prescribe more than one exercise.

Gentle exercises to activate the abdominal wall have been variously described as "bracing," "hollowing," and "pulling in." There appears to be significant confusion about the names and form of these exercises. These exercises have come to mean different things to different people. For the purposes of this discussion, the following operational definitions are used:

Bracing: isometric contraction of the abdominal wall resulting in IAP
Hollowing: visible hollowing of the anterior abdominal wall with elevation (flaring) of the lower ribs
Pulling-in: concentric contraction of the abdominal wall accompanied by a flattening of the abdomen and depression of the lower ribs

Clinical Relevance

EXERCISES FOR MUSCLES OF THE ABDOMINAL WALL: *Contraction of the muscles of the abdominal wall, the internal and external obliques and the transversus abdominis, contribute to spinal stability. Exercises to teach*
(continued)

(Continued)

an individual to increase motor control and endurance of these muscles are important for prevention and rehabilitation of low back pain. However, it is essential that the clinician teach the patient to perform the correct exercise to recruit the intended muscles. Contraction of these muscles can be verified by palpation for a stiffening of the abdominal wall, particularly laterally.

Calibrated intramuscular and surface EMG evidence [28,38] suggests that the various types of curl-ups challenge mainly the rectus abdominis muscles, with little activity in the psoas major, internal and external obliques, and transverse abdominis. Sit-ups (both straight-leg and bent-knee) are characterized by higher psoas major activation and higher low back compression, while leg raises cause even higher activation of the psoas major and also spine compression.

Several relevant observations are made regarding abdominal exercises in these investigations. The challenge to the psoas major is lowest during curl-ups (*Fig. 34.10*), followed by

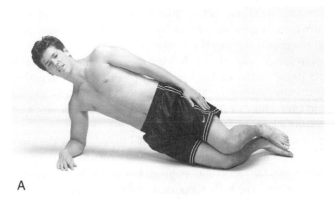

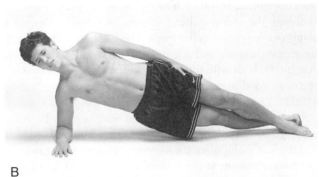

Figure 34.11: The horizontal isometric side bridge or side bridge. Supporting the lower body with the knees on the floor reduces the demand further for those who are more concerned with safety. Supporting the body with the feet increases the muscle challenge, but also the spine load. Progression of the challenge is indicated with the lowest in **(A)** and highest in **(B)**.

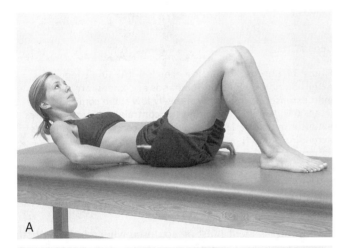

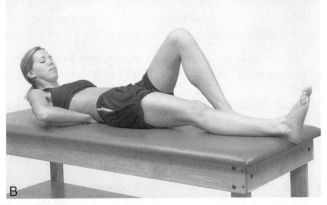

Figure 34.10: **A.** The curl-up is performed by lifting the head and shoulders off the ground with the hands under the lumbar region to help stabilize the pelvis and support the neutral spine. **B.** A variation is to bend only one leg; the straight leg assists in pelvic stabilization and preservation of a "neutral" lumbar curve.

higher levels during the horizontal isometric side support (*Fig. 34.11*). Bent knee sit-ups are characterized by larger psoas major activation than straight leg sit-ups, and the highest psoas major activity is observed during leg raises and hand-on-knee flexor isometric exertions. It is interesting to note that the "press-heels" sit-up that has been hypothesized to activate hamstrings and inhibit psoas major, actually increases psoas major activation. (See normalized EMG data in Table 33.5, Chapter 33.) One exercise not often performed, but that appears to have merit, is the horizontal side bridge. It challenges the lateral obliques without high lumbar compressive loading [5]. In addition, this exercise produces high activation levels in the quadratus lumborum, which appears to be a significant stabilizer of the spine [44], as noted in the previous chapter.

Graded activity in the rectus abdominis muscle and each of the components of the abdominal wall changes with each of these exercises, demonstrating that there is no single best task for the collective "abdominals." Clearly, curl-ups excel at activating the rectus abdominis but produce relatively low oblique activity. Several other clinically relevant findings from Table 33.5 include notions that the psoas major activation is dominated by hip flexion demands. Psoas major activation is relatively high (greater than 25% maximum voluntary contraction, MVC) during pushups, suggesting cautious concern for an individual with an injured low back. Psoas activity is not linked with either lumbar sagittal plane moment or spine compression demands. Thus the often-cited notion that the psoas major is a lumbar spine stabilizer is questionable. Quadratus lumborum activity appears consistent with sagittal and lateral lumbar moments and compression demands, suggesting a larger role in stabilization.

A very wise choice for abdominal exercises, in the early stages of training or rehabilitation, consists of several variations of curl-ups for rectus abdominis and isometric horizontal side support, with the body supported by the knees and the upper body supported by one elbow on the floor. These exercises challenge the abdominal wall in a way that imposes minimal compressive penalty to the spine. The level of challenge with the isometric horizontal side support can be increased by supporting the body with the feet rather than the knees. Specific recommended abdominal exercises are shown: the curl-up with the hands in the low back to stabilize the pelvis and support a neutral lumbar spine together with one hip flexed to assist in "locking the pelvis" to prevent rotation (Fig. 34.9) and the horizontal isometric side support again with the spine in a neutral posture using either the knees or feet for support (Fig. 34.11).

Exercises for the Back Extensors

The search for methods to activate the extensors with minimal spine loading [13] is difficult, since most traditional extensor exercises are characterized by high spine loads that result from externally applied compressive and shear forces. It appears that the single leg extension hold, while on the hands and knees (*Fig. 34.12*) minimizes external loads on the spine but produces an extensor moment on the spine (and small isometric twisting moments) that activates the extensors (one side of lumbar approximately 18% MVC). Activation is sufficiently high on one side of the extensors to facilitate training, but the total spine load is reduced, since the contralateral extensors are producing lower forces (lumbar compression is less than 2,500 N (560 lb). Switching legs trains both sides of the extensors.

In total, seven tasks have been analyzed to facilitate comparison of various extensor tasks [13]. Simultaneous leg extension with contralateral arm raise (the "birddog") increases the unilateral extensor muscle challenge (approximately 27% MVC on one side of the lumbar extensors and 45% MVC on the other side of the thoracic extensors). However, this exercise also increases lumbar compression to well over 3,000 N (672 lb). The often-performed exercise of lying prone on the floor and raising the upper body and legs off the floor is contraindicated for anyone at risk of low back injury or reinjury. In this task the lumbar region pays a high compression penalty to a hyperextended spine (approximately 4,000 N (896 lb) or higher), which transfers load to the facets and crushes the interspinous ligament, noted earlier as an injury mechanism.

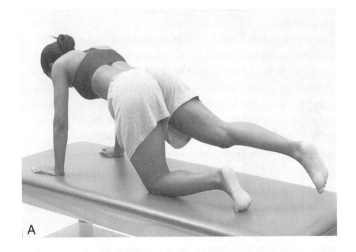

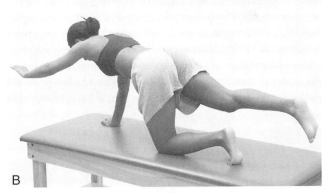

Figure 34.12: Extensor muscle exercises. (A) Single leg extension holds, while on the hands and knees, produces mild extensor activity and relatively low spine compression (<2,500 N; 560 lb). **(B)** Raising the contralateral arm increases extensor muscle activity but also spine compression to levels exceeding 3,000 N.

Should Abdominal Belts Be Worn?

The average patient must be confused when observing both Olympic athletes and those with back injuries wearing abdominal belts. The following results are summarized from a review of the effects of belt wearing [37]:

- Those who have never had a previous back injury appear to have no additional protective benefit from wearing a belt.
- Those who have had an injury while wearing a belt appear to risk a more severe injury. Belts appear to give people the perception they can lift more and may in fact enable them to lift more. Belts appear to increase intraabdominal pressure and blood pressure.
- Belts appear to change the lifting styles of some people to either decrease the loads on the spine or increase the loads on the spine.

In summary, given the assets and liabilities to belt wearing, they are not recommended for routine exercise participation.

Beginner's Program for Stabilization

Specific recommended low back exercises have been shown. The following is an example of an exercise program based on the scientific data reported in this chapter. This program often forms a core set to which additional exercises can be added as patients progress. During the typical rehabilitation program the patient will experience setbacks. When these occur, the patient should return to these core exercises, reestablish slow improvement, and then build the program once again. The four core exercises are:

- Flexion–extension cycles (Fig. 34.9) to reduce spine viscosity, followed by hip and knee mobility exercises [38]. Five or six cycles often suffice to reduce most viscous stresses.
- Anterior abdominal exercises, in this case the curl-up with the hands under the lumbar spine to preserve a neutral spine posture (Fig. 34.10) and one knee flexed but with the other leg straight to stabilize the pelvis on the lumbar spine.
- Lateral musculature exercises are performed—namely, isometric side support, or side bridge, for quadratus lumborum and the obliques of the abdominal wall for optimal stability (Fig. 34.11). The upper leg–foot is placed in front of the lower leg–foot to facilitate longitudinal "rolling" of the torso to challenge both anterior and posterior portions of the wall.
- The extensor program consists of leg extensions and the "birddog" exercises (Fig. 34.12).

"Normal" ratios of endurance times are reported for the torso flexors relative to the extensors (0.99 for men, 0.79 for women) and for the lateral musculature relative to the extensors (0.65 for men and 0.39 for women) [43] to help clinicians identify endurance deficits in specific muscle groups. Finally, as patients progress with these isometric stabilization exercises, conscious simultaneous contraction of the abdominals is recommended to enhance motor control and stability using the deeper abdominal wall that includes the transverse abdominis and internal oblique [49,59].

Notes for Exercise Prescription

The exercise professional must design exercise programs to meet a wide variety of objectives. The following is a list of general caveats to assist in achieving the best prescription [42].

1. While there is a common belief among some "experts" that exercise sessions should be performed at least three times per week, it appears that low back exercises have the most beneficial effect when performed daily [35].
2. The "no pain-no gain" axiom does not apply when exercising the low back, particularly when applied to weight training. Scientific and clinical wisdom suggests the opposite is true.
3. While specific low back exercises have been rationalized in this chapter, general exercise programs that also combine cardiovascular components (e.g., walking) have been shown to be more effective in both rehabilitation and injury prevention [55]. The exercises shown here only make up a component of the total program.
4. Diurnal variation in the fluid level of the intervertebral discs (discs are more hydrated early in the morning after rising from bed) changes the stresses on the disc throughout the day. It is unwise to perform full range spine motion while under load, shortly after rising from bed [1].
5. Low back exercises performed for maintenance of health need not emphasize strength, with high-load low repetition tasks. Instead, more repetitions of less-demanding exercises assist in the enhancement of endurance and strength. There is no doubt that back injury can occur during seemingly low level demands such as picking up a pencil and that the risk of injury from motor control error can occur. While it appears that the chance of motor control errors resulting in inappropriate muscle forces increases with fatigue, there is also evidence documenting the changes in passive tissue loading with fatigue lifting [58]. Given that endurance has more protective value than strength [31], strength gains should not be overemphasized at the expense of endurance.
6. There is no such thing as an ideal set of exercises for all individuals. An individual's training objectives must be identified (e.g., to reduce the risk of injury, optimize general health and fitness, or maximize athletic performance) and the most appropriate exercises chosen. While science cannot evaluate the optimal exercises for each situation, the combination of science and clinical experiential "wisdom" must be used to enhance low back health.
7. Be patient and stick with the program. Increased function and pain reduction may not occur for 3 months [34].

SUMMARY

This chapter reviews the basic factors that explain the loads sustained by the lumbar spine during activity, particularly lifting. In addition, this chapter describes the loading patterns on the passive structures of the lumbar spine during activity as well as the tissues' response to loading. The position of the spine affects the direction of the loads on the spine during activity. Lifting with the lumbar spine extended tends to increase the compressive loads on the spine, while lifting with the trunk flexed increases shear forces on the spine. The lumbar spine tolerates larger compressive forces than shear forces, so strategies to reduce shear forces are discussed.

The information presented in Chapter 33 regarding the muscles of the lumbar spine and the information from the current chapter are applied to the clinical issues surrounding exercise for people with and without a history of low back pain. The best available biomechanical studies are used to generate a list of guidelines for the clinician to follow when developing individual exercise programs. Thus this chapter provides convincing evidence of the clinical benefit of the application of biomechanical analysis to clinical dilemmas.

Acknowledgments

The author wishes to acknowledge the contributions of several colleagues who have contributed to the collection of works reported here: Daniel Juker, M.D.; Craig Axler, M.Sc.; Jacek Cholewicki, Ph.D.; Michael Sharratt, Ph.D.; John Seguin, M.D.; Vaughan Kippers, Ph.D.; and, in particular, Robert Norman, Ph.D. The continual financial support from the Natural Science and Engineering Research Council, Canada, has made this series of work possible.

References

1. Adams MA, Dolan P: Recent advances in lumbar spinal mechanics and their clinical significance. Clin Biomech 1995; 10: 3–19.

2. Adams MA, Hutton WC: Prolapsed intervertebral disc: a hyperflexion injury. Spine 1982; 7: 184–191.

3. Adams MA, Hutton WC: Gradual disc prolapse. Spine 1985; 10: 524–531.

4. Adams P, Muir H: Qualitative changes with age of proteoglycans of human lumbar discs. Ann Rheum Dis 1976; 35: 289.

5. Axler CT, McGill SM: Low back loads over a variety of abdominal exercises: searching for the safest abdominal challenge. Med. Sci. Sports Med. 1997; 29(6): 804–811.

6. Battie MC, Bigos SJ, Fischer LD, et al.: The role of spinal flexibility in back pain complaints within industry: a prospective study. Spine 1990; 15: 768–773.

7. Bedzinski R: Application of speckle photography methods to the investigations of deformation of the vertebral arch. In: Little EG, ed. Experimental Mechanics. New York: Elsevier, 1992.

8. Bogduk N, Macintosh JE: The applied anatomy of the thoracolumbar fascia. Spine 1984; 9: 164–170.

9. Bridger RS, Orkin D, Henneberg M: A quantitative investigation of lumbar and pelvic postures in standing and sitting: interrelationships with body position and hip muscle length. Int J Ind Ergonomics 1992; 9: 235–244.

10. Brinckmann P, Biggemann M, Hilweg D: Prediction of the compressive strength of human lumbar vertebrae. Clin Biomech 1989; 4(suppl 2): S1–S27.

11. Burton AK, Tillotson KM, Troup JDG: Variation in lumbar sagittal mobility with low back trouble. Spine 1989; 14: 584–590.

12. Cady LD, Bischoff DP, O'Connell ER, et al.: Strength and fitness and subsequent back injuries in firefighters. J Occup Med 1979; 21: 269.

13. Callaghan J, Gunning J, McGill SM: A relationship between lumbar spine load and muscle activity during extensor exercises. Phys Ther 1998; 78(1): 8–18.

14. Callaghan JP, Patla A, McGill SM: Low back three-dimensional joint forces, kinematics and kinetics during walking. Clin Biomech 1999; 14: 203–216.

15. Cholewicki J, Greene HS, Polzhofer GR, et al.: Neuromuscular function in athletes following recovery from a recent acute low back injury. J Orthop Sports Phys Ther 2002; 32: 568–576.

16. Cholewicki J, McGill SM: Relationship between muscle force and stiffness in the whole mammalian muscle: a simulation study. J Biomech Eng 1995; 117: 339–342.

17. Cholewicki J, McGill SM: Mechanical stability of the in vivo lumbar spine: implications for injury and chronic low back pain. Clin Biomech 1996; 11: 1–15.

18. Cripton P, Berlemen U, Visarius H, et al.: Response of the lumbar spine due to shear loading, in: Proceedings of the Centers for Disease Control on injury prevention through biomechanics. p. 111. Wayne State University, Detroit, USA. May 4–5, 1995.

19. Daggfeldt K, Thorstensson A: The role of intra-abdominal pressure in spinal unloading. J Biomech 1997; 30: 1149–1155.

20. Dickey JP, Pierrynowski MR, Bednar DA: Deformation of vertebrae in vivo—implications for facet joint loads and spinous process pin instrumentation for measuring sequential spinal kinematics. Presented at the Canadian Orthopaedic Research Society, Quebec City, May 25, 1996.

21. Farfan HF: Mechanical Disorders of the Low Back. Philadelphia: Lea & Febiger, 1973.

22. Fyhrie DP, Schaffler MB: Failure mechanisms in human vertebral cancellous bone. Bone 1994; 15: 105–109.

23. Goel VK, Monroe BT, Gilbertson LG, Brinckmann P: Interlaminar shear stresses and laminae-separation in a disc: finite element analysis of the L3-L4 motion segment subjected to axial compressive loads. Spine 1995; 20: 689–698.

24. Gordon SJ, Young KH, Mayer PJ, et al.: Mechanism of disc rupture—a preliminary report. Spine 1991; 16: 450–456.

25. Gracovetsky S, Farfan HF, Lamy C: Mechanism of the lumbar spine. Spine 1981; 6: 249–261.

26. Hardcastle P, Annear P, Foster D: Spinal abnormalities in young fast bowlers. J Bone Joint Surg 1992; 74B: 421–425.

27. Heylings DJA: Supraspinous and interspinous ligaments of the human lumbar spine. J Anat 1978; 123: 127–131.

28. Juker D, McGill SM, Kropf P, Steffen T: Quantitative intramuscular myoelectric activity of lumbar portions of psoas and the abdominal wall during a wide variety of tasks. Med Sci Sports Exerc 1998; 30: 301–310.

29. King AI: Injury to the thoraco-lumbar spine and pelvis. In: Nahum AM, Melvin JW, eds. Accidental Injury, Biomechanics and Presentation. New York: Springer-Verlag, 1993.

30. Lucas D, Bresler B: Stability of the ligamentous spine. Tech. report no. 40, Biomechanics Laboratory, University of California, San Francisco, 1961.

31. Luoto S, Heliovaara M, Hurri H, Alaranta M: Static back endurance and the risk of low back pain. Clin Biomech 1995; 10: 323–324.

32. Macintosh JE, Bogduk N, Gracovetsky S: The biomechanics of the thoracolumbar fascia. Clin Biomech 1987; 2: 78–83.

33. Malmivaara A, Hakkinen U, Aro T, et al.: The treatment of acute low back pain—bed rest, exercises, or ordinary activity? N Engl J Med 1995; 332: 351–355.

34. Manniche C, Hesselsoe G, Bentzen L, et al.: Clinical trial of intensive muscle training for chronic low back pain. Lancet 1988; Dec 24/31: 1473.

35. Mayer TG, Gatchel RJ, Kishino N, et al.: Objective assessment of spine function following industrial injury: a prospective study with comparison group and one-year follow up. Spine 1985; 10: 482.

36. McGill SM: A myoelectrically based dynamic 3-D model to predict loads on lumbar spine tissues during lateral bending. J Biomech 1992; 25: 395–414.

37. McGill SM: Abdominal belts in industry: a position paper on their assets, liabilities and use. Am Ind Hyg Assoc J 1993; 54: 752–754.

38. McGill SM: The mechanics of torso flexion: situps and standing dynamic flexion manoeuvres. Clin Biomech 1995; 10: 184–192.

39. McGill SM: Biomechanics of low back injury: implications on current practice and the clinic. J Biomech 1997; 30: 465–475.

40. McGill SM: Low back exercises: evidence for improving exercise regimens. Phys Ther 1998; 78: 754–765.

41. McGill SM: Ultimate Back Fitness and Performance, 2nd edition. Backfitpro Inc. 2006 (www.backfitpro.com).

42. McGill SM: Low back exercises: prescription for the healthy back and when recovering from injury. In: American College of Sports Medicine—Resource Manual for Guidelines for Exercise Testing and Prescription. 4th ed. Baltimore: Lippincott Williams & Wilkins, 2001, pp. 120–132.

43. McGill SM, Childs A, Liebenson C: Endurance times for stabilization exercises: clinical targets for testing and training from a normal database. Arch Phys Med Rehab, 1999; 80: 941–944.

44. McGill SM, Juker D, Kropf P: Quantitative intramuscular myoelectric activity of quadratus lumborum during a wide variety of tasks. Clin Biomech 1996; 11: 170–172.

45. McGill SM, Kippers V: Transfer of loads between lumbar tissues during the flexion relaxation phenomenon. Spine 1994; 19: 2190–2196.

46. McGill SM, Norman RW: Partitioning of the L4/L5 dynamic moment into disc, ligamentous and muscular components during lifting. Spine 1986; 11: 666–667.

47. McGill SM, Norman RW: Reassessment of the role of intraabdominal pressure in spinal compression. Ergonomics 1987; 30: 1565–1588.

48. McGill SM, Norman RW: The potential of lumbodorsal fascia forces to generate back extension moments during squat lifts. J Biomed Eng 1988; 10: 312–318.

49. McGill SM: Low back disorders: Evidence-based prevention and rehabilitation. Champaign, IL: Human Kinetics Publishers, 2002.

50. Nachemson A: The load on lumbar discs in different positions of the body. Clin Rel Res 1966; 45: 107–112.

51. Nachemson A: Newest knowledge of low back pain: a critical look. Clin Orthop 1992; 279: 8–20.

52. Nachemson A, Andersson GBJ, Schultz AB: Valsalva manoeuvre biomechanics: effects on lumbar trunk loads of elevated intraabdominal pressure. Spine 1986; 11: 476–479.

53. Nachemson AL: Lumbar interdiscal pressure. Acta Orthop Scand 1960; suppl 43: 1–104.

54. Noyes FR, De Lucas JL, Torvik PJ: Biomechanics of ligament failure: an analysis of strain-rate sensitivity and mechanisms of failure in primates. J Bone Joint Surg 1994; 56A: 236.

55. Nutter P: Aerobic exercise in the treatment and prevention of low back pain. State Art Rev Occup Med 1988; 3: 137.

56. O'Sullivan P, Twomey LT, Allison GT: Evaluation of specific stabilization exercise in the streatment of chronic low back pain with radiologic diagnosis of spondylolysis or spondylolistheses, Spine 1997; 22: 2959–2967.

57. O'Sullivan P, Twomey LT, Allison GT: Altered abdominal back recruitment in patients with chronic back pain following a specific exercise intervention. J Orthop Sports Phys Ther 1998; 27: 114–124.

58. Potvin JR, Norman RW: Can fatigue compromise lifting safety? Proceedings of the NACOB II, the second North American congress on biomechanics, August 24–28, 1992; 153.

59. Richardson CA, Jull GA: Muscle control—pain control. What exercises would you prescribe? Manual Ther 1995; 1: 2–10.

60. Rissanen PM: The surgical anatomy and pathology of the supraspinous and interspinous ligaments of the lumbar spine with special reference to ligament ruptures. Acta Orthop Scand 1960; suppl 46: 7–99.

61. Roaf R: A study of the mechanics of spinal injuries. J Bone Joint Surg 1960; 42B: 810.

62. Saal JA, Saal JS: Nonoperative treatment of herniated lumbar intervertebral disc with radiculopathy: an outcome study. Spine 1989; 14: 431–437.

63. Santaguida L, McGill SM: The psoas major muscle: a three-dimensional mechanical modelling study with respect to the spine based on MRI measurement. J Biomech 1995; 28: 339–345.

64. Sharma M, Langrama NA, Rodriguez J: Role of ligaments and facets in lumbar spine stability. Spine 1995; 20: 887–900.

65. Tesh KM, Dunn J, Evans JH: The abdominal muscles and vertebral stability. Spine 1987; 12: 501–508.

66. Videman T, Nurminen M, Troup JDG: Lumbar spinal pathology in cadaveric material in relation to history of back pain, occupation and physical loading. Spine 1990; 15: 728–740.

67. Wilder DG, Pope MH, Frymoyer JW: The biomechanics of lumbar disc herniation and the effect of overload and instability. J Spine Disord 1988; 1: 16–32.

68. Yingling VR, McGill SM: Anterior shear of spinal motion segments: kinematics, kinetics and resulting injuries. Spine 1999; 24(18): 1882–1889.

Structure and Function of the Bones and Joints of the Pelvis

EMILY L. CHRISTIAN, P.T., PH.D.

CHAPTER CONTENTS

The bones of the pelvic girdle consist of two innominate bones (os coxae, or hip bones) formed by the fusion of three bones, the ilium, ischium, and pubis. In contrast to those of the upper limb, the girdle bones of the lower limb are designed for stability, not mobility (*Table 35.1*). The two innominate bones join to the sacrum dorsally and to one another in the anterior midline to form a robust **osteoligamentous ring**, the pelvis (*Fig. 35.1*). The pelvis joins with the fifth lumbar vertebra above at the lumbosacral junction and below to two femurs (femora) at the hip joints (*Fig. 35.2*).

The function of the bony pelvis is primarily locomotor and therefore somatic (i.e., pertaining to the limbs and body wall). Serving in this capacity, the bony pelvis provides the attachment sites for trunk and lower limb muscles, transmits the superincumbent body weight to the lower limbs (in standing) or ischia (in sitting), and absorbs ground reaction forces in all standing and sitting activities. The bony pelvis functions in a visceral capacity in addition to its somatic one, since several visceral tracts (the pelvic effluents) pass through its caudal end, involving it in micturition, defecation, and, in females, sexual function and childbirth. The purposes of these three chapters on the bony pelvis are to provide an understanding of how specific design features enable it to perform these seemingly divergent functions, to describe changes that occur in pelvic structures over the life span that can have a deleterious effect on function, and to analyze the loads sustained by the pelvis. The specific objectives of this chapter are to

TABLE 35.1: Comparison of Osteological Features of the Limb Girdles

Upper Limb (Pectoral) Girdle	Lower Limb (Pelvic) Girdle
Bones form by both intramembranous and endochondral methods of bone formation	Bones form only by the endochondral method of bone formation
Formed from two elements on each side: clavicle and scapula	Formed from three elements on each side: ilium, ischium, and pubis
The two elements on each side are distinct from each other	The three elements of each side fuse to form two innominate bones
No direct ventral articulation between the two sides	The two innominate bones articulate ventrally at the symphysis pubis
No dorsal articulation	Each innominate bone articulates dorsally with the sacrum
Articulations with the axial skeleton are ventral, small, and highly mobile	Articulations with the axial skeleton are dorsal, robust, and nearly immobile
Joint with proximal member of upper limb is relatively shallow and permits a wide range of motion	Joint with proximal member of lower limb is deeper than that of upper limb and permits a more limited range of motion
Designed for mobility; resilient to mechanical forces	Designed for stability; transmits mechanical forces between spine and lower limb

- Describe the bony features of the fifth lumbar vertebra, sacrum, coccyx, and innominate bones to demonstrate how these features allow the pelvis to provide a stable support for the superincumbent body weight and a sturdy base from which movement of the lower limbs is accomplished
- Discuss the structure and ligamentous support of the lumbosacral articulation to understand its contribution to the transfer of weight to the sacrum and how pathology contributes to its dysfunction
- Discuss the structure, ligaments, and function of each of the articulations between the sacrum and innominate bones and between the two innominate bones and to identify how each ensures stability while permitting movement between specific skeletal elements
- Describe structural alterations in pelvic articulations over time and in subpopulations and the effects these changes impose on pelvic somatic function
- Identify the amount of motion available between the axial and appendicular elements of the bony pelvis as well as between the hemipelves and to discuss the sequelae of alterations in available motion

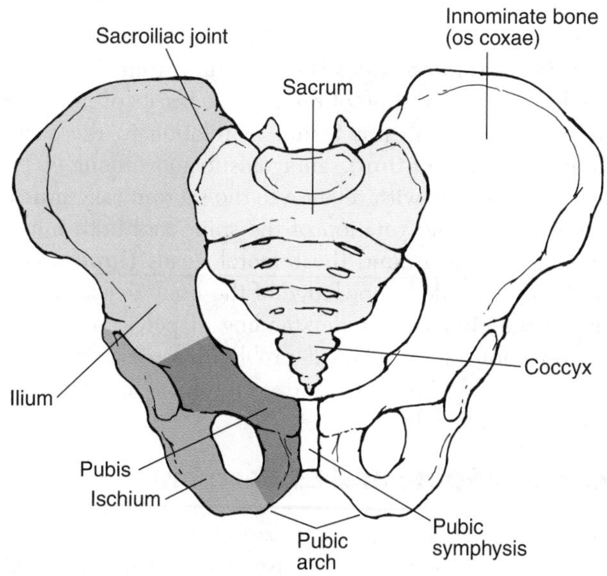

Figure 35.1: Anterior view of the osteoligamentous ring that forms the pelvis. Elements of the ring include the sacrum and innominate bones (os coxae). They are joined posteriorly by two sacroiliac joints and anteriorly at the symphysis pubis. The three bones that fuse to form each innominate bone are indicated.

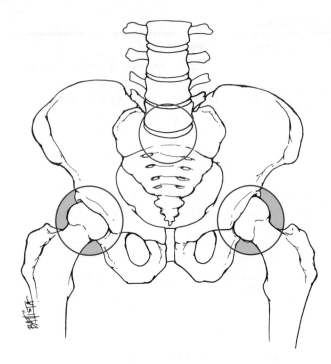

Figure 35.2: The pelvis articulates with the fifth lumbar vertebra above and with paired femora below.

- Describe the alignment of the axial and appendicular elements of the bony pelvis to gain an understanding of how alterations in the normal alignment can result in impaired function and the imposition of potentially harmful loads on adjacent structures
- Compare the bony pelvis of the male and female
- Discuss the role of the bony pelvis in visceral function of the pelvis

OSTEOLOGY OF PELVIC AND ASSOCIATED STRUCTURES

The bony pelvis, consisting of the two innominate bones and the sacrum, provides the transition from the trunk to the lower limb. Motion of the pelvis consists of movement of both innominates as a unit in relation to the sacrum (**symmetrical motion**), antagonistic movement of each innominate bone with relation to the sacrum (**asymmetrical motion**), and rotation of the spine and both innominates as a unit around the femoral heads (**lumbopelvic motion**). Detailed knowledge of the bony pelvis is essential to the clinician's understanding of pelvic motion and appreciation of the clinical problems associated with its mechanical dysfunction. A description of each involved bony structure follows.

Lumbar Spine and L5 Vertebra

Bones of the lumbar spine are discussed in detail in Chapter 32. Their size increases from cranial to caudal, reflecting their role in transmitting the superincumbent body weight to the pelvis for transmission to the lower limbs. Typically, they are wider from side to side than from front to back, are taller anteriorly than posteriorly, and have long, thin transverse processes and short, almost horizontal spinous processes. With the exception of L5, the facets (zygapophyses) of the superior articular processes of the lumbar vertebrae are vertical and directed medially and slightly posteriorly, while those of their inferior articular processes are vertical and directed laterally and slightly anteriorly; the facet (zygapophyseal) joint cavities are oriented, therefore, predominately in the sagittal plane and facilitate flexion and extension. The wedge-shaped (taller anteriorly) vertebral bodies are responsible for the **lordosis** (dorsal concavity) formed by the upper lumbar spine, but the lordotic curvature in the lower part is attributed to both the vertebrae and intervertebral discs (IVDs), both of which are taller anteriorly [136,147].

The fifth lumbar vertebra is transitional from the lumbar to the sacral region and atypical (*Table 35.2*). Several of its features reflect its role in transmitting the weight of the head, upper limbs, and trunk to the sacrum. The most robust of the lumbar vertebrae, it has massive transverse processes that are

TABLE 35.2: Atypical Osteological Features of the Fifth Lumbar Vertebra and Attached Structures

Osteological Features	Attachments
Body: largest and heaviest	Ligaments: anterior and posterior longitudinal, supraspinous
	Muscles: thoracolumbar fascia, psoas major
Body height: greatest discrepancy between anterior and posterior heights	IVDs: thickest of all discs in spine
Articular processes: facets of inferior articular processes oriented in a nearly frontal plane	Zygapophyseal joint capsule
Transverse processes: in contact with entire lateral surface of the pedicle and body; project upward and posterolaterally; shortest	Ligaments: iliolumbar, lumbosacral, intertransverse
	Muscles: thoracolumbar fascia, multifidi, intertransversarii, erector spinae
Spinous process: smallest	Ligaments: interspinous, supraspinous
	Muscles: interspinales, erector spinae

in contact with the entire lateral surface of the pedicle and side of the body (*Fig. 35.3*). The contrast between the anterior and posterior heights of the vertebral body is greatest at L5; this feature, as well as a greater anterior than posterior height of the 5th lumber IVD, contributes to the angle formed at the **lumbosacral junction** (*Fig. 35.4*). The superior articular

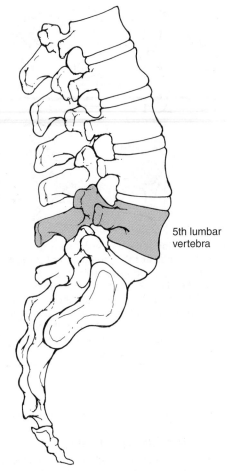

Figure 35.4: Lateral view of the lumbosacral spine. Note that the vertical height of the fifth lumbar vertebral body and intervertebral discs are greater anteriorly than posteriorly. Both of these features contribute to the lumbosacral angle.

processes of L5 are typical, but facets on its inferior articular processes are vertical and project anteriorly and slightly laterally to articulate with superior articular processes of the base of the sacrum (Fig. 35.3); this orientation places the lumbosacral facet joint cavities predominately in the coronal plane. This abrupt change in predominate orientation from the sagittal to the coronal plane contributes significantly to lumbosacral integrity by resisting the shearing stress between the fifth lumbar vertebra, the lowest IVD, and the base of the sacrum [59,136,147].

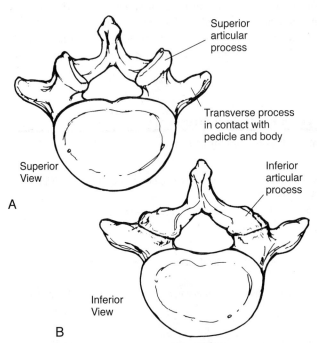

Figure 35.3: The fifth lumbar vertebra. **A.** Superior view. **B.** Inferior view. Note the near-sagittal orientation of the superior articular processes and the near-coronal orientation of the inferior articular processes of this transitional vertebra.

Clinical Relevance

OBLIQUE RADIOGRAPH OF LUMBAR VERTEBRAE:
When viewed on an oblique radiograph, parts of the vertebral arch of L5 (as well as other lumbar vertebrae) and its processes take on the classical appearance of a Scottie dog [101,136] (Fig. 35.5). The oblique view is useful in imaging

(continued)

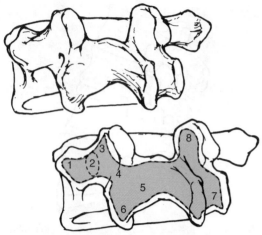

Figure 35.5: Posterior oblique view of the fifth lumbar vertebra demonstrates the parts of the radiographic Scottie dog. The muzzle is formed by the transverse process *(1)*; the eye is the pedicle viewed end on *(2)*; the ear is the superior articular process *(3)*; the neck is the isthmus *(4)*; the body is the lamina and spinous process *(5)*; the foreleg is the inferior articular process *(6)*; the hindleg is the contralateral inferior articular process *(7)*; and the tail is the contralateral lamina and contralateral superior articular process *(8)*.

(Continued)

*the **pars interarticularis (isthmus),** the part of the vertebral arch connecting the superior and inferior articular processes [109]; it coincides with the neck or collar of the Scottie dog. Although not recognized as a vertebral part in the* Nomina Anatomica *(N.A.) [45], its clinical importance and the significance of the oblique radiograph of L5 will become apparent in a later discussion of spondylolisthesis.*

Sacrum

The os sacrum was the sacred bone to the Romans, being the last bone in the body to disintegrate and necessary for resurrection [156,157]. Also known as the vertebra magna, the most atypical of all the vertebrae is an inverted triangle formed from the fusion of five sacral vertebral segments (*Table 35.3*). Its broad base projects anterosuperiorly to articulate with the fifth lumbar vertebra at the lumbosacral junction, and its blunted apex projects posteroinferiorly to articulate with the first coccygeal segment at the **sacrococcygeal junction** (*Fig. 35.6*). The whole of the sacrum is convex dorsally and concave ventrally. Its ventral (pelvic) surface contributes to the posterior wall of the pelvic cavity, while the dorsal surface is subcutaneous.

The sacrum possesses no intervertebral foramina for emerging spinal nerves and has instead four sets of separate dorsal and ventral (pelvic) foramina for passage of the dorsal and ventral primary rami of spinal nerves S1-4. A sacral canal passes through its core and opens at the apex as the sacral hiatus, the site of emergence of the fifth sacral (S5) and coccygeal (Co1) spinal nerves. Sacral bodies are fused along transverse lines in the central third, and fused transverse processes and costal elements form lateral parts that run longitudinally on each side. The piriformis originates from the ventral surface of the sacrum, around the emerging ventral primary rami. Muscles originating from its dorsal surface include the multifidus, erector spinae, and gluteus maximus.

BASE

The base of the sacrum is its broadest part and represents the superior surface of S1. The anterosuperior lip of S1 juts forward as the sacral promontory (*Fig. 35.7*). Facets of the superior articular processes are vertical and project cranially,

---

TABLE 35.3: Osteological Features of the Sacrum and Coccyx and Attached Structures

Osteological Features	Attachments and Associated Structures
Sacrum	
Consists of 5 fused vertebral segments	Ligaments: anterior and posterior longitudinal, dorsal and ventral sacroiliac, sacrotuberous, sacrospinous
	Muscles: piriformis, gluteus maximus, multifidus, erector spinae, coccygeus
A superior base: opening is the sacral canal and facets project superiorly in a nearly coronal plane	Zygapophyseal joint capsules
An inferior apex: opening is the sacral hiatus and sacral cornua project inferiorly to articulate with coccygeal cornua	Ligaments: dorsal, ventral, and lateral sacrococcygeal
No intervertebral foramina: dorsal and ventral sacral foramina instead	Dorsal and ventral primary rami of spinal nerves pass through individual foramina
Coccyx	
Consists of 3–4 rudimentary vertebrae	Ligaments: sacrotuberous, sacrospinous, dorsal sacroiliac, anococcygeal
	Muscles: gluteus maximus, levator ani, coccygeus, external anal sphincter
Coccygeal cornua of Co1 project superiorly to articulate with sacral cornua	Ligaments: dorsal, ventral, and lateral sacrococcygeal, intercoccygeal

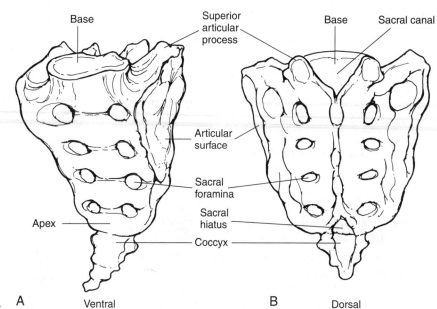

Figure 35.6: The sacrum. **A.** The ventral surface is concave. **B.** The dorsal surface is convex.

posteriorly, and slightly medially to articulate with the facets of the inferior articular processes of L5. This orientation of the lumbosacral facets is important in stabilizing the lumbosacral junction, the point of greatest stress on the entire spine.

LATERAL PART

The lateral part of the sacrum, or ala, is formed by the fusion of sacral transverse processes and costal elements with one

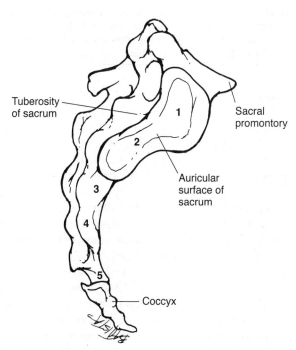

Figure 35.7: Lateral view of the sacrum. Sacral vertebral segments are numbered 1–5; the auricular surface and sacral tuberosity of segments 1–3 participate in the formation of the sacroiliac joints.

Clinical Relevance

POSITION OF THE SACRAL CORNUA: *Sacral cornua are landmarks useful in locating the sacral hiatus for the purpose of injecting an anesthetic agent into the epidural space in caudal epidural blocks [113].*

another, with the remainder of the vertebra, and with each successive level. Each ala is wide at the base of the sacrum and narrow at its apex. In the vast majority of individuals [149], the lateral surface of the combined upper three sacral segments bears an L-shaped auricular surface covered with cartilage for articulation with an L-shaped area on the ilium, also described as auricular, and covered with cartilage. Immediately posterosuperior to the auricular surface is a roughened area, the sacral tuberosity; it approximates an area of similar shape and name on the ilium. Auricular surfaces and tuberosities of both the sacrum and ilium contribute to the formation of the sacroiliac joint (SIJ). The lateral surfaces of the fourth and fifth sacral segments are usually nonarticular; however, S4 may form a part of the sacral auricular surface and contribute to the SIJ [12,149].

APEX

The caudal aspect of the fifth sacral segment, the apex of the sacrum, bears a facet for articulation with the first coccygeal segment. Sacral cornua project caudally on either side of the sacral hiatus, a defect in the vertebral arch of S5 that permits passage of S5 and Co1 spinal nerves (Fig. 35.6B). Along with vascular elements, the sacral hiatus also transmits the coccygeal ligament, the caudal anchor of the spinal cord, formed by contributions of the pial **filum terminale** and arachnoid-dural **filum of the dura** [24].

OSSIFICATION

Primary centers of ossification of the bodies, vertebral arches, and costal elements of the sacrum appear prenatally between the third and eighth months [70,147]; several secondary centers appear later. Fusion of the various parts of each vertebral segment begins at 5 years and continues over the next 18 to 25 years; IVDs between segments may not ossify completely until middle age [147]. Development and ossification of the sacrum occurs later than that of the ilium.

Clinical Relevance

LUMBOSACRAL ANOMALIES: *Being an area of transition from one region of the spine to another, the L5–S1 junction is subject to an unusually high degree of variation and malformation. One author has referred to this region's physiological unstableness [82], and others have described it as being ontogenetically restless [141]. A multitude of anomalous morphological features have been observed. Those that may be tolerated poorly by the individual include partial or complete **sacralization** of L5 (fusion of L5 to the sacrum) or **lumbarization** of the first sacral segment (separation of the first sacral segment from the remaining fused segments) [59,136,147] (Fig. 35.8), congenital absence of a pedicle [117], inequities in the height of the two sides of the base of the sacrum [59], accessory laminae [10], dysplasia of the pars interarticularis (isthmus of the Scottie dog) [141] (Fig. 35.5), aplasia or dysplasia of the superior zygapophyses of the first sacral segment [59,141], and a change in the orientation of one or both of the zygapophyseal facets from coronal to sagittal [28,53] (Fig. 35.9).*

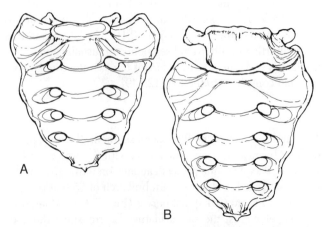

Figure 35.8: Ventral view of anomalous features of lumbar and sacral vertebrae. **A.** Partial lumbarization of the first sacral vertebra. **B.** Partial sacralization of the fifth lumbar vertebra.

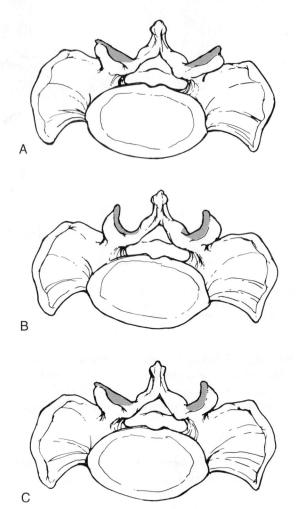

Figure 35.9: Base of the sacrum. The main varieties of superior articular process facet orientation are shown. **A.** Both superior articular facets are flat. **B.** Both superior articular facets are curved. **C.** One facet is flat, the other is curved.

Coccyx

The coccyx, a remnant of the skeleton of the tail [114], is a beaklike bone (Gr. *kokkyx*, cuckoo) represented by three to five fused rudimentary vertebrae, with four being the most common number [113] (*Fig. 35.10*). Its curvature usually follows that of the sacrum (i.e., ventrally concave). The first coccygeal segment has a facet for articulation with the apex of the sacrum and cranially projecting coccygeal cornua for articulation with sacral cornua. A rudimentary IVD is present between the sacrum and coccyx [136].

The coccyx (along with the last two sacral segments) does not transmit weight from above. These bones do, however, provide sites for attachment of several muscles (gluteus maximus, levator ani, coccygeus, sphincter ani externus) and ligaments (sacrospinous, sacrotuberous, long dorsal sacroiliac).

Innominate Bone

Each innominate bone is formed from the union of three separate bones, the ilium, ischium, and pubis (Fig. 35.1).

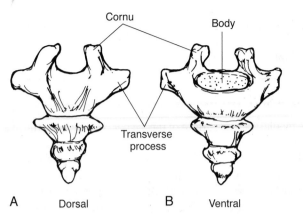

Figure 35.10: The coccyx. **A.** Dorsal surface. **B.** Ventral (pelvic) surface.

The three parts unite at a central point, the acetabulum, from which each of the three bones expand; the ilium superiorly, the ischium posteroinferiorly, and the pubis anteroinferiorly (*Table 35.4*). They are connected by hyaline cartilage until 20–25 years of age, after which they become one bone, the innominate (*Fig. 35.11*). The largest of the three is the ilium, and the smallest is the pubis. Each part has a body; the ala is the upper expanded part of the iliac body, the ischial ramus curves inferiorly and then anteriorly from the ischial body, and superior and inferior pubic rami project posterosuperiorly and posteroinferiorly from the pubic body (*Fig. 35.12*). A large, somewhat oval, obturator foramen is present in the inferior part of the innominate bone. The largest foramen in the body, it is closed completely by the obturator membrane except for a small defect at its anterosuperior margin, the

TABLE 35.4: Osteological Features of the Innominate Bone and Attached Structures

Osteological Features	Attachments and Associated Structures
Ilium	
Iliac crest with outer lip, intermediate area, and inner lip	External oblique, internal oblique, transversus abdominis
ASIS; AIIS	Inguinal ligament and sartorius; straight tendon of rectus femoris
PSIS; PIIS	Gluteus maximus; sacrotuberous ligament
Lateral surface of body	Reflected tendon of rectus femoris
Lateral surface of wing with inferior, anterior, and posterior gluteal lines	Glutei minimus, medius, and maximus
Superior 2/5s of acetabulum and its rim	Capsule of hip joint, ligament of head of femur
Medial surface of wing with iliac fossa	Iliacus
Arcuate line	
Iliac tuberosity	ISIL
Auricular surface	Articular cartilage
Ischium	
Ischial spine	Sacrospinous ligament, superior gemellus, levator ani, coccygeus
Ischial tuberosity	Sacrotuberous ligament, semimembranosus, semitendinosus, biceps femoris, quadratus femoris, adductor magnus, inferior gemellus
Ischial ramus (conjoint ischiopubic ramus when joined with inferior pubic ramus)	Obturator externus, adductor magnus, deep transverse perineus, ischiocavernosus
Posteroinferior 2/5's of acetabulum and its rim	Capsule of hip joint, ligament of head of femur
Body	Obturator internus
Pubis	
Iliopubic eminence	Psoas minor
Superior pubic ramus	Pectineus
Pubic tubercle	Inguinal ligament
Pubic crest	Rectus abdominis
Inferior pubic ramus	Obturator externus, adductor magnus, gracilis, adductor brevis, adductor longus, deep transverse perineus, ischiocavernosus, arcuate pubic ligament
Pecten	Pectineus
Obturator crest and sulcus	Roof of obturator canal
Body	Superior pubic ligament, interpubic disc, pyramidalis
Anteroinferior 1/5 of acetabulum and its rim	Capsule of hip joint, ligament of head of femur
Foramina, Canal, and Notches	
Obturator foramen	Formed by ischium and pubis; largely covered by obturator membrane and obturator internus
Obturator canal	Transmits obturator nerve, artery, and vein
Greater sciatic notch	Between PIIS and ischial spine; transmits pyriformis, gluteal nerves, and vessels
Lesser sciatic notch	Between ischial spine and tuberosity; transmits obturator internus and its nerve, pudendal nerve, and vessels

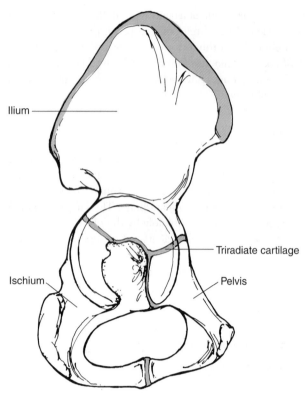

Figure 35.11: Lateral view of the right innominate bone of a child, indicating ossification centers. Note the Y-shaped triradiate cartilaginous stem connecting the three bones of the os coxae in the acetabulum. Cartilage is also present at the ischiopubic junction and along the superior margin of the iliac crest.

obturator canal. Each innominate bone is united to the sacrum posteriorly and to its opposite member anteriorly to form the bony pelvis. The two innominate bones and sacrum receive muscular attachments from the segments above (trunk) and below (lower limbs), while sheltering and supporting the visceral contents of the pelvis.

ILIUM

The ilium is flattened in the sagittal plane and has lateral (gluteal) and medial (pelvic) surfaces. The expanded upper end is the ala (wing), and the lower end is the body. The ala receives fibers from a number of trunk and lower limb muscles. The upper edge of the ala, the iliac crest, represents the caudal limit of the waist. Three ridges—the outer, middle, and inner lips—curve along its upper border and serve as attachment sites for the obliquus externus abdominis, obliquus internus abdominis, and transversus abdominis, respectively.

Clinical Relevance

TRANSVERSE PLANE OF ILIAC CRESTS: *The transverse plane of the iliac crests, or* **supracristal plane,** *is a horizontal one that passes through the IVD between L4 and L5.*

Convenient for assessing the height of the iliac crests in the standing posture, it is also useful for locating the usual site of lumbar puncture [112,136] (Fig. 35.13).

Medial Surface

The medial (pelvic) surface of the ala bears a concavity, the iliac fossa, which gives rise to the iliacus muscle. The posterior part of the medial surface of each ilium has a pair of prominences that mark the site of the SIJ: an anteroinferior L-shaped auricular surface covered with cartilage and a posterosuperior iliac tuberosity. Both the auricular surface and tuberosity articulate with areas of similar shape and name on the ala of the sacrum to form the SIJ. An oblique ridge of bone divides the iliac tuberosity into upper (posterosuperior) and lower (anteroinferior) parts. The interosseous sacroiliac ligament attaches to the lower part; two trunk muscles, the erector spinae and medial fibers of the quadratus lumborum, attach to the upper part. Descending anteriorly from the edge of the auricular surface is the arcuate line; it joins the ilium to the pubis at the iliopubic (iliopectineal) eminence, a roughened area that receives the insertion of the psoas minor when it is present. The inferior end of the medial surface of the body of the ilium marks the position of the upper two fifths of the acetabulum.

Lateral Surface

Three oblique gluteal lines mark the lateral surface of the ala and subdivide it into four areas (Fig. 35.12A). Beginning posteriorly, the gluteus maximus originates between the posterior gluteal line and posterior border of the iliac wing; the gluteus medius from the area between the posterior and anterior gluteal lines; the gluteus minimus (posteriorly) and tensor fasciae latae (anteriorly) from bone between the anterior and inferior gluteal lines; and the reflected tendon of the rectus femoris from the area of bone inferior to the inferior gluteal line, immediately above the acetabulum (Fig. 35.12C). The inferior end of the lateral surface of the body of the ilium forms the upper two fifths of the acetabulum.

Anterior Border

The most anterior point of the iliac crest is the anterior superior iliac spine (ASIS), which receives the inguinal ligament above and the sartorius muscle below. Moving caudally, the anterior border is concave and ends in a large roughened area, the anterior inferior iliac spine (AIIS), which serves as the origin of the tendon of the rectus femoris.

Clinical Relevance

POSITION OF THE ASIS: *The ASIS is an important landmark for measuring leg length. A suspected discrepancy in leg length can be assessed by measuring the distance between the ASIS and the ipsilateral medial or lateral malle*

(continued)

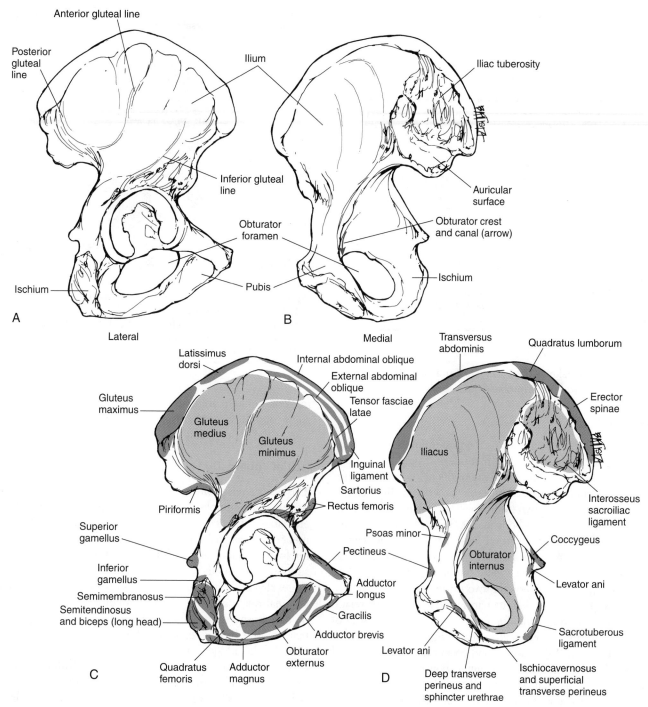

Figure 35.12: Right innominate bone of an adult with osteological features indicated on the lateral (**A**) and medial surfaces (**B**). Sites of attachment of muscles and ligaments are shown on the lateral (**C**) and medial surfaces (**D**).

(Continued)
olus in the supine position and comparing it to the same
measurement obtained from the contralateral limb [98].

Posterior Border

The most posterior point of the iliac crest is the posterior superior iliac spine (PSIS); inferiorly and slightly forward of the PSIS is the posterior inferior iliac spine (PIIS). Fibers of the sacrotuberous ligament are attached to the PSIS and PIIS, while those of the dorsal sacroiliac ligament proceed to the PSIS and posterior end of the medial lip of the iliac crest. Caudal to the PIIS is a deep concavity, the greater sciatic notch, positioned just above the acetabulum; a few fibers of the piriformis originate from its superior margin. Only the superior half of this deep notch is formed by the ilium; its inferior half is formed by the posterior border of the ischium.

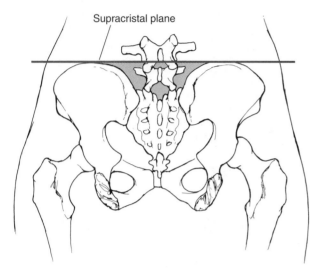

Figure 35.13: The horizontal line through the highest points of the iliac crests passes through the intervertebral disc located between the fourth and fifth lumbar vertebrae; this is the supracristal plane.

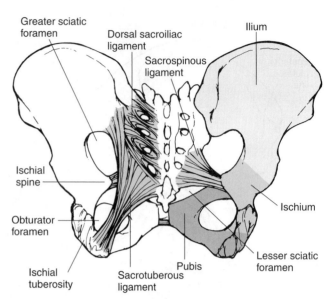

Figure 35.14: Dorsal surface of the pelvis with the three parts of the innominate bone shaded differently; the greater sciatic notch is transformed into a foramen by the sacrospinous ligament; and the lesser sciatic notch is transformed into a foramen by the sacrotuberous ligament.

A dimple in the skin is observable just medial to the PSIS and is especially prominent in obese individuals.

ISCHIUM

The body of the ischium forms the posteroinferior two fifths of the acetabulum. Extending first inferiorly and then anteriorly from its body is the ischial ramus; its union with the inferior pubic ramus is marked by a roughened area, the ischiopubic juncture. The two rami together form the conjoint ischiopubic ramus. The body and ramus of the ischium contribute to the posterolateral wall of the pelvic cavity. Projecting from the posterior border of the ischial body is the sharp ischial spine above and the large, bulbous ischial tuberosity below; between the two is the lesser sciatic notch, a shallower concavity than its partner above. The two sciatic notches are converted into foramina (greater and lesser sciatic) by the sacrospinous and sacrotuberous ligaments, dense ligaments that attach the sacrum and coccyx to the ischium and ilium, thereby reinforcing the union between the axial and appendicular skeletal elements (i.e., SIJ) (*Fig. 35.14*). The sacrospinous ligament is anchored to the ischial spine, and the sacrotuberous ligament to the ischial tuberosity. In addition to these ligamentous structures, many muscles of the pelvis, buttock, and posterior thigh originate from the spine and tuberosity of the ischium. Most of the structures exiting the pelvic cavity pass through the greater sciatic foramen, along with the piriformis; only the obturator internus and its nerve supply, along with the pudendal nerve and internal pudendal vessels, traverse the lesser sciatic foramen.

Ischial Spine

The coccygeus and levator ani originate from the medial surface of the ischial spine (Fig. 35.12D). The superior and

inferior gemelli originate from the lateral surface of the spine and tuberosity, respectively, immediately on either side of the lesser sciatic notch (Fig. 35.12C).

Ischial Tuberosity

This large, posteroinferiorly projecting prominence of the ischium has multiple functions; it serves as the origin of several large muscles of the buttock and thigh, the site of attachment of one extensive ligament that reinforces the SIJ, a shelter for the major nerve of the perineum (pudendal), and a support for the body weight in sitting. Transverse and vertical ridges divide the posterior surface of the tuberosity into four unequal quadrants (*Fig. 35.15*): superolateral for the semimembranosus; superomedial for the semitendinosus and long head of the biceps femoris; inferolateral for the posterior fibers of the adductor magnus; and inferomedial, where it is covered by adipose tissue and the gluteus maximus bursa, for its weight-bearing function. The upper, lateral surface of the ischial tuberosity serves as the origin of the quadratus femoris. The sacrotuberous ligament attaches to the entire medial edge of the tuberosity and extends forward along the ischial ramus as the falciform process (*Fig. 35.16*).

PUBIS

The body of the pubis is compressed in the sagittal plane and has two rami projecting from it, one posterosuperiorly (superior ramus) and one posteroinferiorly (inferior ramus) (Fig. 35.12). The superior ramus is joined to the body of the ilium at the iliopubic (iliopectineal) eminence and the inferior ramus to the ischial ramus at the ischiopubic junction. The bodies of the two pubes project toward the midline as

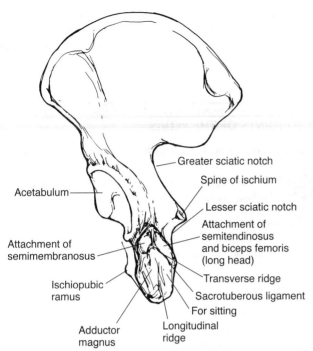

Figure 35.15: Posterolateral aspect of the left os coxae. Two ridges subdivide this caudal part of the ischium: a transverse ridge separates it into upper and lower halves, and a longitudinal ridge divides the lower half. The long hamstrings originate from the upper half; the posterior fibers of the adductor magnus originate from the lateral part of the lower half; and the medial portion of the lower half, used to support the sitting weight, is covered by fat and fibrous connective tissue and a bursa for the gluteus maximus. The upper, lateral surface of the ischial tuberosity gives origin to the quadratus femoris. A ridge along the medial edge of the tuberosity continues forward along the ischiopubic ramus; fibers of the sacrotuberous ligament attach here to form the falciform process.

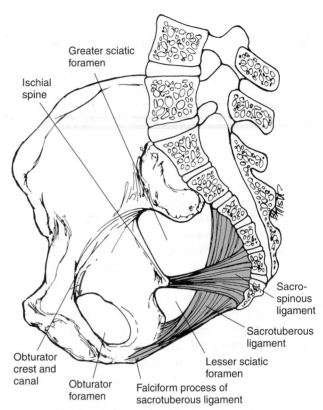

Figure 35.16: Medial view of the right innominate bone. Note the extension of the sacrotuberous ligament along the medial surface of the ischial ramus as the falciform process.

roughened symphyseal surfaces. A fibrocartilaginous disc interposed between the two surfaces is part of the anterior joint between the two innominate bones, the **symphysis pubis.** The posterior surface of the two pubic bodies and interpubic disc form the anterior wall of the pelvic cavity. The adductor longus originates from the anterior surface of the body of the pubis.

Superior Pubic Ramus

The posterior end of the superior pubic ramus, where it joins with the body of the ilium, forms the anteroinferior one fifth of the acetabulum. On the posteroinferior end of the ramus is a slight groove, the obturator sulcus, guarded by a ridge of bone, the obturator crest; the sulcus, crest, and a defect in the obturator membrane, or obturator canal, all mark the site of passage of the obturator nerve and vessels from the pelvic cavity into the medial thigh.

Extending forward along the internal surface of the superior pubic ramus, continuous with the arcuate line of the ilium, is a sharp ridge of bone, the pecten; the arcuate line and pecten together form the linea terminalis. The pecten

terminates at the pubic tubercle; from the tubercle a ridge passes medially, the pubic crest, and terminates at the symphyseal surface. The sacral promontory and ala, linea terminalis, and pubic crest on each side form the **pelvic brim;** it divides the true pelvis (pelvis minor) below from the false pelvis (pelvis major) above. The pecten serves as the origin of the pectineus muscle.

Inferior Pubic Ramus and Ischial Ramus

The inferior ramus of the pubis and ramus of the ischium meet at a point that is approximately equidistant between the anterior limit of the pubis and posterior limit of the ischium; the two parts together form the conjoint ischiopubic ramus. With the inferior margin of the pubic symphysis, the paired inferior pubic rami and ischial rami form the pubic arch (Fig. 35.1). The pubic bodies and ischiopubic rami have a pelvic (medial, posterior) surface that serves as the bony origin for several pelvic and perineal muscles: the levator ani of the pelvic diaphragm from the pubic body, and the urogenital diaphragm, superficial transverse perineal, and ischiocavernosus from the ischiopubic ramus. Their lateral (anterior) surfaces are roughened and mark the site of origin of the medial (adductor) thigh muscles: the anterior fibers of the adductor magnus from the ischiopubic ramus, and the gracilis and adductor brevis from the inferior ramus and body of the pubis.

SACROTUBEROUS LIGAMENT AND PUDENDAL CANAL: *The sacrotuberous ligament that attaches to the medial edge of the ischial tuberosity extends along the medial side of the ischiopubic ramus as the* **falciform process** *[134,147]. This forward extension of the ligament forms the floor of the* **pudendal canal** *(Alcock's canal) and shelters the contents of the canal, the pudendal nerve and internal pudendal vessels, the primary neurovascular elements of the perineum (Fig. 35.17). Nonetheless, contents of the pudendal canal are intimately juxtaposed to the ischiopubic ramus and can be jeopardized when this ramus is fractured and bony fragments impinge upon or sever the neurovascular contents of the canal. More commonly, pressure on the pudendal canal, as experienced in long distance cycling when the seat presses against the medial border of the ischiopubic ramus, can lead to temporary or protracted erectile dysfunction and even impotence in males [4,38,116,148]. Whether these aspects of male sexual dysfunction are vasculogenic (trauma to the internal pudendal vessels), neurogenic (trauma to the pudendal nerve), or a combination of the two continues to be debated [93,143].*

OBTURATOR FORAMEN AND OBTURATOR MEMBRANE

The large, somewhat oval, obturator foramen in the inferior part of the innominate bone is located below the acetabulum and is formed by the body and rami of the ischium and pubis. The obturator foramen is closed almost entirely by the obturator membrane, except for a small anterosuperior defect, the obturator canal, which allows the obturator neurovascular elements to exit the pelvic cavity. The obturator externus originates from most of the obturator membrane's lateral (external) surface, as well as surrounding bone of the pubis and ischium; the obturator internus originates from most of the membrane's medial (internal) surface, along with surrounding bone of the pubis, ischium, and ilium.

PALPATION OF BONY PROMINENCES AND JOINTS OF THE PELVIS

Careful assessment of the low back and pelvis requires precise palpation in an attempt to identify the source of a patient's complaints. Readily palpable structures of the bony pelvis include the following:

- Spinous and transverse processes of L5
- Dorsal sacroiliac ligament
- Dorsal surface of the sacrum
- Coccyx
- ASIS
- Iliac crest
- PSIS
- Sacrotuberous ligament
- Ischial tuberosity
- Conjoint ischiopubic ramus
- Symphysis pubis
- Pubic tubercle
- Superior pubic ramus

OSSIFICATION

Ossification of the innominate bone begins prenatally by three primary centers, one each for the ilium, ischium, and pubis. The center for the ilium appears rostral to the greater sciatic notch in the ninth week, the ischial center in its body by the fourth month, and the center for the pubis in its superior ramus between the fourth and fifth month of intrauterine life [7,37,88]. Significant parts of each of the three bones of the os coxae remain cartilaginous at birth. Most notably, the

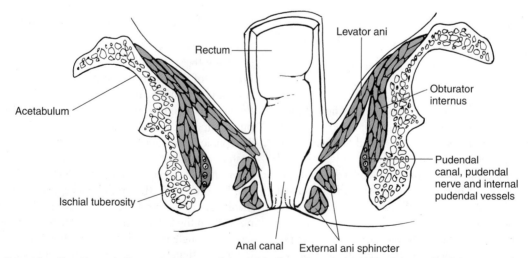

Figure 35.17: Coronal section through the posterior part of the pelvis. Note the relationship of the pudendal nerve and internal pudendal vessels to the medial surface of the ischial ramus.

acetabulum is a cartilaginous cup that has expanding from its center a triradiate stem of cartilage with prongs projecting toward the ilium, ischium, and pubis [147] (Fig. 35.11). Secondary centers of ossification appear at varying times post-natally. Several secondary centers for the ilium, ischium, and pubis appear at puberty and fuse sometime between 15 and 25 years of age. Three secondary centers for the acetabulum join between 16 and 18 years [6,7].

Clinical Relevance

OSSIFICATION AND FUSION OF THE INNOMINATE BONE: *Owing to the lateness of fusion of the bones of the pelvis, certain conditions and activities may be particularly hazardous to adolescents and young adults. Teenage pregnancies are particularly risky, considering the trauma of fetal passage through the pelvic birth canal [150]. In addition, serious consideration should be given to participation by adolescents in certain activities that require sudden acceleration and deceleration, such as sprinting, soccer, football, and basketball [112]. During these activities, avulsion fractures can occur at sites of attachment of muscles to apophyses (a bony prominence without a secondary ossification center), such as the ASIS, AIIS, ischial tuberosity, and ischiopubic ramus.*

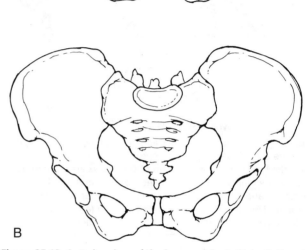

Figure 35.18: Anterior view of the bony pelvis. **A.** Male. **B.** Female.

Sexual Differences

A higher degree of **sexual dimorphism** is apparent in the bones of the pelvis than in other bones of the body (*Fig. 35.18*). Distinctive sex characteristics appear prenatally as early as the third month [18]; pelves are poorly marked prior to puberty but fully developed afterward [86]. Differences between the bony pelves of males and females are related to a number of factors, including, but not limited to, relative differences in stature and body composition resulting from actions of the sex hormones and functions of the pelvis [8,136,147] (*Table 35.5*).

TABLE 35.5: Differences between Female and Male Pelvis That Represent Adaptations for Childbearing

Features of the Male Bony Pelvis	Features of the Female Bony Pelvis
Concavity more conical	Cavity more cylindrical
Sacrum longer and narrower	Sacrum shorter and wider
Sacral concavity shallower	Sacral concavity deeper
>1/3 of the sacral base = the body	>2/3 of the sacral base = the ala

Anterolateral wall of pelvis narrower
  Pubic tubercles closer together
  Distance from the symphysis pubis to the anterior lip of the acetabulum = diameter of the acetabulum
	Anterolateral wall of pelvis wider
	  Pubic tubercles further apart
	  Distance from the symphysis pubis to the anterior lip of the acetabulum > diameter of the acetabulum

Greater sciatic notch narrower	Greater sciatic notch wider
Pubic arch < 90°	Pubic arch ~ 90°
Ischiopubic rami robust and everted	Ischiopubic rami delicate

Ischium relatively and absolutely longer than the pubis
  Ischiopubic index[a] < 90°
	Pubis relatively and absolutely longer than the ischium
	  Ischiopubic index > 90°

[a]Ischiopubic index = (length of pubis × 100) ÷ length of ischium

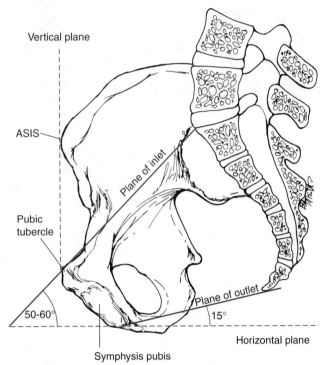

Figure 35.19: The pubic tubercles and anterior superior iliac spines (ASIS) are aligned vertically; the upper surface of the symphysis pubis, the ischial spine, and the tip of the coccyx are aligned horizontally; the plane of the pelvic inlet is approximately 60° off the horizontal; and the plane of the pelvic outlet is approximately 15° off the horizontal. The axis of the pelvic cavity *(arrow)* is oblique, passing through the centers of the inlet and outlet.

In general, estrogen secretion in females stimulates formation of an individual with shorter and lighter bones, lower weight, and lower lean body mass than males [63]; and the requirements of childbirth necessitate a roomier pelvis in females [147]. Subsequently, the sacrum and the innominate bones of females are lighter; bony protuberances are less prominent; and relative widening of the sacral base and pubic body, increasing the angle of the pubic arch, everting the ischial tuberosities, and increasing the forward inclination of the sacrum all contribute to enlargement of the diameters of the pelvic inlet and outlet, thus facilitating parturition. Other

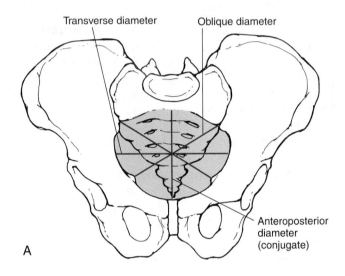

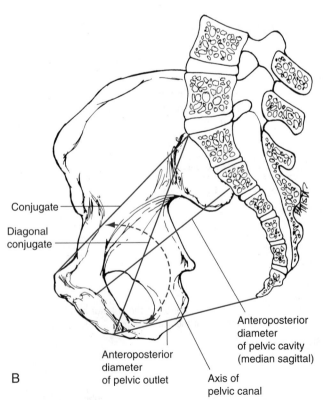

Figure 35.21: A. Diameters of the superior aperture (pelvic inlet). **B.** Anterosuperior diameters of the true (minor) pelvis.

Figure 35.20: The pelvic inlet is bordered by the pelvic brim, formed by the promontory and ala of the sacrum, pecten of the pubis, arcuate line of the ilium (together termed the iliopectineal line, or linea terminalis), and the pubic crest. The junction of the ilium and pubis is marked by the iliopubic eminence.

differences can be seen in the pelvic joints: the acetabulum and auricular surfaces of the ilia and sacrum are smaller [20,149], and the symphyseal surface of the pubic body is shorter [164].

Clinical Relevance

PELVIC DIAMETERS AND TYPES OF PELVES:

*Assessment of the overall size of the female pelvis and the dimensions of its apertures is important in obstetrical practice. Two openings are significant: one is situated above and serves as the **pelvic inlet** (superior aperture), and the other is positioned below and functions as the **pelvic outlet** (inferior aperture) (Fig. 35.19). The size of the pelvic cavity positioned between these two bony boundaries is the limiting factor in obstetric considerations; no attempts are made to account for the fascial and muscular contributions made to this space [135].*

*The **pelvic brim** borders the pelvic inlet (Fig. 35.20). On each side, it is formed posteriorly by the sacral ala, laterally by the arcuate line of the ilium and pecten of the pubis (together forming the linea terminalis), and anteriorly by the pubic crest. The circle is completed in the posterior midline by the sacral promontory and anteriorly by the symphysis pubis. The border of the pelvic outlet is formed anteriorly by the pubic arch, laterally by the ischial tuberosities and sacrotuberous ligaments, and in the posterior midline by the coccyx. The plane of the pelvic inlet is approximately 60° off the horizontal, while the plane of the outlet is nearly horizontal [135] (Fig. 35.19). Owing to the different orientations*

*of the two apertures, the axis of the pelvic cavity, running through the centers of the inlet and outlet, follows a curved course that nearly parallels the sacrococcygeal curvature. During **parturition** (childbirth), the fetus follows this curvature in its passage through the pelvic cavity.*

*For obstetrical purposes, three diameters of the superior aperture of the pelvis are measured commonly to determine the prospective mother's pelvic type prior to delivery (Fig. 35.21). The **true conjugate diameter** is the distance between the superior border of the symphysis pubis to the sacral promontory; the **diagonal conjugate diameter** is similar but has a starting point inferior to the symphysis pubis. The former is measured radiographically, but the latter can be assessed during the vaginal examination. The **transverse diameter,** the greatest distance between symmetrical points on the pelvic brim, is deduced from external pelvic dimensions or the distance between the ischial spines, which are palpable through the vagina. Four types of pelves are described on the basis of the ratio between the transverse and conjugate diameters (Fig. 35.22). These are **gynecoid** (female), **anthropoid** (ape), **android** (male), and **platypelloid** (flat). The transverse diameter is greater than the conjugate in the gynecoid, android, and platypelloid pelves, while the opposite is true in the anthropoid pelvis. Gynecoid and android pelves predominate in Caucasian females, while gynecoid and anthropoid types are more common in Negroid females; few females have platypelloid pelves [8,147]. All pelvic types except the gynecoid type hamper engagement of the fetal head during labor [135].*

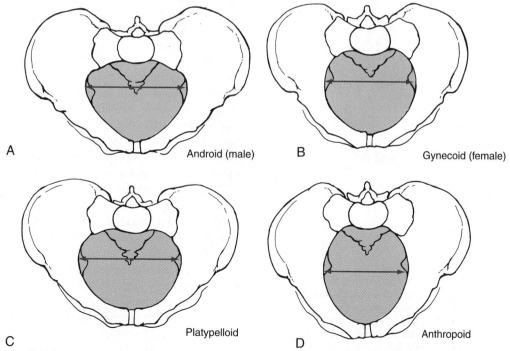

A — Android (male)	B — Gynecoid (female)
C — Platypelloid	D — Anthropoid

Figure 35.22: Shapes of four major types of pelves are based on the ratio between the transverse and conjugate diameters. **A–C.** The transverse diameter is greater than the conjugate. **D.** The opposite is true.

PELVIC JOINTS AND PERIARTICULAR STRUCTURES

In the erect posture, the superincumbent weight of the head, upper limbs, and trunk is transmitted onto the sacrum through the last lumbar vertebra and its disc. Weight is further transmitted through the paired SIJs and distributed to the ischial tuberosities in sitting or the femora in standing. Completed anteriorly with the union of the pubic bodies at the symphysis pubis, this **osteoligamentous ring** is subdivided into two anatomical and functional arches to describe the transmission of forces in the standing posture [3,9, 80,81,147]; a coronal plane passing through the acetabula separates the bony pelvis into **anterior** and **posterior arches** (*Fig. 35.23*). The upper three segments of the sacrum and paired pillars of iliac bone passing from both SIJs to the posterosuperior acetabula form the posterior arch, which serves mainly to transfer weight from above to the lower limbs. The anterior arch is a tie beam or counter arch and consists of the superior pubic rami, pubic bodies, and interpubic disc; it serves the dual function of connecting the anterior ends of the iliac pillars to prevent separation of the posterior arch at the SIJs, as well as acting as a compression strut against the ground reaction forces from the femora below. The sitting arches are somewhat different. Weight is transmitted from above through the SIJs, inferior parts of the iliac pillars, and then to the ischial tuberosities. The tie beam or counter arch for the sitting arch includes the ischial tuberosities, ischiopubic rami, pubic bodies, and interpubic disc [9]. The highest

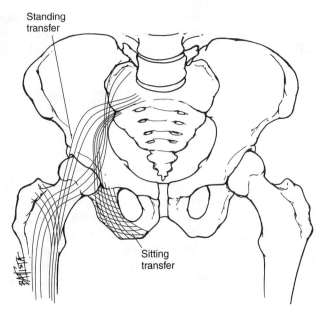

Figure 35.24: Bony trabecular system of the right innominate bone and proximal femur. The transfer of weight via the SIJ is through the arcuate line to the acetabulum in standing, and through the arcuate line to the ischial tuberosities when sitting.

stresses and greatest bone densities of the pelvic bones occur along the lines of the these anterior and posterior arches [34,35,75] (*Fig. 35.24*).

The bones and joints of the pelvis are inherently stable. The line of transmission of both the trunk force from above and the ground reaction forces from below pass anterior to the SIJs (*Fig. 35.25*). The former force tends to tilt the sacrum forward, and the latter tends to rotate the innominate bones backward; both are resisted by the numerous strong ligaments of the pelvic joints, as well as, in the SIJs particularly, the inherent morphology of their articulating surfaces [30,147]. Together, the two forces provide a self-locking, screw-home mechanism for maximal stability [3,59,81,147]. The level of pelvic stability achieved by this arrangement requires thousands of pounds of force to disrupt [30,137]. Furthermore, when large forces are applied to the pelvis, either in vivo or in vitro, the sacrum or ilium often fractures before the ligaments rupture or avulse.

The reader should be warned that many aspects of pelvic joint morphology, mechanics, and pathology have been debated heavily over the years. Most of the questions surrounding these joints appear to have been adequately probed to allow most clinicians and scientists to arrive at well-documented conclusions regarding the issues around which controversy has thrived. Although nagging questions persist, especially as regards the amount and type of motion present at these joints, only a few diehards remain who are skeptical about the other issues. Two things account for the changing perspective toward these joints: first, technological advances in research techniques have produced less-equivocal evidence, and second, the body of evidence from numerous well-designed

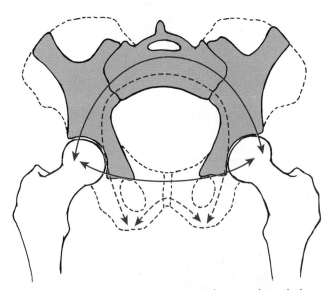

Figure 35.23: In standing, the posterior arch passes through the sacrum, paired iliac pillars, posterosuperior acetabula, and femora, while the anterior (counter) arch passes through the femora, superior pubic rami, pubic bodies, and interpubic disc *(solid lines)*. In sitting, the posterior arch passes through the sacrum, inferior part of the iliac pillars, to the ischial tuberosities, while the anterior (counter) arch passes through the ischial tuberosities, ischiopubic rami, pubic bodies, and interpubic disc *(broken lines)*.

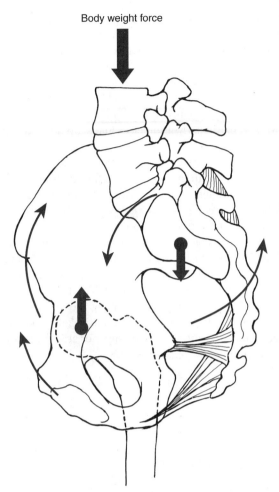

Figure 35.25: Medial aspect of the left hemipelvis. In standing, the sacral promontory tends to tilt down and forward while the ilia tend to tilt backward because the center of gravity passes anterior to the sacroiliac joints (SIJs) and posterior to the hip joints. These tendencies are resisted by the interosseous sacroiliac, sacrotuberous and sacrospinous ligaments, and the inherent morphology of the SIJ.

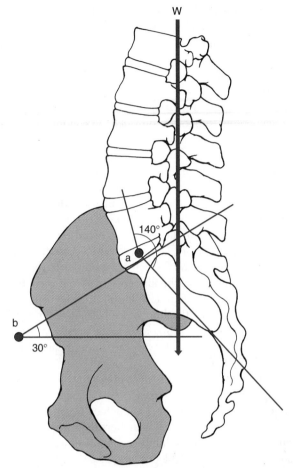

Figure 35.26: The lumbosacral angle (a) is formed by the intersection of lines drawn between the long axis of the fifth lumbar vertebra and the sacrum. It results from a forward sacral inclination (b) and wedge-shaped lower lumbar intervertebral discs and bodies. As the sacral inclination and lumbar lordosis increase, the lumbosacral angle decreases, and vice versa. The sacral inclination is greater in the female, while the lumbosacral angle is greater in the male. W, superincumbent weight.

scientific studies has found its way into clinical and basic science textbooks. Inclusion in this section of all of the studies that have contributed to the knowledge base of the pelvic joints is neither possible nor appropriate. Following a description of each of the joints, the studies most critical to our understanding are offered.

Lumbosacral Junction

The basic components of the L5 and S1 articulations do not differ significantly from the other intervertebral unions. The bodies are joined by an **amphiarthrodial symphysis,** which consists of thin layers of hyaline cartilage on either side of the largest fibrocartilaginous disc in the spine; the disc is taller anteriorly than posteriorly, a matching feature found in the L5 body. The synovial zygapophyseal joints have facets oriented in the coronal plane whose surfaces are more widely separated than those above [147]. The sacrum sits below L5 with its base tilted forward and its apex backward. The **sacral**

inclination thus formed consists of the base of the sacrum being tilted forward off the horizontal by approximately 30° (Fig. 35.26). There is tremendous variability, however, with a reported range of 20 to 90° [58,59,81]; it is greater in the female [9,147]. The **sacral inclination,** as well a wedge-shaped L5 vertebral body and IVD, each contribute to the lumbosacral angle (between the long axes of L5 and the sacrum) [81,136]; it is greater in males.

Clinical Relevance

LUMBOSACRAL ANGLE: *The sacral inclination and the lumbosacral angle are intimately related to the lumbar lordosis. An increase in the sacral inclination along with a decrease in the lumbosacral angle necessitates an increase in the lumbar lordosis.*

Many muscular and ligamentous entities cross and reinforce the lumbosacral junction. The muscles belong to the trunk and lower limbs. Essentially any muscle that moves the trunk across the joints of the lumbar spine stabilizes the joint, including the anterior and anterolateral abdominal wall muscles, posterior abdominal wall muscles, and lumbar deep back muscles. These are described in greater detail in Chapter 33.

Ligamentous support is provided by continuation of the vertebral ligaments that are found at higher levels of the spine and include the anterior and posterior longitudinal, intertransverse, interspinous, and supraspinous ligaments, along with the ligamentum flavum and zygapophyseal capsular elements at the L5–S1 interspace. In addition, the **iliolumbar ligaments** reinforce the junction laterally (*Fig. 35.27*). Each extends from the tip of the transverse process of L5 (and frequently L4) and spreads laterally to connect to the pelvis by way of two bands, both of which pass anterior to the SIJ. An upper band attaches to the iliac crest, where it is continuous above with the thoracolumbar fascia; a lower band (sometimes referred to as the lumbosacral ligament, though not recognized in the N.A. [45]) passes to the upper surface of the sacral ala, where it blends with the anterior sacroiliac ligament [27,91,94,123,147].

The iliolumbar ligament is not present in the newborn; it develops over the first two decades by metaplasia of fibers of the quadratus lumborum and undergoes degeneration from the fourth decade on [94]. Researchers theorize that the ligament develops when the lumbosacral junction is stressed by assumption of the upright posture [27,94] and suggest that the different bands of the ligament serve different functions [27,91]. The lower band is positioned in the coronal plane; it serves to square L5 on the sacrum and thus control lateral

flexion. The upper band runs obliquely backward; it exerts a posterior pull on L5 to prevent anterior slippage during weight bearing, and it controls flexion. The iliolumbar ligaments, as a whole, appear to also control axial rotation [180]. Apparently, the ligament assumes greater functional significance in contributing to lumbosacral stability when the lumbosacral disc degenerates; it may protect the disc from excessive torque, particularly if the facet joints are defective [27].

As already indicated, the lumbosacral junction is a region of high variability, as well as the point of greatest stress in the entire vertebral column. Being one of the levels most subject to internal derangement [33], Kapandji refers to it as the weak link [81]. As a result of the body weight bearing down on L5 and the anterior inclination of the sacrum, an anteroinferior shear stress is produced at the L5–S1 junction; the resultant force vector, acting through the pars interarticularis, is an anterior one [81] (*Fig. 35.28*). Subsequently, L5 tends to slide forward on the sacral promontory. This tendency is resisted, and L5 is restrained, however, by the vertebra's bony hook, formed by its pedicles, pars interarticulares, and inferior articular processes, fitting over the superior articular processes of the sacrum below [59] (Fig. 35.28).

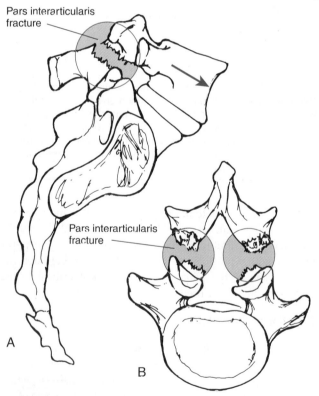

Figure 35.28: The bony hook of L5 consists of its pedicle, pars interarticularis, and inferior articular process; it fits over the superior articular process of the sacrum below. **A.** Disruption of the bony hook mechanism between L5 and S1 can be caused by fracture of the pars interarticularis (spondylolysis) and can result in spondylolisthesis. **B.** Pars interarticularis defect seen from above L5.

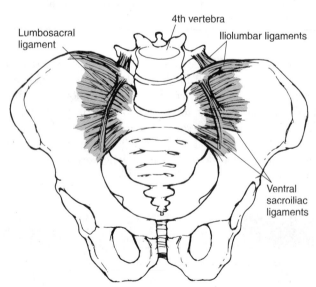

Figure 35.27: Iliolumbar ligaments, both passing anterior to the sacroiliac joint, are shown connecting both the fourth and fifth lumbar vertebrae to the ilium. Although not recognized by the *Nomina Anatomica*, a lumbosacral ligament is shown.

Clinical Relevance

PARS INTERARTICULARIS DEFECTS: *Various anomalies and pathological or congenital conditions, over time and under stress, may weaken or destroy the integrity of the resisting hook mechanism; such defects include congenital aplasia (or dysplasia) of the sacral facets, near-sagittal orientation of one or both of the lumbosacral facet joints (Fig. 35.9), excessive anterior tilt of the sacrum resulting in increased lumbosacral shear, and spondylolysis. Disruption of the pars interarticularis* (**spondylolysis**) *can occur unilaterally (up to 30%), with or without slipping* (**olisthesis**), *and although it has been observed at L3, L4, and L5, it is most frequent at L5 [59,60,100,136]. Although 5% of individuals with this condition are asymptomatic [100],* **spondylolisthesis** *can be a serious consequence of spondylolysis. The Belgian obstetrician Herbineaux [72] is credited with describing the first cases of spondylolisthesis when he noted that, on occasion, a bony prominence on the anterior surface of the sacrum interfered with labor. Because of the location of the spondylolytic defect, the body, pedicles, and superior articular processes slip forward, leaving the inferior articular processes, laminae, and spinous process in their normal position.*

Spondylolisthesis is diagnosed on the oblique radiographic projection; the disrupted pars interarticularis (isthmus) appears as a translucent area in the vicinity of the neck of the Scottie dog, described earlier in this chapter [101] (Fig. 35.5). The degree of slip of L5 on the sacrum is assessed on the lateral radiographic view as a percentage based on a grading system of Myerding [115]: grade 1, 25%; grade 2, 25–50%; grade 3, 50–75%; grade 4, 75–100% overhang (Fig. 35.29). **Spondyloptosis** *occurs when the posterior edge of L5 moves anterior to the sacral promontory [100]. IVD degeneration, cauda equina compression, and severe pain are serious potential sequelae of this disorder [59,61,100,101].*

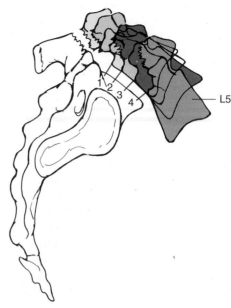

Figure 35.29: Spondylolistheses is graded on the basis of the amount of forward movement of L5 on the sacrum. In grades 1, 2, 3, and 4, some 25, 50, 75, and 100% of the body of L5 is positioned anterior to the sacral promontory, respectively.

Clinical Relevance

COCCYX AND SACROCOCCYGEAL JUNCTION: *During childbirth, the coccyx moves posteriorly, allowing an increase in the diameter of the pelvic outlet, thus facilitating movement of the fetus through the birth canal [113]. Presumably, the movement is passive and secondary to passage of the fetus and made possible by relative relaxation of the ligaments surrounding the coccyx. It is stimulated by an increase in circulating sex hormones and the hormone* **relaxin** *(more on this later) [97,113].*

Most injuries to the coccyx occur in women, probably owing to its more posterior position in the broader pelvic outlet of the female [33]. Injuries can occur during obstetrical and gynecological maneuvers, but most result from other traumas [107,119]. An extension strain or fracture of the coccyx can result from childbirth; flexion injury, fracture, or a direct contusion can result from a fall on an uneven surface or in the half-sitting position (allowing some of the force to be absorbed by the coccyx away from the ischial tuberosities) [33,49,80]. In extremely lean individuals without sufficient gluteal mass, the coccyx may be vulnerable in sitting [130]. **Coccygodynia** *(coccygeal pain; also known as* **coccydynia, coccyalgia**) *from any of the aforementioned mechanisms is always localized to the coccyx. Pain can be experienced with activation of muscular fibers attaching to the coccyx (i.e., gluteus maximus, iliococcygeus and coccygeus). Consequently, walking, especially uphill or upstairs, and sitting, particularly going from standing to seated, are usually painful; defecation and coitus may be noxious in*

Sacrococcygeal Junction

A symphysis consisting of a small fibrocartilaginous IVD sandwiched between thin layers of hyaline cartilage unites the apex of the sacrum and the superior surface of the first coccygeal segment (Fig. 35.7). Anterior, lateral, and posterior sacrococcygeal ligaments complete the union. Successive segments are nodular and generally fused to one another; occasionally, there is a synovial joint between the second and third segments. In the young, all intercoccygeal joints are symphyseal, but they fuse in adulthood, earlier in males than in females; with advancing age, the sacrococcygeal joint fuses [80,147]. The tip of the coccyx is anchored to the overlying skin and can be palpated easily in the intergluteal cleft [113]. Dorsal primary rami of S4-5 and Co1 anastomose with one another and form loops that innervate the sacral apex and coccyx, as well as the overlying skin [147].

*some patients. Muscle pull from the gluteus maximus and anococcygeal musculature may predispose some fractures to nonunion and a **coccygectomy** may be indicated [119,171]. The procedure is, however, highly controversial and not without risk [11,127].*

Sacroiliac Joint (SIJ)

The joints of the pelvic closed kinematic chain have been steeped in controversy since they were first described by Meckel in 1816 [102]. The controversy, involving the SIJ predominately, has raged for centuries and centers around several arthrological features, most significantly its classification, cartilage type, innervation, propensity for movement, and predilection for causing pain. Interest in these joints was generated first by obstetricians, who measured changes in pelvic diameters with different body positions [33,84,167]. With the passage of time, the joints uniting the pelvic ring gained a peripheral place in trauma medicine and rheumatology, but the attention devoted to them as a primary source of mechanical dysfunction and pain has waxed and waned [59]. The SIJs especially fell into disfavor as producers of pain in 1934 when Mixter and Barr demonstrated the key role of the IVD in back pain [110].

Protagonists of the argument that the SIJs are capable of motion and producing pain contend that this joint, being synovial, has a nerve and vascular supply consistent with other joints of its type, is subject to inflammation and radiographically measurable degeneration [47,103], and is capable of limited motion and therefore subject to mechanical dysfunction [5,43,44,59,89,151,173,175]. Others point out the necessity for clinically significant motion somewhere in the pelvic ring to permit widening of the pelvis during delivery [163,176]. Antagonists of these arguments contend that motion at the joint is nearly impossible, considering the complexity of its topography, the magnitude of force required for its disruption, the referred nature of the pain attributed to it, and the flawed nature of the analyses of its motion [47,176]. Clearly, this is an important issue for clinicians, for without motion there will be no dysfunction and no need for manual therapy techniques. What facts, then, can be brought to bear on this enigmatic joint?

STRUCTURE

For centuries, the SIJ was classified variably as a cartilaginous joint (amphiarthrosis) [56,71], a synchondrosis that is ultimately replaced by bone [55], a diarthroamphiarthrodial joint [160], and a cross between a synarthrosis and diarthrosis [129]. Some concluded that the joint is synovial (diarthrodial) but becomes an amphiarthrosis under certain pathological conditions [20,138]. Researchers as early as the 18th and 19th centuries demonstrated that the SIJs are true synovial joints consisting of a joint cavity, synovial membrane, and fluid [40,84,105,165]; nonetheless, some continued to refer to the joint as an amphiarthrosis [50]. In the first three quarters of the 20th century, the SIJ was considered exclusively synovial

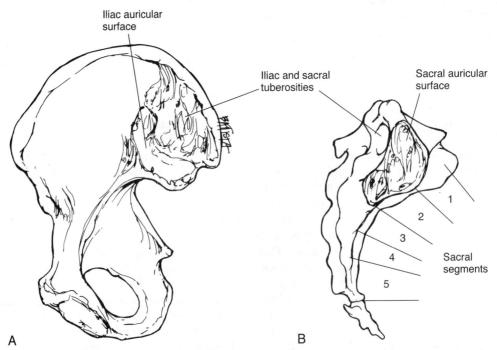

Figure 35.30: Auricular surfaces and tuberosities of the ilium **(A)** and sacrum **(B)** form the sacroiliac joint. The joint has been opened, as a book, to expose each of the bony surfaces that participate in the joint. Sacral segments are numbered 1–5.

[2,32,36,48,52,125,129,142,159,172], a classification reflected by that assigned to it in the 1983 N.A. [45]. The trend today is to include both the **iliac** and **sacral auricular surfaces** and **tuberosities** in the make-up of the SIJ [21,58,59, 147,169]. That is, the auricular surfaces form a **synovial joint,** with a capsule and a cavity filled with fluid, and the tuberosities, connected by an interosseous ligament, constitute a **fibrous** form of a **synarthrosis** (*Fig. 35.30*). Although the synovial part of the joint is usually classified as **plane** [57], its joint surfaces are far from flat or smooth. More prevalent in males than females [161], accessory SIJ articulations are formed frequently from posteriorly positioned supernumerary articular facets [19,44, 64,142,149,161].

The anteroinferior auricular surfaces are complementary L-shaped surfaces, while the tuberosities are paired irregular, pitted areas positioned posterosuperior to the auricular surfaces. The tuberosities are connected by the massive interosseous sacroiliac ligament (*Fig. 35.31*). The L-shaped auricular surfaces have two limbs that point posteriorly and embrace a dorsal concavity [19,149]. The shorter, more vertically oriented cephalic limb consists of the first segment on the sacral side, while the caudal limb is longer, more horizontal, and composed of the second and third segments on the sacral side. The auricular surfaces are strikingly variable, however, both between subjects and from side to side within the same subject; shapes include C- or L-shaped; limbs are long or short and equal or unequal; and the angle formed between the limbs is obtuse or perpendicular [19,21,142,149]. The overall orientation of the joint is obliquely vertical, making it the only weight-bearing joint that is not transverse to the transfer of weight [106].

By all accounts, the cartilage covering the sacral auricular surface differs from that of the ilium. In the vast majority of

reports, the sacral cartilage is hyaline and the iliac cartilage is fibrous [19,131,138,142,159,170]. The one notable and definitive exception is by Paquin et al. [122]. Using microscopic and biochemical methods, they examined the extracellular matrix of cartilage from sacral and iliac auricular surfaces, as well as that from femoral condyles, for comparison. Based on each sample's metachromatic staining (indicating high glycosaminoglycan content), collagen fibril diameter, and exclusive presence of type II collagen peptides [79], they concluded that both sacral and iliac cartilages are hyaline. Cartilage from the two sites differs, however, in the organization of the collagen fibers at the superficial versus the middle and deep zones of the cartilage layer. The latter findings are consistent with other reports indicating a denser aggregate of collagen fibers between chondrocytes in the iliac cartilage than in the sacral side [19,138,170], and probably explain why, using only light microscopic assessment, most past researchers concluded that iliac cartilage is fibrous and not hyaline. The findings of Paquin et al. should not be all that surprising, the literature notwithstanding, when one considers the development of synovial joints. Bones that develop from a cartilaginous anlage (model) have their articulating surfaces covered with hyaline cartilage, while membrane bones develop fibrocartilage at these sites [147]. Both the sacrum and ilium form by endochondral mechanisms, and therefore, their articular surfaces should be covered by hyaline cartilage.

In addition to the differences in their collagen fiber organization, sacral and iliac auricular cartilages are dissimilar in gross appearance, thickness, and the extent to which they undergo degenerative change across their life span. Sacral cartilage is smoother and two to five times thicker than iliac cartilage [19,21,25,122,142,147,163]. The development of the SIJ and its age-related degenerative changes have been well documented [19,20,96,131,138,142,163,164]. The joint develops somewhat differently from other synovial joints, because the ilium significantly antedates the sacrum in development [31,147]. In addition, joint cavitation, which is complete by 12 weeks in most synovial joints [118], begins later and progresses more slowly in the SIJ [142]. A joint cavity appears in the mesenchymal mass between the sacrum and ilium by 7 weeks of intrauterine life, but it does not reach its full extent until 7 or 8 months; a joint capsule is lined by a synovial membrane at 37 weeks [19,31,142]. At birth, joint surfaces are flat and smooth, and the capsule is thin and pliable [19]. During the first 10 years, the auricular surfaces remain flat and, along with a still-pliant capsule, permit gliding motions in all directions. In the teen years, the capsule thickens and complementary unevenness starts to develop on the two auricular surfaces [19,142]. By the early twenties, a convex iliac ridge and a concave sacral depression have formed; they run centrally along the length of the joint surface [19,149]. Although the congruency of the opposing joint surfaces is usually high, eminences are more frequent on the ilium and "almost every conceivable combination of grooves, ridges, eminences, and depressions" [142] is apparent.

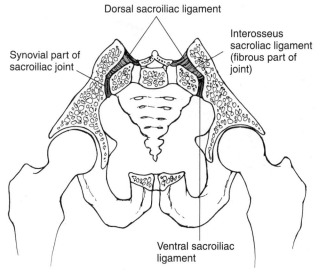

Dorsal sacroiliac ligament

Interosseus sacroiliac ligament (fibrous part of joint)

Synovial part of sacroiliac joint

Ventral sacroiliac ligament

Figure 35.31: Horizontal section through the SIJ, a synovial articulation enclosed by a joint capsule and a fibrous articulation at the interosseous ligament. The short, stout ISIL is the major contributor to sacroiliac integrity.

Auricular surfaces of females are smaller and flatter than those in males [20,149,151,163].

Starting in the middle of the third decade, surfaces of the synovial part of the SIJ begin to show signs of degeneration [19]. Joint degeneration progresses from the fourth through the eighth decade and is characterized by thickening and stiffening of the capsule, severe loss of cartilage thickness, subchondral bone erosion, increasing surface irregularity, intraarticular fibrosis of joint surfaces and, in a few individuals, total ankylosis. The degenerative changes that develop on the iliac side appear first and are more severe than those on the sacral side [19,20,168]; furthermore, they appear at an earlier age and advance more rapidly in males than females [20,21,29,96,131,151,168]. One author [138] reports severe, advanced degenerative changes in over 90% of the SIJs from aged males (over 80 years old).

SUPPORTING STRUCTURES OF THE SIJ

The SIJ is reinforced by some of the strongest and most massive ligaments in the body [6,147,169,175]. Three ligaments are in intimate contact with the joint, and three others, though better termed "accessory," make important contributions to the joint's integrity.

The SIJ capsule is closely attached to the joint's margins; **ventral** and **dorsal sacroiliac ligaments** (VSIL, DSIL) cross the joint, and the **interosseous sacroiliac ligament** (ISIL) connects the sacral and iliac tuberosities (*Figs. 35.31, 35.32*). The VSIL is little more than a thickening of the anterior joint capsule; the cranial part is thin and reinforced by iliolumbar ligament fibers, while the caudal half is well developed below only as far as the iliac arcuate line [147,159]. It assists the symphysis pubis in resisting separation or horizontal movement of the innominate bones at the SIJs. The DSIL is heavier and

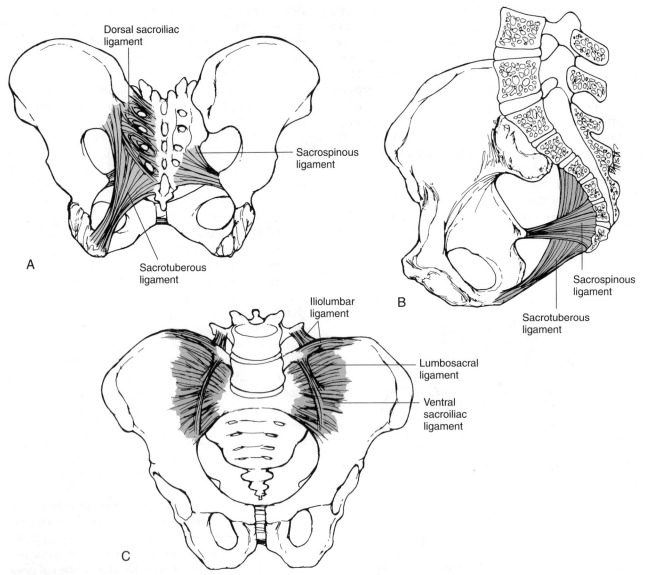

Figure 35.32: Ligaments of the sacroiliac joint. **A.** Dorsal view. **B.** Medial view. **C.** Ventral view.

more extensive than its companion on the ventral surface and, for descriptive and functional purposes, is divided into short and long fibers. Short DSIL fibers are deep and pass infero-medially from the PSIS to the back of the lateral part of the first and second sacral segments. Positioned more superficially, fibers of the long DSIL connect the PSIS to the same area of the third and fourth sacral segments; these fibers are continuous inferolaterally with the sacrotuberous ligament and super-omedially with the posterior lamina of the thoracolumbar fascia [147,159,172]. During incremental loading of the sacrum, the DSIL becomes tense when the base of the sacrum moves backward (**counternutation**) and slackens with movement in the opposite direction (**nutation**) [162]. This is opposite to the tension that develops in the sacrotuberous ligament during movement of the sacrum in the sagittal plane. The ISIL is the major bond between the posterior two thirds of the joint [147]; it connects and fills the space between the sacral and iliac tuberosities. Dorsal primary rami of spinal nerves and blood vessels ramify between the short fibers of the DSIL and the ISIL (*Fig. 35.33*).

The accessory (vertebropelvic) ligaments are the iliolumbar ligament (described earlier in this chapter) connecting L5 to the ilium, and the sacrotuberous and sacrospinous ligaments, passing from the sacrum to the ischium (Fig. 35.32). The sacrotuberous ligament blends with the DSIL as it fans out from the ischial tuberosity, moving upward and medially toward the PSIS, lower sacrum, and coccyx; some of its fibers extend along the ischial ramus as the falciform process. Deep fibers of the gluteus maximus originate from the dorsal surface of this ligament; biceps femoris fibers attach to it as both muscle and ligament fibers anchor themselves to the ischial tuberosity [159]. Deep to, and blended with, the sacrotuberous ligament at its medial attachments, the sacrospinous ligament passes from the ischial spine to the lower sacrum and coccyx. On its deep surface, fibers of the coccygeus (part of the pelvic diaphragm) blend with it. Both the sacrotuberous and sacrospinous ligaments convert the greater and lesser sciatic notches into foramina and resist forward movement of the base of the sacrum under load.

MOTION

Inarguably, the most contentious issue regarding the SIJ is related to the presence, degree, and type of motion available to this joint. The argument has raged for over 2000 years! Hippocrates (460–377 BC) is credited with being first to believe that the SIJ is capable of motion [21,30], but only during pregnancy. Duncan [40,41] was first to provide indirect evidence of SIJ mobility after observing the surface morphology of the joint; he postulated that the sacrum rotated (**nutated** or nodded) around a horizontal axis in the vicinity of the iliac tuberosities. Later, gynecologists made manual measurements of pelvic diameters [84,167]; they attributed the reduction in conjugate diameters from a recumbent to a standing posture to motion at the SIJ. Goldthwaite and Osgood were the first to suggest that the presence of motion at the SIJs was a normal condition for both men and women [52,54] and that the SIJ is a primary source of pain independent of pregnancy [53]. Colachis et al. [30] were the first to make direct measurements of SIJ motion in living subjects; they observed movement of Kirschner wires embedded in the PSISs of the pelvis in nine different body positions.

A multitude of studies designed to assess SIJ mobility were performed during the 19th and 20th centuries; methodologies include morphological observation [19,20,41,149,172], clinical observation [14], mechanical testing [54,92,108], inclinometry [125], conventional radiography [46,173], cineradiography [133], computed tomography [145], stereoradiography [46,132,154], stereophotogrammetry [43], holography [166], the Metrecom skeletal analysis system [144,145], mathematical modeling [51], biomechanical modeling [153], and theoretic consideration [81,176]. *Table 35.6* summarizes findings from a sampling of 20th century studies performed to assess motion of the sacrum relative to the innominates, motion of the innominates relative to one another, and the axes of these motions.

Perusal of the voluminous literature on the subject of SIJ mobility leads to several conclusions:

- SIJs are capable of small amounts of motion.
- Rotation of the sacrum in the sagittal plane between the two innominate bones ranges from 1 to 8°, with the mean between 2 and 3°.
- Translation of the sacrum caudally between the two innominate bones ranges from 0.5 to 8 mm, with a mean between 2 and 3 mm.
- Tremendous variation exists in the amount of motion reported to be available to the SIJs and probably results from a variety of contributive factors, including age, sex, joint surface topography, side-to-side asymmetries in joint structure, ligamentous integrity, degree of joint degeneration, and last but not insignificant, measurement error.

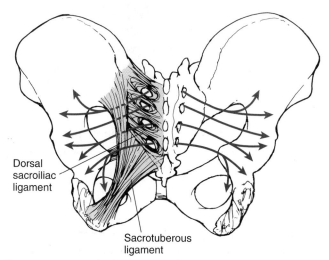

Dorsal sacroiliac ligament

Sacrotuberous ligament

Figure 35.33: Dorsal primary rami of sacral nerves 1–4 ramify between the fibers of the dorsal sacroiliac and ISILs and innervate the joints.

TABLE 35.6: Movement of Sacroiliac Joint

Author(s)	Method(s)	Subjects	Joint Motion Conclusions
Pitkin and Pheasant 1936	Inclinometry	Living subjects	Unilateral antagonistic movement of the ilium around transverse axis through the symphysis pubis averaged 11° (3–19°), or 5.5° on each side
Strachan et al. 1938	Mechanical testing of sacral rotation	Cadavers	During trunk movements, sacral rotation was 1–5° when one ilium was immobilized and the other was fixed to the sacrum
Weisl 1955	Movement of sacral promontory via radiography	Living subjects	Max ventral movement of the sacral promontory was 5.6 ± 1.4 mm with standing from recumbent Axis of angular movement was 5–10 cm below the sacral promontory
Mennell 1960	Changes in distance between PSISs via palpation	Living subjects	PSISs came 0.5 in. closer in horizontal plane
Colachis et al. 1963	Measured distance between Kirschner wires implanted in PSISs	Living subjects	Maximum movement of PSISs was 5 mm with flexion from standing The axis was not fixed
Kapandji 1974	Theorized based on writings of Farabeuf and Bonnaire	None	In nutation the ilia approximate and the iliac tuberosities separate Opposite in counternutation
Frigerio 1974	Biplanar radiography	Cadavers and living subjects	Maximum movement between ilium and sacrum was 12 mm (mean ~2.7 mm) Maximum movement between innominates was 15.5 mm
Egund et al. 1978	Roentgen stereophotogrammetry	Living subjects with hypo- or hypermobile SIJs	Maximum rotation was 2° Axis of sacral rotation was through the iliac tuberosities at the level of S2 Translations were ~2 mm
Wilder et al. 1980	Theoretical best-fit axes of rotation based on topographic analysis of joint surfaces	Dried bony specimens	Joint rotation cannot occur exclusively about any previously proposed axis An important function of the SIJ may be to absorb energy
Reynolds 1980	Stereoradiography	Cadaver	Sacral rotations were 1–2°
Miller et al. 1987	Mechanical testing with one or both ilia fixed	Cadavers	Both ilia fixed: 1.9° rotation, 0.5 mm translation One ilium fixed: rotation 2–7.8× greater and translation 3× greater
Scholten et al. 1988	Biomechanical model	Model	Model relative pelvic motions rarely exceeded 1–2° rotation and 3 mm translation
Sturesson et al. 1989	Stereoradiography	Living subjects	Mean rotation 2.5° ± 0.5° Mean translation 0.7 mm (0.1–1.6 mm)
Smidt et al. 1995	Metrecom skeletal analysis system	Living subjects	Composite sacroiliac motion (relative motion between R/L innominates) was 9° ± 6.5° in oblique sagittal plane and 5° ± 3.9° in transverse plane
Smidt et al. 1997	Computed tomography	Cadavers	Sagittal plane sacral rotation was 7–8° Translation was 4–8 mm

PSISs, posterior superior iliac spines; SIJ, sacroiliac joint.

- In the absence of trauma, the greatest amount of SIJ motion is present in the young, especially the young pregnant female [12].
- The physiological and clinical significance of SIJ motion has been, in the main, ignored by all except obstetricians and clinicians who regularly deal with SIJ syndromes.

In general, three types of motion are available to the innominate bones: **symmetrical motion** is movement of both innominates as a unit in relation to the sacrum; **asymmetrical motion** consists of antagonistic movement of each innominate bone with relation to the sacrum, which includes movement at the symphysis pubis; and **lumbopelvic motion** consists of rotation of the spine and both innominates as a unit around the femoral heads.

Symmetrical Motion

Symmetrical trunk and hip movements result in paired, symmetrical movements at the SIJs [43,138,173,175]. During trunk flexion or bilateral hip flexion, the sacrum **nutates** (L. *nutatio*, nodding) or rotates anteriorly, so that the promontory moves ventrocaudally while the apex moves dorsocranially (*Fig. 35.34*). The sacrum **counternutates,** or moves in the

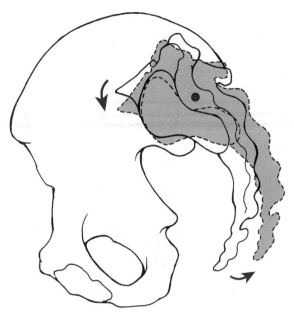

Figure 35.34: Sagittal plane motion of the sacrum. In nutation, the base of the sacrum moves ventrocaudally and its apex moves dorsocranially; this occurs when the sacrum is loaded from above, in trunk flexion, or in bilateral hip flexion. The base of the sacrum moves in the opposite direction during trunk extension and bilateral hip extension, when it counternutates.

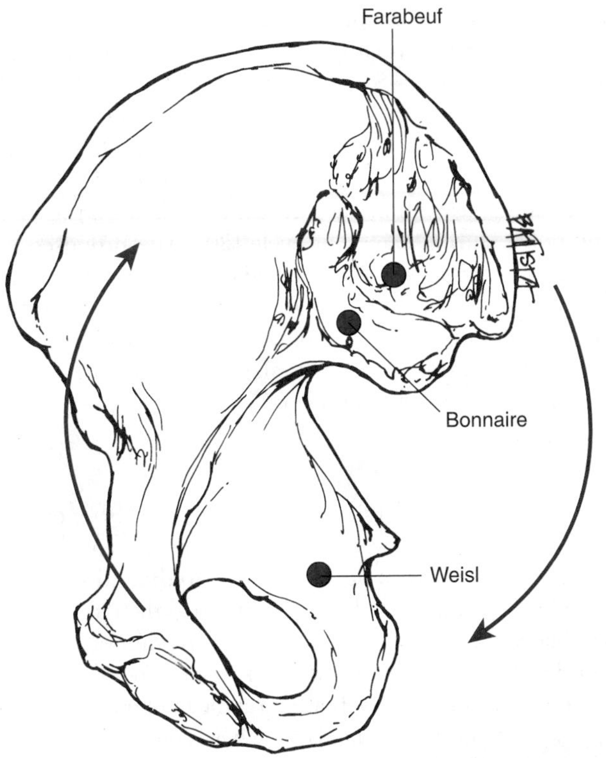

Figure 35.35: Medial view of the innominate bone shows three primary sites proposed as the location of the axis of rotation between the sacrum and the ilium.

opposite direction, during trunk extension or bilateral hip extension. Nutation and counternutation are accompanied by several millimeters of translation. In this type of motion, the innominate bones move symmetrically, as a unit, in the absence of motion at their anterior union, the symphysis pubis [67].

The sacral base always moves further than the apex [173]. Furthermore, it occurs about an instantaneous axis located 5–10 cm below the sacral promontory (*Fig. 35.35*). The combination of rotation and translation is angular movement of the sacrum, during which the iliac crests move closer together while the iliac tuberosities move further apart (*Fig. 35.36*). Sagittal plane angular sacral movement is essentially the same in males as in females, except during pregnancy, when it increases in females. The greatest amount of movement, as much as 5.6 ± 1.4 mm, occurs when going from recumbent to standing and reverses in direction when moving from standing to recumbent [173]. Rotation is accompanied by translation, which results in increased ligamentous tension and absorption of energy [176]. The SIJs thereby function as shock absorbers.

Asymmetrical Motion

A second type of motion occurs at the SIJs when asymmetrical forces are applied to the pelvis, as in static one-legged stance and the one-legged stance that occurs during gait and asymmetrical falls. Application of unbalanced forces to the pelvis results in asymmetrical and antagonistic movements at the SIJs [20,125,175], resulting in **pelvic**

torsion. These movements are always accompanied by movement at the symphysis pubis [67,125], despite the fact that very little movement occurs in the symphysis pubis, except in pregnancy. The experienced clinician can assess manually the end position that results from

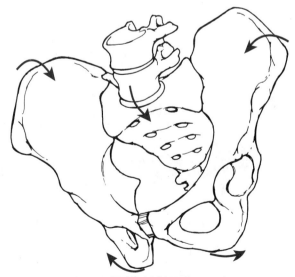

Figure 35.36: Movement of the innominate bones during nutation of the sacrum. The ilia move closer together, and the ischia move farther apart.

movement of one innominate bone relative to the other by palpating the relative prominence of the right and left ASISs and PSISs [33,39,58,90,99,104,152,179]. For instance, if the left ASIS moves upward, the right ASIS and the left PSIS become more prominent while the left ASIS and right PSIS become less prominent (*Fig. 35.37*). Alternating, asymmetrical forces are applied transiently to the pelvis during each gait cycle [20]. The proposed axis for pelvic torsion is transverse and passes through the symphysis pubis [125], though this remains equivocal. Abnormal mobility or instability in either the SIJ or symphysis pubis often is accompanied, however, by a secondary stress lesion in the other [69].

Lumbopelvic Rhythm

The lumbar spine and innominate bones can also move as a unit. Inasmuch as movements of the spine are coupled with those of the pelvis, a **lumbopelvic rhythm** (discussed in Chapter 32), similar to the scapulothoracic rhythm, has been postulated [22] (*Fig. 35.38*). The specific rhythm varies among individuals, but flexion of the trunk from standing combines flexion of the lumbar vertebrae and at the lumbosacral junction with forward rotation of the pelvis on the fixed femora [3,139]. Disturbances in the lumbopelvic rhythm can contribute to low back pain [3,121,139].

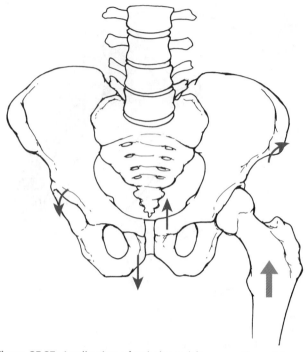

Figure 35.37: Application of unbalanced forces on the pelvis, as in static one-legged stance on the left, results in asymmetrical, antagonistic movement at the SIJs along with movement at the symphysis pubis. This type of movement can be assessed clinically by palpating movement of the ASIS and PSIS.

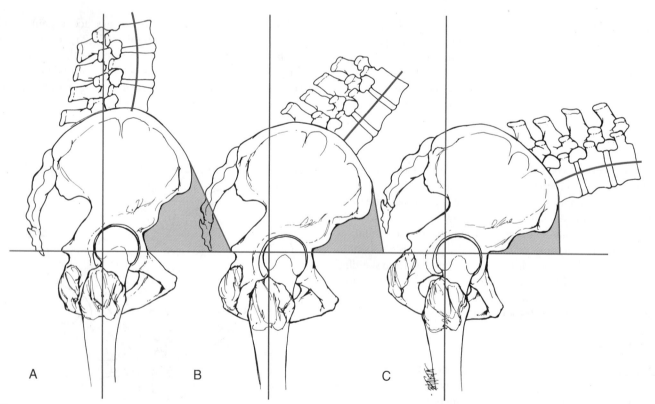

Figure 35.38: Common lumbopelvic rhythm. **A.** Normal standing posture. **B.** During the first 45° of trunk flexion, most motion results from lumbar and sacral flexion causing the sacrum to nutate and the lumbar curve to flatten. **C.** In extreme trunk flexion, the lumbar spine continues to flatten and the pelvis rotates about the femoral heads, while the sacrum paradoxically counternutates.

Clinical Relevance

INFLUENCE OF HORMONES ON MOTION: *Several of the sexually dimorphic features of the SIJs have already been mentioned; none are more functionally and clinically significant than those associated with pregnancy and childbirth. Obstetricians were the first clinicians to show interest in the pelvic joints, noting that during pregnancy and for a period of time following delivery, these joints became more mobile [16,95,105,167]. The pregnancy-induced increase in pelvic mobility lasts up to 4 months postpartum, and the joints become more stable with involution of the uterus [20].*

The changes in pelvic joint mobility are related to ligamentous relaxation stimulated by increased levels of circulating **sex hormones** *during pregnancy and, albeit to a lesser extent, during menstruation [26,39,125]. The hormonally induced changes in pelvic mobility have been confirmed radiographically [1,146,181]. Increased levels of sex hormones as well as the peptide hormone* **relaxin** *produced by the corpus luteum during pregnancy and menstruation are credited by some with the relaxation of pelvic joint ligaments [23,85,97,128]. Controversy continues, however, regarding the exact role of relaxin in contributing to ligamentous relaxation, since serum levels of relaxin do not always correlate with increased peripheral joint laxity [140,174].*

Whatever the cause, relaxation of SIJ ligaments results in a less effective interlocking mechanism between the sacrum and ilia, thereby permitting freer movement at the SIJs and, ultimately, an increase in the diameter of the pelvis. This hormonal effect is not limited to the ligaments of the SIJ; the sacrococcygeal joint and symphysis pubis are affected as well. The result of relaxation at all three sites is a 10–15% increase [113] in the diameter (predominately transverse) of the pelvis and facilitation of movement of the fetus through the pelvic canal [81,95,126,147]. Expediting parturition by increasing pelvic joint mobility does not come without a price, however. That price, according to some, is greater torsional and shear stress, particularly at the SIJ, during pregnancy and for a period of time each month around the menses [3]. In contrast, some researchers and clinicians are convinced that the periodic and cyclical increase in mobility at the female SIJ favors slower development of degenerative changes in the joint [20,138].

INNERVATION

Descriptions of the innervation of the SIJ vary. **Hilton's law of nerves** states that the nerve that innervates a particular muscle also innervates the joint moved by that muscle [158]. This leads to a quandary. On the one hand, the SIJ should have a rich nerve supply, considering its classification as a synovial joint. On the other hand, however, based on the above law, the question is raised as to whether it is innervated to a significant degree, since no muscles are intrinsic to the joint or act on it directly [3,57,59,175]. The classical anatomy texts [147,159,170] and various authors [15,59,74,76,77,87,111,124, 149,177] report innervation of the SIJ from a variety of combinations of cord segments and peripheral nerves; the range for the dorsal part of the joint is by branches of dorsal primary rami of L5–S1-2 and for the ventral part of the joint by the superior gluteal and obturator nerves and branches of ventral primary rami of L4-5–S1-3. More-recent assessment of the joint's innervation, however, using a triad of techniques that include gross and microscopic dissection, routine histology, and immunocytochemistry, on both adult cadaveric and aborted fetal specimens, reveals that the SIJ is innervated exclusively by fine branches from the dorsal primary rami of S1-4 (*Fig. 35.33*) [62,83]; no branches from the sacral plexus, obturator nerve, or superior gluteal nerve are revealed on the ventral surface of the joint, in spite of the intimate relationship between the two as the upper part of the lumbosacral plexus crosses the caudal part of the joint ventrally and is anchored there by fibrous connective tissue [42]. Unmyelinated, finely myelinated, and thickly myelinated fibers are evident, indicating the potential presence of the full spectrum of joint receptors, including those that are activated by painful and mechanical stimuli [13,66,74,87,111].

Clinical Relevance

INNERVATION OF THE SIJ: *Documentation of the SIJ's synovial classification and demonstration of its abundant nerve supply have important clinical application. Clearly, this joint can be a generator of pain. Reports in the literature regarding the precise source of nervous elements to and from the SIJ, however, remain contradictory. On the one hand, one must consider the possibility of individual variation in the innervation pattern of the SIJ. On the other, innervation variability may explain the inconsistent pattern of pain referral observed in individuals with disorders of the SIJ [62,83].*

Symphysis Pubis

The **symphysis pubis** is a median joint that consists of a pair of oval bony surfaces joined by a fibrocartilaginous disc (**pubic disc**) and reinforced by a pair of closely adherent ligaments (*Fig. 35.39*). The symphyseal surfaces of the pubic bodies, shorter and broader in the female than the male, are covered by a thin layer of hyaline cartilage as they project toward one another in the anterior midline to form this **fibrocartilaginous amphiarthrosis** [147,159].

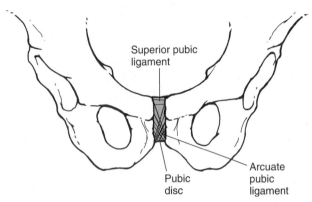

Figure 35.39: Anterior view shows that the symphysis pubis is reinforced by the superior pubic ligament and the arcuate pubic ligament.

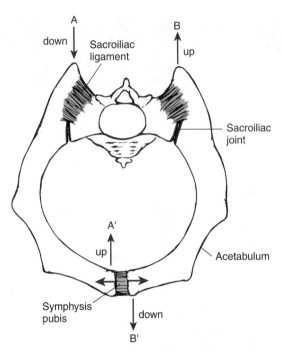

Figure 35.40: Transverse section through the pelvis shows that any transverse movement of the pubes away from each other could contribute to sacroiliac instability. Unpaired antagonistic movement at the SIJs would necessitate some symphysial movement.

Upon removal of the hyaline cartilage, a subchondral contour is exposed that, like the SIJ, consists of complementary ridges and papillae capable of resisting shearing forces. The consistency with which the ridges and papillae increase with age enables forensic scientists to age skeletons on the basis of irregularities of the symphyseal surfaces of pelvic specimens [120,155]. The pubic disc is firmly anchored to each of the hyaline-covered symphyseal surfaces and is usually thicker anteriorly than posteriorly [159]. Thicker overall in the female than the male, the reported normal range is 4–10 mm [175]. In half of specimens, the disc contains an incomplete nonsynovial cavity that rarely appears before the beginning of the second decade and is better-developed in females [147,170]; the cavity may be an area of resorption [147].

Two ligaments reinforce the joint: a **superior pubic ligament** between the two pubic tubercles crosses and is firmly adherent to the disc superiorly; a more robust **arcuate (inferior) pubic ligament** borders the pubic arch as it passes along the disc's inferior edge, between the inferior pubic rami. Several layers of interlacing collagenous fibers derived from aponeuroses of the rectus abdominis and obliquus externus abdominis reinforce the disc anteriorly. Like other amphiarthrodial joints, the symphysis pubis is poorly innervated. Plexuses of afferent nerve terminals penetrate the periphery of the pubic disc only, derived from one or more of the pubic branches of the iliohypogastric, ilioinguinal, and genitofemoral nerves of the lumbar plexus [147].

In most circumstances, movement at the symphysis pubis is slight [147]. Based on elementary physics, however, movement of the symphysis pubis must accompany any unpaired antagonistic movement at one SIJ, unless the axis of SIJ motion is a transverse one that runs through the body of the pubis [125] (*Fig. 35.40*). If the postulated axis does, indeed, pass through the pubic body, unilateral innominate sagittal plane motion would result in only slight torsion at the symphysis pubis.

Clinical Relevance

SYMPHYSIS PUBIS DYSFUNCTION: *Symphysis pubis disruption can occur during pregnancy and for a period of time postpuerperium (the period of 42 days following childbirth) [1,68,178,181], following obstetric and other traumas [17,54,65,78,95], and in athletes, because of repetitive trauma [69,73]. Loss of symphyseal integrity with resultant hypermobility, if significant, contributes further to SIJ instability, even more so in women already experiencing hormonally stimulated SIJ ligamentous laxity [150,169,175]. Malalignment of the symphysis pubis is readily identified radiographically [130]. Horizontal separation of the symphysis pubis in excess of 10 mm and vertical movement of one pubic body in relation to the other by more than 5 mm is considered pathological [65].*

Pathology or Functional Adaptation?

In closing this chapter on pelvic osteology and arthrology, it is appropriate to raise the question of whether certain features of pelvic joint structure and degeneration are functional adaptations or changes in a continuum of changes that lead to pathology. Although the evidence is not unequivocal, several authors support the former, that is, that certain sexually dimorphic features of the pelvis represent functional adaptations to the different roles of the pelvis in males and females [20,21,25,138,163,164].

Two types of evidence support this premise. The first is that the auricular surfaces of SIJs in males have a coarser texture and more ridges and depressions than those in females. Even in advanced age, the ridges and depressions are complementary and generally are covered by intact cartilage [163]. Furthermore, these surface irregularities do not appear until puberty [20], marked by an increase in weight during the growth spurt of adolescence [163]. Furthermore, the male SIJ would be subject to greater torque and therefore higher loads because a male's center of gravity passes more ventral to the SIJ than does the female's [163]. Since these features enhance friction [164], a reasonable conclusion might be that they represent adaptations to the increased body weight and work load generally experienced by males.

The second type of evidence is that the degenerative changes observed in SIJs are more prevalent, are more extensive, and occur earlier in males than in females. As indicated earlier, the SIJ undergoes a progressive loss of mobility with increasing age, with some joints becoming completely or partially ankylosed. In one study of 210 specimens, ankylosis in advanced age was limited to male joints ($n = 105$), where the incidence was 37%; none of the 105 female joints in this study was ankylosed [20]. In the female, apparently, strength at the SIJ is sacrificed for mobility. The joint's ligaments and capsular elements remain comparatively lax in adaptation to its function (i.e., to allow an increase in the pelvic diameter and thereby facilitate the vaginal delivery) [25,169].

SUMMARY

This chapter examines the osteological and arthrological features of the bony pelvis that contribute to its ability to provide a stable support for the body weight while allowing for sufficient motion for the functional requirements of the trunk and lower limbs. The fifth lumbar vertebra is the most robust and angular of the lumbar vertebrae. Its coronally aligned inferior facets and the thick iliolumbar ligaments support the lumbosacral junction against large anterior shear forces. The SIJs are inherently more stable but allow systemic motion, including rotation and translation. Strong ligamentous support and irregular joint surfaces limit mobility and stabilize the SIJ. The pubic symphysis exhibits slight mobility.

The high degree of sexual dimorphism apparent in the bones of the pelvis is described and related to the requirements of childbirth in the female. The female pelvis exhibits a larger medial–lateral diameter and a more posteriorly angled sacrum. Clinically relevant osteological and arthrological variations, malformations, gender differences, and age-related changes of the bony pelvis are detailed, with an emphasis on the controversy involving the SIJ, most significantly its classification, cartilage type, innervation, propensity for movement, and predilection for causing pain.

The following chapter discusses the muscular, nervous, and visceral structures that contribute to the numerous and distinct functions of the pelvis.

References

1. Abramson D, Roberts SM, Wilson PD: Relaxation of the pelvic joints during pregnancy. Surg Gynecol Obstet 1934; 58: 595–613.
2. Albee FH: A study of the anatomy and the clinical importance of the sacroiliac joint. JAMA 1909; 53: 1273–1276.
3. Alderink GJ: The sacroiliac joint: review of anatomy, mechanics, and function. J Orthop Sports Phys Ther 1991; 13: 71–83.
4. Andersen KV, Bovim G: Impotence and nerve entrapment in long distance amateur cyclists. Acta Neurol Scand 1997; 95: 233–240.
5. Bakland O: The "axial sacroiliac joint". Anat Clin 1984; 6: 29–36.
6. Basmajian JV: Articular system. In: Primary Anatomy. Baltimore: Williams & Wilkins, 1976; 75–112.
7. Basmajian JV: Skeletal system. In: Primary Anatomy. Baltimore: Williams & Wilkins, 1976; 21–74.
8. Basmajian JV: Female pelvis. In: Grant's Method of Anatomy. In: Primary Anatomy. Baltimore: Williams & Wilkins, 1980; 227–237.
9. Basmajian JV: Male pelvis. In: Grant's Method of Anatomy. In: Primary Anatomy. Baltimore: Williams & Wilkins, 1980; 207–226.
10. Basmajian JV, Fielding JW, Zickel RE: Accessory lamina. A cause of lumbar nerve root pressure. J Bone Joint Surg 1964; 46-A: 837.
11. Bayne O, Bateman JE, Cameron HU: Influence of etiology on the results of coccygectomy. Clin Orthop 1984; 190: 266–272.
12. Beal MC: The sacroiliac problem: review of anatomy, mechanics, and diagnosis. J Am Osteopath Assoc 1982; 81: 667–679.
13. Bernard TN: The role of the sacroiliac joints in low back pain: basic aspects of pathophysiology, and management. In: Vleeming A, Mooney V, Snijders CJ, et al., eds. Movement, Stability and Low Back Pain. The Essential Role of the Pelvis. New York: Churchill Livingstone, 1997; 73–88.
14. Bogduk N, Twomey LT: Clinical Anatomy of the Lumbar Spine. Edinburgh: Churchill Livingstone, 1987.
15. Bogduk N, Wilson AS, Tynan W: The human lumbar dorsal rami. J Anat 1982; 134: 383–397.
16. Bonnaire E, Bué V: Ann Gynecol Obstet 1900; 52: 296.
17. Borell U, Fernström I: The movements of the sacro-iliac joints and their importance to changes on pelvic dimensions during parturition. Acta Obstet Gynecol Scand 1957; 36: 42–57.
18. Boucher BJ: Sex differences in the fetal pelvis. Am J Phys Anthropol 1957; 15: 581–600.
19. Bowen V, Cassidy JD: Macroscopic and microscopic anatomy of the sacroiliac joint from embryonic life until the eighth decade. Spine 1981; 6: 620–628.
20. Brooke R: The sacro-iliac joint. J Anat 1924; 58: 299–305.
21. Brunner C, Kissling R, Jacob HAC: The effects of morphology and histopathologic findings on the mobility of the sacroiliac joint. Spine 1991; 16: 1111–1117.
22. Cailliet: Low Back Pain Syndrome. Philadelphia: FA Davis, 1988.
23. Calguneri M, Bird HAWA: Changes in joint laxity occurring during pregnancy. Ann Rheum Dis 1982; 41: 126–128.

24. Carpenter MB, Sutin J: Human Neuroanatomy. Baltimore: Williams & Wilkins, 1983.

25. Carter ME, Loewi G: Anatomical changes in normal sacroiliac joints during childhood and comparison with the changes in Still's disease. Ann Rheum Dis 1962; 21: 121–134.

26. Chamberlain WE: The symphysis pubis in the roentgen examination of the sacro-iliac joint. Am J Roentgenol 1930; 24: 621–625.

27. Chow DHK, Luk KDK, Leong JCY, Woo CW: Torsional stability of the lumbosacral junction. Significance of the iliolumbar ligament. Spine 1989; 14: 611–615.

28. Cihak R: Variations of lumbosacral joints and their morphogenesis. Acta Univ Carol Med (Praha) 1970; 16: 145–165.

29. Cohen AS, McNeill JM, Calkins E, et al.: The "normal" sacroiliac joint. Analysis of 88 sacroiliac roentgenograms. Am J Roentgenol 1967; 100: 559–563.

30. Colachis SC, Warden RE, Bechtol CO, Strohm BR: Movement of the sacroiliac joint in the adult male: a preliminary report. Arch Phys Med Rehabil 1963; 44: 490–498.

31. Collins P: Embryology and development. In: Williams PL, ed. Gray's Anatomy: The Anatomical Basis of Medicine and Surgery. New York: Churchill Livingstone, 1995; 91–341.

32. Cunningham D: Textbook of Anatomy. New York: Oxford University Press, 1925.

33. Cyriax J: Textbook of Orthopaedic Medicine. London: Balliere Tindall, 1982.

34. Dalstra M, Huiskes R: Load transfer across the pelvic bone. J Biomech 1995; 28: 715–724.

35. Dalstra M, Huiskes R, Odgaard A, van Erning L: Mechanical and textural properties of pelvic trabecular bone. J Biomech 1993; 26: 523–535.

36. Davies DV: Gray's Anatomy. London: Longmans, 1967.

37. Delaere O, Kok V, Nyssen-Behets C, Dhem A: Ossification of the human fetal ilium. Acta Anat 1992; 143: 330–334.

38. Desai KM, Gingell JC: Hazards of long distance cycling. Br Med J 1989; 298: 1072–1073.

39. DonTigny RL: Function and pathomechanics of the sacroiliac joint. A review. Phys Ther 1985; 65: 35–44.

40. Duncan JM: The behavior of the pelvic articulations in the mechanism of parturition. Dublin Quart J Med Sci 1854; 18: 60.

41. Duncan JM: Researches in Obstetrics. New York: W. Wood and Co., 1868.

42. Ebraheim NA, Lu J, Biyani A, et al.: The relationship of lumbosacral plexus to the sacrum and the sacroiliac joints. Am J Orthop 1997; 26: 105–110.

43. Egund N, Olsson TH, Schmid H, Selnik G: Movements in the sacroiliac joints demonstrated with roentgen stereophotogrammetry. Acta Radiol (Diagn) 1978; 19: 833–846.

44. Ehara S, El-Khoury GY, Bergman RA: The accessory sacroiliac ligament; a common anatomic variant. Am J Roentgenol 1988; 150: 857–859.

45. Federative Committee on Anatomical Terminology: Terminologia Anatomica. International Terminology. New York: Thieme Stuttgart, 1998.

46. Frigerio NA, Stowe RR, Howe JW: Movement of the sacroiliac joint. Clin Orthop 1974; 100: 370–377.

47. Frymoyer J, Akeson W, Brandt J, et al.: Part A: Clinical perspectives. In: Frymoyer J, Gordon SL, eds. New Perspectives in Low Back Pain. Park Ridge, NJ: The American Academy of Orthopedic Surgeons, 1989; 240–242.

48. Gardner E, Gray DJ, O'Rahilly R: Anatomy: A Regional Study of Human Structure. Philadelphia: WB Saunders, 1969.

49. Geckeler EO: Fractures and Dislocations. Baltimore: Williams & Wilkins, 1943.

50. Gerlach UJ, Lierse W: Functional construction of the sacroiliac ligamentous apparatus. Acta Anat (Basel) 1992; 144: 97–102.

51. Goel VK, Svensson NL: Forces on the pelvis. J Biomech 1977; 10: 195–200.

52. Goldthwaite JE: The pelvic articulations: a consideration of their anatomic, physiologic, obstetric and general surgical importance. JAMA 1907; 49.

53. Goldthwaite JE: The lumbo-sacral articulation. Boston Med Surg J 1911; 164: 365–377.

54. Goldthwaite JE, Osgood RB: A consideration of the pelvic articulations from an anatomical, pathological and clinical standpoint. Boston Med Surg J 1905; 152: 593–601.

55. Goss CM: Gray's Anatomy. Philadelphia: Lea & Febiger, 1973.

56. Gray H: Anatomy of the Human Body. Philadelphia: 1924.

57. Grieve EFM: Mechanical dysfunction of the sacro-iliac joint. Int Rehabil Med 1982; 5: 46–52.

58. Grieve GP: The sacro-iliac joint. Physiotherapy 1976; 62: 384–400.

59. Grieve GP: Applied anatomy—regional. In: Common Vertebral Joint Problems. Edinburgh: Churchill Livingstone, 1981; 1–35.

60. Grieve GP: Common patterns of clinical presentation. In: Common Vertebral Joint Problems. Edinburgh: Churchill Livingstone, 1981; 205–302.

61. Grieve GP: Pathological changes—combined regional degenerative. In: Common Vertebral Joint Problems. Edinburgh: Churchill Livingstone, 1981; 125–158.

62. Grob KR, Neuhuber WL, Kissling RO: Die innervation des Sacroiliacalgelenkes beim Menschen. Z Rheumatol 1995; 54: 117–122.

63. Guyton AC, Hall JE: Female physiology before pregnancy and the female hormones. In: Human Physiology and Mechanisms of Disease. Philadelphia: WB Saunders, 1997; 658–669.

64. Hadley LA: Accessory sacroiliac articulations. J Bone Joint Surg 1952; 34A: 149.

65. Hagen R: Pelvic girdle relaxation from an orthopaedic point of view. Acta Orthop Scand 1974; 45: 550.

66. Halata Z, Strasmann T: The ultrastructure of mechanoreceptors in the musculoskeletal system of mammals. In: Zenker W, Neuhuber WL, eds. The Primary Afferent Neuron. New York: Plenum Press, 1990; 51–65.

67. Halliday HV: Applied Anatomy of the Spine. Kirksville, MO: JF Janisch, 1920.

68. Harris NH: Lesions of the symphysis pubis in women. Br Med J 1974; 4: 209–211.

69. Harris NH, Murray RO: Lesions of the symphysis in athletes. Br Med J 1974; 4: 211–214.

70. Harrison RJ: Bones. In: Romanes GJ, ed. Gunningham's Textbook of Anatomy. New York: Oxford University Press, 1972; 75–206.

71. Heisler JC: Practical Anatomy. Philadelphia: 1923.

72. Herbineaux G: Traite sur Divers Accouchments Laborieux et sur les Polypes de la Matrice. Brussels: DeBoubers, 1782.

73. Hesch J: Evaluation and treatment of the most common patterns of sacroiliac joint dysfunction. In: Vleeming A, Mooney V, Snijders CJ, et al., eds. Movement, Stability and Low Back

Pain. The Essential Role of the Pelvis. New York: Churchill Livingstone, 1997; 535–545.

74. Hirsch C, Ingelmark B-E, Miller M: The anatomic basis for low back pain. Acta Orthop Scand 1963; 33: 1–17.

75. Holm NJ: The internal stress pattern of the os coxae. Acta Orthop Scand 1980; 51: 421–428.

76. Ikeda R: Innervation of the sacroiliac joint. Macroscopical and histological studies. Nippon Ika Daigaku Zasshi 1991; 58: 587–596.

77. Jackson HCI, Winkelmann RK, Bickel WH: Nerve endings in the human lumbar spinal column and related structures. J Bone Joint Surg 1966; 48: 1272–1281.

78. Joseph J: The joints of the pelvis and their relation to posture in labour. Midwives Chron Nurs Notes 1988; 101: 63–64.

79. Junqueira LC, Carneiro J, Kelley RO: Basic Histology. Norwalk, CT: Appleton & Lange, 1995.

80. Kane WJ: Fractures of the pelvis. In: Rockwood CA, Green DP, eds. Fractures in Adults. Philadelphia: JB Lippincott, 1984; 1093–1209.

81. Kapandji IA: The Physiology of Joints. Vol. 3. The Trunk and the Vertebral Column. Edinburgh: Churchill Livingstone, 1974.

82. Keith A: Human Embryology and Morphology. London: Edward Arnold, 1948.

83. Kissling RO, Jacob HAC: The mobility of the sacroiliac joints in healthy subjects. In: Vleeming A, Mooney V, Snijders CJ, et al., eds. Movement, Stability and Low Back Pain. The Essential Role of the Pelvis. New York: Churchill Livingstone, 1997; 177–191.

84. Klein K: Zur Mechanik des Ileosacralgelenkes. Z Geburtshilfe Perinatol 1891; 21: 74–118.

85. Kristiansson P, Svardsudd K, von Schoultz B: Serum relaxin, symphyseal pain, and back pain during pregnancy. Am J Obstet Gynecol 1996; 175: 1342–1347.

86. Krogman WM: The Human Skeleton in Forensic Medicine. Springfield, IL: Charles C Thomas, 1962.

87. Lamb DW: The neurology of spinal pain. Phys Ther 1979; 59: 971–973.

88. Laurenson RD: The primary ossification of the human ilium. Anat Rec 1964; 148: 209–211.

89. Lavignolle B, Vital JM, Senegas J, et al.: An approach to the functional anatomy of the sacroiliac joint in vivo. Anat Clin 1983; 5: 169–176.

90. Lee D: The Pelvic Girdle. Edinburgh: Churchill Livingstone, 1989.

91. Leong JC, Luk KDK, Chow DHK, Woo CW: The biomechanical functions of the iliolumbar ligament in maintaining stability of the lumbosacral junction. Spine 1987; 12: 669–674.

92. Lowman CL: Role of iliolumbar ligaments in low back strain. JAMA 1926; 88: 1002–1003.

93. Lue TF, Zeineh SJ, Schmidt RA, Tanagho EA: Neuroanatomy of penile erection: its relevance to iatrogenic impotence. J Urol 1984; 131: 273–280.

94. Luk KDK, Ho HC, Leong JCY: The iliolumbar ligament. A study of its anatomy, development and clinical significance. J Bone Joint Surg Br 1986; 68: 197–200.

95. Lynch FW: The pelvic articulations during pregnancy, labor and puerperium. An x-ray study. Surg Gynecol Obstet 1920; 30: 575–580.

96. MacDonald GR, Hunt TE: Sacroiliac joints: observations on the gross and histological changes in the various age groups. Can Med Assoc J 1952; 66: 157–163.

97. MacLennan AH: The role of the hormone relaxin in human reproduction and pelvic girdle relaxation. Scand J Rheumatol 1991; 20(suppl 88): 7–15.

98. Magee DJ: Orthopedic Physical Therapy. Philadelphia: WB Saunders, 1997.

99. Maitland GD: Vertebral Manipulation. London: Butterworth, 1977.

100. McCulloch J, Transfeldt E: Spondylolysis/spondylolisthesis. In: Macnab's Backache. Baltimore: Williams & Wilkins, 1997; 149–179.

101. McKinnis LN: Lumbosacral spine and sacroiliac joints. In: Fundamentals of Orthopedic Radiology. Philadelphia: FA Davis, 1997; 168–209.

102. Meckel JF: Handbuch der menschlichen Anatomie. Halle, In "Den Buchhandlungen des Hallischen Waisenhauses," Berlin: 1815; 2: 354–356.

103. Meisenbach RO: Sacro-iliac relaxation: with analysis of 84 cases. Surg Gynaecol Obstet 1911; 12: 411.

104. Mennell JB: The Science and Art of Joint Manipulation, Vols. 1 and 2. London: Churchill, 1952.

105. Meyer GH: Ber mechanismus der Symphysis sacro-iliaca. Arch Anat Physiol (Leipzig) 1878; 1: 1–19.

106. Midttun A, Bojsen-Moller F: The sacrotuberous ligament pain syndrome. In: Grieve GP, ed. Modern Manual Therapy of the Vertebral Column. Edinburgh: Churchill Livingstone, 1986; 815–818.

107. Milch H, Milch RA: Fractures of the pelvic girdle. In: Milch H, Milch RA, eds. Fracture Surgery. New York: Paul B. Hoeber, 1959.

108. Miller JAA, Schultz AM, Anderson GBJ: Load-displacement behavior of sacroiliac joints. J Orthop Res 1987; 5: 92–101.

109. Mitchell GAG: Lumbosacral junction. J Bone Joint Surg 1934; 16: 233–254.

110. Mixter WJ, Barr JS: Rupture of the intervertebral disc with involvement of the spinal canal. N Engl J Med 1934; 211: 210–215.

111. Mooney V: Sacroiliac joint dysfunction. In: Vleeming A, Mooney V, Snijders CJ, et al., eds. Movement, Stability and Low Back Pain. The Essential Role of the Pelvis. New York: Churchill Livingstone, 1997; 37–52.

112. Moore KL, Dalley AF: Lower limb. In: Clinically Oriented Anatomy. Philadelphia: Lippincott Williams & Wilkins, 1999; 504–663.

113. Moore KL, Dalley AF: Pelvis and perineum. In: Clinically Oriented Anatomy. Philadelphia: Lippincott Williams & Wilkins, 1999; 332–430.

114. Moore KL, Persaud TVN: The Developing Human, Clinically Oriented Embryology. Philadelphia: WB Saunders, 1998.

115. Myerding H: Spondylolisthesis: surgical treatment and results. Surg Gynecol Obstet 1932; 54: 371–377.

116. Nayal W, Schwarzer U, Klotz T, et al.: Transcutaneous penile oxygen pressure during bicycling. Br J Urol Internat 1999; 83: 623–625.

117. Norman WJ, Johnson C: Congenital absence of pedicle of a lumbar vertebra. Br J Radiol 1973; 46: 631

118. O'Rahilly R, Gardner E: The embryology of moveable joints. In: Sokoloff L, ed. The Joints and Synovial Fluid. New York: Academic Press, 1978; 49–97.

119. Ombregt L, Bisschop P, Veer HJT, Van de Velde T: A System of Orthopedic Medicine. London: Saunders, 1995.

120. Pal GP, Tamankar BP: Preliminary study of age changes in Gujarti (Indian) pubic bones. Indian J Med Res 1983; 78: 694–701.

121. Paquet N, Malouin F, Richards CL: Hip-spine movement interaction and muscle activation patterns during sagittal movement in low back pain patients. Spine 1994; 19: 596–603.

122. Paquin JD, van der Rest M, Marie PJ, et al.: Biochemical and morphologic studies of cartilage from the adult human sacroiliac joint. Arthritis Rheum 1983; 26: 887–895.

123. Pintar FA, Yoganandan N, Myers T, et al.: Biomechanical properties of human lumbar spine ligaments. J Biomech 1992; 25: 1351–1356.

124. Pitkin HC, Pheasant HC: Sacrarthrogenetic telalgia I. A study of referred pain. J Bone Joint Surg 1936; 18: 111–133.

125. Pitkin HC, Pheasant HC: Sacrarthrogenetic telalgia II. A study of sacral mobility. J Bone Joint Surg 1936; 18: 365–374.

126. Porterfield JA, DeRosa C: The sacroiliac joint. In: Gould JA, ed. Orthopedics and Sports Physical Therapy. St. Louis: CV Mosby, 1990; 553–559.

127. Pyper JB: Excision of the coccyx for coccygodynia. A study of the results in twenty-eight cases. J Bone Joint Surg 1957; 39B: 733–737.

128. Quagliarello J, Steinetz BG, Weiss G: Relaxin secretion in early pregnancy. Obstet Gynecol 1979; 53: 62–63.

129. Rauber AA, Kopsch F: Lehrbuch und Atlas der Anatomie des Menschen. Leipzig: 1929.

130. Ravin T: Visualization of pelvic biomechanical dysfunction. In: Vleeming A, Mooney V, Snijders CJ, et al., eds. Movement, Stability and Low Back Pain. The Essential Role of the Pelvis. New York: Churchill Livingstone, 1997; 369–383.

131. Resnick D, Niwayama G, Georgen TG: Degenerative disease of the sacroiliac joint. Invest Radiol 1975; 10: 608.

132. Reynolds HM: Three-dimensional kinematics in the pelvic girdle. J Am Osteopath Assoc 1980; 80: 277–280.

133. Rich EA: Observations noted in 11,000 feet of cineroentgenography film. Cong Rec 1964; 110: 5157–5165.

134. Rosse C, Gaddum-Rosse P: Hollinshead's Textbook of Anatomy. Philadelphia: Lippincott-Raven, 1997.

135. Rosse C, Gaddum-Rosse P: The pelvis. In: Hollinshead's Textbook of Anatomy. Philadelphia: Lippincott-Raven, 1997; 641–680.

136. Rosse C, Gaddum-Rosse P: The vertebral column. In: Hollinshead's Textbook of Anatomy. Philadelphia: Lippincott-Raven, 1997; 109–144.

137. Rothkotter HJ, Berner W: Failure load and displacement of the human sacroiliac joint under in vitro loading. Arch Orthop Trauma Surg 1988; 107: 283–287.

138. Sashin D: A critical analysis of the anatomy and the pathologic changes of the sacro-iliac joints. J Bone Joint Surg 1930; 12: 891–910.

139. Schafer RC: The lumbar spine and pelvis. In: Schafer RC, ed. Clinical Biomechanics, Musculoskeletal Actions and Reactions. Baltimore: Williams & Wilkins, 1987; 446–480.

140. Schauberger CW, Rooney BL, Goldsmith L: Peripheral joint laxity increases in pregnancy but does not correlate with serum relaxin levels. Am J Obstet Gynecol 1996; 174: 667–671.

141. Schmorl G, Junghanns H: The Human Spine in Health and Disease. New York: Grune & Stratton, 1971.

142. Schunke GB: The anatomy and development of the sacro-iliac joint in man. Anat Rec 1938; 72: 313–331.

143. Shafik A: Pudendal artery syndrome with erectile dysfunction: treatment by pudendal canal decompression. Arch Androl 1995; 34: 83–94.

144. Smidt GL, McQuade K, Wei S-H, Barakatt E: Sacroiliac kinematics for reciprocal straddle positions. Spine 1995; 20: 1047–1054.

145. Smidt GL, Wei S-H, McQuade K, et al.: Sacroiliac motion for extreme hip positions. Spine 1997; 22: 2073–2082.

146. Smith-Petersen NM: Clinical diagnoses of common sacro-iliac conditions. Am J Roentgenol 1924; 12: 546–550.

147. Soames RW: Skeletal system. In: Williams PL, ed. Gray's Anatomy. The Anatomical Basis of Medicine and Surgery. New York: Churchill Livingstone, 1995; 425–736.

148. Solomon S, Cappa KG: Impotence and bicycling. A seldom-reported connection. Postgrad Med 1987; 81: 99–100.

149. Solonen KA: The sacroiliac joint in the light of anatomical, roentgenological and clinical studies. Acta Orthop Scand 1957; 28(suppl): 1–127.

150. Stephenson RG, O'Connor LJ: Obstetric and Gynecologic Care in Physical Therapy. Thorofare, NJ: Slack, 2000.

151. Stewart T: Pathologic changes in aging sacroiliac joints. Clin Orthop 1984; 183: 188–196.

152. Stoddard A: Conditions of the sacro-iliac joint and their treatment. Physiotherapy 1958; 44: 97–101.

153. Strachan WF, Beckwith CG, Larson NJ: A study of the mechanics of the sacroiliac joint. J Am Osteopath Assoc 1938; 37: 576–578.

154. Sturesson B, Selvik G, Udén A: Movements of the sacroiliac joints. A roentgen stereophotogrammetric analysis. Spine 1989; 14: 162–165.

155. Suchey JM, Wiseley DV, Green RF, Norguchi TT: Analysis of dorsal pitting in the os-pubis in an extensive sample of modern American females. Am J Phys Anthropol 1979; 51: 517–540.

156. Sugar O: How the sacrum got its name. JAMA 1987; 257: 2061–2063.

157. Swezey RL: The sacroiliac joint. Nothing is sacred. Phys Med Rehabil Clin North Am 1998; 9: 515–519.

158. Taber's Cyclopedic Medical Dictionary: Philadelphia: FA Davis, 1997.

159. Terry RJ, Trotter M: The articulations. In: Schaeffer JP, ed. Morris' Human Anatomy. A Complete Systematic Treatise. New York: Blakiston, 1953; 287–398.

160. Testut JL: Traité d'Anatomie Humaine. Paris: Doin, 1889.

161. Trotter M: Accessory sacroiliac articulations. J Phys Anthropol 1937; 22: 247.

162. Vleeming A, Pool-Goudzwaard AL, Hammudoghlu D, et al.: The function of the long dorsal sacroiliac ligament: its implication for understanding low back pain. Spine 1996; 21: 556–562.

163. Vleeming A, Stoeckart R, Volkers ACW, Snijders CJ: Relation between form and function in the sacroiliac joint. Part I: Clinical anatomical aspects. Spine 1990; 15: 130–132.

164. Vleeming A, Volkers ACW, Snijders CJ, Stoeckart R: Relation between form and function in the sacroiliac joint. Part II: Biomechanical aspects. Spine 1990; 15: 133–136.

165. Von Luschka H: Die Kreuzdarmbeinfuge und die Schambienfuge des Menschen. Virchows Arch Pathol Anat 1854; 7: 299–316.

166. Vukicevic S, Marusic A, Stavljenic A, et al.: Holographic analysis of the human pelvis. Spine 1991; 16: 209–214.

167. Walcher G: Die Conjugata eines engen Beckens ist keine konstante Grösse, sondern lässt sich durch die Körperhaltung der Trägerin verändern. Cbl Gynäk 1889; 13: 892.

168. Walker JM: Age-related differences in the human sacroiliac joint: a histological study; implications for therapy. J Orthop Sports Phys Ther 1986; 7: 325–334.

169. Walker JM: The sacroiliac joint: a critical review. Phys Ther 1992; 72: 903–916.

170. Walmsley R: Joints. In: Romanes GJ, ed. Cunningham's Textbook of Anatomy. London: Oxford University Press, 1972; 207–257.

171. Watson-Jones R: Fractures and Joint Injuries. Baltimore: Williams & Wilkins, 1957.

172. Weisl H: The ligaments of the sacro-iliac joint examined with particular reference to their function. Acta Anat 1954; 20: 201–213.

173. Weisl H: The movements of the sacro-iliac joint. Acta Anat 1955; 23: 80–91.

174. Weiss G: The secretion and role of relaxin in pregnant women. In: Bigazzi M, Greenwood FC, Gasparri F, eds. Biology of Relaxin and its Role in the Human. Amsterdam: Excerpta Medica, 1983, 304–310.

175. Wells PE: Movements of the pelvic joints. In: Grieve GP, ed. Modern Manual Therapy of the Vertebral Column. Edinburgh: Churchill Livingstone, 1986; 176–181.

176. Wilder DJ, Pope MH, Frymoyer JW: The functional topography of the sacroiliac joint. Spine 1980; 5: 575–579.

177. Willard FH: The muscular, ligamentous and neural structure of the low back and its relation to back pain. In: Vleeming A, Mooney V, Snijders CJ, et al., eds. Movement, Stability and Low Back Pain. The Essential Role of the Pelvis. New York: Churchill Livingstone, 1997; 1–35.

178. Wilson JR, Carrington ER: Obstetrics and Gynecology. St. Louis: CV Mosby, 1983.

179. Woerman AL: Evaluation and treatment of dysfunction in the lumbar-pelvic-hip complex. In: Donatelli R, Wooden MJ, eds. Orthopaedic Physical Therapy. New York: Churchill Livingstone, 1989.

180. Yamamoto I, Panjabi MM, Oxland TR, Crisco JJ: The role of the iliolumbar ligament in the lumbosacral junction. Spine 1990; 15: 1138–1141.

181. Young J: Relaxation of pelvic joints in pregnancy: pelvic arthropathy of pregnancy. J Obstet Gynaecol Br Emp 1940; 47: 493–525.

Mechanics and Pathomechanics of Muscle Activity in the Pelvis

EMILY L. CHRISTIAN, P.T., PH.D.
JULIE E. DONACHY, P.T., PH.D.

CHAPTER CONTENTS

The caudal end of the trunk in an upright animal is, of necessity, closed by several layers of pelvic and perineal fascia and striated muscle. Although the fascial contributions to the floor of the pelvic cavity are equal in importance to those made by the muscles from a clinical perspective, this chapter focuses on the muscles' role. Three layers of muscle are positioned at the caudal end of the human funnel-shaped pelvic basin; from deep to superficial, they are the pelvic diaphragm, deep perineal muscles, and superficial perineal muscles. Their various functions include closing the pelvic outlet, permitting transit of the pelvic effluents (urethra, anal canal, and vagina) and controlling their apertures, supporting the pelvic organs, regulating intraabdominal pressure, and contributing to bowel, bladder, and sexual function. Two other muscles contribute to the walls of the pelvic cavity, the piriformis and obturator internus. Any contributions they make to the pelvic cavity, however, are purely ancillary.

Although the muscles of the pelvic floor and perineum are primarily striated and under the control of the somatic nervous system, they differ from other axial or appendicular striated muscles in several ways:

- They frequently contain or blend with structures containing smooth muscle, and subsequently, the combined fiber types receive a visceral (autonomic nervous system, ANS) innervation in addition to a somatic (somatic nervous system, SNS) innervation.
- They are concerned with visceral functions (micturition, defecation, sexual function, parturition, and support of pelvic organs).
- They are innervated by lower motor neurons (LMNs) that are controlled by a special contingent of brainstem and hypothalamic fibers, allowing them to function somewhat independently of conscious cortical control.
- Their contraction does not result in movement at a joint.

The special nature of these multifunctional muscles and the problems associated with their dysfunction should become obvious to the reader following their further description. The specific objectives of this chapter are

- To discuss clinically relevant aspects of the development and anatomy of the pelvic floor
- To describe details of the structure, innervation, and function of the muscles of the pelvic diaphragm
- To describe details of the structure, innervation, and function of the muscles of the perineum
- To discuss neurological aspects of pelvic floor and perineal function
- To describe pertinent aspects of the structure and innervation of pelvic and perineal visceral structures, as well as ways in which their functions are coordinated with those of striated muscle fibers of the pelvic floor and perineum
- To discuss the various dysfunctions of the muscles of the pelvis and perineum relative to aging, gender, nervous degeneration, muscle atrophy, and vaginal delivery

DEVELOPMENTAL ANATOMY OF THE PELVIC FLOOR

Two distinctly human characteristics necessitated changes in the pelvis of *Homo sapiens*. One is that humans give birth to fetuses with uniquely large heads that require wider bony channels of passage to the exterior. The other is assumption of the upright posture. Both characteristics are reflected in changes in the bony pelvis and fibromuscular pelvic floor at the **pelvic outlet,** that is, the tissues interposed between the pelvic cavity and the perineum that form one of several transverse diaphragms in the trunk. Traditionally, anatomists have defined the **pelvic floor** as the fascial and muscular layers of the **pelvic diaphragm,** consisting of the levator ani, coccygeus, and their associated fasciae (see below). Some clinicians include the **perineal musculature** and fasciae (particularly the urogenital diaphragm) in the pelvic floor because they are intimately related, anatomically, neurologically, functionally, and clinically. For the sake of conceptualization, Moore [72] suggests that the pelvic diaphragm be considered the main floor and the urogenital diaphragm the subflooring, thereby suggesting morphological and functional similarity while maintaining autonomy. In the following discussions, pelvic and perineal musculature are considered separate entities.

Little is known about the development of pelvic floor muscles in humans. Although they are thought to develop from somites in a manner similar to those of the anterolateral trunk [19], they bear little resemblance to trunk muscles. The argument is offered that during human development, after all but 3 or 4 of the original 8 to 10 coccygeal segments degenerate [63,91,105], the remaining segments are moved into a position to close the pelvic outlet. This notion is not accepted by Wilson [120], however, who believes that the muscles of the pelvic floor develop independently, with specific attachments and functions.

Changes in the pelvic floor are necessitated by the upright posture of humans. Specializations in the soft tissues of the human pelvic floor are essential for both supporting the weight of abdominopelvic viscera and regulating intraabdominal pressure. Some argue, in fact, that pelvic floor changes are essential for assumption of the upright posture [26,28]. Alterations in the specific fascial and muscular elements were developed to resist increases in intraabdominal pressure that are necessary for a variety of activities: those that involve contraction of the diaphragm during expiration (e.g., speaking, singing, coughing, sneezing, laughing, whistling, and hiccuping); those that involve contraction of the diaphragm and closure of the glottis (**Valsalva's maneuver),** (e.g., straining during lifting, vomiting, urinating, defecating, and delivering a fetus per vaginam); and those that involve contraction of trunk muscles in different body positions and during changes in body position (e.g., standing, walking, leaning over, bending over, and moving from supine to standing). The most striking change in the upright human pelvic floor is loss of muscle and acquisition of tendon and fascia to compensate for that loss in an attempt to withstand constant stress without undue energy expenditure [28]. The postural change and constant stress also necessitate specialization in the metabolic and contractile properties of human pelvic floor muscles. In humans, they consist of type I, fatigue-resistant fibers predominately [24,60,101,111].

MUSCLES OF THE PELVIS AND PERINEUM

From an anatomical perspective, striated muscle fibers located at the caudal end of the trunk are separated traditionally into those that form the posterolateral walls of the pelvic cavity and move the femur, those of the pelvic diaphragm, and those of the perineum. From a functional viewpoint, however, muscles of the pelvic diaphragm and perineum can be divided in two different groups: (*a*) fibers that form sphincters and tether the sphincters (urethral, vaginal, and anal) to the pelvic effluents and (*b*) fibers that flank and attach the pelvic effluents (along with their sphincters) to the perimeter of the bony pelvis. The following descriptions include elements of both perspectives.

Pelvic Muscles Associated with Somatic Function

Two somatic muscles contribute to the formation of the posterior and lateral walls of the pelvic cavity, the piriformis and obturator internus, respectively. Both are related functionally to the lower limb and are primarily external rotators at the hip. They are important muscles of the buttock that exit the pelvic cavity through the greater and lesser sciatic foramina to insert on the greater trochanter of the femur (*Fig. 36.1*). The piriformis is innervated by twigs arising from the sacral plexus inside the pelvic cavity, while the nerve to the obturator internus (and superior gemellus) leaves the pelvic cavity through the greater sciatic foramen and reenters it through the lesser sciatic foramen. Both of these muscles are discussed in greater detail in Chapter 39.

Pelvic Muscles Associated with Visceral Function

The striated musculature of the two sides of the pelvis, along with their associated fasciae, form the **pelvic diaphragm**; it has two parts, the levator ani and coccygeus (*Table 36.1*). In a frontal section through the pelvis, the pelvic diaphragm has the appearance of an inverted tent as it is slung between the two innominate bones. The pelvic diaphragm marks the caudal limit of the pelvic cavity. The pelvic outlet is, therefore, below and outside the pelvic cavity, inasmuch as the pelvic diaphragm spans the interval between the walls of the bony pelvis and not the perimeter of the inferior pelvic aperture [89].

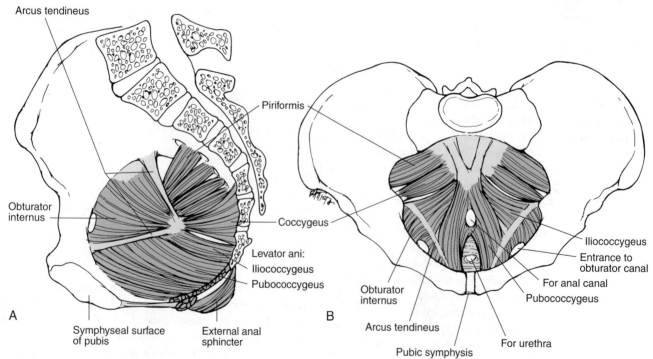

Figure 36.1: Muscles of the pelvic floor of the male. **A.** Medial view. **B.** Superior view.

TABLE 36.1: Muscles of the Pelvis

Muscle	Origin	Insertion	Innervation	Action
Lower limb muscles in wall of pelvic cavity				
Piriformis	Sacral bone lateral to and between pelvic sacral foramina	Tip of greater trochanter	Twigs of ventral primary rami of S1-2	External rotation and abduction of the femur
Obturator internus	Obturator membrane, margins of obturator foramen	Above trochanteric fossa	Nerve to the obturator internus from ventral primary rami of L5 and S1-2	External rotation of the femur
Pelvic floor muscles (pelvic diaphragm)				
Levator ani				
Pubococcygeus	Posterior surface of the body of the pubis and the anterior part of the arcus tendineus	Urethral walls, perineal body, anococcygeal ligament and coccyx	Above by twigs of ventral primary rami of S3-4, below by the pudendal nerve from ventral primary rami of S2-4	Elevates pelvic floor; resists increased intraabdominal pressure; supports contents of pelvic cavity; compresses urethra to control micturition
Levator prostatae	In the male, these are anterior fibers of the pubococcygeus	Fibers swing behind the prostate gland and end in the perineal body		Supports the prostate
Pubovaginalis	In the female, these are anterior fibers of the pubococcygeus	Fibers swing behind the vagina and end in the walls of the vagina and the perineal body; some fibers contribute to the sphincter vaginae		Contributes to sphincteric action around the vagina
Puborectalis	Posterior surface of the body of the pubis	Fibers of both sides meet in the midline at the anorectal junction	Below by the pudendal nerve from ventral primary rami of S2-4	Responsible for the perineal flexure; sphincteric action functions to control anal continence
Illiococcygeus	Posterior part of the arcus tendineus and the ischial spine	Anococcygeal ligament and coccyx	Above by twigs of ventral primary rami of S3-4	Elevates pelvic floor; resists increased intraabdominal pressure; supports contents of pelvic cavity
Coccygeus	Ischial spine	Lateral borders of S4-5 and Co1-2	Above by ventral primary rami of S4-5	Elevates pelvic floor; resists increased intraabdominal pressure; supports contents of pelvic cavity

The **levator ani** is a broad fibromuscular sheet of variable thickness that forms the anterior, larger part of the pelvic diaphragm. All of the pelvic effluents traverse this part of the diaphragm: in the male, the urethra and anus, and in the female, the urethra, vagina, and anus. Each of the parts of the levator ani has the following anatomical features in common: partial or complete origin from the pubic body, arcus tendineus, or ischial spine, and midline union with its mate from the opposite side. The levator ani is divided into three parts: the **pubococcygeus, puborectalis, and iliococcygeus.** The thinnest, weakest part of the levator ani [15], the iliococcygeus, is related closely to the obturator internus through part of its origin, represented by a thickened fascial band of the obturator fascia, the **arcus tendineus** (tendinous arc of the levator ani) [89]. This thin, posterior part of the levator is reinforced by activation of the obturator internus during

straining activities when the hips are rotated externally (e.g., during defecation and parturition [childbirth]) [15].

Several subdivisions of the levator ani make significant contributions to pelvic floor function. Each subdivision contributes muscle fibers to the sphincters and blends with smooth muscle fibers of each of the midline pelvic effluents [73,89,92]. Anterior fibers of the pubococcygeus take several directions: into the walls of the urethra to contribute to the **sphincter urethrae (pubourethralis);** behind the prostate in the male **(levator prostatae);** and behind the vagina in the female **(pubovaginalis)** to contribute to the **sphincter vaginae** of the perineum. Posterior fibers of the pubococcygeus blend with fibers of the rectum and form the **puboanalis** [92]. The puborectalis is a thick bundle of fibers located on the inferior surface of the pubococcygeus. As it swings behind the alimentary passageway at the anorectal junction, it is

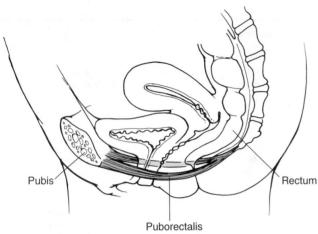

Figure 36.2: Puborectalis is a part of the levator ani that forms a sling around the lower bowel and contributes to the flexure formed at the anorectal junction.

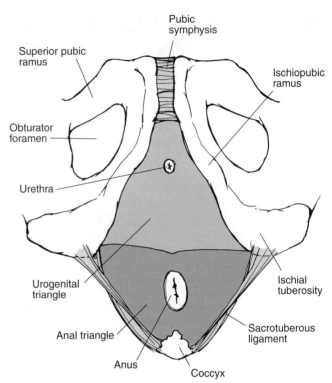

Figure 36.3: Inferior view of the male perineum. The diamond-shaped perineum is bordered on each side by the bodies of the pubes, ischiopubic rami, ischial tuberosities, sacrotuberous ligaments, and coccyx. A line drawn transversely between the ischial tuberosities divides the perineum into an anterior urogenital triangle and a posterior anal triangle.

responsible for the **perineal (anorectal) flexure** (*Fig. 36.2*), an important contributor to anorectal continence. It has been suggested that the fibers of the pubococcygeus that attach to the midline pelvic viscera (e.g., pubourethralis, levator prostatae, pubovaginalis, puboanalis, and puborectalis) could be named more accurately the **pubovisceralis** [65]. This grouping might be helpful in setting apart functionally the muscle fibers of the pelvic diaphragm that are considered to be the most important in maintaining continence and supporting the pelvic organs [66].

The posterior part of the pelvic diaphragm is the **coccygeus,** which could be called the ischiococcygeus if one were consistent with the naming of the other parts of this muscular layer (i.e., pubococcygeus, iliococcygeus, and ischiococcygeus) [89]. The coccygeus differs from the levator ani in several aspects: it is considerably thinner; it has bony connections only; it has no connection with the anococcygeal ligament; and it is innervated *exclusively* by fibers from the ventral primary rami of S1-2, instead of the pudendal nerve, which innervates the levator ani [66,89].

Perineal Muscles

The osteoligamentous frame of the perineum consists of the structures that form the **pelvic outlet,** that is, the pubic arch, ischial rami and tuberosities, sacrotuberous ligaments, and coccyx (*Figs. 35.19–35.21*). The perineum is the diamond-shaped area caudal to the pelvic diaphragm that is subdivided into two triangles (*Fig. 36.3*). The area located anterior to a line drawn between the ischial tuberosities is the **urogenital triangle,** while the **anal triangle** is situated posterior to the same line. Superficial-to-deep dissections of the layers of the perineum of the female and male are shown in *Figure 36.4*.

Striated musculature of the urogenital area is arranged in two layers, deep and superficial (*Table 36.2*). Muscles in the superficial perineal space include the **superficial transverse perineus, bulbospongiosus, and ischiocavernosus;**

those of the deep perineal space include the **deep transverse perineus** and **sphincter urethrae** (*Fig. 36.5*). Subdivisions of the sphincter urethrae include **circular fibers, compressor urethrae,** and the **urethrovaginal sphincter** [73,92] (*Fig. 36.6*). The deep transverse perineus muscle, along with its associated fasciae, is known as the **urogenital diaphragm** (*Figs. 36.7, 36.8*). The perineal musculature of the urogenital area makes significant contributions to a variety of visceral functions: the sphincter urethrae aids in the voluntary control of micturition; the male bulbospongiosus aids in expelling semen or urine from the urethra and contributes to penile erection; the female bulbospongiosus functions as the **sphincter vaginae** (with fibers of the pubovaginalis and urethrovaginal sphincter); and the ischiocavernosus contributes to penile/clitoral erection.

One muscle is located in the anal triangle, the **sphincter ani externus** (*Fig. 36.9*). Surrounding the entire anal canal, it is subdivided traditionally into subcutaneous, superficial, and deep parts (*Fig. 36.10*). Its deep fibers blend with those of the puborectalis and puboanalis, each making a significant contribution to anorectal continence.

Somatic (External) Sphincters

Several bundles of pelvic and/or perineal striated muscle fibers contribute to the sphincters that surround and guard the pelvic effluents. The **external urethral sphincter**

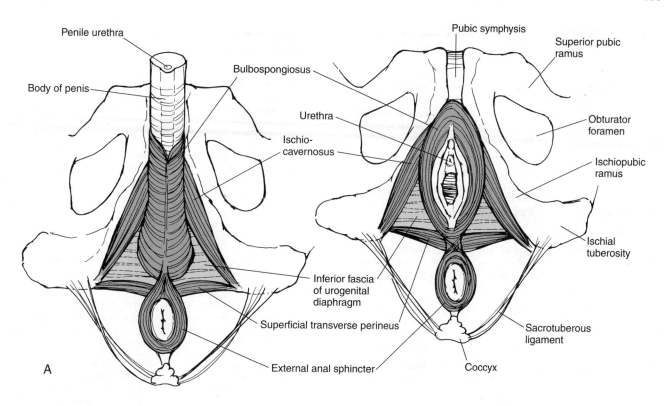

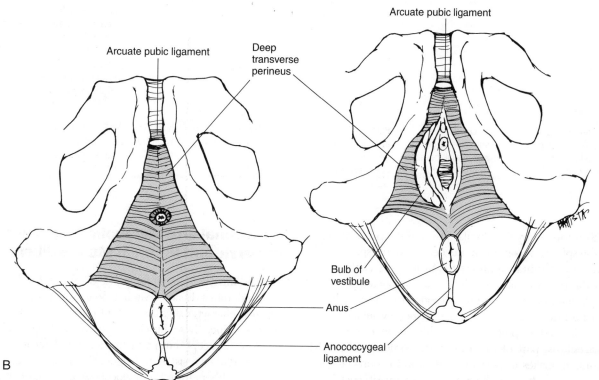

Figure 36.4: The perineum, shown as successively deeper layers of dissection. The male perineum is indicated on the left and the female on the right. **A.** Superficial. **B.** Deep.

TABLE 36.2: Muscles of the Perineum

Muscle	Origin	Insertion	Innervation	Action
Deep perineal muscles				
Deep transverse perineus (with superior and inferior fascial layers, forms the urogenital diaphragm)	Ischiopubic ramus	Two muscles meet in midline, fibers pass to the perineal body; in the female, surrounds vagina	Perineal branch of the pudendal nerve from ventral primary rami of S2-4	Supports and fixes perineal body to aid in supporting pelvic viscera; resists increased intraabdominal pressure
Sphincter urethrae Circular part Compressor urethrae Sphincter urethrovaginalis	Encircles urethra Passes anterior to urethra Female: encircles urethra and vagina	Ischial ramus	Perineal branch of the pudendal nerve from ventral primary rami of S2-4	Compresses urethra to control micturition; in female, the urethrovaginal sphincter compresses the vagina
Superficial perineal muscles				
Superficial transverse perineus	Ischial tuberosity	Two muscles meet in the midline, fibers pass to the perineal body	Perineal branch of the pudendal nerve from ventral primary rami of S2-4	Supports and fixes perineal body to aid in supporting pelvic viscera; resists increased intraabdominal pressure
Ischiocavernosus	Ischiopubic ramus	Male: fascia of the corpora cavernosa Female: fascia of the crura of the clitoris	Perineal branch of the pudendal nerve from ventral primary rami of S2-4	Contributes to erection by forcing blood into body of the penis/clitoris and preventing venous return
Bulbospongiosus	Male: penile raphe, perineal body Female: perineal body	Male: fascia of the corpus spongiosum and corpora cavernosa Female: fascia of the bulb of the vestibule	Perineal branch of the pudendal nerve from ventral primary rami of S2-4	Male: compresses penile bulb to expel urine at the end of micturition and semen during ejaculation; contributes to erection by forcing blood into penile body and preventing venous return Female: contributes to clitoral erection and functions as the sphincter vaginae (with fibers of the pubovaginalis)
Anal muscle				
Sphincter ani externus Subcutaneous part Superficial part Deep part	Circular fibers surround entire anal canal; parallel fibers from the perineal body	Parallel fibers to the anococcygeal ligament; deepest fibers continuous with the puborectalis	Inferior rectal branch of the pudendal nerve from ventral primary rami of S2-4	With the sphincter ani internus and puborectalis, compresses anus to maintain anal continence

(EUS) is formed by the circular fibers of the pubococcygeus and the sphincter urethrae of the deep perineal space. In the female, the **vaginal sphincter** (VS) receives contributions from the pubovaginalis, urethrovaginal sphincter portion of the sphincter urethrae, and bulbospongiosus. And finally, the **external anal sphincter** (EAS) is formed by subcutaneous, superficial, and deep fibers of the sphincter ani externus. The **puborectalis,** part of the levator ani portion of the pelvic diaphragm, makes a special contribution to anorectal continence by maintaining the perineal flexure; it contributes sphincteric function to the EAS by maintaining approximately an 80° posterior flexure at the anorectal junction at all times except during defecation [5,26,73,118]. These muscle fibers constitute somatic sphincters, innervated by somatic efferent and somatic afferent nerve fibers that travel in twigs from the ventral primary rami of S3-4 (from above) or the pudendal nerve containing fibers from the ventral primary rami of S2-4 (from below) to reach their destinations.

Functional and Metabolic Properties of Pelvic and Perineal Muscle Fibers

Striated muscle fibers of the pelvic diaphragm and perineum are predominately slow-twitch, type I fibers with electrophysiological characteristics that differ from those of other striated muscles. Since these muscles are active electrophysiologically at all times except during micturition and defecation [20,80], they need to be resistant to fatigue. Histochemical assessment of muscle fibers from the pubococcygeus, iliococcygeus, and coccygeus from female cadaveric specimens reveal two thirds of them to be type I, slow-twitch, tonic fibers [24]. Density of type II, fast-twitch, phasic fibers is greater in the regions immediately surrounding the urethral and anal orifices (i.e., in the sphincters) [20,33,35]. Constant tonic activity of type I fibers provides support for pelvic organs and keeps the urogenital orifices closed; this aids in unloading connective tissue elements in the pelvic cavity during everyday, routine postural

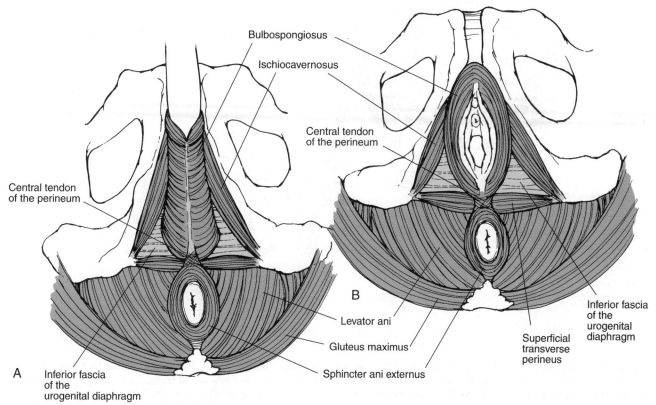

Figure 36.5: Muscles of the perineum. **A.** Male. **B.** Female. Muscles of the anterior half of the perineum (urogenital triangle) are concerned with urogenital function; those of the posterior half contribute to anorectal continence. Note that the bulbospongiosus, superficial and deep transverse perineal muscles, and sphincter ani externus attach to the central tendon of the perineum.

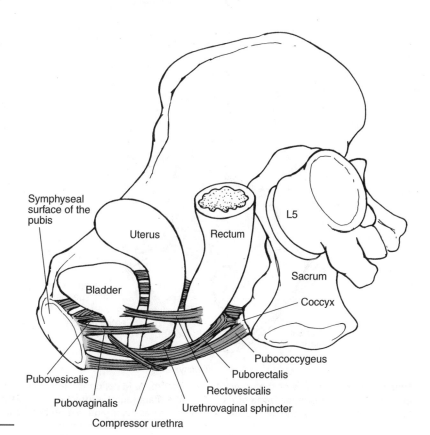

Figure 36.6: Medial view of the muscles that compress the urethra and vagina, including the urethrovaginal sphincter, compressor urethrae, and sphincter urethrae.

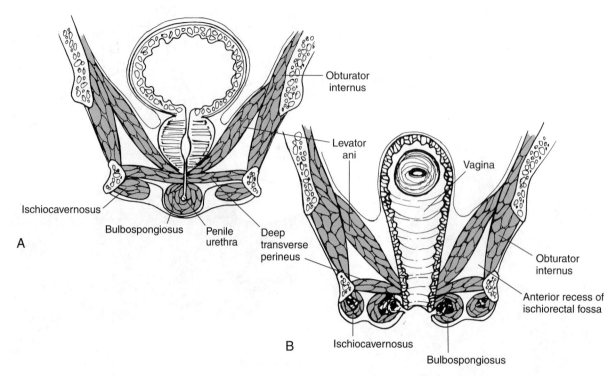

Figure 36.7: Coronal section through the anterior part of the perineum. **A.** Male. **B.** Female. Note the three structures that compose the urogenital diaphragm, the deep transverse perineus muscle along with its inferior and superior fascial layers. Two other perineal muscles are shown, the paired ischiocavernosus and bulbospongiosus. The anterior portion of the pelvic diaphragm (levator ani) is also shown.

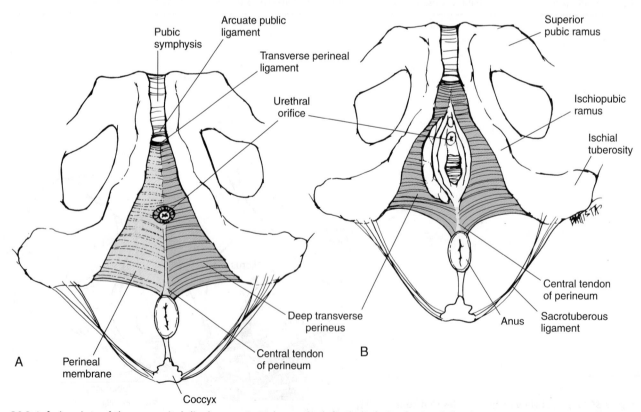

Figure 36.8: Inferior view of the urogenital diaphragm. **A.** Male; on the left, the inferior fascia of the deep transversus perineus (perineal membrane or inferior fascia of the urogenital diaphragm) is intact but has been removed on the right to expose the musculature. **B.** Female; the fascia of the deep transverse perineus has been removed on both sides to expose the muscle fibers.

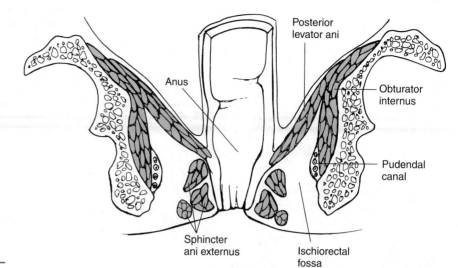

Figure 36.9: Coronal section through the posterior half of the perineum. Note the sphincter ani externus medial to each ischiorectal fossa and the pudendal canal and its contents (pudendal nerve and internal pudendal vessels) on the inferolateral walls of the fossae.

alterations [80,107]. With sudden increases in intraabdominal pressure, type II fibers immediately surrounding the urethral and anal orifices are recruited to maintain their closure. The periurethral and perianal muscle fibers are further characterized as having an extremely slow discharge rate (3–4 cps) during waking and sleeping cycles [47], and studies of their passive length–tension relationships reveal that they are stiffer or develop greater tensions in response to passive tensile force than other striated muscle fibers [61]. This stiffness is attributed to changes in the passive properties of the connective tissue elements surrounding the muscle fibers.

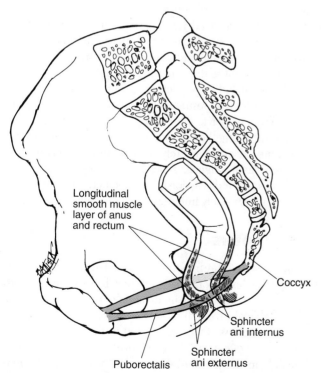

Figure 36.10: Midsagittal section through the lower rectum and anal canal shows the sphincter ani externus and internus. Note the position of the puborectalis and its contribution to the formation of the anorectal angle.

Clinical Relevance

PELVIC AND PERINEAL MUSCLE FIBER TYPES: *A clinician's ability to effect changes in the muscles of the pelvis and perineum depends, in part, upon understanding the metabolic and contractile properties of these very different voluntary muscles and how the principles of exercise physiology affect their training. This knowledge affects directly the choices we make when prescribing exercises, specific activities, and other types of therapeutic interventions for treatment of patients with some types of pelvic floor dysfunction. For maximal effectiveness, clinicians must be aware of several characteristics of these multifunctional muscles: they are composed of voluntary, striated muscle fibers that can be affected by exercise; most of them are type I fibers that discharge tonically and should respond best to endurance exercises (i.e., multiple submaximal contractions); and the predominately type II, phasic fibers that control the sphincters should respond best to high-intensity exercises of short duration [9,10,29,37,46,57,88,90,93,97,98,104].*

Central Tendon of the Perineum

The **central tendon of the perineum (perineal body)** is an important obstetric and gynecological structure of the perineum (*Fig. 36.11*). Located at the central point of the diamond-shaped perineum, it is located at the juncture between the urogenital and anal triangles. In the female, this dense node of tissue is located between the vaginal and anal orifices; in the male, it is in the space between the root of the penis and the anal orifice. The perineal body consists of a triangular fibromuscular condensation that is larger and more

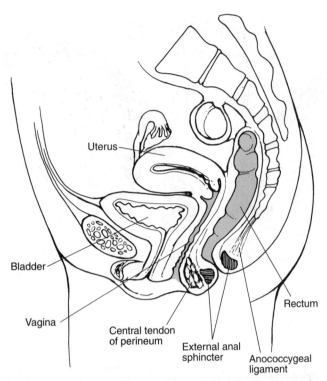

Figure 36.11: Midsagittal section through the female central tendon of the perineum. The central tendon of the perineum (perineal body) is the juncture between the urogenital and anal triangles. In the female it is located between the vaginal and anal orifices.

important clinically in the female than the male [89]. Firmly anchored to it are somatic and visceral fibers from a number of muscles of both the pelvis and perineum, including the pubococcygeus, pubovaginalis, levator prostatae, sphincter urethrae, superficial and deep transverse perinei, sphincter ani externus, bulbospongiosus, sphincter ani internus, and longitudinal (smooth) muscle of the rectum. These muscular connections anchor the perineal body to the pubes, ischia, and coccyx, thereby maintaining the midline position of the urethra, vagina, and anus in the pelvic outlet [92]. Contraction of muscles of the pelvic diaphragm and perineum, through their connection to the perineal body, result in elevation of the pelvic floor [89,92], lending support to pelvic viscera and resisting increases in intraabdominal pressure. Their relaxation allows the pelvic floor to descend, an important component of micturition and defecation.

Clinical Relevance

CENTRAL TENDON OF THE PERINEUM: *Being the lowest and final level of support of pelvic viscera, the perineal body is particularly important in women. Its tearing and separation from the muscles that attach to it during childbirth can lead to disorders collectively referred to as **pelvic floor dysfunction**. Some obstetricians perform an **episiotomy***

(a surgical incision in the perineum) in an attempt to control prophylactically the location and amount of tearing that occurs during parturition [119]. A median episiotomy is an incision through the perineal body, while a mediolateral episiotomy starts in the midline but curves posterolaterally [73]. Routine use of episiotomies is highly debated [77,119]. Some recent evidence indicates that they may actually cause more, rather than less, trauma to the muscles of the pelvic diaphragm and perineum [4,38,64].

NERVOUS CONTROL OF MUSCLES OF THE PELVIS AND PERINEUM

A lengthy discussion of the nervous control of the striated musculature ordinarily is not included in a kinesiology text. However, the muscles of the pelvic diaphragm and perineum are not ordinary. This discussion, therefore, departs from convention for the following reasons:

- To understand how these muscles are structurally and functionally different, it is necessary to discuss their neurological differences.
- Understanding the many functions of these muscles necessitates some information regarding the visceral structures with which they work in concert.
- To describe the ways in which these muscles work in concert with visceral structures requires information regarding their neurological control.
- To establish the need for different clinical interventions between males and females with pelvic dysfunction, it is necessary to substantiate the sexual dimorphism of these muscles, as well as the neurons that control them.
- Clinicians, including physicians, nurses, and therapists, are witnessing a great resurgence of interest in function and dysfunction of pelvic floor and perineal structures. Information regarding the neuromuscular structures in this area is minimized or completely omitted from standard gross anatomy, neuroscience, functional anatomy, and clinical textbooks. Their discussion is included here to ensure exposure to an extremely important area of clinical practice.

Spinal Centers

A century ago, Onufrowicz (who called himself Onuf) described a cluster of small anterior horn cells that are responsible for the somatic innervation of pelvic and perineal somatic (skeletal, striated) musculature [82]. The cell bodies of **Onuf's nucleus** (ON) are located in the ventral horn of spinal cord segments S2-4. Axons of these cells travel predominately in the **pudendal nerve** to reach their destinations (*Figs. 36.12, 36.13*); somatic afferent fibers from receptors in these muscles, as well as perineal skin, also travel in the pudendal nerve and terminate in the **nucleus proprius** (NP) of spinal cord segments S2-4, predominately.

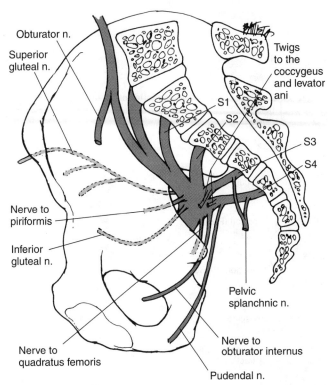

Figure 36.12: Contribution of nerve fibers to the innervation of the pelvic floor from above. Note twigs from the ventral primary rami of S3-4 entering the pelvic diaphragm, as well as the pudendal nerve passing behind and below the coccygeus.

By most accounts, in a wide variety of mammals, neuroanatomical and biochemical differences exist between ONs of males and females [56]. This **sexual dimorphism** is characteristic not only of neurons of ON, but also of the muscles they innervate [18]. Hence, spinal neurons of ON are more numerous, and the musculature of the pelvis and perineum are developed to a greater extent in males than in females [31]. Evidence of sexual dimorphism in the LMNs that innervate the pelvic and perineal musculature, as well as in the muscles themselves, appears early in development and is sex hormone dependent [18]. Furthermore, survival of greater numbers of motor neurons in ON in the presence of androgens may favor the survival of striated muscle fibers in pelvic and perineal musculature of the male; in females, however, greatly reduced androgen secretion may result in attrition of motor neurons by programmed cell death (apoptosis), resulting in fewer pelvic and perineal muscle fibers [18]. Males generally are engaged in activities that require lifting heavier loads and therefore need to be able to resist greater increases in intraabdominal pressures, while females, in their parturient (child-bearing) capacity, acquire increased fascial and ligamentous pelvic floor elements that are necessary to resist the static loads encountered during a lengthy gestational period. In addition, the species-survival roles played by the bulbospongiosus and ischiocavernosus muscles in erection and ejaculation might further explain the male need for more muscle fibers in these perineal muscles, along with a larger motor pool to support their function.

Preganglionic parasympathetic neuronal cell bodies are located in the **sacral autonomic nucleus** (SAN) of spinal cord segments S2-4, while second-order cell bodies for visceral afferent information are located in the **intermediomedial (IMM) nucleus** of the same segments [49]. This arrangement conveniently places the somatic efferent (ON), somatic afferent (NP), parasympathetic visceral efferent (SAN), and visceral afferent (IMM) cell columns for all of the striated and the parasympathetically innervated smooth muscle fibers in the pelvic floor and perineum in the same segments of the spinal cord. Preganglionic neurons responsible for the sympathetically innervated smooth muscle fibers of this region are located in the **intermediolateral (IML) nucleus** of spinal cord segments T11–L2, while second-order cell bodies for visceral afferent information traveling with the sympathetic fibers are located in the IMM nucleus of the same segments (T11–L2) [73].

Supraspinal Centers

Several higher **central nervous system** (CNS) centers contribute to the control of **somatic neurons** (LMNs) and **visceral neurons** (preganglionic autonomic) involved in pelvic and perineal muscular function. Motor neurons located in Brodmann's area 4 of the frontal lobe of the **cerebral cortex** constitute a direct corticospinal projection to ON, the motor pool for the pudendal nerve [71,75]. Other subcortical centers also make significant contributions to the suprasegmental control of ON, most notably the **hypothalamus** and **brainstem reticular formation. Micturition** appears to be the best-defined visceral function of the pelvis and is used as the example in this discussion; presumably, different or similar centers in the same regions of the cerebral cortex, diencephalon, and brainstem are involved in the control of defecation, parturition, and sexual function [26].

The central organization and coordination of micturition depends on two reticular formation centers located in the dorsolateral pontine tegmentum [8,40,41]. A medial region (M-region or Barrington's area) functions as the **pontine micturition center** (PMC), and a lateral region (L-region) functions as the **pontine urinary storage center** (PUSC). In addition to these pontine centers, there are numerous projections from the hypothalamus to the PMC and PUSC and to spinal neurons in the SAN and ON [54].

Degenerative Diseases

Since the neurons of ON innervate striated muscles that are under voluntary control, they are classified as somatic neurons; however, they share features common to visceral efferent neurons. Like the neurons of the phrenic nucleus that innervate striated fibers of the respiratory diaphragm, their constant function is controlled by brainstem centers even in the absence of wakefulness and consciousness [85]. Unlike the LMNs that innervate the vast majority of striated muscles of the body, they receive direct hypothalamic afferents, and their function as well as the muscles they innervate must be

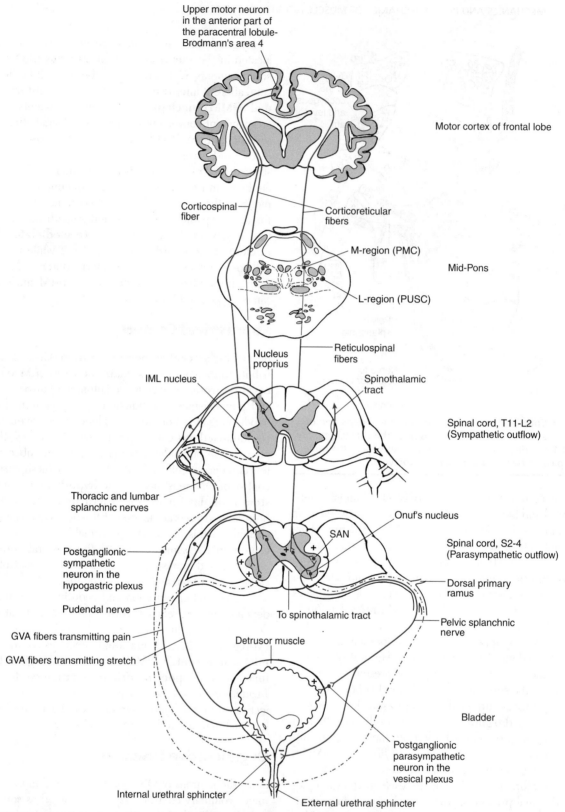

Upper motor neuron
in the anterior part of
the paracentral lobule-
Brodmann's area 4

Motor cortex of frontal lobe

Corticospinal
fiber

Corticoreticular
fibers

M-region (PMC)

Mid-Pons

L-region (PUSC)

Reticulospinal
fibers

Nucleus
proprius

IML nucleus

Spinothalamic
tract

Spinal cord, T11-L2
(Sympathetic outflow)

Thoracic and lumbar
splanchnic nerves

Onuf's nucleus

SAN

Spinal cord, S2-4
(Parasympathetic outflow)

Postganglionic
sympathetic
neuron in the
hypogastric plexus

Dorsal primary
ramus

Pudendal nerve

Pelvic splanchnic
nerve

GVA fibers transmitting pain

To spinothalamic tract

GVA fibers transmitting stretch

Detrusor muscle

Bladder

Postganglionic
parasympathetic
neuron in the
vesical plexus

Internal urethral sphincter

External urethral sphincter

Figure 36.13: Diagram of the descending pathways and peripheral nerve fibers that control micturition and continence. Cortical upper motor neurons as well as those of the L-region excite urethral sphincter motoneurons in ON. The M-region excites GABAergic interneurons that inhibit motoneurons of ON. Preganglionic visceromotor neurons of the IML nucleus and SAN, influenced by the hypothalamus (not shown), are either excitatory or inhibitory to smooth muscle of the bladder (detrusor) and internal urethral sphincter. Visceral afferent fibers that transmit pain travel with the sympathetic division of the autonomic nervous system; those that transmit stretch travel with the parasympathetic division. L-region, pontine urinary storage center (PUSC); M-region, pontine micturition center (PMC); IML nucleus, intermediolateral nucleus (preganglionic sympathetics); SAN, sacral autonomic nucleus (preganglionic parasympathetics); GVA, general visceral afferent; +, excitation; –, inhibition.

coordinated closely with activities of visceral neurons and visceral muscles [95].

Although distinctly somatic [42,86], the cells of ON may be morphologically, biochemically, and functionally different from other somatic motor neurons [32,42,56] and intermediate between a somatomotor and a visceromotor classification [26,52,74,80]. Evidence in support of this position comes from pathological changes observed in neurons in several neurological degenerative diseases. For instance, in the motoneuron diseases poliomyelitis [55], Werdnig-Hoffman disease [110], and amyotrophic lateral sclerosis [3,17,50,52,68], somatic motor neurons are progressively lost, while visceral motor neurons and neurons of ON are spared. In contrast, neurons of ON are selectively vulnerable in visceromotor neuronal disorders such as Shy-Drager syndrome [26,67,69], Hurler's syndrome [110], and Fabry's disease [26]. Other evidence in support of the intermediate classification of cells of ON is that these neurons share several biochemical characteristics with CNS autonomic nuclei [3,11,12,70,74].

Clinical Relevance

STRIATED MUSCLE FIBERS OF THE PELVIC DIAPHRAGM AND PERINEUM: *A variety of data indicate that, physiologically and neurologically, the striated muscles of the pelvic floor and perineum differ from other voluntary, somatic musculature. For these reasons, treatment of their dysfunction by therapists may necessitate a novel approach. To wit, some females, even nulliparous, continent ones are unable to contract their pelvic and perineal muscles voluntarily; others can do so only in concert with other voluntary muscle groups, such as the abdominal and gluteal muscles [84,85]. The decreased voluntary accessibility of these muscles, then, suggests that traditional exercise protocols may not be effective with this population of patients and that clinicians must become more innovative in the ways we approach their rehabilitation.*

The intermediate classification of neurons of ON, between those of somatic and visceral motor neurons, also has significant clinical application. For instance, in certain **motoneuron diseases** *(e.g., amyotrophic lateral sclerosis), incontinence (urinary as well as anorectal) develops as a late sequela of the disease.*

SPECIFIC FUNCTIONS OF PELVIC AND PERINEAL MUSCULATURE

Urinary Continence and Micturition

Essential to an understanding of the role of the voluntary muscle fibers of the pelvic floor and perineum in urinary continence is a brief description of the visceral structures that are involved, specifically, the bladder, bladder neck, and proximal urethra. Each contains smooth muscle fibers that

receive visceral efferent and visceral afferent innervations that are responsible for visceromotor activity and for transmitting stretch.

The **urinary bladder** serves a dual function; it passively stores urine and actively discharges its contents into the urethra. Its wall is composed of a single unit of interlacing bundles of smooth muscle, the **detrusor,** innervated by both divisions of the ANS [14,21,53]. Preganglionic parasympathetic neurons are located in the SAN at spinal cord segments S2-4 and their axons travel in the **pelvic splanchnic nerves (nervi erigentes),** while preganglionic sympathetic neurons are located in the IML nucleus of spinal cord segments T11–L2 and their axons travel in **thoracic** and **lumbar splanchnic nerves** (*Fig. 36.14*). Postganglionic neurons of both divisions of the ANS are located in the **inferior hypogastric (pelvic) plexus** or one of its subdivisions, the **vesical plexus** (*Fig. 36.14*). The dense population of parasympathetic fibers to the detrusor is excitatory, while the sparse sympathetics are vasomotor and inhibitory to the detrusor [14,21,53] (*Table 36.3*). Visceral afferents travel with pelvic splanchnic nerves and transmit stretch and pain, while those that accompany sympathetics carry pain only [27,73].

Smooth muscle in the **bladder neck** and initial part of the **urethra** is histologically, histochemically, and pharmacologically distinct from the cells of the detrusor; furthermore, the area is sexually dimorphic [53]. In the male, circular or truly sphincteric fibers in this region make up an **internal urethral sphincter** (IUS); these fibers receive a dense sympathetic innervation that is excitatory and a sparse parasympathetic innervation that is inhibitory. In the female, however, true sphincteric muscle fibers and the sympathetic nerve fibers are absent. This may be one of the many factors that contribute to a higher incidence of urinary incontinence in females than in males [87,116]. Although the existence of a morphological muscular entity corresponding to an IUS is somewhat controversial [89,121], in both sexes, a bundle of muscle fibers intermingled with collagen and elastic fibers functions as a physiological sphincter to control the passage of urine from the bladder into the proximal urethra [27,89].

Supraspinal, spinal, and peripheral nervous elements, the bladder, urethra, and sphincteric musculature all function in concert to maintain **urinary continence** and allow micturition in the following manner:

- The bladder fills passively between periods of voiding, gradually increasing vesical pressure.
- Urine is retained in the bladder by direct activation of neurons in ON by the PUSC, resulting in tonic activity in the EUS and compression of the urethra.
- Retention of urine by the bladder is facilitated also by activation of neurons in the SAN of S2-4 and IML nucleus of T11–L2 by cells of the paraventricular nucleus of the hypothalamus, resulting in internal urethral sphincter excitation and closure, and detrusor inhibition.
- Urinary continence is maintained as long as vesical pressure does not exceed urethral pressure.

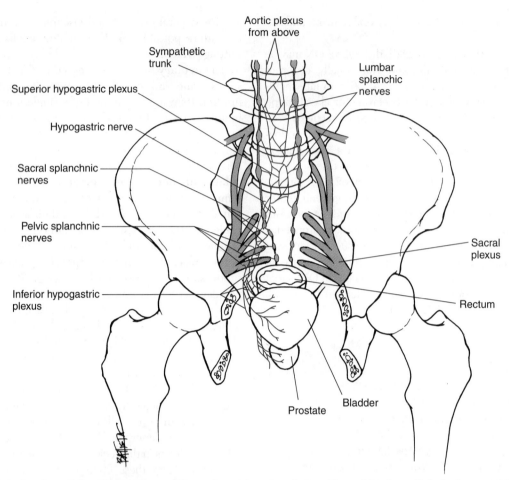

Figure 36.14: Anterior view of the visceral nerves of the male pelvis and perineum. The pelvic plexus (inferior hypogastric plexus) is formed by contributions from parasympathetic pelvic splanchnic nerves and sympathetic fibers that descend through the superior hypogastric plexus (the caudal continuation of the aortic plexus from above). Fibers from both divisions of the autonomic nervous system blend in the pelvic plexus and are distributed to visceral structures in the pelvis and perineum.

TABLE 36.3: Functional Coordination of Visceral and Somatic Musculature of the Pelvis and Perineum

Function	Visceral Efferents, Parasympathetic	Visceral Efferents, Sympathetic	Somatic Efferents via Pudendal Nerve	Visceral Afferents
Urinary continence and micturition	+ to detrusor, − to IUS	− to detrusor, + to IUS	± to EUS	Sense stretch in wall of urinary bladder as it fills
Anal continence and defecation	+ to rectal musculature, − to IAS	− to rectal musculature, + to IAS	± to EAS	Sense stretch in wall of rectum as it fills
Parturition	+ to bulk of uterine musculature	− to musculature of cervix and vagina	+ pelvic and urogenital diaphragms	Sense stretch in walls of uterus and vagina
Sexual	Vasodilation of helicine arteries and penile/clitoral erection	Male: ejaculation with − to detrusor and + to IUS Male & female: detumescence (remission from erection)	Female: + to VS	Male and female: sense degree of vasodilation of helicine arteries Female: sense stretch in walls of vagina

+, excitatory; −, inhibitory; ±, excitation (voluntary contraction) and inhibition (voluntary relaxation); IUS, internal urethral sphincter; EUS, external urethral sphincter, consisting of the sphincter urethrae and fibers of the pubococcygeus surrounding the urethra; IAS, internal anal sphincter; EAS, external anal sphincter with some fibers from the puborectalis; VS, vaginal sphincter, consisting of pubovaginalis, urethrovaginal sphincter portion of the sphincter urethrae and bulbospongiosus.

- When the bladder fills to 400–500 mL (i.e., when vesical pressure exceeds urethral pressure), the micturition reflex is activated.
- The **micturition reflex** consists of the following cascade of events:

    Stretch receptors in the bladder wall are stimulated, and these, in turn, activate visceral afferent fibers that enter the spinal cord via dorsal roots at S2-4 to terminate on second-order neurons in the IMM.

    Axons of neurons in the IMM ascend in the spinoreticular tract to reach the brainstem reticular formation. Spinoreticular fibers (carrying stretch sensations) project to the PMC.

    By way of direct excitation of neurons in the SAN and IML nucleus, along with inhibition of neurons in ON via an interneuron, activity in cells of the PMC results in contraction of the bladder and relaxation of the IUS and EUS.

- Axons of neurons in the IMM nucleus also ascend in the spinothalamic tract to the ventral posterior nucleus of the thalamus; a cortical projection from the thalamus provides a feeling of fullness in the bladder and a conscious desire to urinate.
- The micturition reflex and the cortical projection together culminate in micturition.
- If the micturition reflex occurs when it is inconvenient to urinate, corticospinal fibers can override the reflex for a finite period by directly exciting neurons of ON, thereby increasing the force of contraction of the EUS sufficiently to maintain closure of the urethra until appropriate facilities are available. If however, vesical pressure exceeds the enhanced urethral pressure, micturition occurs, even with maximal voluntary contraction of the EUS.
- Micturition can be facilitated by contraction of the thoracic diaphragm and abdominal muscles to increase intraabdominal pressure (Valsalva's maneuver).

Anorectal Continence and Defecation

Anorectal continence and defecation are controlled and coordinated by the same or similar structures that are involved in urinary continence and micturition, with some major differences [26,73,118]. The sigmoid colon, rectum, and anal canal contain smooth muscle fibers that are innervated by visceral efferent nerve fibers as well as visceral afferent fibers that transmit stretch.

The **rectum** is the middle visceral structure at the caudal end of the alimentary canal, in continuity above with the **sigmoid colon** and below with the **anal canal.** Each is located in a different region; the sigmoid colon is situated in the abdominal cavity, the rectum in the pelvic cavity, and the anal canal in the perineum [121]. The sigmoid colon is the reservoir for fecal material, and the rectum remains empty except when feces enters it to excite defecation [5,23,36,43] or in chronic constipation [5]. The walls of each of these alimentary passageways are composed, in part, of thin inner circular and thick outer longitudinal smooth muscle fibers [5]. Contraction

of the circular fibers results in the pulsatile constrictions of the gut as seen in **peristalsis,** while longitudinal fiber activation produces a shortened segment of bowel. Smooth muscle fibers of the lower part of the alimentary canal are innervated by both divisions of the ANS [5,89,121]. Preganglionic sympathetic neurons are located in the IML nucleus of L1-2. Most postganglionic sympathetic neurons, embedded in ganglia of the superior and inferior mesenteric plexuses of the abdominal cavity, travel in the **superior** and **inferior hypogastric plexuses** to reach the caudal end of the bowel (*Fig. 36.14*). Preganglionic parasympathetic neurons are located in the SAN at spinal cord segments S2-4; their axons travel in the **pelvic splanchnic nerves** to reach postganglionic neurons located in the wall of the bowel segment or the inferior hypogastric plexus [89]. Parasympathetic fibers are excitatory, and sympathetics are inhibitory, to smooth muscle of the bowel. Visceral afferents that travel with pelvic splanchnic nerves (S2-4) transmit stretch as well as pain; those that accompany sympathetic fibers carry pain only [5,73,89].

In the upper two thirds of the anal canal, the circular layer of the muscularis externa (smooth muscle) is thickened and forms the **internal anal sphincter** (IAS). Sympathetic stimulation results in excitation of the IAS, while parasympathetic fibers inhibit it [73]. Under most circumstances, approximately 80–85% of the resting pressure on the anal canal is afforded by the IAS, while the EAS, innervated by somatic fibers of the inferior rectal branch of the pudendal nerve, provides 15–20% [13]. Voluntary recruitment of additional fibers of the EAS and the puborectalis is an effective mechanism for increasing anal pressure beyond the resting state when there are sudden increases in intraabdominal pressure or when defecation must be deferred [62,78,115].

The supraspinal control of **anorectal continence** and **defecation** is less well understood than that of urinary continence and micturition. Although there exists an element of supraspinal (cortical) control, most researchers agree that the greatest contribution to the control of defecation comes from reflex mechanisms [5,26,36,73,89]. Neurons of the spinal cord and autonomic ganglia, smooth muscle of the sigmoid colon, rectum, anal canal and IAS, and striated muscle of the EAS and puborectalis all play a role in the sensorimotor integration of anorectal continence and defecation in the following manner:

- By most accounts, the sigmoid colon serves as the reservoir for fecal material between periods of defecation.
- Activation of neurons in ON and the IML nucleus of the spinal cord results in tonic activity in both the IAS and EAS, as well as the puborectalis, maintaining closure of the anal canal and orifice, except during defecation.
- Excitation of neurons in ON and the IML nucleus, and muscular contractions of the IAS, EAS, and puborectalis is increased during activities in which intraabdominal pressure is increased (e.g., straining to lift a heavy object, forced expiration, coughing, sneezing, parturition); in contrast, the amplitude of the muscular response is decreased when intraabdominal pressure is increased during voluntary straining to defecate.

- Prior to defecation, fecal material moves from the sigmoid colon (and as high as the left colic flexure) into the rectum via peristalsis of the colon [5].
- The stimulus for the initiation of defecation is usually the **intrinsic defecation reflex** [36], stimulated by distention of the rectum after arrival of the feces and activation of visceral afferent fibers by stretch [5,73,89]; an additional mechanism for triggering the arrival of stool in the rectum is the **extrinsic defecation reflex** [105], stimulated by activation of proprioceptors in pelvic floor and perineal muscle fibers, particularly the puborectalis and other fibers of the levator ani [34,39,51,94].
- Completion of the defecation reflex results in relaxation of the IAS; however, voluntary contraction of the EAS prevents further passage of the feces if the time is not convenient for defecation.
- Facilitation of the defecation reflex is afforded by visceral afferent stimulation of the SAN, which, in turn, increases the peristaltic activity in the smooth muscle of the rectum [36].
- If the desire to defecate is strong and the time and place are socially acceptable, defecation commences; ignoring this urge can gradually lead to chronic constipation [36].
- Relaxation of the puborectalis allows some straightening of the perineal flexure and passage of the feces into the anal canal; further relaxation of the puborectalis and reduction of the perineal flexure occurs when one sits [5,26].
- Passage of the feces through the anal canal is allowed by relaxation of the EAS and facilitated by contraction of the thoracic diaphragm and abdominal muscles to increase intraabdominal pressure (Valsalva's maneuver).
- Prior to and during passage of fecal material through the anal canal, the pelvic floor relaxes and descends, and at the same time, longitudinal muscle of the anal canal contracts to shorten it, thus assisting in expulsion of the stool [5].
- The **closing reflex** occurs with contraction of the IAS, EAS, and puborectalis, resulting in closure of the anal orifice and restoration of the perineal flexure.

Clinical Relevance

DEFECATION REFLEXES AND DIGITAL STIMULATION: Using **digital stimulation,** clinicians take advantage of the internal and external defecation reflexes in bowel management of patients with spinal cord injuries and intact reflex cord mechanisms [58]. A gloved, lubricated digit can be inserted into the patient's anorectal passageway and moved in a circular motion for 30–60 seconds to stretch the mucosa and surrounding muscle. This technique stimulates stretch receptors and activates visceral and somatic afferent nerve fibers in and around the lower bowel passageway, resulting in reflex contraction of the smooth muscle of the rectum and bowel emptying.

Sexual Function

Aspects of sexual function that deal with the function and neural control of smooth muscle fibers in the internal and external genitalia and striated muscles of the pelvic floor and perineum are considered here. The prototype for our discussion is the male; differences in sexual function in the female are also addressed. There are four stages of sexual function: **excitation, erection, ejaculation (orgasm),** and **remission.** Function during these stages results predominately from autonomic phenomena; two contain a somatic component.

Excitation occurs with the passage of erotogenic thoughts or with cutaneous stimulation, especially of the erogenous zones, and transmission to the spinal cord via somatic afferents and on to supraspinal centers, particularly the hypothalamus, limbic system, and cerebral cortex. Excitation causes erection of the penis. This is followed by ejaculation of semen, which coincides with the orgasmic phase. In the final stage, remission, the penis returns to the flaccid state (detumescence). The following is a description of the neuroanatomical basis of each of these stages of **sexual function:**

- Erection is a parasympathetic phenomenon; it results from activity in neurons of the SAN, which results in dilation of the helicine arteries of the penis and engorgement of the cavernous spaces of the corpus spongiosum and corpora cavernosa [73,89].
- Activation of striated muscle fibers contributes to erection; turgidity of the erection is increased by pulsatile contractions of the bulbospongiosus and ischiocavernosus muscles secondary to stimulation of neurons in ON.
- Ejaculation results in expulsion of the **semen** (ejaculate; sperm plus seminal fluid) from the external urethral orifice; it has two phases and is controlled by three types of neurons.

  The first phase is passage of the ejaculate into the urethra, and the second phase is passage of the ejaculate out of the urethra through the external urethral orifice. During **emission,** stimulation of the ejaculatory ducts and seminal vesicles by sympathetic neurons in the IML nucleus of L1-2 results in delivery of the ejaculate to the prostatic urethra [73] and prostatic fluid to the ejaculate [6,89].

  During ejaculation, activity in neurons of the IML nucleus of L1-2 maintains closure of the internal urethral sphincter to prevent reflux of the ejaculate into the bladder and leakage of urine [6,73], and neurons of ON activate the EAS to prevent leakage of feces or gas [96]. Activation of parasympathetic neurons in the SAN results in contraction of smooth muscle of the urethra to expel the ejaculate at the external urethral orifice.

  Expulsion of the ejaculate is facilitated by activation of neurons of ON, resulting in pulsatile contractions of the ischiocavernosus and bulbospongiosus [73,96].

- Following ejaculation, the penis returns to a flaccid state (detumescence, remission).

Sympathetic fibers cause constriction of the helicine arteries.

Striated fibers of the bulbospongiosus and ischiocavernosus are relaxed to allow venous return of blood from the cavernous spaces of the penis.

Neuroanatomically, sexual function in the female follows the same pattern as in the male, with one obvious exception. Although the female genital tract secretes fluids similar to those of the male, there is no true ejaculate from the urethra containing fluid or semen; genital tract fluids are deposited in the vestibule. As in the male ejaculatory phase, however, there are pulsatile contractions of the bulbospongiosus and VS during the orgasmic phase in the female.

Parturition

During **gestation,** smooth muscle fibers of the uterus become hypertrophied and stretched. In addition, pelvic floor and perineal structures, including the musculature, increase in bulk and strength to compensate for the erect posture of the expectant mother. Specifically, sphincteric fibers of the EUS, EAS, and VS undergo hypertrophy to maintain urinary and anorectal continence in the presence of the superincumbent fetus, which steadily increases in bulk, and to block egress of the fetus through the cervical canal [1]. The soft tissues that increase in bulk during pregnancy for purposes of support will, of necessity, be stretched or torn during labor and delivery and may even obstruct passage of the fetus [6].

The weak, slow, rhythmic contractions of the uterus that are present throughout most of pregnancy (**Braxton Hicks contractions)** intensify toward the end of pregnancy and, commencing with labor, become sufficiently strong to stretch the cervix and move the fetus through the birth canal [106]. An increase in estrogen relative to progesterone and oxytocin, secreted by the neurohypophysis, are probably responsible for the uterine contractions [6,36]. Afferent nerve fibers from the cervical canal and pelvic floor are involved in the facilitation of neurogenic reflexes that contribute to a reflex urgency in the expectant mother to bear down and expel the fetus (399).

With progression of the labor, a true **positive feedback** is established, one that is thought to be the prime mechanism for the onset and intensification of **labor** [36]. Specifically, descent of the fetus stretches the uterine cervix, and visceral afferents stimulate uterine smooth muscle contractions to push the fetus further into the cervical canal. At the same time, pressure on the pelvic diaphragm and rectum activates somatic afferent fibers that cause contraction of the thoracic diaphragm and abdominal wall muscles, thus increasing intraabdominal pressure and stimulating contraction of the striated muscles of the pelvic diaphragm and perineum to resist the increase in intraabdominal pressure. As labor proceeds, the major impediments to fetal passage are offered by the cervix, pelvic diaphragm, and perineum [6]. As uterine contractions intensify in force and frequency, the

reflexly facilitated muscles at the pelvic outlet are torn to allow egress of the fetus. At this time, periurethral and perianal muscle fibers, as well as the perineal body, can rupture spontaneously.

PELVIC MUSCLE DYSFUNCTION

Pelvic floor dysfunction describes a wide variety of clinical conditions involving impairment, separately or in combination, of the nervous, muscular, and fascial elements of the pelvic floor and perineum. These include disorders of micturition, defecation, and sexual function as well as organ prolapse and pelvic discomfort. Although female gender, parity, and advanced age are recognized risk factors for pelvic floor dysfunction, other factors may put men as well as women at risk at nearly all ages. Interest in this area has escalated sharply in the past 10–20 years, reflected by the number of publications in scientific and clinical journals and the frequency with which this topic is addressed at professional meetings. Data from many of the studies, particularly epidemiological, are difficult to interpret and compare because of discrepancies in the basic definition of the specific disorder, errors, and inconsistencies in study design, and source of subjects [116]. Clearly, more well-designed, longitudinal studies need to be performed to answer the multitude of questions related to pelvic floor dysfunction. The discussion here emphasizes pelvic organ prolapse in women and both varieties of incontinence (urinary and anorectal) because they share etiological features and they involve the neuromuscular elements that are the subject of this chapter. Comprehensive reviews provide more information regarding the causes [87] and epidemiology [116] of pelvic floor dysfunction.

Pelvic Organ Prolapse

Insofar as muscles of the urogenital and pelvic diaphragms along with the pelvic fascia and visceral ligaments support the organs of the pelvic cavity, weakness or rupture can lead to **pelvic organ prolapse,** defined as protrusion of one or more pelvic organs into the vaginal canal [89]. **Uterine prolapse** occurs when the uterine cervix descends into the vagina. **Rectocele, cystocele,** and **urethrocele** refer, respectively, to bulging of the rectum, bladder, or urethra into the posterior or anterior wall of the vagina.

The exact cause of pelvic organ prolapse and the number of women who develop it are unknown [87,116,117]. Weakening or loss of the noncontractile elements (visceral ligaments, fascia) of the pelvic floor and perineum and concomitant loss of pelvic organ support is the traditional explanation [7,89]; however, injury to the pudendal nerve and denervation of muscles of the pelvic diaphragm and perineum have also been implicated in the etiology of prolapse [64,100,109,113]. An estimated 50% of parous women have pelvic organ prolapse to some degree [7]. Conservative treatment of this disorder involves exercises and other techniques to strengthen muscles of the pelvic diaphragm and perineum, and surgery may be indicated in some individuals [87]. The National Center for Health Statistics reports that approximately 400,000 women receive surgical intervention for genitourinary prolapse per annum [79,81].

Urinary Incontinence

In 1988, the National Institutes of Health (NIH) Consensus Conference [76] defined **urinary incontinence** as "the involuntary loss of urine so severe as to have social and/or hygienic consequences." A similar definition has been adopted by the International Continence Society [45]. This disorder is a huge problem, socially, psychologically, and economically. Although the true incidence is unknown, the estimate is 13 million Americans in 1996 at a cost of $15 billion [87], and 10 million in the United Kingdom in 1999 at a cost of £1.4 billion [45]. Urinary incontinence is more common in women than men, in older than younger women, and in multiparous than nulliparous women [30,76,87,116]. Prevalence of urinary incontinence is estimated to be 10–30% in females and 1.5–5% in males, aged 15 to 64 years [30]. Its prevalence in institutionalized individuals can be as high as 50% [30].

Factors contributing to the development of urinary incontinence are numerous. They include prostatectomy in males, changes in hormone status and vaginal delivery in females, and supraspinal neurological lesions, advanced age, functional impairment, and drugs [118] in both sexes. In males, earlier detection of prostate cancer and its surgical treatment has resulted in an increased incidence of postprostatectomy incontinence [25,59,83]. Since parts of the female urinary tract contain estrogen receptors, alterations in levels of circulating estrogen and progesterone during menstruation or with menopause can affect continence [44]. Vaginal delivery can damage the nerves to the pelvic floor as well as the muscles, particularly the EUS [2,64,102,108,109,112]. The resultant urinary incontinence, transient or long term, has been observed in as many as 20–30% of women after their first pregnancy and delivery [99]. Furthermore, compared with males, a smaller motor pool controlling fewer muscle fibers in this area and the absence of an IUS may all contribute to the higher prevalence of urinary incontinence in females. With advancing age, there is a significant loss of striated muscle cells in the pelvic diaphragm, an increase in connective tissue elements, and a decrease in vascularity [16,24]. Neurological lesions of the spinal cord or below the pons can result in **detrusor-sphincter dyssynergia,** characterized by lack of coordination between detrusor contraction and EUS relaxation; lesions above the pons may cause **detrusor hyper-reflexia,** characterized by loss of inhibition to the detrusor [118]. Taken together, the loss of estrogen, one or more vaginal births, the loss of muscle mass and replacement by connective tissue, and the decreasing functional level of many individuals in an ever-enlarging aged population that is increasingly dependent upon medications, one can readily understand the scope of the urinary incontinence problem.

Anorectal Incontinence

Although not considered as widespread a problem as urinary incontinence, **anorectal incontinence** is nonetheless a serious problem. More than any other type of pelvic floor dysfunction, anorectal incontinence causes social withdrawal and mental anguish, and it may be (along with urinary incontinence) the single most important factor in the decision to place an individual in an institution [45,87]. Since patients are extremely embarrassed and reluctant to admit to anorectal incontinence, even to their physicians, accurate epidemiological data regarding the "pelvic floor closet issue of the 1990s" [116] are difficult to come by. In addition, definitions of anorectal incontinence vary from involuntary loss of flatus (gas) to liquid or solid fecal material [87,116]. Prevalence reports range from 1 [114] to 18% [87].

Urinary and anorectal incontinence have some factors common to their development—vaginal delivery, supraspinal neurological lesions, advanced age, functional impairment, and drugs. Iatrogenic or parturient damage to the levator ani, particularly the puborectalis, the EAS, and their nerve fibers, may be causative in many cases of anorectal incontinence [2,22,103,108,109,112].

Role of the Therapist in Management of Pelvic Floor Dysfunction

Conservative management of all types of pelvic dysfunction that involve weakened pelvic and perineal musculature as well as pelvic pain should include a therapist. As recently as two decades ago, therapists regularly saw patients for prenatal and postpartum pelvic floor (Kegel) exercises [48]. That practice generally fell by the wayside when time constraints, reimbursement issues, and flagging interest began to limit evaluation and treatment of this population of patients. The past few years, however, have witnessed a resurgence of clinical and scientific interest in individuals with pelvic floor dysfunction. Increasingly, therapists are making this an important emphasis in their practice and research activities. This trend should continue and escalate as therapists, who are eminently qualified to care for these patients, learn more about the efficacy of therapeutic interventions in this predominately female population.

SUMMARY

This chapter details the structure, function, and innervation of the striated muscles of the pelvis and perineum of both sexes. The three layers of muscle from deep to superficial are the pelvic diaphragm, deep perineal muscles, and superficial perineal muscles. Function and metabolic properties of the fibers that compose these muscles are discussed. The muscles of the pelvic diaphragm and perineum are composed predominantly of fatigue-resistant type I fibers. Type II fibers predominate in the regions immediately surrounding the urethral, vaginal, and anal orifices. The roles of the specific fiber types in controlling the visceral functions of micturition, defecation, sexual function, parturition, and pelvic organ support are discussed.

To facilitate an understanding of the special nature of the pelvic and perineal muscles and the ways they are involved in dysfunction, specifics of their neurological control and coordination of their function with that of pelvic visceral structures are presented. Function of the pelvic musculature exhibits a finely regulated feedback system involving sympathetic and parasympathetic influence for conscious and unconscious control. Specific attention is given to sexual dimorphism of these muscles as well as the neurons that control them. Males exhibit stronger muscles providing better pelvic control during high loads. Females exhibit smaller muscles and more fascial tissue providing better static control, especially during pregnancy. Pelvic dysfunction, more common in women than in men, may involve dysfunction in the muscular, nervous, or fascial components of the pelvis. Numerous clinically significant sequelae of pelvic and perineal musculature dysfunction related to gender, age, vaginal delivery, muscular atrophy, and nervous degeneration are presented.

References

1. Abitol MM: Quadrupedalism, bipedalism, and human pregnancy. In: Vleeming A, Mooney V, Snijders CJ, et al. eds. Movement, Stability and Low Back Pain. New York: Churchill Livingstone, 1997; 395–404.

2. Allen RE, Hosker GL, Smith ARB, Warrell DW: Pelvic floor damage and childbirth: a neurophysiological study. Br J Obstet Gynecol 1990; 97: 770–779.

3. Anneser JM, Borasio GD, Berthele A, et al.: Differential expression of group I metabotropic glutamate receptors in rat spinal cord somatic and autonomic motoneurons: possible implications for the pathogenesis of amyotrophic lateral sclerosis. Neurobiol Dis 1999; 6: 140–147.

4. Argentine Episiotomy Trial Collaborative Group: Routine vs selective episiotomy: a randomized controlled trial. Lancet 1993; 342: 1517–1518.

5. Bannister LH: Alimentary system. In: Williams PL, ed. Gray's Anatomy. The Anatomical Basis of Medicine and Surgery. New York: Churchill Livingstone, 1995; 1683–1812.

6. Bannister LH, Dyson M: Reproductive system. In: Williams PL, ed. Gray's Anatomy. The Anatomical Basis of Medicine and Surgery. New York: Churchill Livingstone, 1995; 1847–1880.

7. Beck RP: Pelvic relaxational prolapse. In: Kase NG, Weingold AB, eds. Principles and Practice of Clinical Gynecology. New York: John Wiley & Sons, 1983.

8. Blok BF, Holstege G: Two pontine micturition centers in the cat are not interconnected directly: implications for the central organization of micturition. J Comp Neurol 1999; 403: 209–218.

9. Bo K, Hagen RH, Kvarstein B, et al.: Pelvic floor muscle exercise for the treatment of female stress urinary incontinence: III. Effects of two different degrees of pelvic floor muscle exercises. Neurourol Urodyn 1990; 9: 489–502.

10. Bo K, Talseth T, Holme I: Single blind, randomized controlled trial of pelvic floor exercises, electrical stimulation, vaginal cones, and no treatment in management of genuine stress incontinence in women. Br Med J 1999; 318: 487–493.

11. Brook GA, Schmitt AB, Nacimiento W, et al.: Distribution of B-50 (GAP-43) mRNA protein in the normal adult human spinal cord. Acta Neuropathol (Berl) 1998; 95: 378–386.

12. Brown JL, Liu H, Maggio JE, et al.: Morphological characterization of substance P receptor-immunoreactive neurons in the rat spinal cord and trigeminal nucleus caudalis. J Comp Neurol 1995; 356: 327–344.

13. Burleigh DE: Pharmacology of the internal anal sphincter. In: Henry MM, Swash M, eds. Coloproctology and the Pelvic Floor. London: Butterworth-Heineman, 1992.

14. Burnstock G: Innervation of bladder and bowel. Ciba Found Symp 1990; 151: 2–18.

15. Bustami FM: A reappraisal of the anatomy of the levator ami muscle in man. Acta Morphol Neerl Scand 1989; 26: 255–268.

16. Carlile A, Davies I, Rigby A: Age changes in the human female urethra: a morphometric study. J Urol 1988; 139: 532–535.

17. Carvalho M, Schwartz MS, Swash M: Involvement of the external anal sphincter in amyotrophic lateral sclerosis. Muscle Nerve 1995; 18: 848–853.

18. Catala M: How sex dimorphism is established in the spinal nucleus of Onuf. Morphologie 1999; 83: 5–8.

19. Collins P: Embryology and development. In: Williams PL, ed. Gray's Anatomy. The Anatomical Basis of Medicine and Surgery. New York: Churchill Livingstone, 1995; 91–341.

20. Critchley HOD, Dixon JS, Gosling JA: Comparative study of the periurethral and perianal parts of the human levator ani muscle. Urol Int 1980; 35: 226–232.

21. De Groat WC: Anatomy and physiology of the lower urinary tract. Urol Clin North Am 1993; 20: 383–401.

22. Delancey JO: Childbirth, continence, and the pelvic floor. N Engl J Med 1993; 329: 1956–1957.

23. Denny-Brown D, Robertson EG: Investigation of nervous control of defaecation. Brain 1935; 58: 256–310.

24. Dimpfl T, Jaeger C, Mueller-Felber W, et al.: Myogenic changes of the levator ani muscle in premenopausal women: the impact of vaginal delivery and age. Neurourol Urodyn 1998; 17: 197–205.

25. Diokno AC: Post prostatectomy urinary incontinence. Ostomy Wound Manage 1998; 44: 54–58, 60.

26. Dubrovsky B, Filipini D: Neurobiological aspects of the pelvic floor muscles involved in defecation. Neurosci Biobehav Rev 1990; 14: 157–168.

27. Dyson M: Urinary system. In: Williams PL, ed. Gray's Anatomy. The Anatomical Basis of Medicine and Surgery. New York: Churchill Livingstone, 1995; 1813–1845.

28. Elftman HO: The evolution of the pelvic floor of primates. Am J Anat 1932; 51: 307–346.

29. Enoka RM: Muscle strength and its development. New perspectives. Sports Med 1988; 6: 146–168.

30. Fantl JA, Newman DK, Colling J: Urinary incontinence in adults: acute and chronic management. In: Anonymous. Clinical Practice Guidelines no. 2, AHCP&R Publ no. 96-1682. Rockville, MD: US Dept of Health & Human Services, Public Health Service, Agency for Health Care Policy and Research, 1996; 1–16.

31. Forger NG, Frank LG, Breedlove SM, Glickman SE: Sexual dimorphism of perineal muscles and motoneurons in spotted hyenas. J Comp Neurol 1996; 375: 333–343.

32. Gibson SJ, Polak JM, Katagiri T, et al.: A comparison of the distributions of eight peptides in spinal cords from normal controls and cases of motor neurone disease with special reference to Onuf's nucleus. Brain Res 1988; 474: 255–278.

33. Gilpin SA, Gosling JA, Smith ARB: The pathogenesis of genitourinary prolapse and stress incontinence of urine: a histological and histochemical study. Br J Obstet Gynaecol 1989; 96: 15–23.

34. Goligher JC, Hughes ESR: Sensibility of the rectum and colon. Its role in the mechanism of anal continence. Lancet 1951; 260: 543–548.

35. Gosling JA, Dixon JS, Critchley HOD: A comparative study of the human external sphincter and periurethral levator ani muscles. Br J Urol 1981; 53: 35–41.

36. Guyton AC: Textbook of Medical Physiology. Philadelphia: WB Saunders, 1991.

37. Hannerz J: Discharge properties of motor units in relation to recruitment order in voluntary contraction. Acta Physiol Scand 1974; 91: 374–384.

38. Henriksen T, Bek K, Hedegaard M, Secher N: Episiotomy and perineal lesions in spontaneous vaginal deliveries. Br J Obstet Gynaecol 1992; 99: 950–953.

39. Holschneider AM: The problem of anorectal continence. In: Rickman PP, Prevost J, eds. Anorectal Malfunctions and Associated Diseases. Baltimore: University Park Press, 1974; 85–97.

40. Holstege G: Some anatomical observations of the projections from the hypothalamus to brainstem and spinal cord: an HRP and autoradiographic tracing study in the cat. J Comp Neurol 1987; 260: 98–126.

41. Holstege G, Griffiths D, De Wall H, Dalm E: Anatomical and physiological observations on supraspinal control of bladder and urethral sphincter muscles in the cat. J Comp Neurol 1986; 250: 449–461.

42. Holstege G, Tan J: Supraspinal control of motoneurons innervating the striated muscles of the pelvic floor including urethral and anal sphincter in the cat. Brain 1987; 110: 1323–1344.

43. Hurst AF: Chronic constipation. London: Oxford University Press, 1919.

44. Iosif S, Batra S, Ek A: Oestrogen receptors in the female lower urinary tract. Am J Obstet Gynecol 1981; 141: 817–820.

45. Jackson S, Shepherd A, Brookes S, Abrams P: The effect of oestrogen supplementation on post-menopausal urinary incontinence: a double-blind placebo-controlled trial. Br J Obstet Gynaecol 1999; 106: 711–718.

46. Johnson VY: How the principles of exercise physiology influence pelvic floor muscle training. J Wound Ostomy Continence Nurs 2001; 28: 150–155.

47. Kawakami M: Electromyographic investigation of the human external sphincter muscles of the anus. Jpn J Physiol 1954; 4: 196–204.

48. Kegel AH: Progressive resistance exercises in the functional restoration of the perineal muscle. Am J Obstet Gynecol 1948; 56: 238–248.

49. Kiernan JA: Barr's The Human Nervous System. Philadelphia: Lippincott-Raven, 1998.

50. Kiernan JA, Hudson AJ: Changes in shapes of surviving motor neurons in amyotrophic lateral sclerosis. Brain 1993; 116: 203–215.

51. Kiesewetter WB, Nixon HH: Imperforate anus. I. Its surgical anatomy. J Pediatr Surg 1967; 2: 60–68.

52. Kihira T, Yoshida S, Yoshimasu F, et al.: Involvement of Onuf's nucleus in amyotrophic lateral sclerosis. J Neurol Sci 1997; 147: 81–88.

53. Klück P: The autonomic innervation of the human urinary bladder, bladder neck and urethra: a histochemical study. Anat Rec 1980; 198: 439–447.

54. Kohama T: Neuroanatomical studies on pontine urine storage facilitatory areas in the cat brain. Part II. Output neuronal structures from the nucleus locus subcoeurleus and the nucleus reticularis pontis oris. Nippon Hinyokika Gakkai Zasshi 1992; 83: 1478–1483.

55. Kojima H, Furuta Y, Fujita M, et al.: Onuf's motoneuron is resistant to poliovirus. J Neurol Sci 1989; 93: 85–92.

56. Koliatsos VE, Price DL, Clatterbuck RE: Motor neurons in Onuf's nucleus and its rat homologues express the p75 nerve growth factor receptor: sexual dimorphism and regulation by axotomy. J Comp Neurol 1994; 345: 510–527.

57. Kraemer WJ, Fleck SJ, Evans WJ: Strength and power training: physiological mechanisms of adaptation. Exerc Sport Sci Rev 1996; 24: 363–397.

58. Kraft C: Bladder and bowel management. In: Buchannan LE, Nawoczenski DA, eds. Spinal Cord Injury. Concepts and Management Approaches. Baltimore: Williams & Wilkins, 1987; 81–98.

59. Krane RJ: Urinary incontinence after treatment for localized prostate cancer. Mol Urol 2000; 4: 279–286.

60. Krier J, Adams T, Meijer R: Physiological, morphological and histochemical properties of cat external anal sphincter. Am J Physiol 1988; 255: G772–G778.

61. Krier J, Ronald M, Percy V: Length tension relationship of striated muscle of cat external anal sphincter. Am J Physiol 1989; 256: 6773–6778.

62. Kuijpers JHC: Anatomy and physiology of the mechanism of continence. Neth J Med. 1990; 37(suppl): 2–5.

63. Larsen WJ: Human Embryology. New York: Churchill Livingstone, 1997.

64. Lavin J, Smith AR: Pelvic floor damage. Mod Midwife 1996; 6: 14–16.

65. Lawson JON: Pelvic anatomy. I. Pelvic floor muscles. Ann R Coll Surg Engl 1974; 54: 244–252.

66. Mandelstam D: The pelvic floor. Physiotherapy 1978; 64: 236–239.

67. Mannen T: Neuropathology of Onuf's nucleus. Rinsho Shinkeigaku 1991; 31: 1281–1285.

68. Mannen T, Iwata M, Toyokura Y, Nagashima K: Preservation of a certain motoneurone group of the sacral cord in amyotrophic lateral sclerosis: its clinical significance. J Neurol Neurosurg Neuropsychiatry 1977; 40: 464–469.

69. Mannen T, Iwata M, Toyokura Y, Nagashima K: The Onuf's nucleus and the external anal sphincter in amyotrophic lateral sclerosis and Shy Drager syndrome. Acta Neuropathol (Berl) 1982; 58: 255–260.

70. Marsala J, Marsala M, Vanicky I, Taira Y: Localization of NADPHd-exhibiting neurons in the spinal cord of the rabbit. J Comp Neurol 1999; 406: 263–284.

71. Merton PA: Electrical stimulation through the scalp of pyramidal tract fibers supplying pelvic floor muscles. In: Henry MH, Swash M, eds. Coloproctology and the Pelvic Floor. London: Butterworths, 1986; 125–129.

72. Moore KL: Clinically Oriented Anatomy. Baltimore: Williams & Wilkins, 1992.

73. Moore KL, Dalley AFI: Clinically Oriented Anatomy. Philadelphia: Lippincott Williams & Wilkins, 1999.

74. Nacimiento W, Topper R, Fischer A, et al.: B-50 (GAP-43) in Onuf's nucleus of the adult cat. Brain Res 1993; 613: 80–87.

75. Nakagawa S: Onuf's nucleus of sacral cord in a South American monkey (Saimiri): its location and bilateral cortical input from area 4. Brain Res 1980; 191: 337–344.

76. NIH Consensus Statement: Urinary incontinence in adults. 1988; 7: 1–11.

77. Niswander KR: Manual of Obstetrics Diagnosis and Therapy. 87. Boston: Little, Brown & Co, 1987.

78. Nivatongs S: The length of the anal canal. Dis Colon Rectum 1981; 24: 600–601.

79. Norton PA, Baker JE, Sharp HC: Genitourinary prolapse and joint hypermobility in women. Obstet Gynecol 1995; 85: 225–228.

80. Olsen AL, Rao SSC: Clinical neurophysiology and electrodiagnostic testing of the pelvic floor. Gastroenterol Clin North Am 2001; 30: 33–54.

81. Olsen AL, Smith VJ, Bergstrom JO: Epidemiology of surgically managed pelvic organ prolapse and urinary incontinence. Obstet Gynecol 1997; 89: 501–506.

82. Onuf B: On the arrangement and function of the cell groups in the sacral region of the spinal cord. Arch Neurol Psychopathol 1900; 3: 387–411.

83. Palmer MH: Postprostatectomy incontinence: the magnitude of the problem. J Wound Ostomy Continence Nurse 2000; 27: 129–137.

84. Pesters UM, Gingelmaier A, Jundt K, et al.: Evaluation of pelvic floor muscle strength using four different techniques. Int Urogynecol J 2001; 12: 27–30.

85. Peschers UM, Vodusek DB, Fanger G, et al.: Pelvic muscle activity in nulliparous volunteers. Neurourol Urodyn 2001; 20: 269–275.

86. Pullen AH, Martin JE, Swash M: Ultrastructure of presynaptic input to motor neurons in Onuf's nucleus: controls and motor neuron disease. Neuropathol Appl Neurobiol 1992; 18: 213–231.

87. Roberts MM, Park TA: Pelvic floor function/dysfunction and electrodiagnostic evaluation. Phys Med Rehabil Clin North Am 1998; 9: 831–851.

88. Rose SJ, Rothstein JM: Muscle mutability. Part 1. General concepts and adaptations to altered patterns of use. Phys Ther 1982; 62: 1773–1787.

89. Rosse C, Gaddum-Rosse P: Hollinshead's Textbook of Anatomy. Philadelphia: Lippincott-Raven, 1997.

90. Rothstein JM: Muscle biology. Clinical considerations. Phys Ther 1982; 62: 1823–1830.

91. Sadler TW: Langman's Medical Embryology. Baltimore: Williams & Wilkins, 1995.

92. Salmons S: Muscle. In: Williams PL, ed. Gray's Anatomy. The Anatomical Basis of Medicine and Surgery. New York: Churchill Livingstone, 1995; 737–900.

93. Salmons S: Exercise, stimulation and type transformation of skeletal muscle. Int J Sports Med 2001; 15: 136–141.

94. Scharli AF: Defecation and continence: some new concepts. Dis Colon Rectum 1970; 13: 81–107.

95. Schroeder HD: Localization of the motoneurons innervating the pelvic muscles of the male rat. J Comp Neurol 1980; 192: 567–587.

96. Shafik A: Pelvic floor muscles and sphincters during erection and ejaculation. Arch Androl 1997; 39: 71–78.

97. Shelley B, Herman H: Methodology for Evaluation and Treatment of Pelvic Floor Dysfunction. Dover, NH: The Prometheus Group, 1994.

98. Sipilä S, Elorinne M, Alen M, et al.: Effects of strength and endurance training on muscle fibre characteristics in elderly women. Clin Physiol 1977; 17: 459–474.

99. Sleep J, Grant A: West Berkshire perineal management trial: three-year follow up. Br Med J 1987; 295: 749–751.

100. Small KA, Wynne JM: Evaluating the pelvic floor in obstetric patients. Aust NZ J Obstet Gynaecol 1990; 30: 41–45.

101. Snooks SJ, Swash M: The innervation of muscles of continence. Ann R Coll Surg Engl 1986; 68: 45–49.

102. Snooks SJ, Swash M, Henry MM: Effect of vaginal delivery on the pelvic floor: a 5-year follow-up. Br J Surg 1990; 77: 1358–1360.

103. Snooks SJ, Swash M, Setchell M, Henry MM: Injury to innervation of pelvic floor sphincter musculature in childbirth. Lancet 1984; 2: 546–550.

104. Solomonow M, Baratta R, Zhou BH, et al.: Historical update and new developments on the EMG-force relationships of skeletal muscles. Orthopedics 1986; 9: 1541–1543.

105. Stephens FD, Durham-Smith EC: Ano-rectal malformations in children. Chicago: Year Book Medical Publishers, 1971.

106. Stephenson RG, O'Connor LJ: Obstetric and Gynecologic Care in Physical Therapy. Thorofare, NJ: Slack, 2000.

107. Strohbehn K: Normal pelvic floor anatomy. Obstet Gynecol Clin North Am 1998; 25: 683–705.

108. Sultan AH, Kamm MA, Hudson CN: Pudendal nerve damage during labour: prospective study before and after childbirth. Br J Obstet Gynaecol 1994; 101: 22–28.

109. Sultan AH, Monga AK, Stanton SL: The pelvic floor sequelae of childbirth. Br J Hosp Med 1996; 55: 575–579.

110. Sung JH, Mastri AR: Spinal autonomic neurons in Werdnig Hoffman disease, mannosidosis and Hurler's syndrome: distribution of autonomic neurons in the sacral cord. J Neuropathol Exp Neurol 1980; 39: 441–451.

111. Swash M: Neurology of the sphincters. Clin Exp Neurol 1987; 23: 1–14.

112. Swash M: The pelvic floor and incontinence. Lancet 1994; 344: 1301.

113. Swash M: Pelvic floor incompetence. In: Rushton DN, ed. Handbook of Neuro-urology. New York: Marcel Dekker, 1994.

114. Szurszewski JH, Holt PR, Schuster M: Proceedings of a workshop entitled "Neuromuscular function and dysfunction of the gastrointestinal tract in aging." Dig Dis Sci 1989; 34: 1135–1146.

115. Toglia MR, Delancey JOL: Anal incontinence and the obstetrician-gynecologist. Obstet Gynecol 1994; 84: 731–740.

116. Visco AG, Figuers C: Nonsurgical management of pelvic floor dysfunction. Obstet Gynecol Clin North Am 1998; 25: 849–866.

117. Wall LL, Delancey JO: The politics of prolapse: a revisionist approach to disorders of the pelvic floor in women. Perspect Biol Med 1991; 34: 486–496.

118. Wester C, Brubaker L: Normal pelvic floor physiology. Obstet Gynecol Clin North Am 1998; 25: 707–722.

119. Wilson JR., Carrington ER, Ledger WJ: Obstetrics and Gynecology. 83. St. Louis, MO: CV Mosby, 1983.

120. Wilson PM: Some observations on pelvic floor evolution in primates. S Afr Med J 1973; 47: 1203–1209.

121. Woodburne RT, Burkel WE: Essentials of Human Anatomy. New York: Oxford University Press, 1994.

Analysis of the Forces on the Pelvis during Activity

Many complaints of pelvic pain are mechanical and may be related to the forces sustained by the pelvis. This chapter examines the forces exerted on the joints and in the bones of the pelvis during activity and the loads sustained during injuries. The unique features of the lumbosacral junction described in Chapter 35 limit the generalizability of the findings in the lumbar spine to the lumbosacral junction, which exhibits its own mechanical challenges. The sacroiliac joints apparently move and also are susceptible to mechanical dysfunctions. The magnitude and direction of the forces across the sacroiliac joint may contribute to patients' complaints. High loads associated with impacts such as those seen in motor vehicle accidents can produce pelvic fractures. An understanding of the forces generated in such collisions may lead to better rehabilitation strategies to minimize the impairments following such injuries. The purposes of this chapter are to examine the loads sustained by the pelvis and its associated joints and to provide a simplified analysis of the forces applied to the region. The specific goals of this chapter are to

- Provide examples of two-dimensional kinetic analysis of the pelvis
- Examine the forces sustained by the lumbosacral junction
- Analyze the forces across the sacroiliac joints
- Investigate the mechanics of pelvic fractures

FORCES SUSTAINED AT THE LUMBOSACRAL JUNCTION

The lumbosacral junction and the L4–L5 junction are the most common sites of disc lesions in the low back [13]. In addition, the lumbosacral junction is susceptible to anterior slippage of L5 on S1, a phenomenon known as **spondylolisthesis** (*Fig. 37.1*) [20]. An understanding of the forces generated at this joint complex helps explain the pathomechanics associated with these disorders. However, fewer studies investigate the forces at the lumbosacral junction than investigate the other segments of the lumbar spine. One analysis of the region identifies 114 individual muscle units capable of exerting unique forces on the lumbosacral junction [25]. Sophisticated analytical tools and many simplifying assumptions beyond the scope of this book are required to solve for the muscle and joint forces in this **indeterminate system,** a system with more unknowns than equations to solve.

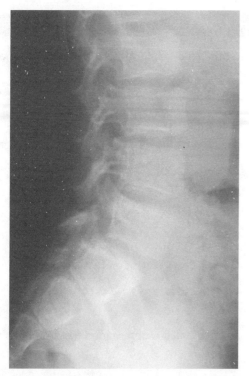

Figure 37.1: Spondylolisthesis of L5 on S1. Radiograph shows that L5 has slipped anteriorly on S1.

(Chapter 1 provides a brief overview of the approaches to solving indeterminate systems.) The following is a greatly simplified analytic model to examine the forces on the pelvis.

Two-Dimensional Example of the Analysis of Forces on the Pelvis

Examining the Forces Box 37.1 presents a two-dimensional analysis of the forces on the lumbosacral junction. This example uses the assumption that all of the muscular and ligamentous forces can be lumped together into a single muscle, M. Because this assumption undoubtedly is false, the results derived from this analysis are, at best, rough estimates of the real loads sustained by the region and probably underestimate the true reaction forces.

The simplified model in Examining the Forces Box 37.1 estimates loads in the single extensor muscle to be approximately 1.12 times body weight, and compressive and shear forces of 1,305 N and 379 N (293 and 85 lb), respectively. These loads are well below the loads to failure reported for the lumbar spine in Chapter 34. However, these loads are generated by lifting a small load (10% body weight) while bending the knees.

Because the L5–S1 junction is so prone to disc lesions and to spondylolisthesis, it is useful to consider what factors might

EXAMINING THE FORCES BOX 37.1

SIMPLIFIED TWO-DIMENSIONAL ANALYSIS OF THE LOADS ON THE LUMBOSACRAL JUNCTION

What are the loads on the lumbosacral junction for a 120-lb (534 N) woman who bends to pick up a 12-lb load (10% of her body weight)? To solve this problem using the basic mechanical tools described in Chapter 1, the muscles and ligaments supporting the lumbosacral region are lumped into a single extensor muscle [26], although Chapter 34 clearly demonstrates that many muscles and ligaments participate together to support the low back during bending activities.

The static equilibrium conditions used to solve this question are

$$\Sigma M = 0$$
$$\Sigma F_X = 0$$
$$\Sigma F_Y = 0$$

The following anthropometric quantities are found in the literature [7,16]:

Weight of the head, arms, and trunk (HAT) is approximately 69% of body weight = 320.4 N

Center of gravity of the HAT weight is approximately 60% of the length from hip joint to top of the head = 0.46 m

Moment arm of the single equivalent extensor muscle = 0.065 m

Angle of flexion of the trunk = 30°

Angle between the plane of the lumbosacral junction and the transverse plane = 30°

Using the static equilibrium equations, first calculate the equivalent extensor muscle force.

$$\Sigma M = 0$$

53.4 N × (0.48 m × sin 30°) + 320.4 N × (0.46 × sin 30°) − (M × 0.065 m) = 0

12.8 Nm + 73.6 Nm = M × (0.065 m)

M = 1132 N, or 1.12 times body weight

Once the muscle force is known, the joint reaction forces at the lumbosacral junction can be determined. A coordinate system oriented in the fifth lumbar vertebra allows direct calculation of the compression and shear forces on L5. The shear forces lie parallel to the

(continued)

EXAMINING THE FORCES BOX 37.1 (Continued)

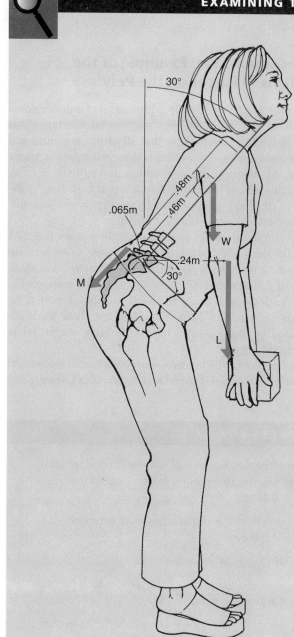

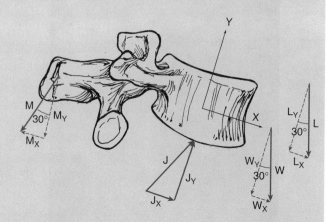

x axis, and the compression forces lie parallel to the y axis.

The shear force on L5 is determined by the following:

$\Sigma F_X = 0$

$J_X - M_X + L_X + W_X = 0$

$J_X - (M \times \sin 30°) + (L \times \sin 30°) + (W \times \sin 30°) = 0$

$J_X - 566\ N + 26.7\ N + 160.2\ N = 0$

$J_X = 379.1\ N$ or approximately 0.71 times body weight

The compression force on L5 is determined by the following:

$\Sigma F_Y = 0$

$J_Y - M_Y - L_Y - W_Y = 0$

$J_Y - (M \times \cos 30°) - (L \times \cos 30°) - (W \times \cos 30°) = 0$

$J_Y - 981\ N - 46.3\ N - 277.8\ N = 0$

$J_Y = 1305.1\ N$, or approximately 2.44 times body weight

increase the compressive or shear forces to dangerous levels. The compressive load is primarily a function of the muscle force needed to support the junction (*Fig. 37.2*). Any increase in the externally applied moment necessitates an increase in muscle force. Picking up a larger load increases the external moment, as does lifting a small load while holding it farther from the body, which increases the moment arm of the load (*Fig. 37.3*). Both cases require increased muscle force, leading to larger compressive forces at the lumbosacral junction.

The orientation of the lumbosacral junction also affects the magnitude of the compression and shear forces because the compression force is approximately perpendicular to the bodies of L5 and S1, and the shear forces are parallel to the plane between the bodies of L5 and S1. Shear forces appear to be more dangerous than compressive loads on the spine. Because the plane of the lumbosacral junction usually is oriented at a larger angle from the horizontal than the rest of the lumbar spine, the lumbosacral junction is particularly susceptible to anterior shear forces [20] (*Fig. 37.4*). As the angle between the plane of the vertebral bodies and the transverse plane increases, the shear component of the weight of the head, arms, and trunk (HAT weight) and any lifted weight also increases.

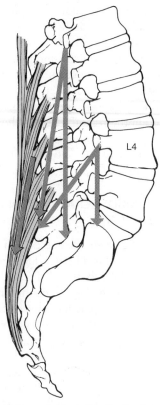

Figure 37.2: Several muscles crossing the lumbosacral junction contract simultaneously during activity, increasing the compressive force on the junction.

Slouched sitting posture also appears to increase the anterior shear forces on the lumbosacral junction when the backrest pushes the HAT weight anteriorly as the sacrum rotates posteriorly (*Fig. 37.5*) [21].

Clinical Relevance

SPONDYLOLISTHESIS: *Spondylolisthesis frequently is asymptomatic but may be painful, especially in active individuals [2,20]. Individuals with spondylolisthesis frequently report pain with increased activity, especially activities that use hyperextension of the low back. In contrast, many other patients with low back pain have increased pain with trunk flexion and report that lumbar extension relieves the symptoms. Although the cause of the back pain is frequently unclear, it is essential that the clinician identify the movements that exacerbate the symptoms and those that relieve the symptoms.*

Loads at the Lumbosacral Junction

There are few studies that specifically examine the loads on the lumbosacral joints during activity. Most of these studies use the same basic approach to calculate the forces in the muscles and ligaments and across the lumbosacral junction as demonstrated in Examining the Forces Box 37.1. However, these studies apply more-sophisticated

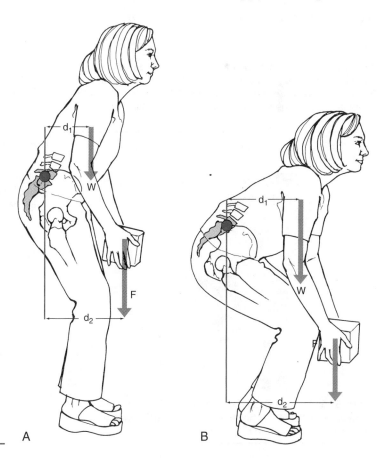

Figure 37.3: A. The external moment (M_{EXT}) on the lumbosacral junction is the sum of the moments due to the weight of the head, arms, and trunk *(W)* and the moment due to the load being lifted *(F)*. An increase in the magnitude of either W or F increases the external moment on the lumbosacral junction. **B.** An increase in the moment arm of the head, arms, and trunk weight *(d_1)* or the moment arm of the load *(d_2)* also increases the external moment (M_{EXT}) on the lumbosacral junction.

A   B

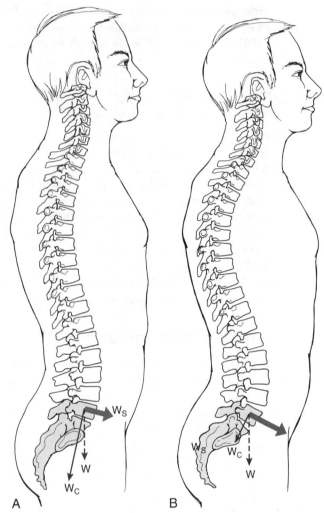

Figure 37.4: A. The anterior shear force component of the weight of the head, arms, and trunk *(W)* on the lumbosacral junction is parallel to the plane of the L5–S1 junction. **B.** As the inclination of the L5–S1 junction increases, the shear component also increases.

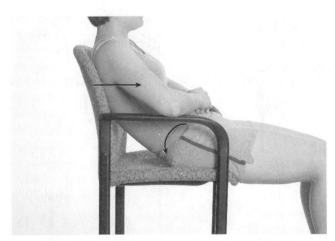

Figure 37.5: Anterior shear force on the lumbosacral joint. The backrest of the chair pushes the trunk anteriorly while the sacrum rotates posteriorly.

mathematical tools to derive more-accurate solutions and to estimate the loads in the individual muscles and ligaments [1,6,17,26]. It is important, however, to recognize that even these studies require simplifying assumptions, and the outcomes from these calculations depend on the accuracy of the assumptions [1,17,26]. Consequently, current studies yield only general approximations of the loads actually generated in the region. Despite the limitations of these studies, their results offer clinicians an insight into the demands of some activities and help clinicians to identify strategies to minimize a patient's complaints.

LOADS IN THE LUMBOSACRAL REGION DURING BENDING AND LIFTING

Peak joint moments between 200 and 250 Nm are reported at the lumbosacral joint while lifting or lowering 10- to 15-kg loads (approximately 22–33 lb) [6,17]. These data are consistent with loads in the lumbar spine reported in Chapter 34. Models that report the joint reaction force on the joint center of the lumbosacral junction show more variability. Estimates of compressive loads on the disc range from 1,200 N (270 lb) to more than 5,500 N (1,236 lb) [1,26,27]. Reported peak anterior shear forces range from approximately 400 to 1200 N (90–270 lb) [26]. Calculations of the joint moments and forces depend on the assumptions made in the model, including the size of the trunk and pelvis, the shape of the lumbar curve, and the muscles and ligaments included in the model as well as the movements of the spine that are studied [1,26]. Additional studies are needed to provide a more precise estimate of the loads sustained by the lumbosacral junction.

Peak compression loads on the lumbar spine reported in Chapter 34 are over 7,000 N (1573 lb) when lifting a 27-kg force (60 lb). However, in the lumbar spine, lifting with the lumbar spine flexed greatly increases the anterior shear forces by inhibiting the contraction of the extensor muscles (see video from Chapter 34). Because spondylolisthesis is a common occurrence at the L5–S1 junction and may produce symptomatic back pain in some individuals, clinicians need similar studies that examine the effects of posture and bending technique on the shear forces on the lumbosacral joint to guide intervention and prevention strategies.

LOADS ON THE LUMBOSACRAL JOINT DURING WALKING

Average peak compression forces at the lumbosacral joint range from 1.7 to 2.52 times body weight, and anterior shear forces range from 0.22 to 0.33 times body weight during preferred speed walking [3,13]. The resultant forces on the lumbosacral facet joints, while smaller than the loads on the disc, are approximately 1.5 times body weight [3]. The reaction forces on both the disc and facet joints peak during the double limb support phases of gait, when the pelvis is tilted anteriorly [15,24] *(Fig. 37.6)*. Because anterior pelvic tilt is associated with an increase in lumbar joint extension (increased lumbar lordosis), trunk hyperextension appears

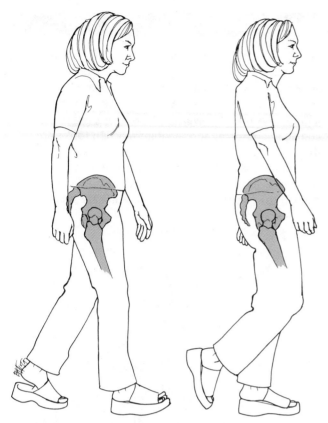

Figure 37.6: During gait, the pelvis is tilted anteriorly more at double limb support than during single limb support.

to increase loads on the L5–S1 junction, which may help explain why some patients report increased low back pain with walking.

FORCES SUSTAINED AT THE SACROILIAC JOINTS

Forces on the sacroiliac joint are even less well studied than those on the lumbosacral junction. Because the joint appears to allow at least small movements, an appreciation of the forces exerted across the joint may improve the clinician's understanding of the pathomechanics of sacroiliac joint dysfunction [11,22].

Overview of the Analytical Model of the Sacroiliac Joint

Like all of the biomechanical analyses demonstrated throughout this text, analysis of the forces at the sacroiliac joint begins with a free-body diagram. The free-body diagram of the sacroiliac joint is complicated by the fact that so many structures affecting the joint actually have no attachment on either the ilium or sacrum. To assist in identifying the relevant loads during single limb stance, the sacrum is considered a part of a rigid body including the head, arms, trunk and non-weight-bearing lower extremity, and the ilium

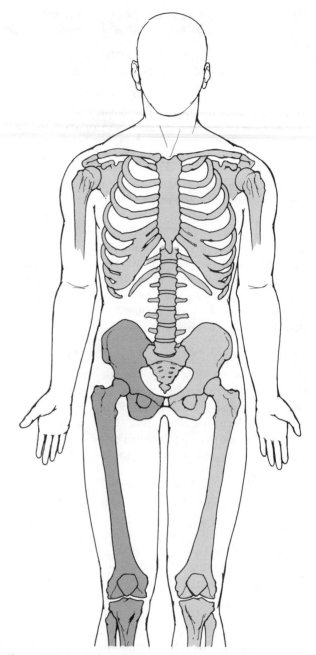

Figure 37.7: To analyze the forces on the sacroiliac joint, it is useful to view the body as two segments, the ilium with the weight-bearing limb and the sacrum with the head, arms, trunk, and the non-weight-bearing lower extremity.

as part of a rigid body including the pelvis and lower extremity on the weight bearing side [8] (*Fig. 37.7*). Determination of the forces on the pelvis in such a model requires the inclusion of hip and trunk muscles as well as pelvic ligaments and the ground reaction force, leading to another indeterminate system, with many more unknowns than equations to solve. Models of the sacroiliac joint report up to approximately 100 unknowns [8,28]. Because the sacroiliac joint exhibits complex three-dimensional motion, a two-dimensional model is insufficient to even approximate the mechanics of the joint [11,22]. *Examining the Forces Box 37.2* outlines the basic

EXAMINATION OF THE FORCES ON THE SACROILIAC JOINT DURING STANCE ON ONE LEG

To consider the forces on the innominate bone of the sacroiliac joint, the lower extremity and innominate bone are lumped together as a single rigid body. Forces on this rigid body are depicted in the free body diagram.

Using the static equilibrium conditions to solve this question yields the following equations:

$$\Sigma M_X = 0 = \Sigma F_{mus\,i} \times ma_{mus\,i} + \Sigma M_{EXT\,x}$$

where $F_{mus\,i}$ is the force in each muscle and ligament, $ma_{mus\,i}$ is the moment arm for that force (i.e., the perpendicular distance between the force and the point of rotation in the y-z plane), and $M_{EXT\,x}$ is the external moments about the x axis applied by the segment weights and ground reaction force.

$$\Sigma M_Y = 0 = \Sigma F_{mus\,i} \times ma_{mus\,i} + \Sigma M_{EXTy}$$

where $F_{mus\,i}$ is the force in each muscle and ligament, $ma_{mus\,i}$ is the moment arm for that force (i.e., the perpendicular distance between the force and the point of rotation in the x-z plane), and M_{EXTy} is the external moments about the y axis applied by the segment weights and ground reaction force.

$$\Sigma M_Z = 0 = \Sigma F_{mus\,i} \times ma_{mus\,i} + \Sigma M_{EXT\,z}$$

where $F_{mus\,i}$ is the force in each muscle and ligament, $ma_{mus\,i}$ is the moment arm for that force (i.e., the perpendicular distance between the force and the point of rotation in the x-y plane) and $M_{EXT\,z}$ is the external moments about the Z axis applied by the segment weights and ground reaction force.

$$\Sigma F_X = 0 = \Sigma F_{mus\,ix} + G_X + J_X$$

where $F_{mus\,ix}$ is the force of each muscle and ligament in the x direction, G_X is the ground reaction force in the x direction, and J_X is the joint reaction force in the x direction.

$$\Sigma F_Y = 0 = \Sigma F_{mus\,iy} + G_Y + J_Y$$

where $F_{mus\,iy}$ is the force of each muscle and ligament in the y direction, G_Y is the ground reaction force in the y direction, W is the weights of the segments that all act in the y direction, and J_Y is the joint reaction force in the y direction.

$$\Sigma F_Z = 0 = \Sigma F_{mus\,iz} + G_Z + J_{Z'}$$

where $F_{mus\,iz}$ is the force of each muscle and ligament in the z direction, G_Z is the ground reaction force in the z direction, and J_Z is the joint reaction force in the z direction.

Knowing the anatomy of the structure through the use of various imaging techniques allows measurement of all of the relevant moment arms. Force plates in the ground measure the ground reaction forces, and limb segment weights are available. Therefore, the muscle and ligament forces and the joint reaction forces are the only unknowns in the equations. However, there are still too many unknowns to be solved by these six equations. Techniques briefly described in Chapter 1 are needed to solve this **statically indeterminate** system.

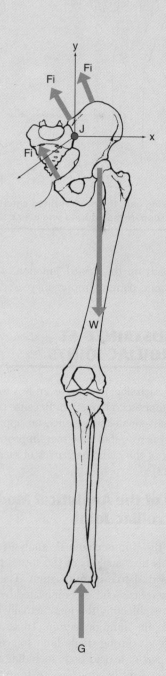

three-dimensional problem to solve for sacroiliac joint forces and the forces in the surrounding muscles and ligaments, but complete analysis is beyond the scope of this book.

Clinical Relevance

STANDING HIP FLEXION TEST FOR SACROILIAC DYSFUNCTION: *One test for dysfunction of the sacroiliac joint complex requires the patient to stand on one leg and flex the opposite hip, bringing the knee toward the chest. A normal response to the test is a posterior rotation of the ilia on the sacrum. A positive response for possible sacroiliac joint complex dysfunction is pain in the area of the sacroiliac joint on the stance side. Motion analysis during the test reveals that patients with pain associated with the sacroiliac joint complex often demonstrate an anterior rotation of the ilium on the sacrum on the weight-bearing side [10]. This test applies the principles of loading at the sacroiliac joint to test the stability of the joint. Single limb stance applies enormous loads through the sacroiliac joint, requiring large stabilizing forces from surrounding ligaments and joints. An inability to maintain stability during single limb stance may be a contributing factor to the patient's complaints.*

Sacroiliac Joint Forces from the Literature

Loads on the sacroiliac joint between 0.85 and 1.1 times body weight are reported for static single leg stance [8]. Forces on the sacroiliac joint over four times body weight are reported at the end of single limb support during gait [4]. Walking requires more muscle activity than static single limb stance, and it is consistent that the calculations show that the sacroiliac joint sustains larger loads during ambulation. Authors report the need for muscular activity and large muscle forces to stabilize the sacroiliac joint during function [14,18,19,22,23,28]. The extensor muscles that attach close to the sacroiliac joint appear to help support the low back and generate forces of more than 6,500 N (1,430 lb) [14]. Although only a few studies examine forces at the sacroiliac joint, the joints appear to sustain large loads, which may contribute to sacroiliac joint dysfunction in some individuals.

MECHANICS OF PELVIC FRACTURES

Most pelvic fractures occur from motor vehicle accidents, usually from side impacts [5]. Lateral impacts load the pelvis through the acetabulum after the lateral aspect of the femur, typically the greater trochanter, is hit. The site of the resulting pelvic fracture(s) depends on the velocity of the impact as well as the magnitude of the force applied. The importance of impact velocity is consistent with the mechanical properties of bone described in Chapter 3, which reports

that bone strength and elasticity depend on the rate at which the bone is loaded. A force of approximately 8,600 N (1,933 lb) applied at a rate consistent with a car traveling about 25 miles per hour produces a fracture of the pubic ramus on the side opposite the impact. More-extensive fractures and even dislocations of the sacroiliac joints and pubic symphysis can result from higher loading rates or greater impact forces. Automotive engineers can use these data to design safety systems such as restraint systems and air bag devices to reduce the injuries sustained in motor vehicle accidents. These data also help practitioners appreciate the extent of trauma that may be sustained by individuals in motor vehicle accidents.

Although acute pelvic fractures are the most common pelvic fracture, stress fractures of the pelvis also occur [9,12]. Fractures of the pubic ramus, usually the inferior ramus, are reported in female military recruits and are associated with the use of an unnaturally long stride, particularly by shorter women and women who train with men [9,12]. Bone density, fitness level, and menses do not appear to predict pelvic fractures, but African American women exhibit stress fractures less frequently than Caucasian women do. Pelvic stress fractures occur most frequently in the narrowest part of the pubic ramus and may be the culmination of repeated loads from the adductor muscles during the gait cycle.

Clinical Relevance

STRESS FRACTURES OF THE PELVIS: *Symptoms of pelvic stress fractures include groin pain, which is also a common symptom in individuals with chronic hip dysfunction. Practitioners may need to consider the presence of pelvic stress fractures in small women, particularly Caucasian women, with complaints of groin pain and who exhibit no direct signs of hip dysfunction. A history of repeated loading, such as running, also is relevant.*

SUMMARY

This chapter examines the loads sustained by the pelvis during single limb stance and during impact loading. An accurate analysis of the loads on the pelvis requires a more sophisticated analysis than that presented in this text, but this chapter reviews the basic application of static equilibrium equations to determine the loads at the lumbosacral junction and at the sacroiliac joints. Estimates of the compressive loads on the lumbosacral junction are as high as 5,500 N (1,236 lb), with estimated shear forces up to 1,200 N (270 lb). Normal walking also produces loads of more than two times body weight at the lumbosacral junction. Forces greater than four times body weight are reported at the sacroiliac joint during gait. High-impact loads such as those incurred during motor vehicle accidents can produce pelvic fractures as well as dislocations of the joints of the pelvis. The pelvis also sustains stress fractures, particularly in Caucasian women with low body mass.

This three-chapter unit on the mechanics of the pelvis completes the discussion of the spine. This unit has repeatedly noted that the pelvis transmits the weight of the head, arms, and trunk to the lower extremities. The following unit on the hip begins the discussion of the lower extremity.

References

1. Anderson CK, Chaffin DB, Herrin GD, Matthews LS: A biomechanical model of the lumbosacral joint during lifting activities. J Biomech 1985; 18: 571–584.
2. Canale ST: Campbell's operative orthopaedics. Philadelphia: Mosby, 1998.
3. Cheng CK, Chen HH, Chen CS, Lee SJ: Influences of walking speed change on the lumbosacral joint force distribution. Biomed Mater Eng 1998; 8: 155–165.
4. Dalstra M, Huiskes R: Load transfer across the pelvic bone. J Biomech 1995; 28: 715–724.
5. Dawson JM, Khmelniker BV, McAndrew MP: Analysis of the structural behavior of the pelvis during lateral impact using the finite element method. Accid Anal Prev 1999; 31: 109–119.
6. de Looze MP, Toussaint HM, van Dieen JH, Kemper HCG: Joint moments and muscle activity in the lower extremities and lower back in lifting and lowering tasks. J Biomech 1993; 26: 1067–1076.
7. Dempster WT: Space requirements of the seated operator. geometrical, kinematic, and mechanical aspects of the body with special reference to the limbs. In: Krogman WM, Johnston FE, eds. Human Mechanics. Philadelphia: Aerospace Medical Division, 1963; 215–340.
8. Goel VK, Svensson NL: Forces on the pelvis. J Biomech 1977; 10: 195–200.
9. Hill PF, Chatterji S, Chambers D, Keeling JD: Stress fracture of the pubic ramus in female recruits. J Bone Joint Surg [Br] 1996; 78–B: 383–386.
10. Hungerford B, Gilleard W, Lee D: Altered patterns of pelvic bone motion determined in subjects with posterior pelvic pain using skin markers. Clin Biomech 2004; 19: 456–464.
11. Jacob HAC, Kissling RO: The mobility of the sacroiliac joints in healthy volunteers between 20 and 50 years of age. Clin Biomech 1995; 10: 352–361.
12. Kelly EW, Jonson SR, Cohen ME, Shaffer R: Stress fracture of the pelvis in female navy recruits: an analysis of possible mechanisms of injury. Milit Med 2000; 165: 142–146.
13. Khoo BCC, Goh JCH, Bose K: A biomedical model to determine lumbosacral loads during single stance phase in normal gait. Med Eng Phys 1995; 17: 27–35.
14. McGill SM: A biomechanical perspective of sacro-iliac pain. Clin Biomech 1987; 2: 145–151.
15. Murray MP: Gait as a total pattern of movement. Am J Phys Med 1967; 48: 290–333.
16. Nemeth G, Ohlsen H: Moment arm lengths of trunk muscles to the lumbosacral joint obtained in vivo with compute tomography. Spine 1986; 11: 158–160.
17. Plamondon A, Gagnon M, Gravel D: Moments at the L5/S1 joint during asymmetrical lifting: effects of different load trajectories and initial load positions. Clin Biomech 1995; 10: 128–136.
18. Pool-Goudzwaard A, Hoek van Dijke G, van Gurp M, et al.: Contribution of pelvic floor muscles to stiffness of the pelvic ring. Clin Biomech 2004; 19: 564–571.
19. Richardson CA, Snijders CJ, Hides JA, et al.: The relation between the transversus abdominis muscles, sacroiliac joint mechanics, and low back pain. Spine 2002; 27: 399–405.
20. Salter RB: Textbook of Disorders and Injuries of the Musculoskeletal System. 3rd ed. Baltimore: Williams & Wilkins, 1999.
21. Snijders CJ, Hermans PFG, Niesing R, et al.: The influence of slouching and lumbar support on iliolumbar ligaments, intervertebral discs and sacroiliac joints. Clin Biomech 2004; 19: 323–329.
22. Snijders CJ, Ribbers MTLM, de Bakker HV, et al.: EMG recordings of abdominal and back muscles in various standing postures: validation of a biomechanical model on sacroiliac joint stability. J Electromyogr Kinesiol 1998; 8: 205–214.
23. Snijders CJ, Vleeming A, Stoeckart R: Transfer of lumbosacral load to iliac bones and legs part 2: loading of the sacroiliac joints when lifting in a stooped posture. Clin Biomech 1993; 8: 295–301.
24. Sutherland DH, Kaufman KR, Moitoza JR: Kinematics of normal human walking. In: Rose J, Gamble JG, eds. Human Walking. Philadelphia: Williams & Wilkins, 1981; 23–44.
25. van Dieen JH: Are recruitment patterns of the trunk musculature compatible with a synergy based on the maximization of endurance? J Biomech 2001; 30: 1095–1100.
26. van Dieen JH, de Looze MP: Sensitivity of single-equivalent extensor muscle models to anatomical and functional assumptions. J Biomech 1999; 32: 195–198.
27. van Dieen JH, Kingma I: Total trunk muscle force and spinal compression are lower in asymmetric moments as compared to pure extension moments. J Biomech 1999; 32: 681–687.
28. Van Dijke GAH, Snijders CJ, Stoeckart R, Stam HJ: A biomedical model on muscle forces in the transfer of spinal load to the pelvis and legs. J Biomech 1999; 32: 927–933.

Kinesiology of the Lower Extremity

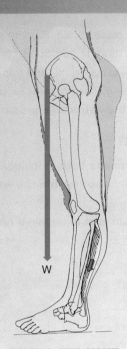

W

UNIT 6: HIP UNIT

UNIT 7: KNEE UNIT

UNIT 8: ANKLE AND FOOT UNIT

The hip marks the proximal end of the lower extremity, whose primary functions are weight bearing and locomotion. Consequently, all of the joints of the lower extremity, including the hip joint, commonly function with the foot in contact with the ground, participating in a **closed chain.** In a closed chain, movement of any segment of the chain produces movement in other links of the chain. Hip position and muscular control at the hip often depend on the location and movement of the trunk on the lower extremity rather than on the movement of the femur on the pelvis.

The functional requirements of the hip itself are quite varied. It is the most mobile joint of the lower extremity, allowing such extreme positions as standing and squatting. In addition to mobility, however, the hip must also possess sufficient stability to support the weight of the head, arms, trunk, and opposite lower extremity during single limb stance and dynamic activities such as walking and jumping. The hip joint successfully combines these seemingly conflicting functions of mobility and stability by its unique bony structure and surrounding soft tissue.

The purposes of the three chapters on the hip are to

- Demonstrate how the structures of the hip promote both mobility and stability
- Discuss how the muscles of the hip move it and also stabilize the weight of the head, arms, and trunk on the hip joint
- Examine how alterations in these structures can lead to impaired function and deleterious loads on the hip and neighboring structures

Structure and Function of the Bones and Noncontractile Elements of the Hip

CHAPTER CONTENTS

This chapter examines the bony structure of the hip and the connective tissues that stabilize it and protect it during movement and weight-bearing activities. The purposes of this chapter are to

- Investigate details of the hip's bony structure to understand how specific characteristics contribute to the stability and mobility of the hip joint
- Study the noncontractile supporting structures of the hip to understand their effects on its stability and mobility
- Examine the normal ranges of motion (ROMs) available at the hip
- Examine the relative alignment of the pelvis and femur and consider its contributions to normal and abnormal mechanics of the hip
- Compare the structure and function of the hip and the glenohumeral joint, its counterpart in the upper extremity

STRUCTURE OF THE BONES OF THE HIP

The hip is composed of two large bones, the innominate bone of the pelvis and the femur. Each of these bones is discussed individually below.

Innominate Bone

The innominate bone contributes the proximal articular surface of the hip. The two innominate bones together form the bony pelvis. The details of the bony pelvis are presented in Chapter 35. For the purposes of the present chapter, the discussion of the innominate bone is limited to those factors that directly apply to the hip. Thus the acetabulum, providing the proximal articular surface of the hip, is discussed in detail.

Located on the lateral aspect of the innominate bone, the acetabulum comprises the Y-shaped junction of the ilium, ischium, and pubis, which forms a deep, spherical socket that holds the head of the femur (*Fig. 38.1*). The orientation of the acetabulum influences the mobility of the hip and the location of weight-bearing forces on the femoral head. An anterior view of the pelvis reveals that the acetabulum faces laterally and slightly inferiorly (*Fig. 38.2*). A superior view of the pelvis demonstrates that the acetabulum also faces anteriorly.

The superior aspect, or roof, of the acetabulum is formed by the ilium, the anterior aspect by the pubis, and the posterior wall by the ischium. The deepest portion of the acetabulum, known as the floor, or acetabular fossa, is rough and nonarticular. The articular, or lunate, surface of the acetabulum consists of a horseshoe-shaped rim ringing the acetabular fossa on its anterior, superior, and posterior aspects [66]. The rim is incomplete inferiorly, leaving a gap between the

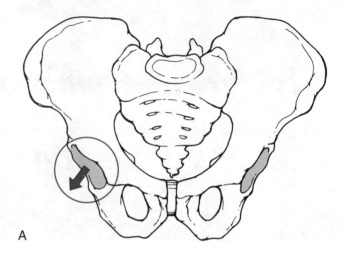

A

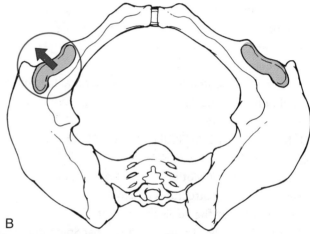

B

Figure 38.2: Orientation of the acetabulum. **A.** Anterior view of the pelvis shows that the acetabulum faces laterally and inferiorly. **B.** Superior view of the pelvis shows that the acetabulum faces anteriorly.

anterior and posterior segments. A transverse acetabular ligament spans the gap, completing the acetabular rim.

The floor of the acetabulum consists of a thin shelf of bone that may be no more than 2–4 mm thick [21]. The density of the subchondral bone increases in the periphery of the acetabulum and appears to peak in the acetabular roof and in the anterior and posterior extremes of the articular surface [47,68]. These variations in bony thickness reflect Wolff's law, which states that a bone's structure responds to the loads placed on it [6]. Weight bearing at the hip joint involves the thicker superior and peripheral aspects of the acetabulum, while the thin, central, deepest part of the socket is unsuited for weight bearing [6,27,68]. Well-organized arrays of trabecular bone surrounding the acetabulum, but particularly superior to it, reinforce the weight-bearing capacity of the socket [44].

A fibrocartilaginous ring, or labrum, deepens the acetabulum, which helps to stabilize the hip joint, increase contact

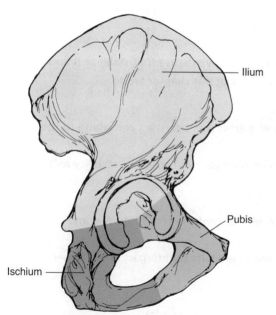

Ilium

Pubis

Ischium

Figure 38.1: The acetabulum is formed by the three bones of the innominate bone, the ilium, ischium, and pubis.

area, and decrease joint stress [8]. These functions are fulfilled while avoiding a loss of mobility since the increased surface area is a compressible ring. Additionally the acetabular labrum appears to seal a pressurized layer of synovial fluid that may protect the articular surfaces from damage [14]. Although magnetic resonance imaging (MRI) of individuals without known hip pathology reveals considerable variability in labral shape and length, and some individuals without hip pain appear to lack some portions of the labrum, labral tears are a recognized source of hip pain [8,37,43]. Labral tears may not only contribute directly to joint pain but also may destabilize the joint and allow increased stress on the articular surfaces, eventually leading to degenerative joint changes [14,31,37].

Clinical Relevance

ACETABULAR LABRAL TEARS: *Labral tears in the hip are a suspected cause of pain in many individuals with chronic hip pain (Fig. 38.3). Frank trauma or repetitive microtrauma from repeated twisting or pivoting motions are likely mechanisms of labral tears. Athletes participating in sports such as soccer or golf are particularly susceptible to labral tears. However, clinical diagnosis is difficult. Suggestive findings include pain with active or passive hip flexion, medial rotation and adduction, and clicking in the hip with these motions. Magnetic resonance arthrography (MRA) has better sensitivity (66–95%) and specificity (71–88%) than clinical tests, but arthroscopic surgery remains the most reliable diagnostic procedure [37,43].*

The relative depth of the acetabulum with its labrum changes during fetal development and early childhood [55]. The ratio of depth to diameter of the acetabulum is greatest in utero and least at or around the time of birth; it gradually increases again throughout childhood. The shallow acetabulum at birth is an important risk factor for congenital hip dislocation. By adulthood, the acetabulum without the labrum is slightly less than a hemisphere [29].

Femur

The femur, normally the largest bone of the body, is composed of a head, neck, and shaft, or body, which ends distally in the femoral condyles. This chapter discusses only those attributes of the femur that apply to the hip, specifically, the head, neck, and proximal end of the body of the femur. The remainder of the femur is discussed in Chapter 41 with the knee.

The head of the femur provides the distal articular surface of the hip joint (*Fig. 38.4*). The head of the femur in the adult forms approximately two thirds of a sphere, although its surface is not actually perfectly spherical. The articular cartilage on the femoral head provides a more spherical shape to the articular surface. Even the healthy femoral head looks slightly flattened on x-ray since the articular cartilage is not visualized by standard x-ray [21]. The femoral head is covered with articular cartilage throughout its surface, with the exception of a small pit (fovea of the head of the femur) on its posteromedial aspect where the ligamentum teres attaches. The articular cartilage of the femoral head is thickest centrally and thins at the periphery of the head [21,29,33].

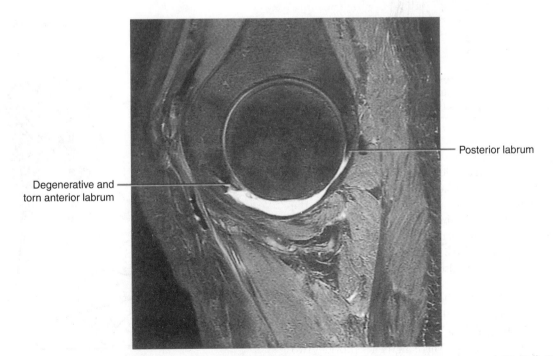

Degenerative and torn anterior labrum

Posterior labrum

Figure 38.3: A magnetic resonance arthrogram shows a labral tear at the hip. (Reprinted from "Arthropscopy, vol. 21, Kelly BT, Weiland DE, Schenker ML, Philippon MJ: Arthroscopic labral repair in the hip: surgical technique and review of the literature, 1496–1504, 2005, with permission from Arthroscopy Association of North America.)

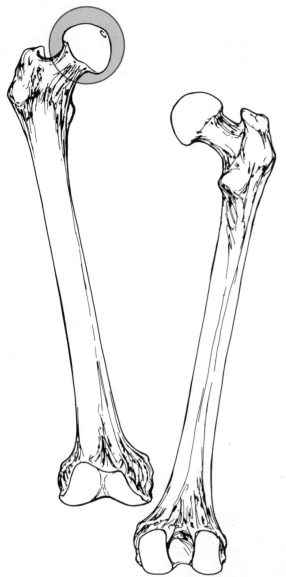

Figure 38.4: The head of the femur forms approximately two thirds of a sphere, although its surface is not perfectly spherical.

The articular cartilage of the femoral head and of the acetabulum is among the thickest in the body. Reported thicknesses range from 0.7 to 3.6 mm, with the greatest thicknesses usually found in the anterosuperior aspect of the acetabulum [12,30]. The acetabular and femoral articular cartilage surfaces exhibit small incongruities in shape, thickness, and stiffness, which may facilitate cartilage lubrication and chondrogenesis. They may also contribute to degenerative changes of the articular cartilage [2,12].

Despite the small incongruities between the femoral head and acetabulum, the bones of the hip joint are generally congruent with each other, and the congruency is improved even more by the articular cartilage. This congruency provides two important benefits. First, the congruency allows larger areas of the joint to articulate with one another throughout the natural ROM of the hip. This means that the loads sustained during weight bearing can be spread across larger surface areas,

thus reducing the **stress** (force/area) the joint must withstand. Additionally, the congruency facilitates stability of the joint throughout the ROM.

The femoral neck extends laterally and posteriorly from the head of the femur and is almost entirely enclosed by the hip joint capsule. The orientation of the head and neck of the femur, like that of the acetabulum, influences hip excursion and weight bearing. An anterior view of the femur reveals that the femoral head faces medially and superiorly in the acetabulum (*Fig. 38.5*). In the frontal plane, the **angle of inclination** refers to the approximately 125° angle between the neck of the femur and the shaft of the femur. A transverse plane view demonstrates that the head of the femur projects anteriorly. The neck forms an angle of approximately 15° with the plane of the femoral condyles.

The femoral neck sustains large bending moments as well as tensile and compressive forces during weight bearing and is reinforced by thickened cortical bone and organized arrays of cancellous, or trabecular, bone [53]. Cancellous bone extends from the shaft of the femur to the neck and head of the femur in organized arrays within the intertrochanteric region and along the superior and inferior aspects of the neck. A medial array of cancellous bone extends from the medial cortex of the femoral shaft to the weight-bearing surface of the femoral head. Another bundle runs on the lateral aspect of the shaft from the base of the greater trochanter and femoral neck to the inferior aspect of the head of the femur (*Fig. 38.6*). The arrangement of cancellous bone in the femur also provides another graphic example of Wolff's law [6].

There are several landmarks on the femur, distal to the hip joint proper, that are relevant to the function of the hip

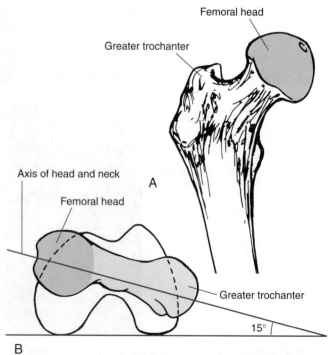

Figure 38.5: Orientation of the femoral head. **A.** Anterior view of the femur reveals that it faces medially and superiorly. **B.** Superior view of the femur reveals that it faces anteriorly.

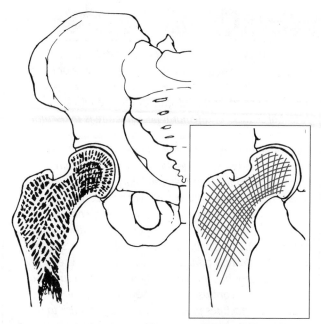

Figure 38.6: The trabecular bone in the proximal femur is highly organized to resist the loads on the femoral head and neck.

(*Fig. 38.7*). Several serve as attachments for muscles of the hip, and some are palpable, providing important landmarks during a physical examination. The base of the neck is distinguished from the shaft of the femur anteriorly by a roughened intertrochanteric line running distally and medially from greater to lesser trochanter. It continues as a spiral line, distal

and medial to the lesser trochanter, and proceeds posteriorly to form the medial lip of the linea aspera.

The greater trochanter is a large prominence on the proximal end of the femoral shaft. It has anterior, lateral, posterior, and superior surfaces and is readily palpable about a hand's length distance distal to the iliac crest. This significant protrusion of bone gives rise to several muscles, including the large gluteal muscles. The location of the greater trochanter distal to the femoral neck lengthens the moment arms of the attached muscles, improving their mechanical advantage to generate joint moments [25,51,60]. The lesser trochanter is posteromedial on the proximal femoral shaft and provides distal attachment for the iliopsoas tendon. Separating the two trochanters posteriorly is the intertrochanteric crest. At the proximal aspect of the crest is the quadrate tubercle. Distal to the crest and greater trochanter is the gluteal tuberosity, which continues distally to form the lateral lip of the linea aspera. Distal to the lesser trochanter, directed toward the medial lip of the linea aspera, is the pectineal line.

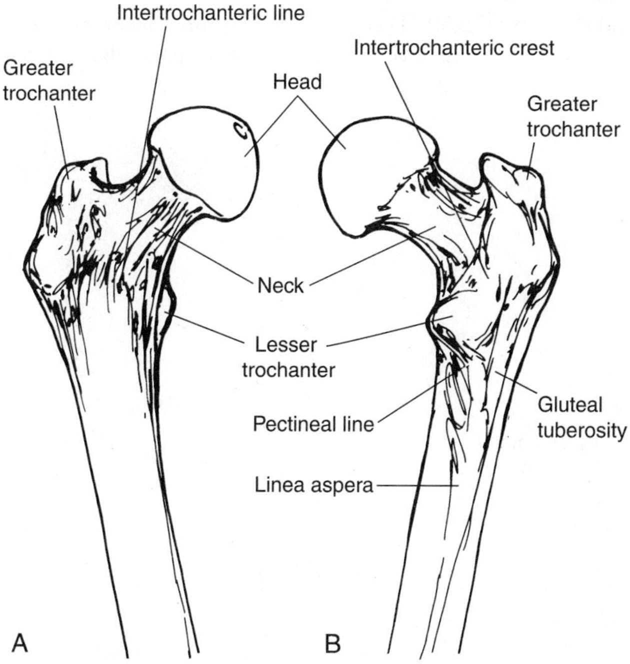

A clear image of each of the bones composing the hip is essential to understanding their relationship to each other as well as to developing the skills to perform a thorough and valid physical examination of the hip. The relevant palpable landmarks surrounding the hip are listed below:

- Anterior superior iliac crest
- Posterior superior iliac crest
- Ischial tuberosity
- Iliac crest
- Greater trochanter
- Greater sciatic notch

STRUCTURE OF THE HIP JOINT

The hip joint is a synovial, ball-and-socket, or triaxial, joint. To meet its antagonistic functions of stability and mobility, the hip has its own unique articular structures including its ligaments and fibrocartilaginous expansion, the labrum. The relative orientation of the proximal femur and acetabulum also influences the mobility and stability available at the hip joint. This section reviews the supporting structures of the hip and their effects on hip motion.

Joint Capsule

As a synovial joint, the hip is supported by a synovial capsule that is attached to the bony rim of the acetabulum proximally and to the intertrochanteric crest and line of the femur distally (*Fig. 38.8*). The capsule of the hip joint is composed primarily of fibers running parallel to its length, the longitudinal fibers. It also possesses a band of fibers oriented circumferentially around the center of the femoral neck [62,71]. This bundle is known as the zona orbicularis, or femoral arcuate ligament [23].

The capsule encloses most of the femoral neck and the entire femoral head. The blood supply to synovial joints is generally provided by a network of blood vessels, or anastomoses, at the attachment of the capsule and bone. The primary blood supply to the femoral head and neck arises from

Figure 38.7: A. Anterior view of the proximal femur reveals important landmarks including the head, neck, and greater and lesser trochanters. **B.** Posterior view of the proximal femur reveals the lesser and greater trochanters, intertrochanteric crest, gluteal tuberosity, pectineal line, and linea aspera.

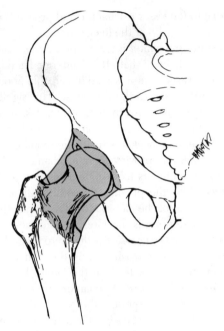

Figure 38.8: The hip joint capsule attaches to the acetabulum proximally and to the intertrochanteric crest and line distally.

the medial and lateral circumflex femoral arteries at the base of the femoral neck that then travel proximally within synovial folds of the capsule reflected onto the femoral neck [71]. Thus most of the vessels supplying the head of the femur must travel the length of the femoral neck to reach the femoral head. The femoral head does receive an artery within the ligament to the head of the femur that attaches to the floor of acetabulum and the pit of the head of the femur. However, anatomists believe that the essential blood supply to the femoral head originates at the base of the femoral neck [20,64].

Iliofemoral, Pubofemoral, and Ischiofemoral Ligaments

The hip joint capsule is reinforced anteriorly by three longitudinal bundles of fibers, the iliofemoral, ischiofemoral, and pubofemoral ligaments, the first two being the most consistent and strongest [22,59,71] (*Fig. 38.9*). The three ligaments originate on their respective bony parts of the acetabular rim and

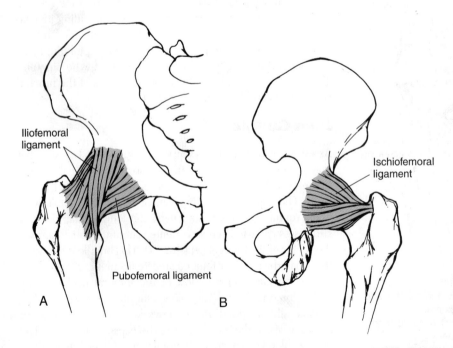

Iliofemoral ligament

Pubofemoral ligament

Ischiofemoral ligament

A   B

Figure 38.9: The iliofemoral, ischiofemoral, and pubofemoral ligaments reinforce the hip joint capsule anteriorly. **A.** Anterior view. **B.** Posterior view.

attach distally on the femur. The iliofemoral ligament arises not only from the iliac portion of the acetabulum but also from the anterior inferior iliac spine (AIIS). It proceeds in two parts along the anterior and superior aspects of the joint, creating the image of a Y, with its base directed toward the AIIS, and its top directed inferolaterally toward the intertrochanteric line. This ligament prevents excessive extension and lateral rotation ROM of the hip joint. In addition, the superior portion limits adduction ROM. The iliofemoral ligament appears to be the strongest ligament of the hip joint, sustaining larger tensile forces before rupturing [22].

The ischiofemoral ligament attaches to the ischial portion of the rim of the acetabulum. A portion of the ligament runs horizontally, reinforcing the capsule posteriorly. Another portion projects superiorly, spiraling over the superior aspect of the femoral neck to attach to the superior and medial aspects of the greater trochanter. These spiral fibers, like the iliofemoral and pubofemoral ligaments, limit excessive hyperextension. The posterior fibers limit medial rotation of the hip [22]. The ischiofemoral ligament also limits adduction ROM when the hip is flexed. The pubofemoral ligament originates from the pubic portion of the acetabular rim and from the superior pubic ramus. It extends along the inferior aspect of the capsule. It, too, limits excessive extension ROM. Additionally, it helps to prevent too much abduction ROM.

Additional Ligaments

The hip also contains an intraarticular ligament known as the ligament to the head of the femur, or ligamentum teres (*Fig. 38.10*). This ligament lies deep within the joint and runs from the acetabular fovea to the pit of the head of the femur.

The ligament carries a small artery from the acetabulum to the femoral head, but although the artery within this ligament may provide some blood supply to the femoral head, it is unlikely to be an adequate blood supply in the absence of arteries from the femoral neck. The ligament itself is believed to provide little mechanical support to the hip, especially in adults [48,59]. However, adaptive changes are reported in this ligament in individuals with avascular necrosis of the femoral head, suggesting that the ligament may bear more load and perhaps provide some support in such individuals [7].

In addition to the ligaments that span the hip joint, the transverse acetabular ligament (TAL) appears to provide some support during weight bearing. Lohe et al. note that the acetabular notch widens during weight bearing [39]. These authors report that the TAL sustains tensile forces as the notch widens. The functional significance of this finding is not known, but this ligament may provide increased shock absorption at the hip during weight bearing.

Hip Joint Stability

The hip is stabilized by its bony configuration and then by its strong capsular and reinforcing ligaments. These ligaments consist of longitudinal and circumferential fibers criss-crossing one another. This fiber arrangement allows the capsule to function much like a Chinese finger puzzle that, when stretched, clamps down on the structures within. As the hip is extended, the fibers of the capsule clamp down on the bony contents within, firmly holding the femoral head in the acetabulum (*Fig. 38.11*). In contrast, hip flexion slackens the joint capsule. Like the glenohumeral joint, the hip may gain additional stability from a negative intraarticular pressure [31].

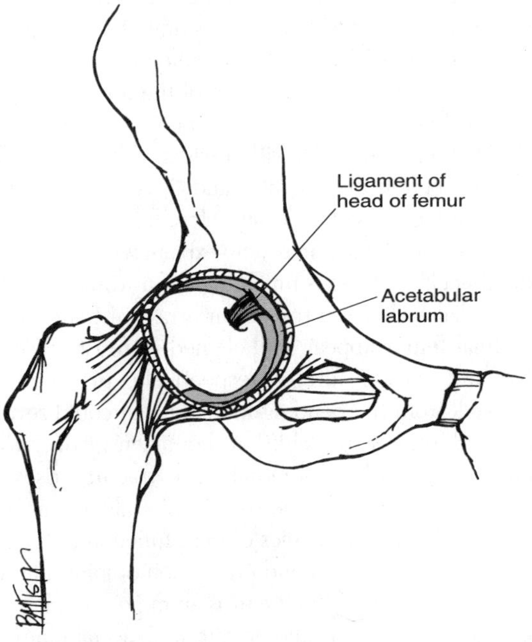

Figure 38.10: The ligament to the head of the femur arises from the floor of the acetabulum and attaches to the fovea on the head of the femur.

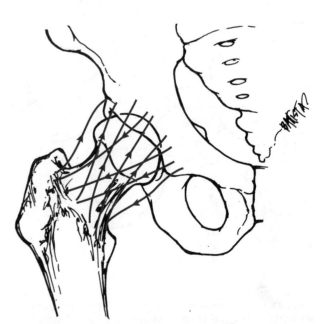

Figure 38.11: The fibers of the capsule and surrounding ligaments function like a Chinese finger puzzle, clamping down on the joint as the joint surfaces are distracted.

ALIGNMENT OF THE ARTICULATING SURFACES

The individual orientation of the acetabular and femoral components has already been described. It is now necessary to understand the relationship of these articulated structures in normal upright stance. This understanding allows investigation of the effects of common hip malalignments. In the normal erect posture, the acetabulum and femoral head are aligned so that the head of the femur is directed slightly anteriorly and superiorly in the acetabulum. This orientation exposes the anterior aspect of the femoral head, leaving a large articular surface available for movement toward flexion (*Fig. 38.12*). The

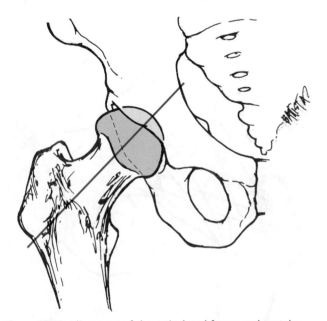

Figure 38.12: Alignment of the articulated femur and acetabulum in the anatomical position. Because the femur faces the anterior–superior aspect of the acetabulum and the acetabulum also faces anteriorly, the anterior surface of the head of the femur is exposed in the anatomical position.

orientation of the femur and acetabulum facilitates advancement of the thigh in front of the trunk (flexion), while limiting the potential for backward movement of the thigh beyond the trunk. Flexion and abduction of the hip move the femoral head toward the deepest part of the acetabulum.

Bony alignment of the femur and acetabulum also affects the loads applied to the hip joint and the rest of the lower extremity. The joint reaction force on the normal proximal femur during upright standing is more vertically aligned than the femoral neck, creating a bending moment on the head and neck of the femur [42,53,60]. The bending moment produces tensile forces on the superior aspect of the femoral neck and compressive forces on the inferior aspect of the neck [1,53] (*Fig. 38.14*). Femoral necks with a wider superior to inferior diameter are better able to withstand the bending moments sustained during weight bearing. Men have wider femoral necks than women, which may help explain why the incidence of femoral neck fractures is much higher in women [11,45].

The medial and lateral trabecular arrays of bone found in the proximal femur appear well aligned to resist these compressive and tensile forces, respectively, protecting the femoral neck from the bending moment that could sever the femoral head from the neck [42]. As bone density decreases in osteoporosis, the risk of femoral neck fracture rises [40]. Clinicians must appreciate the role of joint alignment on the mechanics and pathomechanics of joint function to intervene effectively in the treatment and prevention of joint injuries.

Intrinsic alignment of the femur is an important element in the relationship between the femur and acetabulum. The femoral head is directed toward the superior and anterior aspect of the acetabulum, resulting from the angle of inclination between the femoral neck and shaft in the frontal plane and the

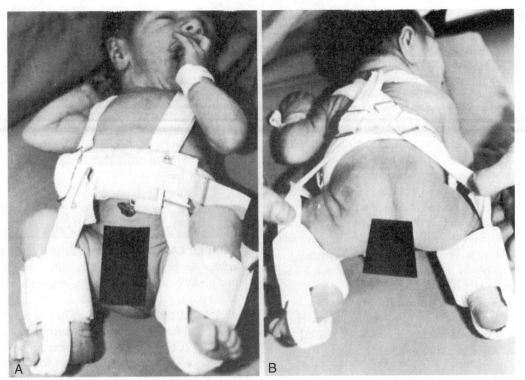

Figure 38.13: The Pavlik splint is one of a variety of splints designed to position the infant's hips in flexion and abduction to facilitate normal development of the femoral head and acetabulum. (From Tecklin JS: Pediatric Physical Therapy. Baltimore: Lippincott Williams & Wilkins, 1999)

transverse plane orientation of the femoral neck. As stated earlier, the angle of inclination is typically reported to be 125°. Yoshioka et al. report an average angle of 131° in a sample of 32 cadaver specimens [72]. A hip with an excessive frontal plane angle is said to have a **coxa valga deformity,** or valgus deformity of the hip (*Fig. 38.15*). This deformity directs the femoral head more superiorly in the acetabulum. Many biomechanical alterations appear to result from a coxa valga [34,42,53]. The

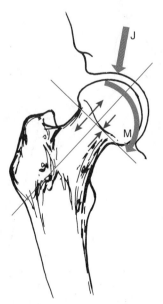

Figure 38.14: The joint reaction force on the femur (*J*) exerts a bending moment (*M*) on the neck of the femur, creating tensile forces on the superior surface of the femoral neck and compressive forces on its inferior surface.

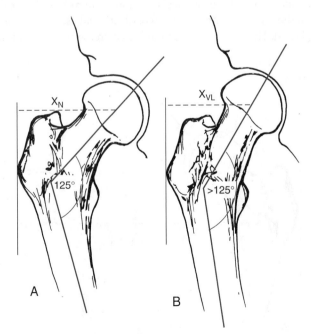

Figure 38.15: Frontal plane alignment of the hip. **A.** The angle of inclination in normal alignment is approximately 125–130°. **B.** In coxa valga, the angle of inclination is greater than normal.

joint reaction force on the femur is more parallel to the femoral neck in coxa valga. This alignment subjects the femoral neck to more compressive forces and less of a bending moment, which may explain why, in coxa valga, cancellous bone in the femoral neck appears to be arranged in columns parallel to the neck rather than in the medial and lateral intersecting bundles seen in well-aligned femora. The perpendicular distance between the hip joint center and the trochanter is decreased in coxa valga, putting the hip abductor muscles at a disadvantage by reducing their moment arm. With decreased moment arms, the hip abductor muscles must generate larger contractile forces to support the hip joint, resulting in increased joint reaction forces [25,60]. In addition, the joint reaction force is displaced laterally in the acetabulum and is applied over a smaller joint surface, leading to increased joint stress. In other words, coxa valga deformities are likely to increase the risk of degenerative joint disease within the hip by increasing the joint reaction force as well as the stress sustained by the femoral head.

In contrast, a **coxa vara deformity** is a decrease in the angle between the shaft and neck of the femur, increasing the bending moment applied to the femoral neck [29,42] (*Fig. 38.16*). The increased bending moment increases the compressive forces on the medial aspect of the femoral neck and the tensile forces laterally, leading to an increase in the medial and lateral trabecular arrays. In addition, a coxa vara deformity moves the trochanter farther from the joint center, effectively lengthening the moment arm of the hip abductors. This puts the hip abductors at a mechanical advantage and may actually reduce the force they are required to exert during stance, thus reducing the joint reaction force. Orthopaedic surgeons use the positive effect of altering the femoral neck alignment and improving the mechanical advantage of the abductor muscles in surgical osteotomies to reduce the loads on the hip for treatment of osteoarthritis and aseptic necrosis [17,25]. However, coxa vara tends to increase the medial pull

on the femur into the acetabulum, which may contribute to erosion of the acetabulum [35,42]. Additionally, an increased advantage for the abductor muscles may be accompanied by fatigue in the antagonist muscles [5]. The moment arm of the joint reaction force may also be increased with a net result of an increased bending moment on the femoral neck. Carpintero et al. suggest that coxa vara is a risk factor for stress fractures of the femoral neck [5]. All things considered, normal frontal plane alignment of approximately 125° appears to minimize the negative consequences of weight bearing on the healthy hip joint.

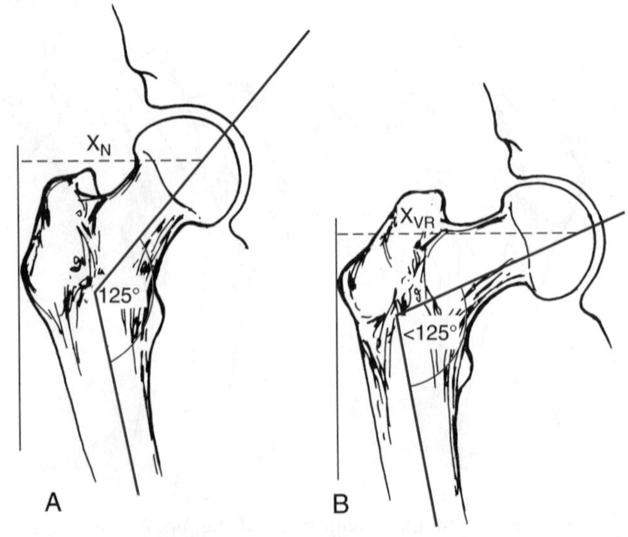

Clinical Relevance

SLIPPED CAPITAL FEMORAL EPIPHYSIS: *A slipped capital femoral epiphysis is a gradual or sudden inferior and posterior displacement of the epiphysis, or growth plate at the base of the femoral head [61]. The mechanisms producing a slipped capital epiphysis help to illustrate the changes in femoral loading with coxa valga and coxa vara (Fig. 38.17). Unlike the adult, the newborn possesses a femoral neck–shaft angle that is significantly larger than 125°. In other words, coxa valga is the "normal" alignment of the hip at birth. This valgus alignment gradually decreases to normal adult values throughout growth. During early development when the femoral neck has a maximum*

(continued)

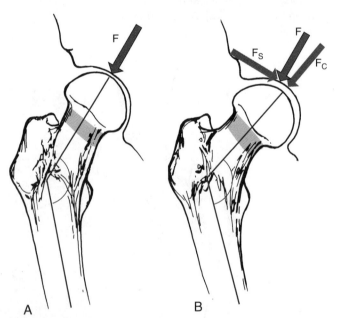

Figure 38.17: Mechanics of a slipped capital epiphysis. **A.** In the young child, the femur exhibits a coxa valga alignment normally, and the capital epiphysis is approximately perpendicular to the joint reaction force (F). **B.** As the child grows, the coxa valga decreases and the epiphysis is no longer perpendicular to the joint reaction force. In this case, the joint reaction force consists of both a compressive force (F_C) and a shear (F_S) force.

Figure 38.16: In a coxa vara deformity, the angle of inclination is less than normal.

(Continued)

valgus alignment, the epiphyseal plate of the femoral head (capital femoral epiphysis) lies approximately perpendicular to the joint reaction force on the head of the femur. In this position the joint reaction force applies a compressive force on the epiphysis. As the valgus decreases, the growth plate lies more oblique to the joint reaction force. Consequently, the joint reaction force exerts both compressive and shear forces on the epiphyseal plate. As the obliquity of the epiphysis increases, the shear force on it also increases. The shear force tends to slide the head of the femur off the epiphysis. If the shear force exceeds the strength of the growth plate, a slipped capital epiphysis results [53]. This disorder is seen most often in adolescent males. Although hormonal imbalances have been implicated in the development of slipped capital epiphysis, other factors including obesity and sudden growth spurts are significant contributors as well, since these increase the joint reaction force and its shear component [56,61].

Transverse plane alignment of the proximal femur also contributes to the function and dysfunction of the hip joint. In the adult, the femoral neck and head face anteriorly with respect to the plane of the femoral condyles in approximately 15° of anteversion (*Fig. 38.18*). However, like frontal plane alignment, transverse plane alignment changes throughout development. Means of 32° and 40° of anteversion at birth are reported [41,54]. Anteversion gradually decreases during growth until adult values of approximately 15° are present later in adolescence, that is, by about 16 years of age. Jenkins et al. report average anteversion of 12° (±3°) in 5 adults using a clinical examination, but 17° (±7°) using MRI [28].

Excessive femoral anteversion places the head of the femur farther anteriorly in the acetabulum than normal (*Fig. 38.19*). Medial rotation of the hip compensates for excessive femoral anteversion by putting the femoral head in a more normal location within the acetabulum. In standing, such compensatory

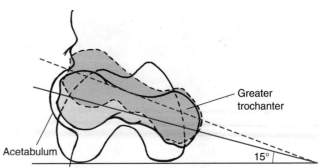

Figure 38.19: Uncompensated excessive femoral anteversion. If there is no compensation for excessive anteversion, the femoral head projects too far anteriorly or even outside the acetabulum.

medial rotation of the hip results in an in-toed posture if accompanied by no other compensation [32] (*Fig. 38.20*). Because individuals with excessive femoral anteversion compensate for it with medial rotation of the hip, subjects with excessive femoral anteversion typically display increased medial rotation ROM and a concomitant decrease in lateral rotation ROM [65]. Children with excessive anteversion frequently choose the "frog sitting" posture over other sitting posture alternatives.

Over time, many individuals with continued excessive femoral anteversion develop a secondary compensation in the

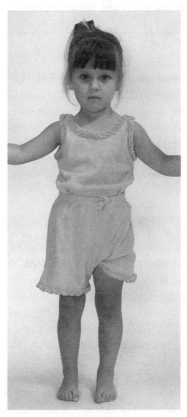

Figure 38.20: To compensate for excessive femoral anteversion, locating the femoral head appropriately in the acetabulum, young children typically rotate the hip medially, producing a pigeon-toed posture.

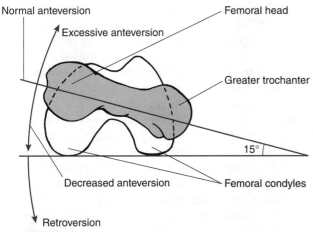

Figure 38.18: Transverse plane orientation of the hip joint. The hip normally exhibits approximately 15° of anteversion.

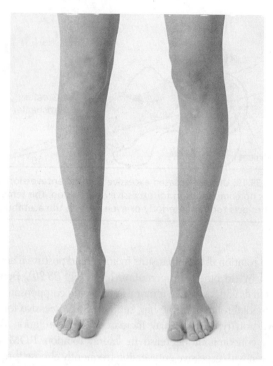

Figure 38.21: To compensate for excessive femoral anteversion, locating the femoral head appropriately in the acetabulum, an adult continues to rotate the hip medially, so that in standing, the knees face medially. However, the tibia also undergoes adaptation by developing lateral torsion, so that in standing, the feet are directed straight ahead and the subject no longer exhibits a pigeon-toed posture.

tibia, **lateral tibial torsion,** which turns the foot laterally with respect to the knee [32]. As a result, the in-toed standing posture disappears. However, close examination of the femoral condyles reveals that the standing posture continues to be characterized by medial rotation of the hip (*Fig. 38.21*). In other words, despite the disappearance of an in-toed posture, the original deformity remains.

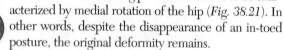

Clinical Relevance

TREATMENT FOR EXCESSIVE FEMORAL ANTEVERSION: *Investigations into common conservative treatments of excessive femoral anteversion reveal no change in anteversion following standard clinical treatments such as shoe modifications, twister cables, and splints [54]. These authors also find no change in alignment with no intervention at all. Conservative treatments are similar to one another in that they apply mechanical forces to the foot and leg to influence the hip. The result of such treatments apparently is an increase in lateral tibial torsion with no change in the femoral anteversion deformity. Many, perhaps most, individuals with excessive femoral anteversion develop secondary tibial torsional deformities spontaneously.*

Investigators recommend that treatment of femoral anteversion be reserved for only those who display functional difficulties associated with the anteversion deformity and suggest that tibial osteotomy be considered for those who show little or no tibial torsion by the age of 7 and have little lateral rotation ROM of the hip.

Retroversion is a transverse plane deformity in which the femoral neck is rotated posterior to the frontal plane, although lower than normal anteversion is also sometimes described as retroversion. Retroversion or less than normal anterversion typically results in increased lateral rotation ROM of the hip and concomitant diminished medial rotation ROM. Excessive out-toeing can be a postural manifestation of retroversion [65]. Retroversion also appears to increase the risk of slipped capital femoral ephiphysis in adolescents [15].

NORMAL MOTION OF THE HIP

Motion of the hip is certainly influenced by the supporting structures detailed in the preceding section. In addition, hip motion is almost inextricably linked to the motion of the low back and pelvis. In this section, the values of normal hip joint motion reported in the literature are presented with a discussion of the structures that are the normal limiters of motion. This is followed by discussions of the contributions by the pelvis and low back to apparent hip motion.

Normal Range of Motion

With the exception of hip flexion ROM, values of "normal" ROM of the hip vary widely in the literature, as demonstrated in *Table 38.1*. Many of the values cited do not include a description of the population from which the values were determined or details of the methodology used to obtain the values. The clinician then is left to determine whether a patient's ROM values are actually "normal." This lack of a clear description of the normal variation of ROM values in a population of individuals without hip pathology, in combination with the absence of a consistent measurement procedure, limits the usefulness of such "normal" ROM values to the clinician. At best, these numbers can offer a general perspective by which to judge the adequacy of a patient's hip ROM. Despite the lack of normative data, the research provides some useful perspectives. Gender has a slight effect on hip ROM [13,69]. Medial rotation ROM appears greater in women and adduction appears greater in men, but other motions appear similar. Aging appears to produce a clinically insignificant reduction in hip ROM in all directions, at least until the age of 80 [13,36,57,69]. Consequently, significant decreases in ROM suggest the existence of a joint impairment.

TABLE 38.1: Hip ROM (°) in Healthy Individuals Reported in the Literature

Reference	Flexion	Extension	Abd	Add	MR	LR
Roaas and Andersson [58][a]	120 ± 8.3	9 ± 5.2	39 ± 7.2	31 ± 7.3	33 ± 8.2	34 ± 6.8
Roach and Miles [57][b]	121 ± 13	19 ± 8	42 ± 11	—	32 ± 8	32 ± 9
Departments of the Army and the Air Force [9]	120	10	45	30	45	45
Boone and Azen [3][c]	122 ± 6.1	9.8 ± 6.8	45.9 ± 9.3	26.9 ± 4.1	47.3 ± 6.0	47.2 ± 6.3
Hislop and Montgomery [24]	120	—	45	15–20	45	45
Gerhardt and Rippstein [16]	125	15	45	15	45	45
Escalante [13][d]	123	—	—	—	—	—
Van Dillen et al. [67][e]	—	−2.5	—	—	—	—

[a]Data from 108 men, aged 30–40 years.
[b]Data from 821 males and 862 females, aged 25–74 years.
[c]Data from 109 males, aged 18–54 years.
[d]Data from 687 individuals, aged 65–79 years.
[e]Data from 25 women and 10 men, aged 31 ± 11 years.

Normal Limiting Structures of Hip ROM

One aid in making clinical judgments about ROM measures is an understanding of the structures that normally limit hip movement. Sources state that hip flexion ROM is limited primarily by soft tissue approximation between the thigh and trunk [52]. However, a review of Table 38.1 reveals that most sources also say that the normal hip flexion ROM is no more than 125°. Few subjects exhibit contact between the thigh and abdomen with 120° of hip flexion ROM. Therefore, other structures appear to contribute to the end of ROM in flexion. These limiting structures are most likely the posterior joint capsule and the gluteus maximus. Soft tissue contact limits hip flexion ROM with greater excursion and in overweight individuals. Obesity is significantly related to decreased hip flexion range [13].

Extension flexibility is limited by the anterior joint capsule with its three reinforcing ligaments. The one-joint hip flexors also provide some limits to extension ROM. The hip adductor muscles and the pubofemoral ligament limit hip abduction excursion; the superior part of the iliofemoral ligament and the hip abductor muscles restrict hip adduction ROM. Finally, lateral rotation flexibility is limited primarily by the anterior capsule and by the iliofemoral and pubofemoral ligaments; medial rotation excursion is checked by the lateral rotator muscles, the posterior capsule, and perhaps by a portion of the ischiofemoral ligament [52,64].

Contribution of the Pelvis to Hip Motion

ROM measurements of the hip are usually taken with the lower extremity functioning in an open chain, in which the femur is moved with respect to the pelvis. **Flexion** is defined as the femur moving toward the anterior aspect of the pelvis and trunk; **extension** is the reverse. **Abduction** is the femur moving toward the lateral aspect of the pelvis, and **adduction**

is the reverse. **Lateral rotation** occurs when the femoral head rotates anteriorly in the acetabulum, and **medial rotation** is the femoral head rotating posteriorly. However, in daily life, the lower extremity functions frequently in a closed chain, so that the pelvis moves on the femur. In upright standing with the femur fixed, an anterior pelvic tilt flexes the hip, since the pelvic motion brings the anterior aspect of the pelvis closer to the femur; a posterior pelvic tilt on a fixed femur extends the hip (*Fig. 38.22*). When the pelvis is elevated on one side in the frontal plane and the lower extremity remains fixed, the lateral aspect of the pelvis on the opposite side moves closer to its respective femur (*Fig. 38.23*). This pelvic position results in abduction of the hip on the side opposite the elevation. The hip on the elevated side is adducted. Finally, in erect standing with both femurs fixed, forward rotation of the pelvis on one side in the transverse plane results in lateral rotation of the hip on the forward side and medial rotation of the opposite hip (*Fig. 38.24*). Understanding the pelvic contribution to hip position is essential to understanding hip movement in activities such as walking, climbing, and dancing. For example, in gait at heel strike, the pelvis is rotated forward in the transverse plane on the side of heel contact, contributing to lateral rotation of the hip on the side with heel contact and to medial rotation of the hip on the opposite side.

Interaction of the Hip Joint and Lumbar Spine in Hip Motion

One of the likely sources of difference in the normal ROMs reported in the literature is the difficulty in separating the contributions of pure hip joint motion from lumbar spine motion. Hip joint motion is measured by determining the position of the thigh relative to the trunk. Unless care is taken to control the movement of the pelvis and thus the

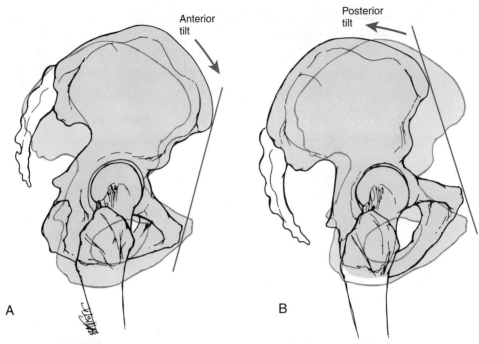

Figure 38.22: Effect of pelvic position on sagittal plane hip position. **A.** An anterior pelvic tilt flexes the hip. **B.** A posterior tilt produces hip extension.

lumbar spine, the measured movements may actually reflect both hip and spine motion. In hip flexion ROM, when the femur has reached the end of its excursion in the acetabulum, posterior tilting of the pelvis continues to move the femur toward the trunk, apparently contributing to additional hip flexion while flattening the lumbar spine (*Fig. 38.25*) [10]. Conversely, an anterior pelvic tilt in the absence of movement at the hip joint contributes to apparent

hip extension while extending the lumbar spine. Trunk side-bending and pelvic movement in the frontal plane can appear to be hip abduction or adduction motion (*Fig. 38.26*). It is important to recognize the pelvic and femoral contributions to hip motion may occur simultaneously, not just sequentially. Therefore, considerable care is needed to distinguish true hip motion from apparent hip motion coming from the pelvis and low back.

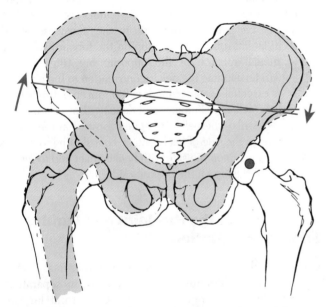

Figure 38.23: When standing with the feet together and the pelvis elevated on one side, the hip on the elevated side is in adduction, and the opposite hip is in abduction.

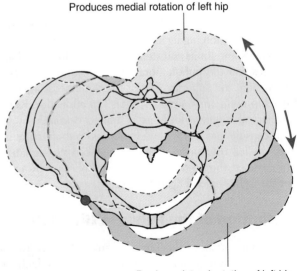

Produces medial rotation of left hip

Produces lateral rotation of left hip

Figure 38.24: When the pelvis rotates over the femur in the transverse plane, the hip on the forward side is laterally rotated, and the hip on the opposite side is medially rotated.

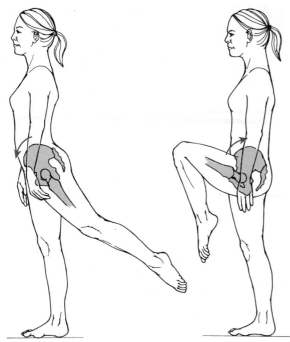

Figure 38.25: **A.** An anterior pelvic tilt can substitute for hip extension. **B.** A posterior pelvic tilt can substitute for hip flexion.

Clinical Relevance

COMPENSATIONS FOR DECREASED HIP MOTION:
Pelvic and lumbar spine movement can provide additional movement between the trunk and thigh in individuals with

limited or absent hip motion. Patients with a fused or painful hip use an anterior pelvic tilt to substitute for hip extension to advance the body over the limb during stance and use a posterior pelvic tilt to assist in advancing the limb during swing [19,70]. The interaction between the hip joint and lumbar spine may also help explain the source of low back pain in some patients [18]. Limited hip mobility may lead to overuse and hypermobility in the low back. Repeat use of lumbar motion to compensate for limited hip motion can produce injury or pain. Therefore, assessment of hip mobility is an important component of the evaluation of an individual with low back pain. Activities such as rising from a chair and squatting require up to 130° of hip flexion [26,49]. Individuals who lack such excursion may use lumbar flexion to get out of a chair or squat to tie a shoe or retrieve an object from the floor.

Hip Motion in Activities of Daily Living

Hip motion is essential to many daily activities, including rising from a chair or toilet, picking up something from the floor, walking, and climbing stairs. Normal walking utilizes approximately 20–30° of flexion, reaching a maximum at about initial contact. Stair climbing utilizes more, approximately 45–65° and slightly less for stair descent [38,46]. Rising from a chair typically requires more than 100° of hip flexion, usually less than the amount of flexion used when bending to tie a shoe or squatting to pick up something from the floor [50].

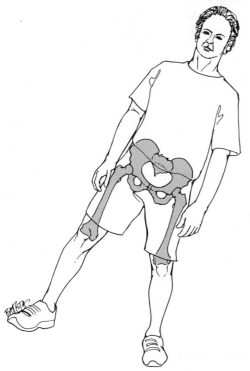

Figure 38.26: A lateral tilt of the trunk and pelvis can substitute for hip abduction.

Clinical Relevance

PRECAUTIONS AFTER TOTAL HIP REPLACEMENT:
Dislocation is one of the most common complications of total hip replacement (THR). A primary cause of dislocation is impingement between the femoral and acetabular components which causes the femoral head to be "pried" out of the acetabulum. Impingement typically occurs with excessive hip flexion, adduction, or medial rotation. Surgeons and therapists carefully instruct the THR patient to avoid these motions, specifically avoiding flexion beyond 90° and any hip adduction or medial rotation. However, such instructions are difficult to follow since rising from a chair typically uses at least 100° of flexion and tying a shoe uses even more. Special adaptations such as chairs with extra cushions or leg extenders, raised toilet seats, extended shoe horns, and elastic shoe laces can be very helpful to a patient who must avoid excessive hip flexion or other motions (Fig. 38.27).

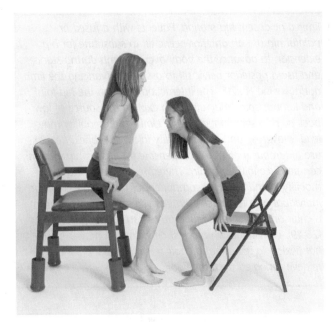

Figure 38.27: Rising from a chair with leg extensions (chair on the left) requires less hip flexion than rising from a standard chair.

COMPARISON OF THE HIP JOINT TO THE GLENOHUMERAL JOINT

Although the hip and glenohumeral joints are the two most notable ball-and-socket, or triaxial, joints of the human body, they possess very different architectures. This helps explain their considerably different functional capabilities. First, the shapes of the articular surfaces are quite different in the hip and glenohumeral joint. While both the head of the femur and head of the humerus are spherical, the femoral head completes almost two thirds of a sphere, while the humerus is only hemispherical. The proximal articular surfaces, the acetabulum and the glenoid fossa, are even more different from one another. The acetabulum is a deep receptacle for the femoral head and has a curvature similar to that of the femoral head itself; with the labrum it covers more than half the femoral head in the articulated joint. In contrast, the glenoid fossa is very shallow, articulating with only a small portion of the humeral head at any instant. These differences help to explain why the glenohumeral joint is more mobile than the hip joint and why the hip joint is more stable than its upper extremity counterpart.

The soft tissue supporting structures of the hip and glenohumeral joints also contribute to the different functional capabilities of these two joints. The articular capsule and reinforcing ligaments of the hip provide substantial passive support to the hip joint, while the capsule and reinforcing ligaments of the glenohumeral joint provide only a portion of the support needed for the integrity of the joint. Recognizing the structural differences that contribute to functional differences between joints can help the clinician understand the underlying pathology in a region and identify a successful intervention strategy.

Clinical Relevance

INSTABILITY IN THE HIP COMPARED TO THE GLENOHUMERAL JOINT: *Instability at the hip is rarely a problem in adults, but glenohumeral joint instability is a relatively common problem in adults. Instability in the hip is more commonly the problem of a young developing hip. However, although strengthening exercises for the glenohumeral joint may be a useful approach to increasing stability, such a strategy is inadequate to restore stability at the hip. The hip's stability depends more on bony architecture and the integrity of noncontractile tissue than on muscular support.*

SUMMARY

This chapter examines how the bony architecture as well as the noncontractile supporting structures of the hip contributes to its functional requirements of stability and mobility. The deep socket formed by the acetabulum and labrum provides inherent stability to the hip joint. A strong joint capsule with reinforcing ligaments offers additional support. The relative alignment of the femur and innominate bone allows considerable joint mobility, especially in flexion, and increases the mechanical advantage of muscles at the hip. Malalignments of the hip alter the mechanics of the hip and may contribute to increased loads and stresses on the joint, leading to joint degeneration.

Hip joint ROM is reported and demonstrates little effect from age. Loss of hip mobility suggests frank joint impairments and may result in excessive motion at the spine and pelvis. Since increased pelvic and lumbar spine motion may result from decreased hip mobility, assessment of hip motion is an essential part of the examination of an individual with low back pain. A grasp of these morphological and functional relationships is essential to understanding normal function of the hip as well as to recognizing and treating dysfunctions of the hip or spine successfully. The following chapter presents the structures that provide further support and, most importantly, active motion at the hip—the muscles.

References

1. Aamodt A, Lund-Larsen J, Eine J, et al.: In vivo measurements show tensile axial strain in the proximal lateral aspect of the human femur. J Orthop Res 1997; 15: 927–931.
2. Athanasiou KA, Agarwal A, Dzida FJ: Comparative study of the intrinsic mechanical properties of the human acetabular and femoral head cartilage. J Orthop Res 1994; 12: 340–349.
3. Boone DC, Azen SP: Normal range of motion of joints in male subjects. J Bone Joint Surg 1979; 61-A: 756–759.
4. Bower C, Stanley FJ, Kricker A: Congenital dislocation of the hip in Western Australia. A comparison of neonatally and post neonatally diagnosed cases. Clin Orthop 1987; 224: 37–44.

5. Carpintero P, Leon F, Zafra M, et al.: Stress fractures of the femoral neck and coxa vara. Arch Orthop Trauma Surg 2003; 123: 273–277.

6. Carter DR, Wong M, Orr TE: Musculoskeletal ontogeny, phylogeny, and functional adaptation. J Biomech 1991; 24: 3–16.

7. Chen HH, Li AFY, Li KC, et al.: Adaptations of ligamentum teres in ischemic necrosis of human femoral head. Clin Orthop 1996; 328: 268–275.

8. Cotten A, Boutry N, Demondion X, et al.: Acetabular labrum: MRI in asymptomatic volunteers. J Comput Assist Tomogr 1998; 22: 1–7.

9. Departments of the U.S. Army and Air Force. US Army Goniometry manual: technical manual no. 8-640; Air Force pamphlet no. 160-14. 1-8-1968. Washington, DC: Departments of the Army and Air Force, 1968.

10. Dewberry MJ, Bohannon RW, Tiberio D, et al.: Pelvic and femoral contributions to bilateral hip flexion by subjects suspended from a bar. Clin Biomech 2003; 18: 494–499.

11. Duan Y, Beck TJ, Wang XF, Seeman E: Structural and biomechanical basis of sexual dimorphism in femoral neck fragility has its origins in growth and aging. J Bone Miner Res 2003; 18: 1766–1774.

12. Eckstein F, Eisenhart-Rothe RV, Landgraf J, et al.: Quantitative analysis of incongruity, contact areas and cartilage thickness in the human hip joint. Acta Anat 1997; 158: 192–204.

13. Escalante A, Lichtenstein MJ, Dhanda R, et al.: Determinants of hip and knee flexion range: results from the San Antonio longitudinal study of aging. Arthritis Care Res 1999; 12: 8–18.

14. Ferguson SJ, Bryant JT, Ganz R, Ito K: The acetabular labrum seal: a poroelastic finite element model. Clin Biomech 2000; 15: 463–468.

15. Fishkin Z, Armstrong DG, Shah H, et al.: Proximal femoral physis shear in slipped capital femoral epiphysis—a finite element study. J Pediatric Orthop 2006; 26: 291–294.

16. Gerhardt JJ, Rippstein J: Measuring and Recording of Joint Motion Instrumentation and Techniques. Lewiston, NJ: Hogrefe & Huber, 1990.

17. Goldie IF, Dumbleton JH: Intertrochanteric osteotomy of the femur. In: Black J, Dumbleton JH, eds. Clinical Biomechanics. A Case History Approach. New York: Churchill Livingstone, 1981; 72–93.

18. Gombatto SP, Collins DR, Sahrmann SA, et al.: Gender differences in pattern of hip and lumbopelvic rotation in people with low back pain. Clin Biomech 2006; 21: 263–271.

19. Gore DR, Murray RM, Sepic SB, Gardner GM: Walking patterns of men with unilateral surgical hip fusion. J Bone Joint Surg 1975; 57-A: 759–765.

20. Harty M: Some aspects of the surgical anatomy of the hip joint. J Bone Joint Surg 1966; 48-A: 197–202.

21. Harty M: Anatomic considerations. Orthop Clin North Am 1982; 13: 667–679.

22. Hewitt J, Glisson R, Guilak F, Vail T: The mechanical properties of the human hip capsule ligaments. J Arthroplasty 2002; 17: 82–89.

23. Hewitt J, Guilak F, Glisson R, Vail T: Regional material properties of the human hip joint capsule ligaments. J Orthop Res 2001; 19: 359–364.

24. Hislop HJ, Montgomery J: Daniel's and Worthingham's Muscle Testing: Techniques of Manual Examination. Philadelphia: WB Saunders, 1995.

25. Iglic A, Antolic V, Srakar F, et al.: Biomechanical study of various greater trochanter positions. Arch Orthop Trauma Surg 1995; 114: 76–78.

26. Ikeda E, Schenkman M, O'Riley P, Hodge WA: Influence of age on dynamics of rising from a chair. Phys Ther 1991; 71: 473–481.

27. Ipavec M, Brand RA, Pedersen DR, et al.: Mathematical modelling of stress in the hip during gait. J Biomech 1999; 32: 1229–1235.

28. Jenkins SEM, Harrington ME, Zavatsky AB, et al.: Femoral muscle attachment locations in children and adults, and their prediction from clinical measurement. Gait Posture 2003; 18: 13–22.

29. Johnston RC: Mechanical considerations of the hip joint. Arch Surg 1973; 107: 411–417.

30. Kawabe K, Konishi N: Three dimensional modeling of cartilage thickness in hip dysplasia. Clin Orthop 1993; 289: 180–185.

31. Kelly BT, Weiland DE, Schenker ML, Philippon MJ: Arthroscopic labral repair in the hip: surgical technique and review of the literature. Arthroscopy 2005; 21: 1496–1504.

32. Kling TF Jr, Hensinger RN: Angular and torsional deformities of the lower limbs in children. Clin Orthop 1983; 176: 136–147.

33. Kurrat HJ, Oberlander W: The thickness of the cartilage in the hip joint. J Anat 1978; 129: 145–155.

34. Kutlu A, Memick R, Mutlu M, et al.: Congenital dislocation of the hip and its relation to swaddling used in turkey. J Pediatr Orthop 1992; 12: 598–602.

35. Laforgia R, Specchiulli F, Solarino G, Nitti L: Radiographic variables in normal and osteoarthritic hips. Bull Hosp Joint Dis 1996; 54: 215–221.

36. Lee LW, Zavarei K, Evans J, et al.: Reduced hip extension in the elderly: dynamic or postural? Arch Phys Med Rehabil 2005; 86: 1851–1854.

37. Lewis CL, Sahrmann SA: Acetabular labral tears. Phys Ther 2006; 86: 110–121.

38. Livingston LA, Stevenson JM, Olney SJ: Stairclimbing kinematics on stairs of differing dimensions. Arch Phys Med Rehabil 1991; 72: 398–402.

39. Lohe F, Eckstein F, Sauer T, Putz R: Structures, strain and function of the transverse acetabular ligament. Acta Anat 1996; 157: 315–323.

40. Lotz JC, Cheal EJ, Hayes WC: Stress distributions within the proximal femur during gait and falls: implications for osteoporotic fracture. Osteoporos Int 1995; 5: 252–261.

41. MacEwen GD: Anteversion of the femur. Postgrad Med 1976; 60: 154–156.

42. Maquet P: Biomechanics of hip dysplasia. Acta Orthop Belg 1999; 65: 302–314.

43. Martin RL, Enseki KR, Draovitch P, et al.: Acetabular labral tears of the hip: examination and diagnostic challenges. JOSPT 2006; 36: 503–515.

44. Martinon-Torres M: Quantifying trabecular orientation in the pelvic cancellous bone of modern humans, chimpanzees, and the kebara 2 neanderthal. Am J Hum Biol 2003; 15: 647–661.

45. Mayhew PM, Thomas CD, Clement JG, et al.: Relation between age, femoral neck cortical stability, and hip fracture risk. Lancet 2005; 366: 129–135.

46. McFadyen BJ, Winter DA: An integrated biomechanical analysis of normal stair ascent and descent. J Biomech 1988; 21: 733–744.

47. Michaeli D, Murphy S, Hipp J: Comparison of predicted and measured contact pressures in normal and dysplastic hips. Med Eng Phys 1997; 19: 180–186.

48. Moore KL: Clinically Oriented Anatomy. Baltimore: Williams & Wilkins, 1980.

49. Mulholland S, Wyss UP: Activities of daily living in non-Western cultures: range of motion requirements for hip and knee joint implants. Int J Rehabil Res 2001; 24: 191–198.

50. Nadzadi ME, Pedersen DR, Yack HJ, et al.: Kinematics, kinetics, and finite element analysis of commonplace maneuvers at risk for total hip dislocation. J Biomech 2003; 36: 577–591.

51. Neumann DA: Biomechanical analysis of selected principles of hip joint protection. Arthritis Care Res 1989; 2: 146–155.

52. Norkin CC, White DJ: Measurement of Joint Motion. A Guide to Goniometry. Philadelphia: FA Davis, 1995.

53. Pauwels F: Biomechanics of the Normal and Diseased Hip: Theoretical Foundation, Technique and Results of Treatment. An Atlas. Berlin: Springer-Verlag, 1976; 30–37.

54. Pizzutillo PT, MacEwen GD, Shands AR: Anteversion of the femur. In: Tonzo RG, ed. Surgery of the Hip Joint. New York: Springer-Verlag, 1984.

55. Ralis Z, McKibbin B: Changes in shape of the human hip joint during its development and their relation to its stability. J Bone Joint Surg 1973; 55B: 780–785.

56. Ramsey PL: Congenital hip dislocation before and after walking age. Postgrad Med 1976; 60: 114–120.

57. Roach KE, Miles TP: Normal hip and knee active range of motion: the relationship to age. Phys Ther 1991; 71: 656–665.

58. Roass A, Andersson GB: Normal range of motion of the hip, knee, and ankle joints in male subjects, 30–40 years of age. Acta Orthop Scand 1982; 53: 205–208.

59. Romanes GJE: Cunningham's Textbook of Anatomy. Oxford: Oxford University Press, 1981.

60. Ruff C: Biomechanics of the hip and birth in early homo. Am J Phys Anthropol 1995; 98: 527–574.

61. Salter RB: Textbook of Disorders and Injuries of the Musculoskeletal System. 3rd ed. Baltimore: Williams & Wilkins, 1999.

62. Schmidt A, Swiontkowski M: Femoral neck fractures. Orthop Clin North Am 2002; 33: 97–111.

63. Sims S: Subtrochanteric femoral fractures. Orthop Clin North Am 2002; 33: 113–126.

64. Singleton MC, LeVeau BF: The hip joint: structure, stability, and stress. Phys Ther 1975; 55: 957–973.

65. Staheli LT: Rotational problems of the lower extremities. Orthop Clin North Am 1987; 18: 503–512.

66. Tillmann B: A contribution to the functional morphology of articular surfaces. Norm Pathol Anat (Stuttg) 1978. 34: 1–50.

67. Van Dillen L, McDonnell M, Fleming D, Sahrmann S: Effect of knee and hip position on hip extension range of motion in individuals with and without low back pain. J Orthop Sports Phys Ther 2000; 30: 307–316.

68. von Eisenhart-Rothe R, Eckstein F, Müller-Gerbl M, et al.: Direct comparison of contact areas, contact stress and subchondral mineralization in human hip joint specimens. Anat Embryol 1997; 195: 279–288.

69. Walker JM, Sue D, Miles-Elkousy N, et al.: Active mobility of the extremities in older subjects. Phys Ther 1984; 64: 919–923.

70. Watelain E, Dujardin F, Babier F, et al.: Pelvic and lower limb compensatory actions of subjects in an early stage of hip osteoarthritis. Arch Phys Med Rehabil 2001; 82: 1705–1711.

71. Williams P, Bannister L, Berry M, et al.: Gray's Anatomy, The Anatomical Basis of Medicine and Surgery, Br. ed. London: Churchill Livingstone, 1995.

72. Yoshioka Y, Siu D, Cooke TDV: Anatomy and functional axes of the femur. J Bone Joint Surg 1987; 69A: 873.

Mechanics and Pathomechanics of Muscle Activity at the Hip

CHAPTER CONTENTS

T he preceding chapter provides an understanding of the roles that the bones and supporting structures play in the function of the hip. This chapter discusses the effects that the surrounding musculature has on the hip joint under normal and pathological conditions.

Muscles that move the hip can be grouped into one-joint and two-joint muscles that *(a)* flex, *(b)* extend, *(c)* abduct, *(d)* adduct, and *(e)* rotate the hip *(Fig. 39.1)*. This chapter focuses on the one-joint muscles of the hip. The two-joint

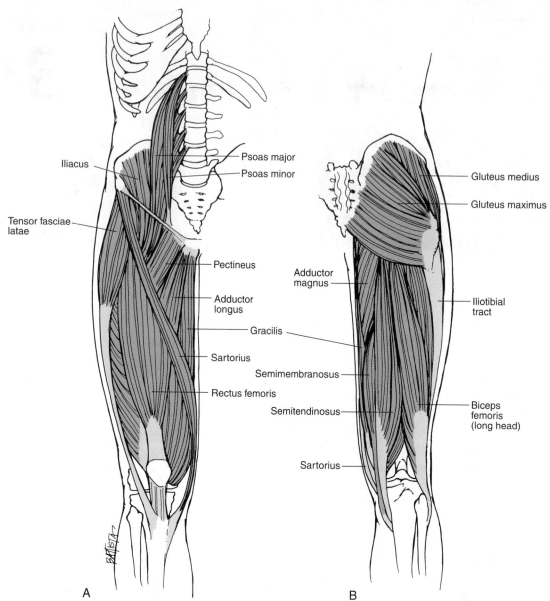

Figure 39.1: Muscles of the hip. **A.** Anterior view of the hip shows the hip flexors and the adductor muscles. **B.** Posterior view of the hip shows the gluteus maximus, medius, and other adductors.

muscles are mentioned briefly and are presented more thoroughly in Chapter 42 with the knee. This separation is, of course, artificial, and the clinician must remember that the two-joint muscles, although obviously important muscles of the knee, also provide important functions at the hip.

The muscles of the hip usually are classified by their actions, a useful and convenient classification. However, this can lead to erroneous oversimplifications unless care is taken to recognize that virtually all hip muscles perform multiple actions, and the "primary" action of some muscles is often unclear. In addition, the position of the hip has large effects on the actions many muscles produce [13,15,23,33]. This chapter groups muscles by their purported primary action, using the standard classification scheme, but also discusses the contribution of each muscle to other movements and the influence of hip position on the muscles' actions. The purposes of this chapter are to

- Describe the actions produced by the one-joint hip muscles and how those actions are influenced by hip position
- Examine the impact of muscle impairments at the hip
- Begin to discuss the functional roles performed by the hip muscles during stance and gait

HIP FLEXORS

The one-joint hip flexors consist of the psoas major, iliacus, and psoas minor, although the latter does not actually cross the hip joint (*Fig. 39.2*). These muscles lie on the posterior wall of the abdomen and inner surface of the greater pelvis. Additional two-joint hip flexors include the rectus femoris, tensor fasciae latae, and sartorius [9,75].

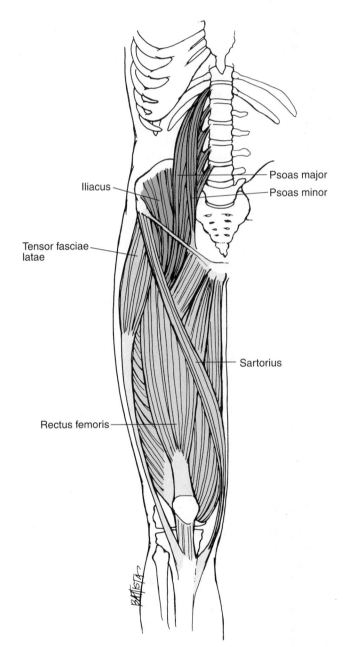

Figure 39.2: One-joint muscles include the psoas major and minor and iliacus. Two-joint hip flexors include the sartorius, tensor fasciae latae, and rectus femoris.

MUSCLE ATTACHMENT BOX 39.1

ATTACHMENTS AND INNERVATION OF THE PSOAS MAJOR

Proximal attachment: On the lateral aspects of the vertebral bodies from T12 to L5 and the intervening intervertebral discs. The muscle also attaches to the bases of the respective transverse processes.

Distal attachment: The lesser trochanter. The tendon of the psoas major, which combines with the tendon of the iliacus, crosses over the superior ramus of the pubis. It is separated from the pelvis and the hip joint by the psoas bursa.

Innervation: Ventral roots of spinal nerves L1–L3(4).

Palpation: Some clinicians report an ability to palpate the muscle belly of the psoas major through a relaxed abdomen [60,68], but in many individuals, this muscle is not palpable.

Psoas Major

Because the psoas major lies deep in the abdomen it is less well studied than some muscles of the hip (*Muscle Attachment Box 39.1*).

ACTIONS

MUSCLE ACTION: PSOAS MAJOR

Action	Evidence
Hip flexion	Supporting
Hip lateral rotation	Supporting
Hip medial rotation	Refuting
Lumbar spine side-bending	Supporting
Lumbar spine flexion	Conflicting
Lumbar spine hyperextension	Conflicting
Lumbar spine stabilization	Supporting

Some of the actions of the psoas major are universally accepted, while others remain controversial. Some of the actions of the psoas major appear clearly contradictory; the following discussion presents the current evidence for each action.

The role of the psoas major as a hip flexor is clear from its location anterior to the mediolateral axis of hip flexion that passes approximately through the center of the femoral head [14]. Although it has a smaller moment arm for flexion than some other hip flexors such as the rectus femoris, sartorius, and tensor fasciae latae, its large physiological cross-sectional area (PCSA) makes it a strong hip flexor [8,15,23,28].

According to one study of eight healthy young adults, resisted hip flexion while standing on the opposite limb recruits the psoas major more vigorously than other exercises and activities designed to elicit maximal contraction [28].

The psoas major is described as a medial rotator of the hip [55] and as a lateral rotator [30]. Analysis of its moment arm reveals a negligible rotation moment arm with the hip in neutral and a slight lateral rotation moment arm with the hip flexed to 90° [13,15]. Additionally, active lateral rotation elicits greater electrical activity of the psoas major than medial rotation, and neither generates more than approximately half the level of activity that hip flexion produces [5,28]. These reports suggest that the psoas major plays only a small role in lateral rotation under normal conditions.

The role of the psoas major in controlling the hip during upright posture remains debatable. The center of mass of the head, arms, and trunk (HAT) lies posterior to the flexion and extension axis of the hip joint, applying an extension moment to the hip [12,51] (Fig. 39.3). Contraction of the psoas major is able to produce a flexion moment to counteract the extension moment [5], but more recent electromyographic EMG data reveal minimal activity (2% of maximum voluntary contraction) of the psoas major during quiet standing, which increases only slightly when standing in trunk hyperextension [28].

Considerable confusion exists regarding the role of the psoas major on the lumbar spine. EMG analysis reveals slight electrical activity of the psoas major during trunk curl-up activities and more activity during sit-up exercises and leg raises from the supine position. The trunk exercises that elicit more activity of the psoas major also use more hip flexion, providing additional evidence that the psoas major is primarily a flexor of the hip.

Analysis of its moment arm and EMG data reveal that the psoas major is an effective lateral flexor of the trunk [28,57]. It contracts concentrically lifting the trunk from the side-lying position and eccentrically when side-bending to the opposite side from a standing position. In contrast, analysis of the moment arms in the sagittal plane reveals small extension moment arms in the upper lumbar region and slight flexion moment arms in the lower lumbar region [57]. The muscle is better aligned to apply significant compressive loads to the lumbar spine than to flex or extend it. This compressive load may be sufficient to assist in stabilization of the spine. Slight activity of the psoas major (<15% maximum voluntary contraction, or MVC) during standing lift activities and ipsilateral side-bending supports its role as a stabilizer of the lumbar spine [28]. The compressive loads applied by psoas major contractions also may explain why individuals with low back pain report pain with hip flexion activities.

Clinical Relevance

PSOAS MAJOR CONTRACTION INCREASES LOW BACK PAIN: *Patients with herniated lumbar discs frequently complain of pain getting in and out of automobiles, especially trying to lift the lower extremity on the painful side or while driving and moving the limb back and forth between accelerator and brake. These maneuvers require active hip flexion and probably involve contraction of the psoas major. Contraction applies compressive loads to the lumbar spine and also pulls on the lumbar intervertebral discs, which may increase the pain. During the acute phase of a low back pain episode, attempts to avoid active hip flexion may help reduce the pain.*

EFFECTS OF WEAKNESS

Weakness of the psoas major decreases the strength of hip flexion. Such weakness could produce difficulties in tasks such as lifting a limb in and out of the bathtub and climbing stairs. Although active hip flexion is an important element of normal locomotion, the amount of force required of the hip flexors during normal gait is relatively small [6,52,59]. Therefore, slight-to-moderate weakness of the psoas major may have an imperceptible impact on locomotion.

A study of 210 women ranging in age from 20 to 79 years reports a steady decline in the cross-sectional area of the psoas major apparent from the fifth decade on [66]. Such loss in

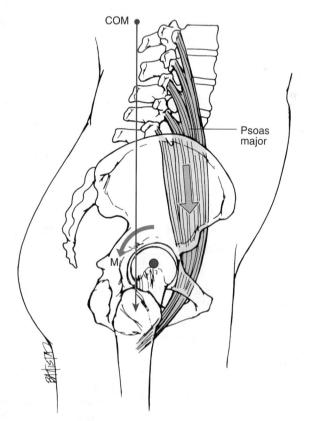

Figure 39.3: In quiet standing, the center of mass (COM) of the HAT creates an extension moment (M) on the hip that can be resisted by contraction of the psoas major.

muscle bulk, presumably accompanied by loss of strength, may contribute to the functional declines documented with age, such as diminished balance and difficulty in stair climbing.

EFFECTS OF TIGHTNESS

Tightness of the psoas major restricts hip extension range of motion (ROM). It may also limit trunk side-bending flexibility. In the upright posture, tightness of the psoas major is often manifested by increased lumbar extension, that is, by an excessive lumbar lordosis. This posture results from the pull on the lumbar vertebrae toward the femur and simultaneous compensation of backward-bending elsewhere in the spine for the individual to keep the eyes on the horizon.

Iliacus

The iliacus is a large muscle with a PCSA equal to or greater than the PCSA of the psoas major [8] (*Muscle Attachment Box 39.2*). It is regarded with the psoas major as the primary hip flexor. Together they are known as the iliopsoas muscle.

ACTIONS

MUSCLE ACTION: ILIACUS

Action	Evidence
Hip flexion	Supporting
Hip lateral rotation	Supporting
Hip medial rotation	Refuting

MUSCLE ATTACHMENT BOX 39.2

ATTACHMENTS AND INNERVATION OF THE ILIACUS

Proximal attachment: The floor of the iliac fossa but also the sacrum and the ligaments of the lumbosacral and sacroiliac joints anteriorly

Distal attachment: Together with the psoas major on the lesser trochanter. Some additional fibers run slightly distally beyond the lesser trochanter and others attach to the anterior aspect of the joint capsule. The expansive proximal attachment indicates that the muscle has a large cross-sectional diameter suggesting that it is a very powerful muscle.

Innervation: The L2 and L3 branches of the femoral nerve

Palpation: The insertion of the iliacus may be palpable in the femoral triangle, medial to the proximal portion of the sartorius.

The primary actions of the iliacus reported in the literature are, like those of the psoas major, contradictory. The iliacus moves the hip joint directly and is an essential flexor of that joint. Because it attaches with the psoas major, the moment arm analyses at the hip are the same for the psoas major and iliacus. Moment arm analysis suggests that the iliacus has little capacity to rotate the hip from the extended position and only a small advantage for lateral rotation once the hip is flexed. Like the psoas major, the iliacus exhibits EMG activity during sit-up and curl-up activities, presumably participating in the hip flexion component of these exercises [18]. It also may provide some support at the hip in upright standing to prevent the HAT weight from hyperextending the hip [5].

EFFECTS OF WEAKNESS

Weakness of the iliacus decreases hip flexion strength. The functional effects are similar to those with weakness of the psoas major. Although these muscles frequently are weak together, in some cases such as in a spinal cord lesion, it is possible for some of the psoas major to be spared while the iliacus is involved.

Although the iliacus may be slightly active to prevent hip hyperextension in quiet standing, the hip contains structures that can support the hip in quiet standing, even in the absence of muscular support. The anterior capsule with its three reinforcing ligaments provides passive limits to hip hyperextension. The subject who lacks muscular control at the hip can stand unsupported by assuming a position of hip hyperextension so that the weight of the HAT generates an extension moment at the hip. By resting in maximum hyperextension, the individual can use the passive support of the ligaments to prevent additional backward bending (*Fig. 39.4*). This is known as **hanging on the ligaments.**

EFFECTS OF TIGHTNESS

Tightness of the iliacus reduces hip extension ROM. In the standing position, tightness of the iliacus results in an anterior pelvic tilt that is accompanied by hyperextension of the lumbar spine, if available, for the individual to maintain vision of the horizon. Therefore, as seen with a tight psoas major, a tight iliacus frequently leads to an increased lumbar lordosis. If, however, the subject lacks hyperextension flexibility in the spine, tightness of the iliacus or psoas major can produce a forward lean and a flattened lumbar spine in upright posture. Van Dillen et al. report decreased hip extension ROM in people with low back pain compared with age- and gender-matched people without back pain [69].

Clinical Relevance

HIP FLEXION CONTRACTURES: *Bilateral hip flexion contractures are common and are an occupational hazard of office workers, truck drivers, and students, that is, of those*

(continued)

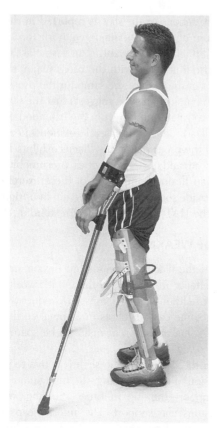

Figure 39.4: In the absence of muscle activity, the anterior hip joint capsule and ilio-, ischio-, and pubofemoral ligaments provide passive resistance to the hyperextension moment at the hip joint, generated by the weight of the HAT.

(Continued)

who spend most of their day sitting. It is not surprising to find hip flexion contractures in sedentary elders [70]. However, individual variations in low back flexibility and strength can markedly affect the resulting compensations. Although stemming from the same musculoskeletal impairment, hip flexor tightness, the varied compensations produce different postural and functional presentations, often leading to disparate musculoskeletal complaints. The individual with a flexible lumbar spine exhibits an excessive lumbar lordosis and may complain of pain from increased loads on the lumbar facet joints (Fig. 39.5). The individual with diminished low back flexibility exhibits a flattened lumbar lordosis and forward lean that may lead to muscle strain and injury to the intervertebral disc from excessive loading.

Unilateral hip flexion contractures also occur, particularly in an individual with an inflammatory process at the hip such as arthritis or following trauma. When only one hip has the contracture or when one hip has a larger contracture than the other hip, the effects on posture may vary. The important factor in understanding the manifestation of a unilateral hip flexion contracture is to determine which attachment site is more displaced. Has the pelvis been pulled toward the femur or has the femur been pulled

toward the pelvis? In the former, the trunk moves in response, and the result is similar to the postures described above in bilateral contractures. In the latter, the lower extremity is drawn toward the trunk, which effectively produces a shortened lower extremity. The patient can respond in a variety of ways to equalize the leg length. Compensations include dropping the pelvis ipsilaterally, plantarflexing the foot on the ipsilateral side, and flexing the knee on the ipsilateral or contralateral side (Fig. 39.6).

Psoas Minor

The psoas minor usually is grouped with the hip flexors but has no attachment on the femur and, consequently, no direct action on the hip (*Muscle Attachment Box 39.3*). It is more accurately described as a trunk muscle. However, because it is so intimately related to the psoas major, it is described here. It is reportedly absent in about 40% of the population [55]. Even when present, its actions cannot be isolated from those of other muscles of the trunk.

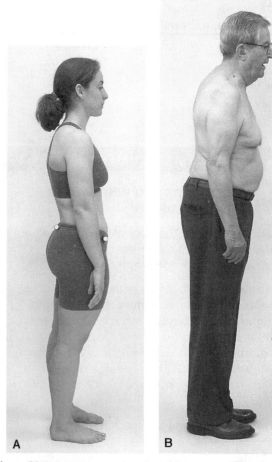

Figure 39.5: Postures associated with bilateral hip flexion contractures. **A.** An individual standing in an anterior pelvic tilt demonstrates an increased lumbar lordosis if the lumbar spine has adequate flexibility. **B.** If an individual lacks adequate lumbar spine flexibility, an anterior pelvic tilt produces a forward lean.

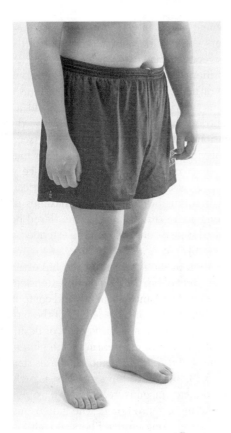

Figure 39.6: Unilateral hip flexion contracture produces a functional leg length discrepancy. In a typical compensation, the individual stands with the ipsilateral knee flexed and foot plantarflexed.

ACTIONS

MUSCLE ACTION: PSOAS MINOR

Action	Evidence
Lumbar spine flexion	Inadequate
Lumbar spine side-bending	Inadequate

MUSCLE ATTACHMENT BOX 39.3

ATTACHMENTS AND INNERVATION OF THE PSOAS MINOR

Proximal attachment: Lateral aspects of the bodies of T12 and L1 and the disc in between

Distal attachment: The iliopubic eminence of the innominate bone and the iliac fascia. Its muscle belly, considerably smaller than that of the psoas major, travels alongside the latter muscle.

Innervation: Ventral ramus of L1

Palpation: Not palpable.

The psoas minor is considerably smaller and weaker than the psoas major. No known investigations exist that examine the role of the psoas minor. Its size and frequent absence suggest that its functions as well as the impairments from weakness or tightness of the psoas minor are minimal.

EXTENSORS OF THE HIP

The gluteus maximus is the primary one-joint hip extensor, although the two-joint hip extensors (the hamstrings) and other one-joint hip muscles included in other muscle groups (adductor magnus) are very important extensors of the hip as well (*Fig. 39.7*).

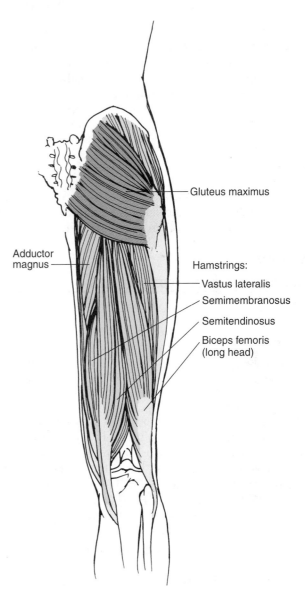

Figure 39.7: The one-joint hip extensor is the gluteus maximus, but other hip extensors include the hamstrings and the adductor magnus.

Gluteus Maximus

The gluteus maximus is a large muscle with a PCSA at least 30% greater that that of the iliopsoas [8] (*Muscle Attachment Box 39.4*). It forms most of the contour of the buttocks.

ACTIONS

MUSCLE ACTION: GLUTEUS MAXIMUS

Action	Evidence
Hip extension	Supporting
Hip lateral rotation	Supporting
Hip abduction	Supporting
Hip adduction	Supporting

The gluteus maximus is a powerful extensor of the hip, with both a large PCSA and a relatively large moment arm [15,39]. Hislop and Montgomery suggest that manual resistance is unable to overcome or "break" the isometric contraction of a gluteus maximus in an individual with normal strength [21]. The function of the gluteus maximus as a hip extensor depends on the position of the body in space as well as the position of the hip joint itself. In the prone position, the gluteus maximus lifts the weight of the lower extremity to extend the hip with a concentric contraction. In quiet standing, because the HAT weight tends to extend the hip, the gluteus maximus is electrically silent [5]. The hip extensors, including the gluteus maximus, contribute postural support when a subject leans forward and the HAT weight creates a

flexion moment at the hip. Under these circumstances, the hip extensors contract eccentrically to control the forward-bending or concentrically to return the individual to an upright position. Yet EMG data from individual subjects reveal little or no activity in the gluteus maximus during forward-bending activities such as bending to lift a 25-lb load [17]. In contrast, the gluteus maximus is active during trunk hyperextension from the prone position [11]. Ascending stairs elicits activity in the hamstrings and adductor magnus along with the gluteus maximus [4,37]. Single-stance wall squats and mini-squats also elicit considerable electrical activity in the gluteus maximus [4]. The gluteus maximus exhibits less activity during active extension from the flexed position and more activity during extension from the extended or hyperextended position [37,77].

Consideration of the structure of the hip extensors helps elucidate the effect of hip position on the extension role of the gluteus maximus. Mechanical analyses and computed tomography (CT) scans to examine the length of the moment arms of the hip extensors from a position of 0° of flexion to 90° of flexion reveal that the moment arm of the gluteus maximus appears greatest at 0° of flexion and decreases steadily to 90° of flexion [15,39,46]. Other hip extensors, namely the hamstrings and adductor magnus, reach their maximum moment arms when the hip is more flexed. The gluteus maximus also consists of relatively long muscle fibers and, although it has a large moment arm in comparison with the hamstrings, it still attaches proximally on the femur [46]. These structural characteristics enhance the gluteus maximus's ability to produce a large joint excursion [23]. The gluteus maximus appears particularly suited to help fully extend or hyperextend the hip joint. These studies suggest that hip extensor recruitment is, at least in part, dictated by the mechanical advantage of the muscles available.

The apparent contradiction in abduction and adduction actions by the gluteus maximus can be explained by dividing the muscle into superior and inferior segments [39]. The superior portion lies superior to the axis of abduction and adduction, while the inferior portion lies inferior to it (*Fig. 39.8*). As a result, the superior portion of the gluteus maximus contributes to abduction of the hip, and its inferior portion contributes to adduction. The whole of the gluteus maximus lies posterior to the axis of medial and lateral rotation, and therefore, the muscle is a lateral rotator of the hip joint with the hip extended [13,15,33]. As the hip flexes, the moment arm for lateral rotation decreases, and by the time the hip reaches 90° of flexion, the superior portion of the gluteus maximus actually has a medial rotation moment arm [13]. EMG data suggest that the addition of active hip abduction or lateral rotation to active hip extension from the extended position significantly increases the electrical activity of the gluteus maximus [11]. Clinicians can enhance gluteus maximus recruitment during exercise by combining hip hyperextension with abduction and lateral rotation.

The role of the gluteus maximus in locomotion has been studied extensively. The gluteus maximus is mildly active

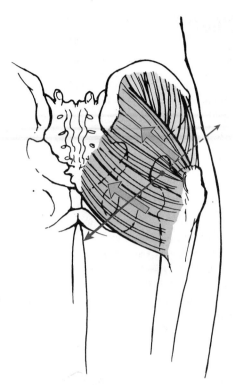

Figure 39.8: The gluteus maximus lies superior and inferior to the axis of abduction and adduction and consequently can contribute to either motion.

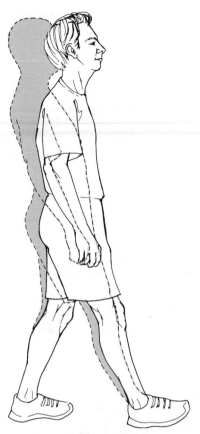

Figure 39.9: The gluteus maximus lurch is characterized by a backward lean of the trunk at heel strike to move the center of mass of the HAT posterior to the hip joint to eliminate the need for the hip extensor muscles.

with the hamstrings during ambulation at the end of swing and the beginning of stance [2,16,37,52,58,76]. These muscles appear to work together to slow the flexion of the hip at the end of swing and to initiate hip extension in early stance by pulling the trunk forward over the stance limb [16,34,36,56,58,76]. Gluteus maximus activity increases substantially with walking up an incline and with running, in which the muscle appears to play an essential role in stabilizing forward trunk lean [34].

WEAKNESS

Weakness of the gluteus maximus results in decreased strength of hip extension and lateral rotation. A classic gait pattern resulting from gluteus maximus weakness, known as the **gluteus maximus lurch,** has been described anecdotally [63] (*Fig. 39.9*). The lurch is a rapid hyperextension of the trunk prior to, and continuing through, heel contact on the side of the gluteus maximus weakness. It has been suggested that the backward "lurch" moves the center of mass of the HAT weight to a position posterior to the hip joint, thus eliminating the need for the gluteus maximus to extend the hip. However, it is also important to recognize that such a significant gait deviation is more likely a result of weakness of other hip extensors in addition to the gluteus maximus.

Clinical Relevance

GLUTEUS MAXIMUS WEAKNESS AND GAIT:
Sutherland et al. report an excessive anterior pelvic tilt and lumbar lordosis seen during ambulation in children with early signs of Duchenne's muscular dystrophy [65]. These authors suggest that weakness of the gluteus maximus explains these gait deviations. The gait pattern documented by Sutherland et al. is similar to, albeit more subtle than, the gluteus maximus lurch described anecdotally and may reflect discrete gluteus maximus weakness.

TIGHTNESS

Tightness of the gluteus maximus limits hip ROM in flexion and medial rotation and, perhaps, adduction, although its effects in the frontal plane are more difficult to ascertain since it appears to be both an abductor and adductor. Athletes such as runners who have strongly developed gluteus maximus muscles can exhibit such tightness. Because hip movement is intimately related to low back movement, tightness of the gluteus maximus may produce excessive movement in the lumbar spine.

Clinical Relevance

GLUTEUS MAXIMUS TIGHTNESS AND LOW BACK PAIN: *Restrictions in hip flexion ROM can require an individual to use excessive trunk flexion during such activities as squatting to pick up an object from the floor or to tie a shoelace. Tightness of the gluteus maximus therefore may be a contributing factor to low back pain.*

ABDUCTORS OF THE HIP

The gluteus medius and gluteus minimus are the primary abductors of the hip, although, as noted in the previous discussion, the gluteus maximus also abducts the hip (*Fig. 39.10*).

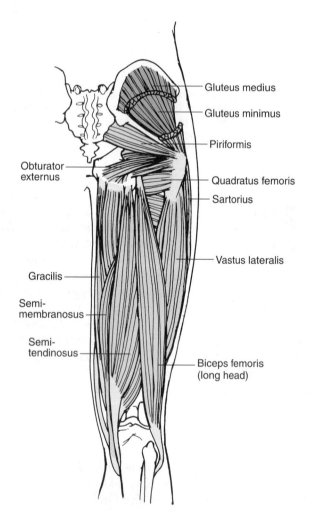

Figure 39.10: The primary hip abductor muscles are the gluteus medius and minimus. The tensor fasciae latae and the sartorius are two-joint muscles that also abduct the hip.

MUSCLE ATTACHMENT BOX 39.5

ATTACHMENTS AND INNERVATION OF THE GLUTEUS MEDIUS

Proximal attachment: The lateral surface of the ala of the ilium between the posterior and anterior gluteal lines

Distal attachment: By tendon to the lateral aspect of the greater trochanter.

Innervation: The superior gluteal nerve, L4,5 and S1

Palpation: Much of the muscle is covered by the gluteus maximus. However, it can be palpated along the posterior surface of the iliac crest at its most superior aspect. It can also be palpated along its length by placing a hand at the iliac crest with the fingers pointing toward the greater trochanter.

Additional two-joint abductor muscles are the tensor fasciae latae and sartorius [9,75]. The gluteus medius and minimus attach to the ala of the ilium and lie on the lateral aspect of the hip and buttocks (*Muscle Attachment Box 39.5*). The electrical activity of the gluteus medius during function is well studied. The gluteus minimus lies deep to the medius and to the tensor fasciae latae and is less well studied (*Muscle Attachment Box 39.6*). Its functional responsibility is usually inferred from knowledge of the gluteus medius. Because these two muscles appear to function together frequently, their functional roles and the effects of weakness and tightness in these muscles are discussed together after discussion of their individual actions.

MUSCLE ATTACHMENT BOX 39.6

ATTACHMENTS AND INNERVATION OF THE GLUTEUS MINIMUS

Proximal attachment: The anterior aspect of the ala of the ilium between the anterior and inferior gluteal lines

Distal attachment: The superior and anterior aspects of the greater trochanter. It lies deep to the gluteus medius but is positioned more anteriorly than the gluteus medius. It cannot be palpated directly.

Innervation: The same as that of the gluteus medius, superior gluteal nerve, L4,5 and S1

Palpation: Not palpable

Gluteus Medius

ACTIONS

MUSCLE ACTION: GLUTEUS MEDIUS

Action	Evidence
Hip abduction	Supporting
Hip medial rotation	Supporting
Hip lateral rotation	Supporting

The gluteus medius undoubtedly is an abductor of the hip. Some authors also report that it medially rotates the hip [21,44] or that the anterior fibers medially rotate the hip and the posterior fibers laterally rotate the hip [30]. Analysis of its moment arms confirms that when the hip is extended, the anterior and middle portions of the gluteus medius are medial rotators of the hip, and the posterior segment laterally rotates the hip [13,15,39]. When the hip is flexed, however, virtually the whole muscle contributes to medial rotation and has little or no capacity to abduct the hip. EMG data show decreased recruitment of the gluteus medius during hip abduction with the hip flexed to 20° [7].

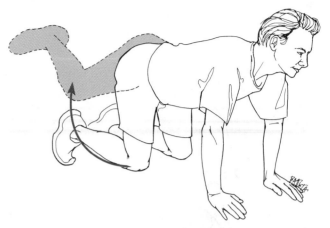

Figure 39.11: The "fire hydrant" exercise, a common exercise for the hip abductors, combines hip abduction with flexion. Since the gluteus medius and minimus muscles are ineffective abductors with the hip flexed, they are unlikely to be strengthened substantially by this exercise.

Clinical Relevance

STRENGTHENING EXERCISES FOR THE GLUTEUS MEDIUS: *Weakness of the gluteus medius produces significant gait deviations and may be associated with hip and knee complaints [19]. Exercises to strengthen the gluteus medius are important and commonly prescribed. One exercise recommended to strengthen the gluteus medius is the "fire hydrant" exercise in which the individual assumes a quadripedal position and lifts one lower extremity with the hip flexed and abducted (Fig. 39.11). Another common exercise uses a weight machine in which the subject sits and abducts the hip against a resistance. Both of these exercises require the subject to abduct the hip when the hip is flexed. However, evidence demonstrates that the gluteus medius is incapable of hip abduction with the hip flexed. The subject is more likely using the gluteus maximus and tensor fasciae latae to abduct the hip. Individuals who want to strengthen the gluteus medius specifically must abduct the hip with the hip extended to ensure recruitment of the gluteus medius. These data demonstrate how a thorough understanding of a muscle's action is essential to prescribe an appropriate exercise regimen.*

Gluteus Minimus

ACTIONS

MUSCLE ACTION: GLUTEUS MINIMUS

Action	Evidence
Hip abduction	Supporting
Hip medial rotation	Supporting
Hip lateral rotation	Supporting

The gluteus minimus is another strong abductor of the hip, although its PCSA is substantially smaller than that of the gluteus medius [8]. Like the gluteus medius, with the hip extended, its anterior portion is a medial rotator of the hip with a larger rotation moment arm than that of the gluteus medius, and its posterior portion is a lateral rotator [13,15]. Hip flexion increases its medial rotation capacity and appears to reduce its ability to abduct the hip. The gluteus minimus also is firmly attached to the hip joint capsule [71]. This attachment may help protect the capsule from impingement by pulling it out of the way of the greater trochanter during active hip abduction. The shoulder, elbow, knee, and ankle exhibit similar mechanisms to protect their sensitive joint capsules.

Functional Role of the Hip Abductors

The broad proximal attachments of both the gluteus medius and gluteus minimus indicate that these muscles are quite strong and are likely to participate in functional activities that require considerable force. Although active abduction of the hip in an open chain is used in activities such as getting on and off a bicycle, the essential role of the abductor muscles occurs during closed chain activities such as walking and running. These activities of bipedal ambulation are characterized by intermittent periods of one-legged stance. During the time of single limb support, the weight of the opposite limb and that of the HAT (the HAT-L weight) exerts an adduction moment on the stance hip, tending to make the body fall onto the unsupported side and adducting the hip on the stance side (*Fig. 39.12*). To hold the pelvis and the weight above it stable, the abductor muscles on the support side pull from their distal attachments on the femur to their proximal pelvic attachments. This pull, if strong enough, holds the pelvis level and prevents its dropping on the unsupported side. Similarly, the hip abductors provide

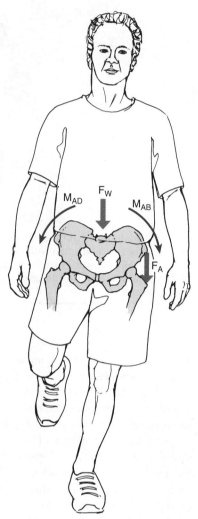

Figure 39.12: During single-limb stance, the force of the weight of the HAT-L (F_W) tends to adduct the stance hip, applying an adduction moment (M_{AD}). The pull of the abductors (F_A) holds the pelvis level, applying an abduction moment (M_{AB}).

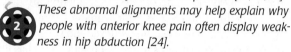

Clinical Relevance

THE ROLE OF THE HIP ABDUCTORS IN MAINTAINING LOWER EXTREMITY ALIGNMENT IN WEIGHT BEARING: *Many upright activities such as stair ascent and descent or stepping on and off a curb require complex stabilization of the hip, knee, and ankle in all three planes of motion. The ability to stabilize the knee and foot in the three planes appears to be in part the responsibility of the hip abductor muscles. Stair descent consists of repeated single limb squats, as an individual lowers body weight onto the lower step by flexing the hip and knee that still bear weight on the upper step. With inadequate stability of the weight-bearing hip, the weight-bearing knee tends to move into more valgus and the foot tends to pronate [10,22,40]. These abnormal alignments may help explain why people with anterior knee pain often display weakness in hip abduction [24].*

Effects of Weakness of the Abductor Muscles

Weakness of the gluteus medius and minimus results in a significant decrease in abduction strength, since they are the primary abductors of the hip. The functional ramifications of such weakness are most apparent in weight-bearing activities, specifically in single-limb support. The functional problem occurs during stance on the side of the weakness. As single-limb support begins and the abductor muscles are too weak to hold the pelvis level, the HAT-L weight tends to cause the pelvis to drop on the unsupported side. Because this is a very unstable phenomenon and puts the subject at risk of falling, most subjects use a typical substitution. To avoid the pelvic drop on the unsupported side, the subject leans the trunk toward the supporting side (*Fig. 39.13*). This lean moves the center of mass of the HAT-L weight to the lateral aspect of the hip joint on the stance side. In this position, the HAT-L weight no longer tends to adduct the hip. In fact, the weight creates a slight abduction moment, thus eliminating the need for active abduction force. The resulting gait pattern is so characteristic of hip abductor weakness it is dubbed a **gluteus medius limp,** although it is likely to involve both the gluteus medius and the gluteus minimus [32,42]. Perhaps the functional deficits resulting from weakness of the gluteus medius and minimus would be described better as an abductor limp. (See video in Chapter 28.)

Clinical Relevance

TRENDELENBURG TEST: *A simple clinical screening procedure for abductor weakness uses single-limb stance and*
(continued)

proximal support to stabilize the femur and help maintain frontal plane alignment of the knee and foot within the lower extremity closed chain [10,22].

A magnetic resonance imaging (MRI) study examines the relative activity of the gluteus medius and gluteus minimus muscles during active abduction in different positions of abduction and during single-limb standing [32]. The authors report that the gluteus minimus demonstrates more activity than the gluteus medius during abduction with the hip abducted to 20° and also during single-limb stance. They also note that while the abduction moment arm of the gluteus medius is longer than that of the gluteus minimus with the hip in the neutral or adducted position, the opposite is true in the abducted position. This study confirms the importance of the gluteus minimus as an abductor and as a support during single-limb stance.

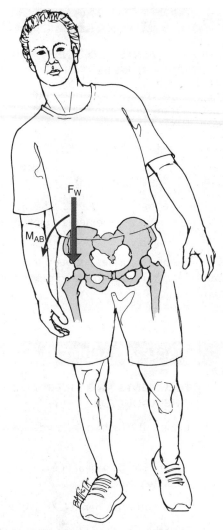

Figure 39.13: Gluteus medius limp. During single-limb stance, an individual with weakness of the hip abductors leans laterally during single-limb stance on the weak side, moving the center of mass of the HAT-L weight to the lateral side of the hip joint, producing an abduction moment (M_{AB}) on the hip.

 (Continued)
*the postural compensation present with abductor weakness. The test is known as the **Trendelenburg test** and uses quiet, single-limb standing. It is positive for abductor weakness on the stance side when the subject leans excessively toward the stance limb or when the pelvis drops on the unsupported side [42].*

Hip abductor weakness is associated with anterior knee pain and the presence of hip osteoarthritis [3,24]. It is not clear whether abductor weakness is a risk factor for or the consequence of these disorders. Additional research is needed to determine if strengthening these muscles can prevent or decrease the pain and dysfunction associated with the disorder. It is clear that clinicians must consider the role of

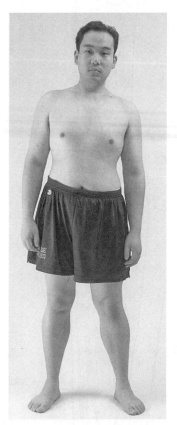

Figure 39.14: Standing posture with one hip abducted. An individual standing with one hip abducted typically lowers the pelvis on the abducted side to allow floor contact.

the hip abductor muscles in treating individuals with lower extremity dysfunction.

Effects of Tightness of the Abductor Muscles

Abductor tightness, although not common, does exist. Tightness of these muscles results in decreased ROM in adduction and, perhaps, in lateral rotation. Such tightness is found in individuals with arthritis whose position of comfort frequently includes hip flexion and abduction. The functional consequences of an abduction contracture are seen most often in upright posture and may include changes in pelvic alignment to maintain erect posture or in the positions of the other joints of the lower extremity to optimize the base of support (*Fig. 39.14*).

ADDUCTORS OF THE HIP

The primary one-joint adductors of the hip include the pectineus, adductor brevis, adductor longus, and adductor magnus (*Fig. 39.15*) (*Muscle Attachment Boxes 39.7–39.9*). The gracilis is a two-joint adductor of the hip. The adductors of the hip share two important characteristics: they all have some attachment to the pubis, and they all receive some innervation

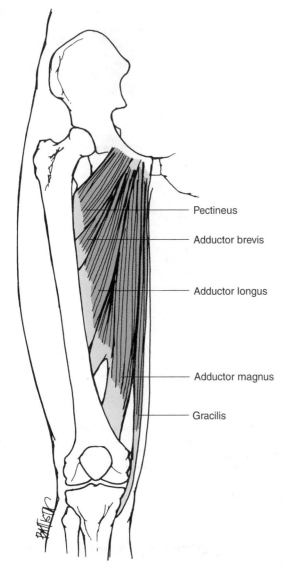

Figure 39.15: The one-joint hip adductor muscles include the pectineus, the adductor brevis and longus, and the adductor magnus. The two-joint adductor is the gracilis.

from the obturator nerve. They are only partially palpable along the medial aspect of the thigh, covered in part by subcutaneous fat and also by the large muscles of the thigh, the hamstrings, and the quadriceps. The role of the adductors in function and the effects of weakness and tightness are discussed as a group following the discussion of their individual actions.

Pectineus

ACTIONS

MUSCLE ACTION: PECTINEUS

Action	Evidence
Hip adduction	Supporting
Hip flexion	Supporting
Hip medial rotation	Supporting

MUSCLE ATTACHMENT BOX 39.7

ATTACHMENTS AND INNERVATION OF THE PECTINEUS

Proximal attachment: The superior ramus of the pubis between the pubic tubercle and the iliopubic eminence

Distal attachment: The pectineal line on the posterior aspect of the femur between the lesser trochanter and the linea aspera.

Innervation: The femoral nerve (L2, 3) and the obturator (L3). However, the nerve supply may be variable [55].

Palpation: The pectineus lies between the psoas major and the adductor longus and cannot be palpated readily.

MUSCLE ATTACHMENT BOX 39.8

ATTACHMENTS AND INNERVATION OF THE ADDUCTOR BREVIS

Proximal attachment: The body and inferior ramus of the pubis

Distal attachment: The pectineal line and the proximal half of the linea aspera.

Innervation: The obturator nerve (L2, 3, 4)

Palpation: The adductor brevis lies posterior to the pectineus and adductor longus and anterior to the adductor magnus and cannot be palpated.

MUSCLE ATTACHMENT BOX 39.9

ATTACHMENTS AND INNERVATION OF THE ADDUCTOR LONGUS

Proximal attachment: The body of the pubis at the intersection of the crest and symphysis

Distal attachment: The medial lip of the linea aspera. The adductor longus attaches more anteriorly on the pubis than any other adductor. It has a prominent long tendon proximally, which gives the muscle its name.

Innervation: The obturator nerve (L2, 3, 4)

Palpation: The proximal tendon is easily palpated in the groin and serves as an important landmark for fitting above-knee prostheses.

The actions of flexion and adduction by the pectineus are consistent with its location at the hip and are supported by analysis of its moment arms [15]. Analysis of the rotation moment arm of the pectineus and EMG data suggest that the muscle also is active in medial rotation with other adductors [1,55,67].

Adductor Brevis

ACTIONS

MUSCLE ACTION: ADDUCTOR BREVIS

Action	Evidence
Hip adduction	Supporting
Hip medial rotation	Supporting
Hip lateral rotation	Refuting
Hip flexion	Supporting
Hip extension	Conflicting

The adductor brevis has one of the largest adduction moment arms of the muscles of the thigh and appears capable of hip adduction with the hip in any position of flexion [15]. Like that of the pectineus, the role of the adductor brevis in rotation is controversial. Anatomy texts report that it either medially rotates the hip [6] or laterally rotates it [44,55]. However, EMG data reveal activity in the adductor brevis only during medial rotation [5]. Moment arm analysis also supports a role only in medial rotation [1]. Moment arm analysis also supports the view that the adductor brevis changes from a hip flexor to an extensor as the hip flexes [15]. Although no EMG studies of the adductor brevis during simple active flexion and extension movements have been found, Basmajian and DeLuca report that during walking, the brevis is most active at toe-off [5]. Since the hip is flexing at toe-off, these data indirectly support the adductor brevis's role as a flexor when the hip is extended.

Adductor Longus

ACTIONS

MUSCLE ACTION: ADDUCTOR LONGUS

Action	Evidence
Hip adduction	Supporting
Hip flexion	Supporting
Hip extension	Refuting
Hip medial rotation	Conflicting
Hip lateral rotation	Conflicting

Mechanical analysis reveals that the muscle possesses an adduction moment arm regardless of sagittal plane hip position [15]. Open chain adduction appears to elicit consistent EMG activity of the adductor longus [5]. Few EMG studies exist, but existing EMG and mechanical data also support the role of the adductor longus as a flexor of the hip, and one study suggests that its role as a flexor exceeds its role as an adductor [5,20]. The adductor longus exhibits a consistent, albeit small, medial rotation moment arm [1,15]. However, EMG data provide contradictory and inconsistent evidence for a role in rotation [5,20,74]. The muscle appears to play a more consistent role in hip flexion and adduction than in rotation.

Adductor Magnus

The adductor magnus rightfully bears the name "magnus," since it is substantially larger than any other adductor muscle, being similar in size to the biceps femoris of the hamstring muscle group [8,72] (*Muscle Attachment Box 39.10*).

ACTIONS

MUSCLE ACTION: ADDUCTOR MAGNUS

Action	Evidence
Hip adduction	Conflicting
Hip extension	Supporting
Hip medial rotation	Conflicting
Hip lateral rotation	Conflicting

Although named an adductor, the role of the adductor magnus in hip adduction remains unclear and probably varies. Some of the confusion lies in the size of the muscle and whether investigators study the muscle as a whole or in segments. Assessment of the muscle's moment arm reveals that the muscle as a whole possesses an adduction moment arm [33]. When segmented, however, the anterior portion exhibits a significant adduction moment arm with the hip in any position of hip flexion. The middle and posterior segments have smaller adduction moment arms and only in portions of the

MUSCLE ATTACHMENT BOX 39.10

ATTACHMENTS AND INNERVATION OF THE ADDUCTOR MAGNUS

Proximal attachment: The inferior ramus of the pubis, the ischial ramus, and the ischial tuberosity

Distal attachment: Along the length of the femur from the quadrate tubercle, along the linea aspera and medial supracondylar line to the adductor tubercle. This broad attachment gives rise to the largest of the adductors, whose size justifies its title "magnus."

Innervation: A branch from the tibial portion of the sciatic nerve, L4 and the obturator nerve, L2, 3, and 4

Palpation: This muscle is most easily palpated at its distal attachment on the adductor tubercle.

hip flexion range. The limited EMG data available provide little additional insight, reporting contradictory results [5,20]. Such contradictions likely arise by recording from different segments of the muscle. More EMG data recorded from all three portions of the muscle may help clarify the role of the adductor magnus in hip adduction.

In contrast, the role of the adductor magnus as a hip extensor is generally well accepted [20,33,39,46]. It is even described as another hamstring muscle [55]. The posterior segment of the adductor magnus has a larger extension moment arm than the gluteus maximus or hamstrings when the hip is extended [15].

EMG data describing the contribution of the adductor magnus to hip rotation also are contradictory [5,20], and again, analysis of the muscle's rotational moment arms helps explain the controversy. Portions of the muscle possess slight medial rotation moment arms, while other segments possess lateral rotation moment arms [1,15]. However, these moment arms are small, and the adductor magnus plays, at most, an accessory role in hip rotation.

Functional Role of the Adductors of the Hip

Despite the areas of disagreement surrounding the individual actions of the adductor muscles, most investigators agree on one important functional role of the adductors—to stabilize the pelvis during weight shifting from one limb to the other. This role is seen during gait as the adductors contract during the transitions from stance to swing and swing to stance [16,52].

The adductors also help stabilize the hip during squatting activities. In squatting to lift something from the floor, an individual typically has the hips slightly abducted (*Fig. 39.16*). Inspection of the ground reaction force reveals that it produces an abduction moment at the hip that must be countered by an adduction moment produced by contraction of the adductor muscles. Anyone who has gardened can probably verify the adductor muscles' role by recalling the muscle soreness in the inner thighs after the spring garden cleanup!

Effects of Weakness

Adductor weakness is not common but may result from an injury to the obturator nerve. Such injuries have been reported following surgeries such as laparoscopic or endoscopic prostatectomies and even rarely following vaginal deliveries [49,62,64]. Symptoms include gait instability and an abducted gait in which the affected limb contacts the ground with the hip excessively abducted [49]. In most cases symptoms resolve with conservative management, including exercise and gait training.

Effects of Tightness

Tightness of the adductors is relatively common and may result from adaptive changes in muscles that are not routinely stretched. Such tightness is likely in sedentary individuals or

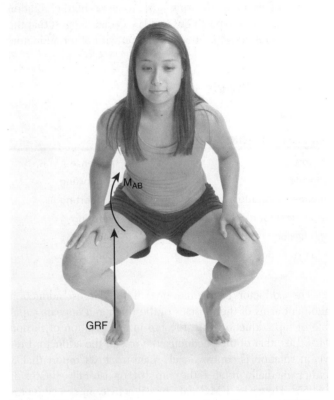

Figure 39.16: During a squat, the ground reaction force (GRF) produces an abduction moment (M_{AB}) on the hip, requiring contraction of the adductors to produce a balancing adductor moment.

in individuals on bed rest who do not receive active or passive exercises. In addition, adductor muscles are commonly affected by central nervous system disorders resulting in spasticity. Examples of such disorders include cerebral vascular accidents (strokes), multiple sclerosis, and cerebral palsy.

In an ambulatory individual, extreme tightness of the adductors of the hip can create significant problems in gait, leading to **scissors gait.** During swing, the limb with the tightness may have difficulty passing the stance limb, causing the individual to trip over the stance limb. The limb with the tightness also may land in front of the opposite limb at the beginning of double-limb support, again presenting a threat of tripping.

Clinical Relevance

ADDUCTOR SPASTICITY IN CHILDREN: *Spasticity of the hip adductors is a common clinical finding in individuals with cerebral palsy. In children, adductor spasticity is an important contributing factor to hip dislocation and hip dysplasia. At birth, the normal alignment of the femur is valgus,* *directing the femoral head toward the superior aspect of the acetabulum when the hip is in the neutral position. Adduction from the neutral position moves the femoral head laterally in the acetabulum. Because the acetabulum is shallowest at birth, prolonged positioning of the hip in adduction can sublux or dislocate the hip joint [53]. The presence of spasticity of the adductors presents significant additional risk for dislocation, and surgical release of spastic muscles around the hip, including the adductors, reduces the dislocating forces, helping to minimize the incidence of dislocation and hip dysplasia [43,54].*

LATERAL ROTATORS OF THE HIP

The lateral rotators of the hip include the piriformis, obturator internus, superior and inferior gemelli, quadratus femoris, and obturator externus (*Fig. 39.17*) (*Muscle Attachment Boxes 39.11–39.15*). These muscles make up the group of short rotators of the hip lying deep to the gluteus maximus, which itself is an important lateral rotator of the hip. None of these muscles can be palpated directly, since they lie deep to the large gluteus maximus. However, the horizontally aligned muscles emerging from the greater sciatic notch may be palpable as a group in the notch through a relaxed gluteus maximus. Their actions and the effects of impairments in these muscle groups are discussed together.

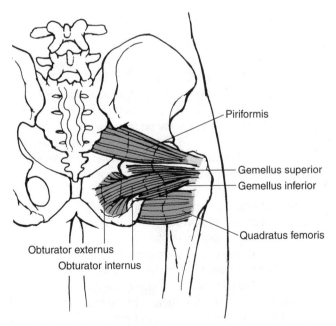

Figure 39.17: The deep lateral rotators of the hip include the piriformis, the superior and inferior gemelli, the obturator internus and externus, and the quadratus femoris.

MUSCLE ATTACHMENT BOX 39.11

ATTACHMENTS AND INNERVATION OF THE PIRIFORMIS

Proximal attachment: The anterior aspect of the sacrum at the level of about S2 through S4. It also has some attachment to the sacrotuberous ligament and to the periphery of the greater sciatic notch as it passes through it, exiting the pelvis. The sciatic nerve usually exits the pelvis alongside the piriformis and emerges at its inferior border.

Distal attachment: The superior and medial aspects of the greater trochanter

Innervation: The ventral rami of L5 and S1,2

Palpation: The piriformis may be palpable indirectly by palpating through the gluteus maximus into the greater sciatic notch.

MUSCLE ATTACHMENT BOX 39.12

ATTACHMENTS AND INNERVATION OF THE OBTURATOR INTERNUS

Proximal attachment: The obturator membrane and the borders of the obturator notch. It exits the pelvis through the lesser sciatic notch.

Distal attachment: The medial aspect of the greater trochanter

Innervation: The nerve to the obturator internus, L5 and S1,2

Palpation: Not directly palpable.

MUSCLE ATTACHMENT BOX 39.13

ATTACHMENTS AND INNERVATION OF THE SUPERIOR AND INFERIOR GEMELLI

Proximal attachment: The inferior aspect of the ischial spine and the superior aspect of the ischial tuberosity, respectively. The two muscles are intimately associated with the obturator internus, one superior and the other inferior to it.

Distal attachment: The medial aspect of the greater trochanter with the obturator internus

Innervation: The nerve to the obturator internus, L5, S1 (superior gemellus) and nerve to the quadratus femoris, L5, S1 (inferior gemellus)

Palpation: Not directly palpable.

MUSCLE ATTACHMENT BOX 39.14

ATTACHMENTS AND INNERVATION OF THE QUADRATUS FEMORIS

Proximal attachment: The lateral border of the ischial tuberosity

Distal attachment: The intertrochanteric crest and quadrate tubercle of the femur. It is a flat, quadrilaterally shaped muscle.

Innervation: The nerve to the quadratus femoris (L4,5, S1)

Palpation: Not palpable.

Group Actions

MUSCLE ACTION: LATERAL ROTATORS

Action	Evidence
Hip lateral rotation	Supporting
Hip abduction	Conflicting
Hip adduction	Conflicting

These muscles are all lateral rotators of the hip, but the position of the hip in the sagittal plane significantly affects their capacity to rotate the hip [13,15]. Moment arm analysis reveals that the quadratus femoris exerts a lateral rotation moment regardless of the hip flexion position [13,15]. With the hip extended, the obturator internus and gemelli also generate lateral rotation moments, but when the hip flexes, their moment arms approach zero so that they generate little or no rotation moment. The piriformis appears to change from a lateral rotator with the hip extended to a medial rotator with the hip flexed. In contrast, the lateral rotation moment arm of the obturator externus increases as the hip flexes. These data

MUSCLE ATTACHMENT BOX 39.15

ATTACHMENTS AND INNERVATION OF THE OBTURATOR EXTERNUS

Proximal attachment: The anterior aspect of the pubic and ischial borders of the obturator foramen and the obturator membrane. The muscle passes posteriorly across the posterior aspect of the femoral neck.

Distal attachment: The intertrochanteric fossa.

Innervation: A division of the obturator nerve (L3,4)

Palpation: Not directly palpable.

reveal that the roles of these deep muscles in rotation are more complex than their title of "lateral rotators" suggests. Clinicians must recognize the influence of hip position on their contribution to rotation. Additionally, a valid assessment of lateral rotation strength requires standard test positions to ensure that the same muscles participate in each test.

Anatomy texts suggest a role for these muscles in abduction and adduction of the hip [44,55]. Biomechanical studies suggest that their contributions to these motions depend on hip position [15]. The piriformis possesses an abduction moment arm regardless of hip position, but the obturator internus can abduct only when the hip is flexed [15,33]. In contrast, the obturator externus and quadratus femoris are capable of hip adduction, but only when the hip is extended or slightly flexed. It is important to note that the PCSA of these muscles is considerably smaller than those of the primary hip abductor and adductor muscles, and consequently, these lateral rotators are far less powerful than the primary hip abductors and adductors. Because of their proximity to the hip joint, virtually surrounding the proximal portion of the joint, the small lateral rotator muscles also may serve as dynamic stabilizers of the hip joint.

Effects of Weakness and Tightness

The gluteus maximus remains the strongest of the lateral rotators, and therefore, discrete weakness of these small muscles may be hard to detect. Like weakness, isolated tightness of the short lateral rotators may be hard to observe. However, the proximity of the sciatic nerve to these muscles, particularly to the piriformis, which may even be pierced by the nerve, makes tightness of these muscles clinically relevant [55]. If tight, these muscles may exert pressure on the sciatic nerve, producing pain radiating into the lower extremity.

Clinical Relevance

PIRIFORMIS SYNDROME: The *piriformis syndrome* refers to pain associated with tightness or spasm of the piriformis muscle that puts pressure on the underlying sciatic nerve, causing radicular symptoms similar to signs of disc pathology. The symptoms can be aggravated by stretching or contracting the piriformis, that is, by medially rotating the hip passively to stretch the muscle or by resisting lateral rotation, causing the piriformis to contract [38]. The clinician uses these passive or resisted movements to elicit the patient's symptoms and to identify piriformis syndrome.

The classic stretch for the piriformis muscle is hip flexion with adduction and medial rotation. Yet laterally rotating the hip has little effect on the stretch of the piriformis. In fact research suggests that sitting with the knees crossed (Fig. 39.18) applies a significant stretch to piriformis of the upper leg despite the fact that the hip is rotated laterally almost 20° [61].

The most common functional use of active medial rotation of the hip occurs during the stance phase of gait when the pelvis rotates over the fixed femur and as the hip moves from the flexed to the extended position. During this period, the abductors contract to support the pelvis in the frontal plane, and the hamstrings are supporting the hip and knee in the sagittal plane. Their activity in medial rotation demonstrates an efficient use of muscles to perform simultaneous tasks.

COMPARISONS OF MUSCLE GROUP STRENGTHS

An understanding of the relative muscle strengths of various muscle groups in the hip provides a helpful perspective for clinicians making judgments about their patients' strengths in the muscles of the hip. This section reviews the data available on the relative strengths of hip muscles in healthy individuals.

Several studies investigate the strength of whole muscle groups of the hip and the effects of joint position on their strength. Data consistently demonstrate that hip flexion strength decreases as the hip flexes from 25 to 130° of flexion, as the muscles go from a lengthened to a shortened position [26,31,73]. Few studies examine hip flexion strength with the hip fully extended, and those studies vary in measurement procedures and results, some demonstrating a continued increase in strength [31,73] and another showing a loss in strength [26]. Any loss in hip flexion strength with the hip extended must be verified by further research but may result from a decrease in the muscles' angle of application.

Most data demonstrate that hip abduction and adduction strength also decreases as the muscles contract from lengthened to shortened positions [31,45,47,50]. The length–tension relationship appears to dictate the force production in hip rotation as well, so that medial and lateral rotation strengths increase as the muscles are lengthened [23,31,41]. These studies emphasize the need to standardize the test positions when assessing hip strength.

Comparisons of the strength of opposing muscle groups also provide useful information to assist clinicians in determining the clinical relevance of muscle strength tests. Hip adduction appears to be stronger than abduction [29,45,48]. However, the position in which the muscles are tested affects the comparisons. Murray and Sepic [45] compare the strength of hip abductor and adductor strength in 80 healthy males and females aged 18 to 55 years with the hip in neutral and in the abducted position. The adductor muscles generate larger isometric torques than the abductor muscles in both hip positions. However, because both the abductors and adductors produce larger isometric moments as they are lengthened, there is less disparity between the muscle groups with the hip in neutral than when the hip is abducted, the position in which the abductor muscles are shortened and the adductors are lengthened. Peak adductor force is larger than peak abductor force, at least partially because the total PCSA of the adductor muscles is larger than that of the abductor muscles [45].

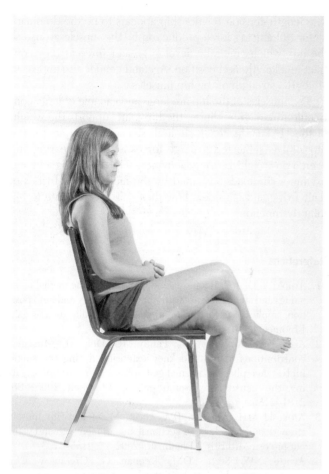

Figure 39.18: Sitting with the legs crossed applies a stretch to the piriformis particularly in the top leg by combining flexion and adduction of the hip.

MEDIAL ROTATORS OF THE HIP

Unlike the other actions of the hip, there are no muscles at the hip whose primary and consistent action is medial rotation of the hip. From the data provided in this chapter, it is evident that the gluteus medius and minimus are capable of medial rotation of the hip, particularly when the hip is flexed. The gluteus maximus and piriformis also may contribute to medial rotation of the hip when the hip is flexed. Some of the hip adductors may generate small medial rotation moments, but their contributions are small and variable.

Another muscle described as a medial rotator of the hip is the tensor fasciae latae, described in more detail with the muscles of the knee [5,9] (Chapter 42). Although EMG activity is reported in the tensor fasciae latae during medial rotation, mechanical analysis reveals no substantial moment arm for hip rotation regardless of hip position [9,15]. The medial hamstrings, the semimembranosus, and semitendinosus also exhibit small medial rotation moment arms with the hip in extension [1]. These data reveal that the muscles that medially rotate the hip depend on hip position and are intimately related to the function of the knee.

Comparisons of hip rotation strength have also been carried out. Several investigators report that with the hip and knee flexed, the standard position for testing the strength of hip rotation, the medial rotators generate more force than the lateral rotators under isometric and concentric conditions [25,35,41]. Jarvis noted a reversal in this relationship when testing with the hip extended and knee flexed in 50 women from 21 to 50 years of age [25]. However, Lindsay et al. also compared strengths with the hip extended and knee flexed and reported that the medial rotators are stronger than the lateral rotators in 60 men and women from 18 to 30 years of age [35]. These differences may be methodological or may represent population differences in the effects of joint position. In either case, the clinician is reminded by these studies that accurate strength assessment at the hip requires careful attention to the position of the joint throughout the test. In addition, it appears that the present level of knowledge prevents any conclusion regarding the relative strength of the hip rotators.

Although only limited data are available, hip strength is greater in men than in women and is greater in younger adults than in older adults [27,45]. Attempts to identify differences between the left and right sides are limited and have produced contradictory results. Neumann et al. reported no significant difference between left and right isometric hip abductor strength overall in 40 healthy right-handed individuals [47]. However, they noted a significantly higher strength in the right than in the left when the hip is positioned in neutral and in adduction. Jarvis found no difference in isometric strength of rotation between left and right sides in 50 healthy women [25]. May, however, reported significantly greater strength on the left than on the right for medial rotation in all positions tested in 25 healthy young men [41]. At the present time there is insufficient data to identify a consistent effect of the side tested on hip strength.

SUMMARY

This chapter details the function of the individual one-joint muscles of the hip. The evidence presented in this chapter reveals that although hip muscles are typically described as flexors, extensors, abductors, adductors, and rotators, the role of each muscle depends greatly upon joint position. A muscle's action depends on its moment arm, which changes with varying joint position. An understanding of the effects of joint position on muscle function allows the clinician to identify optimal positions for exercise.

Muscle impairments at the hip produce significant functional challenges. Weakness in the muscles of the hip may produce specific gait deviations as well as difficulties in activities such as stair climbing and rising from a chair. Muscular tightness at the hip limits hip ROM and may increase the loads on the low back by requiring excessive compensatory lumbar movement.

Strength comparisons reveal that hip position influences the force of contraction of all the muscle groups of the hip.

The length–tension relationship appears to be the dominant factor influencing force production by the muscle groups of the hip, which generally develop greater force as they contract in a lengthened position. Age and gender also appear to affect the strength of the hip muscles.

The muscles of the hip are large and capable of large contractile forces. In addition, the hip joint supports the weight of the HAT-L during single-limb stance. Consequently, the hip joint is subjected to large forces in weight-bearing and even non-weight-bearing activities. The following chapter examines the loads sustained by the hip during activities of daily living and considers how those loads contribute to hip joint dysfunction.

References

1. Arnold A, Delp S: Rotational moment arms of the medial hamstrings and adductors vary with femoral geometry and limb position: implications for the treatment of internally rotated gait. J Biomech 2001; 34: 437–447.
2. Arnold AS, Anderson FC, Pandy MG, Delp SL: Muscular contributions to hip and knee extension during the single limb stance phase of normal gait: a framework for investigating the causes of crouch gait. J Biomech 2005; 38: 2181–2189.
3. Arokoski MH, Arokoski JPA, Haara M, et al.: Hip muscle strength and muscle cross sectional area in men with and without hip osteoarthritis. J Rheumatol 2002; 29: 2185–2195.
4. Ayotte NW, Stetts DM, Keenan G, Greenway EH: Electromyographical analysis of selected lower extremity muscles during 5 unilateral weight-bearing exercises. J Orthop Sports Phys Ther 2007; 37: 48–55.
5. Basmajian JV, DeLuca CJ: Muscles Alive. Their Function Revealed by Electromyography. Baltimore: Williams & Wilkins, 1985.
6. Boccardi S, Pedotti A: Evaluation of muscular moments at the lower limb joints by an on-line processing of kinematic data and ground reaction. J Biomech 1981; 14: 35–45.
7. Bolgla LA, Uhl TL: Electromyographic analysis of hip rehabilitation exercises in a group of healthy subjects. J Orthop Sports Phys Ther 2005; 35: 487–494.
8. Brand RA, Pedersen DR, Friederich JA: The sensitivity of muscle force predictions to changes in physiologic cross-sectional area. J Biomech 1986; 19: 589–596.
9. Carlsoo S, Fohlin L: The mechanics of the two-joint muscles rectus femoris, sartorius and tensor fasciae latae in relation to their activity. Scand J Rehabil Med 1969; 1: 107–111.
10. Claiborne TL, Armstrong CW, Gandhi V, Pincivero DM: Relationship between hip and knee strength and knee valgus during a single leg squat. J Appl Biomech 2006; 22: 41–50.
11. Clark BC, Manini TM, Mayer JM, et al.: Electromyographic activity of the lumbar and hip extensors during dynamic trunk extension exercise. Arch Phys Med Rehabil 2002; 83: 1547–1552.
12. Danis CG, Krebs DE, Gill-Body KM, Sahrmann SA: Relationship between standing posture and stability. Phys Ther 1998; 78: 502–517.
13. Delp SL, Hess WE, Hungerford DS, Jones LC: Variation of rotation moment arms with hip flexion. J Biomech 1999; 32: 493–501.

14. Delp SL, Maloney W: Effects of hip center location on the moment-generating capacity of the muscles. J Biomech 1993; 26: 485–499.

15. Dostal WF, Soderberg GL, Andrews JG: Actions of hip muscles. Phys Ther 1986; 66: 351–361.

16. Eberhart HD, Inman VT, Bresler B: The principal elements of human locomotion. In: Klopsteg PE, Wilson PD, eds. Human Limbs and Their Substitutes. New York: McGraw-Hill, 1954.

17. Fischer FJ, Houtz SJ: EMG of gluteus maximus. Am J Phys Med 1968; 47: 182–191.

18. Flint MM: An electromyographic comparison of the function of the iliacus and the rectus abdominis muscles. J APTA 1965; 45: 248–253.

19. Fredericson M, Cookingham CL, Chaudhari AM, et al.: Hip abductor weakness in distance runners with iliotibial band syndrome. Clin J Sports Med 2000; 10: 175.

20. Green DL, Morris JM: Role of adductor longus and adductor magnus in postural movements and in ambulation. Am J Phys Med 1970; 49: 223–240.

21. Hislop HJ, Montgomery J: Daniel's and Worthingham's Muscle Testing: Techniques of Manual Examination. Philadelphia: WB Saunders, 1995.

22. Hollman JH, Kolbeck KE, Hitchcock JL, et al.: Correlations between hip strength and static foot and knee posture. J Sport Rehabil 2006; 15: 12–23.

23. Hoy MG, Zajac FE, Gordon ME: A musculoskeletal model of the human lower extremity: the effect of muscle, tendon, and moment arm on the moment-angle relationship of musculotendon actuators at the hip, knee, and ankle. J Biomech 1990; 23: 157–169.

24. Ireland ML, Willson JD, Ballantyne BT, Davis IM: Hip strength in females with and without patellofemoral pain. J Orthop Sports Phys Ther 2003; 33: 671–676.

25. Jarvis DK: Relative strength of the hip rotator muscle groups. Phys Ther Rev 1 A.D., 1952; 32: 500–503.

26. Jensen R, Smidt GL, Johnston RC: A technique for obtaining measurements of force generated by hip muscles. Arch Phys Med Rehabil 1971; 52: 207–215.

27. Johnson ME, Mille ML, Martinez KM, et al.: Age-related changes in hip abductor and adductor joint torques. Arch Phys Med Rehabil 2004; 85: 593–597.

28. Juker D, McGill S, Kropf P, Steffen T: Quantitative intramuscular myoelectric activity of lumbar portions of psoas and the abdominal wall during a wide variety of tasks. Med Sci Sports Exerc 1998; 30: 301–310.

29. Kea J, Kramer J, Forwell L, Birmingham T: Hip abduction-adduction strength and one-leg hop tests: test-retest reliability and relationship to function in elite ice hockey players. J Orthop Sports Phys Ther 2001; 31: 446–455.

30. Kendall FP, McCreary EK, Provance PG: Muscle Testing and Function. Baltimore: Williams & Wilkins, 1993.

31. Kulig K, Andrews JG, Hay JG: Human strength curves. Exerc Sports Sci Rev 1984; 12: 417–466.

32. Kumagai M, Shiba N, Higuchi F, et al. Functional evaluation of hip abductor muscles with use of magnetic resonance imaging. J Orthop Res 1997; 15: 888–893.

33. Lengsfeld M, Pressel T, Stammberger U: Lengths and lever arms of hip joint muscles: geometrical analyses using a human multibody model. Gait Posture 1997; 6: 18–26.

34. Lieberman DE, Raichlen DA, Pontzer H, et al.: The human gluteus maximus and its role in running. J Exp Biol 2006; 209: 2143–2155.

35. Lindsay DM, Maitland ME, Lowe RC, Kane TJ: Comparison of isokinetic internal and external hip rotation torques using different testing positions. J Orthop Sports Phys Ther 1992; 16: 43–50.

36. Liu MQ, Anderson FC, Pandy MG, Delp SL: Muscles that support the body also modulate forward progression during walking. J Biomech 2006; 39: 2623–2630.

37. Lyons K, Perry J, Gronley J, et al.: Timing and relative intensity of hip extensor and abductor muscle action during level and stair ambulation. Phys Ther 1983; 63: 1597–1605.

38. Magee DJ: Orthopedic Physical Assessment. Philadelphia: WB Saunders, 1998.

39. Mansour JM, Pereira JM: Quantitative functional anatomy of the lower limb with application to human gait. J Biomech 1987; 20: 1: 51–58.

40. Mascal CL, Landel R, Powers C: Management of patellofemoral pain targeting hip, pelvis, and trunk muscle function: 2 case reports. J Orthop Sports Phys Ther 2003; 33: 642–660.

41. May WW: Maximum isometric force of the hip rotator muscles. J Am Phys Ther Assoc 1996; 46: 233–238.

42. Mendler HM: Relationship of hip abductor muscles to posture. J Am Phys Ther Assoc 1964; 44: 98–102.

43. Miller F, Slomczykowski M, Cope R, Lipton G: Computer modeling of the pathomechanics of spastic hip dislocation in children. J Pediatr Orthop 1999; 19: 486–492.

44. Moore KL: Clinically Oriented Anatomy. Philadelphia: Lippincott Williams & Wilkins, 1999.

45. Murray MP, Sepic SB: Maximum isometric torque of hip abductor and adductor muscles. J Am Phys Ther Assoc 1968; 48: 1327–1335.

46. Nemeth G, Ohlsen H: In vivo moment arm lengths for hip extensor muscles at different angles of hip flexion. J Biomech 1985; 18: 129–140.

47. Neumann DA, Soderberg GL, Cook TM: Comparison of maximal isometric hip abductor muscle torques between hip sides. Phys Ther 1988; 68: 496–502.

48. Nicholas JA, Strizak AM, Veras G: A study of thigh muscle weakness in different pathological states of the lower extremity. Am J Sports Med 1976; 4: 241–248.

49. Nogajski JH, Shnier RC, Zagami AS: Postpartum obturator neuropathy. Neurology 2004; 63: 2450–2451.

50. Olson VL, Smidt GL, Johnston RC: The maximum torque generated by the eccentric, isometric, and concentric contractions of the hip abductor muscles. Phys Ther 1972; 52: 149–158.

51. Opila KA, Wagner SS, Schiowitz S, Chen J: Postural alignment in barefoot and high-heeled stance. Spine 1988; 13: 542–547.

52. Perry J: Gait Analysis, Normal and Pathological Function. Thorofare, NJ: Slack, 1992; 119.

53. Ralis Z, McKibbin B: Changes in shape of the human hip joint during its development and their relation to its stability. J Bone Joint Surg 1973; 55B: 780–785.

54. Ramsey PL: Congenital hip dislocation before and after walking age. Postgrad Med 1976; 60: 114–120.

55. Romanes GJE: Cunningham's Textbook of Anatomy. Oxford: Oxford University Press, 1981.

56. Rose J, Gamble JG: Human Walking. Baltimore: Williams & Wilkins, 1994.

57. Santaguida PL, McGill SM: The psoas major muscle: a three dimensional geometric study. J Biomech 1995; 28: 339–345.

58. Sasaki K, Neptune RR: Differences in muscle function during walking and running at the same speed. J Biomech 2006; 39: 2005–2013.

59. Seireg A, Arvikar RJ: The prediction of muscular load sharing and joint forces in the lower extremities during walking. J Biomech 1975; 8: 89–102.

60. Smith LK, Weiss EL, Lehmkuhl LD: Brunnstrom's Clinical Kinesiology. Philadelphia: FA Davis, 1996; 284.

61. Snijders CJ, Hermans PFG, Kleinrensink GJ: Functional aspects of cross-legged sitting with special attention to piriformis muscles and sacroiliac joints. Clin Biomech 2006; 21: 116–121.

62. Spaliviero M, Steinberg AP, Kaouk JH, et al.: Laparoscopic injury and repair of obturator nerve during radical prostatectomy. Urology 2004; 64: 1030.

63. Steindler A: Kinesiology of the Human Body under Normal and Pathological Conditions. Springfield, IL: Charles C Thomas, 1955.

64. Stolzenburg JU, Rabenalt R, Do M, et al.: Complications of endoscopic extraperitoneal radical prostatectomy: prevention and management. World J Urol 2006; 24: 668–675.

65. Sutherland DH, Olshen R, Cooper L, et al.: The pathomechanics of gait in Duchenne muscular dystrophy. Dev Med Child Neurol 1981; 23: 3–22.

66. Takahashi K, Takahashi HE, Nakadaira H, Yamamoto M: Different changes of quantity due to aging in the psoas major and quadriceps femoris muscles in women. J Musculoskelet Neuronal Interact 2006; 6: 201–205.

67. Takebe K, Vitti M, Basmajian JV: Electromyography of pectineus muscle. Anat Rec 1 A.D., 1974; 180: 281–284.

68. Tixa S: Atlas of Palpatory Anatomy of the Lower Extremities. New York: McGraw-Hill, 1999.

69. Van Dillen LR, McDonnell MK, Fleming DA, Sahrmann SA: Effect of knee and hip position on hip extension range of motion in individuals with and without low back pain. J Orthop Sports Phys Ther 2000; 30: 307–316.

70. Walker JM, Sue D, Miles-Elkousy N, et al.: Active mobility of the extremities in older subjects. Phys Ther 1984; 64: 919–923.

71. Walters J, Solomons M, Davies J: Gluteus minimus: observations on its insertion. J Anat 2001; 198: 239–242.

72. Wickiewicz TL, Roy RR, Powell PL, Edgerton VR: Muscle architecture of the human lower limb. Clin Orthop 1983; 179: 275–283.

73. Williams M, Stutzman L: Strength variation through the range of joint motion. Phys Ther Rev 1959; 39: 145–152.

74. Williams M, Wesley M, Wesley W: Hip rotator action of the adductor longus muscle. Phys Ther Rev 1951; 31: 90–92.

75. Williams P, Bannister L, Berry M, et al.: Gray's Anatomy, The Anatomical Basis of Medicine and Surgery, Br. ed. London: Churchill Livingstone, 1995.

76. Winter DA: The Biomechanics and Motor Control of Human Gait: Normal, Elderly and Pathological. Waterloo, Ontario: University of Waterloo Press, 1991.

77. Worrell T, Karst G, Adamczyk D, et al.: Influence of joint position on electromyographic and torque generation during maximal voluntary isometric contractions of the hamstrings and gluteus maximus muscles. J Orthop Sports Phys Ther 2001; 31: 730–740.

Analysis of the Forces on the Hip during Activity

The previous two chapters presented the structural details of the bones and joints of the hip as well as a functional analysis of its one-joint muscles. Both chapters also discussed relevant hip pathomechanics. The magnitude, direction, and duration of loads sustained by the hip provide links among structure, function, and pathology that affect the joint's activity. This chapter examines the loads that the hip sustains during static and dynamic activities. The purposes of this chapter are to

- Present two-dimensional analyses of the forces sustained by the hip joint during single leg stance
- Investigate the factors that influence the magnitude of the forces on the hip joint
- Examine the loads applied to the hip joint during dynamic activities
- Discuss the stress sustained by the femoral head during activity
- Consider the clinical relevance of force analysis at the hip joint

KINETICS OF SINGLE-LIMB STANCE

Examining the Forces Box 40.1 presents a simplified mathematical analysis of the forces generated during single-limb stance. An understanding of the factors influencing single-limb stance is a prerequisite to understanding the effects on the hip joint of dynamic activities such as walking and running. The task of single-limb stance requires balancing the weight of the head, arms, trunk, and opposite lower extremity (HAT-L weight) over the supporting limb. As discussed in Chapter 1, for an object to remain upright, a vertical line through the object's center of mass must fall within the object's base of support. In the upright human, this means that the center of mass of the HAT-L weight must be vertically aligned over the stance foot. Consequently, the individual shifts the pelvis laterally toward the stance foot, placing the center of mass over the base of support and putting the hip joint of the stance limb in adduction (*Fig. 40.1*). The

HAT-L weight generates an adduction moment on the stance hip, tending to cause the pelvis to drop on the unsupported side, and the abductor muscles pull on the pelvis to counteract the adduction moment. To understand the challenge of single-limb stance, the clinician must answer the following two questions: (*a*) what is the force required of the abductors to support the pelvis? and (*b*) what is the joint reaction force on the head of the femur during this task?

The two-dimensional free-body diagram of the femur in *Examining the Forces Box 40.1* shows the primary forces involved in this task. It is helpful at this point to identify the rotation that each force causes. The ground reaction force, equal to body weight, pushes vertically upward on the stance foot and applies an adduction moment on the hip, tending to rotate the stance limb in a counter-clockwise direction about the hip, or to adduct the hip. The weight of the stance limb acts downward vertically at the limb's center of mass and creates an abduction moment at the hip, tending to rotate the hip

EXAMINING THE FORCES BOX 40.1

2-D ANALYSIS OF SINGLE-LIMB STANCE

The problems:

- What is the force required of the abductor muscles to support single-limb stance?
- What is the force on the femoral head during single-limb stance?

The static equilibrium conditions needed to solve these problems are

$$\Sigma M = 0$$

$$\Sigma F_X = 0$$

$$\Sigma F_Y = 0$$

The following quantities can be defined:

$d_1 \equiv$ perpendicular distance from the point of rotation (hip joint center) to the line of pull of the abductors

$d_2 \equiv$ perpendicular distance from the point of rotation (hip joint center) to the line of force of the weight of the lower extremity

$d_3 \equiv$ perpendicular distance from the point of rotation (hip joint center) to the line of force of the ground reaction force (GRF)

$W_L \equiv$ weight of the lower extremity, approximately one-seventh body weight (W)

$GRF \equiv$ ground reaction force pushing up on the stance foot, equal to body weight (W)

$F \equiv$ force of the abductor muscles

$F_X, F_Y \equiv$ the *x* and *y* components of the abductor force

$J \equiv$ joint reaction force on the head of the femur

$J_X, J_Y \equiv$ the *x* and *y* components of the joint reaction force

Note that the distances defined above can all be measured directly from radiographs and therefore can be regarded as "known" quantities. Body weight is also a "known" quantity. Therefore, the only "unknowns" are the abductor and joint reaction forces. Using these quantities, the static equilibrium equations can be written for single-limb stance. The moment equation is used to determine the abductor force:

$$\Sigma M: (GRF \times d_3) - (W_L \times d_2) - (F \times d_1) = 0$$

Replacing the known values for GRF and L:

$$(W \times d_3) - (1/7 \times W \times d_2) - (F \times d_1) = 0$$

$$6/7 \times W \times (d_3 - d_2) = F \times d_1$$

$$W \times (d_3 - 1/7 \ d_2) \times 1/d_1 = F$$

Note that d_2 is very small and d_3 is approximately twice the size of d_1. These dimensions, available from radiographs, depend upon the size of the individual. However d_1 and d_3 are approximately 1 to 3 inches. Therefore, the magnitude of F ranges from approximately 1.5 to 2 times body weight; that is, the force

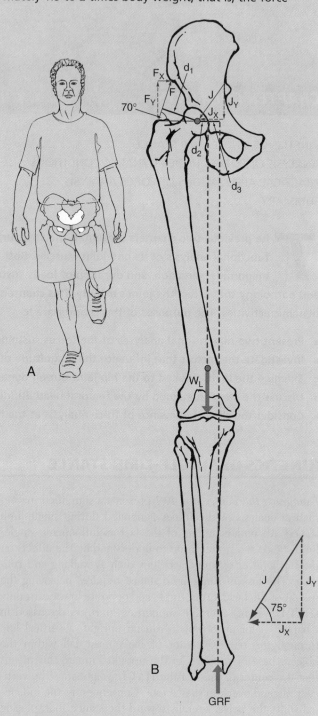

(continued)

EXAMINING THE FORCES BOX 40.1 (*Continued*)

of the abductors required in single-limb stance is 1.5 to 2.0 times body weight.

Assume that F = 1.5W. The remaining static equilibrium equations can be used to determine the force on the head of the femur:

$$\Sigma F_X: F_X + J_X = 0$$

$$J_X = -F_X$$

Note that $F_X = F(\cos 70°)$. Replacing F with F = 1.5 W:

$$J_X = -1.5W (\cos 70°)$$

$$J_X = -0.5W$$

$$\Sigma F_Y: F_Y - W_L + GRF + J_Y = 0$$

Note that $F_Y = F(\sin 70°)$. Replacing F with F = 1.5W, and the other known quantities:

$$J_Y = -(1.5W(\sin 70°)) + 1/7W - W$$

$$J_Y \approx -2.4W$$

Using the Pythagorean theorem:

$$J^2 = J_X{}^2 + J_Y{}^2$$

$$J \approx 2.5W$$

Using trigonometry, the direction of J can be determined:

$$\cos = J_X/J$$

$$\approx 75° \text{ from the horizontal}$$

clockwise. The abductors acting at the greater trochanter apply an abduction moment to the hip. The joint reaction force is assumed to act directly at the joint axis and, therefore, has a moment arm of zero, creating no moment. The HAT-L weight is not included individually in the free body diagram, but is a

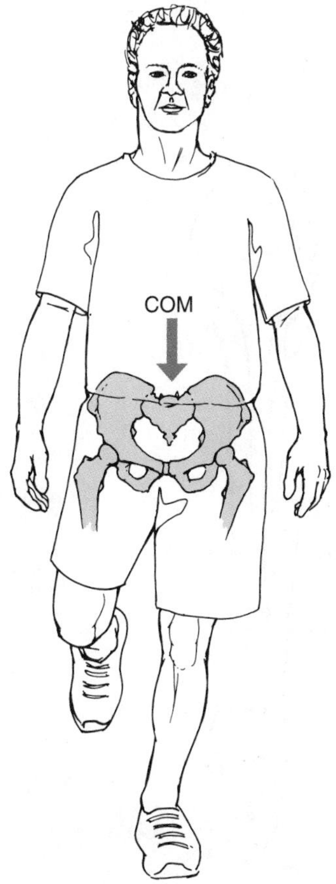

Figure 40.1: In single-limb stance, the individual shifts laterally to keep the center of mass (COM) over the base of support.

part of the joint reaction force, which is affected not only by the HAT-L weight but also by the muscle pull. Application of static equilibrium conditions allows calculation of the force of the abductors needed to remain upright during quiet single-limb stance.

Solutions to this problem reveal that the abductors exert a pull with a force of about twice body weight to support the HAT-L weight during single-limb stance and that the joint reaction force on the head of the femur is approximately 2.5 times body weight. Similar loads during single-leg stance are reported in the literature [2,13,25]. The magnitude of these loads helps the clinician appreciate why the articular cartilage on the femoral head is among the thickest in the body.

The explanation for these large loads lies in the comparison of the moment arms of the ground reaction force and the abductor muscles. The lateral shift used by the subject to keep the center of mass of the HAT-L weight over the foot serves also to move the hip joint (the point of rotation) laterally, farther from the ground reaction force, increasing the moment arm of the ground reaction force. In contrast, the moment arm of the hip abductors remains almost constant and is considerably smaller than that of the ground reaction force, putting the abductors at a mechanical disadvantage and requiring them to generate large contractile forces to balance the effect of the ground reaction force.

Use of a similar analysis allows examination of the effect a cane in the opposite hand has on reducing the load on the hip joint (*Examining the Forces Box 40.2*). The benefit of the cane rests on its effect on the moment arm of the ground reaction force under the foot. The basic task is the same: the subject must stand so that the center of mass falls within the base of support. However, the cane in the opposite hand enlarges the base of support, allowing the subject to stand more erectly (*Fig. 40.2*). Consequently, the stance foot is aligned more closely under the stance hip, and the moment arm of the ground reaction force is smaller than when standing without a

EXAMINING THE FORCES BOX 40.2

2-D ANALYSIS OF SINGLE-LIMB STANCE USING A CANE IN THE CONTRALATERAL HAND

The problems:

- What is the force required of the abductor muscles to support single-limb stance while using a cane in the contralateral hand?
- What is the force on the femoral head during single-limb stance while using a cane in the contralateral hand?

The static equilibrium conditions needed to solve these problems are the same as those in Box 38.1:

$$\Sigma M = 0$$

$$\Sigma F_X = 0$$

$$\Sigma F_Y = 0$$

Assume that the cane bears 15% of the body weight so that the remaining 85% is borne by the stance limb.

The following quantities can be defined:

$d_1 \equiv$ perpendicular distance from the point of rotation (hip joint center) to the line of pull of the abductors

$d_2 \equiv$ perpendicular distance from the point of rotation (hip joint center) to the line of force of the weight of the lower extremity

$d_3 \equiv$ perpendicular distance from the point of rotation (hip joint center) to the line of force of the ground reaction force (GRF)

$W_L \equiv$ weight of the lower extremity, approximately one-seventh body weight (W)

GRF $\equiv$ ground reaction force pushing up on the stance foot, equal to 85% of body weight (W)

$F \equiv$ force of the abductor muscles

$F_X, F_Y \equiv$ the x and y components of the abductor force

$J \equiv$ joint reaction force on the head of the femur

$J_X, J_Y \equiv$ the x and y components of the joint reaction force

Note that the distances defined above can all be measured directly from radiographs and therefore can be regarded as "known" quantities. Body weight is also a "known" quantity. Therefore, the only "unknowns" are the abductor and joint reaction forces. Using these quantities, the static equilibrium equations can be written for single-limb stance. The moment equation is used to determine the abductor force:

$$\Sigma M: (GRF \times d_3) - (W_L \times d_2) - (F \times d_1) = 0$$

Replacing the known values for GRF and W_L:

$$(0.85 \times W \times d_3) + (1/7 \times W \times d_2) - (F \times d_1) = 0$$

$$0.99 \times W \times (d_3 + d_2) = F \times d_1$$

$$0.99W \times (d_3 + d_2) \times 1/d_1 = F$$

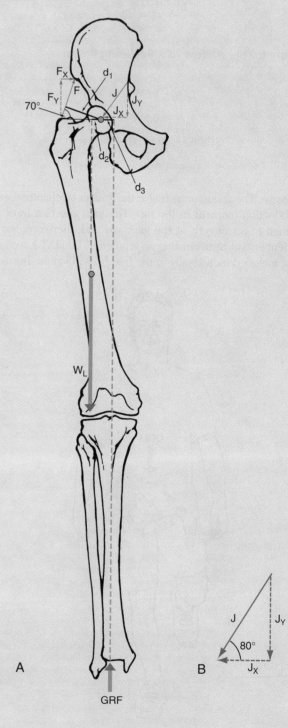

(continued)

EXAMINING THE FORCES BOX 40.2 (*Continued*)

Note that d_2 and d_3 are each very small and their sum is smaller than d_1. As in Box 40.1, these dimensions are available from x-ray data and depend upon the size of the individual and the location of the cane. Assuming that d_1 is almost twice the sum of d_2 and d_3, the magnitude of M is approximately 0.5 times body weight; that is, the force of the abductors required in single-limb stance while using a cane in the opposite hand is approximately one third the force needed without a cane.

Assume that F = 0.5W. The remaining static equilibrium equations can be used to determine the force on the head of the femur:

$$\Sigma F_X: F_X + J_X = 0$$

$$J_X = -F_X$$

Note that $F_X = F(\cos 70°)$. Replacing F with F = 0.5W:

$$J_X = -0.5W (\cos 70°)$$

$$J_X \approx -0.17W$$

$$\Sigma F_Y: F_Y - L + GRF + J_Y = 0$$

Note that $F_Y = F(\sin 70°)$. Replacing F with F = 1.5 W, and the other known quantities:

$$J_Y = -(0.5W(\sin 70°)) + 0.14W - 0.8W$$

$$J_Y \approx -1.12 \ W$$

Using the Pythagorean theorem:

$$J^2 = J_X^2 + J_Y^2$$

$$\mathbf{J \approx 1.13W}$$

Using trigonometry, the direction of J can be determined:

$$\cos = J_X/J$$

$$\approx 80° \text{ from the horizontal}$$

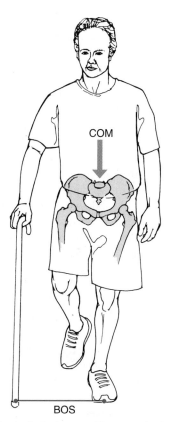

Figure 40.2: In single-limb stance with a cane in the contralateral hand, the individual is able to stand more erectly while keeping the center of mass (*COM*) over the widened base of support (*BOS*).

COM

BOS

cane. Static equilibrium calculations reveal that the use of a cane in the opposite hand reduces the force required of the abductor muscles to approximately 50% of body weight and the joint reaction force to approximately 1.13 times body weight, more than a 50% reduction in the joint reaction force. These data provide concrete support to the admonition offered by Dr. William Blount over a half century ago, "Don't throw away the cane" [7].

Individuals usually learn to use a cane in the hand opposite the impaired side, although casual observation of individuals walking with a cane or a single crutch suggests that many persons use the cane in the hand on the same side as the lower limb problem. It is useful to examine the mechanical implications of using the cane on the contralateral or ipsilateral side. *Figure 40.3* reveals that when the cane is used in the ipsilateral hand, the ground reaction force on the cane actually increases the adduction moment on the hip produced by the HAT-L weight. Thus, for the patient to benefit from the cane on the ipsilateral side, the individual must use other mechanisms to lower the requirements of the abductor muscles and hence reduce the joint reaction force. With the cane on the ipsilateral side, the base of support is even farther lateral to the hip joint than with no cane. Thus the subject must lean farther laterally during ambulation with the cane in the ipsilateral hand than when the cane is in the opposite hand, to put the center of mass over the widened base of support (*Fig. 40.4*). This increased lean of the trunk laterally over the stance foot and cane reduces the HAT-L weight's contribution to the adduction moment and thus reduces the abductor requirement [28]. However, the increased lean requires more work for the rest of the body and may increase the loads on neighboring joints such as the lumbar spine or knee and ankle. Chan et al. report

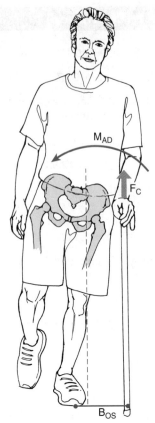

Figure 40.3: In single-limb stance with a cane in the ipsilateral hand, the ground reaction force of the cane exerts an adduction moment (M$_{AD}$) on the trunk.

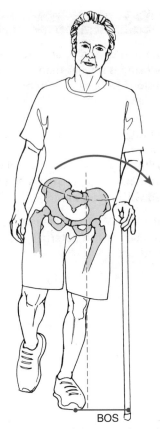

Figure 40.4: Because the base of support is lateral to the hip joint of the stance limb, to benefit from the cane the individual must lean laterally as far as or farther than with no cane at all.

that 14 females with knee osteoarthritis actually generated larger hip abduction muscle moments using the cane on the ipsilateral side than when using the cane on the opposite side or when using no cane at all [8].

The increased lateral lean may also cause the individual to bear more weight on the cane. Increased weight on the cane puts the subject at risk for upper extremity overuse syndromes such as carpal tunnel syndrome. This analysis demonstrates that there are clear and significant benefits to the individual with hip pathology who uses the cane in the contralateral rather than ipsilateral hand. Because the use of the cane in the ipsilateral hand seems so intuitive, this analysis also provides real evidence to help the clinician justify patient instruction in the most appropriate use of the cane.

Clinical Relevance

GAIT TRAINING TO USE A CANE: *Mechanical analysis of the loads on the hip and direct assessment of the electrical activity of the hip abductors during gait demonstrate the benefits of a cane when used in the hand opposite the impaired hip. Careful instruction in the proper use of a cane optimizes the potential benefits of the cane while protecting the patient from injuring other regions such as wrist and hand or low back and knee.*

Mechanical analysis of standing with and without a cane demonstrates that the joint reaction force on the femoral head is largely a function of the muscle force required. Electromyographic (EMG) analysis demonstrates a 30% reduction in activity of the hip abductors during gait with the cane in the contralateral hand compared with walking without a cane [27]. Use of the cane decreases the external moment created by the ground reaction force, thereby reducing the force required of the hip abductors. Chapter 39 discusses the effect of hip abductor weakness and describes the classic **gluteus medius limp.** In this limp, during single-limb support on the weak side, the subject leans laterally over the stance foot, moving the center of mass so that the HAT-L weight creates an abduction moment on the hip, thus eliminating the need for the weakened abductors (*Fig. 40.5*) [42]. The gluteus medius limp demonstrates, again, the benefit of reducing the external moment. Individuals with a painful hip use this same gait pattern to reduce the load on the painful hip by reducing the abductor muscle force [18,19,26]. In this case, the gait pattern is described as **antalgic,** indicating that it results from pain.

In the preceding examples, the force of the abductors is reduced by reducing the external moment. The force required of the abductors also can be reduced by improving the muscles' ability to generate a moment. Specifically, the mechanical advantage of a muscle can be altered by changing its moment arm. In Chapter 38, the effects of coxa vara and coxa valga

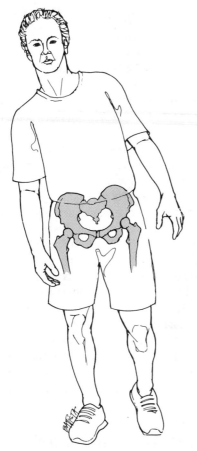

Figure 40.5: In gluteus medius limp, the individual leans laterally while standing on the weak side, moving the center of mass lateral to the hip joint and producing an abduction moment on the stance hip.

advantage and thus a patient's function by reconstructive hip surgery such as osteotomies and even total joint arthroplasties. Joint implants can be designed that influence the abductor mechanical advantage by altering the length of the neck of the femoral component. Similarly, the alignment of the prosthesis as it is implanted can alter the distance from the joint center to the greater trochanter, thereby altering the moment arm of the abductors.

ANALYSIS OF FORCES UNDER DYNAMIC CONDITIONS

The examples provided so far have used analysis of static equilibrium conditions. However, normal walking results in significant increases in forces as a result of the accelerations present in locomotion. Although a more detailed discussion of the principles of dynamic equilibrium used to determine the forces involved in gait are presented in Chapter 48, the conceptual framework is similar to the static equilibrium conditions. The equations of motion for dynamic equilibrium take on the more general form

$$\Sigma \mathbf{F} = m\mathbf{a} \qquad \text{(Equation 40.1)}$$

$$\Sigma \mathbf{M} = I\boldsymbol{\alpha} \qquad \text{(Equation 40.2)}$$

where $\mathbf{F}$ represents the external forces, $\mathbf{M}$ represents the external moments, m is mass, I is moment of inertia, and $\mathbf{a}$ and $\boldsymbol{\alpha}$ represent linear and angular accelerations. Using this approach, several investigators have calculated the loads on the femoral head during normal ambulation. Based on the application of these equations of motion, estimates of peak hip joint reaction forces during gait range from approximately 2.5 to 7 times body weight [1,10,12,34,39]. Investigators also report direct measurements of joint forces using instrumented femoral head prostheses in individuals who undergo hip joint arthroplasty [4–6,15,16,32]. Recognizing that these measurements occur in individuals with joint impairments, the direct measurements suggest that the mathematical analyses may overestimate hip joint forces [15,16]. Yet even the direct measurements demonstrate that the hip sustains loads well in excess of body weight (likely at least two to three times body weight) during normal locomotion. These joint reaction forces increase with fast walking and with running [4,5,34]. Healthy, young adult males and females take an average of 10,000–12,000 step-cycles per day, which can be annualized to almost 2 million step-cycles/year [36,37]. It is no wonder that a painful hip can lead to severe locomotor dysfunction and disability.

An understanding of joint reaction forces provides a useful perspective on the mechanical requirements of daily tasks. However, the concept of a joint reaction force is an oversimplification of the physical situation. Joint reaction forces are generally considered to be applied to a joint at a single point. In reality, the contact forces at a joint are

deformities on the moment arm of the abductors are considered. Coxa valga deformities reduce the moment arm of the abductors, while coxa vara tends to increase the moment arm. The mechanical analyses presented in the current chapter offer a more complete explanation of the mechanisms at work in these clinical situations. A mathematical model demonstrates the result of surgical relocation of the greater trochanter on the moment arm of the abductor muscles and thus on the joint reaction force of the hip [20]. Moving the greater trochanter laterally results in an increase in the abductors' moment arm and, consequently, a considerable increase in the moment generated by a given contraction. This then reduces the amount of muscle force needed to support the HAT-L weight in single-limb support and thus also reduces the joint reaction force. Moving the trochanter medially appears to significantly increase the joint reaction force for similar reasons.

Clinical Relevance

CHANGING MUSCLES' MECHANICAL ADVANTAGE THROUGH SURGERY: *Surgeons apply the basic concepts of mechanical analysis to improve a muscle's mechanical*

applied over a distinct area. Thus the loads generated at the hip as the result of weight bearing and of muscle contractions actually are distributed across the joint surface. A complete discussion of hip joint forces requires discussion of the loads/unit area, or the **stress,** sustained by the hip joint surfaces during activity. Comparative anatomy provides a perspective on the importance of stress as a parameter by which to assess the hip. The human hip is considerably larger than that of apes when normalized for overall body size [22]. This relative increase in joint size results in an improved ability to spread the loads sustained over a larger surface area during stance, thus reducing the stress on the hip. The relative size of the hip joint in humans compared with that in apes appears to be an important structural difference that enhances humans' ability to withstand bipedal ambulation.

Instrumented femoral or acetabular implants installed at the time of a hip joint arthroplasty allow researchers to measure directly the pressures (force/area) on the hip joint surfaces during a variety of activities [2,14,31,35,38,40]. Peak acetabular stresses of approximately 4.0–7.0 MPa are reported on the posterosuperior surfaces of the hip during slow, fast, and free speed walking [23,31]. The high stresses sustained in walking occur in the areas of the hip joint where the articular cartilage is very thick, and very small stresses occur on the anterior lateral surface of the hip where the cartilage is thinner. Direct measurements reveal that the use of a cane reduces peak stresses to 3.0–4.0 MPa, a finding that is consistent with the static analysis described earlier in this chapter. Rising from or descending into a chair and stair climbing increase joint stresses on the hip to approximately 5.0–9.0 MPa [2,40].

Active exercise during the acute phase of rehabilitation following hip fracture generates peak pressures similar to those reported during gait [38]. Non-weight-bearing ambulation appears to produce higher pressures on the hip than touch-down weight bearing in an individual with a femoral head replacement following a hip fracture [14]. It appears that the co-contraction of muscles needed to hold the limb off the ground also approximates the joint surfaces, increasing the contact forces. Stair ascent and descent produce even higher hip joint stresses than walking, with peak stress of 15 MPa reported during descent [31].

Although direct measurement of joint stresses has occurred in only a few individuals and from individuals with specific pathology, studies such as these shed new light on the demands on the hip joint during activity. They offer insights regarding how loads are distributed over a surface, which surfaces sustain large stresses and for how long, and which surfaces bear little or no load. Such evidence helps clarify the relationships among activity, joint loads, and articular integrity. These joint pressure studies also offer an important perspective for the clinician. The data suggest that activities long believed to exert low loads on the hip may actually load the hip quite significantly. These data also provide more information to help therapists develop effective rehabilitation regimens and patient education programs that protect the joint from excessive loads.

Clinical Relevance

HIP JOINT STRESSES AND CLINICAL OUTCOMES IN AVASCULAR NECROSIS: *Avascular necrosis of the femoral head produces painful degenerative changes in the femoral head resulting from death of trabecular and subchondral bone. As the disorder progresses, some of the femoral head is no longer weight bearing and loading occurs over a smaller surface area (increased stress). Treatment includes femoral head arthroplasty and femoral osteotomies to realign the weight-bearing surface so that weight bearing occurs over the undamaged area. In a study of 30 hips that were treated with intertrochanteric osteotomies for avascular necrosis, Dolinar and colleagues report that those individuals with successful outcomes from 9 to 26 years following surgery exhibited an average decrease in peak femoral head stress of 0.2 MPa while those who had an unsuccessful outcome had an average increase in stress of 0.08 MPa [11]. These data suggest that surgical realignment that minimizes the stress on the femoral head may actually improve clinical outcomes. This study demonstrates the direct clinical applicability of biomechanical measures such as bone stress.*

PRACTICAL APPLICATIONS OF FORCE ANALYSIS

Osteoarthritis is the most common rheumatic disease in the world, found in approximately one third of adults aged 65 years or older [3,24,30]. The hip joint is one of the most commonly affected joints [17,21]. Mechanical factors such as the magnitude of the loads on the joints as well as the frequency and duration of loading have long been implicated in degenerative joint disease [33]. The most important risk factors for osteoarthritis of the hip include obesity and occupations that require repeated lifting, providing more evidence linking loads and loading patterns to osteoarthritis [3,9,41]. Thus a common goal of conservative treatment in individuals with arthritis is to reduce the loads on the involved joints. An analysis of forces and pressures applied to the hip offers the clinician direct evidence by which to evaluate such joint protection programs. The examples presented so far provide concrete clinical applications: (*a*) individuals with a painful hip can benefit from the use of a cane in the opposite hand; (*b*) if there are no other problems, using a cane in the ipsilateral hand can worsen the gait in an individual with a painful hip; and (*c*) the femoral head of an individual following hip fracture sustains significant pressures, even during non-weight-bearing ambulation.

The ability to analyze loads on the hip allows the clinician to evaluate most situations and provide advice to help an individual decrease the loads on the hip. For example, carrying a load in the ipsilateral hand reduces the abductor forces used

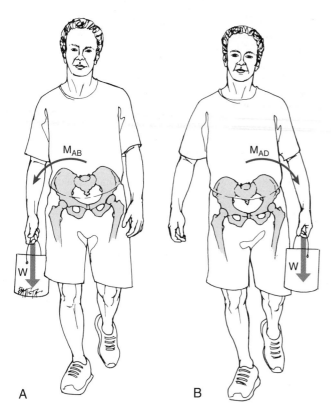

Figure 40.6: A. A weight on the side of the weight-bearing limb produces an abduction moment (M_{AB}) on the stance hip, reducing the force required of the hip abductors. **B.** A weight on the side opposite the weight-bearing limb produces an adduction moment (M_{AD}) on the stance hip, increasing the force required of the hip abductors.

to stabilize the trunk and pelvis and thus decreases the joint reaction force, and carrying loads in the contralateral hand has the opposite effect [27,29]. A brief consideration of the mechanics of the situation reveals that this conclusion is a direct outgrowth of principles of static equilibrium. The load in the ipsilateral hand creates an abduction moment on the stance hip, thereby reducing the need for the abductor muscles (*Fig. 40.6*). Conversely, a load in the contralateral hand creates an adduction moment and increases the need for the abductors. This analysis can be used to evaluate the load on the hip in industrial settings where workers are required to lift or carry loads repetitively. Similarly, the single-limb stance analysis can be applied to situations requiring prolonged asymmetrical support. Thus it behooves the clinician to analyze the mechanics of an activity and use the results of that analysis to optimize an intervention.

SUMMARY

This chapter uses the principles of static equilibrium to analyze the forces involved in the case of single-limb support. The abductor force required during single-limb stance is approximately two times body weight, and the resulting joint

reaction force is approximately 2.5 times body weight. Estimates of the joint reaction force on the femur during locomotion vary but are likely to be two to three times body weight. Mechanical analysis demonstrates that the use of a cane in the opposite hand is quite effective in reducing the joint reaction force on the femoral head. Because the joint reaction force is largely a function of the abductor muscle force, procedures to improve the mechanical advantage of the muscles or strategies to decrease the external moments on the hip are effective in reducing the loads on the hip.

This chapter also examines the stresses applied to the hip and demonstrates that the femoral head sustains large stresses (4–6 MPa) during walking and even during non-weight-bearing gait. Descending stairs generates much larger peak stresses. The chapter also demonstrates that the stresses are applied unevenly across the joint surface and are highest where the articular cartilage is the thickest. Understanding the forces and stresses to which the hip is subjected every day allows the clinician to quantify the impact of structural abnormalities or muscular impairments. These concepts should help guide the clinician to develop more directed, efficient, and successful interventions.

References

1. Anderson D, Hillberry B, Teegarden D, et al.: Biomechanical analysis of an exercise program for forces and stresses in the hip joint and femoral neck. J Appl Biomech 1996; 12: 292–312.
2. Bachtar F, Chen X, Hisada T: Finite element contact analysis of the hip joint. Med Bio Eng Comput 2006; 44: 643–651.
3. Berenbaum F: Osteoarthritis A. Epidemiology, pathology, and pathogenesis. In: Klippel JH, ed. Primer on the Rheumatic Diseases. Atlanta: Arthritis Foundation, 2001; 285–289.
4. Bergmann G, Deuretzbacher G, Heller M, et al.: Hip contact forces and gait patterns from routine activities. J Biomech 2001; 34: 859–871.
5. Bergmann G, Graichen F, Rohlmann A: Hip joint loading during walking and running, measured in two patients. J Biomech 1993; 26: 969–990.
6. Bergmann G, Kniggendorf H, Graichen F, Rohlmann A: Influence of shoes and heel strike on the loading of the hip joint. J Biomech 1995; 28: 817–827.
7. Blount W: "Don't throw away the cane." J Bone Joint Surg 1956; 38: 695.
8. Chan GNY, Smith AW, Kirtley C, Tsang WWN: Changes in knee moments with contralateral versus ipsilateral cane usage in females with knee osteoarthritis. Clin Biomech 2005; 20: 396–404.
9. Cooper C, Campbell L, Byng P, et al.: Occupational activity and the risk of hip osteoarthritis. Ann Rheum Dis 1996; 55: 680–682.
10. Crowninshield RD, Johnston RC, Andrews JG, Brand RA: A biomechanical investigation of the human hip. J Biomech 1978; 11: 75–85.
11. Dolinar D, Antolic V, Herman S, et al.: Influence of contact hip stress on the outcome of surgical treatment of hips affected by avascular necrosis. Arch Orthop Trauma Surg 2003; 123: 509–513.
12. Duda GN, Schneider E, Chao EYS: Internal forces and moments in the femur during walking. J Biomech 1997; 30: 933–941.

13. Genda E, Iwasaki N, Li G, et al.: Normal hip joint contact pressure distribution in single-leg standing—effect of gender and anatomic parameters. J Biomech 2001; 34: 895–905.

14. Givens-Heiss DL, Krebs DE, Riley PO, et al.: In vivo acetabular contact pressures during rehabilitation, Part II: Postacute phase. Phys Ther 1992; 72: 700–710.

15. Heller MO, Bergmann G, Deuretzbacher G, et al.: Musculoskeletal loading conditions at the hip during walking and stair climbing. J Biomech 2001; 34: 883–893.

16. Heller MO, Bergmann G, Kassi JP, et al.: Determination of muscle loading at the hip joint for use in pre-clinical testing. J Biomech 2005; 38: 1155–1163.

17. Hochberg MC: Osteoarthritis. B. Clinical features. In: Klippel JH, ed. Primer of the Rheumatic Diseases. Atlanta: Arthritis Foundation, 2001; 289–293.

18. Hurwitz DE, Foucher K, Sumner DR, et al.: Hip motion and moments during gait relate directly to proximal femoral bone mineral density in patients with hip osteoarthritis. J Biomech 1998; 31: 919–925.

19. Hurwitz DE, Hulet C, Andriacchi T, et al.: Gait compensations in patients with osteoarthritis of the hip and their relationship to pain and passive hip motion. J Orthop Res 1997; 15: 629–635.

20. Iglic A, Antolic V, Srakar F, et al.: Biomechanical study of various greater trochanter positions. Arch Orthop Trauma Surg 1995; 114: 76–78.

21. Ivan D: Pathology for the Health-Related Professions. Philadelphia: WB Saunders, 1996.

22. Jungers W: Relative joint size and hominoid locomotor adaptations. J Hum Evol 1988; 17: 247.

23. Krebs DE, Robbins CE, Lavine L, Mann RW: Hip biomechanics during gait. J Orthop Sports Phys Ther 1998; 28: 51–59.

24. Martin DF: Pathomechanics of knee osteoarthritis. Med Sci Sports Exerc 1994; 26: 1429–1433.

25. McLeish R, Charndey J: Abduction forces in the one-legged stance. J Biomech 1970; 3: 191–209.

26. Murray MP, Gore DR, Clarkson BH: Walking patterns of patients with unilateral hip pain due to osteo-arthritis and avascular necrosis. J Bone Joint Surg 1971; 53A: 259–274.

27. Neumann D: An electromyographic study of the hip abductor muscles as subjects with a hip prosthesis walked with different methods of using a cane and carrying a load. Phys Ther 1999; 79: 1163–1173.

28. Neumann DA: Hip abductor muscle activity as subjects with hip protheses walk with different methods of using a cane. Phys Ther 1998; 78: 490–501.

29. Neumann DA, Cook TM: Effect of load and carrying position on the electromyographic activity of the gluteus medius muscle during walking. Phys Ther 1985; 65: 305–311.

30. O'Sullivan S, Schmitz T: Physical Rehabilitation: Assessment and Treatment. Philadelphia: FA Davis, 1988.

31. Park S, Krebs DE, Mann RW: Hip muscle co-contraction: evidence from concurrent in vivo pressure measurement and force estimation. Gait Posture 1999; 10: 211–222.

32. Pedersen D, Brand R, Davy D: Pelvic muscle and acetabular contact forces during gait. J Biomech 1997; 30: 959–965.

33. Radin EL, Orr RB, Kelman JL, et al.: Effects of prolonged walking on concrete on the knees of sheep. J Biomech 1982; 15: 487–492.

34. Röhrle H, Scholten R, Sigolotto C, Sollbach W: Joint forces in the human pelvis-leg skeleton during walking. J Biomech 1984; 17: 409–424.

35. Rydell N: Intravital measurements of forces acting on the hip-joint. Biomech Related Eng Top 1965; 351–357.

36. Schmalzried TP, Szuszczewicz ES, Northfield MR, et al.: Quantitative assessment of walking activity after total hip or knee arthroplasty. J Bone Joint Surg 1998; 80: 54–59.

37. Sequeira MM, Rickenbach M, Wietlisbach V, et al.: Physical activity assessment using a pedometer and its comparison with a questionnaire in a large population survey. Am J Epidemiol 1995; 142: 989–999.

38. Strickland EM, Fares M, Krebs D, et al.: In vivo acetabular contact pressures during rehabilitation, Part I: Acute phase. Phys Ther 1992; 72: 691–699.

39. Witte H, Eckstein F, Recknagel S: A calculation of the forces acting on the human acetabulum during walking. Acta Anat 1997; 160: 269–280.

40. Yoshida H, Faust A, Wilckens J, et al.: Three-dimensional dynamic hip contact area and pressure distribution during activities of daily living. J Biomech 2006; 39: 1996–2004.

41. Yoshimura N, Sasaki S, Iwasaki K, et al.: Occupational lifting is associated with hip osteoarthritis: a Japanese case-control study. J Rheumatol 2000; 27: 434–440.

42. Zijlstra W, Bisseling R: Estimation of hip abduction moment based on body fixed sensors. Clin Biomech 2004; 19: 819–827.

UNIT 7   KNEE UNIT

The previous unit presents the structure and mechanics of the hip joint. The present unit describes the structure and function of the knee joint as well as factors that contribute to its dysfunction. Like the elbow in the upper extremity, the primary function of the knee is to lengthen and shorten the limb, thus assisting the hip in positioning the foot. For example, the knee shortens the lower extremity to assist in foot clearance during the swing phase of gait and lengthens the limb as it extends toward the ground for the stance phase of gait. However, the knee's role in telescoping the limb is complicated by several factors: (*a*) The knee is weight-bearing; (*b*) it is located between the two longest bones of the body, the femur and tibia; and (*c*) the motion of the foot on the ground causes a twisting motion of the tibia and, consequently, of the knee. These factors require the knee to possess more capabilities than a pure hinge joint has. In fact, the knee exhibits complex three-dimensional motion. The purposes of the unit on the knee are to

- Describe the structure of the bones and articulations of the knee joint and their affects on the mobility and functional capacity of the knee
- Discuss the contribution of the muscles of the knee to the normal mechanics and pathomechanics of the knee
- Examine the forces sustained by the knee during normal function and consider the role of these forces in knee joint pathology

Structure and Function of the Bones and Noncontractile Elements of the Knee

CHAPTER CONTENTS

T he primary function of the knee to alter the length of the lower extremity requires motion of only a simple hinge joint. However, the motion of the tibia caused by the foot on the ground and the location of the knee joint at the center of a long weight-bearing limb place unusual additional demands on the knee joint.

These demands require a delicate balance between the stability needed for weight-bearing and the mobility required for bipedal ambulation. The purposes of this chapter are to

- Discuss the structure of the bones of the knee and how the structure affects the mobility and stability of the knee joint
- Examine the complex three-dimensional movement of the tibiofemoral and patellofemoral articulations
- Examine the normal alignment of the bones of the knee joint
- Consider the articular structures that contribute to the stability of the knee joint
- Review the normal ranges of motion of the knee

BONES OF THE KNEE JOINT

The knee joint is composed of the distal femur, proximal tibia, and the patella. This chapter presents the characteristics of each bone that affect the mechanics of the knee joint, including the femoral shaft and distal femur. The proximal femur is discussed in the preceding unit on the hip (Chapter 38). Similarly, the present chapter describes the proximal tibia. Descriptions of the tibial shaft and distal tibia are furnished in the ankle unit (Chapter 44). Although the fibula does not participate directly in the mechanics of the knee joint, some muscles that cross the knee attach to the fibula. Consequently, the proximal fibula also is described in this chapter.

Shaft and Distal Femur

The shaft of the femur has three surfaces, anterior, medial, and lateral (*Fig. 41.1*). The medial and lateral surfaces are separated from each other posteriorly by the linea aspera, the prominent posterior crest that gives rise to much of the quadriceps femoris muscle. The linea aspera splits distally, contributing to the medial and lateral supracondylar lines and demarcating a posterior surface for attachment of the popliteal muscle. Distally, the femoral shaft flattens in an anterior-posterior direction and widens medially and laterally to form the medial and lateral supracondylar lines. The supracondylar lines terminate in the expanded distal end of the femur, which provides the articular surfaces for the knee joint.

The distal end of the femur consists of two large condyles that are continuous with each other anteriorly but are separated by an intercondylar notch posteriorly. The anterior portions of the articular surfaces of both the medial and lateral condyles combine to provide articulation for the patella. Although this patellar surface is continuous with the rest of the articular surfaces of the medial and lateral condyles, it is distinguished from the tibiofemoral articular surfaces by a very slight mediolateral groove [146]. The articular surface for the patella is concave in the medial-lateral direction with a distinct longitudinal groove through its midline. It is convex in a superior-inferior direction. The anterior surface of the lateral condyle, which articulates with the patella, extends farther anteriorly

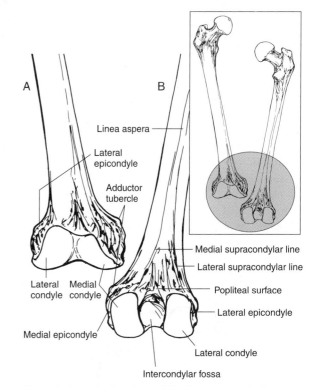

Figure 41.1: **A.** An anterior view of the femur reveals the medial and lateral condyles with their respective epicondyles. **B.** A posterior view of the femur reveals the linea aspera, the medial and lateral supracondylar lines, the popliteal surface, and the intercondylar fossa.

than the anterior surface of the medial condyle, forming a buttress against lateral dislocation of the patella [191].

The medial and lateral condyles are separated from one another by the intercondylar fossa on their distal and posterior surfaces where they articulate with the tibia. The medial and lateral walls of the intercondylar fossa provide attachments for the posterior cruciate ligament (PCL) and anterior cruciate ligament (ACL), respectively. The surfaces of the two condyles are quite different from one another, which helps explain the complex motions of the tibiofemoral articulation. The unique characteristics of each condyle are described below.

MEDIAL CONDYLE

The medial condyle extends farther distally than the lateral condyle. However, because in the normal knee the two condyles lie on the same horizontal plane, the shaft of the femur forms a slight angle with the vertical (*Fig. 41.2*). The proximal surface of the medial condyle is marked by the adductor tubercle, a palpable landmark where the adductor magnus attaches. The medial aspect of the medial femoral condyle offers an easily palpated apex known as the medial epicondyle.

The shape and size of the tibiofemoral articular surface of the medial condyle distinguish it from the lateral condyle and influence the motions of the tibiofemoral articulation. The medial condyle is slightly curved in the transverse plane, as though it lies on a circle that surrounds the lateral condyle (*Fig. 41.3*). The medial condyle's articular surface for the tibia is longer from anterior to posterior than that of the lateral condyle's articular surface. In addition, although the medial condyle is convex from anterior to posterior, its curvature is variable. It is flattest on its most distal surface and is more curved posteriorly [44,81,86,146,191]. The articular surface for the patella also is more curved than the distal surface. **Radius of curvature** describes the curvature of a surface (Chapter 7). In general, the radius of curvature is the radius of the circle from which the articular surface can be derived. Therefore, a flat surface is a segment of a very large circle with a large radius. A curved surface is part of a smaller circle with a smaller radius (*Fig. 7.10*). Thus the radius of curvature of the

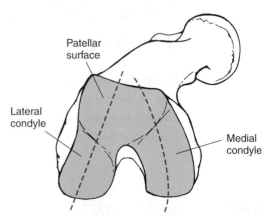

Figure 41.3: A distal view of the femur shows that the medial femoral condyle is curved in the transverse plane, and the lateral femoral condyle projects posteriorly close to the sagittal plane.

medial condyle is greatest distally and is smaller on its posterior surface (*Fig. 41.4*). This asymmetry in curvature contributes to the complex motion between the femur and tibia.

LATERAL CONDYLE

The lateral condyle's articular surface for the tibia projects posteriorly, more in the sagittal plane than the medial condyle. Like the medial condyle, the articular surface presents variable curvatures and, like the medial condyle, is flattest distally. The lateral femoral condyle is flatter distally than the medial condyle and hence has a larger radius of curvature [132]. In the frontal plane, both condyles are slightly convex, but the lateral condyle is flatter than the medial one. The lateral aspect of the lateral condyle forms a prominent projection, the lateral

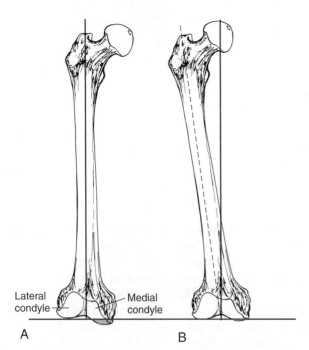

Figure 41.2: A. The larger medial condyle projects beyond the horizontal plane when the femur is vertical. **B.** When the condyles are aligned horizontally as they are in vivo, the femoral shaft is projected laterally.

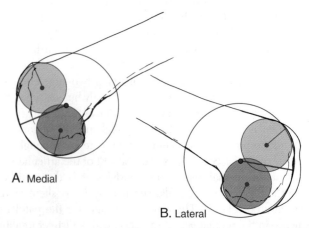

Figure 41.4: The radii of curvature of the medial **(A)** and lateral **(B)** femoral condyles vary across the surface of the condyle, longer distally and shorter anteriorly and posteriorly.

epicondyle, which is an important palpable landmark. The knee joint's axis of flexion and extension passes approximately through the lateral and medial epicondyles [33,179].

Proximal Tibia

The tibia is the second longest bone of the body, exceeded only by the femur. It is characterized by an expanded proximal end that consists of medial and lateral condyles, or plateaus, separated by a nonarticulating intercondylar region (*Fig. 41.5*). This nonarticular region is roughened and consists of an intercondylar eminence and smooth intercondylar areas anterior and posterior to the eminence. Medial and lateral intercondylar tubercles, or spines, project proximally from the eminence. The intercondylar region provides attachment for the medial and the lateral menisci and the ACL and PCL. The anterior surface of the proximal tibia is marked by the tibial tuberosity, readily palpated since it is covered by only skin and the infrapatellar bursa. Just distal to the lateral tibial plateau and lateral to the tibial tuberosity is another tubercle, the tubercle of the lateral condyle of the tibia, also known as Gerdy's tubercle. A facet for the head of the fibula is located on the inferior surface of the lateral condyle. The facet faces laterally, distally, and slightly posteriorly.

ARTICULAR SURFACES OF THE PROXIMAL TIBIA

The articular surfaces of the proximal tibia for the femoral condyles consist of medial and lateral facets on the tibial plateaus. The proximal articular surfaces of the tibia are con-siderably smaller than the respective articular surfaces on the femur. Additionally, the articular surface on the medial tibial plateau is larger than the articular surface of the lateral tibial plateau, decreasing the **stress** (force/area) applied to the medial tibial plateau, which bears more force than the lateral plateau in upright stance [12,148].

The tibia's medial articular surface is slightly concave. However, it has a very large radius of curvature, indicating that it is relatively flat [187,195]. The shape of the lateral articular surface is more variable. It is concave in the medial–lateral direction, but, like the femur, the lateral tibial plateau is flatter than the medial plateau. Although some authors report that the lateral articular surface also is concave in the anterior–posterior direction [191], direct measurements of cadaver knees suggests that the surface actually is flat or even convex throughout most of its anterior–posterior surface [12,50,187,195]. Thus it is apparent that not only do the medial and lateral articular surfaces of the tibia differ from each other, they also differ from the respective articular surfaces of the femur. The differences in shapes of the articular surfaces of the tibiofemoral joint influence the loading pattern across the joint. Although these differences are modulated somewhat by the intervening menisci, which are discussed later in this chapter, the remaining differences among the articular surfaces influence the motion of the tibiofemoral joint.

Effects of the Shapes of the Articular Surfaces on Tibiofemoral Joint Motion

Three factors regarding the shapes of the knee's articular surfaces affect the motion of the tibiofemoral joint:

- The different size of the articular surfaces of the femoral condyles and the tibial condyles
- The different size of the articular surface of the medial femoral condyle and the lateral femoral condyle
- The variation in curvature from anterior to posterior in all of the articular surfaces

Each of these factors has a different impact on the motion that occurs at the tibiofemoral joint, and together they help to explain the complex three-dimensional motion that occurs during flexion and extension of the knee.

DISPARITY BETWEEN THE TIBIAL AND FEMORAL SURFACES

Because there is more articular surface on the femoral side of the knee joint than on the tibial side, pure rolling motion is impossible. As described in Chapter 7, pure rolling occurs when for every point of contact on one surface there is a unique point of contact on the other surface (*Fig. 7.3*). Thus rolling requires equal articular surfaces. If, during knee flexion, the femur underwent pure rolling on the tibia it would roll off the tibial surface (*Fig. 41.6*). During flexion, the contact between the femur and tibia moves progressively posteriorly

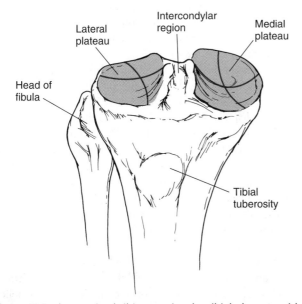

Figure 41.5: The proximal tibia contains the tibial plateaus with their articular facets. The medial articular facet is concave from medial to lateral; the lateral articular facet is concave medial to lateral but slightly convex anterior to posterior.

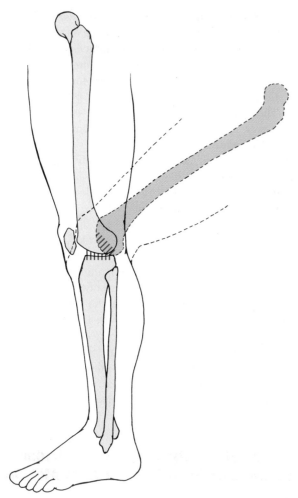

Figure 41.6: If flexion of the knee occurs with pure rolling with no translation of the femur, the femur will "roll off" the tibia.

on the tibia, indicating some rolling [49,170,192,195]. However, the magnitude of the difference in articular surfaces between the tibia and femur dictates that in knee flexion, the femur must undergo additional motions as it rolls into flexion. Conversely, in extension, the contact between femur and tibia moves progressively anteriorly as the knee moves from flexion to extension, but the femur exhibits additional motion as the femur rolls into extension.

DISPARITY BETWEEN THE SIZE OF THE MEDIAL AND LATERAL FEMORAL CONDYLES

Because the lateral femoral condyle has a shorter articular surface for the tibia than the medial condyle, pure flexion and extension movements fail to use the entire articular surface of the medial condyle. Only additional movement in the transverse and frontal planes allows full use of the medial condyle's articular surface.

VARIABILITY OF CURVATURE IN ALL OF THE ARTICULAR SURFACES OF THE TIBIOFEMORAL JOINT

The variability in shape of the individual articular surfaces from anterior to posterior suggests that the relative motion between tibia and femur depends on which part of the condyles are actually in contact. Consequently, the knee's relative motion is a function of its position. Thus the shapes of the femoral and tibial articular surfaces have a direct impact on the relative motion of the tibiofemoral joint [19]. Ligamentous supports also influence tibiofemoral joint motion. The contributions made by these structures are discussed later in this chapter.

Tibiofemoral Motion

The complex shapes and incongruities of the tibiofemoral joint surfaces contribute to intricate three-dimensional movement of the femur and tibia during knee flexion and extension. The classic view of tibiofemoral motion is based on two-dimensional analyses that suggest that knee flexion begins with lateral rotation of the femur and continues with posterior rolling of the femur and concomitant anterior gliding of up to 2 cm [49].

More recent three-dimensional analyses confirm the three-dimensional nature of the tibiofemoral movement during flexion and extension but provide more precise measurements of the frontal and transverse plane movements [33,72,81,193]. These studies demonstrate that lateral rotation of the femur with respect to the tibia accompanies knee flexion reaching approximately 20° of lateral rotation as the knee moves from full extension to at least 90° of flexion (*Fig. 41.7*). In addition, femoral abduction with respect to the tibia also occurs with knee flexion, although this excursion is much smaller, on the order of 5° [134,162]. Extension from the flexed position combines the opposite motions: anterior rolling, medial rotation, and adduction of the femur.

Translation of the femoral condyles also accompanies knee flexion and extension. During flexion the lateral femoral condyle translates posteriorly [38,134,162]. Translation of the medial condyle is less well understood and appears to be less than that of the lateral condyle. The traditional view of femoral or tibial translation during knee flexion and extension appears to require revision. The traditional view, based on two-dimensional analysis, describes knee movement according to the so-called concave-convex rule. The concave–convex rule suggests that a convex surface (the femoral condyles) rolling on a concave surface (the tibial plateaus) will roll in one direction and glide, or translate, in the opposite direction. Applied to the knee, this rule would dictate that during flexion the femoral condyles would roll posteriorly and translate anteriorly. Existing data convincingly refute this belief. Using three-dimensional imaging techniques, investigators consistently demonstrate substantial posterior translation of the lateral femoral condyle during knee flexion. Translation of the medial femoral condyle is reported by some as minimal

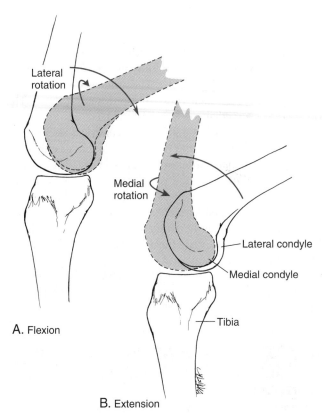

Figure 41.7: A. Flexion of the knee occurs with rolling, lateral rotation and abduction of the femur, and at least some translation. **B.** Extension reverses the motions.

[38], as anterior by some [162], and as posterior by others [68,134]. Some of the posterior translation of the lateral femoral condyle probably reflects lateral femoral rotation but may include independent posterior translation of the femoral condyle. Studies also demonstrate that the contact point on the tibia moves posteriorly during flexion, particularly on the lateral femoral plateau [38].

The confusion regarding knee motion likely stems from the two-dimensional images that were the primary source of information for most of the twentieth century and the erroneous interpretation of femoral rotation as translation. Regardless of the source of the misconception, the twenty-first century understanding of knee motion acknowledges complex three-dimensional motion that consists mainly of flexion or extension with significant longitudinal rotation, slight frontal plane motion, and very slight translation, most of which is posterior.

The timing of the medial or lateral rotation also remains disputed. While the traditional view that rotation occurs only at the beginning of flexion or end of extension has been refuted, some investigators suggest that there is an initial rotation at the beginning of flexion (or end of extension), which then ceases until at least 45° of flexion. Others suggest that the rotation continues smoothly through at least the first 90° of

the motion [193]. The **screw home mechanism** describes the final medial rotation of the femur as the knee reaches full extension. Whether this is a distinct femoral movement or the continuation of the femoral rotation throughout the range is unresolved.

Despite the existing controversies, the tibiofemoral movement during knee flexion and extension exhibits characteristic components:

- During flexion, as the femur rolls into flexion, it rotates laterally with respect to the tibia. Conversely, the femur rotates medially as it rolls into extension.
- Contact between the femur and tibia migrates posteriorly on the tibia during flexion and anteriorly during extension.
- There appears to be some anterior-posterior translation between the tibia and femur during some portions of flexion and extension, although this translation may be small.

Thus far this chapter has described flexion and extension of the knee as motion of the femur on the tibia. Such motion occurs when sitting into, or rising from, a chair. In these cases, the foot is fixed on the floor and the thigh moves over the leg. This is known as a **closed chain** activity. However, during the swing phase of gait, the leg moves more than the thigh. In this case the tibia can be described as moving on the femur. This movement is known as an **open chain** activity, characterized by the foot's ability to move freely in space. Regardless of whether the thigh moves on the leg or the leg on the thigh, the relative motion of femur and tibia remains the same during flexion and extension of the knee. These motions are listed in *Table 41.1*.

It is clear from the description of the motions that occur at the tibiofemoral joint, that the knee does not function as a pure hinge joint. It allows significant motion about the three axes, medial-lateral, anterior-posterior, and longitudinal. Although the motion about the medial-lateral axis far exceeds the motions about the other two axes, all of the motions play a significant role in the function of the tibiofemoral articulation. In addition, the tibiofemoral joint allows translation along all three axes. Although only the anterior-posterior gliding that is limited by the cruciate ligaments is well described, there is potential for a small amount of medial and lateral translation and slight distraction of the joint along its long axis [134,162]. Therefore, the motion of the tibiofemoral joint is an example of a joint with six **degrees of freedom** (DOF), allowing rotation about, and translation along, three axes (*Fig. 41.8*).

TABLE 41.1: Relative Motion of the Femur and Tibia during Knee Flexion and Extension

	Femoral Motion		Tibial Motion	
	Rolling	Rotation	Rolling	Rotation
Flexion	Backward	Lateral	Forward	Medial
Extension	Forward	Medial	Backward	Lateral

Patella

The patella is the largest sesamoid bone in the human body, imbedded in the tendon of the quadriceps femoris muscle. It is triangular, with its **apex** pointing distally (*Fig. 41.9*). Only its posterior surface is articular. The articular surface is oval, with a central ridge that runs from proximal to distal. This ridge creates a medial and larger lateral facet for articulation with the medial and lateral femoral condyles, respectively. A third facet, known as the **odd facet,** or **border facet,** is found on the medial border of the medial facet. The ridge on the posterior surface of the patella glides in the reciprocal groove, or sulcus, on the anterior surface of the distal femur.

Although the patella protects the quadriceps tendon from excessive friction from the femur during knee flexion, its primary function is to increase the angle of application and, consequently, the moment arm of the quadriceps tendon. Estimated reductions of 33 to almost 70% in the quadriceps muscle's moment arm with the knee extended are predicted with removal of the patella [88,186].

Proximal Fibula

The fibula does not participate directly in knee joint function. However, muscles affecting the knee attach to it. Consequently, its proximal end is reviewed here. The slightly enlarged proximal end of the fibula consists of a head and

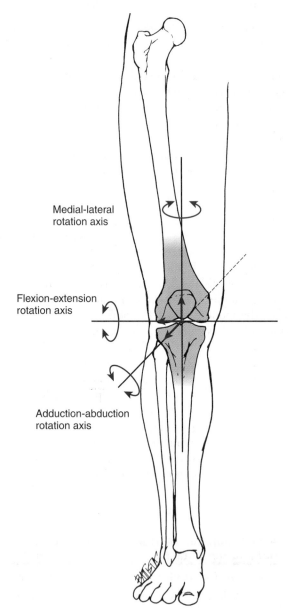

Medial-lateral rotation axis

Flexion-extension rotation axis

Adduction-abduction rotation axis

Figure 41.8: The knee is capable of rotation and translation about three axes and therefore has six degrees of freedom.

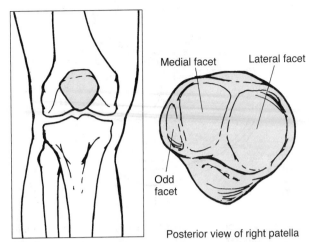

Figure 41.9: The patella is triangular and contains a medial, lateral, and odd facet on its articular surface.

smaller neck. The head contains an articular facet on its medial aspect to articulate with the corresponding facet on the tibia. The proximal end of the fibula ends in a projection known as the styloid process. Both the head and its styloid process are palpable just distal to the lateral aspect of the knee joint.

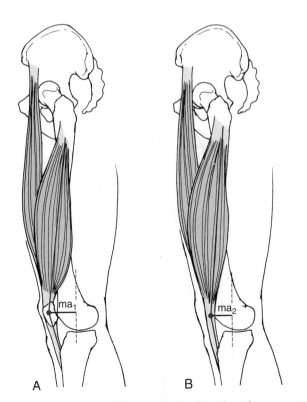

Figure 41.10: A. One role of the patella is to lengthen the moment arm (*ma₁*) of the quadriceps femoris muscle. B. Removal of the patella results in a significant reduction of the muscle's moment arm (*ma₂*), and hence, the moment produced by the muscle.

Palpable Landmarks of the Knee

A thorough examination of the knee depends considerably on the clinician's ability to palpate and identify many of the individual components of the knee. Unlike most joints, many of the connective tissue structures associated with the knee also are directly palpable in addition to the important bony landmarks. The relevant palpable structures of the knee are listed below.

- Medial epicondyle of the femur
- Adductor tubercle of the femur
- Lateral epicondyle of the femur
- Tibial plateaus
- Tibial tubercle
- Tubercle of the lateral condyle of the tibia
- Borders of the patella
- Apex of the patella
- Head of the fibula
- Anterior margins of the menisci
- Medial collateral ligament (MCL)
- Lateral collateral ligament (LCL)

ARTICULAR STRUCTURES OF THE KNEE

The knee joint complex consists of the tibiofemoral and patellofemoral articulations. The proximal tibiofibular joint has an indirect effect on the knee as it functions to absorb motion at the foot and ankle. However, since its motions are best explained in the context of the foot and ankle, it is discussed in full in that chapter. Although the tibiofemoral joint is often described as a hinge joint, it is more precisely a combination of hinge and pivot joints and is sometimes called a **modified hinge joint** [156]. The patellofemoral joint is a gliding joint. The tibiofemoral and patellofemoral articulations share the same supporting structures but also exhibit unique features and motions. The following describes the functionally relevant characteristics of the articular cartilage, the menisci, and the noncontractile supporting structures of the entire knee joint complex.

Organization of the Trabecular Bone and Articular Cartilage Found in the Knee

Like the bony surfaces of the hip, the architecture of the bones involved in the knee appears to follow Wolff's Law [64,65,79,86,122]. The distal femur, proximal tibia, and patella all demonstrate trabecular bone whose organization is correlated with the forces and stresses applied to each bone. The organization observed in each bone suggests that the bones develop according to the forces applied to them and that each bone is specialized to sustain very large loads.

The knee joint also possesses the thickest articular cartilage found anywhere in the body, even thicker than that found in the hip joint (*Fig. 41.11*) [1]. Average thicknesses of between 2 and 3 mm are reported for the patellar and tibial

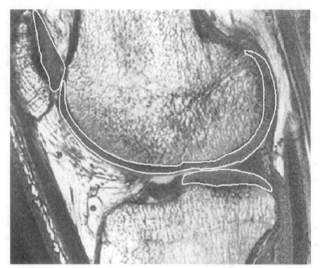

Figure 41.11: Knee joint cartilage. In a lateral view MRI, the manually drawn outline of the articular cartilage of the knee demonstrates the significant thickness of the articular cartilage of the knee, particularly on the patella and tibia. (Reprinted from Clin Biomech, Li G, Park SE, DeFrate LE, et al. The cartilage thickness distribution in the tibiofemoral joint and its correlation with cartilage-to-cartilage contact, 736–744, 2005; 20: with permission.)

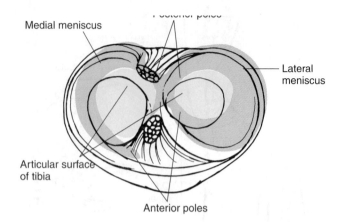

Figure 41.12: Superior view of the menisci shows that the lateral meniscus completes most of a circle, while the medial meniscus forms approximately half a circle. The menisci are attached at their anterior and posterior poles to the tibia.

surfaces, with only slightly less on the distal femur [12,107]. Peak thicknesses of approximately 6 mm are reported on the patella and tibia. The presence of such thick articular cartilage provides further evidence that these articulations sustain large forces. Thick articular cartilage allows considerable deformation of the articulating surface as well. The previous section describes the incongruity between the articular surfaces of the femur and tibia. The curvature of the patella in the superior and inferior directions is larger than the patellar surface of the femur. The compliance of the thick articular cartilage on the patella and the tibia helps improve the congruity between the articulating surfaces of the patellofemoral and tibiofemoral joints [67,143]. Improved congruence increases the area of contact and thus reduces the **stress** (force/area) applied to the surface. The knee exhibits additional specializations that appear designed to help minimize the stress across the tibiofemoral joint, namely, the menisci.

Menisci

STRUCTURE

The two menisci are fibrocartilaginous discs seated on the medial and lateral tibial plateaus [63]. The medial meniscus is larger in diameter than the lateral meniscus, consistent with the larger medial tibial plateau (*Fig. 41.12*). The menisci cover more than 50% of the tibial plateaus, with the lateral covering a greater percentage of the plateau than the medial meniscus [12,51]. As a result, there is more direct contact between the femur and tibia in the medial joint compartment than in the lateral compartment.

When viewed from above, each meniscus forms part of a circle, the medial meniscus completes approximately a half

circle, while the lateral forms almost a complete circle. The anterior and posterior ends of the arcs in each meniscus are known as anterior and posterior poles, or horns. The poles of the lateral meniscus are close to each other, while the poles of the medial meniscus are farther apart. Viewed in the frontal plane, each meniscus is wedge shaped, thicker on its periphery and thin centrally, creating a concave surface for the femoral condyles (*Fig. 41.13*).

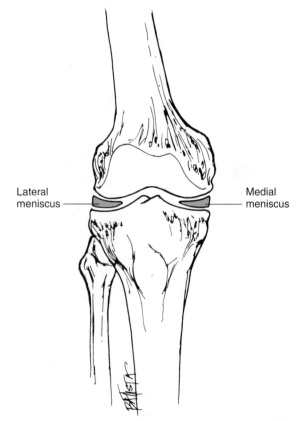

Figure 41.13: In a frontal plane view, the menisci are wedge shaped, thicker on the periphery, creating a concave surface for the femoral condyles.

Although the menisci are frequently described as "washers," they are firmly attached to the tibial plateaus. Ligaments bind both menisci to the tibia at their anterior and posterior horns. In addition, each meniscus attaches to the joint capsule and to the periphery of the tibia by coronary ligaments. The medial meniscus is more firmly attached and also is connected to the MCL. In contrast, the lateral meniscus has no attachment with the LCL. Rather it is attached to the tendon of the popliteus muscle, which may help pull the meniscus posteriorly during knee flexion [23,119]. The lower mobility of the medial meniscus than that of the lateral meniscus may help explain why it is more frequently injured than its lateral counterpart [63].

The menisci receive their nutrition through synovial diffusion and from a blood supply to the horns of the menisci and the peripheral one quarter to one third of each meniscus [56]. Therefore, lesions along the periphery demonstrate healing and even regeneration of meniscus-like tissue. The periphery of the menisci also appears to have sensory innervation that may extend into the more central portion of the discs [11,119]. The sensory function appears to be mostly proprioceptive.

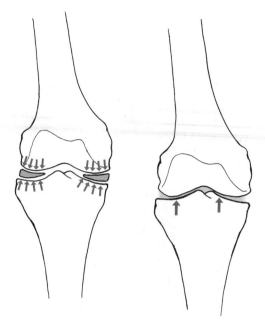

Figure 41.14: The menisci increase the contact area between the tibia and femur. Absence of a meniscus decreases the area of contact between the two bones.

Clinical Relevance

TREATMENT OF MENISCAL TEARS: *A tear in the avascular central region of a meniscus is unable to undergo spontaneous healing. Surgical repair in this region is reported, particularly in young athletes [15,63,160]. Unfortunately, most tears occur in the avascular region of the meniscus [119]. If a surgical repair is not possible, tears in the avascular area of a meniscus usually result in partial meniscectomies, although meniscal transplants may also be considered.*

FUNCTION OF THE MENISCI

Several functions are ascribed to the menisci, including shock absorption [96,184], knee joint lubrication, and stabilization [105,119,137,139]. However, the primary function of the menisci is to increase the contact area between the femur and tibia, thereby reducing the stress sustained by the articular cartilage [51,119,144].

Each meniscus is concave on its superior surface but relatively flattened inferiorly, reflecting the shapes of the femoral condyle and tibial plateau contacting it. Without the menisci, contact between the differently curved femoral condyle and the tibial plateau occurs over a very small area, leading to large stresses applied to the bones (*Fig. 41.14*). The addition of a meniscus between the femoral condyle and tibial plateau approximately doubles the area of contact between the femur and tibia [51]. As a result, the menisci significantly reduce the stress between the femur and tibia. Conversely, removal of a meniscus increases the stresses applied to the tibial plateau and femoral condyle [104,135]. The stresses increase as more meniscal tissue is removed [104].

Clinical Relevance

MENISCECTOMY: *Meniscal tears or progressive degeneration is common and can interrupt the normal function of the knee. A common treatment for a torn meniscus is a complete or partial meniscectomy. However, concern for the long-term consequences of meniscus removal remains. Studies suggest that total removal of a meniscus can lead to accelerated articular cartilage damage [119]. A 15-year follow-up study of 146 patients suggests that accelerated cartilage degeneration is less likely following partial meniscectomies performed arthroscopically [26]. However, other studies continue to report articular degeneration after even partial meniscectomies [115,145]. Because the amount of stress applied to the tibia is related to the amount of meniscal tissue present, these studies suggest a strong link between the stresses applied to a joint and the potential for articular degeneration. This link provides a powerful rationale for identifying treatments that preserve or replace an injured meniscus [32].*

Motion of the Menisci on the Tibia

The complex motion between the femur and tibia applies similarly complex loads to the menisci lying between the two long bones. These forces cause the menisci to deform and to glide on the tibia during knee motion. The motion of the menisci is consistent with their role as washers between the

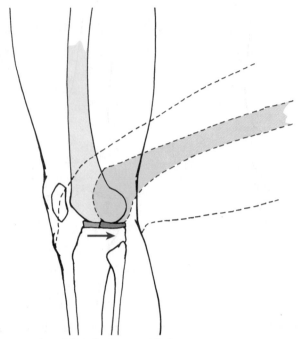

Figure 41.15: The menisci glide posteriorly with knee flexion and anteriorly with knee extension.

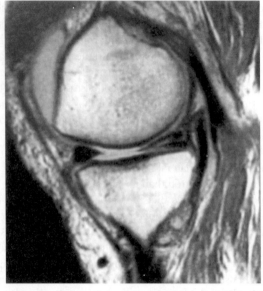

Figure 41.16: Medial meniscus tear. A sagittal view MRI of the medial compartment of the knee reveals a tear of the posterior horn of the medial meniscus. (From Chew FS, Maldjian C, Leffler SG. Musculoskeletal Imaging: A Teaching File, Baltimore: Lippincott Williams & Wilkins; 1999)

two bony surfaces. The menisci move in concert with the rolling femoral condyles (*Fig. 41.15*). As the femur rolls posteriorly in knee flexion, the menisci are pushed posteriorly ahead of the rolling condyles. Similarly, they glide anteriorly ahead of the anteriorly rolling condyles during knee extension [143]. The lateral meniscus moves farther than the medial meniscus because the latter is stabilized by attachments to the medial knee joint capsule, collateral ligament, and the tibial plateau by the coronary ligaments [23,27]. Because the menisci remain attached at their poles as they slide posteriorly and anteriorly on the tibia, they also undergo considerable distortion in shape. This strain may contribute to eventual tears [149].

MENISCAL LESIONS

There are several reasons for the high incidence of meniscal injury. They are located between the two longest bones of the body in a large, weight-bearing joint. Compression forces of several times body weight are reported at the tibiofemoral joint and must be borne by the menisci. In addition, the gliding and rotary motion between the femur and tibia applies large shear forces on the menisci. Finally, the menisci are attached to the tibial plateaus so that the twisting motion of the femur and tibia cause large deformations of the fibrocartilages. All of these factors conspire to cause acute tears and fraying, or fibrillation, of the central border. (*Fig. 41.16*) Fragments from large tears can cause predictable mechanical problems in the knee by becoming dislodged and relocating in the center of the tibial plateau, interrupting the normal rolling and gliding motions of the tibia and femur. A classic complaint of an individual with a meniscal tear is that the joint

"locks," particularly when he or she attempts to extend the knee from a position of weight-bearing, such as rising from a seated position or climbing stairs.

Clinical Relevance

TESTING FOR MENISCAL TEARS: *There are several different clinical tests used to identify a tear in a meniscus. A goal of many of the tests is to dislodge the torn fragment, causing it to interrupt smooth knee motion. A positive test result frequently consists of producing an audible click or a mechanical block to motion [114,176].*

Noncontractile Supporting Structures

The noncontractile supporting structures of the knee include the typical supporting structures, the capsule, and the MCL and LCL. The ACL and PCL provide additional support, playing a role in supporting and guiding the complex translatory and rotary motions of the knee. The capsule also is reinforced posteriorly by additional small ligaments. Each structure is presented below to understand its effects on knee joint stability and mobility. However, it is important to recognize that these supporting structures work in concert to stabilize the knee. Although each ligament appears to serve a primary role in stabilizing some movement, other ligaments provide secondary support [129].

ARTICULAR CAPSULE OF THE KNEE JOINT

The knee joint capsule is the largest joint capsule of the human body [62]. In most joints the two primary layers of the joint, fibrous and synovial, adhere to one another. In the knee, however, these two layers adhere only in parts of the joint. In other areas of the knee, the two layers follow different courses around the joint.

The **fibrous capsule** is attached posteriorly to the posterior margins of the femoral and tibial condyles and spans the intercondylar notch (*Fig. 41.17*). This layer continues medially and laterally, attached along the borders of the articular surfaces of the femur and tibia. Anteriorly, the fibrous layer merges with the tendinous expansions of the vastus medialis and lateralis and attaches to the margins of the patella. These expansions are known as the medial and lateral **patellar retinaculi.** Each retinaculum is reinforced by patellofemoral and patellotibial ligaments. The lateral patellar retinaculum also receives reinforcement from the iliotibial band. The capsule and retinaculi discontinue proximal to the patella, with no anterior attachment on the femur [156,191].

The **synovial layer** of the knee joint capsule is larger and more complex than the fibrous layer. It creates the largest and most extensible synovial cavity in the body, able to hold up to almost a quarter of a cup of fluid without damage [62,173]. Posteriorly, the synovial capsule attaches to the articular margins of the femoral and tibial condyles. However, unlike the fibrous layer, the synovial lining follows the contours of the condyles and thus invaginates in the intercondylar notch. As a consequence, the intercondylar notch and eminence are enclosed by the fibrous capsule but lie outside the synovial space. The superior portion of the posterior synovial lining extends proximally slightly beyond the posterior aspect of the condyles, forming small pouches proximal to each condyle. It may also expand distally and laterally as the popliteal tendon bursa.

The synovial lining continues medially and laterally with the fibrous capsule. Anteriorly, the synovial layer continues with the fibrous layer and attaches to the borders of the patella. However, the synovial lining again diverges from the fibrous layer proximal to the patella. The synovium is attached to the superior border of the patella and the anterior margins of the femoral condyles. It then forms a large pocket that extends proximally a few centimeters between the anterior surface of the femur and the posterior surface of the quadriceps muscle (*Fig. 41.18*). This proximal expansion, known as the suprapatellar pouch, is essential for the full movement of the patella and thus for full excursion of the knee.

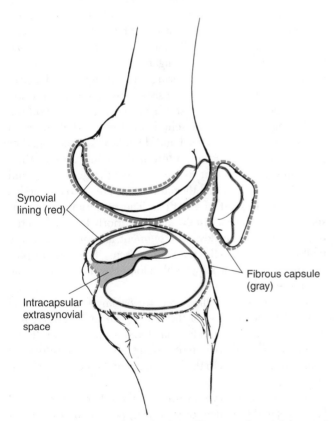

Figure 41.17: The attachments of the fibrous and synovial capsule separate from one another posteriorly, creating an extrasynovial space. The fibrous capsule is absent anteriorly, proximal to the patella.

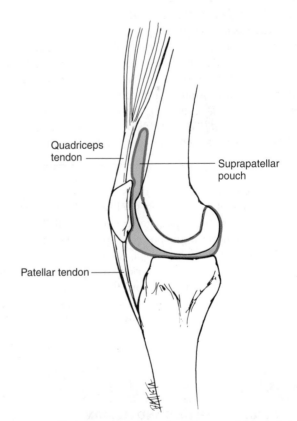

Figure 41.18: The suprapatellar pouch of the synovial capsule is an expansion of the synovial lining proximally between the femur and quadriceps femoris muscle.

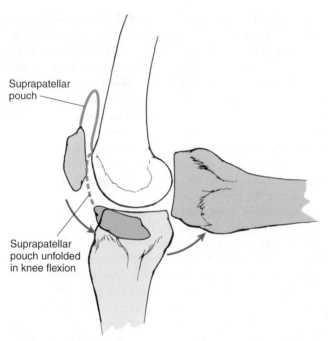

Suprapatellar pouch

Suprapatellar pouch unfolded in knee flexion

Figure 41.19: Distal glide of the patella must accompany knee flexion and requires unfolding of the suprapatellar pouch.

The extensive pouches of the synovial lining complicate the assessment of joint swelling, or effusion. Excess joint fluid is sequestered in the suprapatellar pouch when the knee is extended and moves to the posterior spaces when the knee is flexed. Assessment of knee joint swelling requires that the joint fluid be concentrated anteriorly under the patella. This can be accomplished by positioning the patient with the knee extended to extrude any joint fluid from the posterior spaces. Then manual pressure is used to milk the fluid from the suprapatellar pouch.

The synovial lining of the knee joint is characterized by multiple folds referred to as **plicae** [63]. Some of these folds are large and may become calcified or fibrotic. These folds may also impinge on the patella or femoral condyle, especially during motion. Consequently, the plicae, particularly on the medial side of the joint, may cause knee joint pain producing the **plica syndrome** [14,41].

In conclusion, the capsule of the knee joint is large and complex. It is an essential contributor to the integrity of the knee. However, it may also contribute to impairments in the normal movement of the knee.

COLLATERAL LIGAMENTS

There are two collateral ligaments of the knee, the medial and lateral. These two ligaments provide important reinforcement to the fibrous capsule of the knee joint. The medial (tibial) collateral ligament is more extensive than the lateral (fibular) collateral ligament. It forms a broad, flat, triangular fibrous band covering most of the medial aspect of the joint (*Fig. 41.20*). It consists of two parts, an anterior, more superficial portion and a posterior, deeper portion. Both segments are attached to the medial femoral epicondyle. The superficial and deep layers blend together posteriorly and form the posteromedial joint capsule [155]. The anterior segment is several centimeters long and extends distally and slightly anteriorly to attach to the medial surface of the shaft of the tibia. The posterior segment is shorter and projects distally and posteriorly to attach to the tibial condyle. The posterior segment also attaches to the joint capsule and to the medial meniscus. The anterior border of the ligament is palpable along the medial joint line when the knee is flexed.

The LCL is a cordlike structure passing from the lateral epicondyle to the head of the fibula. The LCL is easily palpated when a varus (adduction) force is applied to a flexed knee. Sitting with one foot resting on the opposite knee applies a varus stress to the knee, making the LCL prominent (*Fig. 41.21*).

Several studies have investigated the role of the collateral ligaments and the effect of knee joint position on their function. As described in Chapter 11, **a valgus force** tends to abduct the distal segment of a joint, and **varus forces** tend to adduct the distal segment. The location of the MCL and LCL on the medial and lateral sides of the joint makes them

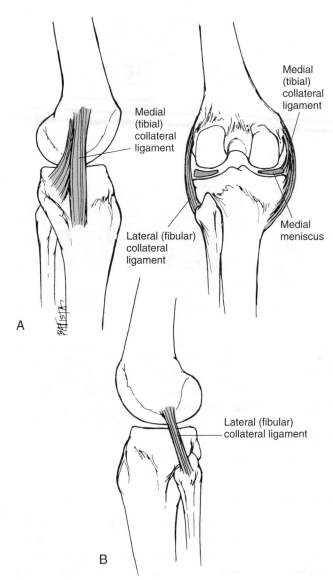

A

B

Figure 41.20: A. The MCL is large, extending distally beyond the tibial condyle as well as anteriorly and posteriorly. Its deep portion attaches to the medial meniscus. **B.** The LCL is a narrow cord from the lateral epicondyle to the head of the fibula.

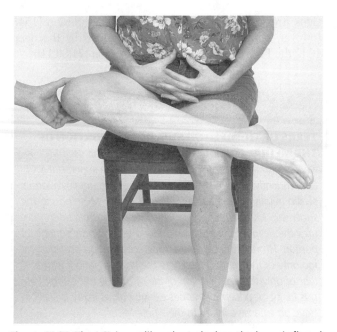

Figure 41.21: The LCL is readily palpated when the knee is flexed and a varus force is applied. The left knee applies a medial force to the right tibia, imparting a varus force to the right knee.

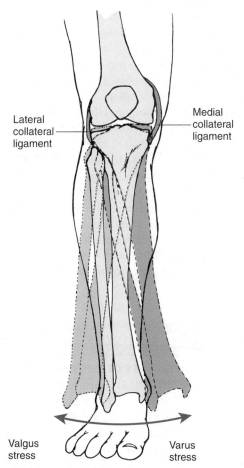

Figure 41.22: The MCL and LCL protect against valgus and varus stresses, respectively.

well-suited to stabilize the knee against valgus and varus stresses, respectively (*Fig. 41.22*). However, other ligaments also contribute to medial and lateral stability. Therefore, there continues to be some controversy regarding the relative importance of the collateral ligaments in supporting the knee against medial and lateral loads [23,139,167]. Although a classic anatomical study by Brantigan and Voshell [23] suggests that there is no significant increase in medial and lateral instability with the sectioning of the collateral ligaments in cadaver specimens, more recent studies indicate that the MCL contributes the primary protection against valgus forces [139,167]. The superficial portion of the medial collateral ligament is considerably stronger than the deep portion, exhibiting almost twice the load to failure, and is composed of longer fibers [153]. It provides the primary support against valgus stresses from 0° to at least 90° of knee flexion [154]. However, significant support also is provided by the deep MCL, the PCL and ACL, and by the menisci [71,80,116].

Clinical Relevance

TEARS OF THE DEEP OR SUPERFICIAL PORTION OF THE MEDIAL COLLATERAL LIGAMENT: *The deep MCL is weaker and consists of shorter fibers than the superficial MCL. Consequently, a valgus movement of the knee applies a larger* **strain** *(relative change in length) to the deep MCL than to the superficial MCL. With a lower* **ultimate strength** *(load to failure), the deep MCL is ruptured more often than the superficial portion. However, because the superficial portion provides the majority of the valgus stability to the knee, a patient with a tear of only the deep portion of the MCL may not exhibit valgus laxity. A patient who does exhibit valgus laxity is likely to have an extensive injury to the whole MCL.*

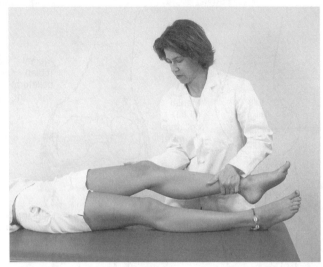

Figure 41.23: Stress tests of the MCL and LCL are performed with the knee slightly flexed. Shown here is the test for the MCL.

Although the LCL provides significant support against varus forces, important support also comes from the popliteal tendon, both cruciate ligaments, the menisci, and the iliotibial band [101,139,167]. Regardless of the combination of ligamentous support, varus and valgus stability of the knee in individuals with intact ligaments depends more on noncontractile tissues rather than muscular support [109]. The collateral ligaments also provide support against medial and lateral rotation of the tibia. The MCL appears to resist both medial and lateral rotations [78,167], while the LCL primarily resists lateral rotations [150,157,167].

The amount of knee flexion influences the roles of the collateral ligaments [23,43,78,109,139,167]. This is not surprising because of the complex structure of the MCL and the irregularity of the femoral condyles. The more extensive MCL is variably affected by knee flexion. The posterior portion of the ligament is stretched more with the knee extended, and the anterior portion is stretched with the knee flexed [23,109]. Although both collateral ligaments appear to be most taut in extension [23,43,89] their relative contribution to medial-lateral stability increases as the knee flexes until at least 30° [139,167].

Clinical Relevance

TESTING THE INTEGRITY OF THE COLLATERAL LIGAMENTS OF THE KNEE: *The standard test for integrity of the MCL and LCL is the manual application of a valgus and varus force, respectively. The test is frequently performed with the knee in 15–30° of flexion (Fig. 41.23). The rationale for the knee flexion stems from studies that demonstrate that in slight knee flexion, the collateral ligaments are the more important stabilizers in the medial and*

lateral directions. Instability medially or laterally with the knee flexed slightly is more likely to indicate damage to a collateral ligament. Medial or lateral instability of the knee with the knee completely extended indicates more-extensive ligamentous damage and perhaps more gross articular damage [77].

CRUCIATE LIGAMENTS

The two cruciate ligaments are essential for normal function of the knee joint and affect both the stability and mobility of the joint. The ACL attaches to the tibia anterior and just lateral to the intercondylar eminence. It attaches to the femur posteriorly on the medial surface of the lateral condyle. The PCL attaches on the posterior surface of the proximal tibia posterior to the intercondylar space and to the posterior aspect of the lateral surface of the medial femoral condyle [55] (*Fig. 41.24*). The PCL has a larger cross-sectional area and is stronger than the ACL [55,178,191]. The two cruciate ligaments are found in the space between the synovial and fibrous layers of the knee joint capsule. Therefore, they are **intracapsular** but **extrasynovial.**

The role of the cruciate ligaments has been studied extensively, and their contributions to knee joint stability are complex [7,13,16,17,23,43,53–55,71,90,130,133,178,197]. Their oblique lines of pull and their complex structures complicate analysis of their functions. Both the ACL and the PCL can be described as consisting of at least two segments. The ACL is composed of an anteromedial and a posterolateral bundle [13,55,178]. Intermediate bundles also are described in the ACL [71,99,158]. The PCL is composed of multiple bundles, most commonly described as an anterior, or anterolateral, bundle and a posterior, or posteromedial, bundle [48,55,85]. Some reports in the literature examine the function of the

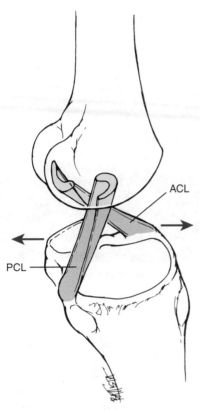

Figure 41.24: The ACL and PCL prevent anterior and posterior glide, respectively, of the tibia on the femur.

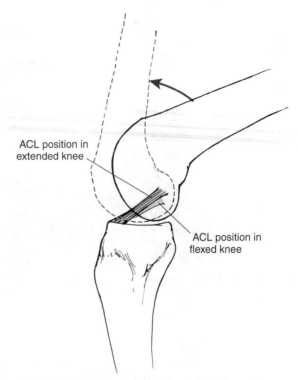

Figure 41.25: The ACL is taut in knee extension.

cruciate ligaments as a whole, while others examine individual segments of the ligaments. This methodological difference helps explain the disagreements found in the literature about the functions of these ligaments.

The ACL limits anterior glide of the tibia on the femur [21,48,143]. However, the degree of anterior laxity resulting from a disruption of the ACL depends on

- The position of knee flexion or extension at which the laxity is assessed
- The portion of the ACL disrupted
- The external load applied to the knee
- The integrity of the surrounding tissue

The effect of knee flexion and extension on the tension in the ACL is well studied, and there is consensus that the ACL is pulled tightest in extension of the knee [16,17,43,54,55, 90,106,133] (*Fig. 41.25*). In fact, disruption of the ACL appears to increase extension or hyperextension ROM [55].

Studies of the restraining role played by discrete portions of the ACL suggest that tension in both the small antero-medial and the larger posterolateral bundles is greatest when the knee is extended. Similarly, tension in both bundles decreases as the knee flexes. However, with increasing flexion, from approximately 30°, tension increases in the anteromedial bundle [13,16,55,99]. Some authors suggest

that sectioning the posterolateral segment of the ACL produces anterior instability when the knee is extended and that anterior instability with the knee flexed to 90° indicates a lesion in the anteromedial bundle of the ACL [53,114]. However, studies investigating the tension or load in these segments in 15° or more of knee flexion report that the anteromedial bundle sustains substantially larger loads than does the posterolateral bundle [158,197]. These data produce an important clinical question: *What test is best at identifying a lesion in the ACL?*

Clinical Relevance

ANTERIOR DRAWER TEST AND THE LACHMAN TEST:
*Two classic tests for ACL integrity are the **anterior drawer test** and the **Lachman test** (Fig. 41.26). The anterior drawer test is performed with the patient's knee flexed to 90°. The examiner attempts to pull the tibia anteriorly on the femur. In the Lachman test, the examiner performs the same maneuver with the patient's knee flexed to 20°. An in vivo study of 20 young adults reports that the Lachman test produces maximum tension through a larger proportion of the entire ACL ligament than does the anterior drawer test. However, more tension occurs in the anteromedial than in the posterolateral bundle in both tests [158]. Thus while the Lachman test may stress more of the overall ACL, it may not be any more specific for the posterolateral bundle of the ACL.*

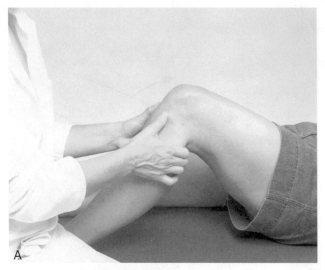

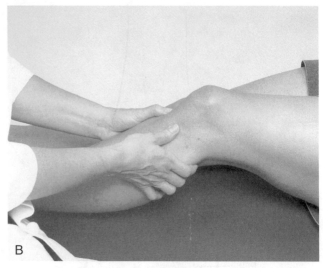

Figure 41.26: Clinical tests of the cruciate ligaments include **(A)** the anterior drawer sign with the knee flexed to approximately 90° and **(B)** Lachman's test with the knee flexed to approximately 20°.

To clarify the role of the ACL and to improve the clinical tests to identify lesions of the ACL, its contributions to rotary stability also have been examined. The ACL is pulled taut with both medial and lateral rotations of the tibia [13]. Some studies indicate that rotations in both directions increase with sectioning of the ACL in cadaver specimens [53,55,167]. Others report only an increase in medial rotation [178], and still others report no significant increase in either direction [75]. There also is evidence to suggest that the ACL's role in stabilizing medial and lateral rotation of the knee depends upon other stresses placed on the knee. Many authors suggest that what appears to be instability in rotation is more accurately described as an anterior subluxation of either the medial or lateral plateau about a long axis or a pivot point in the center of the knee. The addition of varus or valgus stresses as well as compressive loads alters the ligament's ability to limit rotations, or pivots, about the long axis of the knee [30,84,103,117]. Clinical tests assessing both anteromedial and anterolateral subluxations are described for the ACL [77,114].

Clinical Relevance

PIVOT SHIFT TEST OF THE ANTERIOR CRUCIATE LIGAMENT: *The **pivot shift test** is a common test for tears of the ACL. Although there are several versions of the test, it typically adds a medial rotation torque and valgus stress to the anterior force of the original drawer sign [114]. The examiner watches for anterior subluxation of the lateral tibial plateau with a medial pivot of the tibia.*

There appears to be no single, broadly accepted, definitive physical examination maneuver to establish the integrity of the ACL. Clinicians are urged to use more than one test to

evaluate the ACL and to include tests that examine combined, or coupled, motions of the knee [4,77,126,130]. The sensitivity and specificity of an assessment that uses multiple tests are greater than those for individual tests [172]. Continued study using improved three-dimensional motion analysis and imaging techniques is needed to understand fully the complex role of the ACL.

Like the ACL, the PCL has a complex role in stabilizing the knee and contributes to stability in several directions. The PCL limits posterior glide of the tibia on the femur [23,55]. Although the PCL appears to be taut when the knee is extended [54,55,148], studies repeatedly demonstrate that knee flexion increases the tension in the PCL [3,28,37,48] (*Fig. 41.27*). As in the ACL, the position of the knee in the sagittal plane appears to affect the anterior and posterior segments of the PCL slightly differently [3,16,48,178].

The PCL also contributes to varus, valgus, and rotational stability [34,71,80,116,127]. Like the ACL, the PCL is likely to contribute to both medial and lateral rotational stability of the knee, depending on knee position [34,198]. Its role in stabilizing all motions appears coupled with the surrounding ligaments, particularly the MCL and LCL [23,123,127,150, 181,183]. Thus the clinician again must use a combination of test movements to ascertain the integrity of the PCL. In conclusion, it is clear that the cruciate ligaments play a critical role in stabilizing the knee in multiple directions. In addition, it appears that each cruciate ligament is composed of multiple fiber bundles that make slightly different contributions to the function of the whole ligament [3,34,106].

ACCESSORY LIGAMENTS OF THE KNEE

Although the collateral and cruciate ligaments are the primary connective tissue supports in the knee, other smaller ligaments provide some additional support. These are found on the posterior and lateral aspects of the knee. The oblique

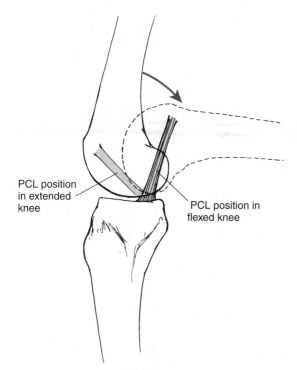

PCL position in extended knee

PCL position in flexed knee

Figure 41.27: The PCL limits maximum flexion of the knee.

popliteal and arcuate popliteal ligaments attach to the lateral joint capsule and are closely associated with the popliteal tendon [191]. They reinforce the LCL, providing additional posterolateral support [127,139,167]. Smaller meniscofemoral ligaments are reported but are inconsistently present. Cadaver data suggest that over 90% of knees contain at least one meniscofemoral ligament [101,124]. Their contributions to overall joint stability remain controversial but they may provide secondary reinforcement to the PCL [5,55,150]. They may also assist and control the motion of the lateral meniscus [61,124].

CONCLUSIONS REGARDING THE CONNECTIVE TISSUE SUPPORT OF THE KNEE

The roles of the collateral and cruciate ligaments are complex and interdependent [136]. The following generalizations are useful in explaining their functions:

- Although the collateral ligaments provide the primary support to control mediolateral stability of the knee joint, the cruciate ligaments supply important secondary support.
- Similarly, the cruciate ligaments stabilize the knee in the anterior and posterior directions but are reinforced by the collateral ligaments.
- Rotary stability is provided by all of the cruciate and collateral ligaments.
- The integrity of the menisci and the articular surfaces also directly affects the stability of the knee joint.

Correct diagnosis of ligamentous injuries is essential to optimizing the function of the knee and to limiting the chances of future joint deterioration resulting from the altered mechanics of a ligament-deficient knee. The functional consequences of injury to any of the primary ligaments of the knee are intimately related to the integrity of the surrounding ligamentous structures.

NORMAL ALIGNMENT OF THE KNEE JOINT

Alignment of the knee is affected by the alignment of the hip, ankle, and foot. This interaction is the result of the knee's location between the ground on which the subject stands and the superimposed weight of the head, arms, trunk, and opposite lower extremity (HAT-L weight). Malalignment of the knee can result from malalignment of the hip, ankle, or foot joints, from muscle imbalances, and from abnormal loads on the knee joint [36,118]. Conversely, there is evidence that knee joint deformities cause abnormal stresses on the joint and can lead to joint degeneration [9,92]. Accurate identification of malalignments of the knee and associated deformities of adjacent joints is an essential part of a thorough musculoskeletal evaluation.

Frontal Plane Alignment

The unique angulation of the knee joint in the frontal plane is considered a hallmark of bipedal ambulation [142,166]. As noted earlier in this chapter, the medial femoral condyle extends farther distally than the lateral femoral condyle. However, in the normally-aligned joint, the distal surfaces of the two condyles lie on the same horizontal plane. Consequently, the shaft of the femur projects laterally from the vertical, putting the knees and feet closer together than the hip joints in normal erect standing. Frontal plane alignment is described by the terms **varus** and **valgus.** Valgus is the alignment in which the angle between the proximal and distal segments opens laterally. In varus alignment, the angle opens medially (*Fig. 41.28*).

The exact value of valgus or varus of the knee depends on the method of measurement. The measure can be made using the **anatomical** or the **mechanical axes** of the knee (*Fig. 41.29*). The anatomical method uses the long axes of the femur and the tibia. The mechanical method uses the mechanical axes of the lower extremity. A radiological study of 120 adults reports approximately 5° of valgus using the anatomical axes [31]. However, values of up to 10° of valgus are reported in individuals without knee pathology [86]. Using the anatomical axes, varus alignment is abnormal in adults and is often associated with degenerative joint disease [9]. However, using the mechanical axes, the normal alignment of the knee is in approximately 2° of varus [31,76]. Location of the mechanical axes requires radiographic assessment.

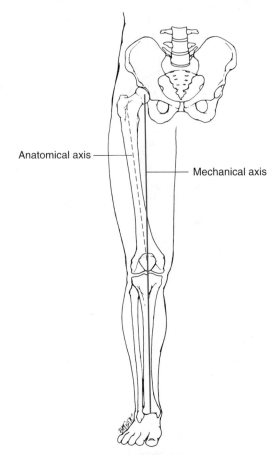

Anatomical axis

Mechanical axis

Figure 41.29: The anatomical axis of the knee is projected through the shafts of the femur and tibia. The mechanical axis projects through the centers of the hip, knee, and ankle joints.

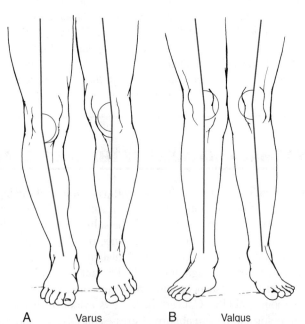

A   Varus   B   Valgus

Figure 41.28: A. In varus alignment of the knee, the angle formed by lines through the femur and tibia opens medially. **B.** In valgus alignment of the knee, the angle formed by lines through the femur and tibia opens laterally.

Therefore, normal frontal plane alignment measured in a physical examination is slight valgus.

Newborns and young children normally exhibit **genu varum** [93]. This varus alignment disappears and is replaced by a valgus alignment that reaches a peak of about 12° by the age of 3 years. There is a gradual reduction of valgus, which finally plateaus at the adult values by the time the child is 6 or 7 years of age. Normal valgus alignment of the knee results in a narrower base of support during stance, requiring less lateral shift to keep the body's center of mass over its base of support during single-limb stance and gait [166] (*Fig. 41.30*).

Sagittal Plane Alignment

Normal erect standing posture of the knee in the sagittal plane consists of a vertically aligned femur and tibia, together forming a 180° angle. However, hyperextension of the knee in standing can occur, and the associated postural alignment is known as **genu recurvatum** (*Fig. 41.31*). It frequently results from muscle imbalances at the ankle or knee. Such a posture applies increased stress to the posterior joint capsule of the knee and to the ACL [110].

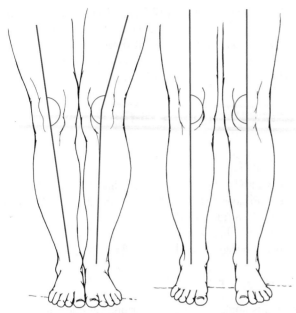

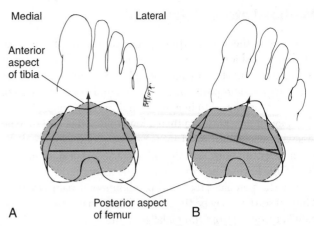

Figure 41.32: **A.** A view of the normally aligned knee in the transverse plane reveals that the femoral and tibial condyles are aligned together along the medial-lateral axis of the knee. **B.** In lateral version of the knee, the tibial condyles are rotated laterally with respect to the femoral condyles.

Figure 41.30: Valgus of the knee allows the feet to be closer together in standing, narrowing the base of support and requiring less lateral shift to stand on one leg.

Transverse Plane Alignment

In a knee free from joint pathology, the tibial plateaus and femoral condyles are aligned so that with the knee extended, the transverse axes of the proximal tibia and distal femur are parallel [42]. This is described as 0° of **version** of the knee (*Fig. 41.32*). In individuals with osteoarthritis of the knee, 5° of lateral tibial version with respect to the femur is reported.

ALIGNMENT OF THE PATELLOFEMORAL JOINT

As noted above, malalignment of the tibiofemoral joint may be the manifestation of altered mechanics at joints proximal and distal to the knee. It may also indicate abnormal stresses on the joint. Finally, malalignment may signify the presence of damaging loads that may precipitate or continue destruction of the joint. Malalignments of the patellofemoral joint may indicate similar scenarios. Consequently, it is essential to recognize the abnormal position of the patella with respect to the femur, to understand and affect the underlying pathomechanics of patellofemoral joint pain.

Alignment of the patella on the femur typically is described in terms of a medial-lateral alignment and a proximal-distal position. These positions are altered by translation of the patella on the femur. In addition, the position of the patella is described in terms of rotations. Several angular orientations are reported in the literature. Some of the most common are described here. **Patellar tilt** describes a rotation about a superior-inferior axis. Additional measures of patellofemoral alignment include the **sulcus angle** and the **congruence angle.** Although patellar translation and patellar tilt are assessed visually in the clinical setting, such observations are reportedly unreliable [140,177,189]. However, assessment of these measures using a variety of radiographic or magnetic resonance imaging (MRI) techniques yields clinically useful information. The descriptions of the patellofemoral joint alignment described below are based on data obtained from radiographic and MRI studies.

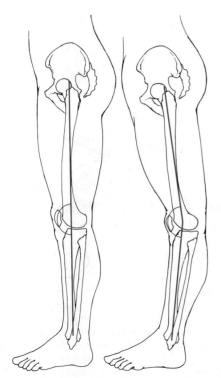

Figure 41.31: Genu recurvatum is sagittal plane alignment of the knee in the hyperextended position.

Medial-Lateral Alignment

In general, the clinical perception is that in the normal patellofemoral joint, the patella lies centered in the trochlear notch, equidistant from the medial and lateral epicondyles [140]. However, reports suggest that slight lateral deviation of the patella as seen with imaging techniques is normal [59,97]. This deviation is no more than a few millimeters and may be less when viewed by MRI [58]. Excessive deviation medially or, more commonly, laterally is known as **medial** or **lateral tracking.** Excessive lateral tracking is associated with chondromalacia patellae [165] and patellofemoral pain [18,196]. These disorders may be the result of abnormal stresses on the patella resulting from the malalignment.

Proximal-Distal Alignment

The proximal-distal position of the patella is described by a ratio of the distance between the patella and the tibia to the length of the patella [2,82,128] (*Fig. 41.33*). The exact distances used vary among specific methods. However, an increase in the ratio, indicating an increase in the distance between the tibia and the patella is noted as **patella alta. Patellar baja (infera)** describes a decrease in the distance between patella and tibia. Both patella alta and baja are associated with anterior knee pain and, like abnormal patellar tracking, are likely to result in abnormal loading of the patellar articular surface [47,73,120,169]. Individuals with patella alta exhibit decreased contact area and increased stress of the patellofemoral joint during fast speed walking [188]. Elevated stress may contribute to pain and degenerative changes in the patellofemoral joint.

Angular Positioning of the Patella

PATELLAR TILT

Patellar tilt is the angle formed by a line drawn through the largest width of the patella and a line touching the most anterior surfaces of the medial and lateral femoral condyles (*Fig. 41.34*). Studies using MRI and computed tomography (CT) suggest that with the knee extended, the patella is positioned in slight lateral tilt [24,138,141].

SULCUS ANGLE

The sulcus angle is the angle formed by lines drawn from the deepest point of the femoral sulcus to the highest point on each condyle. The location on the femur at which the measurement is made alters the angle, indicating that the depth of the sulcus varies over the femoral surface [97]. Reported means vary from approximately 125° to 155°, with no significant difference found between men and women [2,97,174].

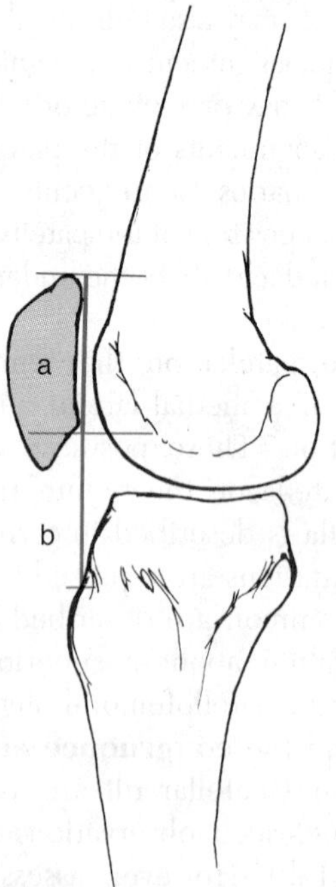

Figure 41.33: The proximal-distal alignment of the patella is described by a ratio of the length of the patella (*a*) and the distance between the distal patella and the tibial tubercle (*b*).

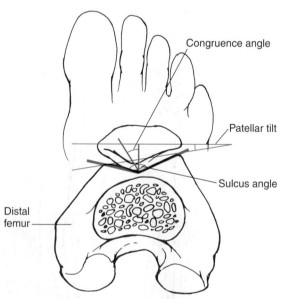

Figure 41.34: Patellar tilt is the angle formed by a line drawn through the largest width of the patella and a line touching the most anterior surfaces of the medial and lateral femoral condyles. The sulcus angle is the angle formed by lines drawn from the deepest point of the femoral sulcus to the highest point on each condyle. The congruence angle is formed by a line bisecting the sulcus angle and another line that projects from the apex of the sulcus angle through the lowest point on the patellar ridge.

CONGRUENCE ANGLE

The congruence angle is a measure of how well the patella fits into the trochlear notch of the femur. It is formed by a line bisecting the sulcus angle and another line that projects from the apex of the sulcus angle through the peak of the patellar ridge. A wide variation in the congruence angle is reported in the literature, from an average of $8° \pm 6°$, larger in women than in men [2], to means of approximately $14°$ to $18°$ [138,196]. Further research establishing normative values for the congruence angle is needed to understand its relationship to patellofemoral joint pathology.

Clinical Relevance

ASSOCIATIONS BETWEEN PATELLAR MALALIGNMENTS AND JOINT PATHOLOGY AND PAIN: *It is commonly believed that pathomechanics contributes to the complaints of pain and dysfunction at the patellofemoral joint. One manifestation of abnormal mechanics at the patellofemoral joint is malalignment. A decrease in patellar tilt is reported in a small sample of individuals with anterior knee pain [196]. An association between an increase in the congruence angle and anterior knee pain also is reported [196]. Patellar alignment also appears to predict lateral patellar subluxations. Escala et al. report odds ratios of 8.7 and 4.5 for increased patellar tilt and patella alta respectively [45]. These data can be interpreted to mean that an individual with increased patellar tilt is 8.7 times as likely to have a lateral subluxation of the patella, and an individual with patella alta is 4.5 times as likely to sublux laterally as individuals without these malalignments. This increased risk may be due to the decreased and laterally displaced contact area between femur and patella found in individuals with lateral subluxation [69].*

All of these associations support the notion that abnormal patellofemoral alignment is involved in patellofemoral joint disorders. However, the exact nature of the relationships remains unclear. Surgical corrections of malalignments are accepted treatment approaches. However, quadriceps strength also is a recognized factor influencing patellar alignment and patellofemoral joint pain. Although malalignments are important clinical findings, clinicians are cautioned to consider them within the context of the entire clinical picture.

In conclusion, malalignments of the tibiofemoral and patellofemoral joints are associated with a number of disorders of the knee joint complex. Further research is needed to define these links clearly enough to establish optimal therapeutic interventions and perhaps to identify effective preventive strategies. An appreciation of the normal alignment of the individual components of the knee joint also is essential to understanding knee motion.

MOTION OF THE KNEE

The motion of the whole knee joint complex is characterized primarily by the flexion and extension of the tibiofemoral joint. However, this apparently simple knee motion involves complex three-dimensional motion of the tibiofemoral joint. In addition, normal knee motion depends upon the motion of the patellofemoral joint.

Normal Range of Motion of the Knee in the Sagittal Plane

The normal ROM of the knee reported in the literature is presented in *Table 41.2*. All ranges are passive except those reported by Roach and Miles [151]. Although reports of hyperextension of the knee are found in the literature, the data presented here demonstrate that significant hyperextension in adult subjects without knee pathology is uncommon. However, hyperextension occurs commonly in young children, then gradually disappears in adolescence [57]. In adults, age and gender appear to have little effect on knee ROM [151,185], but obesity is negatively associated with knee flexion ROM [46].

Studies report that knee excursions during gait range from almost complete extension (approximately $1°$ in midstance) to $65-75°$ in midswing [125,194]. However, many common activities of daily living require more knee flexion. Stair ascent and descent use between 90 and $110°$ of flexion [159,182], rising from a chair requires approximately $90°$ [25], getting in and out of a bath tub requires approximately $130°$ [140], and squatting can use up to $165°$ [159].

Clinical Relevance

KNEE ROM IMPAIRMENTS: *There are many disorders that can lead to reduced knee flexion ROM. The functional significance of such limitations varies in individual patients. Data suggest that only large reductions of flexion ROM will directly affect locomotor patterns. Yet even a slight loss in flexion excursion may have profound repercussions in an individual who must squat or kneel, such as a carpet layer. The clinician must consider the patient's flexibility within the context of the patient's own lifestyle and career requirements to grasp the significance of altered knee flexion ROM.*

Transverse and Frontal Plane Rotations of the Knee

The discussion throughout this chapter clearly indicates that the knee joint allows, actually requires, medial and lateral rotation and abduction and adduction. However, there are limited and varied data describing the normal available ROM in subjects without knee pathology. The challenge in establishing normative values of transverse and frontal plane

TABLE 41.2: Normal ROM of the Knee Reported in the Literature

	Boone and Azen [20][a]	Walker et al. [185][b]	Roach and Miles [151][c]	Roass and Andersson [152][d]	Escalante, et al.[e] [46]
Flexion	141.2 ± 5.3	133 ± 6	132 ± 10	144 ± 6.5	137 ± 15
Hyperextension[f]	−1.1 ± 2.0	−1.0 ± 2	NR[g]	−1.6 ± 2.9	NR

[a]Based on 56 male subjects aged 20 to 54 years.
[b]Based on 30 men and 30 women aged 60 to 84 years.
[c]Based on 1683 men and women aged 25 to 74 years.
[d]Based on 180 knees from 90 male subjects aged 30 to 40 years.
[e]Based on 687 men and women aged 64 to 79 years.
[f]Negative numbers indicate that the mean end range is in flexion rather than hyperextension.
[g]NR: not reported

motion of the knee stems from the technical difficulty of quantifying three-dimensional motion of such small excursions. In addition, these motions are significantly smaller than flexion and extension but are directly influenced by the position of the knee in the sagittal plane [6,23,85,121]. Consequently, only a few studies measure knee motion in all three planes, and these few studies use very different techniques. Some studies assess these motions during walking, while others assess them actively or passively with the subjects at rest. Only one known study describes the loads used to rotate the knee. Therefore, the data provide, at best, a perspective for the clinician to appreciate the relative mobility of the knee.

Despite the limited data it is useful for the clinician to have a general concept of the potential flexibility of the knee in these planes. Reported mean values of total medial and lateral rotation excursion vary from 12° to 80° when the knee is flexed [6,21,23,121,181]. Despite this wide variation in reported means, studies consistently demonstrate a significant decrease in total rotation excursion when the knee is extended [6,23,121,181]. Peak medial and lateral rotation also are approximately equal to one another [121]. However, studies suggest that much less rotation occurs during normal locomotion. Reported total rotations during locomotion range from approximately 8° to 15°, with medial rotation occurring in stance and lateral rotation occurring in the swing phase of gait [91,102,175].

Reports of frontal plane motion of the knee have the same limitations as those reports of rotation. However, the reports of frontal plane motion consistently demonstrate less motion than reported for transverse plane motion. Reports range from approximately 10 to 20° [21,121]. Reported abduction and adduction excursion in gait is even less, approximately 5° [91,102].

Patellofemoral Motion

Proper motion of the patellofemoral joint is critical to the normal function of the tibiofemoral joint. However, the patellofemoral joint is itself subject to pathology. Abnormal movement of the patella during knee flexion and extension is considered by many to be an important contributing factor to patellofemoral disorders [24]. The patella glides distally on the femur during flexion and recoils proximally during knee joint extension. However, its motion during knee flexion and extension is considerably more complex than mere proximal and distal glides. It is important for the clinician to recognize normal and abnormal patellofemoral motion to understand and alter the underlying pathomechanics of knee pain.

When the knee is extended, the patella has only slight contact with the femur [164]. As a result it is freely movable. Although not well studied, the patella appears able to move a few centimeters medially, laterally, and distally in full knee extension with the quadriceps relaxed. Some suggest that the patella should move no more than one half its width in the medial and lateral directions [29]. Medial and lateral translations of the patella with the knee extended are limited by the pull of the retinacular ligaments [39,66]. As flexion begins, the patella slides into the femoral trochlea, and the bony contact greatly reduces its mobility. Although not thoroughly studied, more investigations describe the motion of the patella during knee flexion. The motion consists of both translation and rotation, which are presented separately below.

TRANSLATION OF THE PATELLA DURING KNEE FLEXION

Translations of the patella during flexion and extension of the knee occur in both proximal-distal and medial-lateral directions. The distal glide of the patella during knee flexion is reportedly 5–7 cm, allowed by the unfolding of the suprapatellar pouch [67]. There also is a slight medial translation of the patella at the beginning of flexion [59,94,108,141]. The magnitude and duration of this medial translation remains in dispute. However, there appears to be general agreement that by 30° of knee flexion the patella has begun lateral translation that continues to increase at least until 45° of flexion, when it plateaus.

ROTATION OF THE PATELLA DURING KNEE FLEXION

Rotations of the patella during knee motion include **medial or lateral tilt,** which is defined as it is for the alignment of the patella. The patella also rotates about a medial–lateral

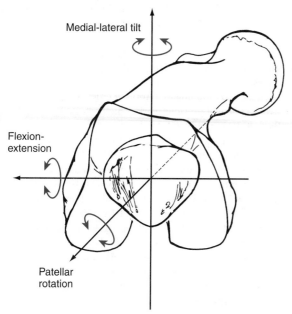

Figure 41.35: The patella is capable of three-dimensional motion with translation along, and rotation about, the cardinal axes.

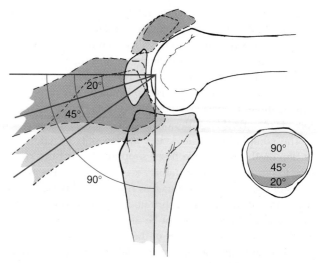

Figure 41.36: The area of contact on the patella increases and moves proximally as the knee flexes to approximately 90°.

axis (*Fig. 41.35*). This motion is termed **flexion** and **extension** of the patella. Finally, the patella undergoes **medial** and **lateral rotation** about an anterior–posterior axis [94]. These motions are inadequately studied; however, there are some consistencies in the literature. The patella appears to be in a slight lateral tilt that increases slightly as the knee flexes [94,141]. The patella also appears to undergo flexion defined as the inferior pole tipping toward the tibia [70,94,108]. Rotations of the patella about the anterior–posterior axis appear negligible [94,108].

These data reveal that the patella undergoes small but systematic movements during knee flexion and extension. The movement of the patella produces significant changes in the location and total area of contact between the patella and the femur. The changes in contact location and area of contact alter the stress applied to the joint surface.

Femoral contact on the patella occurs on the lateral facet at the inferior pole of the patella when the knee is in complete extension. The area of contact steadily increases and includes the medial facet as the knee flexes, moving proximally on the patella [59,67,69,164] (*Fig. 41.36*). The patella contacts the femur on the femoral condyles and patellar surface. Later in flexion, the patella contacts only the femoral condyles, and the odd facet (the medial segment of the patella's medial facet) contacts the lateral aspect of the medial femoral condyle [67].

The large changes in contact location and area between the femur and patella produce large changes in **stress** (force/area). It is believed that abnormal stresses contribute to patellofemoral joint dysfunction.

Clinical Relevance

PATELLOFEMORAL CONTACT AREA WITH PATELLAR SUBLUXATION: *A study of eight individuals with a history of patellar subluxation revealed a significant decrease in contact area between the femur and patella [69]. Perhaps more importantly, the contact area was shifted almost entirely to the lateral femoral condyle during knee flexion from 0–90°. Such changes in patellar movement patterns are likely to produce abnormal stresses and lead to pain and degenerative changes. Careful observation of patellar motion and close evaluation of the structures affecting patellar mobility are essential ingredients to a thorough assessment of the patellofemoral joint.*

SUMMARY

This chapter describes the structure of the bones composing the knee joint. The complex and irregular shapes of these bones are the primary explanation for the complex pattern of movement at the tibiofemoral and patellofemoral articulations during knee flexion and extension. The soft tissue supporting structures of the knee are the primary source of stability of the knee along with the muscles that are presented in the following chapter. The MCL and LCL contribute the primary medial and lateral support, and the cruciate ligaments provide stability in the anterior–posterior directions. However, all four ligaments participate in concert to offer three-dimensional stability.

This chapter also provides a detailed description of the complex motions occurring at the tibiofemoral and patellofemoral joints during flexion and extension of the knee. Although the knee is often described as a hinge joint, its motion includes translations and rotations about the three axes of the body. Flexion occurs with lateral rotation and abduction of the femur with respect to the tibia as well as some translation. Extension reverses these motions. Thus the knee actually exhibits six DOF in its movements. The importance of restoring mobility in all six directions also is noted. The patella also exhibits three-dimensional movements that are essential components of normal knee flexion and extension.

The complexity of the knee's motion puts an enormous burden on the connective tissue supporting structures of the knee to provide sufficient stability even when the knee participates in vigorous activities such as running and twisting. The importance of the muscles surrounding the knee to stabilize and mobilize the knee cannot be understated. The following chapter presents the muscles of the knee and describes their participation in the movement and stability of the knee joint.

References

1. Adam C, Eckstein F, Milz S, Putz R: The distribution of cartilage thickness within the joints of the lower limb of elderly individuals. J Anat 1998; 193: 203–214.

2. Aglietti P, Insall JN, Cerulli G: Patellar pain and incongruence. I: Measurements of incongruence. Clin Orthop 1999; 176: 217–223.

3. Ahmad CS, Cohen ZA, Levine WN, et al.: Codominance of the individual posterior cruciate ligament bundles: an analysis of bundle lengths and orientation. Am J Sports Med 2003; 31: 221–225.

4. Ahmed AM, Burke DL, Duncan NA, Chan KH: Ligament tension pattern in the flexed knee in combined passive anterior translation and axial rotation. J Orthop Res 1992; 10: 854–867.

5. Amis AA, Bull AMJ, Gupte CM, et al.: Biomechanics of the PCL and related structures: posterolateral, posteromedial and meniscofemoral ligaments. Knee Surg Sports Traumatol Arthrosc 2003; 11: 271–281.

6. Andersen HN, Dyhre-Poulsen P: The anterior cruciate ligament does play a role in controlling axial rotation in the knee. Knee Surg Sports Traumatol Arthrosc 1997; 5: 145–149.

7. Ando Y, Fukatsu H, Ishigaki T, et al.: Analysis of knee movement with low-field MR equipment—a normal volunteer study. Radiat Med 1994; 12: 153–160.

8. Andriacchi TP: Dynamics of pathological motion: applied to the anterior cruciate deficient knee. J Biomech 1990; 23: 99-105.

9. Andriacchi TP: Dynamics of knee malalignment. Orthop Clin North Am 1994; 25: 395–403.

10. Andriacchi TP, Birac D: Functional testing in the anterior cruciate ligament-deficient knee. Clin Orthop 1993; 288: 40–47.

11. Assimakopoulos AP, Katonis PG, Afapitos MV, Exarchou EI: The innervation of the human meniscus. Clin Orthop 1992; 275: 232–236.

12. Ateshian GA, Soslowsky LJ, Mow VC: Quantification of articular surface topography and cartilage thickness in knee joints using stereophotogrammetry. J Biomech 1991; 24: 761–776.

13. Bach JM, Hull ML, Patterson HA: Direct measurement of strain in the posterolateral bundle of the anterior cruciate ligament. J Biomech 1997; 30: 281–283.

14. Bae DK, Nam GU, Sun SD, Kim YH: The clinical significance of the complete type of suprapatellar membrane. Arthroscopy 1998; 14: 830–835.

15. Barrett GR, Field MH, Treacy SH, Ruff CG: Clinical results of meniscus repair in patients 40 years and older. Arthroscopy 1998; 14: 824–829.

16. Beynnon B, Yu J, Huston D, et al.: A sagittal plane model of the knee and cruciate ligaments with application of a sensitivity analysis. J Biomech Eng 1996; 118: 227–239.

17. Beynnon BD, Fleming BC: Anterior cruciate ligament strain invivo: a review of previous work. J Biomech 1998; 31: 519–525.

18. Biedert RM, Gruhl C: Axial computed tomography of the patellofemoral joint with and without quadriceps contraction. Arch Orthop Trauma Surg 1997; 116: 77–82.

19. Blacharski PA, Somerset JH: A three-dimensional study of the kinematics of the human knee. J Biomech 1975; 8: 375–384.

20. Boone DC, Azen SP: Normal range of motion of joints in male subjects. J Bone Joint Surg 1979; 61A: 756–759.

21. Brage ME, Draganich LF, Pottenger LA, Curran JJ: Knee laxity in symptomatic osteoarthritis. Clin Orthop 1994; 304: 184–189.

22. Brandsson S, Karlsson J, Eriksson BI, Karrholm J: Kinematics after tear in the anterior cruciate ligament: dynamic bilateral radiostereometric studies in 11 patients. Acta Orthop Scand 2001; 72: 372–378.

23. Brantigan OC, Voshell AF: The mechanics of the ligaments and menisci of the knee joint. J Bone Joint Surg 1941; 23: 44–65.

24. Brossmann J, Muhle C, Schroder C, et al.: Patellar tracking patterns during active and passive knee extension: evaluation with motion-triggered cine MR imaging. Radiology 1993; 187: 205–212.

25. Burdett RG, Habasevich R, Pisciotta J, Simon SR: Biomechanical comparison of rising from two types of chairs. Phys Ther 1985; 65: 1177–1183.

26. Burks RT, Metcalf MH, Metcalf RW: Fifteen-year follow-up of arthroscopic partial meniscectomy. Arthroscopy 1997; 13: 673–679.

27. Bylski-Austrow DI, Ciarelli MJ, Kayner DC, et al.: Displacements of the menisci under joint load: an in vitro study in human knees. J Biomech 1994; 27: 421–431.

28. Carlin GJ, Livesay GA, Harner CD, et al.: In-situ forces in the human posterior cruciate ligament in response to posterior tibial loading. Ann Biomed Eng 1996; 24: 193–197.

29. Carson WG Jr, James SL, Larson RL, et al.: Patellofemoral disorders: physical and radiographic evaluation. Part I: Physical examination. Clin Orthop 1984; 185: 165–177.

30. Chan SC, Seedhom BB: 'Equivalent geometry' of the knee and the prediction of tensions along the cruciates: an experimental study. J Biomech 1999; 32: 35–48.

31. Chao EYS, Neluheni EVD, Hsu RWW, Paley D: Biomechanics of malalignment. Orthop Clin North Am 1994; 25: 379–386.

32. Chen MI: Is it important to secure the horns during lateral meniscal transplantation? A cadaveric study. Arthroscopy 1996; 12: 174–181.

33. Churchill DL, Incavo SJ, Johnson CC, Beynnon BD: The transepicondylar axis approximates the optimal flexion axis of the knee. Clin Orthop 1998; 111–118.

34. Covey DC, Sapega AA, Marshall RC: The effects of varied joint motion and loading conditions on posterior cruciate ligament fiber length behavior. Am J Sports Med 2004; 32: 1866–1872.

35. Crenshaw AH: Campbell's Operative Orthopaedics. St. Louis: Mosby Year Book, 1992.

36. Davids JR, Huskamp M, Bagley AM: A dynamic biomechanical analysis of the etiology of adolescent tibia vara. J Pediatr Orthop 1996; 16: 461–468.

37. DeFrate LE, Gill TJ, Li G: In vivo function of the posterior cruciate ligament during weightbearing knee flexion. Am J Sports Med 2004; 32: 1923–1928.

38. DeFrate LE, Sun H, Gill TJ, et al.: In vivo tibiofemoral contact analysis using 3D MRI-based knee models. J Biomech 2004; 37: 1499–1504.

39. Desio SM, Burks RT, Bachus KN: Soft tissue restraints to lateral patellar translation in the human knee. Am J Sports Med 1998; 26: 59–65.

40. Devita P, Hortobagyi T, Barrier J: Gait biomechanics are not normal after anterior cruciate ligament reconstruction and accelerated rehabilitation. Med Sci Sports Exerc 1998; 30: 1481–1488.

41. Dupont JY: Synovial plicae of the knee. Controversies and review. Clin Sports Med 1997; 16: 87–122.

42. Eckhoff DG: Effect of limb malrotation on malalignment and osteoarthritis. Orthop Clin North Am 1994; 25: 405–414.

43. Edwards RG, Lafferty JF, Lange KO: Ligament strain in the human knee joint. J Basic Eng 1970; 131–136.

44. Elias SG, Freeman MAR, Gokcay EI: A correlative study of the geometry and anatomy of the distal femur. Clin Orthop 1990; 260: 98–103.

45. Escala JS, Mellado JM, Olona M, et al.: Objective patellar instability: MR-based quantitative assessment of potentially associated anatomical features. Knee Surg Sports Traumatol Arthrosc 2006; 14: 264–272.

46. Escalante A, Lichtenstein MJ, Dhanda R, et al.: Determinants of hip and knee flexion range: results from the San Antonio longitudinal study of aging. Arthritis Care Res 1999; 12: 8–18.

47. Fithian DC, Mishra DK, Balen PF, et al.: Instrumented measurement of patellar mobility. Am J Sports Med 1995; 23: 607–615.

48. Fox RJ, Harner CD, Sakane M, et al.: Determination of the in situ forces in the human posterior cruciate ligament using robotic technology. A cadaveric study. Am J Sports Med 1998; 26: 395–401.

49. Frankel VH: Biomechanics of the knee. Orthop Clin North Am 1971; 2: 175–190.

50. Freeman MAR, Pinskerova V: The movement of the normal tibio-femoral joint. J Biomech 2005; 38: 197–208.

51. Fukubayashi T, Kurosawa H: The contact area and pressure distribution pattern of the knee. A study of normal and osteoarthritic knee joints. Acta Orthop Scand 1980; 51: 871–879.

52. Fukubayashi T, Torzilli PA, Sherman MF, Warren RF: An in vitro biomechanical evaluation of anterior-posterior motion of the knee. Tibial displacement, rotation, and torque. J Bone Joint Surg 1982; 64: 258–264.

53. Furman W, Marshall JL, Girgis FG, Girgis DVM: The anterior cruciate ligament. A functional analysis based on postmortem studies. J Bone Joint Surg 1976; 58A: 179–185.

54. Fuss FK: The restraining function of the cruciate ligaments on hyperextension and hyperflexion of the human knee joint. Anat Rec 1991; 230: 283–289.

55. Girgis FG, Marshall JL, Monajem AR: The cruciate ligaments of the knee joint. Clin Orthop 1975; 106: 216–231.

56. Gray JC: Neural and vascular anatomy of the menisci of the human knee. J Orthop Sports Phys Ther 1999; 29: 23–30.

57. Greene WB, Heckman JDE: The Clinical Measurement of Joint Motion. Rosemont, IL: American Academy of Orthopaedic Surgeons, 1994.

58. Grelsamer RP: The medial-lateral position of the patella on routine magnetic resonance imaging: when is normal not normal? Arthroscopy 1998; 14: 23–28.

59. Grelsamer RP, Klein JR: The biomechanics of the patellofemoral joint. J Orthop and Sports Phys Ther 1998; 28: 286–298.

60. Grontvedt T, Heir S, Rossvoll I, Engebretsen L: Five-year outcome of 13 patients with an initially undiagnosed anterior cruciate ligament rupture. Scand J Med Sci Sports 1999; 9: 62–64.

61. Gupte CM, Bull AMJ, Thomas RD, Amis AA: A review of the function and biomechanics of the meniscofemoral ligaments. Arthroscopy 2003; 19: 161–171.

62. Harty M: Knee joint anatomy. Orthop Rev 1976; 5: 23–25.

63. Harty M, Joyce JJ: Arthroscopic surgery: anatomic factors in meniscal injuries. Contemp Orthop 1984; 9: 13–19.

64. Hayes WC, Boyle DJ, Valez A: Functional adaptation in the trabecular architecture of the patella. Trans Orthop Res Soc 1977; 2: 114.

65. Hayes WC, Swenson LW Jr, Schurmans DJ: Axisymmetric finite element analysis of the lateral tibial plateau. J Biomech 1978; 11: 21–33.

66. Heegaard J, Leyvraz PF, Van Kampen A, et al.: Influence of soft structures on patellar three-dimensional tracking. Clin Orthop 1994; 299: 235–243.

67. Hehne JH: Biomechanics of the patellofemoral joint and its clinical relevance. Clin Orthop 1990; 258: 73–85.

68. Hill PF, Vedi V, Williams A, et al.: Tibiofemoral movement 2: the loaded and unloaded living knee studied by MRI. J Bone Joint Surg [Br] 2000; 82B: 1196–1198.

69. Hinterwimmer S, Gotthardt M, von Eisenhart-Rothe R, et al.: In vivo contact areas of the knee in patients with patellar subluxation. J Biomech 2005; 38: 2095–2101.

70. Hinterwimmer S, von Eisenhart-Rothe R, Siebert M, et al.: Patella kinematics and patello-femoral contact areas in patients with genu varum and mild osteoarthritis. Clin Biomech 2004; 19: 704–710.

71. Hollis JM, Takai S, Adams DJ, et al.: The effects of knee motion and external loading on the length of the anterior cruciate ligament (ACL): a kinematic study. J Biomech Eng 1991; 113: 208–214.

72. Hollister AM, Jatana S, Singh AK, et al.: The axes of rotation of the knee. Clin Orthop 1993; 290: 259–268.

73. Holmes SW Jr, Clancy WG Jr: Clinical classification of patellofemoral pain and dysfunction. J Orthop Sports Phys Ther 1998; 28: 299–306.

74. Hooper DM, Morrissey MC, Crookenden R, et al.: Gait adaptations in patients with chronic posterior instability of the knee. Clin Biomech 2002; 17: 227–233.

75. Hsieh YF, Draganich LF, Ho SH, Reider B: The effects of removal and reconstruction of the anterior cruciate ligament on patellofemoral kinematics. Am J Sports Med 1998; 26: 201–209.

76. Hsu RW, Himeno S, Coventry MB, Chao EY: Normal axial alignment of the lower extremity and load-bearing distribution at the knee. Clin Orthop 1990; 255: 215–227.

77. Hughston JC, Andrew JR, Cross MJ, Moschi A: Classification of knee ligament instabilities. Part I The medial compartment and cruciate ligaments. J Bone Joint Surg 1976; 58A: 159–172.

78. Hull ML, Berns GS, Varma H, Patterson HA: Strain in the medial collateral ligament of the human knee under single and combined loads. J Biomech 1996; 29: 199–206.

79. Hurwitz DE, Sumner DR, Andriacchi TP, Sugar DA: Dynamic knee loads during gait predict proximal tibial bone distribution. J Biomech 1998; 31: 1–8.

80. Inoue M, McGurk-Burleson E, Hollis JM, Woo SL: Treatment of the medial collateral ligament injury. I: The importance of anterior cruciate ligament on the varus-valgus knee laxity. Am J Sports Med 1987; 15: 15–21.

81. Iwaki H, Pinskerova V, Freeman MAR: Tibiofemoral movement 1: the shapes and relative movements of the femur and tibia in the unloaded cadaver knee. J Bone Joint Surg [Br] 2000; 82B: 1189–1195.

82. Jakob RP, Von Gumppenberg S, Engelhardt P: Does Osgood-Schlatter disease influence the position of the patella? J Bone Joint Surg 1987; 63B: 579–582.

83. Jomha NM, Borton DC, Clingeleffer AJ, Pinczewski LA: Long-term osteoarthritic changes in anterior cruciate ligament reconstructed knees. Clin Orthop 1999; 358: 188–193.

84. Kanamori A, Woo SL-Y, Ma B, et al.: The forces in the anterior cruciate ligament and knee kinematics during a simulated pivot shift test: a human cadaveric study using robot technology. Arthrosc Assoc North Am 2000; 16: 633–639.

85. Kaneda Y, Moriya H, Takahashi K, et al.: Experimental study on external tibial rotation of the knee. Am J Sports Med 1997; 25: 796–800.

86. Kapandji IA: The Physiology of the Joints. Vol 1, The Upper Limb. Edinburgh: Churchill Livingstone, 1982.

87. Karrholm J, Selvik G, Elmqvist LG, Ansson LI: Active knee motion after cruciate ligament rupture. Acta Orthop Scand 1988; 59: 158–164.

88. Katz BL: Quadriceps femoris strength following patellectomy. Phys Ther 1952; 31: 401–404.

89. Kennedy JC, Hawkins RJ, Willis RB: Strain gauge analysis of knee ligaments. Clin Orthop 1977; 129: 225–229.

90. Kennedy JC, Weinberg HW, Wilson AS: The anatomy and function of the anterior cruciate ligament. J Bone Joint Surg 1974; 56A: 223–235.

91. Kettelkamp DB, Johnston RJ, Schmidt GL, et al.: An electro-goniometric study of knee motion in normal gait. J Bone Joint Surg 1970; 52: 775–790.

92. Kettelkamp DB, Wenger DR, Chao EYS, Thompson L: Results of proximal tibial osteotomy. The effects of tibiofemoral angle, stance-phase flexion-extension, and medial plateau force. J Bone Joint Surg 1976; 58A: 952.

93. Kling JR. TF: Angular deformities of the lower limbs in children. Orthop Clin North Am 1987; 18: 513–527.

94. Koh TJ, Grabiner MD, De Swart RJ: In vivo tracking of the human patella. J Biomech 1992; 25: 637–643.

95. Komistek RD, Dennis DA, Mabe JA, Walker SA: An in vivo determination of patellofemoral contact positions. Clin Biomech 2000; 15: 29–36.

96. Krause WR, Pope MH, Johnson RJ, Wilder DG: Mechanical changes in the knee after meniscectomy. J Bone Joint Surg 1976; 58A: 599–604.

97. Kujala UM, Osterman K, Kormano M, et al.: Patellar motion analyzed by magnetic resonance imaging. Acta Orthop Scand 1989; 60: 13–16.

98. Kumagai M, Mizuno Y, Mattessich SM, et al.: Posterior cruciate ligament rupture alters in vitro knee kinematics. Clin Orthop 2002; 395: 241–248.

99. Kurosawa H, Yamakoshi KI, Yasuda K, Sasaki T: Simultaneous measurement of changes in length of the cruciate ligaments during knee motion. Clin Orthop 1991; 265: 233–240.

100. Kuster M, Blatter G: Knee joint muscle function after patellectomy: how important are the hamstrings? Knee Surg Sports Traumatol Arthrosc 1996; 4: 160–163.

101. Kwak SD, Ahmad CS, Gardner TR, et al.: Hamstrings and iliotibial band forces affect knee kinematics and contact pattern. J Orthop Res 2000; 18: 101–108.

102. Lafortune MA, Cavanagh PR, Sommer HJ, Kalenak A: Three-dimensional kinematics of the human knee during walking. J Biomech 1992; 25: 347–357.

103. Lane JG, Irby SE, Kaufman K, et al.: The anterior cruciate ligament in controlling axial rotation. An evaluation of its effect. Am J Sports Med 1994; 22: 289–293.

104. Lee SJ, Aadalen KJ, Malaviya P, et al.: Tibiofemoral contact mechanics after serial medial meniscectomies in the human cadaveric knee. Am J Sports Med 2006; 34: 1334–1344.

105. Levy IM, Torzilli PA, Warren RF: The effect of medial meniscectomy on anterior-posterior motion of the knee. J Bone Joint Surg 1982; 64A: 883–888.

106. Li G, DeFrate LE, Sun H, Gill TJ: In vivo elongation of the anterior cruciate ligament and posterior cruciate ligament during knee flexion. Am J Sports Med 2004; 32: 1415–1420.

107. Li G, Park SE, DeFrate LE, et al.: The cartilage thickness distribution in the tibiofemoral joint and its correlation with cartilage-to-cartilage contact. Clin Biomech 2005; 20: 736–744.

108. Lin F, Makhsous M, Chang AH, et al.: In vivo and noninvasive six degrees of freedom patellar tracking during voluntary knee movement. Clin Biomech 2003; 18: 401–409.

109. Lloyd DG, Buchanan TS: A model of load sharing between muscles and soft tissues at the human knee during static tasks. J Biomech Eng 1996; 118: 367–376.

110. Loudon JK, Goitz HT, Loudon KL: Genu recurvatum syndrome. J Orthop Sports Phys Ther 1998; 27: 361–367.

111. Lundberg M, Messner K: Ten-year prognosis of isolated and combined medial collateral ligament ruptures. A matched comparison in 40 patients using clinical and radiographic evaluations. Am J Sports Med 1997; 25: 2–6.

112. Lundberg M, Thuomas KA, Messner K: Evaluation of knee-joint cartilage and menisci ten years after isolated and combined ruptures of the medial collateral ligament. Investigation by weight-bearing radiography, MR imaging and analysis of proteoglycan fragments in the joint fluid. Acta Radiol 1997; 38: 151–157.

113. Lysholm M, Ledin T, Odkvist LM, Good L: Postural control—a comparison between patients with chronic anterior cruciate ligament insufficiency and healthy individuals. Scand J Med Sci Sports 1998; 8: 432–438.

114. Magee DA: Orthopedic Physical Assessment. Philadelphia: WB Saunders, 1998.

115. Maletius W, Messner K: The effect of partial meniscectomy on the long-term prognosis of knees with localized, severe chondral damage. A twelve- to fifteen-year followup. Am J Sports Med 1996; 24: 258–262.

116. Markolf KL, Gorek JF, Kabo JM, Shapiro MS: Direct measurement of resultant forces in the anterior cruciate ligament. An in vitro study performed with a new experimental technique. J Bone Joint Surg 1990; 72: 557–567.

117. Matsumoto H, Seedhom BB: Rotation of the tibia in the normal and ligament-deficient knee. A study using biplanar photography. Proc Inst Mech Eng [H] 1993; 207: 175–184.

118. McKellop HA, Llinas A, Sarmiento A: Effects of tibial malalignment on the knee and ankle. Orthop Clin North Am 1994; 25: 415–423.

119. Messner K, Gao J: The menisci of the knee joint. Anatomical and functional characteristics, and a rationale for clinical treatment. J Anat 1998; 193: 161–178.

120. Meyer SA, Brown TD, Pedersen DR, Albright JP: Retropatellar contact stress in simulated patella infera. Am J Knee Surg 1997; 10: 129–138.

121. Mills OS, Hull ML: Rotational flexibility of the human knee due to varus/valgus and axial moments in vivo. J Biomech 1991; 24: 673–690.

122. Milz S, Eckstein F, Putz R: The thickness of the subchondral plate and its correlation with the thickness of the uncalcified articular cartilage in the human patella. Anat Embryol 1995; 192: 437–444.

123. Moglo KE, Shirazi-Adl A: On the coupling between anterior and posterior cruciate ligaments, and knee joint response under anterior femoral drawer in flexion: a finite element study. Clin Biomech 2003; 18: 751–759.

124. Moran CJ, Poynton AR, Moran R, Brien MO: Analysis of meniscofemoral ligament tension during knee motion. Arthroscopy 2006; 22: 362–366.

125. Murray MP: Gait as a total pattern of movement. Am J Phys Med 1967; 46: 290–333.

126. Neeb TB, Aufdemkampe G, Wagener JHD, Mastenbroek L: Assessing anterior cruciate ligament injuries: the association and differential value of questionnaires, clinical tests, and functional tests. J Orthop Sports Phys Ther 1997; 26: 324–331.

127. Nielsen S, Ovesen J, Rasmussen O: The posterior cruciate ligament and rotatory knee instability. An experimental study. Arch Orthop Trauma Surg 1985; 104: 53–56.

128. Norman O, Egund N, Ekelund L, Runow A: The vertical position of the patella. Acta Orthop Scand 1983; 54: 908–913.

129. Noyes FR, Grood ES, Butler DL, Raterman L: Knee ligament tests. What do they really mean? Phys Ther 1980; 60: 1578–1589.

130. Noyes FR, Grood ES, Suntay WJ: Three-dimensional motion analysis of clinical stress tests for anterior knee subluxations. Acta Orthop Scand 1989; 60: 308–318.

131. Noyes FR, Matthews DS: The symptomatic anterior cruciate-deficient knee. J Bone Joint Surg 1983; 65A: 163–174.

132. Nuño N, Ahmed AM: Three-dimensional morphometry of the femoral condyles. Clin Biomech 2003; 18: 924–932.

133. Pandy MG, Shelburne KB: Dependence of cruciate-ligament loading on muscle forces and external load. J Biomech 1997; 30: 1015–1024.

134. Patel VV, Hall K, Ries M, et al.: A three-dimensional MRI analysis of knee kinematics. J Orthop Res 2004; 22: 283–292.

135. Peña E, Calvo B, Martinez MA, et al.: Finite element analysis of the effect of meniscal tears and meniscectomies on human knee biomechanics. Clin Biomech 2005; 20: 498–507.

136. Peña E, Calvo B, Martinez MA, Doblare M: A three-dimensional finite element analysis of the combined behavior of ligaments and menisci in the healthy human knee joint. J Biomech 2006; 39: 1686–1701.

137. Petrosini AV, Sherman OH: A historical perspective on meniscal repair. Clin Sports Med 1996; 15: 445–453.

138. Pinar H: Kinematic and dynamic axial computerized tomography of the normal patellofemoral joint. Knee Surg Sports Traumatol Arthrosc 1994. 1994; 2: 27–30.

139. Piziali RL, Seering WP, Nagel DA, Schurman DJ: The function of the primary ligaments of the knee in anterior-posterior and medial-lateral motions. J Biomech 1980; 13: 777–784.

140. Powers CM, Mortenson S, Nishimoto D, Simon D: Criterion-related validity of a clinical measurement to determine the medial/lateral component of patellar orientation. J Orthop Sports Phys Ther 1999; 29: 372–377.

141. Powers CM, Shellock FG, Pfaff M: Quantification of patellar tracking using kinematic MRI. J Magn Reson Imaging 1998; 8: 724–732.

142. Preuschoft H, Tardieu C: Biomechanical reasons for the divergent morphology of the knee joint and the distal epiphyseal suture in hominoids. Folia Primatol (Basel) 1996; 66: 82–92.

143. Radin EL: Biomechanics of the knee joint. Its implications in the design of replacements. Orthop Clin North Am 1973; 4: 539–546.

144. Radin EL, de Lamotte F, Maquet P: Role of the menisci in the distribution of stress in the knee. Clin Orthop 1984; 185: 290–294.

145. Rangger C, Kathrein A, Klestil T, Glotzer W: Partial meniscectomy and osteoarthritis. Implications for treatment of athletes. Sports Med 1997; 23: 61–68.

146. Rehder U: Morphometrical studies on the symmetry of the human knee joint: femoral condyles. J Biomech 1983; 16: 351–361.

147. Reuben JD, Rovick JS, Schrager RJ, et al.: Three-dimensional dynamic motion analysis of the anterior cruciate ligament deficient knee joint. Am J Sports Med 1989; 17: 463–471.

148. Riegger-Krugh C, Gerhart TN, Powers WR, Hayes WC: Tibiofemoral contact pressures in degenerative joint disease. Clin Orthop 1998; 348: 233–245.

149. Riley PO: Torque action of two-joint muscles in the swing period of stiff-legged gait: a forward dynamic model analysis. J Biomech 1998; 31: 835–840.

150. Ritchie JR, Bergfeld JA, Kambic H, Manning T: Isolated sectioning of the medial and posteromedial capsular ligaments in the posterior cruciate ligament-deficient knee. Influence on posterior tibial translation. Am J Sports Medicine 1998; 26: 389–394.

151. Roach KE, Miles TP: Normal hip and knee active range of motion: the relationship to age. Phys Ther 1991; 71: 656–665.

152. Roass A, Andersson GB: Normal range of motion of the hip, knee, and ankle joints in male subjects, 30–40 years of age. Acta Orthop Scand 1982; 53: 205–208.

153. Robinson JR, Bull AMJ, Amis AA: Structural properties of the medial collateral ligament complex of the human knee. J Biomech 2005; 38: 1067–1074.

154. Robinson JR, Bull AMJ, Thomas RRD, Amis AA: The role of the medial collateral ligament and posteromedial capsule in controlling knee laxity. Am J Sports Med 2006; 34: 1815–1823.

155. Robinson JR, Sanchez-Ballester J, Bull AMJ, et al.: The posteromedial corner revisited: an anatomical description of the passive restraining structures of the medial aspect of the human knee. J Bone Joint Surg Br 2004; 86: 674–681.

156. Romanes GJE: Cunningham's Textbook of Anatomy. Oxford: Oxford University Press, 1981.

157. Rong GW, Wang Y: The role of cruciate ligaments in maintaining knee joint stability. Clin Orthop 1987; 215: 65–71.

158. Rosenberg TD, Rasmussan GL: The function of the anterior cruciate ligament during anterior drawer and Lachman's testing. An in vivo analysis in normal knees. Am J Sports Med 1984; 12: 318–322.

159. Rowe PJ, Myles CM, Walker C, Nutton R: Knee joint kinematics in gait and other functional activities measured using flexible electrogoniometry: how much knee motion is sufficient for normal daily life? Gait Posture 2000; 12: 143–155.

160. Rubman MH, Noyes FR, Barber-Westin SD: Arthroscopic repair of meniscal tears that extend into the avascular zone. A review of 198 single and complex tears. Am J Sports Med 1998; 26: 87–95.

161. Rudolph KS, Eastlack ME, Axe MJ, Snyder-Mackler L: 1998 Basmajian Student Award Paper: Movement patterns after anterior cruciate ligament injury: a comparison of patients who compensate well for the injury and those who require operative stabilization. J Electromyogr Kinesiol 1998; 8: 349–362.

162. Saari T, Carlsson L, Karlsson J, Karrholm J: Knee kinematics in medial arthrosis. dynamic radiostereometry during active extension and weight-bearing. J Biomech 2005; 38: 285–292.

163. Sakane M, Livesay GA, Fox RJ, et al.: Relative contribution of the ACL, MCL, and bony contact to the anterior stability of the knee. Knee Surg Sports Traumatol Arthrosc 1999; 7: 93–97.

164. Salsich GB, Ward SR, Terk MR, Powers CM: In vivo assessment of patellofemoral joint contact area in individuals who are pain free. Clin Orthop Relat Res 2003; 417: 277–284.

165. Salter RB: Textbook of Disorders and Injuries of the Musculoskeletal System. 3rd Ed. Baltimore: Williams & Wilkins, 1999.

166. Saunders JB, Inman VT, Eberhart HD: The major determinants in normal and pathological gait. J Bone Joint Surg 1953; 35: 543–560.

167. Seering WR, Piziali RL, Nagel DA, Schurman DJ: The function of the primary ligaments of the knee in varus-valgus and axial rotation. J Biomech 1980; 13: 785–794.

168. Shaw JA, Eng M, Murray DG: The longitudinal axis of the knee and the role of the cruciate ligaments in controlling transverse rotation. J Bone Joint Surg 1974; 56A: 1603–1609.

169. Singerman R, Davy D, Goldberg V: Effects of patella alta and patella infera on patellofemoral contact forces. J Biomech 1994; 27: 1059–1065.

170. Singerman R: Decreased posterior tibial slope increases strain in the posterior cruciate ligament following total knee arthroplasty. J Arthroplasty 1996; 11: 99–103.

171. Snyder-Mackler L, Delitto A, Bailey SL, Stralka SW: Strength of the quadriceps femoris muscle and functional recovery after reconstruction of the anterior cruciate ligament. A prospective, randomized clinical trial of electrical stimulation. J Bone Joint Surg 1995; 77: 1166–1173.

172. Solomon DH, Simel DL, Bates DW, et al.: Does this patient have a torn meniscus or ligament of the knee? JAMA 2001; 286: 1610–1620.

173. Sperber A, Wredmark T: Tensile properties of the knee-joint capsule at an elevated intraarticular pressure. Acta Orthop Scand 1998; 69: 484–488.

174. Stanford W, Phelan J, Kathol MH, et al.: Patellofemoral joint motion: evaluation by ultrafast computed tomography. Skeletal Radiol 1988; 17: 487–492.

175. Stauffer RN, Laughman RK, Chao EY, Ilstrup DM: Biomechanical evaluation of knee function, before and after total knee replacement. 27th Annual ORS, Nevada, 1981; 55.

176. Stratford PW, Binkley J: A review of the McMurray test: definition, interpretation, and clinical usefulness. J Orthop Sports Phys Ther 1995; 22: 116–120.

177. Tomsich DA, Nitz AJ, Threlkeld AJ, Shapiro R: Patellofemoral alignment: Reliability. J Orthop Sports Phys Ther 1996; 23: 200–215.

178. Trent PS, Walker PS, Wolf B: Ligament length patterns, strength and rotational axes of the knee joint. Clin Orthop 1976; 117: 263–270.

179. Tyston CM, Karpovich PV: Electrogoniometric records of knee and ankle movements in pathologic gait. Arch Phys Med Rehabil 1965; 46: 267–272.

180. van Roermund PM, van Valburg AA, Duivemann E, et al.: Function of stiff joints may be restored by Ilizarov joint distraction. Clin Orthop 1998; 348: 220–227.

181. Veltri DM, Deng XH, Torzilli PA, et al.: The role of the cruciate and posterolateral ligaments in stability of the knee. A biomechanical study. Am J Sports Med 1995; 23: 436–443.

182. Vergis A, Gillquist J: Sagittal plane translation of the knee during stair walking. Comparison of healthy and anterior cruciate ligament-deficient subjects. Am J Sports Med 1998; 26: 841–846.

183. Vogrin TM, Hoher J, Aroen A, et al.: Effects of sectioning the posterolateral structures on knee kinematics and in situ forces in the posterior cruciate ligament. Knee Surg Sports Traumatol Arthrosc 2000; 8: 93–98.

184. Voloshin AS, Wosk J: Shock absorption of meniscectomized and painful knees: a comparative in-vivo study. J Biomed Eng 1984; 5: 157–160.

185. Walker JM, Sue D, Miles-Elkousy N, et al.: Active mobility of the extremities in older subjects. Phys Ther 1984; 64: 919–923.

186. Walker PS: Human joints and their artificial replacements. Springfield, IL: Charles C Thomas, 1977.

187. Walker PS, Hajek JV: The load-bearing area in the knee joint. J Biomech 1972; 5: 581–589.

188. Ward SR, Powers CM: The influence of patella alta on patellofemoral joint stress during normal and fast walking. Clin Biomech 2004; 19: 1040–1047.

189. Watson CJ, Propps M, Galt W, et al.: Reliability of McConnell's classification of patellar orientation in symptomatic and asymptomatic subjects. J Orthop Sports Phys Ther 1999; 29: 378–385.

190. Wendt PP, Johnson RP: A study of quadriceps excursion, torque, and the effect of patellectomy on cadaver knees. J Bone Joint Surg 1985; 67A: 726–732.

191. Williams P, Bannister L, Berry M, et al.: Gray's Anatomy, The Anatomical Basis of Medicine and Surgery, Br. ed. London: Churchill Livingstone, 1995.

192. Wilson DR, Feikes JD, O'Connor JJ: Ligaments and articular contact guide passive knee flexion. J Biomech 1998; 31: 1127–1136.

193. Wilson DR, Feikes JD, Zavatsky AB, O'Connor JJ: The components of passive knee movement are coupled to flexion angle. J Biomech 2000; 33: 465–473.

194. Winter DA, Quanbury AO, Hobson DA, et al.: Kinematics of normal locomotion: a statistical study based on TV data. J Biomech 1974; 7: 479–486.

195. Wisman J, Veldpaus F, Jaussen J, et al.: A three-dimensional mathematical model of the knee joint. J Biomech 1980; 13: 677–685.

196. Witonski D, Goraj B: Patellar motion analyzed by kinematic and dynamic axial magnetic resonance imaging in patients with anterior knee pain syndrome. Arch Orthop Trauma Surg 1999; 119: 46–49.

197. Xerogeanes JW, Takeda Y, Livesay GA, et al.: Effect of knee flexion on the in situ force distribution in the human anterior cruciate ligament. Knee Surg Sports Traumatol Arthrosc 1995; 3: 9–13.

198. Zaffagnini S, Martelli S, Garcia L, Visani A: Computer analysis of PCL fibres during range of motion. Knee Surg Sports Traumatol Arthrosc 2004; 12: 420–428.

Mechanics and Pathomechanics of Muscle Activity at the Knee

CHAPTER CONTENTS

The preceding chapter describes the bony architecture of the knee joint and the connective tissue structures supporting the knee. The present chapter discusses the muscles that move the knee. It is important to recognize that these muscles also provide substantial stabilization, reinforcing the supporting role of the various ligaments. Thus the function and dysfunction of the muscles affect both the mobility and stability of the knee.

The present chapter focuses on the role of these muscles at the knee. However, the vast majority of these muscles cross the hip joint and play an important role at the hip as well. Therefore, the current chapter presents the functions of the muscles that cross the knee as they relate to both the knee and the hip. The specific purposes of this chapter are to

- Explain the normal function of the muscles that cross the knee
- Explore the functional effects of strength and flexibility impairments in these muscles
- Consider the contributions made by these muscles to the pathomechanics of the knee joint
- Describe the relative strengths of these muscle groups

Although there are a variety of ways to classify the muscles crossing the knee, including their location or their innervation, for the purposes of this chapter, the muscles are organized by their actions at the knee. Thus they are grouped as extensors, flexors, medial rotators, and lateral rotators. Each group is presented separately. However, it is important to remain aware that many of the muscles of one group also contribute to the actions of another group.

EXTENSORS OF THE KNEE

The quadriceps femoris muscle represents the primary knee extensor, although the tensor fasciae latae also contributes to knee extension (*Fig. 42.1*). The quadriceps femoris is composed of four separate heads that are discussed individually below.

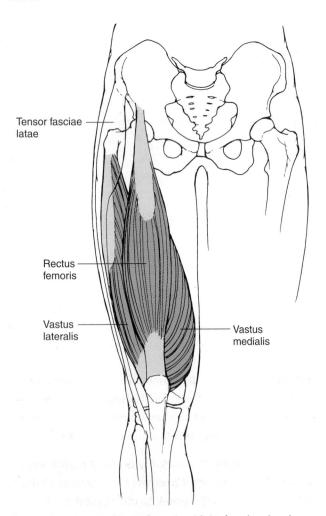

Tensor fasciae latae

Rectus femoris

Vastus lateralis

Vastus medialis

Figure 42.1: The quadriceps femoris with its four heads—the rectus femoris, vastus intermedius, vastus lateralis and vastus medialis—is the primary extensor of the knee, but the tensor fasciae latae also extends the knee.

Rectus Femoris

The rectus femoris is the only head of the quadriceps group that is a two-joint muscle, crossing both the hip and the knee joint (*Muscle Attachment Box 42.1*). It is a bipennate muscle. It also is one of two heads of the quadriceps located centrally on the anterior thigh.

ACTIONS

MUSCLE ACTION: RECTUS FEMORIS

Action	Evidence
Knee extension	Supporting
Hip flexion	Supporting
Hip lateral rotation	Supporting
Hip abduction	Supporting

There is no doubt that the rectus femoris contributes to knee extension and hip flexion [5,53]. However, it is important to understand the circumstances under which the rectus femoris contributes to these motions. The rectus femoris is

MUSCLE ATTACHMENT BOX 42.1

ATTACHMENTS AND INNERVATION OF THE RECTUS FEMORIS

Proximal attachment: Anterior inferior iliac spine and a groove on the ilium, superior to the acetabulum

Distal attachment: The aponeurosis of the quadriceps attaching to the superior border of the patella

Innervation: Femoral nerve, L2–L4

Palpation: The muscle can be palpated proximally between the tendons of the sartorius and tensor fasciae latae and distally between the vastus medialis and vastus lateralis. Subcutaneous fat may make these palpations difficult.

active in knee extension with the hip flexed or extended [23,27,113]. However, studies demonstrate that it is more active during a straight leg raise than when performing an isometric contraction of the quadriceps muscle as a whole in the supine position [107,108]. Electromyographic (EMG) data suggest that the muscle participates in active pure hip flexion only in the middle and end of the flexion range of motion (ROM). However, its activity increases with both lateral rotation and abduction of the hip joint [16]. Biomechanical analysis reveals that the rectus femoris possesses a significant abduction moment arm at the hip [72]. These findings have important implications for the clinician.

Clinical Relevance

EXERCISING THE QUADRICEPS FEMORIS MUSCLE:
A very common exercise to strengthen, or prevent weakness of, the quadriceps femoris muscle is to perform an isometric contraction or to "set" the muscle. The subject is positioned with the knee extended and is instructed to contract the muscle on the anterior surface of the thigh. Data suggest that this exercise is less effective in recruiting the rectus femoris portion of the quadriceps femoris. The clinician must consider additional exercises using hip positions to recruit the rectus femoris optimally.

EFFECTS OF WEAKNESS

Although isolated weakness of the rectus femoris is unusual, it causes a reduction in knee extension strength as well as some decrease in hip flexion strength. The physiological cross-sectional area of the rectus femoris is approximately 15% of the total quadriceps femoris muscle mass [28,118]. Direct electrical stimulation of the rectus femoris suggests that the muscle produces approximately 20–25% of the total extensor torque, during submaximal contractions [128]. Thus the loss of rectus femoris strength alone may produce up to a 25% loss in extension strength.

EFFECTS OF TIGHTNESS

Unlike weakness of the rectus femoris, isolated tightness of the rectus femoris is common, since the position to stretch the muscle (hip extension with knee flexion) is an uncommon position. Tightness of the rectus femoris limits ROM in the combined movements of knee flexion and hip extension. Identification of tightness of the rectus femoris requires examination of knee flexion mobility with simultaneous hip extension. Hip flexion puts the rectus femoris on slack, allowing more knee flexion ROM (*Fig. 42.2*). The role of the rectus femoris in hip abduction and lateral rotation can make assessment of tightness of the rectus femoris difficult. Hip position must be standardized to obtain repeatable measures.

Clinical Relevance

ASSESSING TIGHTNESS OF THE RECTUS FEMORIS:
Tightness of the rectus femoris is assessed typically with the subject prone to extend the hip. The knee is flexed until tension is felt in the anterior thigh from the stretch of the rectus femoris. However, inadvertent abduction of the hip slackens the muscle and may mask the muscle tightness (Fig. 42.3). The clinician must take care to maintain the limb in the sagittal plane while extending the hip and flexing the knee.

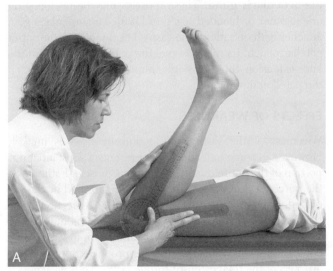
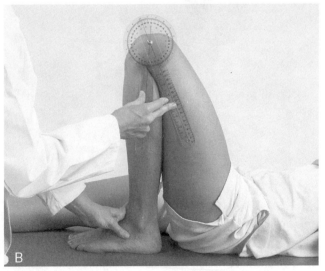

Figure 42.2: A. Tightness of the rectus femoris is assessed by stretching the muscle with combined hip extension and knee flexion. **B.** Allowing the hip to flex puts the rectus femoris on slack and permits full knee-joint flexion.

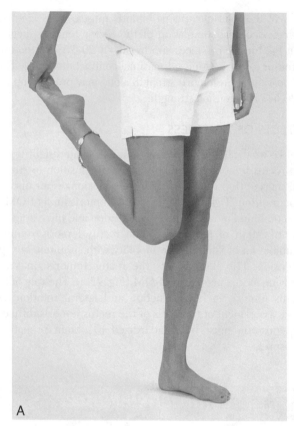

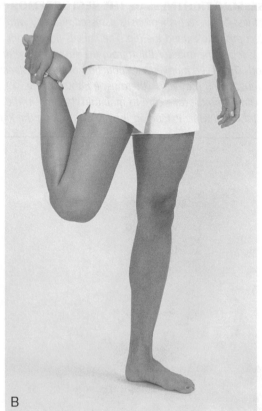

Figure 42.3: **A.** The rectus femoris is stretched by combining hip extension and knee flexion while maintaining the hip in neutral abduction. **B.** Allowing hip abduction puts the rectus femoris on slack and allows more knee flexion.

MUSCLE ATTACHMENT BOX 42.2

ATTACHMENTS AND INNERVATION OF THE VASTUS INTERMEDIUS

Proximal attachment: The anterior and lateral surfaces of the upper two thirds of the femoral shaft. The articularis genu arises from the anterior surface of the lower shaft of the femur.

Distal attachment: The deep portion of the aponeurosis of the quadriceps attaching to the lateral border of the patella and the lateral tibial condyle. The articularis genu inserts into the suprapatellar pouch.

Innervation: Femoral nerve, L2–L4

Palpation: Not palpable in the normal thigh.

Vastus Intermedius

The other centrally positioned quadriceps muscle is the vastus intermedius. It is a unipennate muscle and is the deepest muscle of the quadriceps group [28] (*Muscle Attachment Box 42.2*). It is not palpable in the normal thigh.

ACTIONS

MUSCLE ACTION: VASTUS INTERMEDIUS

Action	Evidence
Knee extension	Supporting

Like the other vasti, the undisputed action of the vastus intermedius is knee extension. EMG studies repeatedly demonstrate activity of the vastus intermedius during knee extension throughout the full excursion of extension. The deepest part of the vastus intermedius is associated with another muscle, the **articularis genu.** These muscles may be distinct from one another or blended together [120]. The articularis genu attaches with or without the vastus intermedius to the suprapatellar pouch. Its role is to pull the pouch proximally during knee extension, thus preventing impingement of the pouch in the patellofemoral joint.

EFFECTS OF WEAKNESS

Weakness of the vastus intermedius by itself is unlikely. However, in some individuals it represents a substantial proportion of the entire quadriceps femoris muscle. Estimates of the percentage of the quadriceps femoris formed by the vastus intermedius based on physiological cross-sectional area range from approximately 15 to 40% of the total muscle bulk [2,8,118]. During direct electrical stimulation in submaximal contractions, the vastus intermedius produces approximately 40–50% of the total extensor torque [128]. Thus weakness of the vastus intermedius results in a substantial decrease in knee extension strength.

EFFECTS OF TIGHTNESS

Tightness of the vastus intermedius, alone, also is unlikely. However, tightness of the vasti together contributes to decreased knee flexion ROM. It is important to recognize that tightness of the three vasti muscles that cross only the knee results in diminished knee flexion ROM regardless of the position of the hip, unlike the rectus femoris, whose tightness is noted when the hip is extended.

Vastus Lateralis

The vastus lateralis is a large, pennate muscle (*Muscle Attachment Box 42.3*). In many individuals it is the largest of the quadriceps femoris muscles [28,35].

ACTIONS

MUSCLE ACTION: VASTUS LATERALIS

Action	Evidence
Knee extension	Supporting

The uncontested action of the vastus lateralis is knee extension. It is active throughout the excursion of knee extension, and the amount of its recruitment is proportional to the amount of resistance to extension [63].

EFFECTS OF WEAKNESS

Weakness of the vastus lateralis reduces knee extension strength. Isolated weakness of the vastus lateralis is not common. However, loss of strength in the vastus lateralis can be expected to produce substantial reductions in extension strength. Estimates based on physiological cross-sectional area suggest that in some individuals, the vastus lateralis may contribute 40% of the extension strength of the knee [28]. However, electrical stimulation of the vastus lateralis during submaximal contractions produced contributions similar to the rectus femoris, approximately 20–25% of the total extension moment [128]. Both of these estimates suggest that weakness in the vastus lateralis produces substantial weakness in knee extension.

EFFECTS OF TIGHTNESS

Isolated tightness of the vastus lateralis is not common. However, tightness limits knee flexion ROM. Tightness may also contribute to an increase in the force of contact between the patella and femur during knee flexion. Thus tightness of the quadriceps may contribute to patellofemoral joint pain.

Vastus Medialis

The vastus medialis is the most studied of the four heads of the quadriceps femoris muscle (*Muscle Attachment Box 42.4*). In the classic study by Lieb and Perry [63], the vastus medialis is described in two parts, the vastus medialis longus (VML) and the vastus medialis oblique (VMO) (*Fig. 42.4*). This division, based on both anatomical and mechanical analysis, has helped to clarify the role of the vastus medialis and to dispel long-held beliefs regarding its functional role. It is estimated that the vastus medialis is approximately 20 to 35% of the overall physiological cross-sectional area of the quadriceps femoris [28,35,118].

ACTIONS

MUSCLE ACTION: VASTUS MEDIALIS

Action	Evidence
Knee extension	Supporting
Patellar stabilization	Supporting

MUSCLE ATTACHMENT BOX 42.4

ATTACHMENTS AND INNERVATION OF THE VASTUS MEDIALIS

Proximal attachment: The VML arises from the distal half of the intertrochanteric line, the medial lip of the linea aspera, the proximal two thirds of the medial supracondylar line, and the medial intermuscular septum. The VMO arises from the tendon of the adductor magnus.

Distal attachment: The quadriceps aponeurosis, attaching to the medial border of the patella and the patellar tendon. The VMO attaches directly into the medial border of the patella.

Innervation: Femoral nerve, L2–L4

Palpation: The vastus medialis is readily palpated on the anteromedial side of the thigh. The oblique portion lies just proximal and medial to the patella.

MUSCLE ATTACHMENT BOX 42.3

ATTACHMENTS AND INNERVATION OF THE VASTUS LATERALIS

Proximal attachment: The intertrochanteric line, the anterior and inferior borders of the greater trochanter, the lateral border of the gluteal tuberosity, and the proximal one half of the lateral lip of the linea aspera and the lateral intermuscular septum

Distal attachment: Quadriceps aponeurosis, attaching to the lateral border and base of the patella and the patellar tendon

Innervation: Femoral nerve, L2–L4

Palpation: The vastus lateralis is palpated on the anterolateral surface of the thigh.

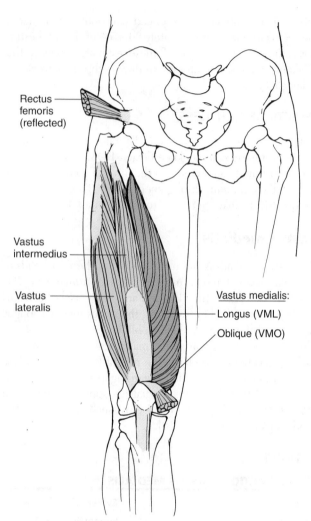

Figure 42.4: The vastus medialis consists of the VML and the VMO.

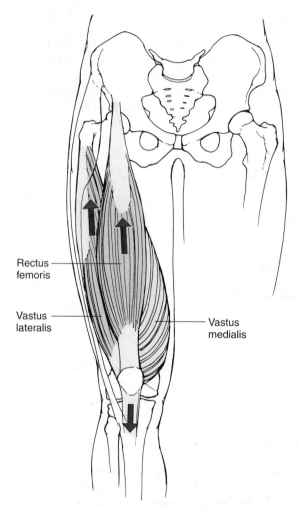

Figure 42.5: The pull of the rectus femoris (RF) and vastus intermedius (VI) is parallel to the shaft of the femur. The line of pull of the vastus lateralis is lateral to the femur. The patellar tendon pulls the patella distally. The sum of these forces is a proximal and lateral pull on the patella.

The role played by the vastus medialis in knee extension was at one time quite controversial [109]. However, repeated analysis of its activity by EMG demonstrates that the vastus medialis is active with the other heads of the quadriceps femoris throughout the entire excursion of active knee extension [63,77,109]. Direct stimulation of the vastus medialis suggests that the vastus medialis provides approximately 10–12% of the total extension torque in submaximal contractions [128]. The myth that the vastus medialis is responsible for the final 15° of knee extension has been refuted convincingly!

The second important function of the vastus medialis is to stabilize the patella during active extension of the knee. To appreciate the importance of this function, it is necessary to examine the overall architecture of the quadriceps femoris muscle. The rectus femoris and the vastus intermedius are centrally located, and their pulls on the patella are exerted along the long axis of the femur. Because the femur deviates laterally from the tibia, they pull proximally and laterally on the patella (*Fig. 42.5*). In addition, the pull of the vastus lateralis on the patella actually is directed slightly laterally with respect to the femur. However, the patellar ligament pulls on

the patella in a distal direction. Addition of these forces on the patella yields a force that is directed laterally on the patella.

The **Q angle** estimates the lateral pull of the quadriceps muscle [90]. It is formed by the intersection of a line drawn from the anterior superior iliac spine (ASIS) of the pelvis to the center of the patella and another drawn from the center of the patella to the center of the tibial tuberosity [1,104] (*Fig. 42.6*). Although estimates of the magnitude of the Q angle found in the healthy population vary, there is general agreement that normal values range from approximately 10 to 20° [1,45,86]. Studies investigating the differences in Q angles between men and women report statistically larger Q angles in women, with values ranging from 15 to 20°. Reported values for men range from approximately 10 to 15°.

In the individual without lower extremity pathology, the Q angle and the measure of valgus of the knee using the long axis of the femur and the tibia are very similar (*Fig. 42.7*). However the Q angle is a function of the location of the tibial tuberosity rather than the shaft of the tibia. Therefore,

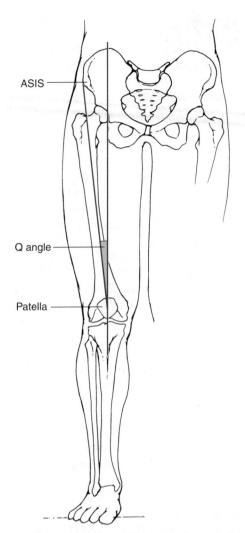

Figure 42.6: The Q angle is formed by a line through the ASIS of the pelvis and the center of the patella and a line from the center of the patella to the tibial tubercle.

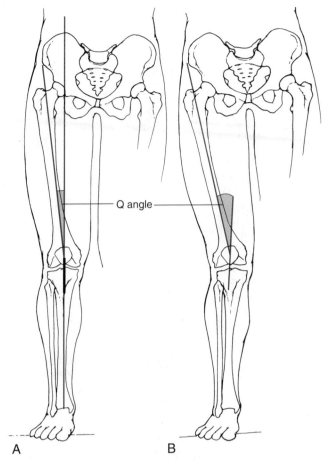

Figure 42.7: A. In normal alignment, the Q angle is approximately equal to the valgus angle of the knee. **B.** Lateral torsion of the tibia can increase the Q angle while the valgus angle remains unchanged.

torsional deformities of the tibia and femur and rotary malalignments of the foot can alter the Q angle without changing the valgus alignment of the knee. (The effects of foot alignment on the mechanics of the knee are examined more closely in Chapter 44.) An increased Q angle indicates an increased lateral pull on the patella and appears to increase the risk of anterior knee pain [1,86].

The Q angle indicates that active contraction of the quadriceps femoris muscle applies a lateral pull on the patella as it pulls the patella proximally and extends the knee. Indeed, reported changes in patellar tilt and congruence angles during contraction of the quadriceps femoris in individuals without knee pathology indicate the tendency of the patella to be pulled laterally, although no true lateral translation is reported [11,123].

There are three systems of protection to stabilize the patella and prevent its lateral deviation [48]. One source of protection is the expanded surface on the lateral condyle of the femur described in the preceding chapter. This bony expansion serves as a buttress against lateral displacement of

the patella. The medial extensor retinaculum also provides passive resistance to the lateral pull on the patella. Finally, dynamic protection is offered by the vastus medialis, particularly by the fibers of the VMO. The fiber arrangement of the VMO makes the muscle ideally suited to provide a stabilizing force, since the fibers run almost completely in a medial and lateral direction and insert directly on the patella (*Fig. 42.8*). Thus the primary function of the VMO appears to be stabilization of the patella against the normal lateral pull of the other heads of the quadriceps femoris muscle.

EFFECTS OF WEAKNESS

Simulated weakness of the vastus medialis in cadaver specimens leads to a lateral shift of the patella during terminal extension [102]. However, the effect of vastus medialis weakness in vivo remains controversial, although some consistency in the data is beginning to emerge. First, it is important to reiterate that the vastus medialis appears to participate with the other heads of the quadriceps femoris muscle throughout knee extension [63]. This participation is independent of the angular position of the knee, the speed of contraction, and the

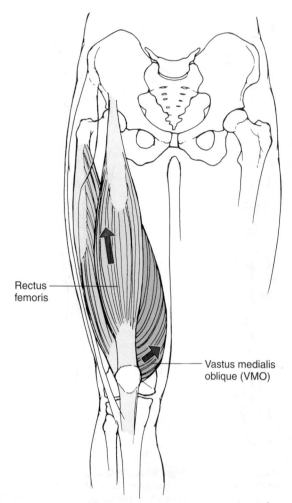

Rectus femoris

Vastus medialis oblique (VMO)

Figure 42.8: The horizontal pull of the VMO on the patella balances the lateral pull of the rest of the quadriceps femoris muscle.

mode of contraction (concentric vs. eccentric) [27,42,77]. Thus it is difficult to identify a scenario in which the vastus medialis is weak in isolation. Weakness of the vastus medialis in conjunction with the rest of the quadriceps femoris muscle leads to decreased strength in knee extension.

Yet there remains a strong clinical impression that weakness of the vastus medialis contributes to anterior knee pain by allowing excessive lateral tracking of the patella. Abnormal lateral displacement of the patella during quadriceps contraction is reported in individuals with anterior knee pain [11]. However, data to demonstrate that specific weakness of the vastus medialis contributes to the abnormal tracking of the patella and thus to anterior knee pain have been elusive. In contrast, quadriceps femoris strength as a whole is correlated with the presence or absence of anterior knee pain [79,98,99]. Quadriceps strength also appears to be a powerful predictor of the success or failure of an intervention regimen for anterior knee pain [85].

EFFECTS OF TIGHTNESS

There are no reports of specific tightness of the vastus medialis. Tightness in conjunction with the rest of the quadriceps femoris muscle decreases knee flexion ROM.

Functional Considerations for the Quadriceps Femoris Muscle

From the preceding discussion, it is clear that the heads of the quadriceps femoris function together to extend the knee. In activities of daily living, contraction of the quadriceps femoris is required primarily to raise and lower the weight of the body while upright. Such activities include getting in or out of a chair or climbing stairs. In contrast, extending the knee during the swing phase of gait requires little or no activity from the quadriceps femoris. This extension occurs primarily as the result of momentum.

Clinical Relevance

EFFECT OF CHAIR HEIGHT ON FUNCTIONALLY IMPAIRED ELDERLY INDIVIDUALS: *More quadriceps force is required to rise from a low chair than from a higher chair (Fig. 42.9). A study of young healthy individuals and frail elders with muscle weakness demonstrates that the elders use a greater percentage of their total strength to rise from the chair [47]. In addition, this study predicts the limit of the chair height from which these individuals can rise. Careful analysis of an individual's home setting and simple alterations in chair height can significantly improve an individual's independence in the home.*

Quadriceps weakness is a strong predictor of impaired performance in many activities of daily living [97]. Quadriceps strength also appears to be a critical factor in rehabilitation of the knee joint following ligamentous injuries [54,82,92, 101,121]. Similarly, knee extension strength is positively correlated with function and negatively correlated with symptoms in individuals with osteoarthritis of the knee [30,32]. There is even evidence that quadriceps strength offers protection from

joint degeneration [75,105]. Thus the clinician is urged to evaluate knee extension strength carefully in patients with lower extremity impairments.

FLEXORS OF THE KNEE

The hamstring muscles represent the primary flexors of the knee (*Fig. 42.10*). However, there are several other muscles capable of flexing the knee. The muscles that contribute to flexion of the knee are: the biceps femoris longus and brevis, semimembranosus, semitendinosus, popliteus, gracilis, sartorius, and gastrocnemius. The hamstrings and popliteus are discussed below. Although the sartorius and gracilis are discussed in a later section of this chapter as rotators of the knee joint, it is important to recognize that these two muscles also undoubtedly participate in knee flexion. The gastrocnemius also produces flexion at the knee. However, it plays an essential role at the ankle and is discussed in Chapter 45 with the other muscles of the leg and foot.

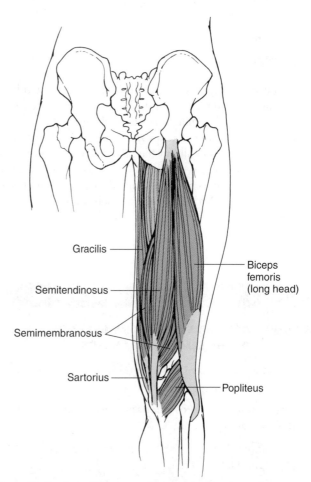

Figure 42.10: The primary knee flexors include the biceps femoris, short head; biceps femoris, long head; semimembranosus; semitendinosus, and popliteus. Additional flexors include the sartorius and gracilis.

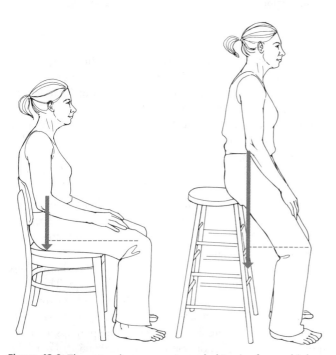

Figure 42.9: The extension moment needed to rise from a high chair is less than that needed to rise from a low chair.

MUSCLE ATTACHMENT BOX 42.5

ATTACHMENTS AND INNERVATION OF THE BICEPS FEMORIS

Proximal attachment: The long head of the biceps femoris attaches to the medial surface of the ischial tuberosity. The short head attaches to the lateral lip of the linea aspera, the proximal half of the lateral supracondylar line, and the lateral intermuscular septum.

Distal attachment: Head of the fibula, the lateral collateral ligament, and the lateral condyle of the tibia

Innervation: The long head is innervated by the tibial division of the sciatic nerve, and the short head is innervated by the common peroneal division of the sciatic nerve, L5, S1, and S2.

Palpation: The tendon of the biceps femoris is readily palpated as it inserts into the fibular head during knee flexion.

Hamstrings

The hamstrings comprise the biceps femoris longus and brevis, forming the lateral mass of the hamstrings, and the semimembranosus and semitendinosus, making up the medial mass (*Muscle Attachment Boxes 42.5–42.7*). All of these muscles flex the knee, and all but the biceps femoris brevis contribute to hip extension. Consequently, their actions and the effects of impairments in strength and flexibility are discussed together. The individual traits of each muscle also are presented.

MUSCLE ATTACHMENT BOX 42.6

ATTACHMENTS AND INNERVATION OF THE SEMIMEMBRANOSUS

Proximal attachment: The lateral facet of the ischial tuberosity

Distal attachment: Posterior and medial surfaces of the medial tibial condyle

Innervation: Tibial division of the sciatic nerve, L5, S1, and S2

Palpation: The muscle belly can be palpated distally on the posterior surface of the knee on either side of the semitendinosus tendon.

MUSCLE ATTACHMENT BOX 42.7

ATTACHMENTS AND INNERVATION OF THE SEMITENDINOSUS

Proximal attachment: Inferior and medial surface of the ischial tuberosity

Distal attachment: Via a flattened aponeurosis to the proximal aspect of the medial surface of the shaft of the tibia

Innervation: Tibial division of the sciatic nerve, L5, S1, and S2

Palpation: The semitendinosus tendon is the most lateral of the muscles on the posteromedial aspect of the knee. It is typically the most prominent tendon in this region.

ACTIONS

MUSCLE ACTION: HAMSTRINGS

Action	Evidence
Knee flexion	Supporting
Hip extension	Supporting
Knee medial rotation	Supporting
Knee lateral rotation	Supporting
Hip medial rotation	Supporting
Hip lateral rotation	Supporting
Hip adduction	Supporting

The role of the hamstring muscles as knee flexors is incontrovertible. However, it is important to recognize that because these muscles attach on both the medial and lateral aspects of the knee joint, pure knee flexion requires activity of both the medial and lateral muscle mass. Contraction of only the medial hamstrings produces knee flexion with medial rotation of the knee; contraction of only the lateral muscle mass produces knee flexion with lateral rotation of the knee joint (*Fig. 42.11*). Yet, EMG studies of lateral and medial rotations of the knee without concomitant knee flexion produce inconsistent activity of the hamstrings [5], emphasizing the importance of the other rotators in moving the knee joint in the transverse plane.

In addition to flexing and rotating the knee, the hamstrings reportedly contribute to the stability of the knee. The hamstrings provide active resistance to anterior glide of the tibia on the femur. Thus they are described as important adjuncts to the anterior cruciate ligament (ACL) and perhaps a critical substitute in the ACL-deficient knee [52,62,65,70,126]. The role of the hamstrings in stabilizing the knee against varus and valgus stresses is less clear. The semimembranosus has an

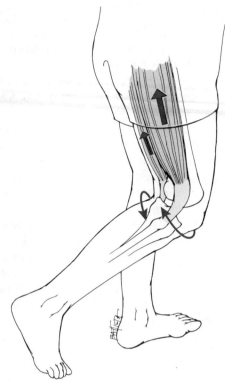

Figure 42.11: When contracting alone, the medial hamstrings produce medial rotation of the knee with knee flexion; the lateral hamstrings produce lateral rotation with knee flexion.

expanded insertion about the medial aspect of the knee, with attachments onto the medial collateral ligament and medial meniscus. Tears of the semimembranosus can accompany medial collateral ligament injuries [6]. Although EMG data are conflicting, there is evidence of hamstring activity during the application of varus and valgus stresses to the knee [3,13,66]. These data suggest that hamstring muscles have the mechanical potential, at least, to help stabilize the knee in the frontal plane.

Clinical Relevance

ROLE OF HAMSTRING MUSCLE ACTIVITY IN THE DYSFUNCTIONAL KNEE: *There is considerable evidence from cadaver studies indicating that the hamstring muscles decrease the strain on the ACL. There also is evidence that individuals with ACL insufficiencies increase the activity of their hamstring muscles in some activities such as hill climbing [52]. Decreased strength in the hamstrings also is associated with poor functional outcomes in individuals following patellectomies [59]. Therefore, while quadriceps strength is well-recognized as important in knee function, careful consideration of hamstring function appears indicated in individuals with disorders of the knees.*

The hamstring muscles also play an essential role in extension of the hip. EMG data reveal that the hamstring muscles are active in hip extension even when the knee is flexed [29]. A study examining the residual hip extension strength after a sciatic nerve block that incapacitated the hamstrings and adductor magnus suggests that the hamstrings provide between 30 and 50% of hip extension strength. Other studies reveal activity in the hamstring muscles during forward bending and lifting [5,87]. Chapter 39 discusses the gluteus maximus and presents data suggesting that it is best suited for hyperextension of the hip. The data presented here suggest that the hamstring muscles play a critical role in hip extension throughout the range of hip motion. EMG evidence also suggests that the hamstring muscles can contribute to adduction of the hip [5]. The biceps femoris longus demonstrates activity during lateral rotation of the hip. Analysis of the medial hamstring muscles' moment arms reveals that with the hip in neutral, the medial hamstrings exhibit very small (<1.0 cm) medial rotation moment arms that increase as the hip laterally rotates [4].

The hamstrings are active during normal locomotion. The most prominent period of activity is at the transition between the swing and stance periods of the gait cycle [25,122] (*Fig. 42.12*). The role of this activity is to slow the extension of the knee in late swing and to help extend the hip in the stance phase. Although a detailed description of

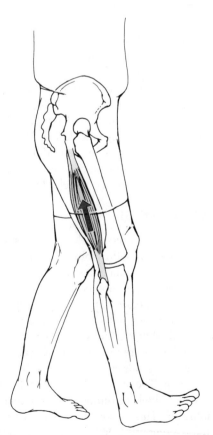

Figure 42.12: The hamstring muscles help to slow the knee's extension and the hip's flexion in the late swing phase of gait.

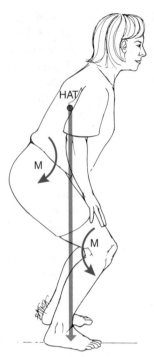

Figure 42.13: The weight of the head, arms, and trunk *(HAT)* when sitting into or rising from a chair produces a flexion moment *(M)* at the knee that must be balanced by quadriceps femoris muscle contraction. The same weight produces a flexion moment *(M)* at the hip that must be balanced by hamstring muscle contraction.

locomotion is found in Chapter 48, it is worth noting that the knee flexion that occurs in late stance and early swing usually occurs without the activity of the hamstrings [25,122]. It also is important to recognize that many activities in the erect posture that require knee flexion such as descending stairs and sitting down use the quadriceps femoris to control the flexion rather than the hamstrings to produce the flexion. The weight of the head, arms, and trunk creates an external flexion moment at the knee that is resisted by an internal extension moment generated by the quadriceps femoris muscle *(Fig. 42.13).*

EFFECTS OF WEAKNESS

Weakness of the hamstring muscles produces a significant loss of knee flexion strength. However, from the preceding discussion, it is clear that knee flexion in the erect posture is often the result of a superimposed weight and controlled by an eccentric contraction of the quadriceps femoris. Consequently, weakness in knee flexion in the erect posture produces little disability. However, weakness of the hamstrings may produce more functional impairment at the hips, where the hamstring muscles provide a substantial part of extension strength. The superimposed weight that creates a flexion moment at the knee during a squat produces a flexion moment at the hip. That flexion moment is resisted by a muscular extension moment generated at least in part by the hamstring muscles. Consequently, weakness of the hamstrings may result in significant difficulty in bending and lifting.

EFFECTS OF TIGHTNESS

The effects of tightness of the hamstrings are complex because all but the biceps femoris brevis cross both the hip and knee joints. As in the rectus femoris, the assessment of tightness in the hamstring muscles must account for their two-joint muscle construction. Tightness of the hamstrings results in limitations in knee extension ROM when the hip is flexed *(Fig. 42.14)* or limited hip flexion with the knee extended. A study of over 200 individuals without lower limb dysfunction reports an average hip flexion ROM of 68.5° ± 6.8° in men and 76.3° ± 9.5° in women with the knee extended [127]. When the hip is extended, the hamstring muscles are put on some slack and allow full knee extension ROM. If the position of the hip has no effect on the range of knee extension, any limitations in knee extension range are the result of one-joint structures such as the joint capsule and ligaments of the knee.

Large amounts of hamstring tightness can produce knee flexion contractures, an inability to reach full knee extension. Knee flexion contractures secondary to hamstring dysfunction are found commonly in individuals with overactivity, or spasticity, of the hamstrings. Overactivity of the hamstring muscles can produce decreased knee extension in late swing and at ground contact during gait [18]. Lesser amounts of hamstring tightness are reportedly associated with a posterior rotation of the pelvis in standing *(Fig. 42.15)*. A posterior rotation of the pelvis tends to flatten the lumbar spine, which may increase the risk of low back pain. However, the associations among hamstring tightness, postural abnormalities, and low back pain are not well-established. Research is needed to identify and explain any links that may exist.

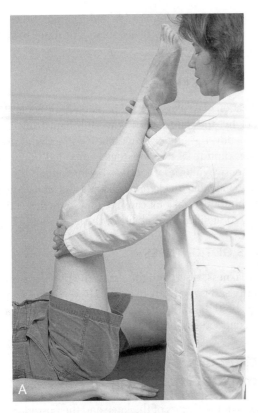

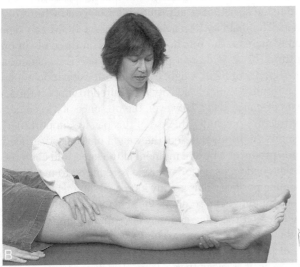

Figure 42.14: A. Hip flexion and knee extension put the hamstrings on stretch so that the knee cannot be fully extended. **B.** Putting the hip in neutral puts the hamstrings on slack, and full knee joint ROM is allowed.

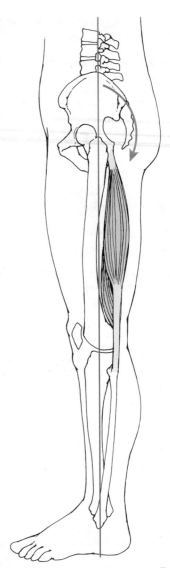

Figure 42.15: Tightness of the hamstrings can pull the pelvis into a posterior pelvic tilt, flattening the lumbar spine.

Mechanics of Two-Joint Muscles at the Knee

The knee is controlled mostly by two-joint muscles that cross either the hip and the knee or the knee and the ankle. Contraction of one of these muscles alone produces movement at all of the joints that the muscle crosses. To isolate movement at a single joint, the two-joint muscle must contract with other muscles, frequently with a one-joint **synergist.**

This is seen at the wrist and finger where the carpi muscles contract with the extrinsic finger muscles to produce pure finger motion (Chapter 15). Such synergists also are available at the knee. The iliopsoas and the hamstrings together produce isolated knee flexion by canceling each other's effect at the hip. Similarly, simultaneous contraction of the gluteus maximus and quadriceps femoris produces knee extension without hip flexion. However, the knee more frequently displays simultaneous contraction of the quadriceps and hamstrings. This unusual pattern of simultaneous contraction of two-joint muscles appears to increase the ability of the knee and hip to generate the large moments needed during many activities. Some of the activities that exhibit this behavior include walking, running, cycling, jumping, bending, and lifting [50,95,114,122]. Co-contraction of the hamstrings and quadriceps also seems to help stabilize the knee and protect the ligamentous structures [66,73]. Although this pattern of a co-contraction increases

MUSCLE ATTACHMENT BOX 42.8

ATTACHMENTS AND INNERVATION OF THE POPLITEUS

Proximal attachment: Lateral aspect of the lateral femoral condyle, popliteus tendon, arcuate ligament, and the fibrous capsule of the knee. The tendon may have an attachment to the lateral meniscus as well.

Distal attachment: A triangular area on the posterior surface of the tibia proximal to the soleal line

Innervation: Tibial nerve, L4, L5, and S1

Palpation: Not easily palpated but may be felt in some people just posterior to the lateral collateral ligament during knee flexion.

the efficiency of producing large muscular moments at both the hip and the knee, it also causes a rise in the loads sustained by the knee.

Popliteus

The popliteus is a small muscle with an unusual pattern of attachments (*Muscle Attachment Box 42.8*). It appears to play a unique role at the knee.

ACTIONS

MUSCLE ACTION: POPLITEUS

Action	Evidence
Knee flexion	Supporting
Tibial medial rotation	Supporting

The physiological cross-sectional area of the popliteus is quite small compared with the rest of the knee flexor muscles [118]. Therefore, its contribution to knee joint flexion torque is small. EMG data reveal only slight activity of the popliteus during knee flexion [5,71]. Its activity increases significantly when knee flexion is accompanied by medial rotation of the tibia, and isolated medial rotation of the knee elicits significant activity in the popliteus [71]. The popliteus also contracts during gait when the tibia is medially rotating.

Studies suggest that the popliteus serves an important role as a dynamic stabilizer of the knee [37,115]. These cadaver studies demonstrate the muscle's ability to reinforce the posterior cruciate ligament, preventing posterior glide of the tibia, as well as rotations into varus and lateral rotation. Finally, the muscle's attachment on the lateral meniscus suggests that it may assist in pulling the meniscus posteriorly during knee flexion, perhaps providing additional protection from tears [10,74]. In summary, the primary role of the popliteus seems

to be to medially rotate the tibia and to protect the integrity of the tibiofemoral joint. It does not contribute substantially to knee flexion strength.

EFFECTS OF WEAKNESS

Identification of weakness in the popliteus is difficult, since it is covered by the large and powerful hamstring muscles. Consequently, the effects of weakness can only be theorized. However, rupture of the popliteus is reported in conjunction with extensive injuries to other posterolateral ligamentous structures including the lateral collateral and arcuate ligaments and the posterolateral joint capsule. Injuries to this entire complex lead to significant instability of the knee joint [37,91,116].

EFFECTS OF TIGHTNESS

As in weakness, discrete tightness of the popliteus is difficult to identify and is not likely to occur. However, the popliteus is likely to be tight with other structures in the presence of a flexion contracture.

Functional Implications of Flexion Contractures of the Knee

Tightness of the flexors of the knee and the posterior connective tissue structures can result in flexion contractures of the knee. The inability to reach full extension ROM can significantly increase the functional demands on the body in erect posture. In normal erect posture, the knee is extended, and the superincumbent weight exerts an extension moment on it. As a result, no muscle activity is required to support the knee in erect stance [111]. However, the presence of a knee flexion contracture precludes the use of this passive support mechanism. With the knee flexed, the weight of the head, arms, and trunk produces a flexion moment at the knee, and contraction of the quadriceps femoris muscle is required to maintain the standing position. This greatly increases the metabolic cost of erect standing. It also alters the magnitude and direction of the forces at the knee and may contribute to further damage of the knee joint complex. The mechanics and pathomechanics of posture are discussed in greater detail in Chapter 47. However, it is clear that a knee flexion contracture significantly increases the challenge of erect posture.

MEDIAL ROTATORS OF THE KNEE

The medial rotators of the knee are the semimembranosus, semitendinosus, and popliteus, which were described in the preceding section, and the sartorius and gracilis, described below (*Fig. 42.16*).

Sartorius

The sartorius is a strap muscle and contains some of the longest muscle fibers found in the human body [46] (*Muscle Attachment Box 42.9*). Reports suggest that the fibers are

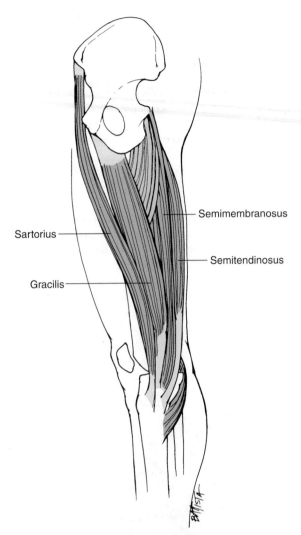

Figure 42.16: The medial rotators of the knee include the sartorius, gracilis, semitendinosus, semimembranosus, and popliteus.

MUSCLE ATTACHMENT BOX 42.9

ATTACHMENTS AND INNERVATION OF THE SARTORIUS

Proximal attachment: Anterior superior iliac spine and the proximal half of the notch below it

Distal attachment: Proximal aspect of the medial surface of the shaft of the tibia.

Innervation: Femoral nerve, L2, and L3

Palpation: The strap-like muscle belly of the sartorius is palpable on the medial aspect of the knee during contraction. It is the most anterior of the pes anserinus muscles.

Palpation: The sartorius is readily palpated at its proximal end. It also is palpated distally, anterior to the tendon of the gracilis.

---

approximately 90% of the length of the muscle [118]. The sartorius is one of the three muscles composing the pes anserinus that crosses the medial aspect of the knee.

ACTIONS

MUSCLE ACTION: SARTORIUS

Action	Evidence
Hip flexion	Supporting
Hip lateral rotation	Supporting
Hip abduction	Supporting
Knee flexion	Supporting
Tibial medial rotation	Insufficient

EMG data and electrical stimulation studies support the role of the sartorius as a hip flexor [2,5,16,72]. Analysis of its moment arms reveals mechanical potential for flexion, abduction, and lateral rotation of the hip [24,72]. Lateral rotation of the hip elicits EMG activity of the sartorius and increases its activity when combined with hip flexion. Hip abduction and abduction with lateral rotation also produce activity of the sartorius. The sartorius has a large moment arm for each motion at the hip. Consequently, despite its small cross-sectional area, the sartorius can generate considerable moments at the hip [72,106].

Knee flexion with the subject prone is accompanied by some sartorius activity, although the activity appears later in the motion than activity of the other muscles such as the hamstrings [16]. This response is consistent with mechanical analyses that show that the muscle's flexion moment arm increases with knee flexion from 0 to 90° [93]. EMG analysis reveals no activity during isolated medial rotation of the knee with the knee slightly flexed and the subject upright [16]. The rotation moment arm of the sartorius changes very little with knee flexion [93]. Studies report activity in early swing with other hip flexors [51,122]. Activity of the sartorius in the early portion of the swing phase of gait is consistent with its role as a hip flexor. Studies differ on the muscle's activity during the stance phase. Although the sartorius is not well studied in locomotion, most studies report activity in early stance, which may reflect its role as a hip abductor with the gluteus medius and minimus [51,122].

EFFECTS OF WEAKNESS

The cross-sectional area of the sartorius is a small fraction of that of the other muscles that flex, abduct, or laterally rotate the hip [64,118]. These muscles include the iliopsoas, glutei, and rectus femoris. Similarly, the hamstrings, the primary flexors of the knee, are much larger and stronger than the sartorius. Consequently, the effects of isolated weakness of the sartorius on the strength of hip and knee flexion may be small.

EFFECTS OF TIGHTNESS

There are no known reports of isolated tightness of the sartorius in the literature. However, it may contribute to a hip flexion contracture, although its size suggests that other muscles may be larger factors in the contracture.

Gracilis

The gracilis is described here because of its role at the knee, although it often is described as part of the hip adductor group (*Muscle Attachment Box 42.10*).

ACTIONS

MUSCLE ACTION: GRACILIS

Action	Evidence
Knee medial rotation	Supporting
Knee flexion	Supporting
Hip adduction	Supporting

The gracilis is rather poorly studied by EMG analysis. However, there are consistent reports that the muscle contributes to both medial rotation and flexion of the knee [5,106]. Analysis of the moment arms of the gracilis support its role as both a flexor and medial rotator of the knee [14,22,93]. Mechanical analyses demonstrate a large adduction moment arm at the hip, with a very small moment arm for lateral rotation.

EFFECTS OF WEAKNESS

The physiological cross-sectional area of the gracilis is very small compared with that of the other knee flexors and hip adductors. However, the gracilis has a substantial moment arm for hip adduction. In addition, it has a large moment arm for knee flexion. Thus the muscle appears capable of generating considerable hip and knee moments; however, there are no known studies that examine the capacity of the gracilis to

MUSCLE ATTACHMENT BOX 42.10

ATTACHMENTS AND INNERVATION OF THE GRACILIS

Proximal attachment: Via a thin aponeurosis from the medial surfaces of the inferior half of the body of the pubis, the inferior pubic ramus, and the ischial tuberosity

Distal attachment: Proximal aspect of the medial surface of the shaft of the tibia.

Innervation: Obturator nerve, L2, and L3

Palpation: The tendon of the gracilis is palpated on the medial aspect of the knee anterior to the semitendinosus tendon during contraction.

generate torque at either the knee or hip. Thus the effects of weakness are unknown.

EFFECTS OF TIGHTNESS

Isolated tightness of the gracilis is unlikely. Tightness is most likely to occur in the presence of tightness of the entire group of hip adductor muscles. The effects of hip adductor tightness are detailed in Chapter 39 but include reduced hip abduction ROM.

Pes Anserinus

The sartorius and gracilis, along with the semitendinosus, insert together forming the pes anserinus. Although these muscles perform the same action at the knee, each has a different function at the hip. Each also has a different innervation. Comparison of these muscles at the knee reveals that the semitendinosus has the largest flexion moment arm, while the sartorius has the smallest [22,93] (*Fig. 42.17*). The semitendinosus also has the largest

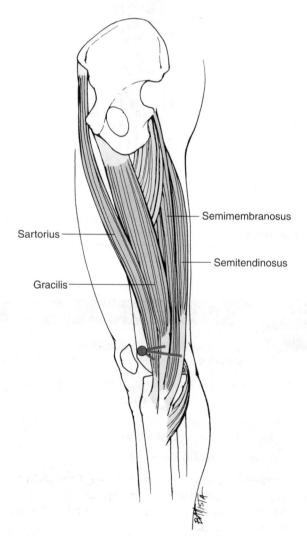

Figure 42.17: The sartorius has the shortest moment arm of the muscles of the pes anserinus, followed by the gracilis, and then the semitendinosus.

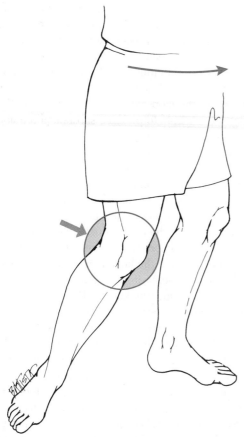

pain of increasing intensity. She denied any specific trauma and reported a gradual onset of pain while playing tennis. She was an elite player, having competed on the professional tour. However, she had discontinued her tennis to begin physical therapy education. She was playing tennis sporadically at the time of the evaluation.

Palpation revealed tenderness on the medial aspect of the knee slightly distal to the joint line. There was no evidence of joint inflammation or joint line tenderness. ROM of the hip and knee joints was full and pain free. Strength of hip flexion, abduction, and medial and lateral rotation was within normal limits and comparable to that of the opposite limb. Similarly, knee flexion and extension strengths were within normal limits and pain free. There was no medial joint instability. However, a valgus stress to the knee produced slight pain. Palpation of the medial collateral ligament was pain free.

Muscle testing of the sartorius by combining resisted hip flexion and abduction with knee flexion produced pain that the patient identified as her chief complaint. Further isolated testing revealed slight discomfort with resisted contractions of the gracilis and semitendinosus muscles. These results suggested that the patient had an inflammation of the pes anserinus bursa that lies deep to the three tendons as they pass over the medial tibial plateau. Her tennis play was consistent with this conclusion, since the activity required repeated rapid movements and pivots on the affected limb. Treatment with ice and rest alleviated the patient's complaints.

Figure 42.18: Many activities that require quick turns such as playing tennis can put large valgus stresses on the knee.

physiological cross-sectional area of the three and thus is able to generate the largest knee flexion moment.

These three muscles together appear to contribute to the dynamic stabilization of the knee against valgus and rotary forces. EMG data reveal increased electrical activity in each of these muscles with the addition of a valgus load to the knee [3,61]. The knee is frequently subjected to such forces. It is intriguing to notice that at least one of these three muscles of the pes anserinus is available to provide support to the knee regardless of the hip position. Similarly, each of the primary motor nerves innervates one of these muscles. Thus there appears to be an organization established to guarantee the availability of some dynamic stabilization of the medial side of the knee. Many sports activities require running and quick turning, including soccer and tennis (*Fig. 42.18*). Such movements require increased stabilization of the knee. When these motions are repeated frequently enough or when the participant is inadequately trained, inflammation of, or around, the pes anserinus can develop.

Clinical Relevance

CASE REPORT: *A 25-year-old female tennis player sought a physical therapy consultation, complaining of medial knee*

LATERAL ROTATORS OF THE KNEE

The lateral rotators of the knee are the biceps femoris longus and brevis, which were described earlier in this chapter, and the tensor fasciae latae described below (*Fig. 42.19*).

Tensor Fasciae Latae

The tensor fasciae latae lies just anterior to the gluteus medius and minimus (*Muscle Attachment Box 42.11*).

ACTIONS

MUSCLE ACTION: TENSOR FASCIAE LATAE

Action	Evidence
Hip flexion	Supporting
Hip abduction	Supporting
Hip medial rotation	Supporting
Knee extension	Supporting
Tibial lateral rotation	Supporting

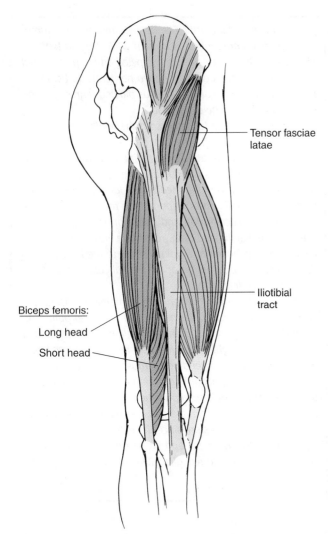

Figure 42.19: The lateral rotators of the knee include the tensor fasciae latae and the biceps femoris, long and short heads.

MUSCLE ATTACHMENT BOX 42.11

ATTACHMENTS AND INNERVATION OF THE TENSOR FASCIAE LATAE

Proximal attachment: Anterior aspect of the lateral surface of the iliac crest and anterior superior iliac spine and from the fascia lata

Distal attachment: Via the iliotibial band (ITB) to the lateral tubercle of the tibia. The ITB also attaches to the lateral condyle of the femur and head of the fibula and blends with the extensor expansion of the vastus lateralis.

Innervation: Superior gluteal nerve, L4, L5, and S1

Palpation: The tensor fasciae latae muscle belly can be palpated at the ASIS of the pelvis during contraction.

EMG data consistently reveal activity of the tensor fasciae latae during hip flexion, abduction, and medial rotation [5,16]. Although the cross-sectional area of the tensor fasciae latae is considerably smaller than that of the iliopsoas or gluteus medius and minimus, it has a large hip abduction moment arm. Its hip flexion moment arm is larger than the moment arm of the iliopsoas [24,46]. Consequently, the tensor fasciae latae is able to produce substantial hip abduction and flexion moments although still not equal to those of the primary abductors or flexors [72].

Reports also reveal electrical activity of the tensor fasciae latae during knee extension which is unchanged by rotation of the knee in either the medial or lateral direction [16,53,80]. In addition, the tensor fasciae latae helps produce lateral rotation of the knee. Like the muscles of the pes anserinus on the medial side of the knee, the tensor fasciae latae provides dynamic stabilization to the knee joint via its attachment into the iliotibial band, increasing its activity in the presence of forces tending to adduct the knee [3,13,61].

During locomotion, activity of the tensor fasciae latae is reported in both the stance and swing phases [36,122]. In the stance period, it most likely contributes to stabilizing the pelvis with the other hip abductors. Chapter 38 demonstrates that medial rotation of the hip can occur either by movement of the femur on the pelvis or by movement of the pelvis on the femur when the lower extremity is fixed. Thus as a medial rotator, the tensor fasciae latae may also help to advance the pelvis on the unsupported side (*Fig. 42.20*). Finally, activity of the tensor fasciae latae during swing occurs with activity of the iliacus and is consistent with the tensor fasciae latae's role as a hip flexor.

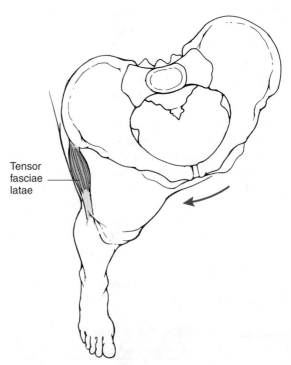

Figure 42.20: In the stance phase of gait, the tensor fasciae latae can pull on the pelvis, causing medial rotation and advancing the pelvis on the opposite side.

EFFECTS OF WEAKNESS

Although the tensor fasciae latae contributes to activities at the hip and knee, its estimated peak force is only approximately 16% of the peak force of the iliopsoas and approximately 12% of the estimated peak force of the gluteus medius [46]. The difference between the estimated peak force of the tensor fasciae latae and the estimated peak in the quadriceps muscles is even larger. Thus isolated weakness of the tensor fasciae latae is unlikely to produce significant disability. A case report of an individual with isolated paralysis of the tensor fasciae latae reports slight but detectable weakness in hip abduction and flexion strength and in medial rotation strength of the hip with the knee extended [80]. A slight reduction in knee extension strength also is reported. Despite these minor weaknesses, the author reports a negative Trendelenburg test result and an unremarkable gait pattern. This case suggests that in the absence of other abnormalities, weakness of the tensor fasciae latae produces little functional loss.

EFFECTS OF TIGHTNESS

Tightness of the tensor fasciae latae reduces the ROM in combined hip extension, adduction, and lateral rotation when the knee is extended. The complex three-dimensional motion at both the hip and the knee resulting from tensor fasciae latae contraction and, therefore, from tightness makes identification of such tightness a clinical challenge.

Clinical Relevance

OBER'S TEST: *The classic test to determine tightness of the tensor fasciae latae is the Ober's test in which the subject's test hip is extended and the amount of adduction available at the hip is observed* (Fig. 42.21). *Although the original test calls for the knee to be flexed, the test is more often performed with the knee extended. One of the challenges of this test for the clinician is to control the limb to prevent medial rotation of the hip, since medial rotation puts the muscle in a slackened position and can produce a false-negative response.*

Tightness of the tensor fasciae latae is associated with both lateral and anterior knee pain. Iliotibial band friction syndrome is an irritation of the iliotibial band (ITB) from repeated rubbing and excess friction between the band and the lateral epicondyle [94]. It is a common complaint in runners and typically is reported during the stance phase of gait when the muscle is active in supporting the hip. Complaints are reportedly diminished by decreasing the amount of knee flexion used during this phase of the gait cycle. Reduction of the knee flexion excursion decreases the stretch on the muscle during active contraction.

Tightness of the tensor fasciae latae and the ITB also are linked to excessive lateral deviation of the patella which is associated with anterior knee pain [38]. Treatments for excessive lateral tracking or excessive lateral tilting of the patella include patellar taping or bracing and surgical release of the lateral patellar retinaculum into which the ITB inserts [38]. The mechanical effects of patellar malalignment and conservative treatments such as bracing are discussed in more detail in Chapter 43.

STRENGTH OF THE FLEXOR AND EXTENSOR MUSCLES OF THE KNEE

Knee joint strength is well recognized as an important factor influencing functional capacity [69,97,100]. Therefore, measurement of muscular strength at the knee is a critical clinical tool. However, the interpretation of strength measurements

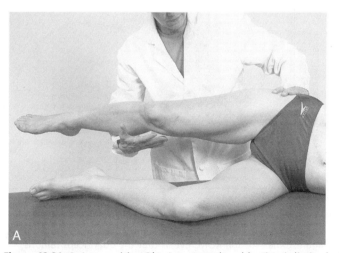
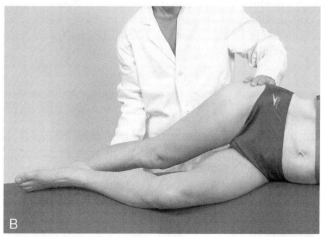

Figure 42.21: A. In a positive Ober's test result, adduction is limited when the hip is held in extension and neutral rotation. **B.** Allowing the hip to roll into medial rotation puts the tensor fasciae latae on slack and allows the hip to adduct, producing a false-negative response to the Ober's test.

may be even more critical in identifying abnormalities and developing strategies to ameliorate the problem. Thus an understanding of the relative strengths of the muscle groups of the knee is particularly useful to the clinician. In addition, appreciation of the factors that affect muscular force production at the knee assists the clinician in distinguishing normal variability from pathology. The data reviewed here are designed to provide a perspective from which the clinician can judge a patient's strength at the knee.

Comparisons between Extension and Flexion Strength at the Knee

It is widely recognized that extension strength at the knee is significantly greater than flexion strength. This finding is consistent with the data that demonstrate that the mass of the extensors is significantly larger than the mass of the flexors [9,118]. Studies demonstrate that the ratio of hamstring strength to quadriceps femoris strength ranges from approximately 0.45 to 0.65. In other words, the maximum strength of the hamstring muscles is approximately 45–65% of the maximum strength of the quadriceps femoris [15,21,33,34,83,84]. This ratio persists throughout the aging process and is present in children from at least the age of six [39,83,84]. However, the magnitude of the ratio is affected by gender and knee joint position, as well as by the speed and mode of contraction. The clinician is cautioned to consider these effects when making judgments about the adequacy of strength in either muscle group. When possible, comparisons with the unaffected limb may be more useful than a target ratio.

Factors Influencing Muscle Strength at the Knee

Age and sex have significant effects on knee joint strength. Reports consistently describe up to 50% less flexion and extension strength in adults over the age of 70 years than in young adults [31,83,84,112]. However, there is less agreement regarding the pattern of strength decline. Some authors report declines from young adulthood to middle age and a larger decline in later years [49,83,84]. Others report less decline until after the age of 50 [31].

Clinical Relevance

DECREASED KNEE STRENGTH IN OLD AGE: *The importance of quadriceps femoris and hamstring strength to rising from a chair, walking up a hill, or getting on and off a toilet is undeniable. The reports of declining strength in the knee musculature with age are worrisome, since they suggest that there may be a concomitant loss in function. It is important for the clinician to recognize the possibility of declining strength in elder patients and to consider the possible functional implications. Fortunately, there is strong*

---

evidence that muscle strengthening is possible at any age [12,81]. Perhaps the loss of strength at the knee with age is preventable, reversible, or at least able to be slowed.

Not surprisingly, men exhibit significantly greater strength than women in both knee flexion and extension [31,76,83,84]. Genetic, hormonal, and cultural factors may all contribute to this difference [76]. Studies are needed to determine if differences in strength contribute to the increased incidence of some musculoskeletal problems in women, such as ACL tears and osteoarthritis.

Effects of Joint Position on Muscle Strength at the Knee

Several studies examine the effects of joint position on knee extension and flexion strength. Chapter 4 describes the basic relationship between joint position and muscle strength in detail. The primary effects result from changes in muscle length and in the moment arm of the muscle. The following presents the available data on the changes in muscle force output at the knee with joint position and provides some data on muscle moment arms to help explain the data.

QUADRICEPS FEMORIS

Most of the studies assessing the effect of joint position on extension strength at the knee report isometric strengths with the subject seated. These data generally demonstrate that quadriceps femoris strength peaks in midrange somewhere between 50 and 80° of knee flexion [21,55,58,96] (*Fig. 42.22*). These findings are explained by the effects of both muscle

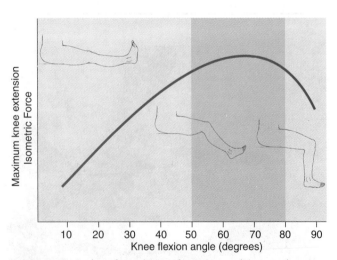

Figure 42.22: A plot of quadriceps femoris muscle strength against knee flexion ROM reveals that the quadriceps femoris generates a maximum force of contraction in the midrange of knee motion, where neither the muscle's length or moment arm are maximized.

length and moment arm. With the hip fixed in flexion, the length of the quadriceps increases as the knee flexes. If the length–tension relationship dominated the results, extension strength would increase with knee flexion and reach a maximum at maximum knee flexion rather than in midrange. Although there is some disagreement in the literature about where the maximum moment arm of the extensor muscles occurs in the ROM of the knee, most studies suggest that the peak occurs at less than 50° of knee flexion [14,57,67,89, 110,117,125]. If the output of the quadriceps femoris were dictated by the muscle's moment arm, maximum extension force would occur earlier in extension. Since peak force occurs somewhere between 50 and 80° of flexion, it appears that like the biceps brachii at the elbow, knee extension strength is a function of both muscle length and moment arm. Hip position can be expected to influence knee extension strength as well but is less well studied.

HAMSTRING MUSCLES

In contrast to the quadriceps femoris muscle, most studies suggest that the hamstring muscles exhibit a steady increase in isometric force output from a position of knee flexion to extension, although most studies examine strength only to 20° of knee flexion [55,58,68,78]. However, some studies show a peak or little change in hamstring strength in the middle range of knee flexion (30–60°) [83,84,124]. Some of the differences in these reports are attributable to differences in hip position, which significantly alters the length of the muscle [58]. Most of the data suggest that hamstring performance is influenced more by muscle length than by moment arm, since the optimal moment arms for the hamstrings occur with the knee flexed [14,67]. However, additional research is needed to resolve the contradictory reports.

These data demonstrate the significant impact on the force production capacity of the knee flexors and extensors made by joint position. The clinician is reminded that valid strength assessments depend on the successful control of factors influencing force production. Therefore, assessment of changes in isometric strength at the knee requires consistency in the joint position used for testing.

SUMMARY

This chapter presents the muscles of the knee and discusses their functions at the knee and hip. These muscles play an obvious role in moving the knee but also contribute significantly to the stability of the knee. In addition, the contribution of these muscles to the pathomechanics of the knee joint is described. Finally, the available data describing the relative strengths of the flexors and extensors of the knee are reviewed. Peak flexion strength is approximately 40–65% of peak extension strength. Joint position, age, and gender all significantly affect knee joint strength.

The muscles that move and stabilize the knee joint are large and capable of producing large contractile forces.

In addition, the knee functions most frequently while bearing at least half, if not all, of a person's body weight. Consequently, the joint surfaces and surrounding connective tissue of the tibiofemoral and patellofemoral joints are subjected to large and repeated loads. The following chapter examines the loads that the knee joint sustains under normal conditions and considers the impact of such loads in pathological conditions.

References

1. Aglietti P, Insall JN, Cerulli G: Patellar pain and incongruence. I: Measurements of incongruence. Clin Orthop 1999; 176: 217–223.
2. Andersson EA, Ma Z, Thorstensson A: Relative EMG levels in training exercises for abdominal and hip flexor muscles. Scand J Rehabil Med 1998; 30: 175–183.
3. Andriacchi TP, Andersson GBJ, Ortengren R, Mikosz RP: A study of factors influencing muscle activity about the knee joint. J Orthop Res 1984; 1: 266–275.
4. Arnold A, Delp S: Rotational moment arms of the medial hamstrings and adductors vary with femoral geometry and limb position: implications for the treatment of internally rotated gait. J Biomech 2001; 34: 437–447.
5. Basmajian JV, DeLuca CJ: Muscles Alive. Their Function Revealed by Electromyography. Baltimore: Williams & Wilkins, 1985.
6. Beltran J, Matityahu A, Hwang K, et al.: The distal semimembranosus complex: normal MR anatomy, variants, biomechanics and pathology. Skeletal Radiol 2003; 32: 435–445.
7. Bevilaqua-Grossi D, Monteiro-Pedro V, de Vasconcelos RA, et al.: The effect of hip abduction on the EMG activity of vastus medialis obliquus, vastus lateralis longus and vastus lateralis obliquus in healthy subjects. J Neuroengineering Rehabil 2006; 3: 13.
8. Boling MC, Bolgla LA, Mattacola CG, et al.: Outcomes of a weight-bearing rehabilitation program for patients diagnosed with patellofemoral pain syndrome. Arch Phys Med Rehabil 2006; 87: 1428–1435.
9. Brand RA, Pedersen DR, Friederich JA: The sensitivity of muscle force predictions to changes in physiologic cross-sectional area. J Biomech 1986; 19: 589–596.
10. Brantigan OC, Voshell AF: The mechanics of the ligaments and menisci of the knee joint. J Bone Joint Surg 1941; 23: 44–65.
11. Brossmann J, Muhle C, Schroder C, et al.: Patellar tracking patterns during active and passive knee extension: evaluation with motion-triggered cine MR imaging. Radiology 1993; 187: 205–212.
12. Brown M: Exercising and elderly person. Phys Ther Pract 1992; 1: 34–42.
13. Buchanan TS, Lloyd DG: Muscle activation at the human knee during isometric flexion-extension and varus-valgus loads. J Orthop Res 1997; 15: 11–17.
14. Buford WL Jr, Ivey M Jr, Malone JD, et al.: Muscle balance at the knee—moment arms for the normal knee and the ACL-minus knee. IEEE Trans Rehabil Eng 1997; 5: 367–379.
15. Calmels PM, Nellen M, van der Borne I, et al.: Concentric and eccentric isokinetic assessment of flexor-extensor torque ratios at the hip, knee, and ankle in a sample population of healthy subjects. Arch Phys Med Rehabil 1997; 78: 1224–1230.

16. Carlsoo S, Fohlin L: The mechanics of the two-joint muscles rectus femoris, sartorius and tensor fasciae latae in relation to their activity. Scand J Rehabil Med 1969; 1: 107–111.

17. Cerny K: Vastus medialis oblique/vastus lateralis muscle activity ratios for selected exercises in persons with and without patellofemoral pain syndrome. Phys Ther 1995; 75: 672–683.

18. Cooney KM, Sanders JO, Concha MC, Buczek FL: Novel biomechanics demonstrate gait dysfunction due to hamstring tightness. Clin Biomech 2006; 21: 59-66.

19. Cowan SM, Bennell KL, Hodges PW, et al.: Delayed onset of electromyographic activity of vastus medialis obliquus relative to vastus lateralis in subjects with patellofemoral pain syndrome. Arch Phys Med Rehabil 2001; 82: 183–189.

20. Cowan SM, Hodges PW, Bennell KL, Crossley KM: Altered vastii recruitment when people with patellofemoral pain syndrome complete a postural task. Arch Phys Med Rehabil 2002; 83: 989–995.

21. Croce RV, Miller JP: Angle- and velocity-specific alterations in torque and semg activity of the quadriceps and hamstrings during isokinetic extension-flexion movements. Electromyogr Clin Neurophysiol 2006; 46: 83–100.

22. Delp SL: Transfer of the rectus femoris: effects of transfer site on moment arms about the knee and hip. J Biomech 1994; 27: 1201–1211.

23. Deutsch H, Lin DC: Quadriceps kinesiology (emg) with varying hip joint flexion and resistance. Arch Phys Med Rehabil 1978; 59: 231–236.

24. Dostal WF, Soderberg GL, Andrews JG: Actions of hip muscles. Phys Ther 1986; 66: 351–361.

25. Dubo HIC, Peat M, Winter DA, et al.: Electromyographic temporal analysis of gait: normal human locomotion. Arch Phys Med Rehabil 1976; 57: 415–420.

26. Earl J, Schmitz R, Arnold B: Activation of the VMO and VL during dynamic mini-squat exercises with and without isometric hip adduction. J Electromyogr Kinesiol 2001; 11: 381–386.

27. Eloranta V: Coordination of the thigh muscles in static leg extension. Electromyogr Clin Neurophysiol 1989; 29: 227–233.

28. Farahmand F, Senavongse W, Amis AA: Quantitative study of the quadriceps muscles and trochlear groove geometry related to instability of the patellofemoral joint. J Orthop Res 1998; 16: 136–143.

29. Fischer FJ, Houtz SJ: EMG of gluteus maximus. Am J Phys Med 1968; 47: 182–191.

30. Fisher NM, Gresham GE, Abrams M, et al.: Quantitative effects of physical therapy on muscular and functional performance in subjects with osteoarthritis of the knees. Arch Phys Med Rehabil 1993; 74: 840–847.

31. Fisher NM, Pendergast DR, Calkins EC: Maximal isometric torque of knee extension as a function of muscle length in subjects of advancing age. Arch Phys Med Rehabil 1990; 71: 729–734.

32. Fisher NM, White SC, Yack HJ, et al.: Muscle function and gait in patients with knee osteoarthritis before and after muscle rehabilitation. Disabil Rehabil 1997; 19: 47–55.

33. Ghena DR, Kurth AL, Thomas M, Mayhew J: Torque characteristics of the quadriceps and hamstring muscles during concentric and eccentric loading. J Orthop Sports Phys Ther 1991; 14: 149–154.

34. Gibson ASC, Lamber MI, Durandt JJ, et al.: Quadriceps and hamstrings peak torque ratio changes in persons with chronic anterior cruciate ligament deficiency. JOSPT 2000; 30: 418–427.

35. Goh JC, Lee PY, Bose K: A cadaver study of the function of the oblique part of vastus medialis. J Bone Joint Surg 1995; 77–B: 225–231.

36. Gottschalk F, Kourosh S, LeVeau B: The functional anatomy of tensor fasciae latae and gluteus medius and minimus. J Anat 1989; 166: 179–189.

37. Harner CD, Hoher J, Vogrin TM, et al.: The effects of a popliteus muscle load on in situ forces in the posterior cruciate ligament and on knee kinematics. A human cadaveric study. Am J Sports Med 1998; 26: 669–673.

38. Harwin SF, Stern RE: Subcutaneous lateral retinacular release for chondromalacia patellae: a preliminary report. Clin Orthop 1981; 156: 207–210.

39. Henderson RC, Howes CL, Erickson KL, et al.: Knee flexor-extensor strength in children. J Orthop Sports Phys Ther 1993; 18: 559–563.

40. Herrington L, Al-Sherhi A: A controlled trial of weight-bearing versus non-weight-bearing exercises for patellofemoral pain. J Orthop Sports Phys Ther 2007; 37: 155–160.

41. Herrington L, Nester C: Q-angle undervalued? The relationship between Q-angle and medio-lateral position of the patella. Clin Biomech 2004; 19: 1070–1073.

42. Herrington L, Pearson S: Does exercise type affect relative activation levels of vastus medialis oblique and vastus lateralis? J Sport Rehabil 2006; 15: 271–279.

43. Herrington L, Pearson S: Does level of load affect relative activation levels of vastus medialis oblique and vastus laterialis? J Electromyogr Kinesiol 2006; 16: 379–383.

44. Hertel J, Earl JE, Tsang KKW, Miller SJ: Combining isometric knee extension exercises with hip adduction or abduction does not increase quadriceps EMG. Br J Sports Med 2004; 38: 210–213.

45. Horton GA, Hall TL: Quadriceps femoris muscle angle: normal values and relationships with gender and selected skeletal measures. Phys Ther 1989; 69: 897–901.

46. Hoy MG, Zajac FE, Gordon ME: A musculoskeletal model of the human lower extremity: the effect of muscle, tendon, and moment arm on the moment-angle relationship of musculotendon actuators at the hip, knee, and ankle. J Biomech 1990; 23: 157–169.

47. Hughes MA, Myers BS, Schenkman ML: The role of strength in rising from a chair in the functionally impaired elderly. J Biomech 1996; 29: 1509–1513.

48. Hungerford DS, Barry M: Biomechanics of the patellofemoral joint. Clin Orthop 1979; 144: 9–15.

49. Hurley M, Rees J, Newham D: Quadriceps function, proprioceptive acuity and functional performance in healthy young, middle-aged and elderly subjects. Age Aging 1998; 27: 55–62.

50. Jacobs R, Bobbert MF, van Ingen Schenau GJ: Mechanical output from individual muscles during explosive leg extensions: the role of biarticular muscles. J Biomech 1996; 29: 513–523.

51. Jaegers SM, Arendzen JH, de Jongh HJ: An electromyographic study of the hip muscles of transfemoral amputees in walking. Clin Orthop 1996; 328: 119–128.

52. Kalund S, Sinkjaer T, Arendt-Nielsen L, Simonsen O: Altered timing of hamstring muscle action in anterior cruciate ligament deficient patients. Am J Sports Med 1990; 18: 245–248.

53. Kendall FP, McCreary EK, Provance PG: Muscle Testing and Function. Baltimore: Williams & Wilkins, 1993.

54. Kim AW, Rosen AM, Brander VA, Buchanan TJ: Selective muscle activation following electrical stimulation of the collateral ligaments of the human knee joint. Arch Phys Med Rehabil 1995; 76: 750–757.

55. Knapik JJ, Wright JE, Mawdsley RH, Braun J: Isometric, isotonic, and isokinetic torque variations in four muscle groups through a range of joint motion. Phys Ther 1983; 63: 938–947.

56. Koutedakis Y, Frischknecht R, Murthy M: Knee flexion to extension peak torque ratios and low-back injuries in highly active individuals. Int J Sports Med 1997; 18: 290–295.

57. Krevolin JL, Pandy MG, Pearce JC: Moment arm of the patellar tendon in the human knee. J Biomech 2004; 37: 785–788.

58. Kulig K, Andrews JG, Hay JG: Human strength curves. Exerc Sport Sci Rev 1984; 12: 417–466.

59. Kuster M, Blatter G: Knee joint muscle function after patellectomy: how important are the hamstrings? Knee Surg Sports Traumatol Arthrosc 1996; 4: 160–163.

60. Laprade J, Culham E, Brouwer B: Comparison of five isometric exercises in the recruitment of the vastus medialis oblique in persons with and without patellofemoral pain syndrome. J Orthop Sports Phys Ther 1998; 27: 197–204.

61. Li G, Kawamura K, Barrance P, et al.: Prediction of muscle recruitment and its effect on joint reaction forces during knee exercises. Ann Biomed Eng 1998; 26: 725–733.

62. Li G, Rudy TW, Sakane M, et al.: The importance of quadriceps and hamstring muscle loading on knee kinematics and in-situ forces in the ACL. J Biomech 1999; 32: 395–400.

63. Lieb FJ, Perry J: Quadriceps function: an anatomical and mechanical study using amputated limbs. J Bone Joint Surg 1968; 50A: 1535–1548.

64. Lieber RL: Skeletal Muscle Structure and Function: Implications for Rehabilitation and Sports Medicine. Baltimore: Williams & Wilkins, 1992.

65. Liu W, Maitland ME: The effect of hamstring muscle compensation for anterior laxity in the ACL-deficient knee during gait. J Biomech 2000; 33: 871–879.

66. Lloyd DG, Buchanan TS, Besier TF: Neuromuscular biomechanical modeling to understand knee ligament loading. Med Sci Sports Exerc 2005; 37: 1939–1947.

67. Lu TW, O'Connor JJ: Lines of action and moment arms of the major force-bearing structures crossing the human knee joint: comparison between theory and experiment. J Anat 1996; 189: 575–585.

68. Lunnen JD, Yack J, LeVean BF: Relationship between muscle length, muscle activity, and torque of the hamstring muscles. Phys Ther 1981; 61: 190–195.

69. MacRae PG, Lacourse M, Moldavon R: Physical performance measures that predict faller status in community-dwelling older adults. J Orthop Sports Phys Ther 1992; 16: 123–128.

70. MacWilliams BA, Wilson DR, DesJardins JD, et al.: Hamstring cocontraction reduces internal rotation, anterior translation, and anterior cruciate ligament load in weight-bearing flexion. J Orthop Res 1999; 17: 817–822.

71. Mann RA, Hagy JL: The popliteus muscle. J Bone Joint Surg 1977; 59: 924–927.

72. Mansour JM, Pereira JM: Quantitative functional anatomy of the lower limb with application to human gait. J Biomech 1987; 20: 1: 51–58.

73. Mesfar W, Shirazi-Adl A: Knee joint mechanics under quadriceps-hamstrings muscle forces are influenced by tibial restraint. Clin Biomech 2006; 21: 841–848.

74. Messner K, Gao J: The menisci of the knee joint. Anatomical and functional characteristics, and a rationale for clinical treatment. J Anat 1998; 193: 161–178.

75. Mikesky AE, Mazzuca SA, Brandt KD, et al.: Effects of strength training on the incidence and progression of knee osteoarthritis. Arthritis Rheum 2006; 55: 690–699.

76. Miller AEJ, MacDougall JD, Tarnopolsky MA, Sale DG: Gender differences in strength and muscle fiber characteristics. Eur J Appl Physiol 1993; 66: 254–262.

77. Mirzabeigi E, Jordan C, Gronley JK, et al.: Isolation of the vastus medialis oblique muscle during exercise. Am J Sports Med 1999; 27: 50–53.

78. Mohamed O, Perry J, Hislop H: Relationship between wire EMG activity, muscle length, and torque of the hamstrings. Clin Biomech 2002; 17: 569–579.

79. Mohr KJ, Kvitne RS, Pink MM, et al.: Electromyography of the quadriceps in patellofemoral pain with patellar subluxation. Clin Orthop Relat Res 2003; 415: 261–271.

80. Muller-Vahl H: Isolated complete paralysis of the tensor fasciae latae muscle. Eur Neurol 1985; 24: 289–291.

81. Mulrow CD, Gerety MB, Kanten D, et al.: A randomized trial of physical rehabilitation for very frail nursing home residents. JAMA 1994; 271: 519–524.

82. Muneta T, Sekiya I, Ogiuchi T, et al.: Objective factors affecting overall subjective evaluation of recovery after anterior cruciate ligament reconstruction. Scand J Med Sci Sports 1998; 8: 283–289.

83. Murray MP, Duthie EH Jr, Gambert SR, et al.: Age-related differences in knee muscle strength in normal women. J Gerontol 1985; 40: 275–280.

84. Murray MP, Gardner GM, Mollinger LA, Sepic SB: Strength of isometric and isokinetic contractions of knee muscles of men aged 20–86. Phys Ther 1980; 60: 412–419.

85. Natri A, Kannus P, Jarvinen M: Which factors predict the long-term outcome in chronic patellofemoral pain syndrome? A 7-yr prospective follow-up study. Med Sci Sports Exerc 1998; 30: 1572–1577.

86. Neely FG: Biomechanical risk factors for exercise-related lower limb injuries. Sports Med 1998; 26: 395–413.

87. Nemeth G, Ekholm J, Arborelius UP, et al.: Hip joint load and muscular activation during rising exercises. Scand J Rehab Med 1984; 16: 93–102.

88. Ng GYF, Zhang AQ, Li CK: Biofeedback exercise improved the EMG activity ratio of the medial and lateral vasti muscles in subjects with patellofemoral pain syndrome. J Electromyogr Kinesiol 2006; e-publication ahead of print.

89. Nisell R: Mechanics of the knee. A study of joint and muscle load with clinical applications. Acta Orthop Scand 1985; 216: 1–42.

90. Noe DA, Mostardi RA, Jackson ME, et al.: Myoelectric activity and sequencing of selected trunk muscles during isokinetic lifting. Spine 1992; 17: 225–229.

91. Noyes FR, Dunworth LA, Andriacchi TP, et al.: Knee hyperextension gait abnormalities in unstable knees. Recognition and preoperative gait retraining. Am J Sports Med 1996; 24: 35–45.

92. Noyes FR, Matthews DS: The symptomatic anterior cruciate-deficient knee. J Bone Joint Surg 1983; 65A: 163–174.

93. Noyes FR, Sonstegard DA: Biomechanical function of the pes anserinus at the knee and the effects of its transplantation. J Bone Joint Surg 1973; 55A: 1241.

94. Orchard JW, Fricker PA, Abud AT, Mason BR: Biomechanics of iliotibial band friction syndrome in runners. Am J Sports Med 1996; 24: 375–379.

95. Pincivero DM, Lephart SM, Karunakara RG: Relation between open and closed kinematic chain assessment of knee strength and functional performance. Clin J Sport Med 1997; 7: 11–16.

96. Pincivero DM, Salfetnikov Y, Campy RM, Coelho AJ: Angle- and gender-specific quadriceps femoris muscle recruitment and knee extensor torque. J Biomech 2004; 37: 1689-1697.

97. Ploutz-Snyder LL, Manini T, Ploutz-Snyder RJ, Wolf DA: Functionally relevant thresholds of quadriceps femoris strength. J Gerontol A. Biol Sci Med Sci 2002; 57: 144–152.

98. Powers CM, Landel R, Perry J: Timing and intensity of vastus muscle activity during functional activities in subjects with and without patellofemoral pain. Phys Ther 1996; 76: 946–955.

99. Powers CM, Perry J, Hsu A, Hislop HJ: Are patellofemoral pain and quadriceps femoris muscle torque associated with locomotor function? Phys Ther 1997; 77: 1063–1075.

100. Robbins AS, Rubenstein LZ, Josephson KR, et al.: Predictors of falls among elderly people. Arch Intern Med 1989; 149: 1628–1633.

101. Rudolph KS, Eastlack ME, Axe MJ, Snyder-Mackler L: 1998 Basmajian Student Award Paper: Movement patterns after anterior cruciate ligament injury: a comparison of patients who compensate well for the injury and those who require operative stabilization. J Electromyogr Kinesiol 1998; 8: 349–362.

102. Sakai N, Luo Z-P, Rand JA, An K-N: The influence of weakness in the vastus medialis oblique muscle on the patellofemoral joint: an in vitro biomechanical study. Clin Biomech 2000; 15: 335–339.

103. Schipplein OD, Trafimow JH, Andersson BJ, Andriacchi TP: Relationship between moments at the L5/S1 level, hip and knee joint when lifting. J Biomech 1990; 23: 907–912.

104. Schulthies SS, Francis RS, Fisher AG, Van De Garaaff KM: Does the Q angle reflect the force on the patella in the frontal plane? Phys Ther 1995; 75: 24–30.

105. Slemenda C, Heilman DK, Brandt KD, et al.: Reduced quadriceps strength relative to body weight: a risk factor for knee osteoarthritis in women? Arthritis Rheum 1998; 41: 1951–1959.

106. Smith LK, Weiss EL, Lehmkuhl LD: Brunnstrom's Clinical Kinesiology. Philadelphia: FA Davis, 1996; 284.

107. Soderberg GL, Cook TM: An electromyographic analysis of quadriceps femoris muscle setting and straight leg raising. Phys Ther 1983; 63: 1434–1438.

108. Soderberg GL, Duesterhaus S, Arnold K, et al.: Electromyographic analysis of knee exercises in healthy subjects and in patients with knee pathologies. Phys Ther 1987; 67: 1691–1702.

109. Speakman HGB, Weisberg MA: The vastus medialis controversy. Physiotherapy 1977; 63: 249–254.

110. Spoor CW, Van Leeuwen JL: Knee muscle moment arms from MRI and from tendon travel. J Biomech 1992; 25: 201–206.

111. Steindler A: Kinesiology of the human body under normal and pathological conditions. Springfield, IL: Charles C Thomas, 1955.

112. Stevens JE, Binder-Macleod S, Snyder-Mackler L: Characterization of the human quadriceps muscle in active elders. Arch Phys Med Rehabil 2001; 82: 973–978.

113. Stratford P: Electromyography of the quadriceps femoris muscles in subjects with normal knees and acutely effused knees. Phys Ther 1981; 62: 279–283.

114. Toussaint HM, vanBaar ME, vanLangen PP, et al.: Coordination of the leg muscles in backlift and leglift. J Biomech 1992; 25: 1279–1290.

115. Veltri DM, Deng XH, Torzilli PA, et al.: The role of the popliteofibular ligament in stability of the human knee. A biomechanical study. Am J Sports Med 1996; 24: 19–27.

116. Veltri DM, Deng XH, Torzilli PA, et al.: The role of the cruciate and posterolateral ligaments in stability of the knee. A biomechanical study. Am J Sports Med 1995; 23: 436–443.

117. Wendt PP, Johnson RP: A study of quadriceps excursion, torque, and the effect of patellectomy on cadaver knees. J Bone Joint Surg 1985; 67A: 726–732.

118. Wickiewicz TL, Roy RR, Powell PL, Edgerton VR: Muscle architecture of the human lower limb. Clin Orthop 1983; 179: 275–283.

119. Wiggin M, Wilkinson K, Habetz S, et al.: Percentile values of isokinetic peak torque in children six through thirteen years old. Pediatr Phys Ther 2006; 18: 3–18.

120. Williams P, Bannister L, Berry M, et al.: Gray's Anatomy, The Anatomical Basis of Medicine and Surgery, Br. ed. London: Churchill Livingstone, 1995.

121. Williams GN, Snyder-Mackler L, Barrance PJ, Buchanan TS: Quadriceps femoris muscle morphology and function after ACL injury: a differential response in copers versus non-copers. J Biomech 2005; 38: 685-693.

122. Winter DA: The Biomechanics and Motor Control of Human Gait: Normal, Elderly and Pathological. Waterloo, Ont: University of Waterloo Press, 1991.

123. Witonski D, Goraj B: Patellar motion analyzed by kinematic and dynamic axial magnetic resonance imaging in patients with anterior knee pain syndrome. Arch Orthop Trauma Surg 1999; 119: 46–49.

124. Worrell T, Karst G, Adamczyk D, et al.: Influence of joint position on electromyographic and torque generation during maximal voluntary isometric contractions of the hamstrings and gluteus maximus muscles. J Orthop Sports Phys Ther 2001; 31: 730–740.

125. Yamaguchi GT, Zajac FE: A planar model of the knee joint to characterize the knee extensor mechanism. J Biomech 1989; 22: 1–10.

126. Yanagawa T, Shelburne K, Serpas F, Pandy M: Effect of hamstrings muscle action on stability of the ACL-deficient knee in isokinetic extension exercise. Clin Biomech 2002; 17: 705–712.

127. Youdas JW, Krause DA, Hollman JH, et al.: The influence of gender and age on hamstring muscle length in healthy adults. J Orthop Sports Phys Ther 2005; 35: 246–252.

128. Zhang LQ, Wang G, Nuber GW, et al.: In vivo load sharing among the quadriceps components. J Orthop Res 2003; 21: 565–571.

Analysis of the Forces on the Knee during Activity

T he preceding two chapters describe the structure of the knee and its impact on the knee's function as well as the mechanics of muscle control across the knee. They emphasize the unusual mechanical demands of the knee, a joint with complex mobility that also sustains large loads as a weight-bearing joint. The knee is controlled by very large muscle groups that stabilize the joint and help move the superimposed weight of the body over a foot fixed on the ground. Consequently, the knee is repeatedly subjected to very large forces throughout a day. The mechanical stresses sustained by the knee are likely contributors to the osteoarthritis so commonly found at the knee. Therefore, it is important for the clinician to be aware of the characteristics of the forces and the factors that influence them. The purposes of this chapter are to

- Present a two-dimensional analysis of the force required of the quadriceps during simple exercises
- Examine the forces and stresses that are applied to the tibiofemoral joint and their relationship to osteoarthritis of the knee
- Consider the loads in the cruciate ligaments as a result of quadriceps femoris and hamstring muscle contraction
- Analyze the forces at the patellofemoral joint under varying exercise strategies

TWO-DIMENSIONAL ANALYSIS OF THE FORCE IN THE QUADRICEPS FEMORIS MUSCLE DURING KNEE EXTENSION

A typical strengthening exercise for the quadriceps femoris muscle is knee extension lifting a weight from the seated position. *Examining the Forces Box 43.1* presents a simple two-dimensional analysis of this exercise. Although this example is an oversimplification of the loads on the knee, it provides an acceptable approximation of the force required

of the quadriceps femoris to hold the leg and foot at a 30° angle of knee flexion with a 10-lb weight at the ankle [6]. The analysis reveals that the extensor muscles must generate a force of 1.08 times body weight (BW) to maintain this position!

Careful examination of the moment arm of the quadriceps femoris muscle compared with the moment arms of the ankle weight and the weight of the leg and foot explains why such a large extensor force is needed. The moment arm of the ankle weight is about 10 times greater than the muscle's moment

EXAMINING THE FORCES BOX 43.1

CALCULATION OF THE QUADRICEPS FEMORIS FORCE NEEDED TO HOLD THE KNEE EXTENDED TO 30° WITH A 10-POUND WEIGHT AROUND THE ANKLE

The following dimensions are based on a female who is 5 feet 8 inches tall (1.72 m) and weighs 140 lb (623 N). The limb segment parameters are extrapolated from the anthropometric data of Braune and Fischer [6]. The geometry of the quadriceps femoris muscle is based on data of Buford et al. [10]. The extension force is assumed to be provided entirely by the quadriceps femoris, with no co-contractions of other muscles.

Weight of the leg and foot: 6% of body weight (BW)
Weight at the ankle: 10 lb (7% BW)

Length of the leg and foot: Approximately 29% of the subject's height: 0.5 m
Center of gravity of the leg and foot: Located at 61% of length of leg and foot from the knee joint
Ankle weight: Located 0.44 m from the knee joint
Moment arm of the quadriceps femoris: 0.04 m

Solve for the quadriceps force (Q):

$$\Sigma M = 0$$

$$(Q \times 0.04 \text{ m}) - (0.06 \text{ BW} \times 0.3 \text{ m} \times (\sin 60°)) - (0.07 \text{ BW} \times 0.44 \text{ m} \times (\sin 60°)) = 0$$

$$(Q \times 0.04 \text{ m}) = (0.06 \text{ BW} \times 0.26 \text{ m}) + (0.07 \text{ BW} \times 0.38 \text{ m})$$

$$Q = 1.06 \text{ BW or } 660 \text{ N}$$

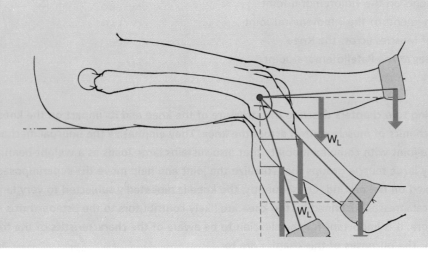

arm. Similarly, the moment arm of the weight of the leg and foot is approximately 6.5 times larger than the moment arm of the quadriceps femoris. The mechanical disadvantage produced by the short moment arm of the quadriceps femoris results in very large force requirements of the muscle.

The example provided in *Examining the Forces Box 43.1* analyzes the force in the quadriceps femoris muscle at a single position of the knee. Changes in the position of flexion and extension of the knee alter the moment arms of the weights and also of the muscle. As the knee extends from 90° to full extension, the moment arms of the ankle weight and the limb weight steadily increase (*Fig. 43.1*). Thus the external moments that must be resisted by the quadriceps muscle increase. As noted in Chapter 42, the moment arm of the quadriceps femoris is greater in extension than in flexion beyond 50°. However, this increase is relatively slight and provides only a small improvement in the mechanical

advantage of the muscle [10,35,43,53,54,67,72]. The increases in the moment arms of the external forces exceed any increased mechanical advantage of the quadriceps femoris. Consequently, the force required of the quadriceps femoris progressively increases from 90° of knee flexion to complete extension [34] (*Fig. 43.2*).

Effect of Mode of Exercise on Quadriceps Femoris Force

The examples described above examine the muscular forces that are required to resist the weight of the leg and foot and any additional applied weights. However, there are many other strengthening devices available that exert resistance on the knee in different ways. Each method may alter the direction of the external force or the mechanics of the muscle output. It is important for the clinician to appreciate the

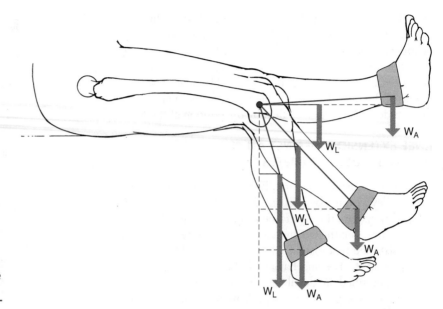

Figure 43.1: Knee extension increases the moment arms of the limb weight (W_L) and the ankle weight (W_A).

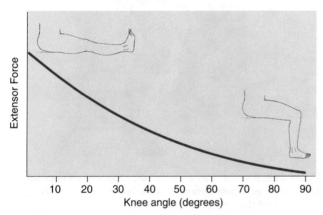

Figure 43.2: Force output of the quadriceps increases as knee extension increases during knee extension against a free weight.

influence that exercise mode has on muscle forces at the knee. This section examines the varying effects of resistance applied by

- A pulley, or cam system
- An isokinetic dynamometer
- A closed-chain exercise

KNEE EXTENSION RESISTANCE DELIVERED BY A PULLEY SYSTEM

The critical difference between resistance from free weights as demonstrated in *Examining the Forces Box 43.1* and a resistance applied through a pulley is the direction of the external force. Weight is a force that, by definition, is exerted in a vertical and downward direction. However, a pulley or cam system is designed to deliver a force that is always directed perpendicular to the limb (*Fig. 43.3*). In this case,

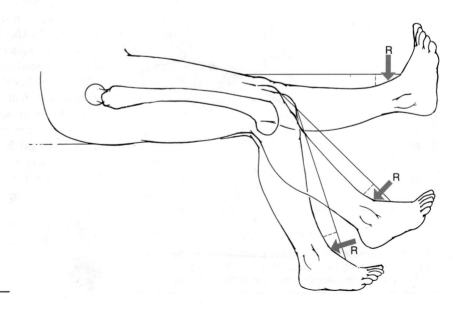

Figure 43.3: A pulley or cam system exerts a perpendicular resistance *(R)* throughout the range of knee extension.

the external moment applied to the knee is constant throughout the range of extension. Since the moment arm of the quadriceps femoris increases slightly in the last half of the extension excursion, the extension muscle force needed to generate the moment is slightly lower in this range. The magnitude of the quadriceps force, then, is affected more by the magnitude of the resistance than by the position of the knee.

KNEE EXTENSION AGAINST AN ISOKINETIC DYNAMOMETER

An isokinetic dynamometer differs from free weights and from pulley systems by allowing a variable resistance. As in the pulley system, the resistance is applied perpendicular to the leg. However, the dynamometer offers an **accommodating resistance** that matches the torque applied by the individual using it. The mechanics of the quadriceps femoris muscle described in detail in Chapter 42 reveal that the extensor muscle generates its peak moment in the middle range of knee flexion, somewhere between approximately 50 and 80° of knee flexion [30,31,53,69]. Therefore, when the individual applies a maximum force to the dynamometer through the range of knee extension, the quadriceps force peaks in midrange [30,53] (*Fig. 43.4*).

KNEE EXTENSION EXERCISES USING A CLOSED-CHAIN FORMAT

A **closed chain** is a mechanical description of a system of links in which both ends of the system are attached to relatively fixed structures [44]. The knee participates in closed-chain activities when the foot is fixed on the ground. Since the hip is connected to a less movable torso superiorly, the knee is situated between two relatively fixed ends and functions in a closed chain. Squats are a common form of closed-chain exercise (*Fig. 43.5*).

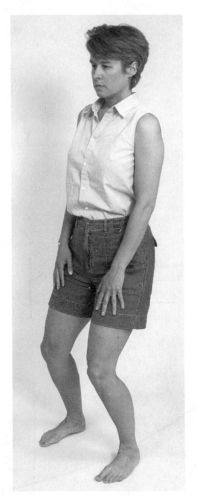

Figure 43.5: A squat is an example of a closed-chain exercise, since the knee moves between two relatively fixed points, the foot and the torso.

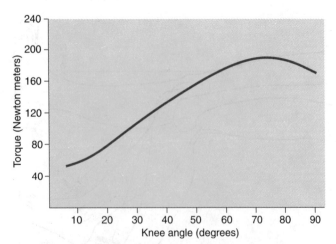

Figure 43.4: Because the quadriceps are strongest in the midrange of knee flexion, quadriceps force during a maximum isokinetic exercise is greatest in the midrange.

Closed-chain exercise exhibits two substantial differences from the other extension-strengthening exercises described so far. First, the resistance is the weight of the head, arms, and trunk (HAT). The other major difference is the relationship between the moment arm of the resistance and the position of the knee joint. In erect standing, the center of mass of the HAT weight lies slightly anterior to the knee joint. In this position, the moment arm of the HAT weight is very small and actually produces a slight extension moment [55]. Consequently, in erect standing, there is no need for activity of the knee extensors. However, as the subject squats, the center of mass of the HAT moves posteriorly, producing a flexion moment arm that increases with the knee flexion angle (*Fig. 43.6*). As the squat increases, the magnitude of the external flexion moment increases, and the force required of the quadriceps femoris muscle increases in concert [15]. Closed-chain activities are common throughout daily life. Rising from a chair, climbing stairs, and getting out of the bathtub are only a few examples of the closed-chain activities undertaken routinely.

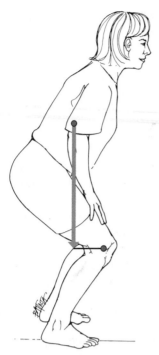

Figure 43.6: In a closed-chain exercise of the knee, the moment arm of the weight of the trunk increases as knee flexion increases.

- Resisted knee extension using a pulley system produces an almost constant quadriceps force (slightly lower, as the quadriceps moment arm decreases somewhat when the knee is flexed less than 50°). The magnitude of the quadriceps force depends primarily on the external force.
- Because isokinetic resistance is accommodating, the quadriceps femoris force reflects the muscle's intrinsic mechanical capacity. Therefore, the peak force of the quadriceps femoris occurs in the midrange of knee flexion.
- Closed-chain exercise requires increasing quadriceps femoris force as flexion of the knee increases.

Several studies report quadriceps muscle force during maximum isometric or isokinetic exercise [3,43,53]. Estimates of the muscle forces generated during maximum efforts vary but are as large as nine times BW [3], or internal moments of approximately 250 Nm [51,59]. For comparison, *Examining the Forces Box 43.2* reproduces the calculations in *Examining the Forces Box 43.1* using internal moments in units of newton-meters (Nm). These calculations reveal that lifting a 10-lb free weight may generate an extension load of approximately 26.3 Nm.

The four exercise modes described here differ from one another in the pattern of quadriceps femoris muscle force required through the range of knee flexion and extension excursion. These patterns are summarized below:

- In exercise with free weights, the required quadriceps femoris force for a given weight peaks when the knee is in full extension.

Clinical Relevance

AVULSION FRACTURE OF THE TIBIAL TUBEROSITY: A CASE STUDY: *Analysis of resisted extension exercises demonstrates the enormous loads that the extensor muscles are capable of generating. Maffulli and Grewal report avulsion fractures sustained by two adolescent male gymnasts during landing maneuvers [36]. These authors report that*

EXAMINING THE FORCES BOX 43.2

CALCULATION OF THE INTERNAL MOMENT AT THE KNEE WHEN HOLDING THE KNEE EXTENDED TO 30° WITH A 10-POUND WEIGHT AT THE ANKLE.

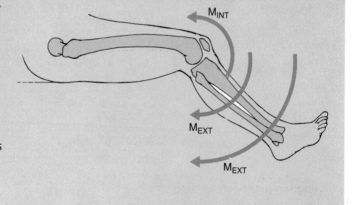

$\Sigma M = 0$

$M_{internal} + M_{external} = 0$

where $M_{internal}$ is the moment created by the quadriceps femoris, $M_{external}$ is the sum of the moments generated by the weight of the leg and foot and the 10-lb weight at the ankle

$M_{internal} = -M_{external}$

$M_{internal} = (0.06 \text{ BW} \times 0.26 \text{ m}) + (0.07 \text{ BW} \times 0.38 \text{ m})$

$M_{internal} = 26.3 \text{ Nm}$

> *both boys displayed greater strength in their uninjured extensors than nonathletic adolescent males. The authors suggest that the force in the quadriceps femoris muscle developed during the landing may have exceeded the strength of the tibial tuberosity's growth plate. These reports are useful in demonstrating the force that the quadriceps femoris muscle is capable of generating. They also serve to warn the clinician that the underlying musculoskeletal system must be capable of sustaining these loads.*

Several studies provide estimates of moments or forces in the extensor muscles during daily activities. In normal locomotion, quadriceps femoris forces of over 400 lb (1800 N) are reported in male subjects [41]. In similar locomotion studies, extensor moments of approximately 30 Nm are reported [33]. Kicking a ball reportedly requires extension moments of approximately 260 Nm [61]. Moments produced during lifting are varied and depend on how the lift is performed but also can be very large [43,48]. Rising from a chair may require moments over 200 Nm but can be reduced by using the upper extremities for additional propulsion [43,49]. These data demonstrate how many activities of daily living require substantial forces from the knee extensor muscles.

FORCES AND MOMENTS ON THE STRUCTURES OF THE KNEE JOINT DURING ACTIVITY

Forces and Moments on the Tibiofemoral Joint

The preceding discussion demonstrates the magnitude of the extensor forces that can be generated. Examples throughout this textbook demonstrate that muscle force is a major contributor to the joint reaction force sustained by any joint. This is certainly the case at the knee. Once the muscle force is determined at a joint, static equilibrium equations can be used to calculate the joint reaction forces at the joint. *Examining the Forces Box 43.3* provides a simple two-dimensional solution for the joint reaction force at the tibiofemoral joint during the free-weight knee extension exercise described in *Examining the Forces Box 43.1*. This example reveals that during the simple knee extension exercise of lifting a 10-lb load, the tibiofemoral joint sustains a joint reaction force of approximately 100% of BW. Since muscle loads are a major contributor to joint reaction forces, it is not surprising that considerably higher loads of up to several times BW are reported during activities such as walking, jogging, lifting, sguatting, and ascending stairs (*Table 43.1*).

EXAMINING THE FORCES BOX 43.3

CALCULATION OF THE REACTION FORCES ON THE TIBIOFEMORAL JOINT WHEN HOLDING THE KNEE EXTENDED TO 30° WITH A 10-POUND WEIGHT AT THE ANKLE.

The results and anthropometric data from Boxes 43.1 and 43.2 are used in this calculation.

ΣF_x:

$J_x - Q \times (\cos 15°) + 0.06 \times BW \times (\sin 30°)$
$\qquad\qquad + 0.07 \times BW \times (\sin 30°) = 0$

where Q = 1.06 BW or 660 N

$\qquad J_x = 598$ N

ΣF_Y:

$J_Y + Q \times (\sin 15°) - 0.06 \times BW \times (\cos 30°)$
$\qquad\qquad - 0.07 \times BW \times (\cos 30°) = 0$

$J_Y = -100.6$ N

Using the pythagorean theorem:

$J^2 = J_x{}^2 + J_Y{}^2$

$J \approx 606.4$ N

$J \approx 0.97$ BW

Using trigonometry, the direction of J can be determined:

$\cos \theta = J_x/J$

$\theta \approx 10°$ from the *x* axis

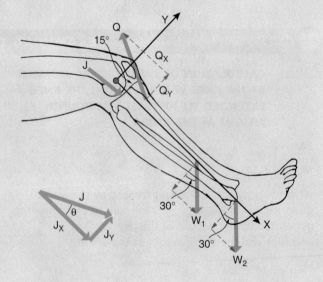

TABLE 43.1: Loads on the Tibiofemoral Joint during Functional Activities (BW = body weight)

Activity	Number of Subjects	Peak Joint Reaction Force	Authors
Level walking	12	3.03 BW	Morrison [41]
Stair climbing	2	4.25 BW	Morrison [40]
Lifting	7	2.12 BW	Nisell [43]
Jogging	3	12.4 BW	Scott and Winter [50]
Squatting	16	7.6 BW	Nagura et al. [42]

The joint reaction force at a joint frequently is reported in terms of its components of axial, or compressive, loading as well as its shear forces in the anterior–posterior and medial–lateral directions. The compressive loads at the knee are far greater than the shear forces [28,42,53,70]. The joint reaction force is of particular interest because it is regarded as an important contributing factor in the development of osteoarthritis (OA). The knee joint is one of the most common weight-bearing joints affected by OA, and knee OA is a leading cause of disability in aging adults [4,16,23,32]. Therefore, it is important for the clinician to recognize the relationship between joint and muscle forces and their possible associations with OA and to consider how exercise affects joint loads [57,68].

The tibiofemoral joint also sustains large moments during functional activities. As noted in Chapter 41, the tibiofemoral joint exhibits 6 degrees of freedom (DOF) and thus sustains forces and moments along and about the medial-lateral, anterior-posterior, and longitudinal axes. Moments about the medial-lateral and anterior-posterior axes are particularly relevant clinically. Moments about the medial-lateral axis tend to produce flexion or extension. An **internal extension moment** produced by the quadriceps balances the **external flexion moment** exerted by the ground reaction force during a squat. In the frontal plane, during normal locomotion the ground reaction force applies an external **adduction moment** on the knee during mid-stance [26]. This adduction moment increases the forces applied to the medial tibial plateau and femoral condyle. The adduction moment increases in individuals with varus alignment of the knee and is associated with degenerative changes of the medial side of the knee joint, *medial compartment knee osteoarthritis.*

In contrast, an individual who lacks adequate hip and knee joint stabilization in the frontal plane may sustain large external abduction moments during weight bearing. Excessive **abduction moments** are associated with medial knee pain and tears of the anterior cruciate ligament [22].

Clinical Relevance

ADDUCTION AND ABDUCTION MOMENTS ON THE KNEE: *The knee joint typically sustains large adduction moments during the stance phase of gait. Adduction moments lead to increased loading of the medial tibial plateau and femoral condyle. Factors such as malalignment and footware may increase the adduction moment. Excessive adduction moments may contribute to the development and progression of knee osteoarthritis, particularly in the medial compartment, leading to the characteristic genu varum deformity (Fig. 43.7). High tibial osteotomies and the use of walking assists such as braces and canes can reduce the adduction moment, relieve pain, and perhaps protect the joint from additional damaging loads [11,45].*

Excessive abduction moments on the knee may be produced during weight bearing when the frontal plane alignment of the knee is compromised by weak abductors of the hip (Fig. 43.8). Weak hip abductors are a common finding in individuals with anterior knee pain or a torn ACL. The increased abduction moment may contribute to excessive Q-angles or produce excessive loads in the ACL. Treatments to increase hip abduction strength may lead to decreased abduction moments and damaging loads on the ligaments. An understanding of the frontal plane moments applied to the knee will allow clinicians to develop more effective prevention and treatment strategies for joint degeneration and trauma.

One important element in linking joint forces and moments with subsequent joint degeneration is the area over which the force is applied. The ability of a joint to sustain joint reaction forces depends not only on the magnitude of the reaction force, but also on its location and how it is dispersed across the joint surface. As defined in Chapter 2, the area over which a force is applied determines the **stress** (F/area) applied to the structure. The incongruity of the articular surfaces of the tibiofemoral joint directly affects the contact area of the knee and, consequently, the stress applied to the tibial surfaces. Chapter 41 describes the articular surfaces of the knee joint in detail. Studies indicate that the normal medial compartment of the knee bears more of the joint reaction force than the lateral compartment [24,29,41]. However, the overall articular surface is greater on the medial side of the joint than on the lateral surfaces [27,47]. Reports differ over which tibial condyle sustains larger stress [27,47,62,63]. Reported magnitudes of peak stress vary from 4 to 9 MPa under static loading conditions, compared with 4 to 7 MPa at the hip during level walking [19,47]. Additional research is needed to characterize the stresses at the knee in individuals with and without pathology.

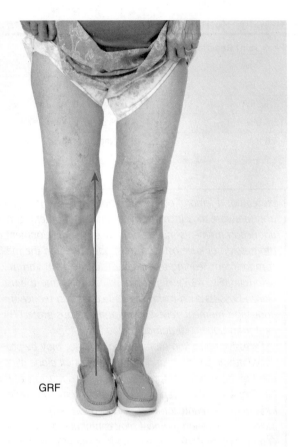

Figure 43.7: Genu varum. Excessive adduction moments may contribute to the development and progression of the varus deformity of the knee that is characteristic of medial compartment knee osteoarthritis.

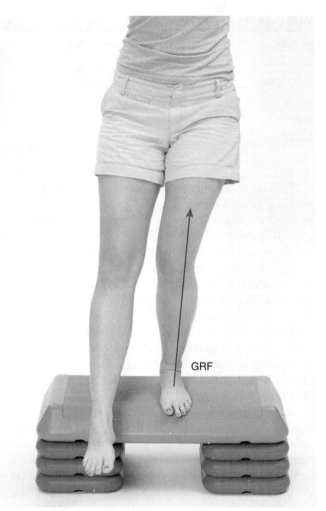

Figure 43.8: Valgus stresses on the knee. Weakness of the hip abductors may lead to excessive abduction moments at the knee because of inadequate frontal plane stability of the femur.

Clinical Relevance

ALTERING THE STRESSES APPLIED TO THE KNEE: *Obesity is a significant risk factor for knee OA [17]. This finding is logical, since body weight is a contributor to the compression forces on the knee. However, other factors including lower extremity alignment and walking patterns also affect the stresses at the knee [58]. Surgical treatments to realign the knee are designed specifically to alter the stresses at the knee [65,66]. However, the use of canes and other assistive devices may improve the loading pattern on the knee [11,39]. In the absence of a cure for OA, an understanding of the links among activity, knee joint loads, and arthritis may lead to more effective treatments and prevention strategies.*

Forces on the Ligaments of the Tibiofemoral Joint

The analysis of tibiofemoral joint forces presented in *Examining the Forces Box 43.3* reveals that the pull of the quadriceps femoris muscle during contraction can be

decomposed into a compressive and a shear component (*Fig. 43.9*). The compressive component contributes to the large axial forces at the tibiofemoral joint described above. The anterior shear force also has important clinical implications. The pull of the muscle in the anterior direction tends to slide the tibia anteriorly on the femur. Anterior shear forces equal to body weight are reported during a vigorous quadriceps contraction [43]. The anterior cruciate ligament (ACL) provides the primary resistance to anterior translation of the tibia. Therefore, contraction of the quadriceps applies a significant pull on the ACL.

Clinical Relevance

FORCES IN THE ACL DURING CONTRACTION OF THE QUADRICEPS FEMORIS MUSCLE: *Biomechanical models and cadaver studies demonstrate that quadriceps activity increases the pull on the ACL [5,51,60]. These findings create a challenge for the clinician. Chapter 42 reveals that*

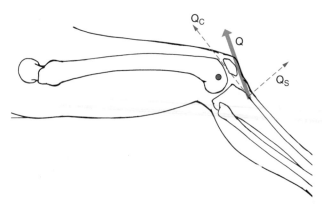

Figure 43.9: The quadriceps femoris force *(Q)* can be decomposed into compressive *(Q_C)* and shear *(Q_S)* forces.

> *quadriceps muscle activity is an important stabilizing force, particularly in the presence of ligamentous injury. Therefore, muscle strengthening is an important component of rehabilitation following injury. Yet a torn or reconstructed ACL may incur further disruption if subjected to excessive loads. Vigorous quadriceps activity, especially with the knee extended, produces large and potentially damaging forces on the ACL [12]. Studies demonstrate that closed-chain exercises generate smaller loads on the ACL than open-chain exercises [60,71]. Consequently, patients undergoing rehabilitation following injury to the ACL are instructed in quadriceps strengthening exercises using closed-chain exercises, or they use a restraining device to limit the amount of anterior glide of the tibia during open-chain exercise (Fig. 43.10).*

Co-contraction of Muscles across the Knee

In the biomechanical analyses presented thus far in this chapter, only the quadriceps femoris muscle is active. However, Chapter 42 indicates that in many activities of daily living, the hamstrings muscles contract with the quadriceps femoris muscle. Indeed, such co-contraction is often used to protect the ACL from excessive pull of the quadriceps femoris. The hamstrings exert a posterior shear force on the tibia during contraction and actually lessen the force on the ACL particularly when the knee is flexed [1,5,13,37,51]. *(Fig. 43.11).*

Clinical Relevance

CLOSED-CHAIN EXERCISES FOR INDIVIDUALS WITH ACL DEFICIENCIES: *Closed-chain exercises such as leg presses and step-up or step-down exercises elicit significant co-contractions of the quadriceps and hamstring muscles. Consequently, they are a routine part of a rehabilitation program for the ACL [44]. However, co-contraction of*

> *muscles produces a significant increase in the compressive component of the joint reaction force [28,70]. Clinicians must remain aware of both the benefits and risks of various exercise regimens to prescribe a program that optimizes the benefits while minimizing the detrimental effects.*

Forces and Stresses at the Patellofemoral Joint

The extraordinarily thick articular cartilage found on the patella suggests that the patella is subjected to very large joint forces. The primary source of the large joint reaction forces at the patellofemoral joint is the large muscle force of the quadriceps femoris generated in so many activities in daily life. The quadriceps pulls proximally on the tibia by pulling on the patella and on the patellar tendon. From the perspective of the patella, the quadriceps pulls proximally on the patella while the patellar ligament pulls distally on the patella *(Fig. 43.12)*. If the patella functions as a pulley, as is frequently described, the magnitude of the proximal pull on the patella equals the magnitude of the distal pull. Although there is now evidence demonstrating that these magnitudes are not equal, this assumption is a justifiable simplification frequently used to estimate the force on the patella at the patellofemoral joint [9,25,38].

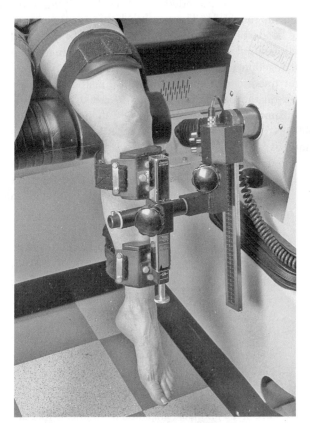

Figure 43.10: A subject exercising the quadriceps femoris on an isokinetic exercise device can use an antishear attachment to protect the ACL.

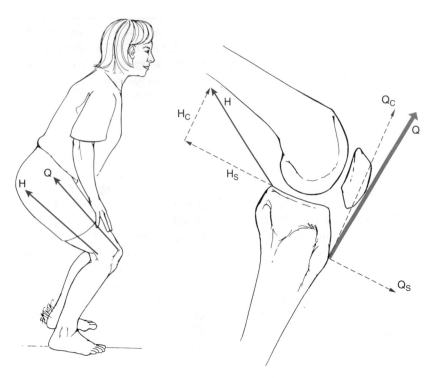

Figure 43.11: During co-contraction of the quadriceps and hamstrings, the pull of the hamstrings *(H)* applies a posterior shear force *(H_s)* that protects the ACL from the shear force of the quadriceps *(Q_s)*. *Q* is the force of the quadriceps muscle and *H_c* and *Q_c* are the compressive components of the hamstring and quadriceps muscle force, respectively.

Examining the Forces Box 43.4 provides a simplified calculation of the forces on the patella generated when holding the knee extended to 30° while holding a 10-lb weight at the ankle. The results of the calculations estimate loads of approximately 83% BW (515 N) on the patellofemoral joint. Not surprisingly, the patellofemoral joint reaction forces are larger in activities that generate larger quadriceps femoris forces. Estimated compressive forces on the patella range from over 800 N (180 lb) to approximately body weight in level walking [7,43] to over 5000 N (1125 lb) in running [18] and in dancers' jump landings [52].

The directions of pull of the quadriceps and patellar tendon also are important in determining the load on the patella. The more flexed the knee, the more the patella is pulled into the femur. Conversely, the more extended the knee, the more the patella is pulled parallel to the femur (*Fig. 43.13*). This knowledge can be applied to understand the effects of various knee-strengthening protocols.

Clinical Relevance

PATELLOFEMORAL JOINT FORCES IN THREE DIFFERENT EXERCISES: *The forces in the quadriceps during knee extension with a free weight, using a cam system and during a closed-chain exercise are reported earlier in this chapter. The patellofemoral joint forces also vary in these exercises (Fig. 43.14). With a free weight, the patellofemoral joint forces are small in knee flexion when the quadriceps force is small. However, in this exercise, the patellofemoral joint reaction force also is small in knee extension, despite a large quadriceps force, because the patella is pulled parallel to the femur, producing very little compression. In resisted knee extension using a cam system, a relatively constant quadriceps force is produced, even at 90° of flexion. Therefore, the patellar joint force reflects the angle of knee flexion, large with knee flexion and steadily decreasing with knee extension. Finally, in closed-chain knee extension, the quadriceps femoris force increases with knee flexion, and the patella is pulled more into the femur as the knee is flexed. Therefore, the patellofemoral joint force increases as knee flexion increases in the closed-chain exercise [64]. Clinicians must be mindful of these relationships when designing exercise regimens for knee strengthening.*

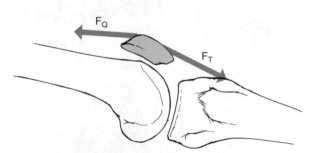

Figure 43.12: It is a justifiable simplification to assume that the pull of the quadriceps tendon *(F_Q)* and the patellar tendon *(F_T)* are equal, because the patella acts somewhat like a pulley for the quadriceps complex.

EXAMINING THE FORCES BOX 43.4

CALCULATE THE FORCES ON THE PATELLA WHEN HOLDING THE KNEE EXTENDED TO 30° WITH A 10-POUND WEIGHT AT THE ANKLE.

Assume that there is equal force (672.8 N) in the quadriceps femoris muscle (Q) and the patellar tendon (Q_T). Use a coordinate system aligned so that the x axis is parallel to PT. Angles of application of the quadriceps femoris muscle and the patellar tendon are based on data from Nisell [43] and Matthews et al. [38].

ΣF_x:

$J_x + 672.8\ N - (672.8\ N \times \cos 45°) = 0$

$J_x = -197.06\ N$

ΣF_Y: $J_Y - (672.8\ N \times \sin 45°) = 0$

$J_Y = 475.74\ N$

Using the pythagorean theorem:

$J^2 = J_x^2 + J_Y^2$

$J \approx 514.94\ N$

$J \approx 0.83\ BW$

Using trigonometry, the direction of J can be determined:

$\cos \theta = J_Y/J$

$\theta \approx 22°$ from the y axis

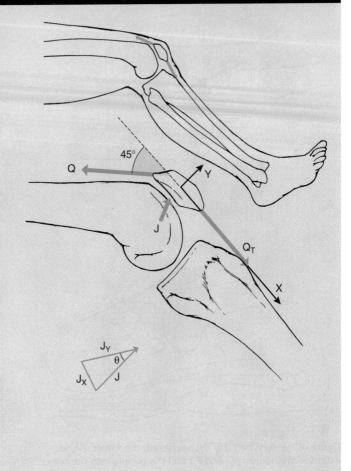

Although joint reaction forces are important to consider in designing an exercise program, the stresses on a joint are also important to consider. This is particularly true at the patellofemoral joint, where the contact surfaces change dramatically through the range of knee flexion. As noted in Chapter 41, there is little contact between the patella and femur when the knee is completely extended and only the inferior portion of the patella contacts the femur in early knee flexion. The area of contact increases as the knee flexes to about 90° [21,38]. The change in contact area on the patella has dramatic effects on the stress applied to the patellofemoral joint. When the knee is completely extended in the free-weight exercise, the quadriceps muscle force is large. However, if there is no contact between patella and femur, there is no stress on the patella. By 15 to 30° of knee flexion there is contact between the patella and femur but over a small area. In the free-weight exercise, the muscle force remains high, and consequently, the patellofemoral stress is quite high. In comparison, the closed-chain exercise actually generates smaller patellofemoral joint stresses with the knee

slightly flexed, because the force of the quadriceps femoris muscle is smaller [56]. The reverse is true with the knee flexed to 90°. The patellofemoral stresses are higher in the closed-chain exercises than in the free-weight exercise with the knee flexed to 90° because of the differences in quadriceps muscle force. As a result, closed-chain exercises in slight knee flexion frequently are recommended to strengthen the quadriceps femoris muscle while avoiding large stresses to the patellofemoral joint [14,44]. *Table 43.2* presents a comparison of the muscle forces and patellofemoral joint forces and stresses developed in the four extensor-strengthening exercises discussed throughout this chapter.

Patellofemoral joint stresses of approximately 3 MPa are reported in normal walking and up to approximately 6 MPa in stair ascent and descent [7,8]. Some individuals with patellofemoral joint pain exhibit decreased patellofemoral joint contact area, which may contribute to increased stress and patellofemoral joint pain. Understanding the relationship between joint stresses and function allows the clinician to consider treatment alternatives to reduce stress and increase function.

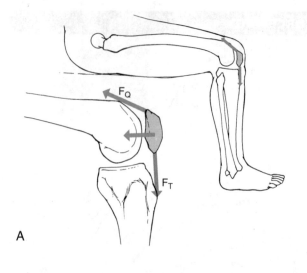

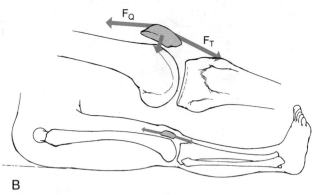

Figure 43.13: A. When the knee is flexed, the forces of the extensor mechanism (F_Q and F_T) pull the patella into the femur. **B.** When the knee is extended, the forces of the extensor mechanism pull the patella almost parallel to the femur.

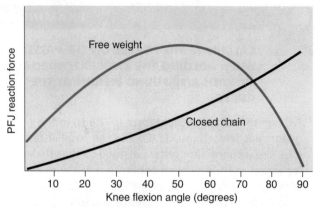

Figure 43.14: The mode of exercise affects the joint reaction forces on the patella between 0 and 90° of flexion. During knee extension against a free weight, the reaction force peaks in midrange of knee flexion; it peaks at 90° of knee flexion in a closed-chain exercise.

Clinical Relevance

PATELLAR BRACING OR TAPING TO REDUCE LATERAL TRACKING: *The use of taping or bracing to reduce patellofemoral joint pain is a common treatment approach. The premise of such treatment is that the tape or brace applies a medial force on the patella to decrease its lateral tracking. Studies consistently report decreased anterior knee pain and improved function with such treatments [2]. Yet studies provide little or no evidence for patellar realignment. Powers et al. demonstrates that patellar bracing while not repositioning the patella increases the contact area between patellar and femoral articular surfaces [46]. These data suggest that patellar taping or bracing may be effective, not because it repositions the patella but because it reduces patellofemoral joint* **stress.**

TABLE 43.2: Comparison of the Mechanics of Quadriceps-Strengthening Exercises between 0 and 90° of Knee Flexion

	Free Weight Resistance	Pulley-System Resistance	Isokinetic Resistance	Closed-Chain Resistance
Knee position with maximum muscle force	0°	Almost constant	Midrange	90°
Knee position with minimum muscle force	90°	Almost constant	0°	0°
Knee position with maximum PFJ force	Midrange	90°	90°	90°
Knee position with minimum PFJ force	0°	0°	0°	0°
Knee position with maximum PFJ stress	Early to midrange flexion	90°	90°	Midrange flexion or 90°[a]
Knee position with minimum PFJ stress	0°	Midrange	0° or midrange	0°
Comments	Quadriceps femoris pull from midrange to 0° extension increases load on ACL	Quadriceps femoris pull from midrange to 0° extension increases load on ACL	Quadriceps femoris pull from midrange to 0° extension increases load on ACL	Co-contraction of extensor and flexors helps protect ACL

PFJ, patellofemoral joint; ACL, anterior cruciate ligament.
[a]Investigators differ in the joint position of maximum PFJ stress [20].

SUMMARY

This chapter uses simple two-dimensional analysis to demonstrate the forces sustained by the quadriceps femoris muscle during exercise and activity. These data are then used to estimate the loads on the tibiofemoral joint and the ACL in similar activities. Finally, the force in the quadriceps femoris muscle also is used to approximate the forces sustained by the patellofemoral joint. The examples provided demonstrate that these structures withstand very large loads. The quadriceps generates loads approximately equal to body weight during low resistance, open-chain exercises and loads several times body weight in maximum resistance exercises. Tibiofemoral joint reaction forces range from approximately 100% BW to more than 1200% BW during jogging. Patellofemoral joint reaction forces over 5000 N (1125 lb) are reported in running and jumping activities.

This chapter also examines the loads on the tibiofemoral and patellofemoral joints in terms of the stress (F/area). Factors influencing the stress on these joints include magnitude of the external loads, joint alignment, and joint position. Since the joints of the knee are commonly affected by OA, an appreciation of the loads and stresses to which the structures of the knee are subjected can help the clinician modify interventions to minimize joint stress.

Throughout this chapter commonly prescribed exercises for quadriceps femoris strengthening are used to demonstrate the concepts of muscle force and joint loads. These data directly influence the clinical decisions necessary when designing a rehabilitation program for an individual with knee pathology. However, in a larger sense, these exercises illustrate how biomechanical analysis of joints informs the practice of rehabilitation. This same approach is useful in studying the mechanics and pathomechanics of the foot and ankle, which are presented in the following unit.

References

1. Aalbersberg S, Kingma I, Ronsky JL, et al.: Orientation of tendons in vivo with active and passive knee muscles. J Biomech 2005; 38: 1780–1788.
2. Aminaka N, Gribble PA: A systematic review of the effects of therapeutic taping on patellofemoral pain syndrome. J Athl Train 2005; 40: 341–351.
3. Baltzopoulos V: Muscular and tibiofemoral joint forces during isokinetic concentric knee extension. Clin Biomech 1995; 10: 208–214.
4. Berenbaum F: Osteoarthritis A. Epidemiology, pathology, and pathogenesis. In: Klippel JH, ed. Primer on the Rheumatic Diseases. Atlanta: Arthritis Foundation, 2001; 285–289.
5. Bottinelli R, Pellegrino MA, Canepari M, et al.: Specific contributions of various muscle fibre types to human muscle performance: an in vitro study. J Electromyogr Kinesiol 1999; 9: 87–95.
6. Braune W, Fischer O: Center of gravity of the human body. In: Krogman WM, Johnston FE, eds. Human Mechanics; Four Monographs Abridged AMRL-TDR-63-123. Wright-Patterson Air Force Base, OH: Behavioral Sciences Laboratory, 6570th Aerospace Medical Research Laboratories, Aerospace Medical Division, Air Force Systems Command, 1963; 1–57.
7. Brechter JH, Powers CM: Patellofemoral stress during walking in persons with and without patellofemoral pain. Med Sci Sports Exerc 2002; 34: 1582–1593.
8. Brechter JH, Powers CM: Patellofemoral joint stress during stair ascent and descent in persons with and without patellofemoral pain. Gait Posture 2002; 16: 115–123.
9. Buff H, Jones LC, Hungerford DS: Experimental determination of forces transmitted through the patello-femoral joint. J Biomech 1988; 21: 17–23.
10. Buford WL Jr, Ivey M Jr, Malone JD, et al.: Muscle balance at the knee—moment arms for the normal knee and the ACL-minus knee. IEEE Trans Rehabil Eng 1997; 5: 367–379.
11. Chan GNY, Smith AW, Kirtley C, Tsang WWN: Changes in knee moments with contralateral versus ipsilateral cane usage in females with knee osteoarthritis. Clin Biomech 2005; 20: 396–404.
12. DeMorat G, Weinhold P, Blackburn T, et al.: Aggressive quadriceps loading can induce noncontact anterior cruciate ligament injury. Am J Sports Med 2004; 32: 477–483.
13. Draganich LF, Jaeger RJ, Kraij AR: Coactivation of the hamstrings and quadriceps during extension of the knee. J Bone Joint Surg 1989; 71: 1075–1081.
14. Escamilla RF: Knee biomechanics of the dynamic squat exercise. Med Sci Sports Exerc 2001; 33: 127–141.
15. Escamilla RF, Fleisig GS, Zheng N, et al.: Biomechanics of the knee during closed kinetic chain and open kinetic chain exercises. Med Sci Sports Exerc 1998; 30: 556–569.
16. Ettinger WH Jr, Afable RF: Physical disability from knee osteoarthritis: the role of exercise as an intervention. Med Sci Sports Exerc 1994; 26: 1435–1440.
17. Felson DT, Anderson JJ, Naimark A, et al.: Obesity and knee osteoarthritis: the Framingham Study. Ann Intern Med 1988; 109: 18–24.
18. Flynn TW, Soutas-Little RW: Patellofemoral joint compressive forces in forward and backward running. J Orthop Sports Phys Ther 1995; 21: 277–282.
19. Fukubayashi T, Kurosawa H: The contact area and pressure distribution pattern of the knee. A study of normal and osteoarthritic knee joints. Acta Orthop Scand 1980; 51: 871–879.
20. Grelsamer RP, Klein JR: The biomechanics of the patellofemoral joint. J Orthop Sports Phys Ther 1998; 28: 286–298.
21. Hehne JH: Biomechanics of the patellofemoral joint and its clinical relevance. Clin Orthop 1990; 258: 73–85.
22. Hewett TE, Myer GD, Ford KR, et al.: Biomechanical measures of neuromuscular control and valgus loading of the knee predict anterior cruciate ligament injury risk in female athletes: a prospective study. Am J Sports Med 2005; 33: 492–501.
23. Hochberg MC: Osteoarthritis. B. Clinical features. In: Klippel JH, ed. Primer of the Rheumatic Diseases. Atlanta: Arthritis Foundation, 2001; 289–293.
24. Hsu RW, Himeno S, Coventry MB, Chao EY: Normal axial alignment of the lower extremity and load-bearing distribution at the knee. Clin Orthop 1990; 255: 215–227.
25. Huberti HH, Hayes WC, Stone JL, Shybut GT: Force ratios in the quadriceps tendon and ligamentum patellae. J Orthop Res 1984; 2: 49–54.
26. Hunt MA, Birmingham TB, Giffin JR, Jenkyn TR: Associations among knee adduction moment, frontal plane ground reaction force, and lever arm during walking in patients with knee osteoarthritis. J Biomech 2006; 39: 2213–2220.

27. Hurwitz DE, Sumner DR, Andriacchi TP, Sugar DA: Dynamic knee loads during gait predict proximal tibial bone distribution. J Biomech 1998; 31: 1–8.

28. Kellis E, Baltzopoulos V: The effects of the antagonist muscle force on intersegmental loading during isokinetic efforts of the knee extensors. J Biomech 1999; 32: 19–25.

29. Kettelkamp DB, Chao EY: A method for quantitative analysis of medial and lateral compression forces at the knee during standing. Clin Orthop 1972; 83: 202–213.

30. Knapik JJ, Wright JE, Mawdsley RH, Braun J: Isometric, isotonic, and isokinetic torque variations in four muscle groups through a range of joint motion. Phys Ther 1983; 63: 938–947.

31. Kulig K, Andrews JG, Hay JG: Human strength curves. Exerc Sport Sci Rev 1984; 12: 417–466.

32. Lawrence RC, Helmick CG, Arnett FC: Estimates of the prevalence of arthritis and selected musculoskeletal disorders in the United States. Arthritis Rheum 1998; 41: 778–799.

33. Lehmann JF, Ko MJ, deLateur BJ: Knee moments: origin in normal ambulation and their modification by double-stopped ankle-foot orthoses. Arch Phys Med Rehabil 1982; 63: 345–351.

34. Lieb FJ, Perry J: Quadriceps function: an anatomical and mechanical study using amputated limbs. J Bone Joint Surg 1968; 50A: 1535–1548.

35. Lu TW, O'Connor JJ: Lines of action and moment arms of the major force-bearing structures crossing the human knee joint: comparison between theory and experiment. J Anat 1996; 189: 575–585.

36. Maffulli N, Grewal R: Avulsion of the tibial tuberosity: muscles too strong for a growth plate. Clin J Sport Med 1997; 7: 129–132.

37. Markolf KL, O'Neill G, Jackson SR, McAllister DR: Effects of applied quadriceps and hamstrings muscle loads on forces in the anterior and posterior cruciate ligaments. Am J Sports Med 2004; 32: 1144–1149.

38. Matthews LS, Sonstegard DA, Henke JA: Load bearing characteristics of the patellofemoral joint. Acta Orthop Scand 1977; 48: 511–516.

39. Mendelson S, Milgrom C, Finestone A, et al.: Effect of cane use on tibial strain and strain rates. Am J Phys Med Rehabil 1998; 77: 333–338.

40. Morrison JB: Function of the knee joint in various activities. Biomech Eng 1969; 4: 573–580.

41. Morrison JB: The mechanics of the knee joint in relation to normal walking. J Biomech 1970; 3: 51–61.

42. Nagura T, Matsumoto H, Kiriyama Y, et al.: Tibiofemoral joint contact force in deep knee flexion and its consideration in knee osteoarthritis and joint replacement. J Appl Biomech 2006; 22: 305–313.

43. Nisell R: Mechanics of the knee. A study of joint and muscle load with clinical applications. Acta Orthop Scand 1985; 216: 1–42.

44. Palmitier RA, An KA, Scott SG, Chao EYS: Kinetic chain exercise in knee rehabilitation. Sports Med 1991; 11: 402–413.

45. Papachristou G: Photoelastic study of the internal and contact stresses on the knee joint before and after osteotomy. Arch Orthop Trauma Surg 2004; 124: 288–297.

46. Powers CM, Ward SR, Chan LD, et al.: The effect of bracing on patella alignment and patellofemoral joint contact area. Med Sci Sports Exerc 2004; 36: 1226–1232.

47. Riegger-Krugh C, Gerhart TN, Powers WR, Hayes WC: Tibiofemoral contact pressures in degenerative joint disease. Clin Orthop 1998; 348: 233–245.

48. Schipplein OD, Trafimow JH, Andersson BJ, Andriacchi TP: Relationship between moments at the L5/S1 level, hip and knee joint when lifting. J Biomech 1990; 23: 907–912.

49. Schultz AB, Alexander NB, Ashton-Miller JA: Biomechanical analyses of rising from a chair. J Biomech 1992; 25: 1383–1392.

50. Scott SH, Winter DA: Internal forces at chronic running injury sites. Med Sci Sports Exerc 1990; 22: 357–369.

51. Shelburne K, Pandy MG: A musculoskeletal model of the knee for evaluating ligament forces during isometric contractions. J Biomech 1997; 30: 163–176.

52. Simpson KJ, Jameson EG, Odum S: Estimated patellofemoral compressive forces and contact pressures during dance landings. J Appl Biomech 1996; 12: 1–14.

53. Smidt G: Biomechanical analysis of knee flexion and extension. J Biomech 1973; 6: 79–92.

54. Spoor CW, Van Leeuwen JL: Knee muscle moment arms from MRI and from tendon travel. J Biomech 1992; 25: 201–206.

55. Steindler A: Kinesiology of the human body under normal and pathological conditions. Springfield, IL: Charles C Thomas, 1955.

56. Steinkamp LA, Dillingham MF, Markels MD, et al.: Biomechanical considerations in patellofemoral joint rehabilitation. Am J Sports Med 1993; 21: 438–444.

57. Stuart MJ, Meglan DA, Lutz GE, et al.: Comparison of intersegmental tibiofemoral joint forces and muscle activity during various closed kinetic chain exercises. Am J Sports Med 1996; 24: 792–799.

58. Tetsworth K, Paley D: Malalignment and degenerative arthropathy. Orthop Clin North Am 1994; 25: 367–377.

59. Thomee R, Grimby G, Svantesson U, Osterberg U: Quadriceps muscle performance in sitting and standing in young women with patellofemoral pain syndrome and young healthy women. Scand J Med Sci Sports 1996; 6: 233–241.

60. Toutoungi DE, Lu TW, Leardini A, et al.: Cruciate ligament forces in the human knee during rehabilitation exercises. Clin Biomech 2000; 15: 176–187.

61. Wahrenberg H, Lindbeck L, Ekholm J: Knee muscular moment, tendon tension force and EMG during a vigorous movement in man. Scand J Rehabil Med 1978; 10: 99–106.

62. Walker PS, Hajek JV: The load-bearing area in the knee joint. J Biomech 1972; 5: 581–589.

63. Wallace AL, Harris ML, Walsh WR, Bruce WJM: Intraoperative assessment of tibiofemoral contact stresses in total knee arthroplasty. J Arthroplasty 1998; 13: 923–927.

64. Wallace DA, Salem GJ, Salinas R, Powers CM: Patellofemoral joint kinetics while squatting with and without ab external load. JOSPT 2002; 32: 141–148.

65. Weidenhielm L, Svensson OK, Brostrom L: Surgical correction of leg alignment in unilateral knee osteoarthrosis reduces the load on the hip and knee joint bilaterally. Clin Biomech 1995; 10: 217–221.

66. Weidenhielm MD, Svensson OK, Brostrom L, Rudberg U: Change in adduction moment about the knee after high tibial osteotomy and prosthetic replacement in osteoarthritis of the knee. Clin Biomech 1992; 7: 91–96.

67. Wendt PP, Johnson RP: A study of quadriceps excursion, torque, and the effect of patellectomy on cadaver knees. J Bone Joint Surg 1985; 67A: 726–732.

68. Wilk KE, Escamilla RF, Fleisig GS, et al.: A comparison of tibiofemoral joint forces and electromyographic activity during open and closed kinetic chain exercises. Am J Sports Med 1996; 24: 518–527.

69. Williams M, Stutzman L: Strength variation through the range of joint motion. Phys Ther Rev 1959; 39: 145–152.

70. Witonski D, Goraj B: Patellar motion analyzed by kinematic and dynamic axial magnetic resonance imaging in patients with anterior knee pain syndrome. Arch Orthop Trauma Surg 1999; 119: 46–49.

71. Yack HJ, Collins CE, Whieldon TJ: Comparison of closed and open kinetic chain exercise in the anterior cruciate ligament-deficient knee. Am J Sports Med 1993; 21: 49–54.

72. Yamaguchi GT, Zajac FE: A planar model of the knee joint to characterize the knee extensor mechanism. J Biomech 1989; 22: 1–10.

UNIT 8

ANKLE AND FOOT UNIT

T he foot and ankle represent the final component of the lower extremity and function together to make habitual bipedal stance and locomotion possible. Just as the wrist and hand are the working unit of the upper extremity, the ankle and foot complex greatly enhances the functional capacity of the lower extremity. Although there are a great number of similarities between the wrist and hand of the upper extremity and the ankle and foot of the lower extremity, the peculiar functional demands of persistent weight bearing induce unique characteristics in the ankle/foot complex. In addition, because the ankle and foot function much of the time in contact with the ground, they complete a closed chain with the rest of the lower extremity. Consequently, the ankle/foot complex has a substantial effect on the knee and even on the hip and spine.

The ankle/foot complex must be stable enough to bear the weight of the rest of the body and also must participate in the advancement of the body over the fixed foot during locomotion. As a result, the muscles of the leg and foot play an essential role in stabilizing the ankle/foot complex during loading but also in propelling and controlling the advancement of the body over the foot during locomotion. As the ankle and foot participate in locomotion they sustain very large loads that may contribute to some of the clinical complaints reported by patients.

The purposes of this three-chapter unit on the ankle and foot complex are to

- Discuss the structure of the bones and joints of the ankle and foot and how these features contribute to the role of weight bearing and propulsion
- Discuss the role of muscles in the mechanics and pathomechanics of the ankle and foot
- Analyze the forces to which the ankle and foot are subjected, particularly during weight-bearing activities

Structure and Function of the Bones and Noncontractile Elements of the Ankle and Foot Complex

CHAPTER CONTENTS

A lthough the bones of the foot bear some resemblance to those of the hand, their unique features have a substantial impact on the mobility and stability of the ankle, as well as the weight-bearing capacity of the entire complex. The supporting structures within the ankle and foot also bear some similarities to those of the wrist and hand, and the differences between these two anatomical units reflect the differences in functional demands.

The purpose of this chapter is to discuss the bones and joints of the ankle/foot complex and how these influence the function of the lower extremity. Specifically, the objectives of the current chapter are to

- Discuss the functionally relevant structural features of the bones of the ankle and foot
- Describe the architecture and supporting structures of the joints of the ankle and foot
- Review the motions available at the individual joints of the ankle and foot
- Describe how the joints of the foot function together to produce total foot motion in the open and closed chain
- Describe the normal alignment of the foot and ankle
- Present the normative data on range of motion (ROM) available at the ankle and foot

BONES OF THE ANKLE AND FOOT

The ankle/foot complex comprises the distal tibia and fibula, the seven tarsal bones, and the digits, consisting of five metatarsals and fourteen phalanges (*Fig. 44.1*). Their unique characteristics contribute substantially to the functional capabilities of the ankle/foot complex.

Shaft and Distal Tibia

TIBIAL SHAFT

The proximal tibia is described in Chapter 41 in the knee unit. The shaft of the tibia continues from the tibial plateaus and tibial tuberosity (*Fig. 44.2*). The anterior border of the tibia extends from the tibial tuberosity distally to the anterior aspect of the medial malleolus. It is superficial and easily palpated until its distal end. Most individuals who are capable of upright walking recognize the anterior border of the tibia as the "shin" that bumps painfully into chair legs or other obstacles. The

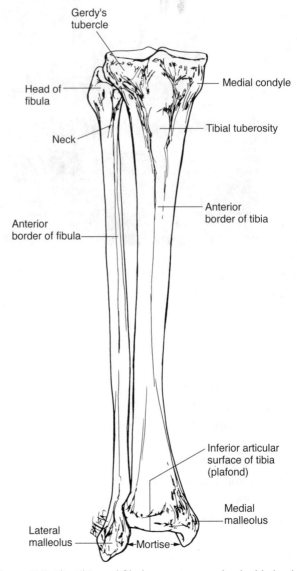

Figure 44.2: The tibia and fibula possess several palpable landmarks and together form the cavity, or mortise, for the talus.

medial surface of the tibia also is palpable the length of the tibia. The posterior surface, from the interosseous border laterally to the medial border, contains the soleal line that runs obliquely from the articular surface of the head of the fibula medially to the medial border of the tibia, approximately one-third of the length of the tibia from its proximal end.

DISTAL TIBIA

The shaft of the tibia ends distally in an inferiorly and medially projecting mass, the medial malleolus, which is readily palpated. The lateral surface of the medial malleolus provides an articular surface for the medial aspect of the talus. It is vertically aligned and almost flat, so it bears little weight. This articular surface on the tibia is continuous with the distal tibial surface, which also offers an articular surface for the talus. The articular surface of the distal tibia, known as the **plafond,** is saddle shaped, concave in an anterior–posterior direction

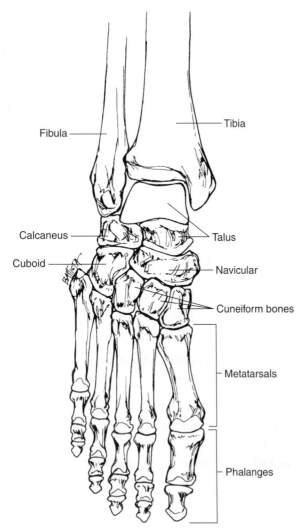

Figure 44.1: The ankle/foot complex consists of the tibia, fibula, seven tarsal bones, five metatarsal bones, and fourteen phalanges.

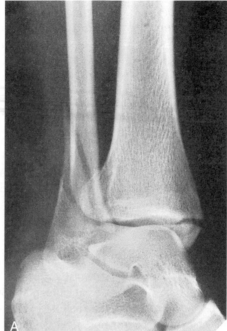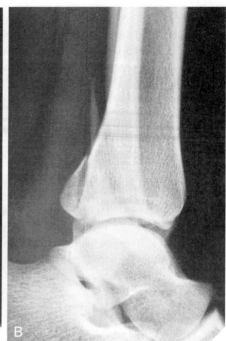

Figure 44.3: Tri-malleolar fracture. A tri-maleollar fracture includes fractures of the medial and lateral malleoli **(A)** and a fracture of the posterior surface of the distal tibia, the third maleollus **(B)**. (Reprinted with permission from Greenspan A. Orthopedic Imaging: A Practical Approach, 4th ed. Philadelphia, Lippincott Williams & Wilkins 2004.)

and convex in a medial–lateral direction. This surface bears approximately 90% of the load through the ankle [14,28].

The lateral aspect of the distal tibia provides the articular surface for the distal fibula. The posterior surface of the distal tibia continues from the articular surface for the fibula to the medial malleolus and is marked by a groove for the tendon of the posterior tibialis, which also marks the medial malleolus. The posterior margin of the distal tibia is sometimes referred to as the **third malleolus** because it projects distally beyond the superior surface of the talus and contributes to the stability of the ankle joint [145,174].

Clinical Relevance

TRI-MALLEOLAR FRACTURE: *A tri-malleolar fracture consists of fractures of the medial and lateral malleoli and the posterior margin of the tibia, the third malleolus (Fig. 44.3). Fracture of the posterior portion of the tibia can include a portion of the articular surface of the distal tibia. As in any fracture, involvement of the articular surface increases the complexity of the fracture and its morbidity.*

Alignment of the Tibia

In adults, the distal portion of the tibia is laterally rotated in the transverse plane with respect to the proximal end of the tibia, creating a normal **lateral,** or **external, tibial torsion** [87,154,169] *(Fig. 44.4)*. Lateral torsion of the tibia moves the medial malleolus anteriorly and consequently influences the position of the foot with respect to the leg, affecting posture and gait. Tibial torsion is measured in a variety of ways, including by the angle between a line through the tibial plateaus and

a line through the medial and lateral malleoli [30,87,169]. Like femoral torsion, tibial torsion changes throughout development, beginning in slight lateral torsion or even medial torsion at birth and gradually progressing to 20–40° of lateral torsion by adulthood [112,152,154,156,169,197].

Clinical Relevance

TORSIONAL DEFORMITIES OF THE TIBIA: *Medial torsion of the tibia is the second most common cause of an in-toeing posture, following only excessive femoral anteversion [34]. (Torsional deformities of the femur are discussed in*

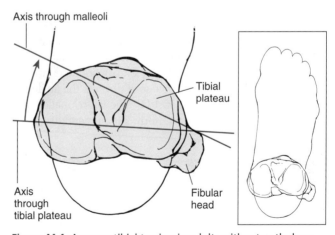

Figure 44.4: Average tibial torsion in adults without pathology, indicated by an angle between a line through the tibial plateaus and the medial and lateral malleoli, ranges from 20 to 40° of lateral torsion.

Chapter 38.) Excessive lateral or external tibial torsion defor-mities are associated with increased Q angles and recurrent patellar dislocations [15,30]. Skeletal malalignments in the lower extremity can contribute to abnormal loading patterns anywhere in the lower extremity, and clinicians should con-sider tibial torsion when assessing skeletal alignment of the lower extremity.

Fibula

The fibula is a long, thin bone extending from just distal to the knee to the ankle joint and contains a head, shaft, and lateral malleolus (*Fig. 44.2*). The fibula provides muscle attachment in the leg and also participates in the ankle articulation allow-ing complex movements of the foot.

HEAD OF THE FIBULA

The head of the fibula is slightly enlarged, with a medial artic-ular facet for the tibia. The apex of the fibular head projects proximally and, with the head, is readily palpable distal to the knee joint. The head of the fibula provides attachment for the biceps femoris tendon of the hamstrings and the lateral col-lateral ligament of the knee and thus plays a role at the knee. The peroneal nerve lies close to the posterior aspect of the fibular head and can be compressed against the fibula by restrictive structures such as a tight cast.

SHAFT OF THE FIBULA

The shaft of the fibula comprises three surfaces, an anterior one that gives rise to the extensor muscles of the foot, a lateral surface providing attachment for the peroneal muscles, and the largest surface, the posterior surface, where the flexor muscles gain attachments. The shaft is palpable distally only for a few centimeters as it blends with the lateral malleolus.

LATERAL MALLEOLUS

The fibula ends in an expansion projecting distally and poste-riorly. Its medial surface provides an articular surface for the talus and is convex from superior to inferior. The plane of the articular surface of the lateral malleolus is oriented laterally and inferiorly so that some of the load through the ankle can be shared by the fibula [74,155,172]. The lateral malleolus is easily palpated anteriorly, posteriorly, laterally, and distally.

Clinical Relevance

FRACTURES OF THE DISTAL TIBIA AND FIBULA: *The distal tibia and fibula are second only to the distal radius in their frequency of fractures. Collectively known as **Pott's fractures,** they frequently result from a sprained ankle pro-ducing an **avulsion fracture** in which the stretched liga-*

ment or tendon applies a tensile force on the bone causing it to fail. Fractures of the distal tibia and fibula also result from shear forces that slide the talus along on the surface of the tibia or fibula.

Tarsal Bones

The foot is joined to the leg by a complex organization of bones that allow considerable mobility while still ensuring adequate stability for weight bearing and ambulation. The tarsal bones show considerably more variation among them-selves than do the carpal bones of the hand.

TALUS

The talus joins the foot to the leg, which helps account for its irregular shape. It is an unusual bone lacking any direct mus-cle attachments [150,191]. Articular cartilage covers more than half its surface with articular facets on its superior, infe-rior, medial, lateral, and anterior surfaces. Consequently, movement of the talus is governed by the forces applied to it by proximal bony attachments, the tibia and fibula, and its dis-tal articulation with the calcaneus.

The talus consists of a large, proximal body and a distal head, with a neck joining the two parts (*Fig. 44.5*). The body of the talus articulates with the tibia superiorly and medially,

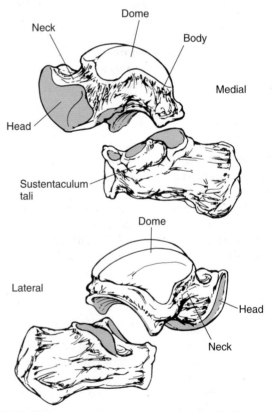

Figure 44.5: The talus and calcaneus compose the hindfoot and possess reciprocal facets for their articulation to each other.

with the fibula laterally, and with the calcaneus inferiorly. The superior, or dorsal, surface of the body, also known as the **talar dome,** or **trochlea,** is trochlear in shape, convex in an anterior–posterior direction, and concave in a medial–lateral direction to fit congruently with the distal surface of the tibia. The anterior aspect of this superior surface is slightly wider than the posterior aspect [142,171,191]. In addition, the lateral ridge, or condyle, of the trochlea is slightly larger than the medial ridge, or condyle [73,171]. This asymmetry in the medial and lateral aspects of the articular surface helps to explain the motion of the ankle, which occurs in an oblique plane close to the sagittal plane.

The medial and lateral surfaces of the talar body are continuous with the superior surface and provide articular surfaces for the medial and lateral malleoli, respectively. These surfaces roughly parallel the articular surfaces of the respective facets on the malleoli [171]. The inferior, or plantar, surface of the body of the talus has a large posterior facet for articulation with the posterior facet on the superior surface of the calcaneus. The body of the talus is grooved posteriorly and medially by the tendon of the flexor hallucis longus.

The head of the talus is a smoothly curved, convex surface projecting distally for articulation with the navicular. The head is almost entirely covered with articular cartilage. Three facets mark the articular surface on the plantar aspect of the talar head. The posterior and largest of the three provides articulation with the sustentaculum tali of the calcaneus. Another facet lying anterior and lateral to the posterior facet also articulates with the calcaneus. The third facet, positioned medially, rests on the calcaneonavicular ligament.

The neck of the talus joins the head to the body of the talus. Both the neck and head project inferiorly and medially from the body of the talus, contributing to the contour of the medial longitudinal arch of the foot. The neck is roughened on its dorsal and plantar surfaces by ligamentous attachments. The sulcus tali is a prominent groove on the medial side of the plantar surface that, together with the calcaneus, forms the sinus tarsi.

The head and neck of the talus are readily palpated. The medial aspect of the head can be palpated just proximal to the tubercle of the navicular, particularly with the foot pronated [77]. The clinician finds the neck of the talus medially between the tendons of the anterior and posterior tibialis tendons and laterally just medial to the sinus tarsi [178].

CALCANEUS

The calcaneus, the largest of the tarsal bones, serves important functions in the foot. As the "heel bone," it sustains large impact forces at heel contact in locomotion; it provides a long moment arm for the tendo calcaneus (Achilles tendon), thus sustaining large tensile forces; and it transmits the weight of the body from the hindfoot to the forefoot.

The calcaneus can be divided into three segments: posterior, middle, and anterior. A large posterior facet that articulates with the posterior facet on the talus covers the superior surface of the middle segment. The superior surface of the

anterior segment possesses two facets, a middle and an anterior facet, which frequently communicate with one another. The middle facet covers the superior surface of a palpable shelf, the sustentaculum tali, which projects from the medial surface of the calcaneus and supports the head of the talus. The small, anterior facet also supports the talar head. A deep groove, the sulcus calcanei, separates the posterior and middle facets on the superior surface of the calcaneus. This groove combines with the corresponding groove on the plantar surface of the talus to form the sinus tarsi.

Clinical Relevance

SINUS TARSI: *The sinus tarsi is a depression palpated readily on the lateral aspect of the dorsum of the foot. The neck of the talus and the anterior talofibular ligaments are palpated within the sinus tarsi. Tenderness within the sinus tarsi may indicate an injury to either of these structures. The sinus tarsi also contains a venous plexus that is frequently torn in a sprained ankle, producing the almost instantaneous golf ball–sized swelling that appears after an acute sprain.*

The posterior third of the calcaneus serves to lengthen the moment arm of the Achilles tendon that attaches to the posterior surface of the bone. The distal aspect of the posterior surface continues onto the plantar surface and is the only portion of the calcaneus that contacts the ground during weight bearing (*Fig. 44.6*). The plantar surface is marked by a calcaneal tuberosity where intrinsic muscles and the plantar aponeurosis attach. The lateral and medial surfaces of the posterior third of the calcaneus are palpable and assist the clinician in identifying the alignment of the foot. The anterior surface of the calcaneus contains a slightly curved, saddle-shaped facet for articulation with the cuboid.

The calcaneus possesses a thin shell of cortical bone that encloses a sparse but highly organized array of trabecular

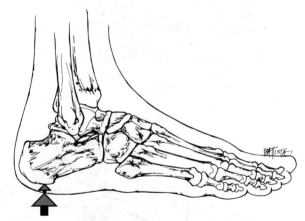

Figure 44.6: In weight bearing, the calcaneus is aligned so that only its posterior aspect contacts the ground and directly sustains ground reaction forces.

bone [55]. The relatively sparse cancellous bone within the calcaneus leaves space that is filled by blood. This high fluid content helps the calcaneus to function as a hydrodynamic shock absorber during impact [49,55].

Clinical Relevance

CALCANEAL FRACTURES: *The calcaneus is the most commonly fractured tarsal bone [55], which can produce significant impairments and functional disabilities [16,95,138,181]. Calcaneal fractures typically result from high-impact loading such as in a motor vehicle accident or from a fall onto the heels from a large height [16,196]. They frequently are intraarticular fractures and occur by large compression loads between the talus and calcaneus (Fig. 44.7). These fractures are difficult to treat and often lead to significant disability.*

NAVICULAR

The navicular is a crescent-shaped bone with a concave posterior surface that is congruent with the head of the talus (*Fig. 44.8*). Three relatively flattened facets for the three

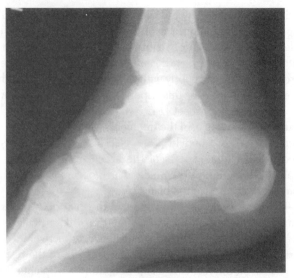

Figure 44.7: Calcaneal fracture. The lateral radiograph shows a fracture of the calcaneus in which the posterior facet is compressed into the body of the calcaneus. (Reprinted with permission from Chew FS, Maldjian C, LEffler SG. Musculoskeletal Imaging: A Teaching File. Philadelphia Lippincott Williams & Wilkins 1999)

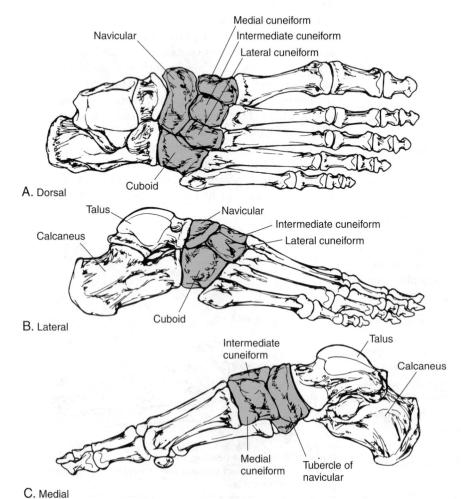

Figure 44.8: The bones of the midfoot include the navicular, cuboid, and three cuneiform bones. **A.** Dorsal view. **B.** Lateral view. **C.** Medial view.

cuneiform bones cover the navicular's convex anterior surface. The medial surface of the navicular ends in a prominent tuberosity that is a useful landmark for clinicians, lying approximately 2 or 3 cm distal to the medial malleolus and anterior to the sustentaculum tali of the calcaneus. Supination of the foot facilitates palpation of the tubercle of the navicular [77]. The lateral surface of the navicular may be nonarticular or may bear a small facet for articulation with the cuboid. The dorsal and plantar surfaces are roughened for ligamentous attachments.

CUBOID

The cuboid is named for its six-sided shape. Its posterior surface is slightly curved for the saddle-shaped facet of the calcaneus, and facets for the bases of the fourth and fifth metatarsal bones flatten its anterior surface. Medially, it bears a flattened facet for the lateral cuneiform and perhaps a small facet for the navicular. The peroneus longus forms a groove on the lateral and plantar surfaces, which meet at the tuberosity of the cuboid occasionally palpable on the plantar surface of the foot.

THREE CUNEIFORM BONES

The three cuneiform bones help form the transverse arch of the foot. The medial cuneiform, the largest of the three, is slightly kidney-shaped and wider on its plantar aspect than its dorsal surface. The middle (intermediate) and lateral cuneiform bones are wedge-shaped, with the apex facing in a plantar direction. The wedge shape of the middle and lateral cuneiforms allows these bones to function as keystones to assist in stabilizing the transverse arch of the foot. The cuneiform bones possess articular facets on their proximal and distal surfaces for articulation with the navicular bone proximally and with the medial three metatarsal bones distally. The medial and lateral cuneiform bones extend distally farther than the middle, forming a socket into which the base of the second metatarsal fits. The cuneiform bones bear facets on their medial and lateral surfaces for articulation with one another and with the cuboid. The dorsal surfaces of the cuneiform bones are palpable through the dorsal skin of the foot but bear no readily identifiable landmarks.

Bones of the Digits

The bones of the digits are very similar to the bones of the fingers, consisting of five metatarsal bones and fourteen phalanges (*Fig. 44.9*).

METATARSAL BONES

The metatarsal bones, like their counterparts in the hand, are miniature long bones consisting of a base, shaft, and head. The metatarsals are generally similar to one another, with a few distinguishing characteristics that influence the mechanics and pathomechanics of the foot and toes. The metatarsal of the great toe is shorter than the second or third metatarsals

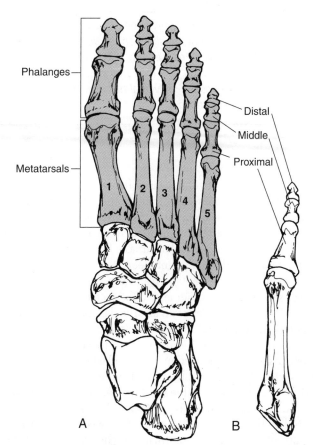

Figure 44.9: The bones of the digits are the metatarsal and phalangeal bones of the five toes. **A.** Dorsal view. **B.** Lateral view of the bones of the fifth toe.

and is the thickest of all the metatarsal bones. Applying Wolff's law, which states that a bone's structure responds to its function (Chapter 3), the robust circumference of the great toe's metatarsal suggests that the bone is specialized to sustain large loads, such as those generated in bipedal ambulation. The ground reaction force on the foot progresses through the medial side of the foot during gait, applying large forces on the great toe.

The second metatarsal is the thinnest and longest of all the metatarsal bones although it projects distally approximately the same distance as the first and third metatarsals. The metatarsal to the second toe extends farther proximally and is securely wedged in by the three cuneiform bones and by the first and third metatarsal bones. The metatarsal of the fifth toe also projects proximally and forms a palpable tuberosity that provides attachment for the peroneus brevis tendon.

Clinical Relevance

METATARSAL LENGTH: *In the normal foot, the metatarsal heads of the medial three toes lie approximately in the same frontal plane. Some individuals have an unusually short first* *metatarsal bone or, conversely, a long second metatarsal bone. This produces uneven stress on the distal ends of the metatarsals, particularly as the body rolls over the foot during walking and running. The increased stress may produce pain and disability as the individual has difficulty rolling evenly over the metatarsals.*

The bases of all five metatarsal bones are similar to each other. Unlike its counterpart in the thumb that has a saddle-shaped base, the metatarsal of the great toe has flattened facets on its base similar to the bases of the other metatarsals. These facets provide articular surfaces for the cuneiform and cuboid bones and for adjacent metatarsal bones.

The heads of the metatarsals of the lateral four toes are quite similar to each other and to the metacarpals of the fingers. They are biconvex, with an articular surface that is continuous on the plantar, distal, and dorsal surfaces. The head of the first metatarsal is larger than those of the other metatarsals and is grooved medially and laterally on the plantar surface by sesamoid bones that improve the mechanical advantage of muscles of the great toe and protect the surface of the metatarsal head. The metatarsal heads are readily palpated on the plantar surface of the foot, where they form the "ball" of the foot. In normal upright standing, all five metatarsal heads contact the floor [56].

PHALANGES

The phalanges are very similar to, albeit shorter than, the phalanges of the fingers. There are three in each of the lateral four (lesser) toes and two in the great toe. Each has a proximal base and a distal head. The bases of the proximal phalanges are biconcave to accommodate the heads of the metatarsals. The bases of the middle and distal phalanges possess a central ridge to fit the trochlear-shaped heads of the proximal and middle phalanges.

Structural Organization of the Foot

The foot can be described by functional units—typically the **hindfoot, midfoot,** and **forefoot**—although some authors include the midfoot in the forefoot. The hindfoot consists of the talus and calcaneus, and the remaining tarsal bones compose the midfoot [129]. The forefoot is composed of the metatarsals and phalanges. The digits also can be described in motion segments, known as **rays** (*Fig. 44.10*). The **first ray** includes the metatarsal of the great toe and the medial cuneiform bone [44]. The **second** and **third rays** contain the second and third metatarsals, respectively, and their proximal cuneiform bones. The **fourth** and **fifth rays** consist only of the fourth and fifth metatarsal, respectively.

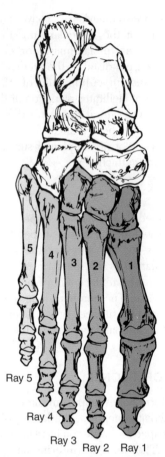

Figure 44.10: The functional units of the foot consist of the first ray, including the metatarsal of the great toe and the medial cuneiform; the second ray, composed of the second metatarsal and the middle cuneiform; the third ray, composed of the third metatarsal and the lateral cuneiform; and the fourth and fifth rays, consisting of only the fourth and fifth metatarsals, respectively.

JOINTS AND SUPPORTING STRUCTURES OF THE LEG AND FOOT

The movement of the foot with respect to the leg is the sum of motions among the tibia, the fibula, the tarsal bones, and the metatarsals. To appreciate the contributions of each joint, it is important to understand the movements of which the foot is capable. Terminology describing foot motion is both confusing and inconsistent, although consistency within the clinical and biomechanical literature is beginning to emerge. *Figure 44.11* presents the axes and motions that operationally define the motions of the foot. **Dorsiflexion** and **plantarflexion** occur in the sagittal plane about a medial–lateral axis. **Eversion** and **inversion** occur in the frontal plane about the long axis of the foot, which lies within the second metatarsal of the foot. **Abduction** and **adduction** occur in the transverse plane about a longitudinal axis through the leg, typically described as parallel to the long axis of the tibia [21,85].

Although the motions of the foot and ankle are defined operationally by motions within the cardinal planes of the body, the actual motions of the ankle and foot occur about

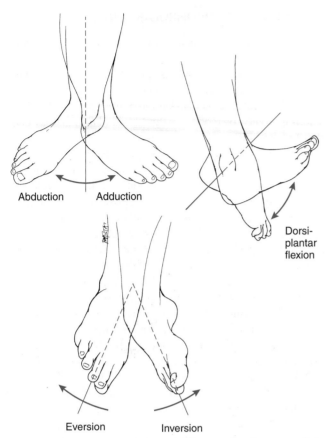

Figure 44.11: Dorsiflexion and plantarflexion occur about a medial–lateral axis; eversion and inversion occur about a long axis through the foot; and abduction and adduction occur about a long axis through the tibia.

TABLE 44.1: Terminology Convention for Triplanar Motion of the Ankle and Foot

	Pronation	Supination
Sagittal plane component	Dorsiflexion	Plantarflexion
Frontal plane component	Eversion	Inversion
Transverse plane component	Abduction	Adduction

the terminology described here is becoming the norm, some authors continue to use other conventions. *Table 44.2* provides variations in terminology that are found in the literature.

Joints and Supporting Structures between the Tibia and Fibula

The tibia and fibula are joined proximally and distally at the proximal and distal tibiofibular joints (*Fig. 44.12*).

PROXIMAL TIBIOFIBULAR JOINT

The proximal tibiofibular joint is a gliding, synovial joint supported by a synovial joint capsule and reinforced by anterior and posterior ligaments to the head of the fibula. The interosseous membrane supports both the proximal and distal tibiofibular joints. Although in close proximity to the knee joint, the joint functions primarily with the distal tibiofibular joint to accommodate the rotation of the tibia during knee motion and the triplanar motion of the foot [74,137]. Loss of the proximal tibiofibular joint through fibular head resection typically results in little residual dysfunction. Consequently, the fibular head is regarded as a good harvest site for articular cartilage to use in osteochondral autografts [33]. Osteochondral autografts are used to repair small localized defects in articular cartilage.

DISTAL TIBIOFIBULAR JOINT

The distal tibiofibular joint is a **fibrous joint,** or **syndesmosis.** The primary support of the distal tibiofibular joint is the interosseous ligament that is an extension of the interosseous membrane. It also is supported by the anterior and posterior tibiofibular ligaments as well as by the interosseous membrane. The medial collateral ligament of the ankle provides additional support to the joint. The distal tibiofibular joint provides essential stability to the ankle joint. Any instability at the distal tibiofibular joint may lead to chronic ankle dysfunction [182].

axes that lie oblique to the cardinal planes. Consequently, these joints exhibit motions that occur outside the cardinal planes but pass through all three cardinal planes. As a result, motions of the foot are described as **triplanar motions** [143,193].

Since the motions of the foot are triplanar, they can be described as the sum of individual motions in all three planes, even if those motions cannot occur independently. The most typical motions exhibited by joints of the ankle and foot combine either dorsiflexion, eversion, and abduction or plantarflexion, inversion, and adduction. These motions are known as **pronation** and **supination,** respectively [85] (*Table 44.1*). Clinicians are cautioned that inconsistency in terminology within the literature creates considerable confusion. Although

TABLE 44.2: Variation in Terminology Describing Ankle and Foot Pronation

	This Textbook	Inman [70]	Alternative Terminology found in the Literature
Sagittal plane component	Dorsiflexion	Dorsiflexion	
Frontal plane component	Eversion	Eversion or pronation (used interchangeably)	Pronation [96]
Transverse plane component	Abduction	Abduction	External rotation [90,96,194]

HIGH ANKLE SPRAINS: *Sprains of the distal tibiofibular joint are known as "high ankle sprains." They occur typically in athletes participating in running sports that require quick cuts and turns, including American football, soccer, and skiing. Unlike typical inversion ankle sprains, high ankle sprains more often occur with ankle/foot abduction, eversion, and/or dorsiflexion, that is, with pronation. High ankle sprains, although less common than inversion ankle sprains, typically require considerably more recovery time.*

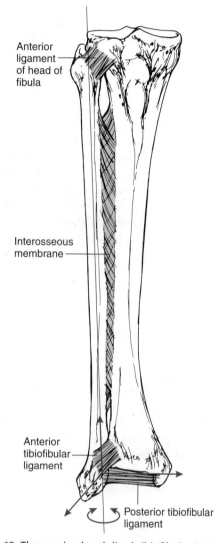

Figure 44.12: The proximal and distal tibiofibular joints are supported by anterior and posterior ligaments at both joints, by the interosseous membrane, and distally by a synovial capsule and interosseous ligament. Both joints allow translation and rotation about a long axis through the fibula. The distal tibiofibular joint allows translation superiorly and inferiorly, anteriorly and posteriorly, and medially and laterally. In addition, the fibula rotates laterally about its own long axis.

MOTION OF THE TIBIOFIBULAR JOINTS

The tibiofibular joints function together just as the radioulnar joints and temporomandibular joints do. The motion available between the tibia and fibula is quite limited, allowing slight rotation of the fibula about a longitudinal axis as well as slight proximal–distal and medial–lateral translations [74,137,155]. The importance of motion at the tibiofibular joints has been debated, leading to differing treatment approaches to the treatment of distal fibular fractures. Surgical screws that cross the distal tibiofibular joint ensure an anatomically accurate reduction of the fracture but limit the mobility of the fibrous joint.

One aspect of the controversy surrounding tibiofibular motion focuses on the width of the superior surface of the talus. As noted earlier, the anterior aspect of the superior surface is slightly wider than the posterior surface. Ankle dorsiflexion moves the anterior aspect of the talar articular surface into the cavity formed by the distal tibia and fibula. Ankle plantarflexion inserts the thinner posterior aspect into the cavity. The varying widths of the talus in contact with the distal tibia and fibula have suggested that the tibia and fibula must separate during dorsiflexion and has led to the assumption that restricted tibiofibular joint motion limits dorsiflexion ROM. Extensive anatomical analysis suggests that the mortise spreads only slightly, if at all, during ankle dorsiflexion but that the fibula does rotate laterally slightly during dorsiflexion [26,74,122]. Studies report minimal or no decrease in dorsiflexion ROM in ankles with immobile distal tibiofibular joints [11,122]. Yet some patients with no motion available at the distal tibiofibular joint report pain and functional limitations. A study using cadaver specimens demonstrates a decrease in contact area between the talus and tibia when the distal tibiofibular joint is surgically immobilized [128]. Perhaps some of the complaints reported by patients with restricted tibiofibular joint mobility arise as a result of increased joint **stress** (force/area) at the ankle joint.

MOBILIZATION OF THE DISTAL TIBIOFIBULAR JOINT: *The mobility of the tibiofibular joint can become restricted during immobilization of the ankle, even with no direct ankle pathology. Gentle remobilization of the distal tibiofibular joint is a frequently applied intervention to relieve pain and improve function. Individuals whose activities demand large ankle and foot mobility may require increased tibiofibular joint mobility. But even in individuals who are moderately sedentary, increased mobility of the distal tibiofibular joint may increase functional ability by restoring the normal contact area between the tibia and talus, thereby decreasing joint stress and increasing comfort during weight-bearing activities. Well-controlled outcome studies are needed to verify the clinical value of such intervention.*

Joints of the Foot

The movement of the foot on the leg reflects motion at the ankle, intertarsal joints, and tarsometatarsal joints and is affected by the motion of the toes. Weight-bearing activities require motion of the foot on the leg or the leg on the foot and thus involve virtually all of the joints of the foot. An understanding of the motion of the foot requires an understanding of each joint individually but also the interaction that occurs among the joints of the foot.

STRUCTURE AND SUPPORTING ELEMENTS OF THE ANKLE JOINT

The ankle joint consists of articulations between the talus and the tibia and fibula, which, bound together at the distal tibiofibular joint, form a cavity, or **mortise,** for the talus. The primary articular surface is on the superior surface of the talus and on the distal surface of the tibia. The anterior joint line is palpated 1 or 2 cm proximal and anterior to the tip of the medial malleolus [57].

The participating articular surfaces of the ankle possess very similar, although not identical, curvatures [91,171]. This congruity helps stabilize the ankle, contributes to a relatively simple, hingelike motion, and increases the contact area of the joint to decrease the joint stress [173]. Data from cadaver experiments suggest that the articular surfaces themselves contribute the primary stabilizing force for inversion and eversion when the ankle is weight bearing [173,179].

Despite the congruent joint surfaces of the ankle, the contact area on the talus changes and moves with joint loads and joint position [14,29,74]. With the ankle in the neutral position, loading occurs on the superior aspect of the talus. The area of contact increases from approximately 10% to approximately 15% with loads of 490 N (110 lb) and 980 N (220 lb), respectively, as the articular cartilage deforms more with larger loads [14]. The area of contact moves anteriorly in dorsiflexion and posteriorly in plantarflexion. Similarly, inversion moves contact to the medial aspect of the talus and to the tibial facet, while eversion moves the contact to the lateral aspect of the talus and to the fibula [14,29]. The articular cartilage of the ankle is thinner and stiffer than the cartilage found at the knee and hip [158,159]. The ankle's inherent congruency may diminish the need for thick articular cartilage, and the cartilage's stiffness may help protect the ankle from degenerative joint disease.

Clinical Relevance

OSTEOARTHRITIS OF THE ANKLE: *Despite its role in weight bearing, the ankle joint rarely develops osteoarthritis spontaneously [65,195]. On the other hand, once there is trauma that alters the joint alignment, joint degenerative changes almost always follow [145,195]. Changes in the relative alignment of the talus, tibia, and fibula produce large changes in the contact areas and stresses between the articular surfaces during weight bearing, probably contributing to the development of degenerative changes.*

A synovial capsule and collateral ligaments provide noncontractile support to the ankle joint. The joint capsule is characterized by numerous pleats anteriorly and posteriorly that fold and unfold to allow the relatively free motion of dorsiflexion and plantarflexion [57,142] (*Fig. 44.13*). The medial and lateral collateral ligaments reinforce the capsule. Both the medial and lateral collateral ligaments consist of three major bands, with additional smaller and more variable components as well [113,114] (*Table 44.3*).

The medial collateral, also known as the deltoid, ligament is larger than the lateral ligament and contains deep and

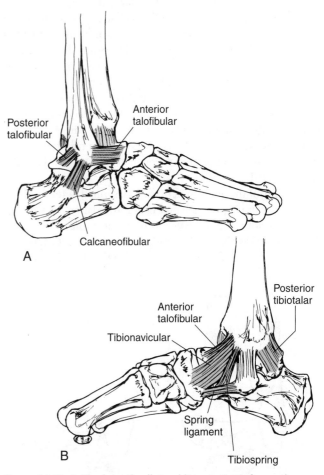

Figure 44.13: A. The lateral collateral ligament reinforces the capsule laterally and consists of the anterior talofibular, calcaneofibular, and posterior talofibular ligaments. **B.** The deltoid ligament consisting of the superficial tibiospring and tibionavicular ligaments and the deep posterior tibiotalar ligament reinforces the ankle joint capsule medially. Both collateral ligaments may contain additional fibers not shown here.

TABLE 44.3: Components of the Collateral Ligaments of the Ankle [113,114]

	Medial Collateral (Deltoid) Ligament	Lateral Collateral Ligament
Primary ligamentous bands	Tibiospring (superficial) Tibionavicular (superficial) Posterior tibiotalar (deep)	Anterior talofibular Calcaneofibular Posterior talofibular
Additional variable fibrous bands	Posterior tibiotalar (superficial) Tibiocalcaneal (superficial) Anterior tibiotalar (deep)	Lateral talocalcaneal Posterior intermalleolar

superficial portions. Of the primary bands of the medial collateral ligament, the deep (posterior tibiotalar) segment runs from tibia to talus, providing direct support to the tibiotalar joint, while the superficial fibers (tibiospring and tibionavicular) extend from the tibia to the navicular and calcaneus, affecting the subtalar articulation as well as the ankle. The lateral collateral ligament also consists of major bands that support the ankle joint directly (the anterior and posterior talofibular ligaments) and a band that crosses both the ankle and subtalar joints (the calcaneofibular ligament).

The collateral ligaments, along with the articular surfaces, help stabilize the ankle and subtalar joints and guide the motion of the ankle [90]. Like other collateral ligaments at the knee and elbow, the precise role that each ligament plays is complex, and controversies remain. However, the ligaments appear to function primarily to limit extremes of movement [73,179]. The deltoid ligament helps support the medial side of the ankle and subtalar joint against laterally directed forces on the foot **(valgus stresses),** while the lateral collateral ligament protects these joints from medially directed forces **(varus stresses)** on the foot. The specific contributions made by each ligamentous segment depends on the position of the ankle [18,101,139,172].

Stability of the ankle joint often is described in terms of the anterior, posterior, medial, and lateral translation, or **shift,** of the talus within the mortise and by the amount of medial or lateral **talar tilt** about an anterior–posterior axis, which occurs when force is applied (*Fig. 44.14*). The deltoid ligament is

positioned to limit lateral tilt and lateral shift of the talus. Some studies report that lateral talar tilt increases significantly when the entire deltoid ligament is cut [52,172,173], while others report a small or inconsistent increase [29]. The lateral malleolus and lateral supporting structures also appear to provide important limits to lateral talar shift by acting as a buttress against the movement [26,52]. The lateral collateral ligament, especially the anterior talofibular and calcaneofibular ligaments, prevent excessive medial tilt of the talus [6,8,38].

Anterior glide of the talus is limited by the lateral malleolus and lateral collateral ligaments and by the deltoid ligament, although the lateral supporting structures appear to be primary [22,80]. Posterior glide of the lateral malleolus is limited primarily by the posterior talofibular and calcaneofibular ligaments [53]. Plantar- and dorsiflexion alter the tension within the individual components of the collateral ligaments. Anterior glide of the talus is greatest with the ankle close to neutral and is more restricted when the ankle is either dorsiflexed or plantarflexed [22,23]. Plantarflexion stretches the anterior talofibular component of the lateral collateral ligament and the anterior tibiotalar and tibionavicular portions of the deltoid ligament; dorsiflexion relaxes these same ligaments [5,18,101,125,139,168]. Most investigators report that dorsiflexion stretches the calcaneofibular ligament while plantarflexion puts it on slack [5,18,125,139,172]. Others, however, suggest that the ligament maintains an almost constant length through the range of plantar- and dorsiflexion and thus provides lateral stability to the ankle regardless of position, helping to guide the ankle motion through the entire ROM [90,101,168]. Clinicians assessing the stability of the ankle and the integrity of surrounding ligaments are advised to maintain a consistent ankle position when performing any mobility tests to ensure reliable test results.

ANKLE JOINT MOTION

The ankle joint basically functions as a hinge joint rotating about an axis that lies close to the malleoli [73,163]. However, several biomechanical studies determine that the precise axis of rotation varies throughout the ankle's ROM [14,100, 147,161]. These studies demonstrate that slight translation accompanies the ankle's rotation. The tibia translates anteriorly during dorsiflexion and posteriorly during plantarflexion. Such translation helps to explain the change in contact area between the tibia and talus that occurs during plantar- and dorsiflexion [14]. Two-dimensional analysis reveals that translation of the tibia produces a change in the **instant center of rotation (ICR)** of the ankle joint so that the ICR moves

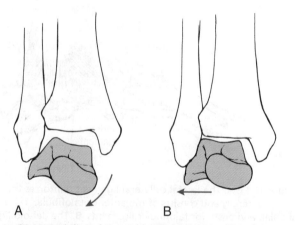

Figure 44.14: Stability of the ankle joint is assessed by examining **(A)** the talar tilt, which is medial or lateral rotation of the talus about an anterior-posterior axis, and **(B)** talar shift, which is the translation of the talus in a medial or lateral direction.

posteriorly with plantarflexion, anteriorly with dorsiflexion, medially with inversion, and laterally with eversion. (Chapter 7 discusses ICR in more detail.)

Clinical Relevance

MANUAL THERAPY OF THE ANKLE JOINT: *Gentle mobilization consisting of anterior and posterior glides of the talus using manually applied pressure form a common intervention for treatment of a stiff ankle. This treatment is consistent with the goal of restoring the normally occurring translation during ankle dorsiflexion and plantarflexion. A randomized clinical trial of anterior–posterior joint mobilizations of the ankle demonstrates better outcomes with mobilization intervention than with treatment without mobilization [47].*

Ankle dorsiflexion and plantarflexion also are accompanied by talar rotation and fibular glide and rotation [63,90,97, 110,172]. Studies suggest that the talus and fibula both rotate laterally with respect to the tibia as the ankle dorsiflexes. This movement is consistent with the shape of the talus. The lateral condyle of the talus is slightly larger than the medial condyle, producing lateral rotation of the talus during its posterior rotation during dorsiflexion. These data demonstrate that although the ankle joint is considered a classic hinge joint, its motion is considerably more complex. In addition, the talus reportedly rocks medially and laterally within the mortise, contributing one third of the supination and pronation of the hindfoot [62,175].

The preceding description of ankle motion reveals the ankle exhibits three-dimensional motion and six degrees of freedom, with rotations about and translations along medial-lateral, anterior-posterior, and longitudinal axes [162,192]. This complexity of joint motion may contribute to the limited success that engineers and surgeons have had in developing successful total joint arthroplasties of the ankle.

Despite the translations and rotations of the talus and the variability of the axes reported during ankle motion, for clinical measurements of ankle ROM, the use of an axis that passes through the two malleoli appears to be a valid simplification to measure motion. This single axis of the ankle is oblique, passing from medial to lateral in a posterior and inferior direction [73] (*Fig. 44.15*). The obliquity of the ankle joint axis produces ankle motion that takes place in a plane perpendicular to the joint axis rather than in any of the cardinal planes of the body [73,78,193]. When the foot rotates in an upward direction about this axis, the obliquity causes the foot to move slightly laterally with respect to the leg and to rotate the plantar surface of the foot laterally. Using the terminology described earlier for leg–foot motions, the ankle dorsiflexes, abducts, and everts; in other words, the foot pronates. It is useful to note that the foot could achieve this same position by

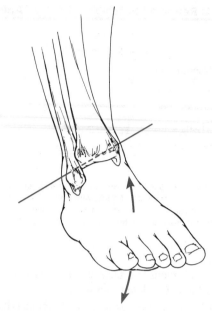

Figure 44.15: To measure the ROM of the ankle, a simplified axis is assumed that runs laterally, inferiorly and posteriorly from the medial to the lateral malleolus.

using a ball-and-socket joint that allows rotation about three separate axes. However, a ball-and-socket joint requires a more complex musculoligamentous system for support and control. Although ankle motion combines dorsiflexion, abduction, and eversion or plantarflexion, adduction, and inversion, the ankle's motion occurs very close to the sagittal plane, and consequently, the ankle's motion consists mostly of dorsiflexion and plantarflexion [161,192].

Range of Motion of the Ankle

Passive and active ROMs reported in the literature are found in *Table 44.4*. These values show considerable variability, attributable at least in part to the magnitude of the force pushing the joint to end range [117]. The largest dorsiflexion range is reported in a study in which the subjects stood and used full body weight to reach end range [141]. Other studies use only manual pressure to achieve the end range. Data suggest that women exhibit greater ankle ROM than men [3,124,184]. Reports disagree regarding the effects of age on ankle ROM in adults, but comparing data across studies suggests that ROM decreases with increased age in adults [10,124,147,184]. Children exhibit more ankle ROM than adults [10,50,124].

STRUCTURE AND SUPPORTING ELEMENTS OF THE SUBTALAR JOINT

The subtalar joint is defined functionally as the joint formed by all three articulating facets of the calcaneus and the matching facets on the talus [129,150,183], although anatomy textbooks often refer only to the articulation between the posterior

TABLE 44.4: Reported Passive and Active Ankle ROM

	Dorsiflexion with Knee Flexed (°)	Plantarflexion (°)
American Academy of Orthopaedic Surgeons [48][a]	20	50
Gerhardt and Rippstein [41][b]	20	45
Roass and Andersson [141][c]	15 ± 5.8	40 ± 7.5
Astrom and Arvidson [3][d]	43 ± 7	49 ± 7
Walker et al. [184][e]	10 ± 5	34 ± 8
Boone and Azen [10][f]	12.2 ± 4.1	54.3 ± 5.9

[a] Passive ROM.
[b] Active ROM.
[c] Mean and standard deviation of passive ROM in 190 ankle joints in men aged 30 to 40 years.
[d] Mean and standard deviation of 121 adults with a mean age of 35 years. Measured with the subjects in weight bearing.
[e] Mean and standard deviation of active ROM in 30 men and 30 women aged 75 to 84 years.
[f] Mean and standard deviation of active ROM in 56 males aged 20 to 54 years.

facets of the calcaneus and talus as the subtalar joint, including the anterior and middle facets in the talocalcaneonavicular joint [142,191]. This textbook uses the functional definition of the subtalar joint including all articulations between the calcaneus and talus.

The subtalar joint is critical to bipedal ambulation and acts to translate the motion of the tibia to the foot or, conversely, to translate the rotation of the foot to the tibia. This translation allows humans to walk smoothly over uneven surfaces and to pivot on one foot, rapidly changing the direction of progression (*Fig. 44.16*). To accomplish this role, the subtalar joint must allow apparently complex motion while remaining stable during weight bearing.

The larger posterior articulation between the talus and calcaneus is saddle-shaped, allowing slight three-dimensional motion, while the anterior facets are flatter, allowing gliding motion. The bony configuration of the joint provides inherent stability to the joint that is amplified by strong reinforcing ligamentous structures. Two joint capsules provide initial support to the subtalar joint, one surrounding the large posterior facet, and another surrounding the anterior and middle facets (*Fig. 44.17*). This latter capsule also surrounds the articulation between the talus and navicular. Two thickenings reinforce the posterior capsule, the medial and lateral talocalcaneal ligaments [183]. The two capsules of the subtalar joint are adjacent to one another in the sinus tarsi. These adjacent capsular surfaces blend together and are reinforced, forming the thick interosseous ligament (*Fig. 44.18*). A cervical ligament attaches to the calcaneus and talus at the lateral border of the sinus tarsi. The interosseous ligament is an important support

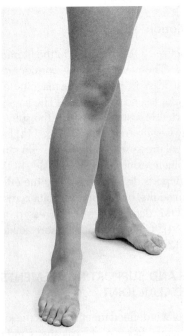

Figure 44.16: Motion of the subtalar joint allows an individual to pivot or accommodate to uneven ground.

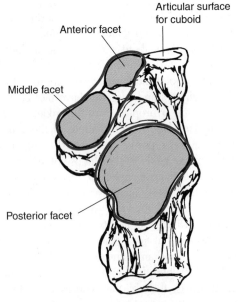

Figure 44.17: The subtalar joint contains two joint capsules, one surrounding the posterior facets of the talus and calcaneus and the other surrounding the anterior and middle facets of the talus and calcaneus as well as the proximal articulating surface of the navicular.

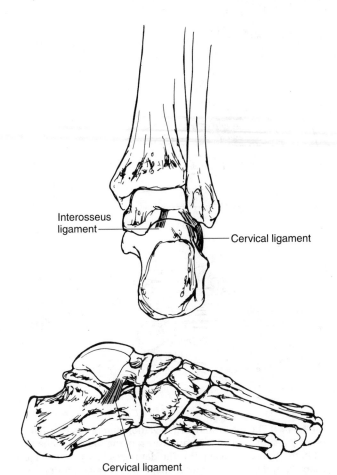

Figure 44.18: The interosseous ligament of the subtalar joint is formed by a thickening of the adjacent walls of the subtalar joint capsules and lies deep in the sinus tarsi. More superficially in the sinus tarsi lies the cervical ligament of the subtalar joint.

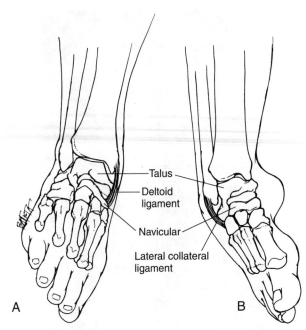

Figure 44.19: **A.** Eversion of the ankle and hindfoot is limited by the deltoid ligament. **B.** Inversion is resisted by the lateral collateral ligament and cervical ligament. The interosseous ligament resists both eversion and inversion.

of the subtalar joint, and its effectiveness is unaltered by ankle or subtalar joint position [101,170]. It appears to restrict supination more than pronation [89]. The cervical ligament also provides important support, preventing excessive supination [170].

The collateral ligaments of the ankle also contribute important support to the subtalar joint, preventing excessive motion. Cadaver measurements reveal stretch of the posterior tibiotalar, tibiocalcaneal, and tibionavicular components of the deltoid ligament with eversion of the foot [101] (*Fig. 44.19*). The lateral collateral ligament limits inversion of the ankle and subtalar joints [18,139,170]. The calcaneofibular component of the lateral collateral ligament provides strong limits to inversion throughout plantar- and dorsiflexion of the ankle, while the anterior talofibular ligament limits inversion most effectively when the ankle is plantarflexed [58,106]. Tests of the strength of the lateral collateral ligament reveal that the anterior talofibular component exhibits the smallest load to failure, with estimates of average peak loads to failure ranging

from 140 to 297 N (31.5–67 lb) [4,39]. Estimates of loads in the calcaneofibular ligament range from 205 to 598 N (46–134 lb).

Clinical Relevance

INVERSION ANKLE SPRAINS: *Most ankle sprains occur with the foot in inversion, straining the lateral structures of the foot and ankle. The most common ligament injured in an inversion sprain is the anterior talofibular ligament, stretched in combined ankle plantarflexion and subtalar supination. Common mechanisms for such an injury are landing on someone else's foot when jumping for a basketball or volleyball or tripping while descending stairs (Fig. 44.20). In each instance, the foot typically is forced rapidly and forcefully into plantarflexion and inversion, rupturing the weakest of all the ankle and subtalar joint ligaments, the anterior talofibular ligament.*

Motion of the Subtalar Joint Complex

Although the motion of the subtalar joint has been studied for well over half a century, there continues to be debate about the nature of its motion. Many authors describe it as a hinge joint whose axis lies oblique to both the foot and the leg [148,149,175]. Yet some biomechanical studies suggest that motion at the subtalar joint occurs about multiple axes [92,161,162,192].

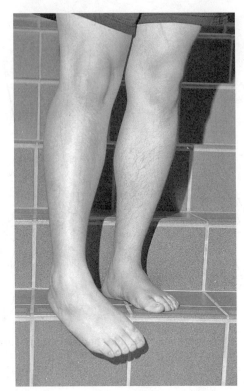

Figure 44.20: Vigorous plantarflexion and inversion that occurs by landing in a hole or tripping on a step is a classic mechanism to produce an inversion sprain.

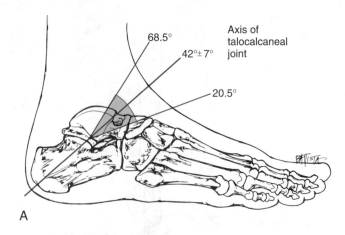
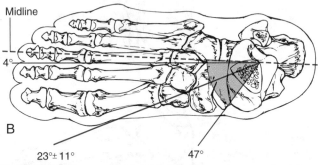

Figure 44.21: The mean standard deviation and range of orientation of the subtalar joint axis are shown in the sagittal plane (A) and in the transverse plane (B). The data reveal large intersubject variability in the axis orientation. (Reprinted with permission from Stiehl JB, ed. Inman's Joints of the Ankle. 2nd ed. Baltimore: Williams & Wilkins, 1991.)

Clinical Relevance

SUBTALAR JOINT–A HINGE OR MULTIAXIAL JOINT?:

Clinicians may ponder the importance of determining the precise number of axes about which the subtalar joint rotates. The fact that engineers appear to be the avid investigators of the question may suggest that the question is esoteric and clinically irrelevant. Yet many patients with rheumatoid arthritis have significant erosive damage to the subtalar joint, making weight-bearing activities painful and difficult. One treatment to improve function and decrease pain is fusion of the subtalar joint, but a better understanding of the true biomechanical nature of the subtalar joint may lead engineers and clinicians to develop joint arthroplasties that preserve the function of the foot while eliminating the pain of a diseased subtalar joint.

Despite the controversy regarding the precise axes of motion at the subtalar joint, there is remarkable agreement about the location and direction of the primary axis of the subtalar joint. This axis lies within, and approximately parallel to, the body of the calcaneus, projecting almost 45° from posterior to anterior and almost 25° medial to the long axis of the foot [92,149] (*Fig. 44.21*). Investigators also agree that there is considerable variability in these numbers among individuals without pathology.

Regardless of whether the subtalar joint rotates about one or multiple axes, it, like the ankle, rotates about axes that differ from the orthogonal axes of the foot. Thus the subtalar joint motion passes through the cardinal planes of the body and is triplanar. Hinge motion of the subtalar joint is classically compared to a **mitered hinge** (*Fig. 44.22*). The motion of the subtalar joint consists of pronation and supination, with unique contributions from the three components of each motion. The specific orientation of the axes of the subtalar joint defines the actual contributions of each motion. When the primary axis lies closer to the long axis of the foot, inversion and eversion constitute the primary components of subtalar motion, but when the axis is closer to the long axis of the leg, the adduction and abduction contributions increase [121] (*Fig. 44.23*). Studies show that the subtalar joint contributes most of the inversion–eversion and adduction–abduction motion of the hindfoot, while contributing minimally to plantarflexion and dorsiflexion [92,97–99,107,162].

Range of Motion of the Subtalar Joint

Table 44.5 presents the reported ROMs found in the literature. ROMs for the subtalar joint typically are reported in terms of the frontal plane components of supination and

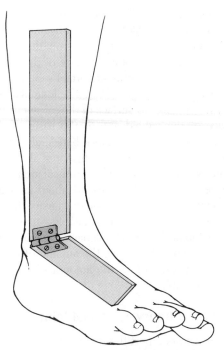

Figure 44.22: The mitered-hinge model helps demonstrate the role of the subtalar joint in transferring motion of the foot to the leg or the motion of the leg to the foot.

TABLE 44.5: Reported Ranges of Motion of the Subtalar Joint (in degrees)

	Inversion	Eversion
Gerhardt and Rippstein [41]	20	10
McPoil and Cornwall [108][a]	18.7 ± 5.2	12.2 ± 4.0
Walker et al. [184][b]	30 ± 10	12 ± 6
Milgrom et al [111][c]	32 ± 7.4	3.9 ± 4.1
	21.4 ± 5.4	3.4 ± 3.1
Roass and Andersson [141][d]		
	27.6 ± 4.6	27.7 ± 6.9

[a] Mean and standard deviation of ROM in 9 men and 18 women; mean age, 26.1 ± 4.8 years.
[b] Mean and standard deviation of active ROM in 30 men and 30 women aged 75 to 84 years.
[c] Mean and standard deviation of passive ROM in 272 males aged 18 to 20 years.
[d] Mean and standard deviation of passive ROM in 190 right subtalar joints in men aged 30 to 40 years.

strongly upon the ankle position maintained during the measurement [111]. Clinicians are cautioned that ROM measures of subtalar motion may have limited clinical use unless acceptable reliability is established.

TRANSVERSE TARSAL JOINT

The transverse tarsal joint consists of the talonavicular and calcaneocuboid joints. It is also known in some clinical literature as **Chopart's joint.**

Talonavicular Joint

The talonavicular joint consists of the well-curved talar head articulating with the reciprocally concave posterior surface of the navicular. The capsule that encloses the anterior articulation between the talus and calcaneus also supports the talonavicular articulation. Additional supports include the talonavicular ligament that crosses the dorsal surface of the joint, the dorsal calcaneonavicular ligament (the medial branch of the bifurcate ligament), and, most importantly, the plantar calcaneonavicular, or spring, ligament (*Fig. 44.25*). The spring

pronation—namely, inversion and eversion—which are determined by the angle formed by a line drawn along the long axis of the leg and a line through the posterior aspect of the calcaneus [48,126] (*Fig. 44.24*). The reported values of subtalar ROMs exhibit considerable variability, and studies report poor intertester reliability [12,131,164,180]. One study demonstrates that the inversion ROM measurement depends

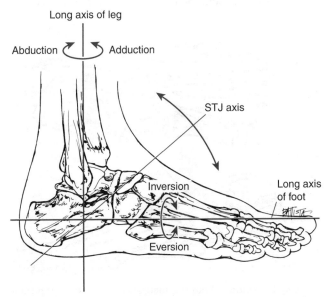

Figure 44.23: When the axis of the subtalar joint lies closer to the long axis of the foot, motion at the subtalar joint (*STJ*) consists mostly of inversion and eversion. When the axis lies closer to the long axis of the leg, the abduction–adduction component increases.

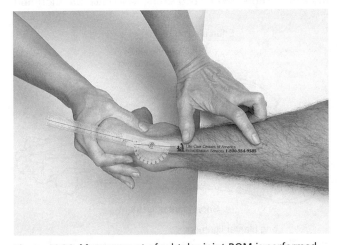

Figure 44.24: Measurement of subtalar joint ROM is performed by measuring the frontal plane component of pronation and supination (eversion and inversion).

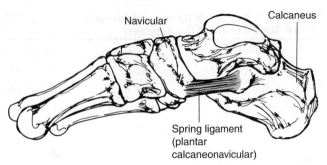

Figure 44.25: The primary supporting structure of the talonavicular joint is the spring ligament.

ligament contains a fibrocartilaginous facet for the head of the talus and acts as a sling for the talar head [25].

The substantial curvature of the talus and navicular allows considerable mobility at the talonavicular joint. Like most of the joints of the foot, motion at this joint is triplanar, consisting of pronation and supination. Fewer studies exist examining the specific motion of the talonavicular joint, but available data reveal that it is quite mobile and contributes significantly to leg–foot motion. Studies suggest that it contributes significantly to plantarflexion of the foot on the leg [85,97,127]. Lundberg et al. report that approximately 12% of the first 30° degrees of plantarflexion is attributable to talonavicular joint motion [97]. The talonavicular joint also exhibits substantial abduction or adduction and eversion or inversion during pronation and supination [85,98,107,127]. The mobility of the talonavicular joint is similar to that of the subtalar joint [97].

Calcaneocuboid Joint

The calcaneocuboid joint is a saddle joint supported by a synovial joint capsule and by several reinforcing ligaments (*Fig. 44.26*). Dorsally, the joint receives support from the bifurcate ligament composed of the dorsal calcaneonavicular and dorsal calcaneocuboid ligaments. On its plantar surface, the joint is supported by two strong ligaments, the short and

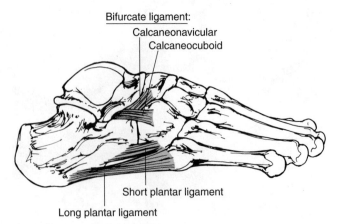

Figure 44.26: The supporting structures of the calcaneocuboid joint consist of the bifurcate ligament and the long and short plantar ligaments.

long plantar ligaments. The short plantar ligament (also known as the plantar calcaneocuboid ligament) lies deep to the long plantar ligament and travels from the anterior aspect of the calcaneus to the plantar surface of the cuboid. It is a very strong ligament that is an important support to the lateral longitudinal arch of the foot [191]. The long plantar ligament extends from the plantar surface of the calcaneus to the plantar surface of the cuboid and to the bases of the second through fourth or fifth metatarsal bones, although its distal attachment is variable [186]. This ligament also provides substantial support for the lateral longitudinal arch.

Discrete motion of the calcaneocuboid joint is less well studied than the other joints of the tarsus. Data from 10 cadaver specimens reveal significantly less motion at the calcaneocuboid joint than at the talonavicular joint, with the latter exhibiting more than twice the amount of pronation and supination and three times the amount of dorsiflexion and plantarflexion [127].

Motion of the Transverse Tarsal Joint

Some investigators report the motion of the transverse tarsal joint as a whole [46,105,143]. Biomechanical analyses suggest that the navicular and cuboid move as a unit [107]. When considered as a whole, two axes of motion are described, a longitudinal axis that is similar to the primary axis of the subtalar joint and an oblique axis that is more similar to the axis of the ankle [46,105] (*Fig. 44.27*). Regardless of whether one considers the transverse tarsal joint as two separate joints or as a single unit, data consistently demonstrate that the midfoot contributes to pronation and supination of the foot. By considering the axes of the transverse tarsal joint as a whole, the clinician is reminded that the joints of the midfoot amplify the motion of the ankle and hindfoot. Motion about the longitudinal axis of the transverse

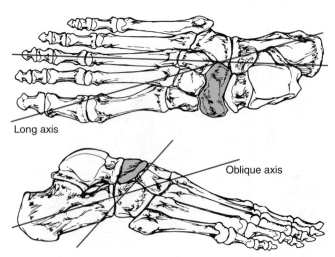

Figure 44.27: Motion about the theoretical long axis of the transverse tarsal joint contributes more eversion and inversion of the foot, while motion about the theoretical oblique axis of the transverse tarsal joint contributes mostly dorsiflexion and plantarflexion of the foot.

tarsal joint contributes to the inversion and eversion motion of the subtalar joint. Motion about the oblique axis adds to the plantarflexion and dorsiflexion provided by the ankle joint.

Clinical Relevance

TRANSVERSE TARSAL JOINT MOTION: *Together the talonavicular and calcaneocuboid joints are quite mobile and amplify the motion of the ankle and subtalar joints. Dorsiflexion is a component of pronation and consequently, pronation of the transverse tarsal joint can provide additional "functional" dorsiflexion ROM in an individual with a flexible midfoot (Fig. 44.28). However, the use of large midfoot motion during activities that require dorsiflexion ROM such as squatting, jumping, walking, or running may lead to excessive stress to structures on the medial side of the foot such as the posterior tibialis tendon, or to abnormal loads to the knee.*

DISTAL INTERTARSAL JOINTS

The distal intertarsal joints include those between the navicular and the cuneiform bones, between the cuboid and lateral cuneiform, and among the cuneiform bones themselves. These articulations are supported by joint capsules that frequently communicate with one another and by dorsal and plantar ligaments that run between adjacent bones. Although poorly studied, the motion appears to be limited to only a few degrees but contributes to the pronation and supination of the rest of the foot [96,127].

Clinical Relevance

TARSAL COALITION: *Tarsal coalition* is an abnormal connection between tarsal bones, leading to decreased mobility between the affected bones. The connections may be bony, cartilaginous, or fibrous and may be partial or complete. Because the joints among the tarsal bones provide important amplification of the motion at the ankle and subtalar joints, any loss of tarsal motion may lead to excessive motion elsewhere, including the ankle and hindfoot. A retrospective analysis of 223 acute ankle sprains suggests that tarsal coalitions may be a risk factor for ankle sprains [166].

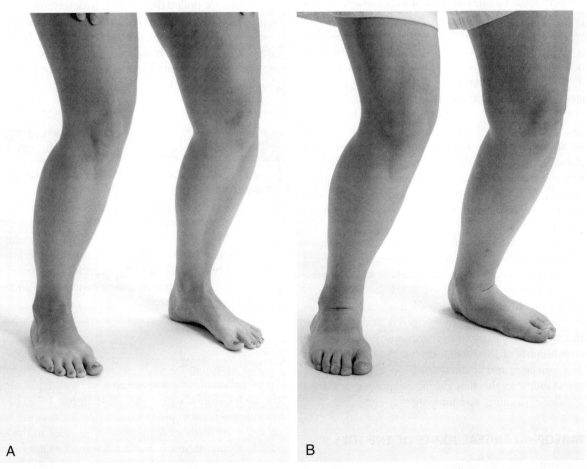

A

B

Figure 44.28: Functional dorsiflexion. The ankle is the primary source of dorsiflexion ROM while the joints of the hindfoot and midfoot contribute slight additional dorsiflexion ROM **(A).** If the midfoot is too flexible, its excessive pronation provides substantial dorsiflexion ROM **(B).**

TARSOMETATARSAL AND INTERMETATARSAL JOINTS OF THE TOES

The tarsometatarsal joints of the toes, also known as the **Lisfranc's joint,** are gliding joints with limited mobility [148,191]. The articulations are supported by joint capsules that typically form three separate joint spaces, one enclosing the articulation between the medial cuneiform and metatarsal of the great toe, another enclosing the second and third metatarsals with the middle and lateral cuneiform bones, and the lateral joint space encircling the cuboid and the fourth and fifth metatarsal bones. The synovial spaces also expand to include the intermetatarsal joints of the metatarsals within each joint capsule. Dorsal and plantar ligaments, the latter of which are thick and strong to support the arches of the foot, reinforce the joint capsules. The cuneometatarsal ligaments of the great and second toes are particularly strong and appear to provide the primary support to these joints [115].

The mobility of the tarsometatarsal joints varies across the toes. There is considerable variability in the reported mobility of the tarsometatarsal joint of the great toe. Studies of the mobility in the sagittal plane report 0–4° of total excursion [37,127,136,185]. Total linear excursion in the sagittal plane of approximately 15 mm also is reported [44]. Reports suggest that increased dorsal mobility of the first tarsometatarsal joint accompanies hallux valgus deformities of the great toe and may be associated with forefoot deformities [42,43,72]. Although some suggest that the first tarsometatarsal joint allows motion in the frontal and transverse planes as well, attempts to measure this motion are limited, and the available data suggest that the joint exhibits less than 5° of frontal plane motion [82,127,146,185]. Other motions appear to be negligible [185]. The motions of the tarsometatarsal joint of the great toe are small in the transverse and frontal planes, but they combine with the great toe's sagittal plane motion differently from the triplanar motions at the ankle, subtalar joint, and midfoot. The first ray combines plantarflexion with abduction and eversion and, therefore, does not contribute to pronation or supination [62,72].

Motion at the second tarsometatarsal joint is even more limited than at the first. Limited motion here results from the tightly wedged base of the second metatarsal among the cuneiforms and first metatarsal. Mobility increases from the third to the fifth tarsometatarsal joints as the bases become progressively less tightly wedged in and the articular surfaces become progressively more curved [127]. The relative immobility of the medial side of the foot provided by the bony surfaces and ligamentous support produces the necessary stability to the foot during propulsive activities such as walking, running, and jumping.

METATARSOPHALANGEAL JOINTS OF THE TOES

The architecture of the metatarsophalangeal joints of the toes is remarkably similar to that of the metacarpophalangeal joints of the fingers. The joints are biaxial, supported by a joint capsule, collateral ligaments, and a fibrous plantar plate covering

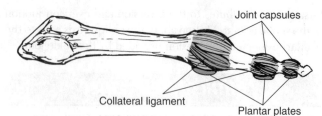

Figure 44.29: Supporting structures of the metatarsophalangeal joints of the toes include the capsule, collateral ligaments, and the plantar plate.

the plantar surface of the joints. Like the joint capsules in the fingers, the capsules of the toes are reinforced dorsally by the extensor tendons and by collateral ligaments that extend from the dorsal aspects of the medial and lateral surfaces of the metatarsal heads toward the plantar aspects of the medial and lateral sides of the proximal phalanges (*Fig. 44.29*).

The plantar plate serves a similar purpose in the toes as in the fingers, protecting the articular surface of the metatarsal heads. The weight-bearing function of the foot makes the plantar plate particularly important in the toes. The plates are attached to the metatarsal heads and the bases of the phalanges and are pulled distally with hyperextension of the toes to protect the distal aspect of the articular surface. Their function is critical to protecting the metatarsal heads during ambulation, when the body rolls over the stance foot, pushing the toes into hyperextension while the foot participates in propelling the body forward (*Fig. 44.30*).

Clinical Relevance

CLAW AND HAMMER TOE DEFORMITIES OF THE TOES: *Claw toe deformities of the toes are similar to claw deformities in the fingers, characterized by hyperextension of the metatarsophalangeal joints of the toes with flexion of the toes (Fig. 44.31). The hyperextension of the metatarsophalangeal joints pull the plantar plate distally, leaving the weight-bearing head of the metatarsal bone unprotected and producing pain as the patient bears weight on the exposed metatarsal heads.*

Two sesamoid bones lie imbedded in the tendon of the flexor hallucis brevis and are attached to the plantar plate of the metatarsophalangeal joint of the great toe. These bones provide additional protection to the metatarsal head and increase the angle of application of muscles to the great toe [140]. Hyperextension injuries to the metatarsophalangeal joint of the great toe, also known as **turf toe,** can produce fractures of the sesamoid bones, ruptures of the plantar plate, or tears in the capsular and collateral ligaments, causing significant pain and dysfunction [135].

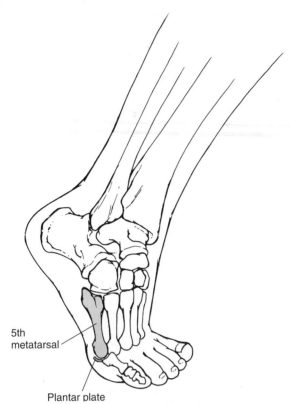

5th metatarsal

Plantar plate

Figure 44.30: Hyperextension of the toes that occurs normally late in the stance phase of gait pulls the plantar plate distally over the distal ends of the metatarsal heads.

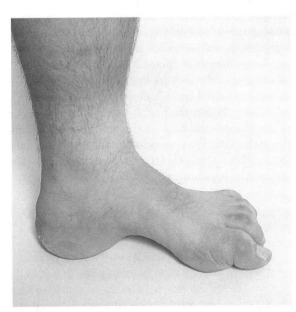

Figure 44.31: Claw toe deformities include hyperextension of the metatarsophalangeal joints and flexion of the interphalangeal joints pulling the plantar plate distally, allowing weight bearing on the exposed metatarsal heads.

Motion of the Metatarsophalangeal Joints

The metatarsophalangeal joints of the toes are biaxial joints but exhibit motion primarily in the sagittal plane. Studies of the kinematics of these joints focus on the motion at the great toe. Flexion and extension occur about a moving joint axis, indicating that the motions include rotation and translation [148]. It is likely that the remaining metatarsophalangeal joints also combine rotation and translation during flexion and extension. The great toe displays deviation in the transverse plane with slight rotation motion in the frontal plane in the familiar **hallux valgus** deformity in which the proximal phalanx deviates laterally on the metatarsal head [103]. Some individuals are able to spread the toes, exhibiting abduction at the metatarsophalangeal joints of the toes, but such excursion apparently is not studied, and its clinical significance is unknown.

Studies examine the available sagittal plane mobility of the metatarsophalangeal joint. Reports of mean hyperextension (dorsiflexion) excursion at the great toe's metatarsophalangeal joint range from 55 to 96° [13,51,66,120,160]. Seventeen to 34° of flexion (plantarflexion) are also reported [13,160]. Cadaver studies of the flexion and extension mobility of the second through fifth metatarsophalangeal joints report 60–100° of hyperextension ROM, decreasing from the second to the fifth toe [94,119]. These studies report flexion from 15–35° at these joints. Toe hyperextension mobility bears considerable clinical significance, since reports of the hyperextension used during locomotion as the body rolls over the foot vary from 40 to 90° [9,104,120].

Clinical Relevance

HALLUX RIGIDUS: *Limited hyperextension mobility of the metatarsophalangeal joint of the great toe, known as **hallux rigidus**, can produce pain and significant functional limitations and disability. Inability to hyperextend the great toe alters normal walking and running patterns, since these activities require the ability to roll over the toes, hyperextending the great toe to at least 40°. Hallux rigidus usually results from degenerative joint disease at the metatarsophalangeal joint and progresses insidiously, leading to progressive pain and disability. Conservative management includes shoe modifications to protect the toe, but severe cases often require surgery.*

INTERPHALANGEAL JOINTS OF THE TOES

The interphalangeal joints of the toes are simple hinge joints like those in the fingers. They are supported by a joint capsule, collateral ligaments, and a plantar plate. The plantar plate serves a purpose similar to that of the palmar plate at the metacarpophalangeal joints, protection of the underlying articular surface. Their motions are poorly studied, but the proximal interphalangeal joints exhibit less than 90° of flexion, with little or no extension [119,191]. Flexion mobility decreases from the second to the fifth toe. The distal interphalangeal joints of the lateral four toes and perhaps the interphalangeal joint of the great toe exhibit some hyperextension mobility, but normative data are not available.

Motion of the Whole Foot

The preceding discussion reveals that most of the joints of the foot contribute to the same triplanar motions of the foot, pronation and supination. Consequently, when the joints move in the same direction, the total motion of the foot is increased. Conversely, individuals with restricted motion at one joint may develop increased mobility at a nearby joint to maintain overall mobility of the foot. In addition, pronation and supination of the foot affect the mechanical properties of the whole foot [45,121,165]. Pronation of the hindfoot increases the passive mobility of the sagittal plane motion of the forefoot, and supination of the hindfoot decreases that mobility [7]. Pronation of the foot after ground contact in gait allows the foot to accommodate to the walking surface. Supination of all of the joints of the foot makes the foot more rigid and occurs later in the stance phase of gait to help stabilize the foot as the body rolls over it [116,157,193].

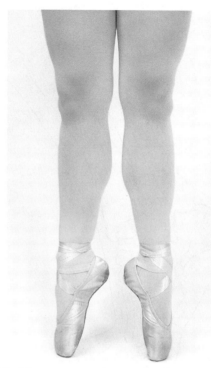

Figure 44.32: What appears to be 90° of plantarflexion allowing a dancer to dance en pointe actually requires plantarflexion from the ankle and throughout the foot.

Clinical Relevance

DANCING EN POINTE: *A ballerina dancing en pointe appears to be able to plantarflex the ankle 90° (Fig. 44.32). Since such motion is not physiologically possible at the ankle, it is clear that mobility throughout the rest of the intertarsal and metatarsal joints contributes sufficient plantarflexion to allow the toes of the foot to be in line with the long axis of the leg, allowing the dancer to balance on the toes.*

PLANTAR FASCIA

The individual ligaments described to this point support specific joints. The foot also contains a structure that functions to support the entire foot. The plantar fascia of the foot provides essential stabilization to the skin on the plantar surface and helps maintain the shape of the whole foot. It exhibits a complex web of attachments extending from the calcaneal tuberosity to the skin, metatarsal and phalangeal bones, and intervening ligaments [191]. Its thick, deep portion, known as the **plantar aponeurosis,** possesses remarkable tensile strength (1000–1500 N, 225–337 lb), almost twice the strength of the strongest ligament in the foot, the deltoid ligament [86].

The plantar aponeurosis spans the arches of the foot and plays a critical role in supporting them. Weight bearing lowers the medial longitudinal arch and stretches the plantar aponeurosis [151]. Studies of full and partial transection of the aponeurosis consistently demonstrate a decrease in arch height when the aponeurosis is compromised [2,19,118,157,176].

Plantar fascia releases also produce large increases in strains in other ligaments of the foot, particularly the spring and long plantar ligaments [19,24]. Although plantar fascia releases may be indicated to relieve chronic foot pain, the resultant changes in other structures of the foot suggest that all possible conservative measures should be tried before resorting to surgery.

The extensive attachments of the plantar fascia also suggest a special dynamic role in locomotion. Plantarflexion of the ankle rotates the calcaneus toward the ground, lowering the arch and stretching the aponeurosis (*Fig. 44.33*). Similarly, hyperextension of the toes applies tension to the aponeurosis by pulling on its distal end. During the push-off phase of gait, an individual rolls over the foot, hyperextending the metatarsophalangeal joints of the toes and simultaneously plantarflexing the ankle. Thus the aponeurosis is pulled taut to stabilize the foot as it bears the load of the body moving over the stance foot toward the opposite foot [20,32,61].

Clinical Relevance

PLANTAR FASCIITIS—A CASE REPORT: *A 40-year-old woman entered physical therapy complaining of medial arch pain. The woman reported that she was training for a 5-km (3.2 miles) race and had noticed a gradual onset of pain in the bottom of her foot, particularly upon rising from bed in the morning. Physical examination revealed a patient*
(continued)

(Continued)

*with a normally aligned foot and a rather high medial arch. The patient also exhibited limited dorsiflexion ROM on the painful side. The patient noted that she had become rather careless about her ankle stretching routine despite training more vigorously, concentrating on increased speed. The therapist surmised that the patient's faster running required increased dorsiflexion ROM at the ankle and increased hyperextension ROM of the metatarsophalangeal joints of the toes. However, the patient lacked adequate ankle ROM, so the joints of the hindfoot and midfoot compensated by providing more dorsiflexion range. The increased dorsiflexion motion in the midfoot stretched the plantar fascia that was also being stretched by increased toe hyperextension and by higher impact loads on the foot with increased running speed. The cumulative effect of these factors produced an inflammatory response in the aponeurosis, **plantar fasciitis.** Treatment included rest and vigorous stretching. Over time the patient was able to resume training without pain as long as she stretched regularly.*

Closed-Chain Motion of the Foot

Discussion of the foot thus far has focused on the movement of the foot with respect to the leg, in which the foot functions in an **open chain.** Yet the foot often functions while fixed to the ground, with the superincumbent body moving over it, functioning in a **closed chain.** Many complaints of pain and dysfunction in the foot, ankle, knee, or hip arise from closed-chain activities such as running, jumping, or dancing. It is essential

for the clinician to understand the mechanics of foot function whether the foot is fixed to the ground or moving above it.

The role of the subtalar joint in transforming movements of the foot to the leg or vice versa becomes critical in closed-chain activities. When the foot is fixed to the ground, the foot pronates and supinates by allowing the proximal segments to move on the distal segments. Thus pronation of the subtalar joint occurs by the tibia and talus moving on the calcaneus. Pronation with the foot fixed on the ground produces medial rotation of the tibia, which carries the talus medially within the mortise [62,69,129]. As the talus moves medially, the calcaneus everts and pulls the cuboid and navicular into abduction and eversion.

Thus the motion of the hindfoot is **coupled** to the motion of the leg and the forefoot. The extent to which foot motion is directly coupled with tibial motion remains unclear. In walking as the foot pronates the tibia medially rotates and as the foot supinates the tibia laterally rotates. Yet neither the magnitude nor timing of foot motion directly parallels tibial motion [132]. Studies suggest that some of the motion of the foot is absorbed within the foot rather than transmitted directly to the tibia. Running appears to increase the correlations between foot and tibial motions, suggesting more direct coupling of the motion between the foot and the leg [27,132].

As noted earlier in this chapter, pronation of the foot tends to make the foot more flexible [45,121,165]. In addition, medial rotation of the tibia accompanies flexion of the knee (Chapter 41), so pronation of the foot tends to facilitate knee flexion [54,147]. Consequently, pronation of the foot during weight bearing may help the lower extremity accommodate to the ground by enhancing its flexibility and shock absorption capabilities. Foot pronation is the normal response of the foot at contact during locomotion [68]. In contrast, supination of the subtalar joint with the foot on the ground produces lateral rotation of the tibia with inversion of the calcaneus, cuboid, and navicular; it tends to extend the knee, making the foot and rest of the lower extremity more rigid [54,69,147]. Supination normally occurs during locomotion in midstance as the body is moving over the foot and push-off begins [68].

A common clinical perception is that inadequate or excessive pronation or supination may contribute to complaints of foot, knee, hip and even back pain by interfering with the coupling between the foot and the rest of the lower extremity during weight bearing [121]. However studies investigating the relationship between excessive pronation and anterior knee pain report little association [60,93,133]. Like low back pain, anterior knee pain is likely to be associated with multiple, interdependent mechanical factors that together help explain the presence or absence of pain. Such factors may include the coupling of foot and leg motion, foot alignment, knee and patellofemoral joint alignment, strength and flexibility at the foot and knee, and even body weight and height. A better understanding of the interactions among these factors and others will help clinicians address the underlying mechanical flaws when treating lower extremity dysfunctions.

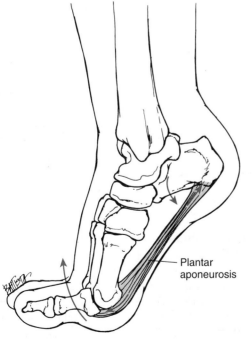

Figure 44.33: The plantar aponeurosis is stretched by plantarflexion of the calcaneus and by hyperextension of the toes.

Plantar aponeurosis

FOOT ALIGNMENT

Because the foot functions primarily in a closed chain while bearing significant loads, foot alignment is implicated in many disorders of the lower extremity. To understand the potential impact of foot alignment on lower extremity function, the clinician requires an understanding of the normal alignment of the foot and the factors that influence that alignment.

Arches of the Foot

The articulated foot exhibits three distinct arches, a **medial** and a **lateral longitudinal arch** and the **transverse arch** (*Fig. 44.34*). The medial longitudinal arch includes the calcaneus, talus, navicular, medial cuneiform, and first metatarsal bone. The lateral longitudinal arch consists of the calcaneus, cuboid, and fifth metatarsal bones. The transverse arch is formed by the cuboid and cuneiform bones and continues at the bases of the metatarsals. The transverse arch disappears in the normal foot at the heads of the metatarsal bones so that all five metatarsal heads contact the ground in normal weight bearing [56].

The arches serve several purposes: they protect the nerves, blood vessels, and muscles on the plantar surface of the foot from compression during weight bearing; they help the foot to absorb shock during impact with the ground; and they help

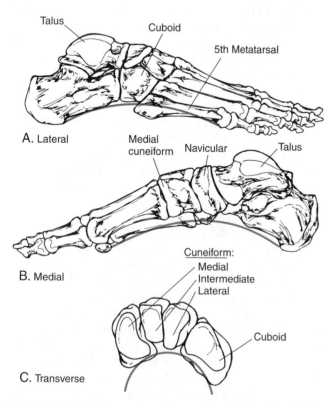

Figure 44.34: The foot possesses three arches: **(A)** lateral and **(B)** medial longitudinal arches and **(C)** a transverse arch.

store mechanical energy then release it to improve the efficiency of locomotion [78,144]. The arches of the foot develop in parallel with gait during childhood and continue to form until a child is 8 or 10 years of age [35,59]. Integrity of the arches depends primarily on ligamentous support with assistance from bony alignment and additional support from extrinsic muscles of the foot [67,102]. The middle and lateral cuneiform bones are shaped and positioned to play the role of keystone in the transverse arch. Their wedge shape, wider dorsally than on their plantar surface, helps prevent their descent through the arch [78].

The plantar fascia, long and short plantar ligaments, the spring ligament, the collateral ligaments of the ankle, and the interosseous ligament of the subtalar joint all contribute important soft tissue support to the arches of the foot. Sectioning these ligaments in cadaver specimens produces altered joint kinematics of the joints that form the arches, and sequential sectioning progressively lowers the arches [67,81,83,84,176]. These studies demonstrate that support of the arches depends on several structures, with no single structure providing the primary support.

Arch height is measured directly by determining the height of the navicular or the dorsum of the foot from the ground during weight-bearing [188]. The **arch index** provides an indirect measure of the integrity of the arch by examining the amount of contact with the ground made by the midfoot [17]. A flat foot, or **pes planus**, refers to a diminished medial longitudinal arch, and a **pes cavus** indicates an abnormally high medial longitudinal arch. Both arch abnormalities appear to predispose individuals to specific musculoskeletal injuries [189,190].

Clinical Relevance

RUNNING INJURIES: *Arch abnormalities in runners are associated with different injury patterns [189]. In a study of 40 runners with histories of running injuries, the runners with high arches reported more ankle and bony injuries, while those with low arches reported more knee and soft tissue injuries. Screening athletes for arch abnormalities may lead to better preventive measures including instructing individuals in appropriate footwear, the use of shoe modifications, and athlete education.*

Loading causes complex movements of the joints of the foot leading to a decrease in the arch height. The primary motion is pronation of the foot, with dorsiflexion, eversion, and abduction of the navicular and calcaneus on the talus (pronation) [18,82,151]. In addition, both the calcaneus and first metatarsal become more horizontally aligned, contributing to the flattening of the arch [82,180,187]. Consistent with the pronation of the calcaneus and navicular, the tibia and talus rotate medially [63,64]. This normal response to loading

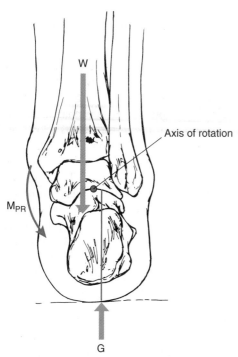

Figure 44.35: The medial alignment of the talus on the calcaneus produces a pronation moment (MP_{PR}) on the hindfoot due to the ground reaction force (G) and the weight of the body (W).

occurs because the ground reaction force on the calcaneus lies lateral to the axis of rotation of the subtalar joint, producing a pronation moment on the foot [129] (*Fig 44.35*). An excessively flattened arch produces increased excursions within the foot and tibia and can even lead to subluxations of joints of the foot [1,36,83].

Pes planus and pes cavus describe the qualitative shape of the arch, and arch height and arch index quantify the magnitude of the arch. However, none of these descriptions provides insight into the mechanisms that lead to the abnormal arch. Arch deformities result from disruptions of the supporting ligaments as well as from muscle weakness or tightness leading to direct impairments of the arch. In some individuals, the foot position is the dynamic compensation for other bony malalignments.

Subtalar Neutral Position

The concept of the **subtalar neutral position** is central to understanding postural compensations in the foot. It is operationally defined as the position of the subtalar joint that is neither pronated nor supinated [143]. Subtalar neutral position appears to maximize the area of contact between the talus and calcaneus, and movements away from the subtalar neutral position into pronation or supination decrease the contact areas [14,29].

Subtalar neutral position is determined with the subject either weight-bearing or non-weight-bearing by palpating the medial and lateral aspects of the talar head to identify the

position in which the talus articulates symmetrically with the navicular. The position is measured by using the same reference lines used to measure subtalar ROM (Fig. 44.22). The angle made by a line bisecting the leg and another bisecting the posterior aspect of the calcaneus quantifies the subtalar neutral position [130,134]. Medial deviation of the calcaneus with respect to the leg constitutes a **varus** deformity, while **valgus** indicates a lateral deviation of the hindfoot on the leg. Varus and valgus also apply to forefoot alignment, although the forefoot position is referenced to the hindfoot [40].

Although a commonly used clinical assessment, the reliability of subtalar neutral measurements remains in question, with some studies demonstrating satisfactory intertester and intratester reliability [76,108,134,180], and other studies reporting unacceptable levels of reliability [31,130]. Recognizing the limits in reliability, reported values of subtalar neutral position in individuals without foot pathology vary from 1–2° of varus [3,108] to less than 1° of valgus [131].

Clinical Relevance

FOOT ORTHOSES FOR TREATMENT OF A VARUS HINDFOOT DEFORMITY: *In upright stance with the tibias approximately vertical, a medially aligned hindfoot, or hindfoot with a varus deformity, must pronate excessively to contact the ground fully (Fig. 44.36). The greater the varus deformity, the more pronation is required to contact the ground. Consequently, an individual with a varus hindfoot may pronate excessively or through a prolonged period*

(*continued*)

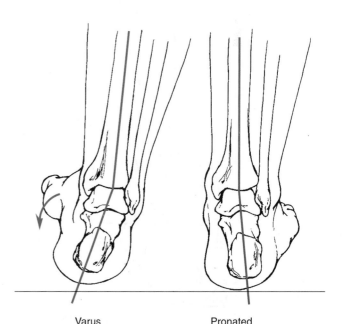

Varus   Pronated

Figure 44.36: A varus hindfoot deformity in standing requires excessive pronation for the foot to come into full contact with the ground.

(Continued)

during the gait cycle [177]. To prevent the excessive prona-tion, some clinicians use orthotic devices that build up, or **post,** *the medial aspect of the foot to provide a mechanical block to pronation [71] (Fig. 44.37). Conversely, supination provides compensation for a valgus deformity of the hind-foot or forefoot. Lateral posting attempts to limit the com-pensatory supination.*

Orthotic devices to control the foot's compensatory movements resulting from foot deformities are common interventions for foot and knee pain [28,88]. The use of foot orthoses to treat knee pain is based on an under-standing of the natural coupling between foot pronation or supination and tibial rotation and knee motion in closed-chain movement. Medial wedge orthoses are report-ed to decrease pain in individuals with patellofemoral joint pain [75]. Yet the common clinical belief that excessive pronation is a risk factor for anterior knee pain lacks strong scientific evidence [60,93,133]. In contrast, gait stud-ies demonstrate that medial wedges exhibit a small but significant ability to control medial rotation of the tibia that occurs with excessive pronation [109,123,167]. Biomechanical studies also suggest that medial or lateral wedges may alter the loading patterns at the knee [153]. In light of the continued debate regarding the reliability of subtalar neutral measures and the limited understanding of the precise coupling among the motions of the foot and leg, clinicians must exercise caution in interpreting foot alignment data and seek additional evidence for the effec-tiveness of orthotic therapy.

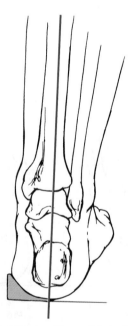

Figure 44.37: A foot orthosis with medial posting raises the ground to the foot, allowing full contact between the foot and the ground without excessive pronation.

SUMMARY

This chapter describes the structure of the bones and joints and how that structure influences the motions of the individ-ual joints of the ankle and foot. Most of the joints of the foot and ankle are hinge or gliding joints, but their alignment pro-duces triplanar motion known as pronation and supination. With the exception of the tarsometatarsal joint of the great toe, the joints of the ankle, hindfoot, and midfoot can pronate together, making the foot more flexible, or supinate together to increase the rigidity of the foot. These movements are essential to the normal loading and unloading of the foot dur-ing locomotion. Hyperextension mobility at the metatar-sophalangeal joints of the toes also is essential in gait to allow the body to roll over the foot. This chapter also describes the movements that occur when the foot functions in a closed chain, pronation of the foot producing medial rotation of the tibia and flexion of the knee and supination producing the opposite.

Several ligaments provide essential support to the joints of the ankle and foot. The ankle joint capsule and collateral lig-aments are particularly important in supporting the ankle and subtalar joints, the latter also being supported by the interosseous ligament. The spring ligament and long and short plantar ligaments are important supporting structures for the midfoot. The plantar plates provide important protec-tion to the articular surfaces of the toes, particularly the metatarsophalangeal joints.

The normal shape and alignment of the foot also are described. Specifically, the tibia normally exhibits lateral tor-sion, and the hindfoot is very close to 0° subtalar neutral posi-tion. The foot maintains a medial and lateral longitudinal and a transverse arch. Although the primary support of the arch-es is ligamentous, muscles provide dynamic support to the arches of the foot. The muscles of the ankle and foot are pre-sented in the following chapter.

References

1. Ananthakrisnan D, Ching R, Tencer A, et al.: Subluxation of the talocalcaneal joint in adults who have symptomatic flatfoot. J Bone Joint Surg (Am) 1999; 81: 1147–1154.
2. Arangio GA, Chen C, Salathe EP: Effect of varying arch height with and without the plantar fascia on the mechanical proper-ties of the foot. Foot Ankle Int 1998; 19: 705–709.
3. Astrom M, Arvidson T: Alignment and joint motion in the nor-mal foot. J Orthop Sports Phys Ther 1995; 22: 216–222.
4. Attarian DE, McCrackin HJ, DeVito DP, et al.: Biomechanical characteristics of the human ankle ligaments. Foot Ankle 1985; 6: 54–58.
5. Bahr R, Pena F, Shine J, et al.: Ligament force and joint motion in the intact ankle: a cadaveric study. Knee Surg Sports Traumatol Arthrosc 1998; 6: 115–121.
6. Bahr R, Pena F, Shine J, et al.: Mechanics of the anterior drawer and talar tilt tests. A cadaveric study of lateral ligament injuries of the ankle. Acta Orthop Scand 1997; 68: 435–441.
7. Blackwood CB, Yuen TJ, Sangeorzan BJ, et al.: The midtarsal joint locking mechanism. Foot Ankle Int 2005; 26: 1074–1080.

8. Boardman DL, Liu SH: Contribution of the anterolateral joint capsule to the mechanical stability of the ankle. Clin Orthop 1997; 341: 224–232.

9. Bojsen-Moller F, Lamoreux L: Significance of free dorsiflexion of the toes in walking. Acta Orthop Scand 1979; 50: 471–479.

10. Boone DC, Azen SP: Normal range of motion of joints in male subjects. J Bone Joint Surg 1979; 61A: 756–759.

11. Bostman OM: Distal tibiofibular synostosis after malleolar fractures treated using absorbable implants. Foot Ankle 1993; 14: 38–43.

12. Buckley RE, Hunt DV: Reliability of clinical measurement of subtalar joint movement. Foot Ankle Int 1997; 18: 229–232.

13. Buell T, Green DR, Risser J: Measurement of the first metatarsophalangeal joint range of motion. J Am Podiatr Med Assoc 1988; 78: 439–448.

14. Calhoun JH, Eng M, Ledbetter BR, Viegas SF: A comprehensive study of pressure distribution in the ankle joint with inversion and eversion. Foot Ankle 1994; 15: 125–133.

15. Cameron JC, Saha S: External tibial torsion. An underrecognized cause of recurrent patellar dislocation. Clin Orthop 1996; 328: 177–184.

16. Canale ST: Campbell's Operative Orthopaedics. St. Louis: Mosby, 1998.

17. Cavanagh PR, Rodgers MM: The arch index: A useful measure from footprints. J Biomech 1987; 20: 547–551.

18. Cawley PW, France EP: Biomechanics of the lateral ligaments of the ankle: an evaluation of the effects of axial load and single plane motions on ligament strain patterns. Foot Ankle 1991; 12: 92–99.

19. Cheung JT, An KN, Zhang M, et al.: Consequences of partial and total plantar fascia release: a finite element study. Foot Ankle Int 2006; 27: 125–132.

20. Cheung JTM, Zhang M, An KN: Effect of achilles tendon loading on plantar fascia tension in the standing foot. Clin Biomech 2006; 21: 194–203.

21. Close JR, Inman VT, Poor PM, Todd FN: The function of the subtalar joint. Clin Orthop 1967; 50: 159–179.

22. Corraza F, Leardini A, O'Connor JJ, et al.: Mechanics of the anterior drawer test at the ankle: the effects of ligament viscoelasticity. J Biomech 2005; 38: 2118–2123.

23. Corraza F, O'Connor JJ, Leardini A, et al.: Ligament fibre recruitment and forces for the anterior drawer test at the human ankle joint. J Biomech 2003; 36: 363–372.

24. Crary JL, Hollis JM, Manoli A: The effect of plantar fascia release on strain in the spring and long plantar ligaments. Foot Ankle Int 2003; 24: 245–250.

25. Davis WH, Sobel M, DiCarlo EF, et al.: Gross, histological, and microvascular anatomy and biomechanical testing of the spring ligament complex. Foot Ankle Int 1996; 17: 95–102.

26. Deland JT, Morris GD, Sung IH: Biomechanics of the ankle joint. A perspective on total ankle replacement. Foot Ankle Clin 2000; 5: 747–759.

27. Dierks TA, Davis I: Discrete and continuous joint coupling relationships in uninjured recreational runners. Clin Biomech 2007; 22: 581–591.

28. Donatelli R, Hurlbert C, Conaway D, St Pierre R: Biomechanical foot orthotics: a retrospective study. JOSPT 1988; 10: 205–212.

29. Earll M, Wayne J, Brodrick C, et al.: Contribution of the deltoid ligament to ankle joint contact characteristics: a cadaver study. Foot Ankle Int 1996; 17: 317–324.

30. Eckhoff DG, Johnson KK: Three-dimensional computed tomography reconstruction of tibial torsion. Clin Orthop 1994; 302: 42–46.

31. Elveru RA, Rothstein JM, Lamb RL: Goniometric reliability in a clinical setting: subtalar and ankle joint measurements. Phys Ther 1988; 68: 672–677.

32. Erdemir A, Hamel AJ, Fauth AR, et al.: Dynamic loading of the plantar aponeurosis in walking. J Bone Joint Surg 2004; 86: 546–552.

33. Espregueira-Mendes JD, Vieira da Silva M: Anatomy of the proximal tibiofibular joint. Knee Surg Sports Traumatol Arthrosc 2006; 14: 241–249.

34. Fabry G, Cheng LX, Molenaers G: Normal and abnormal torsional development in children. Clin Orthop 1994; 302: 22–26.

35. Forriol F, Pascual J: Footprint analysis between three and seventeen years of age. Foot Ankle 1990; 11: 101–104.

36. Franco AH: Pes cavus and pes planus: analyses and treatment. Phys Ther 1988; 67: 688–694.

37. Fritz GR, Prieskorn D: First metatarsocuneiform motion: a radiographic and statistical analysis. Foot Ankle Int 1995; 16: 117–123.

38. Fujii T, Luo ZP, Kitaoka HB, An KN: The manual stress test may not be sufficient to differentiate ankle ligament injuries. Clin Biomech (Bristol, Avon) 2000; Oct 15: 619–623.

39. Funk JR, Hall GW, Crandall JR, Pilkey WD: Linear and quasilinear viscoelastic characterization of ankle ligaments. J Biomech Eng 2000; 122: 15–22.

40. Garbalosa JC, McClure MH, Catlin PA, Wooden M: The frontal plane relationship of the forefoot to the rearfoot in an asymptomatic population. JOSPT 1994; 20: 200–206.

41. Gerhardt JJ, Rippstein J: Measuring and Recording of Joint Motion Instrumentation and Techniques. Lewiston, NJ: Hogrefe & Huber, 1990.

42. Glasoe WM, Allen MK, Ludewig PM: Comparison of first ray dorsal mobility among different forefoot alignments. JOSPT 2000; 30: 612–623.

43. Glasoe WM, Allen MK, Saltzman CL: First ray dorsal mobility in relation to hallux valgus deformity and first intermetatarsal angle. Foot Ankle Int 2001; 22: 98–101.

44. Glasoe WM, Allen MK, Yack HJ: Measurement of dorsal mobility in the first ray: elimination of fat pad compression as a variable. Foot Ankle Int 1998; 19: 542–546.

45. Glasoe WM, Yack HJ, Saltzman CL: Anatomy and biomechanics of the first ray. Phys Ther 1999; 79: 854–859.

46. Gray GW: When the feet hit the ground everything changes: program outline and prepared notes—a basic manual. Toledo. OH: American Physical Rehabilitation Network, 1984.

47. Green T, Refshauge K, Crosbie J, Adams R: A randomized controlled trial of a passive accessory joint mobilization on acute ankle inversion sprains. Phys Ther 2001; 81: 984–994.

48. Greene WB, Heckman JDE: The Clinical Measurement of Joint Motion. Rosemont, IL: American Academy of Orthopaedic Surgeons, 1994.

49. Grimm MJ, Williams JL: Measurements of permeability in human calcaneal trabecular bone. J Biomech 1997; 30: 743–745.

50. Grimston SK, Nigg BM, Hanley DA, Engsberg JR: Differences in ankle joint complex range of motion as a function of age. Foot Ankle 1993; 14: 215–222.

51. Halstead J, Redmond AC: Weight-bearing passive dorsiflexion of the hallux in standing is not related to hallux dorsiflexion during walking. J Orthop Sports Phys Ther 2006; 36: 550–556.

52. Harper MC: Deltoid ligament: an anatomical evaluation of function. Foot Ankle 1987; 8: 19–22.

53. Harper MC: Posterior instability of the talus: an anatomic evaluation. Foot Ankle 1989; 10: 36–39.

54. Harris GF: Analysis of ankle and subtalar motion during human locomotion. In: Stiehl JB, ed. Inman's Joints of the Ankle. Baltimore: Williams & Wilkins, 1991; 75–84.

55. Harty M: Anatomic considerations in injuries of calcaneus. Orthop Clin North Am 1973; 4: 179–183.

56. Harty M: Metatarsalgia. Surgery 1973; 136: 105–106.

57. Harty M: Ankle arthroscopy: anatomical features. Orthopedics 1985; 8: 1538–1540.

58. Heilman AE, Braly WG, Bishop JO, et al.: An anatomic study of subtalar instability. Foot Ankle 1990; 10: 224–228.

59. Hennig EM, Rosenbaum D: Pressure distribution patterns under the feet of children in comparison with adults. Foot Ankle 1991; 11: 306–311.

60. Hetsroni I, Finestone A, Milgrom C, et al.: A prospective biomechanical study of the association between foot pronation and the incidence of anterior knee pain among military recruits. J Bone Joint Surg 2006; 88B: 905–908.

61. Hicks JH: The mechanics of the foot. II The plantar aponeurosis and the arch. J Anat 1954; 88: 25–31.

62. Hicks JH: The mechanics of the foot. I. The joints. J Anat 1953; 87: 345–357.

63. Hintermann B, Nigg BM: In vitro kinematics of the axially loaded ankle complex in response to dorsiflexion and plantarflexion. Foot Ankle Int 1995; 16: 514–518.

64. Hintermann B, Sommer C, Nigg BM: Influence of ligament transection on tibial and calcaneal rotation with loading and dorsi-plantarflexion. Foot Ankle Int 1995; 16: 567–571.

65. Hochberg MC: Osteoarthritis. B. Clinical features. In: Klippel JH, ed. Primer of the Rheumatic Diseases. Atlanta: Arthritis Foundation, 2001; 289–293.

66. Hopson MM, McPoil TG, Cornwall MW: Motion of the first metatarsophalangeal joint. J Am Podiatr Med Assoc 1995; 85: 198–204.

67. Huang C-K, Kitaoka HB, An K-N, Chao EYS: Biomechanical evaluation of longitudinal arch stability. Foot Ankle Int 1993; 14: 353–357.

68. Hunt AE, Smith RM, Torode M: Extrinsic muscle activity, foot motion and ankle joint moments during the stance phase of walking. Foot Ankle Int 2001; 22: 31–41.

69. Huson A: Biomechanics of the tarsal mechanism. J Am Podiatr Med Assoc 2000; 90: 12–17.

70. Inman VT: The joints of the ankle. Baltimore: Williams & Williams, 1976.

71. Johanson MA, Donatelli R, Wooden MJ, et al.: Effects of three different posting methods on controlling abnormal subtalar pronation. Phys Ther 1994; 74: 149–161.

72. Johnson CH, Christensen JC: Biomechanics of the first ray. Part I. The effects of peroneus longus function: a three-dimensional kinematic study on a cadaver model. J Foot Ankle Surg 1999; 38: 313–321.

73. Johnson JE: Axis of rotation of the ankle. In: Stiehl JB, ed. Inman's Joints of the Ankle. Baltimore: Williams & Wilkins, 1991; 21–30.

74. Johnson JE: Shape of the trochlea and mobility of the lateral malleolus. In: Stiehl JB, ed. Inman's Joints of the Ankle. Baltimore: Williams & Wilkins, 1991; 15–20.

75. Johnston LB, Gross MT: Effects of foot orthoses on quality of life for individuals with patellofemoral pain syndrome. J Orthop Sports Phys Ther 2004; 34: 440–448.

76. Jonson SR, Gross MT: Intraexaminer reliability, interexaminer reliability, and mean values for nine lower extremity skeletal measures in healthy naval midshipman. J Orthop Sports Phys Ther 1997; 25: 253–263.

77. Joyce JJ, Harty M: Surgical anatomy and exposures of the foot and ankle. In: AAOS Instructional Course Lectures. St. Louis: CV Mosby, 1970; 1–11.

78. Kapandji IA: The physiology of the joints. Vol 2, the lower limb. Edinburgh: Churchill Livingstone, 1970.

79. Ker RF, Bennett MB, Bibby SR, et al.: The spring in the arch of the human foot. Nature 1987; 325: 147–149.

80. Kerkhoffs GMMJ, Blankevoort L, van Poll D, et al.: Anterior lateral ankle ligament damage and anterior talocrural-joint laxity: an overview of the in vitro reports in literature. Clin Biomech 2001; 16: 635–643.

81. Kitaoka HB, Ahn T-K, Luo ZP, An K-N: Stability of the arch of the foot. Foot Ankle Int 1997; 18: 644–648.

82. Kitaoka HB, Lundberg A, Luo ZP, An KN: Kinematics of the normal arch of the foot and ankle under physiologic loading. Foot Ankle Int 1995; 16: 492–499.

83. Kitaoka HB, Luo Z-P, An K-N: Three-dimensional analysis of flatfoot deformity: cadaver study. Foot Ankle Int 1998; 19: 447–451.

84. Kitaoka HB, Luo ZP, An K: Mechanical behavior of the foot and ankle after plantar fascia release in the unstable foot. Foot Ankle Int 1997; 18: 8–15.

85. Kitaoka HB, Luo ZP, An K-N: Three-dimensional analysis of normal ankle and foot mobility. Am J Sports Med 1997; 25: 238–242.

86. Kitaoka HB, Luo ZP, Growney ES, et al.: Material properties of the plantar aponeurosis. Foot Ankle Int 1994; 15: 557–560.

87. Kling TF Jr, Hensinger RN: Angular and torsional deformities of the lower limbs in children. Clin Orthop 1983; 176: 136–147.

88. Klingman RE, Liaos SM, Hardin KM: The effect of subtalar joint posting on patellar glide position in subjects with excessive rearfoot pronation. J Orthop Sports Phys Ther 1997; 25: 185–191.

89. Knudson GA, Kitaoka HB, Lu CL, et al.: Subtalar joint stability. Talocalcaneal interosseous ligament function studied in cadaver specimens. Acta Orthop Scand 1997; 68: 442–446.

90. Leardini A, O'Connor JJ, Catani F, Giannini S: Kinematics of the human ankle complex in passive flexion; a single degree of freedom system. J Biomech 1999; 32: 111–118.

91. Leardini A, O'Connor JJ, Catani F, Giannini S: A geometric model of the human ankle joint. J Biomech 1999; 32: 585–591.

92. Leardini A, Stagni R, O'Connor JJ: Mobility of the subtalar joint in the intact ankle complex. J Biomech 2001; 34: 805–809.

93. Livingston LA, Mandigo JL: Bilateral rearfoot asymmetry and anterior knee pain syndrome. J Orthop Sports Phys Ther 2003; 33: 48–54.

94. Loh JS, Lim BH, Wan CT, et al.: Second metatarsophalangeal joint. Clin Orthop Rel Res 2004; 421: 199-204.

95. Lowery RB, Calhoun JH: Fractures of the calcaneus: part 1: anatomy, injury mechanism, and classification. Foot Ankle Int 1996; 17: 230–235.

96. Lundberg A: Kinematics of the ankle and foot: in vivo roentgen stereophotogrammetry. Acta Orthop Scand Suppl 1989; 60: 1–23.

97. Lundberg A, Goldie I, Kalin B, Selvik G: Kinematics of the ankle/foot complex: plantarflexion and dorsiflexion. Foot Ankle 1989; 9: 194–200.

98. Lundberg A, Svensson OK, Bylund C, et al.: Kinematics of the ankle/foot complex-part 2: pronation and supination. Foot Ankle 1989; 9: 248–253.

99. Lundberg A, Svensson OK, Bylund C, Selvik G: Kinematics of the ankle/foot complex-part 3: influence of leg rotation. Foot Ankle 1989; 9: 304–309.

100. Lundberg A, Svensson OK, Nemeth G, Selvik G: The axis of rotation of the ankle joint. J Bone Joint Surg 1989; 71B: 94–99.

101. Luo Z-P, Kitaoka HB, Hsu H-C, et al.: Physiological elongation of ligamentous complex surrounding the hindfoot joints: in vitro biomechanical study. Foot Ankle Int 1997; 18: 277–283.

102. Mann R, Inman VT: Phasic activity of intrinsic muscles of the foot. J Bone Joint Surg 1964; 46A: 469–481.

103. Mann RA: The great toe. Orthop Clin North Am 1989; 20: 519–533.

104. Mann RA, Hagy JL: The function of the toes in walking, jogging and running. Clin Orthop 1979; 142: 24–29.

105. Manter JT: Movements of the subtalar and transverse tarsal joints. Anat Rec 1941; 80: 397–410.

106. Martin LP, Wayne JS, Monahan TJ, Adelaar RS: Elongation behavior of calcaneofibular and cervical ligaments during inversion loads applied in an open kinetic chain. Foot Ankle Int 1998; 19: 232–239.

107. Mattingly B, Talwalkar V, Tylkowski C, et al.: Three-dimensional in vivo motion of adult hind foot bones. J Biomech 2006; 39: 726–733.

108. McPoil TG, Cornwall MW: The relationship between three static angles of the rearfoot and the pattern of rearfoot motion during walking. JOSPT 1996; 23: 370–375.

109. McPoil TG, Cornwall MW: The effect of foot orthoses on transverse tibial rotation during walking. J Am Podiatr Med Assoc 2000; 90: 2–11.

110. Michelson JD, Helgemo SL: Kinematics of the axially loaded ankle. Foot Ankle Int 1995; 16: 577–582.

111. Milgrom C, Gilad M, Simkin A, et al.: The normal range of subtalar inversion and eversion in young males as measured by three different techniques. Foot Ankle Int 1985; 6: 143–145.

112. Milner CE, Soames RW: A comparison of four in vivo methods of measuring tibial torsion. J Anat 1998; 193: 139–144.

113. Milner CE, Soames RW: Anatomy of the collateral ligaments of the human ankle joint. Foot Ankle Int 1998; 19: 757–760.

114. Milner CE, Soames RW: The medial collateral ligaments of the human ankle joint: anatomical variations. Foot Ankle Int 1998; 19: 289–292.

115. Mizel MS: The role of the plantar first metatarsal cuneiform ligament in weightbearing on the first metatarsal. Foot Ankle 1993; 14: 82–84.

116. Morris JM: Biomechanics of the foot and ankle. Clin Orthop 1977; 122: 10–19.

117. Moseley AM, Crosbie J, Adams R: Normative data for passive ankle plantarflexion-dorsiflexion flexibility. Clin Biomech 2001; 16: 514–521.

118. Murphy GA, Pneumaticos SG, Kamaric E, et al.: Biomechanical consequences of sequential plantar fascia release. Foot Ankle Int 1998; 19: 149–152.

119. Myerson MS, Shereff MJ: The pathological anatomy of claw and hammer toes. J Bone Joint Surg 1989; 71–A: 45–49.

120. Nawoczenski DA, Baumhauer JF, Umberger BR: Relationship between clinical measurements and motion of the first metatarsophalangeal joint during gait. J Bone Joint Surg Am 1999; 81: 370–376.

121. Nawoczenski DA, Saltzman CL, Cook TM: The effect of foot structure on the three-dimensional kinematic coupling behavior of the leg and rear foot. Phys Ther 1998; 78: 404–416.

122. Needleman RL, Skrade DA, Stiehl JB: Effect of the syndesmotic screw on ankle motion. Foot Ankle 1989; 10: 17–24.

123. Nester CJ, van der Linden ML, Bowker P: Effect of foot orthoses on the kinematics and kinetics of normal walking gait. Gait Posture 2003; 17: 180–187.

124. Nigg BM, Fisher V, Allinger TL, et al.: Range of motion of the foot as a function of age. Foot Ankle Int 1992; 13: 336–343.

125. Nigg BM, Skarvan G, Frank CB, Yeadon MR: Elongation and forces of ankle ligaments in a physiological range of motion. Foot Ankle 1990; 11: 30–40.

126. Norkin CC, White DJ: Measurement of Joint Motion. A Guide to Goniometry. Philadelphia: FA Davis, 1995.

127. Ouzounian TJ, Shereff MJ: In vitro determination of midfoot motion. Foot Ankle Int 1989; 10: 140–146.

128. Pereira DS, Koval KJ, Resnick RB, et al.: Tibiotalar contact area and pressure distribution: the effect of mortise widening and syndesmosis fixation. Foot Ankle Int 1996; 17: 269–274.

129. Perry J: Anatomy and biomechanics of the hindfoot. Clin Orthop 1983; 177: 9–15.

130. Picciano AM, Rowlands MS, Worrell T: Reliability of open and closed kinetic chain subtalar joint neutral positions and navicular drop test. JOPST 1993; 18: 553–558.

131. Pierrynowski MR, Smith SB: Rear foot inversion/eversion during gait relative to the subtalar joint neutral position. Foot Ankle Int 1996; 17: 406–412.

132. Pohl MB, Messenger N, Buckley JG: Forefoot, rearfoot and shank coupling: effect of variations in speed and mode of gait. Gait Posture 2007; 25: 295–302.

133. Powers CM, Chen PY, Feischl SF, et al.: Comparison of foot pronation and lower extremity rotation in persons with and without patellofemoral pain. Foot Ankle Int 2002; 23: 634–640.

134. Powers CM, Maffucci R, Hampton S: Rearfoot posture in subjects with patellofemoral pain. JOSPT 1995; 22: 155–160.

135. Prieskorn D, Graves S, Yen M, et al.: Integrity of the first metatarsophalangeal joint: a biomechanical analysis. Foot Ankle Int 1995; 16: 357–362.

136. Prieskorn DW, Mann RA, Fritz G: Radiographic assessment of the second metatarsal: measure of first ray hypermobility. Foot Ankle Int 1996; 17: 331–333.

137. Radakovich M, Malone T: The superior tibiofibular joint: the forgotten joint. J Orthop Sports Phys Ther 1982; 3: 129–132.

138. Randle JA, Kreder HJ, Stephen D, et al.: Should calcaneal fractures be treated surgically? A meta-analysis. Clin Orthop 2000; 377: 217–227.

139. Renstrom P, Wertz M, Incavo S, et al.: Strain in the lateral ligaments of the ankle. Foot Ankle 1988; 9: 59–63.

140. Richardson EG: Injuries to the hallucal sesamoids in the athlete. Foot Ankle 1987; 7: 229–244.

141. Roass A, Andersson GB: Normal range of motion of the hip, knee, and ankle joints in male subjects, 30–40 years of age. Acta Orthop Scand 1982; 53: 205–208.

142. Romanes GJE: Cunningham's Textbook of Anatomy. Oxford: Oxford University Press, 1981.

143. Root ML, Orien WP, Weed JH: Clinical biomechanics: normal and abnormal functions of the foot. Los Angeles: Clinical Biomechanics Corp, 1977.

144. Salathe EP Jr, Arangio GA, Salathe EP: The foot as a shock absorber. J Biomech 1990; 23: 655–659.

145. Salter RB: Textbook of Disorders and Injuries of the Musculoskeletal System. 3rd ed. Baltimore: Williams & Wilkins, 1999.

146. Saltzman CL, Brandser EA, Anderson CM, et al.: Coronal plane rotation of the first metatarsal. Foot Ankle Int 1996; 17: 157–161.

147. Sammarco GJ, Burstein AH, Frankel VH: Biomechanics of the ankle: a kinematic study. Orthop Clin North Am 1973; 4: 75–96.

148. Sammarco GJ, Hockenbury RT: Biomechanics of the foot and ankle. In: Nordin M, Frankel VH, eds. Basic Biomechanics of the Musculoskeletal System. Philadelphia: Lippincott Williams & Wilkins, 2001; 222–255.

149. Sangeorzan BJ: Biomechanics of the subtalar joint. In: Stiehl JB, ed. Inman's Joints of the Ankle. Baltimore: Williams & Wilkins, 1991; 65–74.

150. Sangeorzan BJ: Subtalar Joint: Morphology and Functional Anatomy. In: Stiehl JB, ed. Inman's Joints of the Ankle. Baltimore: Williams & Wilkins, 1991; 31–38.

151. Sarrafian SK: Functional characteristics of the foot and plantar aponeurosis under tibiotalar loading. Foot Ankle 1987; 8: 4–18.

152. Sayli U, Bolukbasi S, Atik OS, Gundogdu S: Determination of tibial torsion by computed tomography. J Foot Ankle Surg 1994; 33: 144–147.

153. Schmalz T, Blumentritt S, Drewitz H, et al.: The influence of sole wedges on frontal plane knee kinetics, in isolation and in combination with representative rigid and semi-rigid ankle-foot-orthoses. Clin Biomech 2006; 21: 631–639.

154. Schneider B, Laubenberger J, Jemlich S, et al.: Measurement of femoral antetorsion and tibial torsion by magnetic resonance imaging. Br J Radiol 1997; 70: 575–579.

155. Scranton PE, McMaster JH, Kelly E: Dynamic fibular function. Clin Orthop 1976; 118: 76–81.

156. Seber S, Hazer B, Kose N, et al.: Rotational profile of the lower extremity and foot progression angle: computerized tomographic examination of 50 male adults. Arch Orthop Trauma Surg 2000; 120: 255–258.

157. Sharkey NA, Ferris L, Donahue SW: Biomechanical consequences of plantar fascial release or rupture during gait: part I—disruptions in longitudinal arch conformation. Foot Ankle Int 1998; 19: 812–820.

158. Shepherd DE, Seedhom BB: The 'instantaneous' compressive modulus of human articular cartilage in joints of the lower limb. Rheumatology (Oxford.) 1999; 38: 124–132.

159. Shepherd DE, Seedhom BB: Thickness of human articular cartilage in joints of the lower limb. Ann Rheum Dis 1999; 58: 27–34.

160. Shereff MJ, Bejjani FJ, Kummer FJ: Kinematics of the first metatarsophalangeal joint. J Bone Joint Surg 1986; 68A: 392–398.

161. Siegler S, Chen J, Schneck CD: The three-dimensional kinematics and flexibility characteristics of the human ankle and subtalar joints-part 1: kinematics. J Biomech Eng 1988; 110: 364–373.

162. Siegler S, Udupa JK, Ringleb SI, et al.: Mechanics of the ankle and subtalar joints revealed through a 3D quasi-static stress MRI technique. J Biomech 2005; 38: 567-578.

163. Singh AK, Starkweather KD, Hollister AM, et al.: Kinematics of the ankle: a hinge axis model. Foot Ankle 1992; 13: 439–446.

164. Smith-Oricchio K, Harris BA: Interrater reliability of subtalar neutral, calcaneal inversion and eversion. JOSPT 1990; 12: 10–15.

165. Snook AG: The relationship between excessive pronation as measured by navicular drop and isokinetic strength of the ankle measurements. Foot Ankle Int 2001; 22: 234–240.

166. Snyder RB, Lipscomb AB, Johnston RK: Relationship of tarsal coalitions to ankle sprains in athletes. J Sports Med 1981; 9: 313–317.

167. Stacoff A, Reinschmidt C, Nigg BM, et al.: Effects of foot orthoses on skeletal motion during running. Clin Biomech (Bristol, Avon) 2000; 15: 54–64.

168. Stagni R, Leardini A, Ensini A: Ligament fibre recruitment at the human ankle joint complex in passive flexion. J Biomech 2004; 37: 1823–1829.

169. Staheli LT: Rotational problems of the lower extremities. Orthop Clin North Am 1987; 18: 503–512.

170. Stephens MM, Sammarco GJ: The stabilizing role of the lateral ligament complex around the ankle and subtalar joints. Foot Ankle 1992; 13: 130–136.

171. Stiehl JB: Anthropomorphic studies of the ankle joint. In: Stiehl JB, ed. Inman's Joints of the Ankle. Baltimore: Williams & Wilkins, 1991; 1–6.

172. Stiehl JB: Biomechanics of the ankle joint. In: Stiehl JB, ed. Inman's Joints of the Ankle. Baltimore: Williams & Wilkins, 1991; 39–64.

173. Stormont DM, Morrey BF, Kain-Nan A, Cass J: Stability of the loaded ankle: relation between articular restraint and primary and secondary static restraints. Am J Sports Med 1985; 13: 295–300.

174. Tanaka A, Okuzumi H, Kobayashi I, et al.: Age-related changes in natural and fast walking. Percept Motor Skills 1995; 80: 217–218.

175. Taylor KF, Bojescul JA, Howard RS, et al.: Measurement of isolated subtalar range of motion: a cadaver study. Foot Ankle Int 2001; 22: 426–432.

176. Thordarson DB, Kumar PJ, Hedman TP, Ebramzadeh E: Effect of partial versus complete plantar fasciotomy on the windlass mechanism. Foot Ankle Int 1997; 18: 16–20.

177. Tiberio D: Pathomechanics of structural foot deformities. Phys Ther 1988; 68: 1840–1849.

178. Tixa S: Atlas of Palpatory Anatomy of the Lower Extremities. New York: McGraw-Hill, 1999.

179. Tochigi Y, Rudert J, Amendola A, et al.: Tensile engagement of the peri-ankle ligaments in stance phase. Foot Ankle Int 2005; 26: 1067–1073.

180. Torburn L, Perry J, Gronley JK: Assessment of rearfoot motion: passive positioning, one-legged standing, gait. Foot Ankle Int 1998; 19: 688–693.

181. Tufescu TV, Buckley R: Age, gender, work capability, and worker's compensation in patients with displaced intraarticular calcaneal fractures. J Orthop Trauma 2001; 15: 275–279.

182. Uchiyama E, Suzuki D, Kura H, et al.: Distal fibular length needed for ankle stability. Foot Ankle Int 2006; 27: 185–189.

183. Viladot A, Lorenzo JC: The subtalar joint: embryology and morphology. Foot Ankle 1984; 5: 54–66.

184. Walker JM, Sue D, Miles-Elkousy N, et al.: Active mobility of the extremities in older subjects. Phys Ther 1984; 64: 919–923.

185. Wanivenhaus A, Pretterklieber M: First tarsometatarsal joint: anatomical biomechanical study. Foot Ankle 1989; 9: 153–157.

186. Ward KA, Soames RW: Morphology of the plantar calcaneocuboid ligaments. Foot Ankle Int 1997; 18: 649–653.

187. Wearing SC, Urry S, Periman P, et al.: Sagittal plane motion of the human arch during gait: a videofluoroscopic analysis. Foot Ankle Int 1998; 19: 738–742.

188. Williams DS III, McClay IS: Measurements used to characterize the foot and the medial longitudinal arch: reliability and validity. Phys Ther 2000; 80: 864–871.

189. Williams DS III, McClay IS, Hamill J: Arch structure and injury patterns in runners. Clin Biomech 2001; 16: 341–347.

190. Williams DS III, McClay IS, Hamill J, Buchanan T: Lower extremity kinematic and kinetic differences in runners with high and low arches. J Appl Biomech 2001; 17: 153–163.

191. Williams P, Bannister L, Berry M, et al.: Gray's Anatomy, The Anatomical Basis of Medicine and Surgery, Br. ed. London: Churchill Livingstone, 1995.

192. Wong Y, Kim W, Ying N: Passive motion characteristics of the talocrural and the subtalar joint by dual Euler angles. J Biomech 2005; 38: 2480–2485.

193. Wright DG, Desai SM, Henderson WH: Action of the subtalar and ankle joint complex during the stance phase of walking. J Bone Joint Surg (Am) 1964; 46A: 361–382.

194. Wu G, Siegler S, Allard P, et al.: ISB recommendation on definitions of joint coordinate systems of various joints for the reporting of human joint motion-part 1: ankle, hip and spine. J Biomech 2002; 35: 543–548.

195. Wynarsky GT, Greenwald AS: Mathematical model of the human ankle joint. J Biomech 1983; 16: 241–251.

196. Yoganandan N, Pintar FA, Seipel R: Experimental production of extra- and intra-articular fractures of the os calcis. J Biomech 2000; 33: 745–749.

197. Yoshioka Y, Siu DW, Scudamore RA, Cooke TDV: Tibial anatomy and functional axes. J Orthop Res 1989; 7: 132–137.

Mechanics and Pathomechanics of Muscle Activity at the Ankle and Foot

CHAPTER CONTENTS

The preceding chapter discusses the bony components of the ankle and foot and describes the architectural organization of the foot. That chapter also identifies the importance of the ligamentous structures in supporting the foot at rest. While the muscles of the leg and ankle play only a limited role in supporting the static foot, they are essential for the proper function of the foot in its most important role, locomotion. The current chapter presents the function of the muscles in the leg and foot and the effects of their impairments.

Specifically, the purposes of this chapter are to

- Examine the actions of the individual muscles of the ankle and foot
- Consider the effects of impaired strength and extensibility of these muscles
- Briefly discuss the roles these muscles play during locomotor activities
- Compare the strengths of the different muscle groups measured in individuals without impairments

The muscles of the ankle and foot include both extrinsic and intrinsic muscles as found in the wrist and hand. The extrinsic muscles are conveniently organized into an anterior group that dorsiflexes the ankle and contributes to extension of the toes, a posterior group that contributes to plantarflexion of the ankle and flexion of the toes, and a lateral group that pronates the foot. Most of these muscles cross several joints of the foot, and an understanding of each muscle's action and function requires careful attention to the muscle's action at each joint.

Individual roles for each intrinsic muscle of the foot are less clear. This chapter briefly presents the actions of individual intrinsic muscles and discusses the current understanding of the function of the whole group.

Terminology to describe the actions of the muscles of the ankle and foot is confusing. The last chapter presents the notion of triplanar motion and defines pronation and supination as the combined motions of dorsiflexion, eversion, and abduction or plantarflexion, inversion, and adduction, respectively. Yet the literature typically describes the actions of the muscles of the leg and foot in terms of single-plane movements such as dorsiflexion or inversion [35,76,95]. To avoid continual reinterpretation of the literature, this chapter adheres to the traditional terminology. The reader is reminded that a single-plane motion is only one component of the overall triplanar movement. For example, the peroneus brevis everts the foot and thus can also be described as a pronator of the foot.

Finally, one of the primary functional responsibilities of the muscles of the leg and foot is to control the foot and facilitate the movement of the body over the foot during locomotion, and no discussion of the mechanics of these muscles is complete without reference to their role in gait. The mechanics of normal locomotion are described in detail in Chapter 48. Therefore, the role that these muscles play during locomotion is described only briefly in the current chapter.

DORSIFLEXORS OF THE ANKLE

The dorsiflexor muscles of the ankle are found in the anterior compartment of the leg and include the anterior tibialis, the extensor hallucis longus, the extensor digitorum longus, and the peroneus tertius (*Fig 45.1*). All lie anterior to the axis of the ankle joint and thus dorsiflex the ankle [56,95]. Their roles at the other joints of the foot depend on their location with respect to each joint. The dorsiflexor group provides two important functions during locomotion: During the swing phase when the foot is off the ground, the dorsiflexor muscles help lift the foot and toes off the ground to provide adequate ground clearance. The second function occurs at, and immediately after, ground contact, when the dorsiflexors oppose the plantarflexion moment imparted to the foot by the ground reaction force and control the descent of the foot onto the ground (*Fig. 45.2*). During swing, the muscles contract concentrically and isometrically; following contact, the contraction is primarily eccentric.

All of the dorsiflexor muscles are stabilized at the ankle by the extensor retinaculum, which prevents the tendons from pulling away from the ankle joint, or **bowstringing**, as the ankle dorsiflexes. (See Chapter 17 for more information about bowstringing.)

Anterior Tibialis

The anterior tibialis is the largest dorsiflexor muscle, with a physiological cross-sectional area that is as much as twice the physiological cross-sectional area of the rest of the dorsiflexor muscles combined [11,94] (*Muscle Attachment Box 45.1*).

ACTIONS

MUSCLE ACTION: ANTERIOR TIBIALIS

Action	Evidence
Ankle dorsiflexion	Supporting
Inversion of foot	Supporting

The role of the anterior tibialis in dorsiflexion of the ankle is undisputed. Reports of its maximum dorsiflexion moment arm range from approximately 30 to 70 mm [10,38,45,49,59,85] (*Fig. 45.3*). In contrast, less agreement exists regarding its ability to invert the foot. Some suggest that the muscle lies so close to the axis of the subtalar joint, that its effect on that joint is

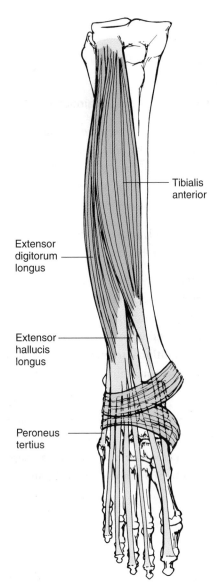

Figure 45.1: The dorsiflexor muscles of the foot include the anterior tibialis, the extensor hallucis longus, the extensor digitorum longus, and the peroneus tertius.

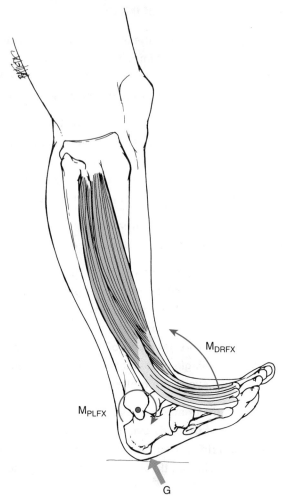

Figure 45.2: The dorsiflexor muscles must generate an extension (dorsiflexion) moment (M_{DRFX}) to balance the flexion (plantarflexion) moment (M_{PLFX}) applied by the ground reaction force (G).

negligible [54]. Others report a small inversion moment on the subtalar joint [15]. A comprehensive study using cadaver specimens and live subjects investigated the contribution of the anterior tibialis during inversion of the whole foot, not just inversion at the subtalar joint [3]. This study demonstrates that while the anterior tibialis never contracts alone to invert the foot, it actively contracts during inversion of the foot in most individuals. Other investigators also note that the activity of the anterior tibialis in inversion is variable [7]. A biomechanical analysis to measure its inversion moment arm estimates lengths of approximately 10 mm or less, considerably smaller than its dorsiflexion moment arm and the inversion moment arm of the posterior tibialis and flexor hallucis longus, which may explain its variable activity during inversion [45]. Just as the anterior tibialis contracts eccentrically to control plantarflexion of the ankle at heel strike in gait, its ability to invert

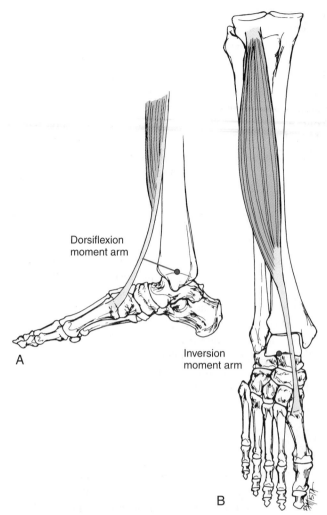

Figure 45.3: The tibialis anterior exhibits a large dorsiflexion moment arm **(A)**, but has a much smaller moment arm for inversion **(B)**.

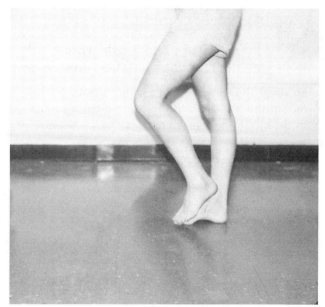

Figure 45.4: Drop foot. Significant weakness of the anterior tibialis can lead to a "drop foot" during the swing phase of gait, when the muscle is needed to lift the foot for toe clearance.

the foot may help control the pronation that occurs normally just after heel strike. Regardless of the extent of the tibialis anterior's participation in inversion, it is important to recognize that the anterior tibialis is able to produce some combination of dorsiflexion and inversion (i.e., pronation and supination) because it is a multijointed muscle, producing dorsiflexion (pronation) at the ankle and inversion (supination) at the subtalar and transverse tarsal joints.

The anterior tibialis's contribution to active inversion explains its ability to provide dynamic support to the medial longitudinal arch. As noted in the previous chapter, the primary support to the arches of the feet during quiet stance is ligamentous. Yet individuals with flattened arches exhibit increased activity of the anterior tibialis as well as other muscles of the leg during dynamic functions [7]. This increased activity may indicate an attempt to increase the stability of the foot.

EFFECTS OF WEAKNESS

Although there are other dorsiflexor muscles, its size and mechanical advantage make the anterior tibialis the strongest of the dorsiflexors. With the ankle positioned in neutral, electrical stimulation of the anterior tibialis produced 42% of the total dorsiflexion torque produced by a maximum voluntary contraction of all of the dorsiflexors [57]. Thus weakness of the anterior tibialis severely weakens, but does not eliminate, active ankle dorsiflexion. Loss of the anterior tibialis alone impairs the ability to control the foot after heel contact during normal locomotion. Inability to control the foot may cause the individual to slap the ground with the foot immediately after contact, often producing an audible **foot slap.** Weakness of the anterior tibialis in conjunction with weakness of the other dorsiflexor muscles may lead to an inability to lift the foot away from the ground during the swing phase of gait. Inadequate dorsiflexion during swing produces a **foot drop** in which the foot dangles toward the ground as the limb advances, making ground clearance difficult (*Fig. 45.4*). In addition, isolated weakness of the anterior tibialis leaves the peroneus longus, its antagonist, unopposed, producing plantarflexion of the first metatarsal [45].

EFFECTS OF TIGHTNESS

Tightness of the anterior tibialis develops in the absence of adequate plantarflexion strength. The forefoot is pulled medially, accentuating the medial longitudinal arch and producing a **cavus foot.**

MUSCLE ATTACHMENT BOX 45.2

ATTACHMENTS AND INNERVATION OF THE EXTENSOR HALLUCIS LONGUS

Proximal attachment: Middle half of the medial surface of the fibula and the adjacent anterior surface of the interosseous membrane

Distal attachment: Dorsal aspect of the base of the distal phalanx of the hallux

Innervation: Deep peroneal nerve (L5, S1)

Palpation: The tendon is easily palpated on the dorsum of the foot and ankle, but the muscle belly lies deep to the anterior tibialis and extensor digitorum longus and cannot be palpated directly.

Extensor Hallucis Longus

The extensor hallucis longus has a smaller physiological cross-sectional area than either the anterior tibialis or the extensor digitorum longus [11,94] (*Muscle Attachment Box 45.2*).

ACTIONS

MUSCLE ACTION: EXTENSOR HALLUCIS LONGUS

Action	Evidence
Extension of the metatarso-phalangeal and interphalangeal joints of great toe	Supporting
Ankle dorsiflexion	Supporting
Inversion of foot	Inadequate

The role of the extensor hallucis at the great toe is clear. The extensor hallucis longus provides the only active extension force to the interphalangeal joint and the primary active extension force to the metatarsophalangeal joint. The extensor hallucis longus has only a slightly smaller moment arm for dorsiflexion at the ankle than the anterior tibialis and, consequently, also contributes to active ankle dorsiflexion. In contrast, although some authors report that the extensor hallucis longus contributes to inversion of the foot [43], it crosses very close to the axis of the subtalar joint, and its contribution to the subtalar joint is unclear [56]. A study of cadaver specimens and live subjects demonstrates a slight ability to supinate the whole foot and reveals electromyographic activity of the extensor hallucis longus during some supination activities of the whole foot, such as lifting the medial side of the foot from the ground when standing [3].

EFFECTS OF WEAKNESS

Weakness of the extensor hallucis longus weakens extension at the metatarsophalangeal and interphalangeal joints of the great toe. Since it is the only extensor at the interphalangeal

joint, weakness in interphalangeal joint extension is diagnostic for extensor hallucis longus weakness.

During normal locomotion, an individual contacts the ground with the heel of the foot first. The ground reaction force applies a plantarflexion moment to the whole foot, which is resisted by all of the dorsiflexors. Weakness of the extensor hallucis longus diminishes an individual's ability to control the descent of the medial portion of the foot, particularly the great toe. Patients with weakness of the extensor hallucis longus also report that the toe tends to fold under the foot when they are pulling on socks or shoes and can cause tripping.

EFFECTS OF TIGHTNESS

Tightness of the extensor hallucis longus pulls the metatarsophalangeal joint of the great toe into extension, which, as in the fingers and thumb, tends to produce flexion at the interphalangeal joint as the flexor hallucis longus is stretched, and a **claw toe deformity** emerges. Hyperextension of the great toe pulls the plantar plate distally, exposing the metatarsal head to excessive loads and producing pain. Similarly, hyperextension of the metatarsophalangeal joint pulls the interphalangeal joint into the toe box of a shoe, causing pain and calluses, or corns, on the dorsal surface of the interphalangeal joint.

Clinical Relevance

CLAW DEFORMITIES OF THE TOES: *Claw toe deformities in a foot with sensation are quite painful. Claw deformities in a foot without sensation put the individual at risk of skin breakdown as the result of increased pressure under the metatarsal heads and between the dorsal surfaces of the toes and the shoe.*

Extensor Digitorum Longus

The extensor digitorum longus has a physiological cross-sectional area greater than that of the extensor hallucis longus but may be only half the area of the anterior tibialis [11, 94]. (*Muscle Attachment Box 45.3*).

ACTIONS

MUSCLE ACTION: EXTENSOR DIGITORUM LONGUS

Action	Evidence
Extension of the metatarso-phalangeal joints of lateral four toes	Supporting
Extension of PIP and DIP joints of lateral four toes	Supporting
Ankle dorsiflexion	Supporting
Eversion of foot	Supporting

MUSCLE ATTACHMENT BOX 45.3

ATTACHMENTS AND INNERVATION OF THE EXTENSOR DIGITORUM LONGUS

Proximal attachment: Lateral surface of the lateral condyle of the tibia, proximal two thirds to three quarters of the medial surface of the fibula, deep fascia, and adjacent anterior surface of the interosseous membrane

Distal attachment: Extensor hood mechanism on the dorsum of the metatarsophalangeal joints and proximal phalanges of the four lateral toes. A central slip inserts to the base of the middle phalanx, and two collateral strips insert to the base of the distal phalanx.

Innervation: Deep peroneal nerve (L5, S1)

Palpation: The tendons are readily palpated along the dorsum of the foot and across the lateral four metatarsophalangeal joints.

MUSCLE ATTACHMENT BOX 45.4

ATTACHMENTS AND INNERVATION OF THE PERONEUS TERTIUS

Proximal attachment: Distal one third or more of the medial surface of the fibula and adjoining surface of the interosseous membrane (This muscle is a partially separated portion of the extensor digitorum longus.)

Distal attachment: Medial part of the dorsal surface of the base of the fifth metatarsal bone

Innervation: Deep peroneal nerve (L5, S1)

Palpation: If present, the tendon is palpated on the dorsolateral surface of the foot as it inserts into the base of the fifth metatarsal bone.

hallucis longus tightness, the resulting claw toe deformities are painful and functionally limiting.

Peroneus Tertius

The peroneus tertius is part of the extensor digitorum longus and is absent in about 5% of the population (*Muscle Attachment Box 45.4*). When present, it is visible on the lateral aspect of the dorsum of the foot. It is the smallest of the dorsiflexor muscles [11].

ACTIONS

MUSCLE ACTION: PERONEUS TERTIUS

Action	Evidence
Ankle dorsiflexion	Supporting
Eversion of foot	Supporting

The role of the peroneus tertius in ankle dorsiflexion and foot eversion are well accepted [76,84,95]. However, its size and variable presence suggests that it plays only an accessory role in these movements.

EFFECTS OF WEAKNESS

Weakness of the peroneus tertius occurs in conjunction with weakness of the extensor digitorum longus and the other dorsiflexor muscles. Consequences of isolated weakness, albeit unlikely, are probably minimal.

EFFECTS OF TIGHTNESS

Like weakness, isolated tightness of the peroneus tertius is unlikely, and the consequences of concomitant tightness of the extensor digitorum longus are greater than any potential consequences of peroneus tertius tightness.

Reports agree that the extensor digitorum longus is the primary extensor of the metatarsophalangeal joints of the lateral four toes and, with the intrinsic muscles of the foot, contributes to extension of the proximal and distal interphalangeal joints of these toes [43,68,76,95]. Similarly, its participation in ankle dorsiflexion is well accepted [43,68,76,95]. The extensor digitorum longus possesses a dorsiflexion moment arm similar to those of the anterior tibialis and extensor hallucis longus.

Several authors report that the extensor digitorum longus participates in eversion of the foot [30,43,84], and its location lateral to the axis of the subtalar joint measured in cadavers supports this view [56]. Data from live subjects reveal a consistent role in active eversion [3].

EFFECTS OF WEAKNESS

As the primary extensor to the metatarsophalangeal joints of the lateral toes, weakness of the extensor digitorum longus decreases an individual's ability to lift the toes from the ground during the swing phase of gait and, like the extensor hallucis longus, to control the descent of the toes onto the ground as the heel contacts the ground.

EFFECTS OF TIGHTNESS

Tightness of the extensor digitorum longus produces effects on the lateral toes similar to those produced by tightness of the extensor hallucis longus on the great toe. The metatarsophalangeal joints are hyperextended, and typically, the proximal and distal interphalangeal joints flex as the result of the stretch on the flexor digitorum longus. As with extensor

SUPERFICIAL MUSCLES OF THE POSTERIOR COMPARTMENT

The superficial muscles of the posterior compartment include the gastrocnemius, soleus, and plantaris muscles (*Fig. 45.5*). These three muscles form the bulk of the calf musculature and give the calf its characteristic shape. Although many other muscles contribute to the total plantarflexion torque available at the ankle, estimates suggest that these three muscles contribute 60–87% of the total plantarflexion torque [13, 24, 66, 80].

   The gastrocnemius and soleus insert jointly on the posterior surface of the calcaneus by way of the tendo calcaneus (Achilles tendon) and together form the triceps surae. The plantaris may also join the Achilles tendon. The functions of these three muscles at the ankle and hindfoot are similar and depend on their common attachment to the Achilles tendon. To appreciate the behavior of the superficial muscles of the posterior compartment, it is useful to examine the mechanics of the Achilles tendon.

Achilles Tendon

The Achilles tendon is the thickest and strongest tendon of the body [95]. Its attachment onto the posterior surface of the calcaneus gives the triceps surae muscles a large moment arm and a significant mechanical advantage in plantarflexion [45, 51,78,85] (*Fig. 45.6*). Estimates of the plantarflexion moment arm of the Achilles tendon vary from approximately 5 to 6 cm.

   Reports of the effects of ankle position on Achilles tendon length are conflicting. Some studies report that the plantarflexion moment arm of the Achilles tendon is maximum when the ankle is in neutral [60,85]. However, others report that the moment arm increases as the ankle plantarflexes [24,45,78]. All reports agree that the Achilles tendon possesses the largest moment arm of all the muscles that cross the ankle. [45,85]. The Achilles tendon also possesses an inversion moment arm, at least when the foot is in the neutral or pronated position. So both the grastrocnemius and soleus potentially contribute to inversion of the hindfoot [3,45,98].

   The strength and stiffness of the Achilles tendon contribute to the overall stiffness of the ankle and increase the efficiency of gait by enabling the tendon to store energy as it is stretched like a spring during the stance phase of gait. [18,79,87]. The Achilles tendon exhibits up to approximately 5–6% **strain** (percent change in length) during vigorous plantarflexion contractions and normal gait [48,52]. The elasticity

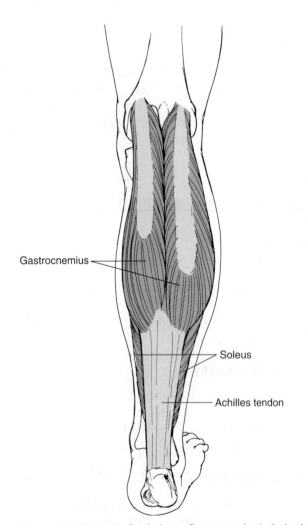

Figure 45.5: The superficial plantarflexor muscles include the gastrocnemius, soleus, and the plantaris (not pictured).

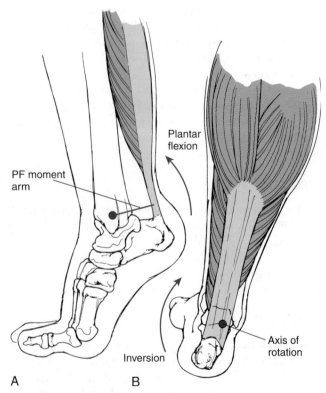

Figure 45.6: The Achilles tendon has a large moment arm for plantarflexion **(A)** and a small moment arm for inversion **(B)**.

of the Achilles tendon provides passive energy to activities such as walking, running and jumping and plays an important role in maximizing the efficiency of these activities [37,48,50].

Cadaver data suggest that the ultimate strength of the Achilles tendon is approximately 4600 N (1034 lb) at low loading rates and increases with loading rate [96]. Despite its, size and strength, the Achilles tendon is the most frequently ruptured tendon in the body, and the incidence of rupture is increasing [23,96]. One reason for the high incidence of injury may be related to the vascular supply to the tendon, which is reduced in the tendon's midsection, between its attachments to the muscle bellies and to the calcaneus [12].

Clinical Relevance

ACHILLES TENDON RUPTURES: *Achilles tendon ruptures are more common in sedentary individuals who participate in sporadic, physically strenuous activity. During his first term as vice-president of the United States, Mr. Al Gore ruptured his Achilles tendon playing tennis, a typical scenario. Clinicians may help to reduce the incidence of such injuries by actively instructing individuals to gradually increase their level of physical activity and to avoid sudden bursts of intense activity without appropriate preconditioning.*

Gastrocnemius

The gastrocnemius is the superficial muscle of the calf, and its two muscle bellies are easily identified on the posterior surface of the leg (*Muscle Attachment Box 45.5*).

MUSCLE ATTACHMENT BOX 45.5

ATTACHMENTS AND INNERVATION OF THE GASTROCNEMIUS

Proximal attachment: Medial head: Upper and posterior part of the medial femoral condyle behind the adductor tubercle and from a slightly raised area on the popliteal surface of the femur above the medial condyle

Lateral head: Upper and posterior part of the lateral surface of the lateral femoral condyle and lower part of the corresponding supracondylar line

Distal attachment: Posterior surface of the calcaneus via the tendo calcaneus

Innervation: Tibial nerve (S1, S2)
Palpation: The gastrocnemius muscle bellies are palpated as two almost symmetrical muscle masses in the proximal one half of the posterior leg.

ACTIONS

MUSCLE ACTION: GASTROCNEMIUS

Action	Evidence
Ankle plantarflexion	Supporting
Inversion of foot	Supporting
Knee flexion	Supporting

Investigators agree that the gastrocnemius plays a major role in plantarflexion of the ankle. It functions with the soleus to lift the weight of the body when rising onto the forefoot [3,7,30,43]. It is active during the stance phase of gait to assist in forward progression and to control the forward glide of the body over the stance foot [67]. It also helps to stabilize the ankle as the individual rolls over and off the foot in late stance [35,82,83]. The inversion moment arm of the Achilles tendon supports the role of the gastrocnemius in inversion.

The gastrocnemius crosses the knee and has a significant moment arm for flexion of the knee. The moment arm increases from almost zero when the knee is extended to more than 3 cm when the knee is flexed beyond 90° [14,45] (*Fig. 45.7*). This allows the gastrocnemius to generate a substantial flexion moment at the knee, although the hamstrings are the primary flexors of the knee.

Clinical Relevance

TESTING KNEE FLEXION STRENGTH: *Because the gastrocnemius is capable of producing knee flexion, it is important for the clinician to detect any substitutions made by the gastrocnemius when testing the strength of the hamstrings (Fig. 45.8). The clinician must ensure that the ankle remains relaxed when testing the strength of the hamstring muscles specifically.*

EFFECTS OF WEAKNESS

The gastrocnemius provides substantial plantarflexion force, and loss of the gastrocnemius produces a large decrease in plantarflexion strength. Decreased plantarflexion strength hampers an individual's ability to rise up on toes or climb hills or ladders, and normal locomotion is impaired significantly [73].

EFFECTS OF TIGHTNESS

Tightness of the gastrocnemius may limit an individual's dorsiflexion range of motion (ROM), but because it crosses the knee and the ankle, its effect on ankle ROM depends on knee position. A clinician identifies tightness of the gastrocnemius by examining dorsiflexion ROM with the patient's knee extended, putting the gastrocnemius on stretch, and with the knee flexed, putting the muscle on slack (*Fig. 45.9*). Most individuals exhibit less dorsiflexion ROM with the knee extended

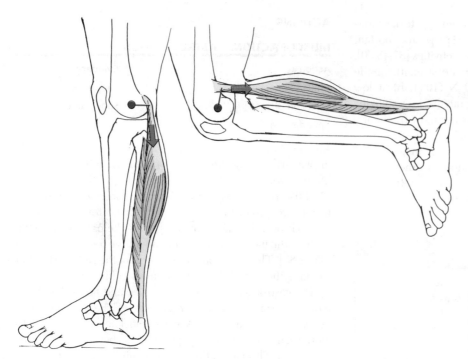

Figure 45.7: The moment arm of the gastrocnemius at the knee is smaller when the knee is extended than when the knee is flexed to 90°.

than with the knee flexed [75,80]. Reports of peak dorsiflexion ROM with the knee extended range from 10 to 18° in individuals without pathology [62,64,75]. Moseley uses normative data from 300 male and female subjects without pathology to suggest that dorsiflexion of less than 4° with the knee extended indicates hypomobility [62]. Normal upright standing posture requires the ability to reach neutral dorsiflexion with the knee extended. Extreme tightness of the gastrocnemius causes the individual to stand on the forefoot without heel contact or to stand with the knees flexed. Normal locomotion uses

approximately 5° of dorsiflexion with the knee extended, and tightness of the gastrocnemius muscle may impair an individual's ability to roll over the foot later in the stance phase of locomotion [44,47,65]. Using a mechanical simulation of gastrocnemius tightness, Matjacic et al suggest that gastrocnemius tightness results in a significant increase in knee flexion at initial contact and midstance [58].

Soleus

The soleus lies deep to the gastrocnemius and possesses the largest physiological cross-sectional area of all of the muscles of the leg (*Muscle Attachment Box 45.6*). Its physiological cross-sectional area is approximately twice that of the gastrocnemius [11,94].

ACTIONS

MUSCLE ACTION: SOLEUS

Action	Evidence
Ankle plantarflexion	Supporting
Inversion of foot	Supporting

Like the gastrocnemius, the soleus is undoubtedly a plantarflexor [7,30,43,76,95]. With its large cross-sectional area, it is capable of large forces. The soleus is composed mostly of type I muscle fibers, while the gastrocnemius consists of approximately half type I and half type II fibers [40,61,63,80]. Electromyographic activity of the soleus is apparent in low-resistance plantarflexion, while activity of the gastrocnemius appears with increased resistance [28]. Similarly, high-velocity contractions with the knee extended recruit the gastrocnemius more than the soleus [81,88]. However, when the knee

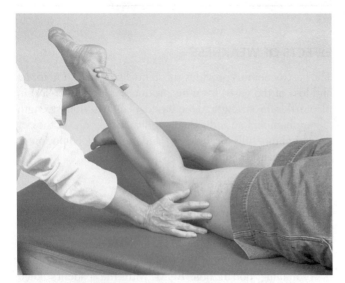

Figure 45.8: Active plantarflexion during resisted knee flexion suggests that the subject is using the gastrocnemius as a knee flexor to enhance knee flexion strength.

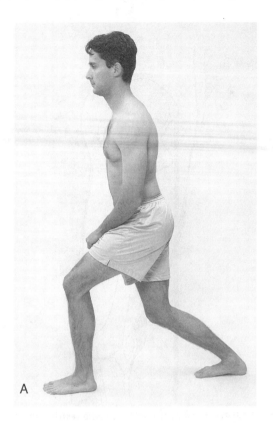

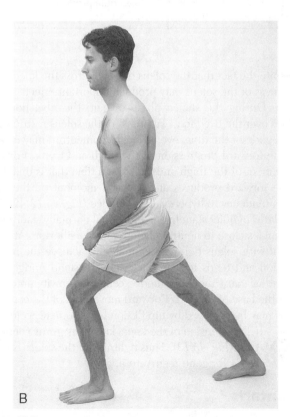

Figure 45.9: A. With the knee flexed, the gastrocnemius is on slack, and ankle dorsiflexion ROM is limited only by the soleus and the joint capsule. B. With the knee extended, the gastrocnemius is stretched, and ankle dorsiflexion ROM is reduced.

MUSCLE ATTACHMENT BOX 45.6

ATTACHMENTS AND INNERVATION OF THE SOLEUS

Proximal attachment: Posterior surface of the head and proximal 1/4 to 1/3 of the shaft of the fibula, soleal line and middle 1/3 of the medial border of the tibia, and a fibrous band between the tibia and fibula

Distal attachment: Posterior surface of the calcaneus via the tendo calcaneus

Innervation: Tibial nerve (S1, S2)

Palpation: The soleus is palpable just deep to the medial and lateral borders of the gastrocnemius as the muscle bellies of the gastrocnemius insert into the Achilles tendon *(Fig. 45.10)*.

is flexed, the soleus is recruited regardless of plantarflexion velocity. Increasing the pedaling speed during cycling appears to produce greater activation of the gastrocnemius with little change in soleus recruitment [81].

These studies suggest that the soleus and gastrocnemius play related but distinct roles in lower extremity function. The soleus appears well suited to play a larger role in such phasic

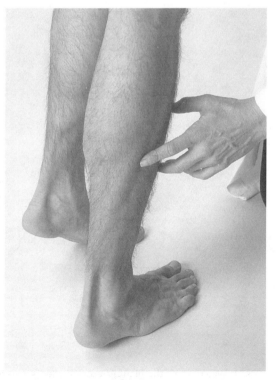

Figure 45.10: The soleus is palpated along the distal borders of the gastrocnemius bellies as they insert into the Achilles tendon.

activities as controlling upright posture, while the gastrocnemius is critical in high-velocity and forceful activities such as jumping [7,19]. Both the gastrocnemius and soleus muscles are active during the stance phase of gait, although the activity of the soleus begins earlier, and the activity of the gastrocnemius lasts longer [35,82]. The soleus and gastrocnemius both contribute to forward progression in stance, but the soleus helps to decelerate the leg as the body glides forward over the fixed foot during midstance [67]. Like the gastrocnemius, the soleus with its insertion into the Achilles tendon has a small inversion moment arm, suggesting that the soleus can contribute to inversion of the hindfoot [3,45].

EFFECTS OF WEAKNESS

Weakness of the soleus produces a significant loss in plantarflexion strength with resulting impairments in locomotion. Weakness of the soleus impairs the ability to control the leg as the body glides over the stance foot, and excessive ankle dorsiflexion during stance may result. In addition, an individual with weakness of the soleus has difficulty rolling onto the forefoot later in stance and, consequently, may exhibit a late heel rise [73] (*Fig. 45.11*).

EFFECTS OF TIGHTNESS

Tightness of the soleus also restricts dorsiflexion ROM; however, unlike tightness of the gastrocnemius, the resulting **plantarflexion contracture** is independent of knee position.

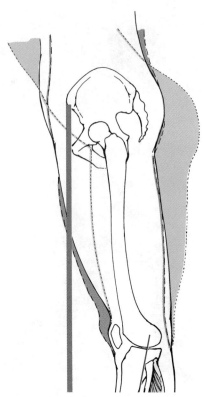

Figure 45.12: Tightness of the soleus muscle restricts the forward progression of the tibia during stance. The forward progression of the thigh and trunk over the fixed tibia produces an extension moment (M_{EXT}) on the knee joint.

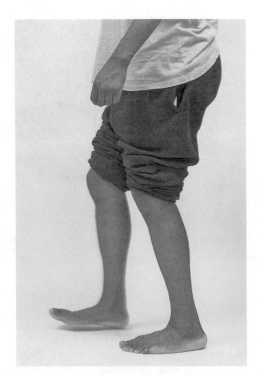

Figure 45.11: Weakness of the plantarflexor muscles is manifested in the latter half of the stance phase of gait by inadequate roll off and often a late heel rise.

Despite the fact that the soleus does not cross the knee joint, tightness of the soleus may produce important effects on the knee. During the stance phase of gait, the tibia normally glides over the fixed foot. Tightness of the soleus restricts forward glide of the tibia, even though momentum may continue the forward progression of the thigh and trunk. Forward movement of the thigh and trunk on a tibia that is unable to move forward produces an extension moment on the knee and a tendency to hyperextend the knee (*Fig. 45.12*) [29,58]. Similarly, in quiet standing an individual normally stands with the ankles close to neutral plantar- and dorsiflexion. An individual with soleus tightness is unable to achieve the neutral position and tends to lean backward. To stand upright, the individual must move the body's center of gravity anteriorly over the base of support. Forward movement of the center of mass may be achieved by hip flexion but also may occur with hyperextension of the knee, known as **genu recurvatum** (*Fig. 45.13*). Thus tightness of the soleus is a risk factor for genu recurvatum.

Plantaris

The plantaris is a small muscle that lies between the gastrocnemius and soleus muscles (*Muscle Attachment Box 45.7*). Cadaver studies suggest that it is absent in 5–10% of the population [91,95], although examination of 40 individuals

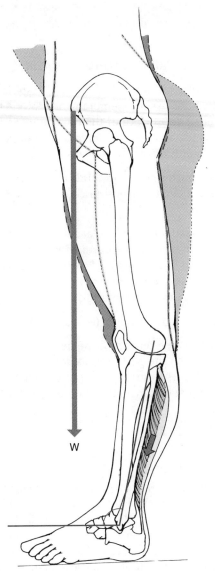

Figure 45.13: Tightness of the soleus may contribute to a genu recurvatum (hyperextension) deformity of the knee by holding the ankle in plantarflexion, tending to cause the individual to lean backward. To keep the center of mass over the base of support, an individual leans forward. The forward lean may occur at the hips or at the knee. Forward lean at the knee produces genu recurvatum.

undergoing surgical repair of a ruptured Achilles tendon revealed absence of the plantaris in 24 (60%) of the subjects [36].

ACTIONS

MUSCLE ACTION: PLANTARIS

Action	Evidence
Ankle plantarflexion	Inadequate
Inversion of foot	Inadequate
Knee flexion	Inadequate

MUSCLE ATTACHMENT BOX 45.7

ATTACHMENTS AND INNERVATION OF THE PLANTARIS

Proximal attachment: Lower part of the lateral supracondylar ridge, adjacent part of the popliteal surface of the femur, and oblique popliteal ligament

Distal attachment: Posterior surface of the calcaneus via the tendo calcaneus

Innervation: Tibial nerve (S1, S2)

Palpation: Not palpable

Although the plantaris crosses the knee and ankle in line with the medial gastrocnemius, its size and variable presence suggests that it provides no unique function at the ankle and foot.

EFFECTS OF WEAKNESS AND TIGHTNESS

Impairments of the plantaris cannot be identified clinically.

Clinical Relevance

"TENNIS LEG": *An injury known as tennis leg is characterized by the sudden, acute onset of pain in the posteromedial aspect of the upper calf, usually following sudden and rapid weight bearing on the leg, such as a fall off a curb or a lunge for a tennis ball. Historically, these complaints were attributed to an isolated tear of the plantaris muscle. The inability to perform a clinical test to assess the integrity of the muscle prevented verification of the injury. More recently, the complaints have been associated with a tear of the medial head of the gastrocnemius. Only one known case report verifies the occurrence of an isolated tear of the plantaris muscle, confirmed at surgery [26].*

DEEP MUSCLES OF THE POSTERIOR COMPARTMENT

The deep muscles of the posterior compartment of the leg include the posterior tibialis, flexor digitorum longus, and flexor hallucis longus (*Fig. 45.14*). These muscles wrap around the medial aspect of the ankle and foot, where they are easily palpated. The tendons of the posterior tibialis, flexor digitorum longus, and flexor hallucis longus are contained with the neurovascular bundle in the **tarsal tunnel** formed by the deltoid ligament and the flexor retinaculum [41]. Entrapment of the nerve or tendons is reported as they enter or exit the tarsal tunnel.

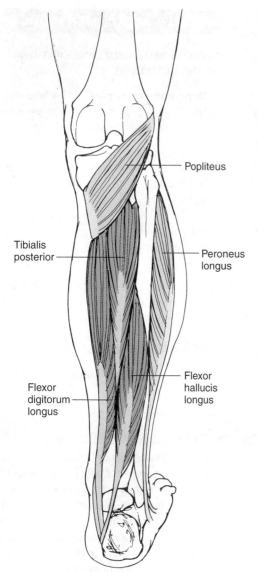

Figure 45.14: The deep muscles of the posterior compartment of the leg include the posterior tibialis, the flexor digitorum longus, and the flexor hallucis longus.

MUSCLE ATTACHMENT BOX 45.8

ATTACHMENTS AND INNERVATION OF THE POSTERIOR TIBIALIS

Proximal attachment: Medial part: Posterior surface of the interosseous membrane and lateral area on the posterior surface of the tibia between soleal line above and the junction of the middle and lower thirds of the shaft below

Lateral part: Upper two thirds of posterior fibular surface, deep transverse fascia, and intermuscular septa

Distal attachment: Navicular tuberosity and plantar surface of medial cuneiform with tendinous bands to tip and distal margin of the sustentaculum tali [76], all tarsal bones except the talus, and bases of the middle three metatarsals

Innervation: Tibial nerve (L4, L5)

Palpation: The tendon of the posterior tibialis is palpated along the posterior border of the medial malleolus. The muscle belly can be palpated just posterior to the medial surface of the shaft of the tibia.

Posterior Tibialis

The posterior tibialis is the deepest of the deep muscles of the posterior compartment of the leg [95] (*Muscle Attachment Box 45.8*). Its physiological cross-sectional area is more than the physiological cross-sectional area of the other two deep muscles combined [11,94].

ACTIONS

MUSCLE ACTION: POSTERIOR TIBIALIS

Action	Evidence
Inversion of foot	Supporting
Ankle plantarflexion	Supporting

The posterior tibialis has an inversion moment arm at the subtalar joint of almost 3 cm, almost three times that of the anterior tibialis [45]. Its size and large moment arm make it the primary inverter of the subtalar joint, and electromyographic data support this role [3]. Similarly, its extensive attachment on the other tarsal bones contributes to its effectiveness in inverting the whole foot [55]. In contrast, its plantarflexion moment arm at the ankle is approximately 1 cm and approaches zero when the ankle is plantarflexed [85]. The posterior tibialis with the other deep muscles of the posterior compartment produces some plantarflexion torque, but its primary action is inversion [66].

The posterior tibialis also appears to contribute to the dynamic support of the medial longitudinal arch [16,42]. The preceding chapter reports that the ligaments of the foot are the primary support of the arches of the foot during static posture. However, muscles provide additional support to the foot during activity such as locomotion. The posterior tibialis helps control the descent of the arch during loading and contributes to the restoration of the arch later in stance [69,82].

EFFECTS OF WEAKNESS

Weakness of the posterior tibialis impairs inversion strength, producing at least a 50% reduction in strength [42]. The posterior tibialis is an important stabilizer of the forefoot, and weakness impairs an individual's ability to rise up on the toes, even with intact plantarflexor muscles, because the foot is unstable. Weakness also produces an imbalance with the everter muscles, and the foot tends to evert and abduct; that is, it tends to pronate [25,55,89]. Patients with posterior tibialis tendon dysfunction (PTTD) exhibit increased pronation at the hindfoot and forefoot, reflecting the muscle's extensive role in supporting most of the foot [89]. PTTD is a primary cause of acquired flat feet and alters the normal movement of the tarsal bones during weight bearing and gait [31,69]. Factors associated with increased risk of PTTD are obesity, aging, hypertension, diabetes, and vascular insufficiency within the tendon [31]. A preexisting flat foot deformity also appears to be a risk factor for a rupture of the posterior tibialis. [16]. Arai et al. report increased resistance to glide of the posterior tibialis around the medial malleolus in specimens with flat feet [4]. The increased frictional force on the posterior tibialis tendon may contribute to the tendon's increased risk of rupture in individuals with flat feet.

MUSCLE ATTACHMENT BOX 45.9

ATTACHMENTS AND INNERVATION OF THE FLEXOR DIGITORUM LONGUS

Proximal attachment: Medial part of the posterior surface of the tibia inferior to the soleal line and the fascia covering tibialis posterior

Distal attachment: Plantar surface of the base of the distal phalanx of the lateral four digits

Innervation: Tibial nerve (L5, S1, S2)

Palpation: The tendon of the flexor digitorum longus is palpated just posterior to the posterior tibialis tendon at the medial malleolus.

Clinical Relevance

POSTERIOR TIBIALIS RUPTURE: *Spontaneous rupture of the posterior tibialis tendon produces pain and significant functional limitations. It frequently occurs after a prolonged episode of chronic tendinitis. Its association with preexisting foot deformities, obesity, aging, and hypertension suggests that treatments to control the flat foot such as orthotic devices to limit pronation may help to reduce the stress on the posterior tibialis tendon and may help prevent rupture. Outcome studies are needed to determine the efficacy of such interventions.*

EFFECTS OF TIGHTNESS

Tightness of the posterior tibialis pulls the foot into inversion and adduction of the forefoot and may include slight plantarflexion, producing a **varus** or an **equinovarus deformity** of the foot. Such deformities are often found in individuals with spasticity of the posterior tibialis or with an imbalance between the posterior tibialis and the everters of the foot [77].

Flexor Digitorum Longus

The flexor digitorum longus has a cross-sectional area similar to that of the flexor hallucis longus, and considerably smaller than that of the posterior tibialis [11,94] (*Muscle Attachment Box 45.9*). It is palpable just posterior to the posterior tibialis tendon as it wraps around the medial malleolus.

ACTIONS

MUSCLE ACTION: FLEXOR DIGITORUM LONGUS

Action	Evidence
Flexion of the metatarsophalangeal, PIP and DIP joints of the lateral four toes	Supporting
Ankle plantarflexion	Supporting
Inversion of foot	Supporting

The flexor digitorum longus clearly flexes the joints of the toes and is the sole muscle able to flex the distal interphalangeal joints of the toes.

Clinical Relevance

MANUAL MUSCLE TESTING OF THE FLEXOR DIGITORUM LONGUS: *An isolated manual muscle test to assess the strength of the flexor digitorum longus requires manual resistance to flexion of the distal interphalangeal joints of the toes. Because this muscle is the only muscle capable of flexing these joints, weakness in flexion of the distal interphalangeal joint confirms flexor digitorum longus weakness.*

Although flexion of the toes is the open-chain activity of the flexor digitorum longus, in the closed-chain activity of locomotion, the muscle functions to stabilize the toes and foot against the ground reaction force that tends to extend, or dorsiflex, the toes and midfoot as the body rolls over the foot (*Fig. 45.15*).

Assessment of plantarflexion moment arms at the ankle reveals that the flexor digitorum longus has a larger plantarflexion moment arm than the posterior tibialis. However, its small size limits its potential to produce plantarflexion. Although the data are limited, the flexor digitorum longus appears to have a substantial inversion moment arm and participates consistently with the posterior tibialis during inversion of the foot [3].

EFFECTS OF WEAKNESS

Weakness of the flexor digitorum longus produces weakness in toe flexion, most clearly identified at the distal interphalangeal joints. Functionally, weakness of the flexor digitorum longus produces difficulty in stabilizing the foot and toes during stance and is manifested by delayed or limited heel rise as the body rolls over the foot.

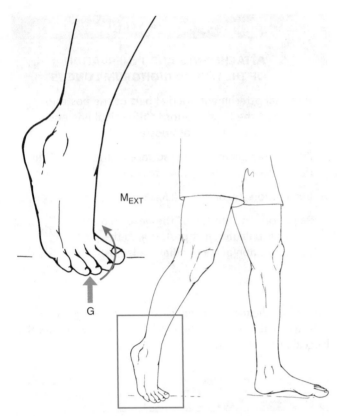

Figure 45.15: The ground reaction force (G) applies an extension moment (M_{EXT}) on the toes as the body rolls off the stance foot.

MUSCLE ATTACHMENT BOX 45.10

ATTACHMENTS AND INNERVATION OF THE FLEXOR HALLUCIS LONGUS

Proximal attachment: Distal two thirds of the posterior surface of the fibula, the adjacent interosseous membrane, and the fascia covering the tibialis posterior

Distal attachment: Plantar aspect of the base of the distal phalanx of the hallux

Innervation: Tibial nerve (L5, S1, S2)

Palpation: The tendon of the flexor hallucis longus is palpated posterior and slightly distal to the medial malleolus.

EFFECTS OF TIGHTNESS

Tightness of the flexor digitorum longus impairs extension ROM of the toes. It can occur with tightness of the extensor digitorum longus and contributes to the claw toe deformities described earlier.

Flexor Hallucis Longus

The flexor hallucis longus lies deeper and posterior to the tendons of the posterior tibialis and flexor digitorum longus (*Muscle Attachment Box 45.10*).

ACTIONS

MUSCLE ACTION: FLEXOR HALLUCIS LONGUS

Action	Evidence
Flexion of the metatarsophalangeal, interphalangeal joints of the great toe	Supporting
Ankle plantarflexion	Supporting
Inversion of foot	Supporting

The flexor hallucis longus is the primary flexor of the great toe and is the only muscle to flex the interphalangeal joint of the great toe. Like the flexor digitorum longus, manual muscle testing at the interphalangeal joint isolates the flexor

hallucis longus and identifies weakness in that muscle. The flexor hallucis longus possesses a larger plantarflexion moment arm than the posterior tibialis or flexor digitorum longus and contributes plantarflexion torque to the ankle [45,85,95]. Although the soleus and gastrocnemius are the primary plantarflexors of the ankle, some individuals appear to recruit the flexor hallucis longus as an important plantarflexor as well [17]. Individuals who have sustained an Achilles tendon rupture recruit the flexor hallucis longus more than the soleus during submaximal contractions of both the injured and uninjured ankles. Whether this recruitment pattern is the result of the injury or a motor pattern that predisposes an individual to injury is unclear. But these data reinforce the role of the flexor hallucis longus as an ankle plantarflexor.

Although some studies report that it is similar in size to the flexor digitorum longus [11,94], others suggest that the flexor hallucis longus is larger and stronger than the flexor digitorum longus [66,93]. In contrast, the flexor hallucis longus has the smallest inversion moment arm of the three muscles and contributes variably to inversion of the foot [3,45].

EFFECTS OF WEAKNESS

Weakness of the flexor hallucis longus weakens flexion of the great toe and probably contributes to decreased plantar flexion strength. Weakness may also contribute to slight inversion weakness. A case report of a strain or partial rupture in a 42-year-old man documents pain and weakness in toe flexion and plantarflexion [33].

EFFECTS OF TIGHTNESS

Tightness of the flexor hallucis longus limits extension of the joints of the toes particularly when the ankle is dorsiflexed. Plantarflexing the ankle puts the muscle on slack and allows more toe extension [33].

Tightness of the flexor hallucis longus also is implicated in a claw deformity of the great toe.

Tightness of the flexor hallucis longus may also contribute to foot pain in the medial longitudinal arch. Runners occasionally develop pain along the flexor hallucis longus tendon as the result of repeatedly stretching the contracting muscle during the push off phase of running.

Clinical Relevance

RUNNING STRETCHES: *Most runners are familiar with the need to stretch the plantarflexor muscles before and after running. However the flexor hallucis longus is frequently ignored during those stretches. Runners need to learn to include stretching the big toe into hyperextension at the MTP joint to help avoid irritation of the flexor hallucis longus tendon. Stretches must stabilize the ankle and metatarsal of the great toe in neutral in order to provide adequate stretch to the flexor hallucis longus tendon.*

MUSCLES OF THE LATERAL COMPARTMENT OF THE LEG

The peroneus longus and brevis lie on the lateral aspect of the leg and are palpable as they curve around the lateral malleolus (*Fig. 45.16*). Although not the only everters of the foot, they appear to be the primary everters, contributing an estimated 65% of the total work capacity of the everters [13].

Peroneus Longus

The peroneus longus is palpable through much of its length along the lateral aspect of the leg (*Muscle Attachment Box 45.11*).

ACTIONS

MUSCLE ACTION: PERONEUS LONGUS

Action	Evidence
Eversion of foot	Supporting
Ankle plantarflexion	Supporting
Plantarflexion of first ray	Supporting

The peroneus longus clearly everts the foot, exhibiting an eversion moment arm of 1–3 cm and a larger physiological cross-sectional area than the peroneus brevis [11,45,94]. Cadaver studies reveal that it possesses a plantarflexion moment arm, although considerably smaller than that of the Achilles tendon [45,85]. In vivo, it appears to play only a secondary role in plantarflexion of the ankle [3,13].

The peroneus longus plays an important role in stabilizing the forefoot by plantarflexing the first ray, although this role

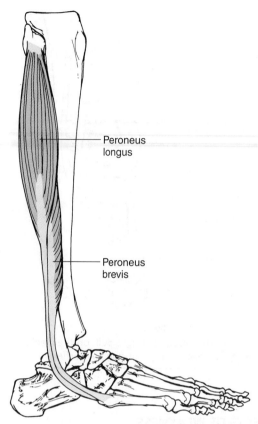

Figure 45.16: The muscles of the lateral compartment consist of the peroneus longus and brevis.

frequently is ignored [56,90] (*Fig. 45.17*). This function is apparent during gait, as the peroneus longus is active in midstance to stabilize the forefoot as the body moves over the foot [9,22,35,82].

MUSCLE ATTACHMENT BOX 45.11

ATTACHMENTS AND INNERVATION OF THE PERONEUS LONGUS

Proximal attachment: Fibers from the lateral condyle of the tibia, head and proximal two thirds of the lateral surface of the fibula, and anterior and posterior crural intermuscular septa

Distal attachment: Lateral side of the base of the first metatarsal bone and medial cuneiform by two slips and occasionally a third slip to the base of the second metatarsal bone [95]

Innervation: Superficial peroneal nerve (L5, S1)

Palpation: The peroneus longus muscle belly is palpated just distal to the head of the fibula. The tendon is palpated just posterior to the lateral malleolus.

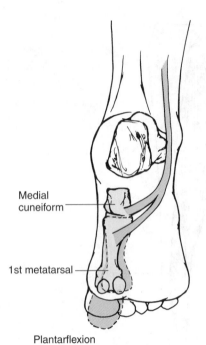

Figure 45.17: The peroneus longus pulls on the medial cuneiform and first metatarsal bone, producing plantarflexion of the first ray.

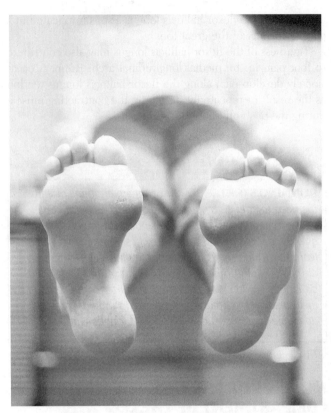

Figure 45.18: Plantarflexed first ray. This individual with Charcot Marie Tooth disorder has severely plantarflexed first rays resulting from significant muscle weakness and imbalance with tightness of the peroneus longus bilaterally. Note the large calluses on the metatarsal heads of the great toes.

EFFECTS OF WEAKNESS

Weakness of the peroneus longus contributes to weakness in eversion of the foot. Consequently, the inverters, particularly the posterior tibialis, pull the foot into inversion or inversion with plantarflexion, and a varus, or equinovarus, deformity results [6,77].

EFFECTS OF TIGHTNESS

The peroneus longus is a multijointed muscle, affecting the ankle, hindfoot, and forefoot, but tightness in the peroneus longus is most apparent distally. Although tightness may limit inversion ROM of the subtalar joint, tightness is manifested primarily by a plantarflexed first ray [56]. In weight bearing the plantarflexed first ray may produce excessive loading on the metatarsal head of the great toe, which can lead to pain and large callus formation under the first metatarsal head (*Fig. 45.18*). Weight bearing in upright stance with a plantarflexed first ray also produces a supination moment on the foot (*Fig. 45.19*). Consequently, individuals with a plantarflexed first ray as a result of tightness in the peroneus longus tendon may exhibit a supinated foot in stance [1,56]. Thus a person may stand with the foot supinated as the result of either tightness or weakness of the peroneus longus.

Peroneus Brevis

The peroneus brevis lies anterior to the peroneus longus (*Muscle Attachment Box 45.12*).

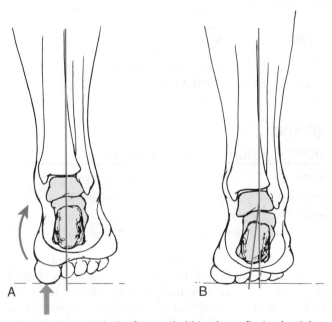

Figure 45.19: A. With the first ray held in plantarflexion by tightness of the peroneus longus, the ground reaction force during stance produces a supination moment on the foot. **B.** If supination ROM is available, the individual with tightness of the peroneus longus is likely to stand in supination.

MUSCLE ATTACHMENT BOX 45.12

ATTACHMENTS AND INNERVATION OF THE PERONEUS BREVIS

Proximal attachment: Distal two thirds of the lateral surface of the fibula and the anterior and posterior crural intermuscular septa

Distal attachment: Lateral tubercle on the base of the fifth metatarsal bone

Innervation: Superficial peroneal nerve (L5, S1)

Palpation: The peroneus brevis tendon is palpated as it emerges from posterior to the lateral malleolus and travels toward the base of the fifth metatarsal. The muscle belly may be palpated proximal to the malleolus and posterior to the peroneus longus tendon.

ACTIONS

MUSCLE ACTION: PERONEUS BREVIS

Action	Evidence
Eversion of foot	Supporting
Ankle plantarflexion	Supporting

The peroneus brevis is unquestionably an everter of the foot, affecting the subtalar and transtarsal joints of the foot [55,76,95]. It has a moment arm similar to and perhaps slightly larger than that of the peroneus longus. Like the peroneus longus, the peroneus brevis also possesses a small but measurable moment arm for plantarflexion [45,85].

Clinical Relevance

INVERSION SPRAINS OF THE ANKLE: *Most ankle sprains occur as the result of a sudden, forceful medial twist of the ankle, producing an* **inversion sprain.** *This movement applies a vigorous tensile force to the ligaments and tendons on the lateral aspect of the ankle, including the peroneus brevis. These ligaments and tendons, in turn, apply tensile forces to their attachments. Chapter 3 notes that bone sustains larger compressive forces than tensile forces before failure. When the ultimate failure strength of the tendon or ligament exceeds the ultimate strength of the bone, the tendon or ligament pulls a piece of bone from the rest of the bone, producing an* **avulsion fracture,** *instead of a torn tendon or ligament. An inversion sprain frequently produces an avulsion fracture of the fifth metatarsal at its tuberosity by pulling the peroneus brevis from its distal attachment.*

EFFECTS OF WEAKNESS

Weakness of the peroneus brevis decreases eversion strength and contributes to an imbalance between the inverter and everter muscles. Consequently, weakness of the peroneus brevis increases the relative contribution of the inverters and leads to a varus hindfoot deformity [25,56,77].

EFFECTS OF TIGHTNESS

Although rare, tightness of the peroneus brevis may contribute to valgus deformities of the foot. However, other factors such as weakness of the posterior tibialis or overactivity of the extensor digitorum longus also are important contributors to valgus deformities of the foot.

INTRINSIC MUSCLES OF THE FOOT

The intrinsic muscles of the foot exhibit many similarities with the intrinsic muscles of the hand. However, although the data are limited, the intrinsic muscles of the foot appear to function as a single large group, at least during weight-bearing activities. Therefore, this chapter briefly presents the reported actions of the individual intrinsic muscles and then discusses the group function. The intrinsic muscles are organized into four layers and are described here by layer, starting with the most superficial.

First Muscular Layer in the Foot

The first muscular layer is just deep to the plantar aponeurosis described in Chapter 44. This layer contains the abductor hallucis, flexor digitorum brevis, and the abductor digiti minimi (*Fig. 45.20*).

ABDUCTOR HALLUCIS

MUSCLE ACTION: ABDUCTOR HALLUCIS

Action	Evidence
Abduction of metatarsophalangeal joint of great toe	Insufficient
Flexion of metatarsophalangeal joint of great toe	Insufficient

The reported action of the abductor hallucis is flexion and abduction of the metatarsophalangeal joint of the great toe (*Muscle Attachment Box 45.13*). Unlike its counterpart in the thumb, the abductor hallucis has no attachment into an extensor hood mechanism and, therefore, has no direct action on the interphalangeal joint.

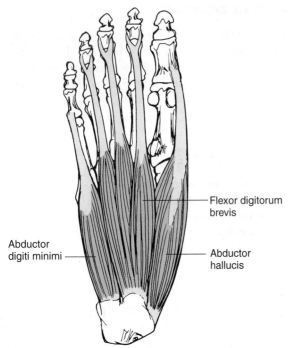

Figure 45.20: The first layer of intrinsic muscles includes the abductor hallucis, flexor digitorum brevis, and abductor digiti minimi.

FLEXOR DIGITORUM BREVIS

MUSCLE ACTION: FLEXOR DIGITORUM BREVIS

Action	Evidence
Flexion of metatarsophalangeal joints of lateral four toes	Insufficient
Flexion of proximal interphalangeal joints of lateral four toes	Insufficient

The insertion of the flexor digitorum brevis is almost identical to that of its homologue in the hand, the flexor digitorum

MUSCLE ATTACHMENT BOX 45.13

ATTACHMENTS AND INNERVATION OF THE ABDUCTOR HALLUCIS

Proximal attachment: Flexor retinaculum, medial process of the calcanean tuberosity, plantar aponeurosis, and intermuscular septum

Distal attachment: Medial side of the base of the proximal phalanx of the hallux

Innervation: Medial plantar nerve (S1, S2)

Palpation: The abductor hallucis is palpated on the medial aspect of the foot.

MUSCLE ATTACHMENT BOX 45.14

ATTACHMENTS AND INNERVATION OF THE FLEXOR DIGITORUM BREVIS

Proximal attachment: Medial process of the calcanean tuberosity, central part of the plantar aponeurosis, and intramuscular septa

Distal attachment: By two tendons (having been perforated by the long flexor tendons) to the middle phalanx of the four lateral digits

Innervation: Medial plantar nerve (S1, S2)

Palpation: Not palpable

superficialis (*Muscle Attachment Box 45.14*). Its apparent action is similar, flexion of the metatarsophalangeal and proximal interphalangeal joints.

ABDUCTOR DIGITI MINIMI

MUSCLE ACTION: ABDUCTOR DIGITI MINIMI

Action	Evidence
Abduction of metatarsophalangeal joint of little toe	Insufficient
Flexion of metatarsophalangeal joint of little toe	Insufficient

Like the abductor hallucis, the abductor digiti minimi lacks an attachment to an extensor hood mechanism (*Muscle Attachment Box 45.15*). Consequently, its reported actions are limited to flexion and abduction of the metatarsophalangeal joint of the little toe.

MUSCLE ATTACHMENT BOX 45.15

ATTACHMENTS AND INNERVATION OF THE ABDUCTOR DIGITI MINIMI

Proximal attachment: Both processes of the calcanean tuberosity, plantar surface of the bone between them, lateral part of the plantar aponeurosis, and intermuscular septum

Distal attachment: Lateral side of the base of the proximal phalanx of the fifth toe

Innervation: Lateral plantar nerve (S1, S2, S3)

Palpation: The abductor digiti minimi is palpated on the lateral aspect of the foot.

MUSCLE ATTACHMENT BOX 45.16

ATTACHMENTS AND INNERVATION OF THE FLEXOR DIGITORUM ACCESSORIUS

Proximal attachment: Medial head: Medial concave surface of the calcaneus below the groove for the tendon of flexor hallucis longus. Lateral head: Calcaneus distal to the lateral process of the calcanean tuberosity, long plantar ligament

Distal attachment: Lateral border of the tendon of flexor digitorum longus

Innervation: Lateral plantar nerve (S1, S2, S3)

Palpation: Not palpable

Second Muscular Layer in the Foot

The second muscular layer of the foot contains the flexor digitorum accessorius and the lumbricals.

FLEXOR DIGITORUM ACCESSORIUS

MUSCLE ACTION: FLEXOR DIGITORUM ACCESSORIUS

Action	Evidence
Flexion of proximal and distal interphalangeal joints of the lateral four toes	Insufficient

The flexor digitorum accessorius is unique to the foot and is a necessary development, coincident with the development of bipedal ambulation (*Muscle Attachment Box 45.16*). Contraction of the flexor digitorum longus pulls the toes medially, since the muscle enters the foot from its medial aspect. The pull of the flexor digitorum accessorius on the tendons of the flexor digitorum longus redirects the force on the toes, producing flexion of the toes in the sagittal plane (*Fig. 45.21*). The pull of the flexor digitorum accessorius on the flexor digitorum longus provides a vivid example of vector addition.

LUMBRICALS

MUSCLE ACTION: LUMBRICALS

Action	Evidence
Flexion of metatarsophalangeal joints of lateral four toes	Insufficient
Extension of interphalangeal joints of lateral four toes	Insufficient

The lumbricals of the foot are almost identical to those in the hand with the exception that they travel and attach to the medial sides of the toes, while the lumbrical muscles in the hand lie on the lateral (radial) side of the fingers (*Muscle Attachment Box 45.17*). The apparent actions also are similar: flexion of the metatarsophalangeal joints and extension of the interphalangeal joints by their pull on the extensor hood mechanism.

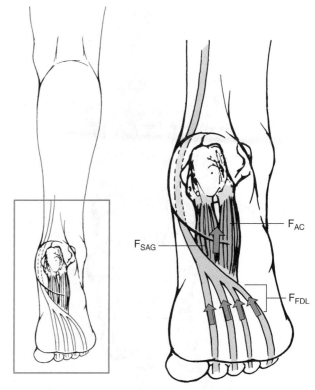

Figure 45.21: The pull of the flexor accessorius (F_{AC}) on the tendons of the flexor digitorum longus adds to the force (F_{FDL}) of the flexor digitorum longus to produce a flexion force (F_{SAG}) on the toes in the sagittal plane.

MUSCLE ATTACHMENT BOX 45.17

ATTACHMENTS AND INNERVATION OF THE LUMBRICALS

Proximal attachment: Four small muscles that arise from the tendons of the flexor digitorum longus tendons. They each arise from the sides of two adjacent tendons except for the first, which arises only from the medial border of the first tendon.

Distal attachment: Proximal phalanges via tendinous fibers inserting on the medial side of the dorsal hood of the four lateral digits

Innervation: First lumbrical: Medial plantar nerve (S1, S2)

Lateral three lumbricals: Lateral plantar nerve (S2, S3) [76], deep branch of lateral plantar nerve (S2, S3) [95]

Palpation: Not palpable

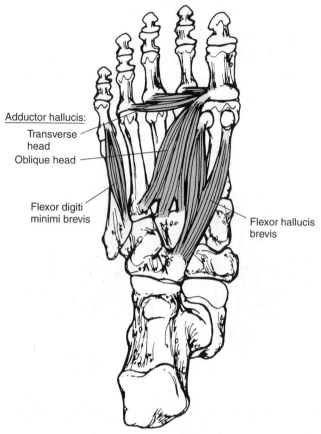

Figure 45.22: The third layer of the intrinsic muscles includes the flexor hallucis brevis, adductor hallucis, and flexor digiti minimi brevis.

Third Muscular Layer in the Foot

The third muscular layer consists of the flexor hallucis brevis, the adductor hallucis, and the flexor digiti minimi brevis (*Fig. 45.22*).

FLEXOR HALLUCIS BREVIS

MUSCLE ACTION: FLEXOR HALLUCIS BREVIS

Action	Evidence
Flexion of metatarsophalangeal joint of great toe	Insufficient

The two tendons of the flexor hallucis brevis each contain a sesamoid bone that increases the angle of pull of the muscle as it inserts onto the proximal phalanx of the great toe (*Muscle Attachment Box 45.18*). The muscle appears well positioned to contribute to flexion of the metatarsophalangeal joint of the great toe.

Clinical Relevance

SESAMOID BONES OF THE GREAT TOE: *The sesamoid bones of the great toe, imbedded in the tendon of the flexor hallucis brevis, increase the mechanical advantage of the*

MUSCLE ATTACHMENT BOX 45.18

ATTACHMENTS AND INNERVATION OF THE FLEXOR HALLUCIS BREVIS

Proximal attachment: Medial part of the plantar surface of the cuboid, adjacent part of the lateral cuneiform, tendon of posterior tibialis, and the medial intermuscular septum

Distal attachment: Base of the proximal phalanx of the hallux

Innervation: Medial plantar nerve (S1, S2)

Palpation: Not palpable

muscle and protect the underlying metatarsal head. In normal walking and running, an individual pivots over these two bones as the body rolls over the foot. Pathology related to these bones can contribute to severe foot pain. Such pathology includes stress fractures and inflammation known as sesamoiditis. Muscle imbalances, abnormal movement patterns, and overuse may contribute to the pathology.

ADDUCTOR HALLUCIS

MUSCLE ACTION: ADDUCTOR HALLUCIS

Action	Evidence
Adduction of metatarsophalangeal joint of great toe	Insufficient
Flexion of metatarsophalangeal joint of great toe	Insufficient

The adductor hallucis has two heads, the oblique and transverse [71] (*Muscle Attachment Box 45.19*). The oblique head is several times larger than the transverse head [5].

MUSCLE ATTACHMENT BOX 45.19

ATTACHMENTS AND INNERVATION OF THE ADDUCTOR HALLUCIS

Proximal attachment: Oblique head: Plantar surface of the base of second, third, and fourth metatarsal bones and fibrous sheath of the tendon of peroneus longus. Transverse head: Plantar metatarsophalangeal ligaments of the third, fourth, and fifth digits and the deep transverse metatarsal ligaments between them

Distal attachment: Lateral sesamoid bone and lateral side of the base of the proximal phalanx of the hallux

Innervation: Deep branch of the lateral plantar nerve (S2, S3)

Palpation: Not palpable

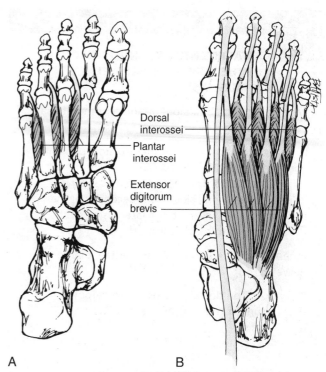

A   B

Figure 45.23: The plantar and dorsal interossei form the fourth layer of the intrinsic muscles of the foot. The extensor digiti brevis is palpable on the dorsal surface of the foot. **A.** Plantar view containing the plantar interossei. **B.** Dorsal view containing the dorsal interossei and the extensor digitorum brevis.

MUSCLE ATTACHMENT BOX 45.20

ATTACHMENTS AND INNERVATION OF THE FLEXOR DIGITI MINIMI BREVIS

Proximal attachment: Medial part of the plantar surface of the base of the fifth metatarsal bone and sheath of peroneus longus

Distal attachment: Lateral side of the base of the proximal phalanx of the fifth digit and some deeper fibers to the lateral part of the distal half of the fifth metatarsal bone [95]

Innervation: Superficial branch of the lateral plantar nerve (S2, S3)

Palpation: Not palpable

It reportedly adducts and flexes the metatarsophalangeal joint of the great toe. Surgeons often release this muscle during surgery to correct a hallux valgus deformity.

MUSCLE ACTION: FLEXOR DIGITI MINIMI BREVIS

Action	Evidence
Flexion of metatarsophalangeal joint of little toe	Insufficient

The flexor digiti minimi reportedly produces flexion of the metatarsophalangeal joint of the little toe (*Muscle Attachment Box 45.20*).

Fourth Muscular Layer in the Foot

The fourth and deepest layer of the foot contains the plantar and dorsal interossei (*Fig. 45.23*).

MUSCLE ACTION: PLANTAR INTEROSSEI

Action	Evidence
Addition of metatarsophalangeal joints of lateral three toes	Insufficient
Flexion of metatarsophalangeal joints of lateral three toes	Insufficient
Extension of interphalangeal joints of lateral three toes	Insufficient

The three plantar interossei are very similar to their counterparts in the hand, the palmar interossei (*Muscle Attachment Box 45.21*). Lying on the medial side of the lateral three toes, they adduct the metatarsophalangeal joints, pulling the toes toward the reference toe, the second toe. Like the palmar interossei, they contribute to metatarsophalangeal joint flexion and by their insertion into the extensor hood, contribute to interphalangeal joint extension.

MUSCLE ACTION: DORSAL INTEROSSEI

Action	Evidence
Abduction of metatarsophalangeal joints of middle three toes	Insufficient
Flexion of metatarsophalangeal joints of middle three toes	Insufficient
Extension of interphalangeal joints of middle three toes	Insufficient

The four dorsal interossei are capable of producing metatarsophalangeal joint abduction of the second toe in the medial

MUSCLE ATTACHMENT BOX 45.21

ATTACHMENTS AND INNERVATION OF THE PLANTAR INTEROSSEI (3 MUSCLES)

Proximal attachment: Base and medial side of the third, fourth, and fifth metatarsal bones

Distal attachment: Medial side and base of the proximal phalanx of the same toe and the dorsal digital expansion [95]

Innervation: Deep branch of the lateral plantar nerve (S2, S3)

Palpation: Not palpable

MUSCLE ATTACHMENT BOX 45.22

ATTACHMENTS AND INNERVATION OF THE DORSAL INTEROSSEI (4 MUSCLES)

Proximal attachment: Sides of adjacent metatarsal bones by two heads

Distal attachment: Bases of the proximal phalanx and dorsal digital expansion. The first inserts into the medial side of the second toe; the second inserts to the lateral side of the second toe; the third and fourth insert to the lateral side of the third and fourth toes, respectively.

Innervation: Deep branch of the lateral plantar nerve (S2, S3)

Palpation: The dorsal interossei are palpated on the dorsum of the foot between adjacent metatarsals.

MUSCLE ATTACHMENT BOX 45.23

ATTACHMENTS AND INNERVATION OF THE EXTENSOR DIGITORUM BREVIS

Proximal attachment: Anterior superolateral surface of the calcaneus, the interosseous talocalcaneal ligament, and inferior extensor retinaculum

Distal attachment: Dorsal aspect of the base of the proximal phalanx of the hallux (sometimes referred to as the extensor hallucis brevis) and lateral sides of the tendons of the extensor digitorum longus to the second, third, and fourth toes

Innervation: Lateral terminal branch of the deep peroneal nerve (L5, S1) [95], (S1, S2) [76]

Palpation: The muscle belly of the extensor digitorum brevis is the only muscle belly on the dorsum of the foot and is palpated just distal to the ankle and lateral to the tendons of the extensor digitorum longus.

and lateral direction as well as abduction of the third and fourth toes (*Muscle Attachment Box 45.22*). In addition, they apparently can produce flexion of the metatarsophalangeal joints and extension of the interphalangeal joints.

Extensor Digitorum Brevis

MUSCLE ACTION: EXTENSOR DIGITORUM BREVIS

Action	Evidence
Extension of interphalangeal joints of medial four toes	Insufficient
Extension of interphalangeal joints of middle three toes	Insufficient

The extensor digitorum brevis sends tendons to the medial four toes (*Muscle Attachment Box 45.23*). The most medial tendon extends to the great toe and is sometimes known as the extensor hallucis brevis. This tendon crosses only the metatarsophalangeal joint that it helps to extend. The other three slips of the extensor digitorum brevis blend with the tendons of the extensor digitorum longus and, therefore, assist with extension of all three joints of these toes.

Group Effects of the Intrinsic Muscles of the Foot

Although some individuals are able to actively abduct their toes and even isolate the lumbricals and interossei by flexing the metatarsophalangeal joints while extending the interphalangeal joints of the toes, most individuals are incapable of fine motor control of the toes. Studies of the intrinsic muscles of the foot suggest that these muscles function as a group during weight-bearing activities [7,53]. The classic study by Mann and Inman, now over 40 years old, remains the cornerstone of current understanding of the role of the intrinsic muscles [53]. This study demonstrates activity of the whole group during the stance phase of gait, as the foot is supinating. This activity is interpreted as a contribution to the stabilization of the foot as the body rolls over it onto the opposite foot. Individuals with excessive pronation exhibit increased activity of the intrinsic muscles of the foot, apparently to provide additional support to a foot that remains too flexible. Finally, this study and others repeatedly demonstrate that the intrinsic muscles of the foot are quiet during normal quiet standing, confirming the notion that static foot alignment is supported primarily by inert tissues [7,97].

Weakness of the intrinsic muscles contributes to a loss of muscle balance in the foot and leads to an accentuated medial longitudinal arch and claw toe deformities [1,25].

COMPARISONS OF GROUP MUSCLE STRENGTH

An understanding of the relative strengths of the major muscle groups of the ankle and foot helps the clinician make clinical judgments of strength impairments in the leg. Most of the studies of strength in the muscles of the leg focus on the strength of plantarflexion and dorsiflexion. These studies reveal, as expected, that plantarflexion is significantly stronger than dorsiflexion [20,34,92]. These comparisons consistently demonstrate that the plantarflexors produce at least three times more peak torque than the dorsiflexors (*Table 45.1*).

TABLE 45.1: Comparisons of Peak Plantar and Dorsiflexion Torques

	Subjects	Peak Plantarflexion Torque (Nm)[a]	Peak Dorsiflexion Torque
Gadeberg et al. [20]	6 women, 12 men (age, 29–64 years)	117 ± 26	32 ± 8
Vandervoort and McComas [92]	11 men	171 ± 34	43.5 ± 6.5
	11 women (age, 20–32 years)	113 ± 35	26.6 ± 4.5

[a]Measured with the knee flexed to between 70 and 80°.

Such a difference in peak torque is consistent with the large difference in total muscle mass between the two groups, which shows a three- to fourfold difference in cross-sectional area [20]. The strength comparisons reported in *Table 45.1* are based on plantarflexion torque measurements made with the knee flexed. Studies suggest that peak plantarflexion torque increases by 10–20% when measured with the knee extended [46,80].

Several factors influence the peak plantar- and dorsiflexion torque produced. Plantar- and dorsiflexion torques are greater in men than in women and both decrease steadily with age [21,32,39,86,92]. Joint position also affects torque measurements by altering muscle length and moment arm. (Chapter 4 describes these effects in detail.) The length of the muscle appears to be the greater influence on isometric peak plantarflexion torque, which occurs with the ankle positioned just short of maximum dorsiflexion [8,70,80]. In contrast, peak dorsiflexion occurs with the ankle in approximately 10° of plantarflexion [34,57]. Studies demonstrate that the moment arms of the dorsiflexors are longest when the ankle is at neutral or slightly dorsiflexed, and shortest when the ankle is plantarflexed [45,49,78,85]. In contrast, the length of the dorsiflexor muscles is shortest in dorsiflexion and longest in plantarflexion. The peak torque output of the dorsiflexors appears to be affected by both muscle length and angle of application, so that, like the biceps brachii at the elbow and the quadriceps femoris at the knee, peak dorsiflexion torque occurs with the ankle in a midposition where neither angle of application nor muscle length is optimal, but where their combined effect produces the largest torque output.

Fewer studies compare the strength of the inverter and everter muscles of the foot. Although they report no direct comparison, Paris and Sullivan report peak forces of 75.22 ± 20.99 N (17 ± 4.7 lb) and 74.73 ± 21.09 N (16.8 ± 4.7 lb) for inversion and eversion, respectively, when the ankle is in neutral dorsiflexion [72]. Other studies reporting concentric and eccentric strengths find little or no difference between the two groups. Studies report torques of 27 Nm and 24 Nm for inversion and eversion, respectively at 60°/sec and 16 Nm for both groups at 120°/sec [2,27]. After lateral ankle sprains, eversion strength appears reduced compared with inversion strength [2,74]. Perhaps a goal of rehabilitation following ankle sprains should be to restore the equality of strength between the everter and inverter muscles.

Table 45.2 presents the physiological cross-sectional areas of the muscles that can invert and those that can evert the foot reported by Brand for a single male subject [11]. If only the posterior tibialis as the primary muscle of inversion is compared with only the primary everters, peroneus longus and brevis, the latter have a slight advantage in size. However, the moment arm of the posterior tibialis is larger than those of the peroneus longus and brevis, and thus it is not surprising that strength of these two groups is similar. Recruitment of additional muscles to invert or evert the foot changes these relationships.

Clinical Relevance

STRENGTH TESTING OF INVERSION AND EVERSION: *Data suggest that the strength of inversion and eversion of the foot is similar. However, if the subject is allowed to use toe muscles during one or both motions, the group strengths are altered. To monitor a patient's change in strength, the clinician must use caution to ensure that the same procedure is followed and that the same muscles participate during each test.*

TABLE 45.2: Physiological Cross-Sectional Areas (PCAs) of Muscles That Invert and Evert the Foot

Inverters	PCA (cm²)	Everters	PCA (cm²)
Posterior tibialis	26.27	Peroneus longus	24.65
Flexor digitorum longus	6.4	Peroneus brevis	19.61
Flexor hallucis longus	18.52	Extensor digitorum longus	7.46
Anterior tibialis	16.88	Peroneus tertius	4.14

SUMMARY

This chapter presents the muscles that move the ankle and joints of the foot. The extrinsic muscles of the foot are organized according to their function and data are presented to explain their relative contributions to the motions of the ankle and foot. It is demonstrated that while the anterior tibialis is the strongest dorsiflexor muscle, other muscles contribute significantly to dorsiflexion torque. Similarly, the posterior tibialis and the peroneus longus and brevis are the primary inverter and everters, respectively, but additional muscles make important contributions to both motions. The gastrocnemius and soleus together contribute most of the plantarflexion moment, but other muscles provide some plantarflexion as well. Strength comparisons reveal that plantarflexion is considerably stronger than dorsiflexion. Inversion and eversion strengths are more similar to each other, although contributions from muscles affecting the toes can alter that comparison.

The role of these muscles in normal locomotion is presented, and the effects of impairments on normal locomotion discussed. Details of normal locomotion are presented in Chapter 48. However, before proceeding to discussions of posture and gait, it is useful to examine the loads to which the foot is subjected during activities such as quiet standing, walking, and running. Chapter 46 discusses the forces applied to the foot by the surrounding muscles and limb segments during various activities of daily life.

References

1. Alexander IJ, Johnson KA: Assessment and management of pes cavus in Charcot-Marie-Tooth disease. Clin Orthop 1989; 246: 273–281.
2. Amaral de Noronha M, Borges NG: Lateral ankle sprain: isokinetic test reliability and comparison between invertors and evertors. Clin Biomech 2004; 19: 868–871.
3. Ambagtsheer JBT: The function of the muscles of the lower leg in relation to movements of the tonsus. Acta Orthop Scand 1978; 172: 1–196.
4. Arai K, Ringleb SI, Zhao KD, et al.: The effect of flatfoot deformity and tendon loading on the work of friction measured in the posterior tibial tendon. Clin Biomech 2007; 22: 592–598.
5. Arakawa T, Tokita K, Miki A, et al.: Anatomical study of human adductor hallucis muscle with respect to its origin insertion. Ann Anat 2003; 185: 585–592.
6. Barnes MJ, Herring JA: Combined split anterior tibial-tendon transfer and intramuscular lengthening of the posterior tibial tendon: results in patients who have a varus deformity of the foot due to spastic cerebral palsy. J Bone Joint Surg 1991; 73A: 734–738.
7. Basmajian JV, DeLuca CJ: Muscles Alive. Their Function Revealed by Electromyography. Baltimore: Williams & Wilkins, 1985.
8. Bobbert MF, van Ingen Schenau J: Isokinetic plantar flexion: experimental results and model calculations. J Biomech 1990; 23: 105–119.
9. Bohne WHO, Lee K, Peterson MGE: Action of the peroneus longus tendon on the first metatarsal against metatarsus primus varus force. Foot Ankle Int 1997; 18: 510–512.
10. Bonnefoy A, Doriot N, Senk M, et al.: A non-invasive protocol to determine the personalized moment arms of knee and ankle muscles. J Biomech 2007; 40: 1776–1785.
11. Brand RA, Pedersen DR, Friederich JA: The sensitivity of muscle force predictions to changes in physiologic cross–sectional area. J Biomech 1986; 19: 589–596.
12. Carr AJ, Norris SH: The blood supply of the calcaneal tendon. J Bone Joint Surg 1989; 71B: 100–101.
13. Clarke HD, Kitaoka HB, Ehman RL: Peroneal tendon injuries. Foot Ankle Int 1998; 19: 280–288.
14. Croce RV, Miller JP, St Pierre P: Effect of ankle position fixation on peak torque and electromyographic activity of the knee flexors and extensors. Electromyogr Clin Neurophysiol 2000; 40: 365–373.
15. Czerniecki JM: Foot and ankle biomechanics in walking and running: a review. Am J Phys Med Rehabil 1988; 67: 246–252.
16. Dyal CM, Feder J, Deland JT, Thompson FM: Pes planus in patients with posterior tibial tendon insufficiency: asymptomatic versus symptomatic foot. Foot Ankle Int 1997; 18: 85–88.
17. Finni T, Hodgson JA, Lai AM, et al.: Muscle synergism during isometric plantarflexion in Achilles tendon rupture patients and in normal subjects revealed by velocity-encoded cine phase-contrast MRI. Clin Biomech 2006; 21: 67–74.
18. Fukunaga T, Kubo K, Kawakami Y, et al.: In vivo behaviour of human muscle tendon during walking. Proc R Soc Lond B Biol Sci 2001; 268: 229–233.
19. Furlani J, Vitti M, Costacurta L: Electromyographic behavior of the gastrocnemius muscle. Electromyogr Clin Neurophysiol 1978; 18: 29–34.
20. Gadeberg P, Anderson H, Jakobsen J: Volume of ankle dorsiflexors and plantarflexors determined with stereological techniques. J Appl Physiol 1999; 86: 1670–1675.
21. Gajdosik RL, Vander Linden DW, Williams AK: Concentric isokinetic torque characteristics of the calf muscles of active women aged 20 to 84 years. JOSPT 1999; 29: 181–190.
22. Glasoe WM, Yack HJ, Saltzman CL: Anatomy and biomechanics of the first ray. Phys Ther 1999; 79: 854–859.
23. Gravlee JR, Hatch RL: Achilles tendon rupture: a challenging diagnosis. J Am Board Fam Pract 2000; 13: 371–373.
24. Gregor RJ, Komi PV: A comparison of the triceps surae and residual muscle moments at the ankle during cycling. J Biomech 1991; 24: 287–297.
25. Guyton GP, Mann RA: The pathogenesis and surgical management of foot deformity in Charcot-Marie-Tooth disease. Foot Ankle Clin 2000; 5: 317–326.
26. Hamilton W, Klostermeier T, Lim EVA, Moulton JS: Surgically documented rupture of the plantaris muscle: a case report and literature review. Foot Ankle Int 1997; 18: 522–523.
27. Hartsell HD, Spaulding SJ: Eccentric/concentric ratios at selected velocities for the invertor and evertor muscles of the chronically unstable ankle. Br J Sports Med 1999; 33: 255–258.
28. Herman R, Bragin SJ: Function of the gastrocnemius and soleus muscles. Phys Ther 1967; 47: 105–113.
29. Higginson JS, Zajac FE, Neptune RR, et al.: Effect of equines foot placement and intrinsic muscle response on knee extension during stance. Gait Posture 2006; 23: 32–36.
30. Hislop HJ, Montgomery J: Daniel's and Worthingham's Muscle Testing: Techniques of Manual Examination. Philadelphia: WB Saunders, 1995.
31. Holmes GB, Mann RA: Possible epidemiological factors associated with rupture of the posterior tibial tendon. Foot Ankle 1992; 13: 70–79.

32. Horstmann T, Maschmann J, Mayer F, et al.: The influence of age on isokinetic torque of the upper and lower leg musculature in sedentary men. Int J Sports Med 1999; 20: 362–367.

33. Howard PD: Differential diagnosis of calf pain and weakness: flexor hallucis longus strain. JOSPT 2000; 30: 78–84.

34. Hoy MG, Zajac FE, Gordon ME: A musculoskeletal model of the human lower extremity: the effect of muscle, tendon, and moment arm on the moment-angle relationship of musculotendon actuators at the hip, knee, and ankle. J Biomech 1990; 23: 157–169.

35. Hunt AE, Smith RM, Torode M: Extrinsic muscle activity, foot motion and ankle joint moments during the stance phase of walking. Foot Ankle Int 2001; 22: 31–41.

36. Incavo SJ, Alvarez RG, Trevino SG: Occurrence of the plantaris tendon in patients sustaining subcutaneous rupture of the achilles tendon. Foot Ankle 1987; 8: 110–111.

37. Ishikawa M, Komi PV, Grey MJ, et al.: Muscle-tendon interaction and elastic energy usage in human walking. J Appl Physiol 2005; 99: 603–608.

38. Ito M, Akima H, Fukunaga T: In vivo moment arm determination using B-mode ultrasonography. J Biomech 2000; 33: 215–218.

39. Jan MH, Chai HM, Lin YF et al.: Effects of age and sex on the results of an ankle plantar-flexor manual muscle test. Phys Ther 2005; 85: 1078–1084.

40. Johnson MA, Polgar J, Weightman D, Appleton D: Data on the distribution of fibre types in thirty-six human muscles: an autopsy study. J Neurol Sci 1973; 18: 111–129.

41. Joyce JJ, Harty M: Surgical anatomy and exposures of the foot and ankle. In: AAOS Instructional Course Lectures. St. Louis: CV Mosby, 1970; 1–11.

42. Kaye RA, Jahss MH: Tibialis posterior: a review of anatomy and biomechanics in relation to support of the medial longitudinal arch. Foot Ankle 1991; 11: 244–247.

43. Kendall FP, McCreary EK, Provance PG: Muscle Testing and Function. Baltimore: Williams & Wilkins, 1993.

44. Kerrigan DC: Gender differences in joint biomechanics during walking: normative study in young adults. Am J Phys Med Rehabil 1998; 77: 2–7.

45. Klein P, Mattys S, Rooze M: Moment arm length variations of selected muscles acting on talocrural and subtalar joints during movement: an in vitro study. J Biomech 1996; 29: 21–30.

46. Kulig K, Andrews JG, Hay JG: Human strength curves. Exerc Sport Sci Rev 1984; 12: 417–466.

47. Kuster M, Sakurai S, Wood GA: Kinematic and kinetic comparison of downhill and level walking. Clin Biomech 1995; 10: 79–84.

48. Lichtwark GA, Wilson AM: Is Achilles tendon compliance optimized for maximum muscle efficiency during locomotion? J Biomech 2007; 40: 1768–1775.

49. Maganaris CN: In vivo measurement-based estimations of the moment arm in the human tibialis anterior muscle-tendon unit. J Biomech 2000; 33: 375–379.

50. Maganaris CN, Baltzopoulos V, Sargeant AJ: Human calf muscle responses during repeated isometric plantarflexions. J Biomech 2006; 39: 1249–1255.

51. Maganaris CN, Baltzopoulos V, Sargeant AJ: In vivo measurement-based estimations of the human Achilles tendon moment arm. Eur J Appl Physiol 2000; 83: 363–369.

52. Maganaris CN, Paul JP: Tensile properties of the in vivo human gastrocnemius tendon. J Biomech 2002; 35: 1639–1646.

53. Mann R, Inman VT: Phasic activity of intrinsic muscles of the foot. J Bone Joint Surg 1964; 46A: 469–481.

54. Mann RA: Biomechanical approach to the treatment of foot problems. Foot Ankle 1982; 2: 205–212.

55. Mann RA: Posterior tibial tendon dysfunction: treatment by flexor digitorum longus transfer. Foot Ankle Clin 2001; 6: 77–87.

56. Mann RA, Missirian J: Pathophysiology of Charcot-Marie-Tooth disease. Clinical Orthopaedics and Related Research 1988; 234: 221–228.

57. Marsh E, Sale DG, McComas AJ, Quinlan J: Influence of joint position on ankle dorsiflexion in humans. Journal of Applied Physiology: Respiration, Environment, Exercise Physiology 1981; 51: 160–167.

58. Matjacic Z, Olensek A, Bajd T: Biomechanical characterization and clinical implications of artificially induced toe-walking: differences between pure soleus, pure gastrocnemius and combination of soleus and gastrocnemius contractures. J Biomech 2006; 39: 255–266.

59. Menegaldo LL, de Toledo Fleury A, Weber HI: Moment arms and musculotendon lengths estimation for a three-dimensional lower-limb mode. J Biomech 2004; 37: 1447–1453.

60. Miller JA: Locomotor advantages of Neandertal skeletal morphology at the knee and ankle. J Biomech. 1998; 31: 355–361.

61. Monster AW, Chan H, O'Connor D: Activity patterns of human skeletal muscles: relation to muscle fiber type composition. Science 1978; 200: 314–317.

62. Moseley AM, Crosbie J, Adams R: Normative data for passive ankle plantarflexion-dorsiflexion flexibility. Clin Biomech 2001; 16: 514–521.

63. Moss CL: Comparison of the histochemical and contractile properties of human gastrocnemius muscle. J Orthop Sports Phys Ther 1991; 13: 322–327.

64. Mueller MJ, Minor SD, Schaaf JA, et al.: Relationship of plantar-flexor peak torque and dorsiflexion range of motion to kinetic variables during walking. Phys Ther 1995; 75: 684–693.

65. Murray MP: Gait as a total pattern of movement. Am J Phys Med 1967; 46: 290–333.

66. Murray MP, Guten GN, Baldwin JM, Gardner GM: A comparison of plantar flexion torque with and without triceps surae. Acta Orthop Scand 1976; 17: 122–124.

67. Neptune RR, Kautz SA, Zajac FE: Contributions of the individual ankle plantar flexors to support, forward progression and swing initiation during walking. J Biomech 2001; 34: 1387–1398.

68. Neviaser TJ: Adhesive capsulitis. Orthop Clin North Am 1987; 18: 439–443.

69. Niki H, Ching RP, Kiser P, Sangeorzan BJ: The effect of posterior tibial tendon dysfunction on hindfoot kinematics. Foot Ankle Int 2001; 22: 292–300.

70. Out L, Vrijkotte TGM, van Soest AJ, Bobbert MF: Influence of the parameters of a human triceps surae muscle model on the isometric torque-angle relationship. J Biomech Eng 1996; 118: 17–25.

71. Owens S, Thordarson DB: The adductor hallucis revisited. Foot Ankle Int 2001; 22: 186–191.

72. Paris DL, Sullivan SJ: Isometric strength of rearfoot inversion and eversion in nonsupported, taped, and braced ankles assessed by a hand-held dynamometer. JOSPT 1992; 15: 229–235.

73. Perry J: Gait Analysis, Normal and Pathological Function. Thorofare, NJ: Slack, 1992.

74. Pontaga I: Ankle joint evertor-invertor muscle torque ratio decrease due to recurrent lateral ligament sprains. Clin Biomech 2004; 19: 760–762.

75. Riener R, Edrich T: Identification of passive elastic joint moments in the lower extremities. J Biomech 1999; 32: 539–544.

76. Romanes GJE: Cunningham's Textbook of Anatomy. Oxford: Oxford University Press, 1981.

77. Root L: Varus and valgus foot in cerebral palsy and its management. Foot Ankle 1984; 4: 174–179.

78. Rugg SG, Gregor RJ, Mandelbaum BR, Chiu L: In vivo moment arm calculations at the ankle using magnetic resonance imaging (MRI). J Biomech 1990; 23: 495–501.

79. Salathe EP Jr, Arangio GA, Salathes EP: The foot as a shock absorber. J Biomech 1990; 23: 655–659.

80. Sale D, Quinlan J, Marsh E, et al.: Influence of joint position on ankle plantarflexion in humans. J Appl Physiol 1982; 52: 1636–1642.

81. Sanderson DJ, Martin PE, Honeyman G, et al.: Gastrocnemius and soleus muscle length, velocity, and EMG responses to changes in pedaling cadence. J Electromyogr Kinesiol 2006; 16: 642–649.

82. Shiavi R: Electromyographic patterns in adult locomotion: a comprehensive review. J Rehabil Res Dev 1985; 22: 85–98.

83. Simon SR, Mann RA, Hagy JL, Larsen LJ: Role of the posterior calf muscles in normal gait. J Bone Joint Surg 1978; 60A: 465–472.

84. Smith LK, Weiss EL, Lehmkuhl LD: Brunnstrom's Clinical Kinesiology. Philadelphia: FA Davis, 1996.

85. Spoor CW, vanLeewen JL, Meskers CGM, et al.: Estimation of instantaneous moment arms of lower-leg muscles. J Biomech 1990; 23: 1247–1259.

86. Sunnerhagen KS, Hedberg M, Henning GB, et al.: Muscle performance in an urban population sample of 40- to 79-year-old men and women. Scand J Rehabil Med 2000; 32: 159–167.

87. Svantesson U, Carlsson U, Takahashi H, et al.: Comparison of muscle and tendon stiffness, jumping ability, muscle strength and fatigue in the plantarflexors. Scand J Med Sci Sports 199; 8: 252–256.

88. Tamaki H, Kitada K, Akamine T, et al.: Electromyogram patterns during plantarflexions at various angular velocities and knee angles in human triceps surae muscles. Eur J Appl Physiol 1997; 75: 1–6.

89. Tome J, Nawoczenski DA, Flemister A, et al.: Comparison of foot kinematics between subjects with posterior tibialis tendon dysfunction and healthy controls. J Orthop Sports Phys Ther 2006; 36: 635–644.

90. Tynan MC, Klenerman L, Helliwell TR, et al.: Investigation of muscle imbalance in the leg symptomatic forefoot pes cavus: a multidisciplinary study. Foot Ankle Int 1992; 13: 489–501.

91. Vanderhooft E: The frequency of and relationship between the palmaris longus and plantaris tendons. Am J Orthop 1996; 25: 38–41.

92. Vandervoort AA, McComas AJ: Contractile changes in opposing muscles of the human ankle joint with aging. J Appl Physiol 1986; 61: 361–367.

93. Wapner KL, Hecht PJ, Shea JR, Allardyce TJ: Anatomy of second muscular layer of the foot: considerations for tendon selection in transfer for achilles and posterior tibial tendon reconstruction. Foot Ankle Int 1994; 15: 420–423.

94. Wickiewicz TL, Roy RR, Powell PL, Edgerton VR: Muscle architecture of the human lower limb. Clin Orthop 1983; 179: 275–283.

95. Williams P, Bannister L, Berry M, et al.: Gray's Anatomy, The Anatomical Basis of Medicine and Surgery, Br. ed. London: Churchill Livingstone, 1995.

96. Wren TAL, Yerby SA, Beaupre GS, Carter DR: Mechanical properties of the human achilles tendon. Clin Biomech 2001; 16: 245–251.

97. Wu LJ: Nonlinear finite element analysis for musculoskeletal biomechanics of medial and lateral plantar longitudinal arch of virtual Chinese human after plantar ligamentous structure failures. Clin Biomech 2007; 22: 221–229.

98. Zifchock RA, Piazza SJ: Investigation of the validity of modeling the Achilles tendon as having a single insertion site. Clin Biomech 2004; 19: 303–307.

Analysis of the Forces on the Ankle and Foot during Activity

T he feet are the platform on which human beings stand and from which they propel themselves along the earth during locomotion, in a game of basketball, while jumping over a stream, or during any number of activities throughout the day. Central to all of these tasks is the ability of the foot to bear large loads. The purpose of this chapter is to examine the loads sustained by the structures of the foot during weight-bearing activities and how these loads contribute to complaints patients report in the clinic. Specifically the objectives of this chapter are to

- Review the applications of a two-dimensional analysis to calculate loads on joints of the foot
- Examine the loads sustained by the muscles and joints of the ankle and foot during function
- Investigate the reported loads applied to the plantar surface of the foot during weight-bearing activities

TWO-DIMENSIONAL ANALYSIS OF THE FORCES IN THE FOOT

Several studies estimate the loads exerted on the ankle and joints of the foot during weight-bearing activities. Analyses at the ankle and the great toe provide opportunities to review the methods of two-dimensional analysis to estimate muscle and joint reaction forces.

Two-Dimensional Analysis at the Ankle

A two-dimensional analysis of the forces on the ankle while standing on tiptoes demonstrates the important role that the calcaneus plays during upright stance (*Examining the Forces*

Box 46.1). The plantarflexor muscles provide the necessary force to lift the body weight from the floor, and the calcaneus provides a large moment arm for the plantarflexors, enhancing their mechanical advantage. The ground reaction force produces an external extension, or dorsiflexion, moment (M_{EXT}) of 47.4 Nm that requires an internal, plantarflexion moment of equal magnitude produced by the plantarflexor muscles. Assuming that each foot bears half the body weight, standing on tiptoes requires that the plantarflexor muscles in each foot generate a force that is approximately 1.2 times body weight. A smaller moment arm for the plantarflexor muscles would require a larger force of contraction. It is worth noting that as the individual rises higher onto the toes, the moment arm of the ground reaction force decreases so

CALCULATION OF FORCES AT THE ANKLE WHILE STANDING ON TIPTOES

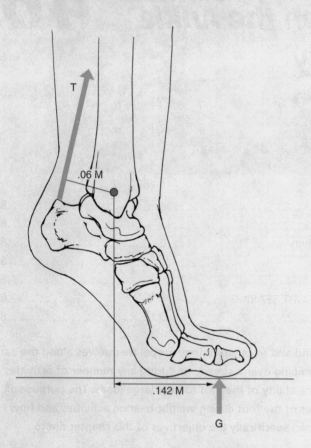

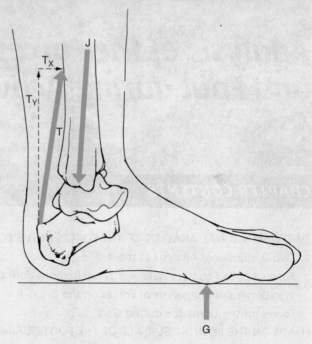

ΣF_X:

$$J_X + T_X = 0$$
$$J_X = -T_X$$

where $T_X = T (\cos 80°)$

$$J_X = -T (\cos 80°)$$
$$J_X = -137 \text{ N}$$

ΣF_Y:

$$J_Y + T_Y + 334 \text{ N} = 0$$

where $T_Y = T (\sin 80°)$

$$J_Y = -334 \text{ N} - 782 \text{ N}$$
$$J_Y = -1116 \text{ N}$$

Using the pythagorean theorem:

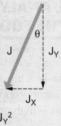

$$J^2 = J_X{}^2 + J_Y{}^2$$
$$J = 1124 \text{ N}$$
$$\mathbf{J \approx 1.7 \text{ BW}}$$

Using trigonometry, the direction of J can be determined:

$$\sin \theta = J_X/J$$

$$\boldsymbol{\theta \approx 7° \text{ from the vertical}}$$

The following dimensions are based on an individual who is approximately 5 feet 10 inches tall (1.75 m) and weighs 150 lb (668 N). The limb segment parameters are extrapolated from the anthropometric data of Braune and Fischer [3] and Winter [30]. The plantarflexion force is assumed to be provided entirely by the triceps surae (T).

   Length of foot (L): 0.2 m
   Moment arm of triceps surae: 0.06 m [15,21]
   Ground reaction force (G) is half body weight: 334 N
   Moment arm of ground reaction force: 0.142 m

$$\Sigma M = 0$$
$$(G \times 0.142 \text{ m}) - (T \times 0.06 \text{ m}) = 0$$
$$47.4 \text{ Nm} = T \times 0.06 \text{ m}$$
$$T = 790 \text{ N}$$

$$\mathbf{T = 1.2 \text{ BW}}$$

Calculate the joint reaction forces (J) on the talus. Assume that the force of the triceps surae is applied to the foot at an angle of 80° and the ground reaction force is vertical.

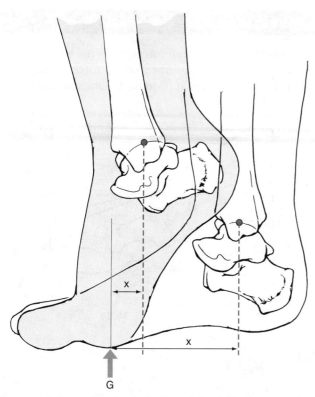

Figure 46.1: Increasing plantarflexion of the ankle decreases the dorsiflexion moment arm (x) of the ground reaction force (G).

degenerative changes within the tendon reduce the ultimate strength of the tendon so that the loads sustained during high-speed movements such as lunging for a tennis ball or tripping are certainly sufficient to exceed the tolerance of a weakened Achilles tendon and produce a rupture.

Mathematical models that calculate joint reaction forces at the ankle joint during gait suggest that the ankle sustains peak compressive loads three to five times body weight [18,25,26]. Loads of more than 10 times body weight are reported during running [22]. Despite these very large loads applied to the ankle with every step, the ankle appears rather immune to degenerative changes unless they are precipitated by joint trauma. Chapter 44 demonstrates that the talocrural articulation is quite congruent, which appears to help reduce joint stresses. In addition, studies demonstrate that the contact area between the talus and the tibia and fibula is greatest and stress (force/area) is minimized with the ankle plantarflexed [6,17]. Peak ankle joint forces during walking and running occur with the ankle joint plantarflexed, and although the ankle joint sustains large peak joint reaction forces, the stresses appear to be small enough to avoid degeneration of the articular surfaces.

Clinical Relevance

ANKLE OSTEOARTHRITIS: *Osteoarthritis of the ankle is uncommon and occurs typically as a result of ankle injuries. Such degenerative changes are likely the result of changes in stress applied to the joint surfaces. Lloyd et al. demonstrate that talar shifts of 1 mL produce a 40% reduction in contact area at the tibiotalar joint [14]. Talar shifts may occur in the unstable ankle following ankle sprains. These data suggest that there is a strong biomechanical rationale for rehabilitation or surgical intervention to restore ankle stability and joint congruity following severe ankle injuries. Such an intervention may help reduce the risk of degenerative joint disease later in life.*

that the required force from the plantarflexor muscles decreases [13] (*Fig. 46.1*). Despite the advantage of the plantarflexors and the reduced moment arm of the ground reaction force, the joint reaction force on the ankle during tiptoe stance is almost twice body weight. The large joint reaction force reflects the difference in moment arms of the plantarflexors and ground reaction force, the latter still larger than the former.

Forces Applied to the Ankle and Tarsal Regions during Activity

Activities that generate larger ground reaction forces, such as standing on one foot, in which the ground reaction force equals full body weight, or walking, when accelerations cause the ground reaction force to rise above body weight, generate even larger muscle and joint forces at the ankle. Several studies examine the loads at the ankle while walking at normal speeds. Estimated internal plantarflexion moments during normal locomotion range from 83 to 117 Nm [20,23].

In vivo determination of tendo calcaneus (Achilles tendon) forces during gait reveal average peak forces of 1430 N ± 500 N (321 ± 112 lb) [9]. A biomechanical model of the foot predicts peak forces in the Achilles tendon that are almost four times the weight of the body [10]. A report of the Achilles tendon's load to failure at high loading rates reveals that the loads sustained during walking fall well below the average ultimate strength of 5579 ± 1143 N (1253 ± 257 lb) [31]. Yet

Studies also examine the forces sustained elsewhere in the foot. Data collected from cadaver specimens during loading of the foot and ankle suggest that the subtalar joint sustains loads up to 2000 N (450 lb), or over four times body weight, and stresses from 3 to 4 MPa during axial loading or simulated gait [10,19,29]. Contact forces and stresses are reportedly smaller but still several times body weight at the calcaneocuboid and talonavicular joints.

Two-Dimensional Analysis of Forces on the Great Toe

Rising up on the forefoot also applies large loads to the bones and joints of the toes and particularly to the metatarsophalangeal joint of the great toe, since most individuals locate the load under the great toe during the final stages of stance [2,16,28,32]. *Examining the Forces Box 46.2* presents a

EXAMINING THE FORCES BOX 46.2

CALCULATION OF THE JOINT REACTION FORCE AT THE FIRST METATARSO-PHALANGEAL JOINT DURING GAIT

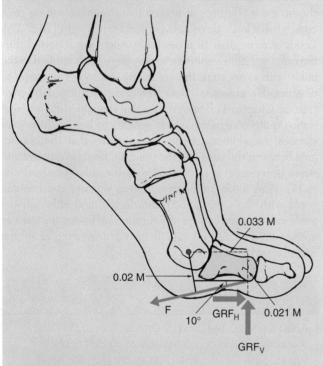

The following dimensions are based on an individual who is approximately 5 feet 3 inches tall (1.6 m) and weighs 125 lb (556 N). The limb segment parameters are extrapolated from the literature [3,15,21,30]. The plantarflexion force on the great toe is assumed to be provided entirely by the flexor hallucis longus (F). The ground reaction force has both vertical (GRF$_V$) and horizontal (GRF$_H$) components.

> Moment arm of flexor hallucis longus: 0.02 m
> Vertical ground reaction force (GRF$_V$): 240 N
> Moment arm of vertical ground reaction force: 0.033 m
> Horizontal ground reaction force (GRF$_H$): 40 N
> Moment arm of horizontal ground reaction force: 0.021 m

$\Sigma M = 0$

$(GRF_V \times 0.033 \text{ m}) + (GRF_H \times 0.021 \text{ m})$
$\qquad - (F \times 0.02 \text{ m}) = 0$

$240 \text{ N} \times (0.033) + (40 \text{ N} \times 0.021 \text{ m}) = F \times 0.02 \text{ m}$

$8.76 \text{ Nm} = F \times 0.02 \text{ m}$

Note that the internal moment (M$_{INT}$) = 8.76 Nm

$F = 438 \text{ N}$

$F = 0.79 \text{ BW}$

Calculate the joint reaction forces (J) on the base of the proximal phalanx. Assume that the force of the flexor hallucis longus is applied to the phalanx at an angle of 10°.

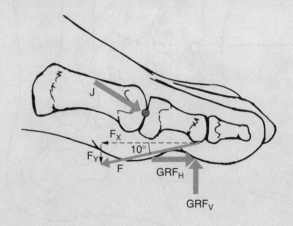

ΣF_X:

$\qquad GRF_H + J_X - F_X = 0$

$\qquad J_X = F_X - 40 \text{ N}$

where $F_X = F (\cos 10°)$

$\qquad J_X = 431 \text{ N} - 40 \text{ N}$

$\qquad J_X = 391 \text{ N}$

ΣF_Y:

$\qquad GRF_V + J_Y - F_Y = 0$

where $F_Y = F (\sin 10°)$

$\qquad J_Y = -240 \text{ N} + 76.1 \text{ N}$

$\qquad J_Y = -164 \text{ N}$

Using the pythagorean theorem:

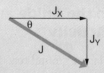

$\qquad J^2 = J_X{}^2 + J_Y{}^2$

$\qquad J = 424 \text{ N}$

$\qquad \textbf{J} \approx \textbf{0.76 BW}$

Using trigonometry, the direction of J can be determined:

$\qquad \cos \theta = J_X/J$

$\qquad \boldsymbol{\theta \approx 23° \text{ from the horizontal}}$

two-dimensional analysis of the loads on the base of the proximal phalanx of the great toe as the body rolls over the foot during locomotion. During the late stages of stance as the body passes over the stance foot, the stance foot applies a backward and downward force on the ground, and the ground reaction force is upward (GRF_V) and forward (GRF_H). The ground reaction force tends to extend, or dorsiflex, the metatarsophalangeal joint of the great toe. The extension moment applied by the ground reaction force is balanced by a flexion moment produced by the flexor muscle force (F). Using estimates of the ground reaction force from the literature, the flexor muscles in this sample problem generate 438 N (98 lb), or approximately 79% of body weight, to stabilize the great toe during roll off [30]. The joint reaction force determined for this phase of gait is 424 N (95 lb), or approximately 76% body weight.

Forces on the Great Toe during Gait

Published estimates of the joint reaction force at the metatarsophalangeal joint of the great toe during normal locomotion vary widely and range from approximately 30% to almost 100% of body weight [12,16,28,32]. These variations originate, in part, from differences in the models used to calculate the forces. However, all of the studies also report large interindividual variability. A major contributor to the calculation is the magnitude of the ground reaction force on the toe, which depends on walking form and walking speed. Older individuals appear to have smaller ground reaction forces because they walk more slowly [32]. In running, which produces much larger ground reaction forces, the external moment to dorsiflex the metatarsophalangeal joint reaches reported peaks ranging from 60 to 100 Nm [27].

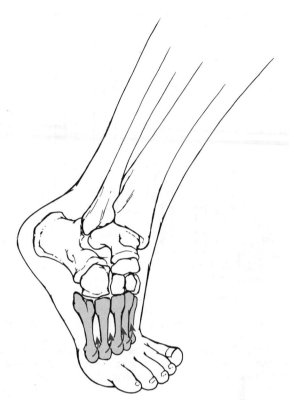

Figure 46.2: The loads on the metatarsal heads during gait produce bending moments in the metatarsal bones that may contribute to stress fractures.

LOADS ON THE PLANTAR SURFACE OF THE FOOT DURING WEIGHT BEARING

This chapter demonstrates that the structures of the foot sustain large loads during weight-bearing activities, especially locomotor activities. These loads are directly related to the contact forces between the foot and the ground. While walking, the foot collides with the ground at every step, and each collision is even more vigorous in running. The foot possesses many special structures to sustain such repeated collisions, including the fat pad on the plantar surface of the heel, the plantar aponeurosis, the plantar plates of the metatarsophalangeal and interphalangeal joints, as well as the special bony architecture of the foot. The magnitude and location of the loads applied to the plantar surface of the foot contribute to many complaints of foot pain and dysfunction, from sore feet and blisters to diabetic ulcers. An understanding of factors that contribute to the loading characteristics of the foot helps clinicians identify ways to minimize the detrimental effects of these loads.

Loading on the foot is typically described by **pressure** that, like stress, equals the force/area, where the measured force is perpendicular to the measuring device. In studies of the foot, pressure is a close approximation of the vertical stress on the foot. Investigation of the loading pattern of the foot reveals, as expected, that the largest vertical loads and pressures are applied to the heel at ground contact [7]. Peak

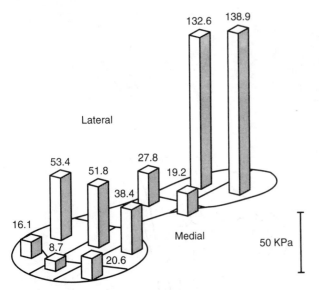

Figure 46.3: Although most of the plantar surface of the foot sustains substantial pressures during the stance phase of gait, the largest pressures are found at the heel, metatarsal heads, and the great toe. (Redrawn with permission from Sammarco GJ, Hockenbury RT: Biomechanics of the foot and ankle. In: Nordin M, Frankel VH, eds. Basic Biomechanics of the Musculoskeletal System. Philadelphia: Lippincott Williams & Wilkins, 2001.)

pressures on the heel of approximately 13 to 14 MPa are reported during standing (*Fig. 46.3*). The fat pad of the heel is specially equipped to absorb such high stresses.

Although almost the entire plantar surface of the foot is exposed to pressure in most individuals, the next highest peaks occur at the metatarsal heads, with the greatest pressures on the second metatarsal (approximately 5.0 MPa). Such high pressures likely contribute to the high incidence of stress fractures of the second metatarsal bone in runners and military recruits [8,24]. The hallux sustains the largest pressures of the five toes (approximately 2.0 MPa). The foot also withstands large shear stresses during gait, as high as 8.5 MPa [11]. Several factors influence the pressures and shear stresses applied to the foot, including its shape, arch height, and supporting muscles. Individuals with pes cavus, an excessively high medial longitudinal arch, report an increased prevalence of foot pain compared to individuals with normal arch height [5]. Not surprisingly, these individuals also demonstrate increased plantar pressures on the rearfoot and an increased duration of high pressures on the rearfoot and forefoot. These changes in stress are consistent with a decrease in contact area on the foot because of the elevated arch (stress = force/area). Walking speed also appears to affect plantar pressures. Increased walking speed reportedly increases pressures under the heel, forefoot, and toes in healthy elders [4].

Footwear affects plantar pressures as well. Some shoes increase the contact area between the foot and ground, thereby decreasing stress. The structure of the shoe and the interface between the foot and the shoe, including the sock, can alter the plantar pressures and shear forces on the foot. The popularity of

jogging has stimulated an entire industry that has led to numerous innovations in the design and construction of footwear to enhance the foot's ability to withstand these high-impact loads.

Clinical Relevance

SKIN ULCERS IN THE INSENSITIVE FOOT: *Individuals who lack sensation to the foot are at high risk for skin breakdown on the plantar surface of the foot. The data on the pressures applied to the foot during normal walking indicate that even the normal foot has discrete areas of high stress. A high-arched foot may have increased stress under the metatarsal heads, while a foot with excessive pronation may sustain increased stress on the medial aspect of the forefoot. Areas of high stress typically produce pain, and under normal circumstances, the individual takes action to reduce the pain, perhaps by wearing more comfortable shoes or decreasing the load on the feet by resting. However, an individual who lacks sensation may be unaware of the areas of high or excessive stress and therefore do nothing to reduce the stress.*

Prolonged stress can cause vascular changes within the stressed tissue and lead to tissue damage that, in some cases, may prove catastrophic. Some individuals with impaired sensation also exhibit a compromised vascular system. For example, an individual with diabetes mellitus may develop a peripheral neuropathy with resulting muscle weakness, sensory loss, and vascular changes in the feet and a common clinical scenario unfolds. As the patient continues to ambulate, the gait pattern gradually changes because of the weakness, and areas of high stress on the plantar surface of the foot during gait develop [1]. With the gradual diminution of sensation, the individual is unaware of the areas of high stress on the bottom of the foot, and the continued stresses lead to skin breakdown. The patient's impaired peripheral vascular system inhibits healing, and the ulcer fails to heal. Infection may set in, and in the worst case, the patient faces amputation. By understanding the normal pattern of loading on the foot and the factors that produce abnormally high stresses, clinicians can help prevent the catastrophic skin lesions by teaching the patient to identify areas of high stress and by recommending shoe modifications to alter the stress patterns under the foot.

SUMMARY

This chapter uses examples of two-dimensional analysis to demonstrate the magnitude of the loads sustained by the ankle and metatarsophalangeal joint of the great toe. Although these examples are oversimplifications of the three-dimensional nature of the forces on these joints as well as the anatomical structures that exert loads at the joints, they provide the clinician with a perspective to appreciate the normal wear-and-tear that the foot withstands with every step. A review of the literature reveals that all of the structures of the foot sustain large loads that are even larger during activities that produce large ground reaction forces, such as running and jumping. The chapter also demonstrates that the high loads applied to the foot may contribute to pathological processes within the foot that produce pain and disability. Examples in which the loads on the foot contribute directly to pathology include stress fractures of the metatarsals and skin ulcers in an insensitive foot that sustains excessive plantar pressures. This chapter concludes the presentation of the mechanics and pathomechanics of the bones, joints, and muscles of the lower extremity. The remaining two chapters of this text apply the current understanding of the structure and function of the musculoskeletal system to the examination of their contributions to two functions that are central to the function of human beings, upright posture and locomotion.

References

1. Abboud RJ, Rowley DI, Newton RW: Lower limb muscle dysfunction may contribute to foot ulceration in diabetic patients. Clin Biomech 2000; 15: 37–45.
2. Blanc Y, Balmer C, Landis T, Vingerhoets F: Temporal parameters and patterns of the foot roll over during walking: normative data for healthy adults. Gait Posture 1999; 10: 97–108.
3. Braune W, Fischer O: Center of gravity of the human body. In: Krogman WM, Johnston FE, eds. Human Mechanics: Four Monographs Abridged AMRL-TDR-63-123. Wright-Patterson Air Force Base, OH: Behavioral Sciences Laboratory, 6570th Aerospace Medical Research Laboratories, Aerospace Medical Division, Air Force Systems Command, 1963; 1–57.
4. Burnfield JM, Few CD, Mohamed OS, et al.: The influence of walking speed and footwear on plantar pressures in older adults. Clin Biomech 2004; 19: 78–84.
5. Burns J, Crosbie J, Hunt A, et al.: The effect of pes cavus on foot pain and plantar pressure. Clin Biomech 2005; 20: 877–882.
6. Calhoun JH, Eng M, Ledbetter BR, Viegas SF: A comprehensive study of pressure distribution in the ankle joint with inversion and eversion. Foot Ankle 1994; 15: 125–133.
7. Cavanagh PR, Rodgers MM, Iiboshi A: Pressure distribution under symptom-free feet during barefoot standing. Foot Ankle 1987; 7: 262–276.
8. Donahue SW, Sharkey NA: Strains in the metatarsals during the stance phase of gait: implications for stress fractures. J Bone Joint Surg 1999; 81A: 1236–1244.
9. Finni T, Komi PV, Lukkariniemi J: Achilles tendon loading during walking: application of a novel optic fiber technique. Eur J Appl Physiol Occup Physiol 1998; 77: 289–291.
10. Giddings VL, Beaupre GS, Whalen RT, Carter DR: Calcaneal loading during walking and running. Med Sci Sports Exerc 2000; 32: 627–634.
11. Hosein R, Lord M: A study of in-shoe plantar shear in normals. Clin Biomech (Bristol, Avon) 2000; 15: 46–53.
12. Jacob HAC: Forces acting in the forefoot during normal gait-an estimate. Clin Biomech 2001; 16: 783–792.
13. Kerrigan DC, Riley PO, Rogan S, Burke DT: Compensatory advantages of toe walking. Arch Phys Med Rehabil 2000; 81: 38–44.
14. Lloyd J, Elsayed S, Hariharan K, et al.: Revisiting the concept of talar shift in ankle fractures. Foot Ankle Int 2006; 27: 793–796.
15. Maganaris CN, Baltzopoulos V, Sargeant AJ: In vivo measurement-based estimations of the human Achilles tendon moment arm. Eur J Appl Physiol 2000; 83: 363–369.
16. McBride ID, Wyss UP, Cooke TDV, et al.: First metatarsophalangeal joint reaction forces during high-heeled gait. Foot Ankle 1991; 11: 282–288.
17. Michelson JD, Checcone M, Kuhn T, Varner K: Intra-articular load distribution in the human ankle joint during motion. Foot Ankle Int 2001; 22: 226–233.
18. Procter P, Paul JP: Ankle joint biomechanics. J Biomech 1982; 15: 627–634.
19. Reeck J: Support of the talus: a biomechanical investigation of the contributions of the talonavicular and talocalcaneal joints, and the superomedial calcaneonavicular ligament. Foot Ankle Int 1998; 19: 674–682.
20. Robon MJ, Perell KL, Fang M, Guererro E: The relationship between ankle plantarflexor muscle moments and knee compressive forces in subjects with and without pain. Clin Biomech 2000; 15: 522–527.
21. Rugg SG, Gregor RJ, Mandelbaum BR, Chiu L: In vivo moment arm calculations at the ankle using magnetic resonance imaging (MRI). J Biomech 1990; 23: 495–501.
22. Scott SH, Winter DA: Internal forces at chronic running injury sites. Med Sci Sports Exerc 1990; 22: 357–369.
23. Scott SH, Winter DA: Talocrural and talocalcaneal joint kinematics and kinetics during the stance phase of walking. J Biomech 1991; 24: 743–752.
24. Sharkey NA, Ferris L, Smith TS, Matthews DK: Strain and loading of the second metatarsal during heel-lift. J Bone Joint Surg [Am] 1995; 77: 1050–1057.
25. Simonsen EB, Dyhre-Poulsen P, Voigt M, et al.: Bone-on-bone forces during loaded and unloaded walking. Acta Anat [Basel] 1995; 152: 133–142.
26. Stauffer RN, Chao EYS, Brewster RC: Force and motion analysis of the normal, diseased, and prosthetic ankle joint. Clin Orthop 1977; 127: 189–196.
27. Stefanyshyn DJ, Nigg BM: Mechanical energy contribution of the metatarsophalangeal joint to running and sprinting. J Biomech 1997; 30: 1081–1085.
28. Stokes IA, Hutton WC, Stott JR: Forces acting on the metatarsals during normal walking. J Anat 1979; 129: 579–590.
29. Wang CL, Cheng CK, Chen CW, et al.: Contact areas and pressure distributions in the subtalar joint. J Biomech 1995; 28: 269–279.
30. Winter D: Biomechanics and Motor Control of Human Movement. New York: John Wiley & Sons, 1990.
31. Wren TAL, Yerby SA, Beaupre GS, Carter DR: Mechanical properties of the human achilles tendon. Clin Biomech 2001; 16: 245–251.
32. Wyss UP: Joint reaction forces at the first MTP joint in a normal elderly population. J Biomech 1990; 23: 977–984.

Posture and Gait

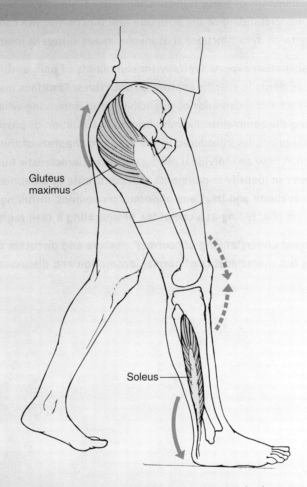

Gluteus
maximus

Soleus

PART V

The first part of this textbook presents the basic principles needed to understand the mechanics and pathomechanics of the musculoskeletal system and presents the mechanical properties of the individual components of the musculoskeletal system. Most of the text then examines the structural and functional properties of the individual joint complexes in the body. This final portion of the textbook applies this knowledge to the analysis of two intrinsically human functions, erect standing and bipedal locomotion. The goals of this final segment are to:

- discuss the biomechanical demands of these two functions
- demonstrate how a basic understanding of the structure and function of the components of the musculoskeletal system leads to the ability to analyze functions that involve many different joint complexes

Patients seek help from rehabilitation experts typically for complaints of pain or difficulty in performing a task rather than with complaints of impairments in specific anatomical structures. Clinicians must be able to observe the activity in question, analyze the biomechanical demands of the activity, and determine what, if any, impairments contribute to the pathomechanics producing the complaints. Examination and evaluation of posture and gait require an understanding of the basic biomechanical principles introduced in the first two chapters of this book and use knowledge of muscle and joint function to explain how an individual produces these characteristic human behaviors. Clinicians who can evaluate posture and gait and can identify impairments that contribute to an abnormal movement pattern will be able to apply these same skills to evaluate and treat any abnormal movement, including activities as diverse as lifting boxcar hitches, performing a grand plié, typing at a computer, or operating a cash register at the local supermarket.

Chapter 47 describes the current understanding of "correct" posture and discusses the mechanisms to control the posture. Chapter 48 presents the characteristics of normal locomotion and discusses the factors that influence it.

Characteristics of Normal Posture and Common Postural Abnormalities

P osture is the relative position of the parts of the body, usually associated with a static position. Clinicians evaluate posture with the underlying assumptions that abnormal posture contributes to patients' complaints and that many impairments within the neuromusculoskeletal system are reflected in an individual's posture. Thus clinical interpretation of an individual's posture requires blending a description of an individual's posture with an understanding of the person's physical condition and complaints.

Posture in erect standing is the focus of much clinical attention, but postures in sitting and during activities, such as lifting or assembly line work, also may contribute to musculoskeletal complaints. This chapter focuses on standing posture, but the issues considered to understand erect standing posture are applicable to any other posture as well. It is important to recognize that even seemingly static postures such as erect standing exhibit small, random movements, and typically, humans move in and out of several postures. As a result, assessment of a single posture may be insufficient to understand the link between posture and a patient's complaints.

Analysis of posture is a well-established clinical tradition and forms a basic part of the physical examination for many different health disciplines. Despite the frequency with which such evaluations are carried out, there remains a surprising lack of unanimity in the description of "normal" posture. Although faulty posture has been associated with such diverse complaints as headaches, respiratory and digestive problems, and back pain throughout the centuries, the direct consequences of faulty posture are not well documented. The purposes of this chapter are to describe the current understanding of normal posture and to describe some common postural faults. Specifically, the objectives of this chapter are to

- Describe the alignment of the body in erect standing posture and its variability
- Discuss the current understanding of the muscles needed to control erect standing posture
- Describe common postural faults
- Briefly discuss the purported consequences of postural faults

NORMAL POSTURE

Posture is evaluated by examining its stability and also by describing the relative alignment of adjacent limb segments.

Postural Sway

Normal erect standing posture is often compared to the movement of an inverted pendulum in which the base is fixed and the pendulum is free to oscillate over the fixed base (*Fig. 47.1*). Although erect standing appears static to the casual observer, it is characterized by small oscillations in which the body sways anteriorly, posteriorly, and side to side; and the body's **center of mass**, approximately located just anterior to the body of the first sacral vertebra, inscribes a small, irregular circle within the base of support [8,42]. This normal **postural sway** in erect standing also is described by the movement of the **center of pressure**, which is related to, but distinct from, the location of the body's center of mass [29,50]. The center of pressure locates the center of the distributed pressures under both feet. In contrast, a vertical line through the center of mass locates the center of mass within the entire base of support. The normal sway of the body during quiet standing moves the center of mass and the center of pressure of the body anteriorly and posteriorly up to 7 mm [8,42,50,67]. Side-to-side excursions of the centers of mass and pressure are only slightly less than those in the anterior–posterior direction [8].

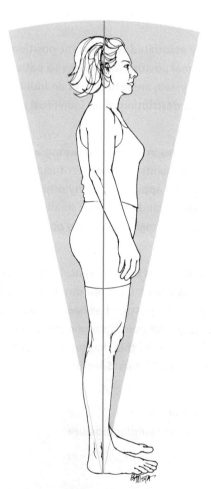

Figure 47.1: Standing posture often is modeled as an inverted pendulum in which the body sways over the fixed feet.

Clinical Relevance

ASSESSING STABILITY IN QUIET STANDING: *Stability in quiet standing is assessed in different populations to better understand why some individuals are at increased risk for falling. Changes in the magnitude or frequency of postural sway determined by the oscillations of either center of pressure or center of mass are reported in healthy elders and in individuals with impairments such as hemiparesis, sensory deficits, flat and high-arched feet, and vestibular dysfunctions [8,42,50,63].*

Segmental Alignment in Normal Posture

SAGITTAL PLANE ALIGNMENT OF THE BODY IN NORMAL POSTURE

Although both **ideal posture** and **normal posture** have been described in the clinical literature, the criteria for the ideal posture remain hypothetical [31,58]. Ideal posture is variously described as the posture that requires the least amount of muscular support, the posture that minimizes the stresses on the joints, or the posture that minimizes the loads in the supporting ligaments and muscles [1,31]. In the absence of a clear understanding of the meaning of the "ideal" posture, careful measurements of the positions assumed by individuals without known musculoskeletal impairments or complaints provide a perspective on the typical, if not ideal, alignment of limb segments.

Table 47.1 presents the relative orientation of landmarks in the sagittal plane with respect to the ankle joint from two studies examining the posture of individuals without any known musculoskeletal impairment or complaint [8,48]. *Fig. 47.2* presents the relative location of the landmarks with respect to a line through the center of mass, which lies approximately 4 to 6 cm anterior to the ankle joint [8,48]. The two studies report similar relative alignments, and both also agree somewhat with the "ideal posture" described by Kendall et al. [31]. The relatively large standard deviations at the superior landmarks reported by Danis et al. are consistent with the normal postural sway that occurs in quiet standing.

TABLE 47.1: Alignment in the Sagittal Plane of Body Landmarks with Respect to the Ankle during Erect Standing

	Opila et al. [48][a]		Danis [8][b]	
	Description of Landmark	Location[c] (cm)	Description of Landmark	Location[c] (cm)
Ankle	Lateral malleolus		Calculated joint center	
Knee	Lateral epicondyle of Femur	5.1	Calculated joint center	4.24 ± 2.14
Hip	Greater trochanter	5.4	Calculated joint center	5.42 ± 2.86
Shoulder	Acromioclavicular joint	3.0	Acromion process	1.89 ± 3.01
Head/neck	Just inferior to the external auditory meatus	5.4	Approximately the atlanto-occipital joint	4.84 ± 4.03

[a]Based on 19 unimpaired males and females aged 21 to 43 years. Originally reported with respect to the body's center of gravity.
[b]Based on 26 unimpaired males and females aged 22 to 88 years. Originally referenced to the ankle joint.
[c]Positive numbers indicate that the landmark is anterior to the ankle joint.

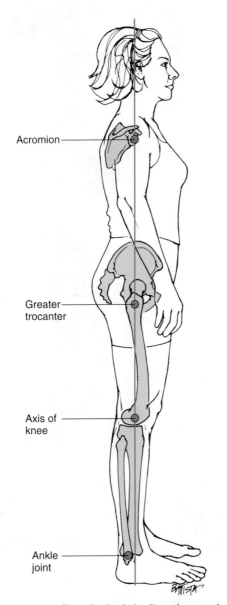

Acromion

Greater trocanter

Axis of knee

Ankle joint

Figure 47.2: In erect standing, the body is aligned approximately so that a line through the body's center of mass passes very close to the ear, slightly anterior to the acromion process of the scapula, close to the greater trochanter, slightly anterior to the knee joint, and anterior to the ankle joint.

Trunk and Pelvic Alignment

The data presented in Table 47.1 describe the sagittal plane orientation of many body parts in erect standing but provide little information regarding the normal alignment of the spine and pelvis. The adult spine is characterized by a **kyphosis** in the thoracic and sacral regions in which the curves are convex posteriorly and a **lordosis** in the cervical and lumbar regions in which the curves are concave posteriorly. At birth, the spine is entirely kyphotic, and consequently, the thoracic and sacral curves are **primary curves.** Development of head control by approximately 4 months of age induces the development of a cervical lordosis, and a child's progression to upright standing and bipedal ambulation lead to the formation of the lumbar lordosis. Hence these curves are known as **secondary curves** and do not develop in the absence of acquisition of the respective skill.

The most common means of characterizing the curvatures of the spine use a radiographic method to assess the total curve of a region. The **Cobb angle** describes the angle formed by the surfaces of the superior and inferior vertebrae of a spinal region (*Fig. 47.3*). Mean Cobb angles of 20 to 70° are reported for the lumbar region and 20 to 50° for the thoracic region [19,27,66,70]. These data demonstrate wide disparities and are influenced by the measurement procedures used in each investigation, but also reflect the wide spectrum of spinal curvatures found in a population with no known pathology. Despite the differences reported in the literature, some consistent findings are found. The studies that examine both the thoracic and lumbar curves consistently report a larger lumbar lordosis than thoracic kyphosis [2,19,28,53,64]. Both thoracic and lumbar curves appear to increase during growth and development [39]. There is general agreement that the peak or apex of the thoracic curve occurs at approximately the midthoracic region, most often at T7, and the apex of the lumbar curve typically is located at either L3 or L4 [2,17,19,64].

Although the Cobb method is the most frequently used method of quantifying spinal curves, it requires radiographic assessment and is not part of a routine physical examination.

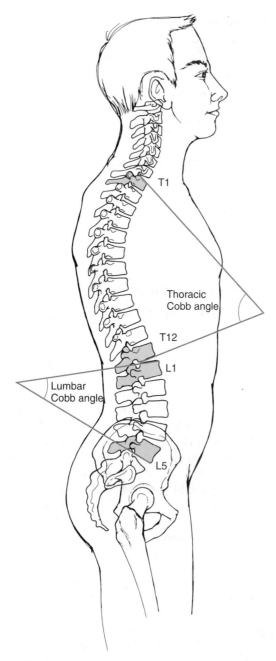

Figure 47.3: Cobb angles in the thoracic and lumbar spines are determined radiographically by determining the angles formed between the superior surface of the most superior vertebra of the region and the inferior surface of the most inferior vertebra of the region.

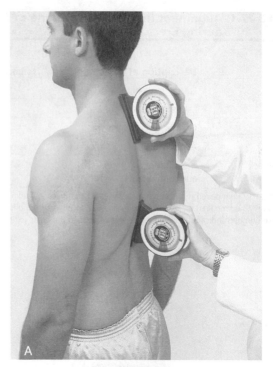

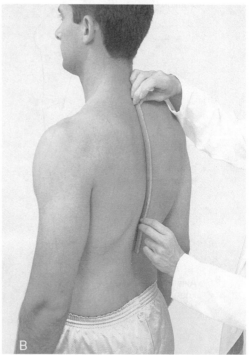

Figure 47.4: Surface methods to assess spinal curves. **A.** Clinicians use inclinometers to measure the curvature of spinal regions from surface palpations. **B.** Flexible rulers are used to trace the curvature in a spinal region, and the tracing can be quantified mathematically.

Methods to evaluate the spinal curves from surface assessment include the use of inclinometers to define the angulation, and flexible rulers and computer-assisted surface digitizers to trace the shape of the spinal curvature [18,46,62,77] (*Fig. 47.4*). The surface curvature methods yield different measurements from radiographic methods and may differ among themselves, depending upon the mathematical analyses used to describe the curves [46,59]. No current surface curvature methods offer normative data defining the range of curvature values found in a healthy population. Based on current knowledge, clinicians lack well-accepted criteria for normal curvatures of the spine in the sagittal plane using surface methods and continue to rely on qualitative assessments of the spinal curves [40].

Clinical Relevance

MONITORING CHANGES IN FORWARD-HEAD POSTURE: *Forward-head posture is associated with a wide range of patient complaints including headaches, vertigo, temporomandibular joint pain, and neck and shoulder pain. A typical physical examination of a patient with any of these complaints includes assessment of postural alignment (Fig. 47.5). Although objective procedures to quantify head position exist [18,24], the clinician often resorts to visual observation of head posture, assessing head alignment as normal or noting a "mild," "moderate," or "severe" forward head position. In the presence of an abnormal forward-head posture, the clinician typically initiates an intervention to improve or normalize the posture. However, without operational definitions of the postural deviations, it is difficult to identify changes in posture objectively and to associate any changes in the patient's complaints with changes in posture. Third-party payers are challenging the value of interventions to alter posture. Well-controlled outcome studies to measure the effectiveness of postural interventions are needed, and these studies demand more precise and more objective measures of postural alignment.*

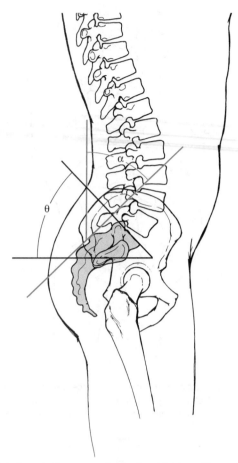

Figure 47.6: Sacral alignments determined from radiographs typically measure the angle between the superior surface of the sacrum and the horizontal (θ) or an angle between the posterior surface of the sacrum and the vertical (α).

Orientation of the pelvis is a common postural evaluation performed in conjunction with the assessment of spinal curves. Pelvic alignment is determined from the orientation of the sacrum or by the orientation of pelvic landmarks. Most measurements based on sacral alignment derive from radiographic assessment and report the angle made between a vertical or horizontal reference line and either the superior or posterior surface of the sacrum [27,66] (*Fig. 47.6*). The angle between the horizontal and the superior surface of the first sacral vertebra is known as the **sacral slope. Pelvic incidence** is another radiologic parameter that relates the sacral slope to the location of the femoral heads.

Orientation of the pelvis from surface landmarks is reported as the angle formed between the horizontal and a line connecting the posterior superior iliac spine with the anterior superior iliac spine [5,16,77] (*Fig. 47.7*). Typical measurements of sacral and pelvic orientation are reported in *Table 47.2*. Measurements based on the orientation of the sacrum are larger than those based on the pelvis, and the two measurement procedures show only slight-to-moderate correlations with each other [20].

Clinical literature suggests interdependence among the spinal curves and pelvic alignment [31]. An increased lordosis purportedly accompanies an increased thoracic kyphosis. Similarly, an anterior pelvic tilt reportedly accompanies an increased lumbar lordosis, while a decreased lumbar lordosis

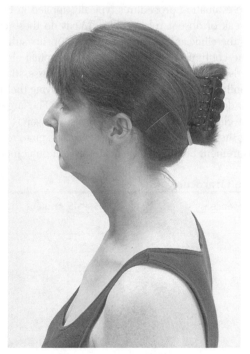

Figure 47.5: Forward-head alignment observed in the clinic is often assessed qualitatively as mild, moderate, or severe.

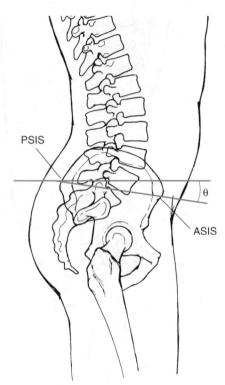

PSIS

θ

ASIS

Figure 47.7: Pelvic alignment from surface landmarks is defined by the angle between a line drawn through the anterior superior iliac spine (ASIS) and the posterior superior iliac spine (PSIS) and the horizontal (θ).

between the thoracic kyphosis and the lordosis between L5 and S1. Although additional research is required, these data suggest some association between the thoracic and lumbar curves, but their interdependence may be a function of age and the specific morphology of an individual's spine.

Studies investigating the relationship of pelvic alignment and lumbar lordosis also yield conflicting results. Studies that use radiographic measures consistently demonstrate an association between pelvic tilt as measured by sacral alignment and lumbar lordosis measured by the Cobb method [11,16,53]. These studies demonstrate the expected positive associations between an anterior tilt of the sacrum and an increased lordosis and between posterior tilting and a flattening of the lordosis (*Fig. 47.8*). Both sacral slope and pelvic incidence have strong positive correlations with the lumbar lordosis, and pelvic incidence appears to be increased in individuals with spondylolisthesis at L5-S1 [4,53]. Yet studies using surface methods to assess pelvic and spinal alignment in static posture fail to demonstrate any significant correlation between pelvic alignment using pelvic landmarks and the amount of lumbar lordosis using inclinometers or flexible rulers [55,62,63]. In contrast, studies using surface methods to assess the association between pelvic tilt and lumbar position during active movement demonstrate that posterior pelvic rotations do appear to decrease the lumbar lordosis [8,30]. Controversy continues regarding the effect of an active anterior pelvic tilt and the lordosis, with studies showing an increased lordosis with an anterior tilt [7,30] and others showing no change [8].

The studies reported here present confusing results for clinicians. On the one hand, radiographic data support the generally accepted clinical impression that pelvic alignment and spinal curves are related, but assessments of those relationships using the evaluation procedures typically applied in the clinic reveal weak or absent relationships. What do these conflicts mean to the clinician? Existing evidence appears sufficient to justify the continued belief that pelvic and spinal alignments are interdependent. However, current clinical assessment tools may be influenced enough by soft tissue overlying the skeleton that they do not reflect true bony alignment. The larger question that clinicians and researchers must answer is whether knowing the alignment of the pelvis and the spine, regardless of measurement technique, affects treatment outcomes.

is reportedly associated with a posterior pelvic tilt. There is limited evidence to support these purported relationships, and the existing relationships may be more complex than those reflected by the popular beliefs. The assessment procedures as well as the populations studied appear to affect the strength of the associations reported. A study of 100 adults over the age of 40 years reports a correlation between the thoracic kyphosis measured between T5 and T12 and the total lumbar lordosis but finds no association between the kyphosis in the upper thorax and the lumbar lordosis [16]. A study of 88 adolescents reports no relationship between the thoracic kyphosis from T3 to T12 and the total lumbar lordosis [53]. However, the same study does find correlations

TABLE 47.2: Measurements of Pelvic Orientation Reported in the Literature

	Sacral Orientation	Pelvic Incidence	ASIS–PSIS Angle
Voutsinas and MacEwen [66]	56.5 ± 9.3[a]		
During et al. [13]	40.4 ± 8.8[b]		
Jackson and McManus [27]	50.4 ± 7.7[c]		
Boulay et al. [4]		53.0 ± 9°[d]	
Levine and Whittle [35]			11.3 ± 4.3
Crowell et al. [5]			12.4 ± 4.5

[a]Based on the angle made by the superior surface of the sacrum and the horizontal.
[b]Based on the angle made by the posterior surface of the sacrum and the vertical.
[c]Based on the angle made by the superior surface of the sacrum and the horizontal.
[d]Based on the angle between a line perpendicular to the superior surface of the sacrum and a line from the superior surface of the sacrum to the center of the hip joint.

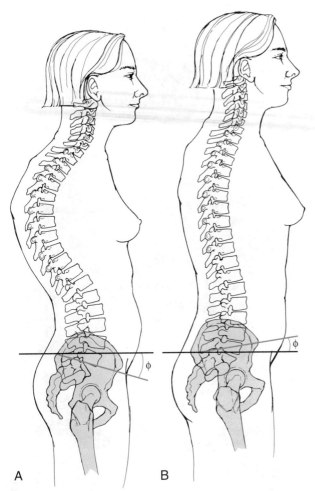

Figure 47.8: An anterior pelvic tilt, which enlarges the angle (φ) formed by the horizontal and a line through the anterior superior iliac spine, is believed to lead to an increased lumbar lordosis **(A)** and a posterior pelvic tilt in which the angle (φ) decreases and produces a decreased lumbar lordosis **(B)**. Data supporting these beliefs conflict.

Clinical Relevance

IS POSTURE REEDUCATION A USEFUL INTERVENTION STRATEGY FOR A PATIENT WITH LOW BACK PAIN?: *A patient with low back pain provides a good model to examine the role posture plays in some treatment strategies. The patient reports pain with lumbar extension and in quiet standing and decreased pain with forward bending and sitting. Radiographs demonstrate a spondylolisthesis at L4–L5.* **Spondylolisthesis** *is an anterior displacement of one vertebra on the vertebra below, and decreasing the lumbar curve would decrease the forces that tend to increase the displacement. Although the evidence regarding the effect of pelvic alignment on lumbar curvature is conflicting, the clinician chooses to proceed with a*

program to teach the patient to stand maintaining a posterior pelvic tilt to flatten the lumbar curve. The clinician teaches the patient abdominal strengthening exercises and posterior pelvic tilts. The patient learns to stand while contracting the abdominal muscles and the gluteus maximus, rotating the pelvis posteriorly. The patient reports pain relief.

This case provides an example of the commonly reported anecdotal evidence supporting the use of postural education to treat patients' complaints. Anecdotal evidence by itself, however, is insufficient to determine the effectiveness of the intervention, since many factors besides pelvic alignment may contribute to the reduction in symptoms, including the placebo effect. Without well-controlled biomechanical studies to determine the mechanical effects of pelvic alignment on low back posture and without similarly well-controlled effectiveness studies, the role of postural interventions in rehabilitation remains a firmly held belief.

FRONTAL AND TRANSVERSE PLANE ALIGNMENT IN NORMAL ERECT POSTURE

In the frontal and transverse planes, normal posture suggests a general right–left symmetry, with the head and vertebral column aligned vertically, hips and shoulders at an even height, the knees exhibiting symmetrical genu valgum within normal limits, and symmetrical placement of the upper and lower extremities in the transverse plane (*Fig. 47.9*). Gangnet and colleagues using three-dimensional radiography report very slight (<5°) deviations of the vertebrae to the left with similarly slight rotations to the right in a sample of 34 asymptomatic adults during upright standing [17].

Scoliosis describes a postural deformity of the vertebral column that is most apparent in the frontal plane but includes both frontal and transverse plane deviations. The curve is named according to its location in the spine and the side of its frontal plane convexity. For example, a right thoracic curve indicates that the curve is located in the thoracic region of the spine and its convexity is on the right side.

Scolioses can be either structural or functional. A **functional scoliosis** results from soft tissue imbalances, but a **structural scoliosis** includes bony changes as well as soft tissue asymmetries. As noted in Chapter 29, **idiopathic scoliosis** is the most common form of scoliosis. It is a structural scoliosis that is found most frequently in adolescent girls. The curve usually involves at least two spinal regions, and the curves typically are compensated, so that adjacent regions have opposite convexities (*Fig. 47.10*). A structural scoliosis in the thoracic region is accompanied by a rib hump on the same side as the convexity as a result of the coupled movements of the thoracic spine and their effects on the joints of the ribs. (Chapter 29 reviews the mechanics producing a rib hump.)

A popular theory in rehabilitation suggests that hand dominance induces muscle imbalances that lead to functional

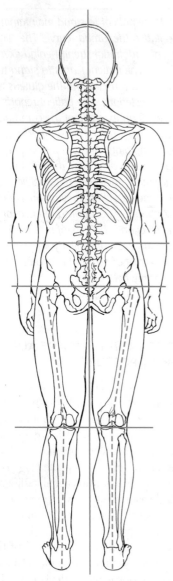

Figure 47.9: Normal alignment of the head and trunk in the frontal plane is characterized by a vertically aligned head and vertebral column, with shoulder, pelvis, hips, and knees at the same height, and the knees and feet exhibiting valgus and subtalar neutral positions within normal limits.

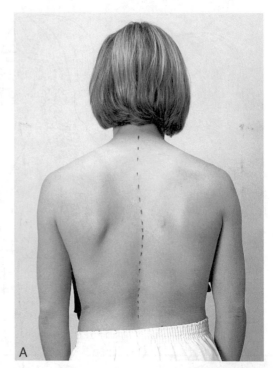

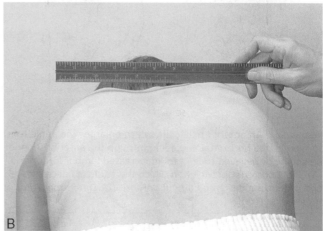

Figure 47.10: **A.** An individual exhibits a right thoracic left lumbar idiopathic scoliosis. **B.** When flexed forward, the individual exhibits a rib hump on the right, the side of the thoracic convexity.

scolioses and asymmetry in shoulder and hip alignment [31]. Few objective studies exist that test this hypothesis, but a study of 15 females aged 19 to 21 years reports no statistically significant differences in frontal plane alignment of the scapula between the dominant and nondominant sides, although 11 of 15 subjects demonstrated a lower right shoulder [57]. Horizontal distances between the medial border of the scapula and the vertebral column range from 5 to 9 cm [7,52,57]. Although asymmetry in hip height, or pelvic obliquity, also is allegedly associated with hand dominance, there is no known direct evidence to support or refute the contention [31].

The relative alignment of the hip, knee, and foot in the frontal and transverse planes during erect standing is discussed in some detail in the respective chapters dealing with each joint

(Chapters 38, 41, and 44, respectively). *Figure 47.11* provides a brief review of the characteristic alignments. Because the lower extremities participate in a closed chain during erect standing, lower extremity malalignments may indicate local deformities but also may reflect compensations for more remote malalignments. Findings from a postural assessment lead a clinician to hypothesize underlying impairments. Direct assessment of joints can identify the impairments that contribute to or explain the postural malalignments. A single contracture at either the hip, knee, or ankle may produce the same posture as the individual compensates for the functional limb length discrepancy produced by the contracture (*Fig. 47.12*). An understanding of the mechanisms contributing to faulty posture requires careful assessment of each joint.

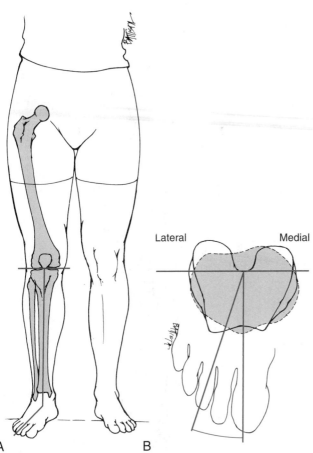

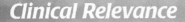

Figure 47.11: In normal alignment, the femoral condyles are aligned in the frontal plane so that the hip is in neutral rotation and the feet exhibit out-toeing of approximately 15–25°. **A.** Frontal view. **B.** Superior view.

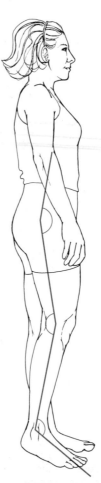

Figure 47.12: Flexion contractures of the hip or knee functionally shorten the lower extremity, and a common compensation is plantarflexion to lengthen the limb so that the individual can stand with the pelvis level. A plantarflexion contracture produces a functionally lengthened lower extremity so that an individual with a plantarflexion contracture may stand with a flexed hip and/or knee to restore symmetry and stand with a level pelvis. The resulting postures look approximately the same although the precipitating factors differ.

Clinical Relevance

RELATING POSTURAL FINDINGS TO IMPAIRMENTS OF THE NEUROMUSCULOSKELETAL SYSTEM: A CASE REPORT: *A 45-year-old male with rheumatoid arthritis was evaluated in the clinic with hip, knee, and foot pain bilaterally. An evaluation of his standing posture revealed a pelvic obliquity, right side higher than left, a slightly plantarflexed right ankle, and increased out-toeing on the left (Fig. 47.13). Many possible impairments could explain these findings, and the clinician's initial hypotheses included a structural leg length discrepancy and a plantarflexion contracture. A thorough examination of all of the joints of the lower extremities was required before an explanation for the posture emerged. The patient demonstrated bilateral hip flexion contractures. In addition, range of motion assessments revealed that the patient had a complex contracture of the left hip, holding it flexed, laterally rotated, and abducted. The patient stood*

with an anterior pelvic tilt and increased lordosis, consistent with the hip flexion contractures, but the lateral rotation and abduction contractures on the left effectively shortened the left lower extremity while turning the toes outward. The patient stood with the left hip in obligatory abduction secondary to the abduction contracture, while the right hip was adducted, and consequently, the pelvis was higher on the right. Correction of standing posture required reduction of the contractures of both the left and right hip. Although conservative treatment failed to reduce the contractures on the left, a total hip replacement on the left restored normal joint alignment, and standing posture was immediately improved.

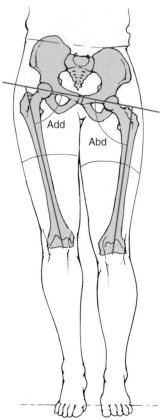

Figure 47.13: A patient with an abduction contracture of the left hip stands with the left hip abducted. To maintain an upright posture with the feet close together, the individual adducts the right hip, producing a pelvic obliquity in the frontal plane. The left hip is abducted and the right hip is adducted. The right ankle plantarflexes to equalize limb length.

Muscular Control of Normal Posture

Examples throughout this textbook demonstrate that ground reaction forces and body segment weights apply external moments to the joints, which are balanced by internal moments supplied by the surrounding muscles and noncontractile connective tissue. The alignment of the body's center of mass relative to joint axes in quiet standing defines the external moments applied to the joints during erect standing. These external moments then are balanced by either active or passive support to maintain the upright posture against the ever-present gravitational forces tending to press the body into the ground. Examination of the external moments applied to the joints of the lower extremities, trunk, and head by the ground reaction forces helps explain the forces needed to support these joints (*Fig. 47.14*). Using the data from the studies presented in Table 47.1, the sagittal plane external moments on many joints of the body are presented in *Table 47.3*. Biomechanical analysis of these moments and electromyographic (EMG) studies combine to help explain the mechanisms used to maintain upright posture.

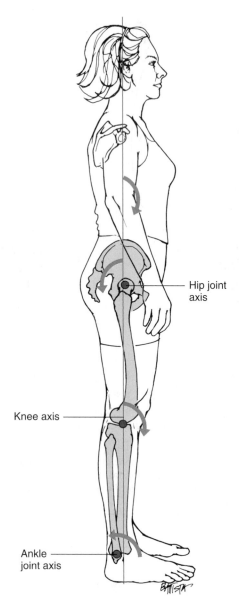

Figure 47.14: In quiet standing, the ground reaction force applies a dorsiflexion moment at the ankle, extension moments at the knee and hip, and flexion moments on the spine.

Although the external moments described in Table 47.3 are the predominant moments applied during quiet standing, it is important to recall that standing posture is dynamic and that even so-called quiet standing is characterized by oscillations of the body over the fixed feet. Panzer et al. report that during quiet standing, the EMG activity of muscle groups is less than 10% of each group's activity during a maximum voluntary contraction (MVC) [50]. These investigators also note that many of these muscle groups exhibit sudden, brief activity levels of 30–45% of their MVC and suggest that these sudden bursts may reflect a muscle group's response to the sway of the body's center of mass.

Because the body's center of mass generates a dorsiflexion moment on the ankle during quiet standing, the plantar flexor

TABLE 47.3: External Moments Applied to the Joints Based on the Center of Mass Line

	Opila et al. [40][a] External Moment	Danis [6][b] External Moment
Ankle	Dorsiflexion	Dorsiflexion[c]
Knee	Extension	Extension
Hip	Extension	Extension
Back	Flexion	Flexion
Head/neck	Flexion	Approximately zero[d]

[a]Based on 19 unimpaired males and females aged 21 to 43 years. Originally reported with respect to the body's center of gravity.
[b]Based on 26 unimpaired males and females aged 22 to 88 years. Referenced to the ankle joint.
[c]Moment is reported directly in the study but is derived from the available data.
[d]Although the moment arm is 0.03 cm, the standard deviation is almost 4 cm, suggesting that some individuals sustain a flexion moment, and others sustain an extension moment.

muscles generate a plantarflexion moment to maintain static equilibrium. EMG data demonstrate activity of both the soleus and the gastrocnemius during quiet standing [1,50]. Brief, intermittent, and slight EMG activity is also found in the dorsiflexor muscles, apparently in response to postural sway [1,50]. Research suggests that plantar flexion fatigue in young healthy adults produces an anterior shift of the center of pressure in quiet standing as well as an increase in postural sway [67].

In contrast to the ankle, the knee exhibits minimal muscle activity during quiet standing [1,50]. In erect posture, the ground reaction force applies an extension moment to the knee allowing it to maintain extension using its passive constraints, including the collateral and anterior cruciate ligaments. Reports of slight electrical activity in the quadriceps muscles (4–7% of MVC) and hamstrings (1% of MVC) are consistent with the use of passive supports to sustain the extended knee during quiet standing [50]. However, like the muscle activity at the ankle, larger brief bursts of activity in the quadriceps and hamstrings muscles may reflect the muscles' response to sway.

Few studies examine activity of the hip musculature during erect posture. The ground reaction force produces an extension moment at the hip, and EMG data reveal activity of the iliacus in quiet standing, exerting a stabilizing flexion moment [1]. Understanding the role of muscles and ligaments in generating the internal moments needed to balance the external moments exerted by body weight and ground reaction forces allows the clinician to intervene to provide postural stability in the absence of muscular support.

Clinical Relevance

MAINTAINING ERECT POSTURE IN THE PRESENCE OF MUSCLE WEAKNESS: A PATIENT WITH PARAPLEGIA: *A patient with a spinal cord injury resulting in loss of muscle function from the level of L2 is beginning rehabilitation. Functional goals include standing for stimulation of bone growth and limited ambulation. Weakness secondary to the spinal cord injury begins at the hip flexors*

and extends throughout the rest of the lower extremities. To teach the individual safe and efficient standing, the clinician uses an understanding of the effects of external moments on the joints of the lower extremities and a recognition of the passive structures that are available to support the joints.

The individual lacks muscular support at the hip, knee, and ankle, but the astute clinician knows that the hip possesses strong anterior ligaments, the iliofemoral, pubofemoral, and ischiofemoral ligaments. By maintaining the hip in hyperextension, the individual can "hang on" these anterior ligaments, even in the absence of the hip flexors. Similarly, the knee normally maintains extension in erect standing without muscular support, since the body's center of mass falls anterior to the knee joint and exerts an extension moment on the knee. As long as the knee remains extended, no additional muscular support is needed. Thus the individual can stand in hip and knee hyperextension using passive supports at these joints.

Stable erect posture requires that the body's center of mass remain over the base of support. To maintain hip and knee hyperextension while keeping the body's center of mass over the base of support, the individual's ankles assume a dorsiflexed position, and the ground reaction force applies an external dorsiflexion moment (Fig. 47.15). With no muscle support at the ankle, the individual with weakness from the hips distally requires external support from an orthosis to exert a plantarflexion moment at the ankle, balancing the external dorsiflexion moment. Thus the individual can stand with minimal external support to stabilize the lower extremity by using the external moments generated by the ground reaction force to apply external moments at the knee and hip that can be balanced by passive joint structures.

For the individual described in this case to stand with minimal external support, he or she must be able to assume a position of hip and knee hyperextension. Flexion contractures at the hips or knees or plantarflexion contractures at the ankle produce disastrous results, preventing the individual from positioning the joints to use passive supports (Fig. 47.16).

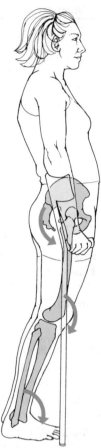

Figure 47.15: Standing posture of an individual with weakness at the hip, knees, and ankles. By hyperextending the hip joints, the individual uses the passive restraint of the anterior ligaments of the hip joint to support the hip. Hyperextension of the knee increases the extension moment at the knee that is supported by passive structures of the knee. To maintain hyperextension of the hip and knees while keeping the center of mass over the base of support, the ankles dorsiflex, producing a dorsiflexion moment that is withstood by an externally applied plantarflexion moment using an orthotic device.

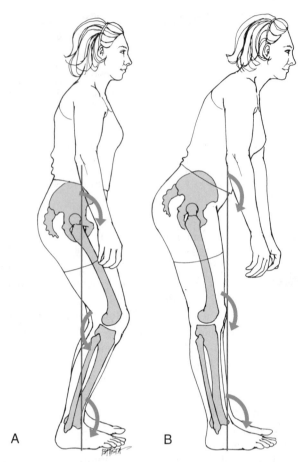

Figure 47.16: Effect of sagittal plane contractures on standing posture and the external moments applied to the hip, knees, and ankles. **A.** Flexion contractures at either the hip or knee cause an individual to stand in a flexed position at both the hips and knees, generating external flexion moments at both joints. Consequently, the individual is unable to use the passive supports at the hip and knee joints. **B.** Plantarflexion contractures at the ankles prevent an individual from moving the center of mass over the base of support while still maintaining hip and knee hyperextension. To relocate the center of mass over the base of support, the patient flexes the hip joints, thus requiring muscular support to support the hip joints.

The weight of the trunk exerts an external flexion moment on the back, requiring an extension moment to maintain erect posture. EMG data show low-level activity of the erector spinae and multifidus with intermittent bursts of increased activity [1,50,69]. The cervical region also sustains an external flexion moment because the head's center of mass is anterior to the joints of the cervical spine. Active contraction of cervical extensors maintains upright posture of the head and neck, but as in the trunk, EMG data reveal that only slight activity is required to hold the head erect. Although few studies examine activity in the cervical muscles during quiet standing, data show activity in the semispinalis muscles with no activity in the splenius muscles [61].

The role of the abdominal muscles during quiet standing continues to be debated. EMG studies of the abdominal muscles identify activity, particularly in the internal oblique muscle, with some activity in the external oblique muscle during quiet standing [1,14,51,56]. Yet studies that investigate the association between abdominal muscle strength as measured by leg-lowering maneuvers and postural alignment of the pelvis report either no association [68] or weak associations in females and no association in males [76]. The leg-lowering exercise often used to assess abdominal strength recruits the rectus abdominis more than the oblique abdominal muscles in most individuals and, consequently, may not reflect the ability of the oblique abdominal muscles to participate in postural support [51]. Contraction of the muscles of the abdominal wall appears to stabilize the pelvis and prevent excessive anterior pelvic tilt during prone hip hyperextension [47]. Chapter 34 discusses the role of the abdominal muscles in stabilizing the spine. The data presented here suggest that the oblique abdominal muscles are important in erect posture, although their role may be to function with the transversus abdominis muscle to stabilize the spine rather than to position the pelvis.

The role played by muscles to maintain shoulder position during quiet standing also lacks definitive conclusions. Inman et al. demonstrate active contraction of the levator scapulae along with the upper trapezius and upper portion of the serratus anterior muscles in quiet standing, suggesting that these muscles are providing upward support for the shoulder girdle and upper extremity [26]. However, Johnson et al. note that only the levator scapulae and the rhomboid major and minor muscles can directly suspend the scapula [30]. EMG studies show that in the presence of voluntary relaxation of the upper trapezius in quiet standing, there is an increase in EMG activity of the two rhomboid muscles but a decrease in activity in the levator scapulae [49]. These data support the notion that the rhomboid muscles can and do support the upright position of the shoulder girdle, at least under certain circumstances. Whether the levator scapulae contributes additional support remains debatable.

POSTURAL MALALIGNMENTS

Health care providers evaluate posture on the premise that postural malalignments contribute to altered joint and muscle mechanics, producing impairments that lead to pain [24,31]. Complaints attributed to postural deviations of the head and spine include circulatory, respiratory, digestive, and excretory dysfunctions; headaches; backaches; depression; and a generalized increased susceptibility to disease [6,24,44,45]. Pain in the back and lower extremities also is attributed to abnormal alignment in the hips, knees, and feet [12,33,34,37,72].

Despite the presumption of associations between postural abnormalities and patients' complaints, studies examining these associations vary in their findings. Correlations between the incidence of reported head, neck, and shoulder pain are reported in people with forward head, rounded shoulders, and increased thoracic kyphoses [24]. Studies investigating the association between low back postural deviations and low back pain draw variable conclusions, with some reporting little or no difference in posture between those with and without low back pain [9,13,75], and others finding differences between the two groups [27,28,53]. Malalignments of the patellofemoral joint are associated with a variety of pain syndromes at the knee [25,41,55]. Considerably more research is required to determine the role that postural abnormalities play in musculoskeletal complaints and to determine the effectiveness of treatments directed toward improving posture to reduce pain.

Typical postural deviations are listed and defined in *Tables 47.4 and 47.5 (Fig.47.17)*. These postural abnormalities are presumed to produce excessive or abnormally located **stresses** (force/area) on joint surfaces or to contribute to altered muscle mechanics by putting some muscles on slack while stretching others [31]. Although evidence supports these effects in some cases, evidence is lacking for others [11,34,37]. Determining the role posture plays in the pathomechanics of musculoskeletal disorders requires continued research in basic anatomy and biomechanics, as well as well-controlled outcome studies examining the effectiveness of treatments directed toward posture reeducation.

Muscle Imbalances Reported in Postural Malalignments

A commonly held clinical perception is that postural malalignments produce adaptive changes in the muscles surrounding the malaligned joints. Specifically, it is believed that muscles on one side of the joint are held in a lengthened position and the antagonistic muscles are maintained in a shortened position. Clinicians also suggest that these length changes produce joint impairments including weakness and

TABLE 47.4: Common Postural Abnormalities in the Sagittal Plane

Postural Deviation	Description
Forward head	The mastoid process lies anterior to the body of C7
Forward shoulders	The acromion process lies anterior to the body of C7, or the scapula tilts anteriorly
Excessive/flattened thoracic kyphosis	The sagittal plane curve of the thorax is excessive or inadequate
Excessive/flattened lumbar lordosis	The sagittal plane curve of the lumbar spine is excessive or inadequate
Anterior/posterior pelvic tilt	The angle made by a line through the ASIS and PSIS and the horizontal increases/decreases from an angle of approximately 10–15°
Forward/backward translation of the pelvis	Determined by the location of the greater trochanter with respect to the vertical line through the center of mass, which in normal alignment passes approximately through the trochanter
Genu recurvatum	Angle between the mechanical axes of the leg and thigh in the sagittal plane is greater than 0°

TABLE 47.5: Common Postural Abnormalities in the Frontal and Transverse Planes

Postural Deviation	Description
Head tilt	The line through the center of the head deviates from the midsagittal plane
Asymmetrical shoulder height	Measured by the height of the acromions or the inferior angles of the scapulae
Scoliosis	Frontal plane deviation of the vertebral column as assessed by the spinous processes
Pelvic obliquity	Asymmetrical height of the pelvis as measured by the iliac crests
Asymmetrical hip height	Measured by the height of the greater trochanters or gluteal folds
Genu varum/valgus	Angle between the mechanical axes of the leg and thigh in the frontal plane
Foot pronation/supination	Indicated by several different measures including (1) the frontal plane alignment of the heel and leg, (2) the height of the navicular relative to the medial malleolus and the head of the first metatarsal, and (3) the subtalar neutral position
In-toeing/out-toeing	The angle between the long axis of the foot and the malleoli is less than/greater than approximately 20°

limited range of motion that contribute to a patient's complaints. Although these hypotheses are logical and may still prove true, few studies to date identify clear associations between malalignments and joint impairments [11,43]. Borstad reports that individuals with tight pectoralis minor muscles demonstrate a rounded shoulder posture as defined by the distance between the sternal notch and the coracoid

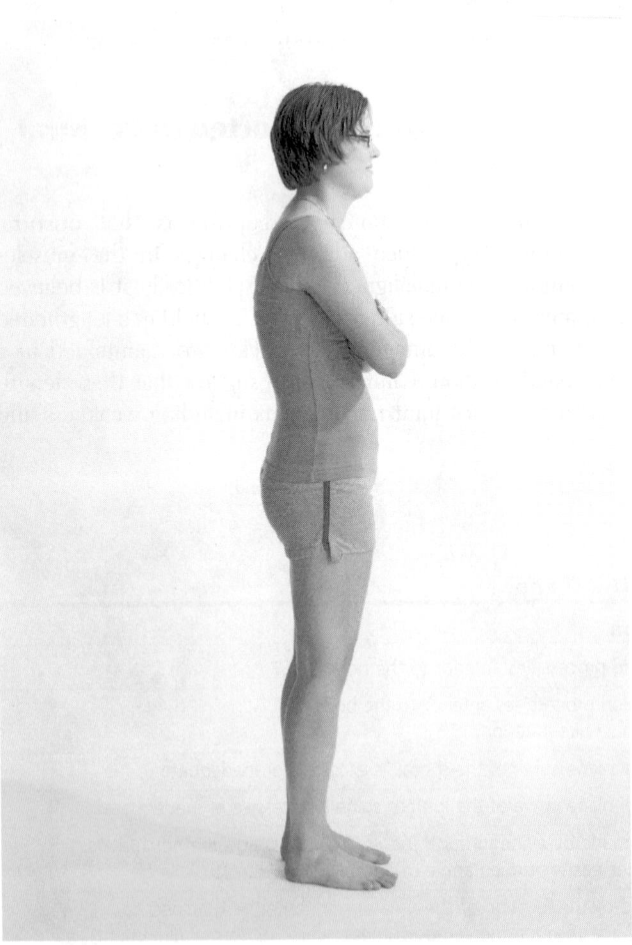

Figure 47.17: Excessive curves. This individual displays a common but abnormal posture, characterized by excessive sagittal plane curves of the spine.

process accompanied by internal rotation of the scapula [3]. Although these findings link muscle changes with postural malalignments, they still do not relate the postural deviations to joint impairments or functional deficits. Additional research is needed to determine what links exist among postural abnormalities, muscle impairments, and patients' complaints.

As noted in Chapter 4, studies in animals demonstrate that prolonged length changes in muscles produce structural changes in muscle, although those changes depend upon many factors besides length. These additional mitigating factors include age, fiber arrangement within the muscles, and fiber type within the muscle [36,38]. In general, prolonged stretch of a muscle induces protein synthesis and the production of additional sarcomeres [21,22,60,71,73]. The lengthened muscle hypertrophies, and as a result, peak contractile force increases with prolonged stretch [36,38]. The structural remodeling that accompanies prolonged lengthening appears to maintain the muscle's original length–tension relationship so that, although the muscle has a larger peak torque, it generates the peak torque at a different joint position. The clinical literature describes **stretch weakness** in which a muscle that has been held in a stretched position long enough to remodel appears weak when tested in the traditional test position [23,31]. For example, at the shoulder, stretch weakness suggests that a posture characterized by rounded shoulders applies a prolonged stretch to the middle trapezius, which undergoes the structural adaptations that lead to weakness when assessed in the traditional manual muscle test position. Although the changes described here are logical and plausible, they remain unproved.

Animal studies examining prolonged shortening reveal that shortening produced by immobilization appears to accelerate atrophy, and muscles demonstrate a loss of sarcomeres [21,60,73]. Studies examining the effect of prolonged length changes in muscle reveal that the relationship between muscle length and muscle performance is complex, requiring independent investigation of the relationship with each muscle. The complexity of the association helps explain the absence of clearly defined associations.

Attempts to confirm the expected muscle impairments with postural abnormalities have failed to yield clear relationships.

Individuals with idiopathic scoliosis exhibit atrophy of the muscles of the posterior thorax, particularly on the concave side, and a higher percentage of type I muscle fibers than normal on the convex side of the deformity [15,74,78]. The muscles of the thorax on the concave side of the curve are likely shortened, while those on the convex side are lengthened; yet both muscle groups exhibit atrophy. Although this atrophy may precede the development of the scoliosis, the expected adaptive changes with prolonged lengthening apparently are lacking. Similarly, attempts to relate scapular alignment and muscle performance fail to reveal consistent associations [3,11]. However, the scapula moves in a complex, three-dimensional way, and studies so far may not accurately reflect the effects of scapular malalignment on muscle length. These data demonstrate the need for careful anatomical, biomechanical, and clinical studies to identify and explain any detrimental effects of postural malalignment.

Because of the lack of definitive studies that link postural malalignments with patient complaints, impairments, and disabilities, clinicians continue to argue the significance and utility of postural examinations [54]. Boulay et al. use a statistical model to suggest that biomechanical efficiency in posture depends on several interdependent factors [4]. They suggest, for example, that an individual with a given pelvic incidence has a range of sacral slopes, lumbar lordoses, and thoracic kyphoses that can be combined to achieve biomechanical economy. If, however, the individual's lordosis falls outside the range of acceptable values, then his or her posture may lead to impairments and dysfunction. Such an interdependent and dynamic postural adaptation suggests that clinicians may need to consider clusters of postural alignments and perhaps identify thresholds beyond which malalignments should be treated.

SUMMARY

This chapter describes the relative alignment of body segments identified in healthy adults during quiet standing. In the absence of a validated description of "ideal posture," the documented alignments provide clinicians with a view of the variability of alignments found in individuals without musculoskeletal complaints. Although individuals demonstrate a wide spectrum of alignments, the overall image of upright posture shows a head well balanced over the pelvis, which in turn is well balanced over the feet. Using these alignments, the chapter also demonstrates the external moments applied to the joints of the lower extremities and trunk during upright standing. The external moments are balanced by internal moments generated by muscle contractions and noncontractile connective tissue support. EMG data are consistent with the mechanical data, demonstrating low levels of activity in the plantar flexors, hip flexors, and erector spinae muscles of the lumbar and cervical regions. Additional activity in the oblique abdominal muscles is consistent with their role as stabilizers of the spine. In addition, other muscle groups such as the dorsiflexor muscles, the quadriceps, and the hamstrings demonstrate

very brief bursts of activity that may be required to control the small, but persistent sway of the body that occurs throughout quiet stance.

Postural alignment is commonly assessed clinically, and some abnormal postures are associated with musculoskeletal abnormalities and clinical complaints. However, many of the commonly held beliefs regarding the associations between postural abnormalities and musculoskeletal impairments lack objective evidence. Although these associations may well exist, additional research is required to identify such relationships and to demonstrate the effectiveness of treating postural deviations to reduce pain or other impairments.

References

1. Basmajian JV, DeLuca CJ: Muscles Alive. Their Function Revealed by Electromyography. Baltimore: Williams & Wilkins, 1985.
2. Bernhardt M, Bridwell KH: Segmental analysis of the sagittal plane alignment of the normal thoracic and lumbar spines and thoracolumbar junction. Spine 1989; 14: 717–721.
3. Borstad J: Resting position variables at the shoulder: evidence to support a posture-impairment association. Phys Ther 2006; 86: 549–557.
4. Boulay C, Tardieu C, Hecquet J, et al.: Sagittal alignment of spine and pelvis regulated by pelvic incidence: standard values and prediction of lordosis. Eur Spine J 2006; 15: 415–422.
5. Crowell RD, Cummings GS, Walker JR: Intratester and intertester reliability and validity of measures of innominate bone inclination. J Orthop Sports Phys Ther 1994; 20: 88–97.
6. Culham E, Jimenez HA, King CE: Thoracic kyphosis, rib mobility, and lung volumes in normal women and women with osteoporosis. Spine 1994; 19: 1250–1255.
7. Culham E, Peat M: Functional Anatomy of the Shoulder Complex. J Orthop Sports Phys Ther 1993; 18: 342–350.
8. Danis CG, Krebs DE, Gill-Body KM, Sahrmann SA: Relationship between standing posture and stability. Phys Ther 1998; 78: 502–517.
9. Day JW, Smidt GL, Lehmann T: Effect of pelvic tilt on standing posture. Phys Ther 1984; 64: 510–516.
10. Delisle A, Gagnon M, Sicard C: Effect of pelvic tilt on lumbar spine geometry. IEEE Trans Rehabil Eng 1997; 5: 360–366.
11. DiVeta J, Walker M, Skibinski B: Relationship between performance of selected scapular muscles and scapular abduction in standing subjects. Phys Ther 1990; 70: 470–476.
12. Donatelli R, Hurlbert C, Conaway D, St. Pierre R: Biomechanical foot orthotics: a retrospective study. J Orthop Sports Phys Ther 1988; 10: 205–212.
13. During J, Goudfrooij H, Keesen W, et al.: Toward standards for posture—postural characteristics of the lower back system in normal and pathologic conditions. Spine 1985; 10: 83–87.
14. Floyd WF, Silver PHS: Electromyographic study of patterns of activity of the anterior abdominal wall muscles in man. J Anat 1950; 84: 132–145.
15. Ford DM, Bagnall KM, McFadden KD, et al.: Paraspinal muscle imbalance in adolescent idiopathic scoliosis. Spine 1984; 9: 373–376.
16. Gajdosik RL, Simpson R, Smith R, Dontigny RL: Intratester reliability of measuring the standing position and range of motion. Phys Ther 1985; 65: 169–174.

17. Gangnet N, Dumas R, Pomero V, et al.: Three-dimensional spinal and pelvic alignment in an asymptomatic population. Spine 2006; 31: E507–E512.

18. Garrett TR, Youdas JW, Madson TJ: Reliability of measuring forward head posture in a clinical setting. J Orthop Sports Phys Ther 1993; 17: 155–160.

19. Gelb DE, Lenke LG, Bridwell KH, et al.: An analysis of sagittal spinal alignment in 100 asymptomatic middle and older aged volunteers. Spine 1995; 2: 1351–1358.

20. Gilliam J, Brunt D, MacMillan M, et al.: Relationship of the pelvic angle to the sacral angle: measurement of clinical reliability and validity. J Orthop Sports Phys Ther 1994; 20: 193–199.

21. Goldspink G: The influence of immobilization and stretch in protein turnover of rat skeletal muscle. J Physiol 1977; 264: 267–282.

22. Goldspink G: Changes in muscle mass and phenotype and the expression of autocrine and systemic growth factors by muscle in response to stretch and overload. J Anat 1999; 194: 323–334.

23. Gossman MR, Sahrmann SA, Rose SJ: Review of length-associated changes in muscle. Phys Ther 1982; 62: 1799–1807.

24. Griegel-Morris P, Larson K, Mueller-Klaus K, Oatis CA: Incidence of common postural problems in the cervical, shoulder and thoracic regions and their association with muscle imbalance and pain. Phys Ther 1992; 72: 425–431.

25. Holmes SW Jr, Clancy WG Jr: Clinical classification of patellofemoral pain and dysfunction. J Orthop Sports Phys Ther 1998; 28: 299–306.

26. Inman VT, Saunders M, Abbott LC: Observations on the function of the shoulder joint. J Bone Joint Surg 1944; 26: 1–30.

27. Jackson RP, Mcmanus AC: Radiographic analysis of sagittal plane alignment and balance in standing volunteers and patients with low back pain matched for age, sex and size. Spine 1994; 19: 1611–1618.

28. Jackson RP, Phipps T, Hales C, et al.: Pelvic lordosis and alignment in spondylolisthesis. Spine 2003; 28: 151–160.

29. Jian Y, Winter DA, Ishac MG, Gilchrist L: Trajectory of the body COG and COP during initiation and termination of gait. Gait Posture 1993; 1: 9–22.

30. Johnson GR, Spalding D, Nowitzke A, Bogduk N: Modelling the muscles of the scapula morphometric and coordinate data and functional implications. J Biomech 1996; 29: 1039–1051.

31. Kendall FP, McCreary EK, Provance PG: Muscle Testing and Function. Baltimore: Williams & Wilkins, 1993.

32. Kim Y, Bridwell KH, Lenke LG, et al.: An analysis of sagittal spinal alignment following long adult lumbar instrumentation and fusion to L5 or S1: can we predict ideal lumbar lordosis? Spine 2006; 31: 2343–2352.

33. Klingman RE, Liaos SM, Hardin KM: The effect of subtalar joint posting on patellar glide position in subjects with excessive rearfoot pronation. JOSPT 1997; 25: 185–191.

34. Laforgia R, Specchiulli F, Solarino G, Nitti L: Radiographic variables in normal and osteoarthritic hips. Bull Hosp Joint Dis 1996; 54: 215–221.

35. Levine D, Whittle MW: The effects of pelvic movement on lumbar lordosis in the standing position. J Orthop Sports Phys Ther 1996; 24: 130–135.

36. Lieber RL: Skeletal Muscle Structure and Function: Implications for Rehabilitation and Sports Medicine. Baltimore: Williams & Wilkins, 1992.

37. Loudon JK, Goitz HT, Loudon KL: Genu recurvatum syndrome. J Orthop Sports Phys Ther 1998; 27: 361–367.

38. Loughna PT: Disuse and passive stretch cause rapid alterations in expression of developmental and adult contractile protein genes in skeletal muscle. Development 1990; 109: 217–223.

39. Mac-Thiong JM, Berthonnaud E, Dimar JR, et al.: Sagittal alignment of the spine and pelvis during growth. Spine 2004; 29: 1642–1647.

40. Magee DA: Orthopedic Physical Assessment. Philadelphia: WB Saunders, 1998.

41. Meyer SA, Brown TD, Pedersen DR, Albright JP: Retropatellar contact stress in simulated patella infera. Am J Knee Surg 1997; 10: 129–138.

42. Murray MP, Seireg A, Sepic SB: Normal postural stability and steadiness: quantitative assessment. J Bone Joint Surg 1975; 57A: 510–516.

43. Neumann DA, Soderberg GL, Cook TM: Comparison of maximal isometric hip abductor muscle torques between hip sides. Phys Ther 1988; 68: 496–502.

44. Nicholson GG, Gaston J: Cervical headache. J Orthop Sports Phys Ther 2001; 31: 184–193.

45. Nicolakis P, Nicolakis M, Piehslinger E, et al.: Relationship between craniomandibular disorders and poor posture. Cranio 2000; 18: 106–112.

46. Norton BJ, Hensler K, Zou D: Comparisons among noninvasive methods for measuring lumbar curvature in standing. J Orthop Sports Phys Ther 2002; 32: 405–413.

47. Oh JS, Cynn HS, Won JH, et al.: Effects of performing an abdominal drawing-in maneuver during prone hip extension exercises on hip and back extensor muscle activity and amount of anterior pelvic tilt. J Orthop Sports Phys Ther 2007; 37: 320–324.

48. Opila KA, Wagner SS, Schiowitz S, Chen J: Postural alignment in barefoot and high-heeled stance. Spine 1988; 13: 542–547.

49. Palmerud G, Sporrong H, Herberts P, Kadefors R: Consequences of trapezius relaxation on the distribution of shoulder muscle forces: an electromyographic study. J Electromyogr Kinesiol 1998; 8: 185–193.

50. Panzer VP, Bandinelli S, Hallett M: Biomechanical assessment of quiet standing and changes associated with aging. Arch Phys Med Rehabil 1995; 76: 151–157.

51. Partridge MJBS, Walters CE: Participation of the abdominal muscles in various movements of the trunk in man: an electromyographic study. Phys Ther Rev 1959; 39: 791–800.

52. Peterson DE, Blankenship KR, Robb JB, et al.: Investigation of the validity and reliability of four objective techniques for measuring forward shoulder posture. J Orthop Sports Phys Ther 1997; 25: 34–42.

53. Roussouly P, Gollogly S, Berthonnaud E, et al.: Sagittal alignment of the spine and pelvis in the presence of L5-S1 isthmic lysis and low-grade spondylolisthesis. Spine 2006; 31: 2484–2490.

54. Sahrmann SA: Does postural assessment contribute to patient care? J Orthop Sports Phys Ther 2002; 32: 376–379.

55. Singerman R, Davy D, Goldberg V: Effects of patella alta and patella infera on patellofemoral contact forces. J Biomech 1994; 27: 1059–1065.

56. Snijders CJ, Slagter AHE, van Strik R, et al.: Why leg crossing? The influence of common postures on abdominal muscle activity. Spine 1995; 18: 1989–1993.

57. Sobush DC, Simoneau GG, Dietz KE, et al.: The Lennie test for measuring scapular position in healthy young adult females: a reliability and validity study. J Orthop Sports Phys Ther 1996; 23: 39–50.

58. Steindler A: Kinesiology of the human body under normal and pathological conditions. Springfield, IL: Charles C Thomas, 1955.

59. Stokes IA, Bevin TM, Lunn RA: Back surface curvature and measurement of lumbar spinal motion. Spine 1987; 12: 355–361.

60. Tabary JC, Tabary C, Tardieu C, et al.: Physiological and structural changes in the cat's soleus muscle due to immobilization at different lengths by plaster casts. J Physiol 1972; 224: 231–244.

61. Takebe K, Vitti M, Basmajian JV: The function of the semispinalis capitis and splenius capitis. Anat Rec 1974; 179: 477–480.

62. Tillotson KM, Burton AK: Noninvasive measurement of lumbar sagittal mobility. Spine 1991; 16: 29–33.

63. Tsai LC, Yu B, Mercer VS, et al.: Comparison of different structural foot types for measures of standing postural control. J Orthop Sports Phys Ther 2006; 36: 942–953.

64. Vedantam R, Lenke LG, Keeney JA, Bridwell KH: Comparison of standing sagittal spinal alignment in asymptomatic adolescents and adults. Spine 1998; 23: 211–215.

65. Vialle R, Levassor N, Rillardon L, et al.: Radiographic analysis of the sagittal alignment and balance of the spine in asymptomatic subjects. J Bone Joint Surg 2005; 87: 260–267.

66. Voutsinas SA, MacEwen GD: Sagittal profiles of the spine. Clin Orthop 1986; 210: 235–242.

67. Vuillerme N, Forestier N, Nougier V: Attentional demands and postural sway: the effect of the calf muscles fatigue. Med Sci Sports Exerc 2002; 34: 1907–1912.

68. Walker ML, Rothstein JM, Finucane SD, Lamb RL: Relationships between lumbar lordosis, pelvic tilt, and abdominal muscle performance. Phys Ther 1987; 67: 512–521.

69. Waters RL, Morris JM: Effect of spinal supports on the electrical activity of muscles of the trunk. J Bone Joint Surg 1970; 52A: 51–60.

70. White AA III, Panjabi MM: Practical biomechanics of scoliosis and kyphosis. In: Cooke DB, ed. Clinical Biomechanics of the Spine. Philadelphia: JB Lippincott, 1990; 127–163.

71. Williams P, Kyberd P, Simpson H, et al.: The morphological basis of increased stiffness of rabbit tibialis anterior muscles during surgical limb-lengthening. J Anat 1998; 193: 131–138.

72. Witonski D, Goraj B: Patellar motion analyzed by kinematic and dynamic axial magnetic resonance imaging in patients with anterior knee pain syndrome. Arch Orthop Trauma Surg 1999; 119: 46–49.

73. Yang H, Alnaqeeb M, Simpson H, Goldspink G: Changes in muscle fibre type, muscle mass and IGF-I gene expression in rabbit skeletal muscle subjected to stretch. J Anat 1997; 190: 613–622.

74. Yarom R, Robin GC: Studies on spinal and peripheral muscles from patients with scoliosis. Spine 1979; 4: 12–21.

75. Youdas JW, Garrett TR, Egan KS, Therneau TM: Lumbar lordosis and pelvic inclination in adults with chronic low back pain. Phys Ther 2000; 80: 261–275.

76. Youdas JW, Garrett TR, Harmsen S, et al.: Lumbar lordosis and pelvic inclination of asymptomatic adults. Phys Ther 1996; 76: 1066–1081.

77. Youdas JW, Suman VJ, Garrett TR: Reliability of measurements of lumbar spine sagittal mobility obtained with the flexible curve. J Orthop Sports Phys Ther 1995; 21: 13–27.

78. Zetterberg C, Aniansson A, Grimby G: Morphology of the paravertebral muscles in adolescent idiopathic scoliosis. Spine 1983; 8: 457–462.

Characteristics of Normal Gait and Factors Influencing It

CHAPTER CONTENTS

Habitual bipedal locomotion is a uniquely human function and influences an individual's participation and interaction in society. Impairments in gait are frequent complaints of persons seeking rehabilitation services and are often the focus of an individual's goals of treatment. Rehabilitation experts require a firm understanding of the basic mechanics of normal locomotion to determine the links between impairments of discrete segments of the musculoskeletal system and the patient's abnormal movement patterns in gait.

Therapists and other rehabilitation experts are called upon daily to analyze a patient's movements and determine the cause of the abnormal, often painful, motion. A thorough understanding of normal locomotion and the factors that influence it, as well as an understanding of the functions of the components of the musculoskeletal system, provides a framework for evaluation and treatment of locomotor dysfunctions. This chapter describes the general characteristics of normal locomotion and introduces the clinician to the basic concepts central to all movement analysis.

Normal human locomotion consists of stereotypical movement patterns that are immediately recognizable. Yet most individuals also are able to distinguish the gait of close friends and associates by the sound of their footsteps in the hallway. The purpose of this chapter is to describe the common characteristics of normal human locomotion and their variability and to provide insight into how impairments within the musculoskeletal system may be manifested in altered gait patterns. The specific objectives of this chapter are to

- Describe the basic components of the gait cycle
- Present the temporal and distance characteristics of normal gait

- Detail the angular displacement patterns of the joints of the lower extremity, the trunk, and the upper extremities
- Describe the patterns of muscle activity that characterize normal locomotion
- Briefly discuss the methods for determining muscle and joint loads sustained during normal locomotion and present the findings from representative literature
- Briefly consider the energetics of normal locomotion and the implications of gait abnormalities on the efficiency of gait

Gait has been studied for millennia, and the last 50 years have seen an explosion in the research examining the characteristics of gait and the factors that control it. The current chapter is, of necessity, an overview of the characteristics of locomotion that are useful to a clinician and that demonstrate the effect of the integrity of the musculoskeletal system on gait. Several textbooks dealing only with locomotion provide details regarding the movement and methods of its assessment, and insight into the central nervous system's role in controlling and modifying the movement of gait [31,134,147,184].

THE GAIT CYCLE, THE BASIC UNIT OF GAIT

Gait is a cyclical movement that, once begun, possesses very repeatable events that continue repetitively until the individual begins to stop the motion. The steady-state movement of normal locomotion is composed of a basic repeating cycle, the **gait cycle** (*Fig. 48.1*). The cycle is traditionally defined as the movement pattern beginning and ending with ground contact of the same foot. For example, using the right foot as the reference foot, the gait cycle begins when the right foot contacts the ground (usually with the heel) and ends when it contacts the ground again. Thus a gait cycle consists of the time the reference foot is on the ground (**stance**) and the time it is off the ground (**swing**). The movement of both limbs that occurs during the gait cycle is known as the **stride**.

The **stance phase** of gait makes up approximately 60% of the gait cycle, so that the remaining 40% consists of the swing phase. The gait cycle with respect to the right limb is slightly out of phase with the gait cycle of the left limb. At contact on the right, the left limb is just ending its stance phase. At approximately 10% of the gait cycle on the right, the left limb leaves the ground and begins its swing phase, returning to the ground at approximately 50% of the gait cycle of the right limb. Thus the gait cycle is characterized by two brief periods, each lasting approximately 10% of the gait cycle, in which both limbs are in contact with the ground. These are periods of **double limb support,** and the remaining cycle consists of **single limb support.**

The stance phase can be divided into smaller periods associated with specific functional demands and identified by distinct events (*Fig. 48.2*) [136]. The period immediately following ground contact is known as **contact response,** or **weight acceptance,** and ends when the whole foot flattens on the ground. During contact response, the limb absorbs the shock of impact and becomes fully loaded. The **foot flat** event that

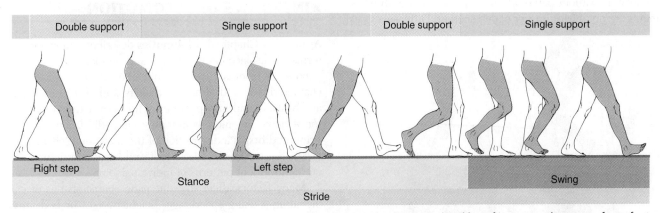

Figure 48.1: The gait cycle of a single lower extremity consists of a stance and swing period and lasts from ground contact of one foot to the subsequent ground contact of the same foot. It includes two steps that are defined as the period from ground contact of one foot to the ground contact of the opposite foot. A single gait cycle includes two periods of double limb support and two periods of single limb support.

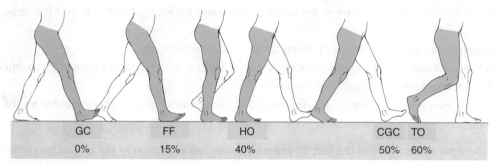

Figure 48.2: The stance phase is divided into smaller phases that are demarcated by specific events. *GC,* ground contact; *FF,* foot flat; *HO,* heel off; *CGC,* contralateral ground contact, *TO,* toe off.

ends contact response occurs at approximately 15% of the normal gait cycle. It is important to recognize that loading response includes double limb support and continues into single limb support. The period following loading response is **midstance,** also known as **trunk glide,** since during this period the trunk glides over the fixed foot, moving from behind the stance foot to in front of it. **Heel off** ends trunk glide at approximately 40% of the gait cycle and begins **terminal stance,** which ends at 50% of the gait cycle when contralateral ground contact occurs. The final stage of stance, from 50 to 60% of the gait cycle, is **preswing** and is characterized by double limb support. It ends with **toe off.**

The swing phase also is divided into early, middle, and late periods, although it lacks distinctive events to delineate these phases (*Fig. 48.3*). **Early swing** continues from 60% to approximately 75% of the gait cycle and is characterized by the rapid withdrawal of the limb from the ground. **Midswing** continues until approximately 85% of the gait cycle and consists of the period in which the swing limb passes the stance limb. **Late,** or **terminal, swing** finds the swing limb reaching toward the ground, preparing for contact.

Although normal gait is often assumed to be symmetrical, substantial evidence exists to refute that assumption [15,68,106,151]. Although the differences are small among ambulators without pathology, the right and left limb movements are not mirror images of one another. Differences exist in timing and movement patterns, in muscle activity, and in the loads applied to each limb [55,150]. Asymmetry appears greatest at slower walking speeds [57]. When evaluating the gait patterns of individuals with asymmetrical impairments, clinicians must remember that small asymmetries in gait are normal, particularly when walking slowly.

Consideration of the basic functional tasks of the swing and stance phase of gait provides a framework for characterizing the movements in each phase of gait. While the overriding goal of locomotion is forward progression, the stance and swing phases contribute to that goal in different ways. The stance phase has three tasks in locomotion: providing adequate support to avoid a fall, absorbing the shock of impact between the limb and the ground, and providing adequate forward and backward force for forward progress [35,183]. The basic tasks of the swing phase are safe limb clearance, appropriate limb placement for the next contact, and transfer of momentum. By keeping these tasks in mind, the clinician can understand the importance of discrete movements of limb segments or the specific sequencing of muscle activity and can begin to appreciate the significance of specific joint impairments.

KINEMATICS OF LOCOMOTION

As noted in Chapter 1, **kinematics** describes a movement in terms of displacement, velocity, and acceleration. The vast majority of kinematic analyses of gait examines displacement characteristics, and although velocity and acceleration data are available and may provide useful information, this chapter reviews the more commonly cited displacement data. Presented first is a description of the movement characteristics of the stride as a whole followed by descriptions of discrete movement patterns of individual joints.

Many factors affect the kinematic characteristics of gait, including walking speed, age, height, weight or body mass index, strength and flexibility, pain, and aerobic conditioning. Walking speed and age have large and important effects on gait and are discussed later in this chapter. Unless noted otherwise, the data reported come from trials in which the subjects walk at their self-selected, comfortable, or **free,** speed.

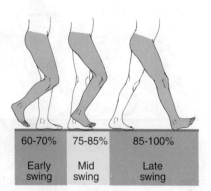

Figure 48.3: The swing phase is divided into early swing, when the limb is pulled away from the ground; midswing, as the swing limb passes the stance limb; and late swing, when the swing limb extends toward the ground.

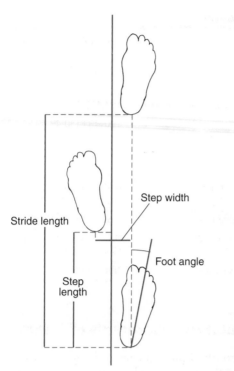

Figure 48.4: Several distance measures help describe a typical gait cycle.

Temporal and Distance Parameters of a Stride

A **stride** consists of the movement of both limbs during a gait cycle and contains two steps. A **step** is operationally defined as the movement of a single limb from ground contact of one limb to ground contact of the opposite limb (*Fig. 48.4*). The literature demonstrates that there is considerable difference in step and stride characteristics among subjects and even among trials of the same subject [53,133,171]. Despite this normal variability, these parameters are capable of distinguishing between individuals with and without impairments [83,176].

DISTANCE CHARACTERISTICS OF THE STRIDE

The typical distance parameters of gait are defined in *Table 48.1*. A representative range of values also is presented from the literature [24,65,82,101,104,120,122,131,133].

Stride and step lengths depend directly upon standing height, so measures of absolute step or stride length, although frequently reported, are difficult to interpret. These measures can be normalized by standing height or lower extremity length to compare values from different individuals [30,81]. Estimates of normalized stride length vary from approximately 60 to 110% of standing height [24,30]. Judge et al. report a mean step length of 74 ± 4% of leg length in young healthy adults [81]. Step width and foot angle are less frequently reported but provide an indication of the size of the base of support.

TEMPORAL CHARACTERISTICS OF THE STRIDE

The temporal characteristics of the stride are defined in *Table 48.2* [43,49,59]. Included in this list is walking speed, or gait velocity, although this is typically computed over several strides. The normal gait cycle at free speed lasts approximately 1 second, and walking speed is between 3 and 4 miles per hour (4.8–6.4 km/h) or approximately 1.3 m/sec. Walking speed is a function of both **cadence** (steps/minute) and step length. An increase in either cadence or step length contributes to increased walking speed [7,62,101,119,159,176].

Walking speed affects swing and stance time differently. Increased walking speed decreases the overall duration of the gait cycle, but the decrease in cycle duration results in a greater decrease in stance time than in swing time [7,119]. As stance time decreases with less change in swing time, double limb support time decreases, and single limb support time increases. The difference between running and walking is the absence of a double limb support phase in running. The ratio between swing and stance time increases toward 1 with increasing walking speed.

Many gait disorders lead to altered time and distance parameters, typically decreased speed and stride length and, in the case of unilateral disorders, altered swing and stance times with abnormal swing–stance ratios. Such measures are relatively easy to obtain in the clinic and serve as useful outcome measures, sensitive to change. On the other hand, many different disorders produce similar temporal and distance characteristics. For example, a patient with unilateral hip pain and a patient with hemiparesis secondary to a stroke both walk with decreased velocity, and both demonstrate decreased single limb support time on the affected side and increased double limb support time [119]. These parameters

TABLE 48.1: Distance Parameters of Stride in Young Healthy Adults

Parameter	Definition	Range of Values Reported in the Literature
Stride length	The distance between ground contact of one foot and the subsequent ground contact of the same foot	1.33 ± 0.09 to 1.63 ± 0.11 m [65,82,101,104,120,122,131]
Step length	The distance between ground contact of one foot and the subsequent ground contact of the opposite foot	0.70 ± 0.01 to 0.81 ± 0.05 m [65,120,159]
Step width (also known as base of support)[a]	The perpendicular distance between similar points on both feet measured during two consecutive steps [25,104]	0.61 ± 0.22 to 9.0 ± 3.5 cm [104,120,122,159,169]
Foot angle	Angle between the long axis of the foot and the line of forward progression	5.1 ± 5.7 to 6.8 ± 5.6° [104]

[a]Step width is defined variably in the literature. Some measures incorporate the angle of the foot on the ground.

TABLE 48.2: Temporal Parameters of Stride in Young, Healthy Adults

Parameter	Definition	Values From the Literature
Stride time	Time in seconds from ground contact of one foot to ground contact of the same foot	1.00 ± 0.23 to 1.12 ± 0.07 [104,120,122,131]
Speed (also known as velocity)	Distance/time, usually reported in m/sec	0.82–1.60 ± 0.16 [49,65,81,82,101, 104,119,122,131,159]
Cadence	Steps per minute	100–131 [30,43,49,81,82,104,119, 122,159]
Stance time	Time in seconds that the reference foot is on the ground during a gait cycle	0.63 ± 0.07 to 0.67 ± 0.04 [104,120,122]
Swing time	Time in seconds that the reference foot is off the ground during a gait cycle	0.39 ± 0.02 to 0.40 ± 0.04 [104,120,122]
Swing/stance ratio	Ratio between the swing time and the stance time	0.63–0.64 [82,122]
Double support time	Time in seconds during the gait cycle that two feet are in contact with the ground	0.11 ± 0.03 to 0.141 ± 0.03 [104,119,120]
Single support time	Time in seconds during the gait cycle that one foot is in contact with the ground	Not reported

distinguish between normal gait and abnormal walking patterns but are unlikely to identify the differences in gait patterns between the two patients, even though such differences often are easily detected by an observer. Thus temporal and distance parameters may be helpful in tracking a patient's progress but are insufficient to characterize a gait pattern fully and to identify the mechanisms driving the movement pattern. Patterns of joint excursions, however, can help the clinician to identify the differences in gait patterns between individuals with similar temporal and distance characteristics.

Clinical Relevance

EFFECTS OF STANDING HEIGHT ON DISTANCE AND TEMPORAL CHARACTERISTICS OF GAIT: *Two friends agreed to participate in a 2-day Breast Cancer Walk. The walk consisted of a 26.2-mile walk the first day and a 13.1-mile walk the following day. The friends trained for the walk by walking together several times per week, distances ranging from 4 to 20 miles. One friend was 5 feet 8 inches tall and the other 5 feet 2 inches tall. Both were active, healthy individuals of the same age. Neither had any known musculoskeletal problems or gait deviations.*

At the beginning of the official walk, all participants received pedometers. The friends completed the first day without difficulty, walking together the entire distance. At the end of the day they checked their pedometers and one reported 65,000 steps and the other 48,000 steps. Was one pedometer broken?! The friends walked the second day together again and finished without incident. At the end of the 2-day walk the pedometers read 99,500 and 63,000 steps! Not surprisingly, the shorter friend was wearing the pedometer that read 99,500. That individual had taken over 50% more steps than the taller friend. Since they walked together the entire time, the shorter friend must have used a higher cadence (steps/minute) to stay with the taller friend.

Angular Displacements of Joints

The growth of photography in the mid- to late 19th century allowed the systematic observation of discrete movements of each joint during the complex activity of normal locomotion [5]. Over the last 50 years improved photographic techniques and the development of the computer have led to ever more precise monitoring of the three-dimensional motion of individual segments. The sagittal plane motions of the joints of the lower extremity are the most thoroughly studied and best understood, at least in part because sagittal plane motions are the largest and easiest to measure. In contrast, frontal and transverse plane motions of the joints of the lower extremities and the three-dimensional motions of the upper extremities and trunk are less frequently studied. Joint displacement data reveal intra- and intersubject variability in all planes, although the variability is greater in the frontal and transverse planes than in the sagittal plane and across subjects than between cycles of a single individual [16,42,63,82]. The smaller excursions in the frontal and transverse planes are particularly sensitive to differences in measurement procedure, which accounts for some of the increased variability of these motions [75,145]. Despite the variability in magnitudes of the movements, the patterns and sequencing of joint movements in gait are remarkably consistent across trials and across subjects [14,34,35,119].

SAGITTAL PLANE MOTIONS

The classic studies by Murray remain the foundation for understanding sagittal plane motion of the lower extremity [119,120,122,123] (*Fig. 48.5*). More-recent studies confirm the overall patterns of motion for the hip, knee, and ankle, although there is variation in the reported maximal joint positions. Because studies demonstrate both intra- and intersubject variability, the reader is cautioned that the pattern of motion is the focus of the following discussion rather than the specific magnitudes [45,82,184]. Values of peak excursion are mentioned to provide an image of the motion rather than to define an absolute norm.

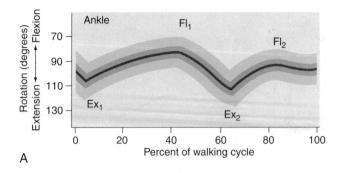

A

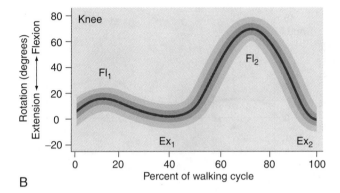

B

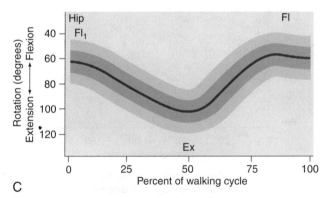

C

Figure 48.5: Sagittal plane excursions of the ankle, knee, and hips. Plots indicate mean and 2 standard deviations. (Reprinted with permission from Murray MP: Gait as a total pattern of movement. Am J Phys Med 1967; 46: 290–333.)

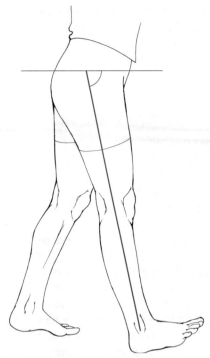

Figure 48.6: In most locomotion studies the hip excursion is described as the angle between the length of the thigh and a room-fixed coordinate system.

flexing again, reaching maximum flexion late in swing, at 80–85% of the gait cycle. The cycle repeats at ground contact.

The knee exhibits a slightly more complex movement pattern, landing in extension, albeit usually a few degrees short of maximum extension, at ground contact. The knee flexes 10 to 20° immediately after contact, reaching maximum flexion at about 15% of the gait cycle when the subject achieves foot flat. At foot flat the knee begins to extend and reaches maximum extension at about 40% of the gait cycle as the heel rises from the ground. Flexion of the knee begins again and reaches a maximum of approximately 70° in midswing (approximately 75% of the gait cycle). Knee extension resumes, and the knee reaches maximum knee extension just before ground contact [23,88,100,119,149].

Ankle motion also exhibits several reversals in direction. Ground contact occurs with the ankle close to neutral in either slight plantarflexion or slight dorsiflexion [88,99,119]. Following contact, the ankle plantarflexes an additional 5 or 10°, reaching a maximum at about 5% of the gait cycle. As the body glides over the stance foot, the ankle dorsiflexes, reaching a maximum just after the knee reaches full extension. Ankle plantarflexion resumes, and the ankle reaches maximum plantarflexion of approximately 20° just following toe off. In swing, the ankle dorsiflexes slightly but may remain in slight plantarflexion throughout swing.

Pelvic motions in the sagittal plane are small, with no consistent definition of neutral. However, studies suggest that the pelvis anteriorly tilts whenever either hip is extending [120,122,157,179]. The anterior pelvic tilt contributes to the

The hip exhibits a single cycle of motion. Beginning at ground contact, the hip is in maximum flexion (approximately 25°) and gradually extends, reaching maximum hip hyperextension (approximately 10°) at close to 50% of the gait cycle, when contralateral ground contact occurs [88,99,119,184]. The magnitude of apparent hip hyperextension excursion depends on the point of reference. As noted in Chapter 38, a normal hip exhibits little or no hyperextension range of motion. Consequently, the hyperextension reported at the hip during locomotion is the result of pelvic motions in the transverse and sagittal planes. In most studies, the reported hip hyperextension reflects the orientation of the thigh with the trunk or with the room-fixed reference frame as seen in *Fig. 48.6.* After reaching maximum extension, the hip begins apparent hip hyperextension that occurs in late stance. Upper extremity sagittal plane motion also shows a rhythmic oscillation that is related to the movement of the lower extremities. At free walking speed, flexion of the shoulder and elbow parallel flexion of the opposite hip [119,123,175].

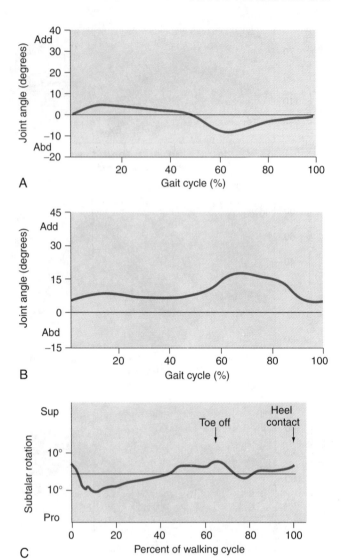

Figure 48.7: Frontal plane excursions of the hip (A), knee (B), and foot (C) are much smaller than sagittal plane excursions but show characteristic patterns of movement.

Clinical Relevance

ASSOCIATED MOVEMENTS IN AN INDIVIDUAL FOLLOWING STROKE: *Close examination of the sagittal plane motions of the hip, knee, and ankle reveal that only for a very brief instant following toe off are these three joints moving in the same direction with respect to the ground. Just following toe off, all three joints are pulling the foot away from the ground, the hip and knee are flexing, and the ankle is dorsiflexing. At other points in the gait cycle the joints move independently, so that one or two joints move the foot toward the ground as the other(s) pull it away from the ground. A common impairment found in patients following stroke is an inability to disassociate movements, and as a result, a patient is compelled to move all three joints of the lower extremity together in the same direction. For example, to flex the knee, the patient may flex the knee and hip and dorsiflex the ankle simultaneously in a **flexion pattern**, or **synergy**, or extend the knee while simultaneously extending the hip and plantarflexing the ankle in an **extension pattern**, or **synergy**. Such obligatory movements interfere with the normal timing and sequencing of joint movements in gait. For instance, in late swing, as the patient extends the knee toward the ground, the hip tends to extend, and the ankle plantarflex, producing a foreshortened step and an abnormal foot position at ground contact. A flexion pattern produces similar conflicts as the hip begins to flex in terminal stance. At this time, the hip and knee should be flexing while the ankle continues to plantarflex. A flexion pattern stops the ankle plantarflexion and interferes with the normal roll off of late stance.*

FRONTAL PLANE MOTIONS

Frontal plane excursions are less well studied and more varied than sagittal plane movements (*Fig. 48.7*). Hip position in the frontal plane is affected by the motion of the pelvis over the femur and by the orientation of the femur as the subject translates toward the opposite foot to keep the center of mass over the base of support. The hip lies close to neutral abduction at ground contact and then adducts during weight acceptance as the pelvis drops on the contralateral side [9,78,79,82] (*Fig. 48.8*). Adduction is amplified as the subject shifts toward the stance side to keep the center of mass over the foot. Adduction continues until late stance, when loading begins on the opposite limb. At that instance, the pelvis drops on the side in late stance, and the hip moves into abduction (*Fig. 48.9*). Reported knee motion in the frontal plane is slight, with estimates ranging from approximately 2 to 10° of adduction, peaking in early swing [9,23,82,100].

Frontal plane motion of the foot recorded during walking reflects the inversion and eversion component of supination and pronation of the foot. Although the position of the hindfoot at ground contact is variable and the magnitude of the reported excursions differs among reports, data consistently demonstrate a motion pattern following ground contact characterized by eversion, consistent with pronation, continuing until mid to late stance when the hindfoot begins inverting or supinating [29,91,115,138,139,189]. Forefoot motion is similar to hindfoot motion, although forefoot pronation during stance begins after hindfoot pronation has begun [74,139,189].

TRANSVERSE PLANE MOTIONS

Transverse plane motions of the limbs and trunk also demonstrate more variability and smaller excursions than those seen in the sagittal plane (*Fig. 48.10*). Transverse plane rotations of the hip are a function of the transverse plane motion of the pelvis as well as the transverse plane motion of the femur

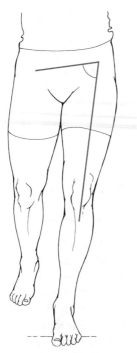

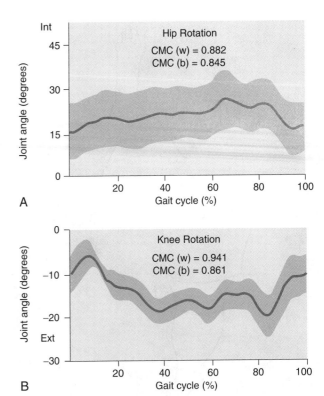

A

B

Figure 48.8: At weight acceptance, the individual shifts laterally to keep the center of mass close to the stance foot, and the pelvis drops on the unsupported side. The stance hip is in adduction.

Figure 48.10: Transverse plane motions of the hip and knee. (Reprinted with permission from Kadaba MP, Ramakrishnan HK, Wootten ME, et al.: Repeatability of kinematic, kinetic, and electromyographic data in normal adult gait. J Orthop Res 1989; 7: 849–860.)

(Fig. 48.11). Pelvic rotation in the transverse plane accompanies hip flexion, so that the pelvis rotates forward on the side of the flexing hip, reaching maximum forward rotation at approximately ground contact [51,82,89,119]. Forward rotation of the pelvis contributes to lateral rotation of the hip. At the same time, the

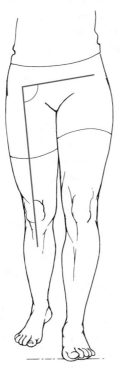

Figure 48.9: During weight acceptance, the hip drops on the unsupported side, which is abducted.

opposite hip is in maximum extension, and the relative backward position of the pelvis on that side allows the hip to appear hyperextended. The transverse plane alignment of the pelvis on the extended hip tends to medially rotate the extended hip.

Independent femoral movement provides its own contribution to hip position. At ground contact, the femur is aligned close to neutral but rotates medially from contact to midstance. Lateral femoral rotation then begins and continues into mid swing when medial rotation resumes. Hip joint position is the sum of the pelvic contribution and the femoral contribution to joint position. Although there is disagreement about the hip position at ground contact among the reported data, there is good consistency regarding the direction of the hip motion, medial rotation from ground contact to mid- or late stance and then lateral rotation until late swing or ground contact [78,79,82,129].

The knee, too, exhibits transverse plane motion with medial rotation following ground contact and gradual lateral rotation from midstance through most of swing, although there is more disagreement about knee motion in swing [9,23,82,100,129]. Transverse plane motion of the knee is linked to the motion of the foot and to the sagittal plane motion of the knee, particularly during stance, when the lower extremity functions in a closed chain. As the foot pronates, the tibia medially rotates and allows the knee to flex. This coupled motion assists in shock absorption during

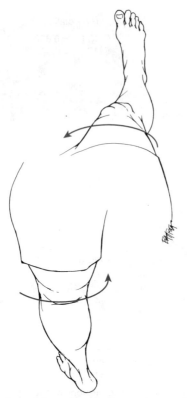

Figure 48.11: The pelvic position in the transverse plane and the femoral rotation in the transverse plane both contribute to the transverse plane hip joint position during the gait cycle. At ground contact the femur is medially rotating, but the forward alignment of the pelvis contributes to lateral rotation of the hip. At heel off the opposite is true.

loading response [137]. Later in stance, the foot supinates as the tibia rotates laterally, and the knee extends while the body rolls forward onto the opposite limb.

MOTIONS OF THE TRUNK

Studies of the head and trunk reveal that these segments undergo systematic translation and rotation in three dimensions and exhibit both intrasubject and intersubject variability [97,174]. The trunk exhibits slight flexion and extension during the gait cycle, is more erect or extended during single limb support, and is more flexed during double limb support [32,97]. Frontal plane motion of the trunk is consistent with the need to keep the center of mass over the stance foot. So the trunk leans slightly to the stance limb at each step [97,119,157,174]. In the transverse plane, the rotation of the trunk is opposite the rotation of the pelvis, with the trunk rotating forward on the side in which the shoulder is flexing [97,119,157].

Clinical Relevance

THE TRUNK'S CONTRIBUTION TO SMOOTH GAIT:
The gait pattern of a toddler learning to walk is characterized by large lateral leans with little forward rotation of the

trunk and shoulders [11]. As the child matures, the pattern becomes smoother and more stable, and trunk rotation moves out of phase with the pelvis. The coupling motion of the trunk and pelvis contributes to the efficiency and stability of gait. Patients who lack the ability to rotate the trunk separately from the pelvis, such as patients with Parkinson's syndrome or patients with low back pain, may lose gait efficiency and expend more energy to walk.

MUSCLE ACTIVITY DURING LOCOMOTION

Studies that examine the electrical activity of muscles during locomotion have played a central part in defining the role of muscles in producing and controlling locomotion. Data from Winter and Yack [188] demonstrate the normalized electromyographic (EMG) data for 16 muscles recorded in up to 19 subjects (*Fig. 48.12*). These data reveal important principles regarding muscle activity during gait. First, the duration of large bursts of activity for most muscles is quite brief, and most of these bursts occur at the transitions between swing and stance or between stance and swing. These data demonstrate the considerable variability in muscle activity across individuals. Studies also demonstrate variability within a single individual, although there is less than across individuals [22,76,82,188].

Despite the variability of muscle activity, certain consistent functions for specific muscle groups emerge from the EMG data [76,82,92,161,180]. In order to understand the role muscles play during gait it is important to recall that each lower extremity functions in both an open and closed kinetic chain, open through the swing phase and closed through the stance phase. Consequently, a muscle contraction can affect not only the joint crossed by that muscle, but also joints throughout the chain.

The gluteus maximus and hamstrings are active prior to and following ground contact, exerting a deceleration force on the hip and knee at the end of swing. Their activity also helps to initiate hip extension during early stance. By controlling the femur the gluteus maximus also helps to accelerate the knee toward extension during early single-limb support [10].

The gluteus medius contracts just before ground contact and continues its activity through most of stance, until loading begins on the opposite side. The activity of the hip abductors provides essential frontal plane stability to the pelvis throughout stance and adds to hip and knee extension support in mid to late stance [2,10]. The hip flexors contract in late stance and continue their activity into early swing to slow hip extension and initiate hip flexion [10,61]. The iliopsoas also contributes to the flexion velocity of the knee in midstance [58].

Muscle activity at the knee is characterized by co-contraction of the hamstrings and quadriceps for approximately the first 25% of the gait cycle, during loading response and early midstance. During this period, the knee is flexing and then extending, and the quadriceps activity is essential in controlling

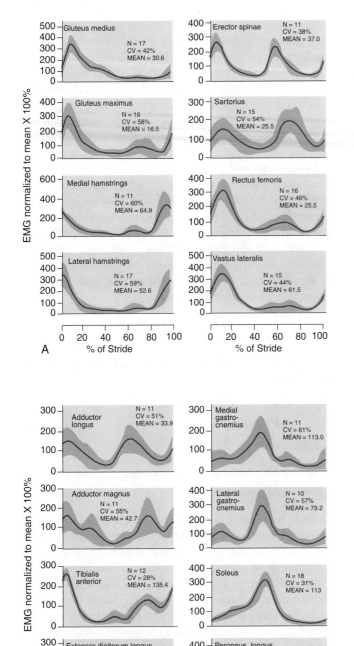

Figure 48.12: Electrical activity of lower extremity muscles during gait. (Reprinted with permission from Winter DA, Yack HJ: EMG profiles during normal human walking: stride-to-stride and inter-subject variability. Electroencephalogr Clin Neurophysiol 1987; 67: 402–411.)

beginning of stance [8,125]. Most of swing proceeds with no muscle activity at the knee joint.

The ankle also exhibits co-contraction of the dorsiflexor and plantarflexor muscles. Dorsiflexors of the ankle exhibit slight activity throughout swing to hold the foot away from the ground. The activity continues at ground contact and through the loading response, controlling the descent of the foot onto the ground. The plantarflexor muscles gradually increase their activity from ground contact through most of stance, with the greatest burst of activity from heel off to toe off as the body rolls over the plantarflexing foot. Through the mechanics of the closed chain, the plantarflexors also help control the hip and knee joints [10,162]. The plantarflexor muscles provide the majority of support to the lower extremity during the latter portion of the stance phase [2]. With the iliopsoas, the gastrocnemius contributes to the flexion velocity of the knee [58].

Review of the muscle activity of these large muscle groups demonstrates that much of the activity is characterized by an eccentric contraction followed by a concentric contraction. For example, the gluteus maximus contracts eccentrically as the hip flexes late in swing and then contracts concentrically as the hip begins to extend. The same pattern is found in the gluteus medius, hip flexors, quadriceps, and dorsiflexors. The plantarflexors also exhibit lengthening and then shortening, although at least some of the change in length is a passive stretch and shortening in the tendo calcaneus (Achilles tendon), so the actual change in muscle fiber length may be small [52]. The hamstrings also begin their activity with an eccentric contraction in late swing, but their subsequent length is more difficult to discern, since at loading response the hip is extending while the knee is flexing. The overall length change in the hamstrings during loading response may be negligible. The lengthening contractions that begin many muscles' activity in gait decelerate each joint, and then the subsequent concentric contractions begin the joint's forward movement.

This pattern of eccentric then concentric contraction is known as the **stretch-shortening cycle** and is used by most muscles during gait as an efficient means of generating muscle force and storing energy (see Chapter 4 for more details). Some of the energy stored by the stretched muscle is released during the muscle's lengthening to help propel a limb segment without requiring additional muscle contraction [126]. Thus normal gait utilizes muscle contractions in a very efficient way to generate force and produce movement.

It is worth noting that at most joints, the motion occurring during the concentric contraction continues after the contraction ceases. For example, the hip continues to extend long after the peak activity of the gluteus maximus and hamstrings, and the hip flexes after cessation of hip flexor activity. Similarly, the knee continues to extend without significant quadriceps activity, and the ankle continues to dorsiflex after the burst of dorsiflexor activity early in stance. Thus the chief functions of the muscles of the lower extremity during

this movement. Some individuals exhibit activity of either the quadriceps, especially the rectus femoris, or hamstrings at the transition from stance to swing, but this activity is both variable and smaller in magnitude than the activity at the

locomotion are to slow one motion and to provide an initial burst, or pull, in the opposite direction. How motion continues in the absence of active muscle contraction is related to the kinetics of the movement.

Clinical Relevance

MUSCLE WEAKNESS AND CHANGES IN GAIT: *Muscles play complex roles during gait, including controlling and propelling the individual joint(s) they cross as well as supporting and propelling joints throughout the lower limbs. Consequently, weakness of even a single muscle can produce significant changes in movement patterns throughout the lower extremities [95,162]. For example, in the presence of significant quadriceps weakness the individual will avoid knee flexion while bearing weight on the affected limb. In order to avoid knee flexion, however, the individual must alter other joint movements as well. The subject may avoid the ankle dorsiflexion position as a means of ensuring the knee remains extended or avoid the use of the plantarflexor muscles because they contribute to acceleration of the knee. Similarly, weakness in hip musculature may alter hip, knee, or ankle joint movements.*

KINETICS OF LOCOMOTION

Kinetics examines the forces, moments, and power generated during a movement and, in the case of locomotion, includes the moments generated by the muscles, the forces applied across joints, and the mechanical power and energy generated. A discussion of the kinetics of gait allows consideration of the efficiency of gait.

Joint Moments and Reaction Forces

As indicated in the preceding sections, gait consists of complex cyclical movements occurring in a coordinated sequence that is controlled by muscle activity. In addition, gait entails the repetitive impact loading of both lower extremities in each gait cycle. Thus it is easy to recognize that normal locomotion produces large forces between the foot and the ground, requires significant muscle forces, and generates large joint reaction forces. Many impairments in gait are related to an individual's inability to generate sufficient muscular support or to sustain the large reaction forces of gait.

DYNAMIC EQUILIBRIUM

Researchers and clinicians have long been interested in the forces sustained by the muscles and joints during normal and abnormal locomotion [17,110,168]. Chapter 1 of this text describes the principles used to determine the loads in muscles and on joints during activity. Newton's first law defines the conditions of **static equilibrium** ($\Sigma F = 0$, $\Sigma M = 0$), stating that an object remains at rest (or in uniform motion)

unless acted upon by an unbalanced external force. Throughout this text, two-dimensional examples of static equilibrium problems are provided to analyze the forces in the muscles and on joints during static tasks or in tasks where acceleration is negligible. However, during gait, limb segments undergo large linear accelerations, and joints exhibit large angular accelerations. As a result, the assumption used in static equilibrium analysis, that acceleration is negligible, is not valid when applied to gait.

Newton's second law of motion, $\Sigma F = ma$, states that the unbalanced force on a body is directly proportional to the acceleration of that body. The specific relationships between the accelerations and the forces and moments can be determined by applying the principles of **dynamic equilibrium.** The conditions of dynamic equilibrium are very similar to the conditions of static equilibrium. To determine the forces on an accelerating body in a two-dimensional analysis, the following conditions must be satisfied:

$$\Sigma \mathbf{F_X} = ma_X, \ \Sigma \mathbf{F_Y} = ma_Y,$$
$$\Sigma \mathbf{M} = I \times \boldsymbol{\alpha} \qquad \text{(Equation 48.1)}$$

In three-dimensional analysis, the conditions for dynamic equilibrium are

$$\Sigma \mathbf{F_X} = ma_X, \ \Sigma \mathbf{F_Y} = ma_Y,$$
$$\Sigma \mathbf{F_Z} = ma_Z \qquad \text{(Equation 48.2)}$$

and

$$\Sigma \mathbf{M_X} = I \times \boldsymbol{\alpha_X}, \ \Sigma \mathbf{M_Y} = I \times \boldsymbol{\alpha_Y},$$
$$\Sigma \mathbf{M_Z} = I \times \boldsymbol{\alpha_Z} \qquad \text{(Equation 48.3)}$$

where $\mathbf{F}_i$ is the force in the ith direction, $\mathbf{a}_i$ is the linear acceleration in the ith direction, $\mathbf{M}_i$ is the moment about the ith axis, $\boldsymbol{\alpha}_i$ is the angular acceleration in the ith direction, and I is the moment of inertia. The moment of inertia indicates a body's resistance to angular acceleration and depends on the body's mass and distribution of mass. The larger the mass and the farther the mass is from the body's center of mass, the larger is the body's moment of inertia. Elite gymnasts tend to possess short and compact bodies (smaller moments of inertia) that allow high angular accelerations producing rapid rotations about horizontal bars and in tumbling routines. The acceleration quantities in each of the equations of dynamic equilibrium, ma_i and $I \times \boldsymbol{\alpha}_i$, are known as **inertial forces** and are intuitively explained by the awareness that it takes more force to push a car to start or stop its rolling, that is, to accelerate or decelerate it, than it takes to keep the car rolling.

Solutions to the conditions of dynamic equilibrium, also known as **equations of motion,** require knowledge of several parameters, including mass and moment of inertia. Mass is usually determined from tables derived from cadaver measurements, as demonstrated in examples throughout this textbook [40]. Similarly, these tables provide means to calculate moments of inertia of a limb or limb segment from easily obtained anthropometric measurements, although methods also exist to compute the moment of inertia of some segments directly [25,155]. Regardless of the method chosen, the properties of mass and moment of inertia can be estimated and entered into the equations of motion to allow solutions.

Theoretically, the equations of motion in dynamic equilibrium can be used to calculate a body's acceleration from all of the forces on the body. This approach is useful to determine the response of an airplane or rocket to an applied force. However, in the case of human movement, where forces cannot be measured directly, the equations of motion are used more often to determine the forces on the body when the accelerations are known. This approach, known as **inverse dynamics,** allows estimation of the forces on the human body and requires direct determination of the acceleration. Application of inverse dynamics in static equilibrium is straightforward because the accelerations are, by definition, zero, and the examples of two-dimensional analysis throughout this book demonstrate the use of inverse dynamics.

Chapter 1 reminds the reader that acceleration is the change of velocity over time, and velocity is the change in displacement over time. Therefore, if a body's displacement is known over time, then velocity and acceleration can be determined. Precise calculations of velocity and accelerations of the body or of any limb segment requires careful measurement of the displacement, which can be accomplished by a number of techniques including high-speed cinematography, videography, or electromagnetic tracking devices [99,119,124,140]. Appropriate signal processing of the displacement data and mathematical calculations yield satisfactory estimations of velocity and accelerations of the body of interest. A thorough discussion of the methods and challenges in these techniques is beyond the scope of this book; suffice it to say that the necessary acceleration values are available, so that the equations of motion can finally be solved for the applied forces.

Examining the Forces Box 48.1 provides an example of the equations of motion for the leg–foot segment during the swing phase of gait. Using anthropometric data from Dempster [40], the mass (m) and moment of inertia (I) are entered directly into the calculations. Videographic data are

---

EXAMINING THE FORCES BOX 48.1

EQUATIONS OF MOTION IN TWO DIMENSIONS FOR THE LEG–FOOT SEGMENT DURING EARLY SWING

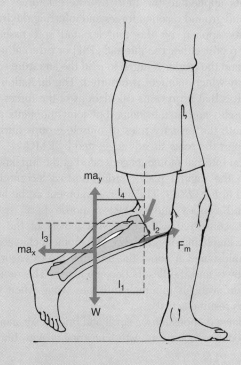

m = the mass of the leg and foot combined

W = the weight of the leg and foot combined

F_M = the muscle force

J = the joint reaction force

I_1 = the moment arm of the weight of the leg–foot

I_2 = the moment arm of the muscle

I_3 = the moment arm of the inertial force ($-ma_X$)

I_4 = the moment arm of the inertial force ($-ma_Y$)

Since the limb segment accelerates during gait, the dynamic equilibrium conditions apply:

$$\Sigma F_X = ma_X, \; \Sigma F_Y = ma_Y, \; \Sigma M = I \times \alpha$$

where: a_X, a_Y, and α are the x and y components of the linear accelerations and angular accelerations, respectively. These equations can be rewritten as

$$\Sigma F_X - ma_X = 0, \; \Sigma F_Y - ma_Y = 0, \; \Sigma M - I \times \alpha = 0$$

where $(-ma_X)$, $(-ma_Y)$, and $(-I \times \alpha)$ are known as inertial forces. The inertial forces contribute to moments about the knee joint so that taking moments about the knee, the motion equation is

$$(W \times I_1) + (F_M \times I_2) - [(-ma_X) \times I_3] - [(-ma_Y) \times I_4] = I \times \alpha$$

Since the accelerations and anthropometric parameters, W and I, can be measured or determined from available data, the equation can be solved for the muscle force, F. Once the muscle force is determined, the joint reaction forces, J_X and J_Y are calculated from:

$$\Sigma F_X = ma_X$$
$$F_{MX} + J_X = ma_X$$
$$\Sigma F_Y = ma_Y$$
$$F_{MY} + J_Y - W = ma_Y$$

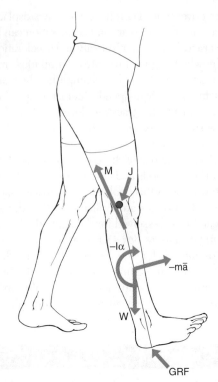

Figure 48.13: Free body diagram of the leg–foot segment during stance includes the forces: weight of the leg-foot (*W*), joint reaction force (*J*), muscle force (*M*), ground reaction force (*GRF*), inertial forces –*ma* and –*Iα*, where m = mass, a = linear acceleration, I = moment of inertia, and α = angular acceleration.

collected at a rate of 60 Hz (hertz, or cycles per second) and manipulated so that the linear and angular accelerations of the leg–foot segment are determined for every 1/60 of a second and entered into the equations. The equations of motion are solved repeatedly for the muscle force (F) at each increment of time. A similar procedure is applied to the stance phase of gait, but the external forces on the foot also include the ground reaction forces (*Fig. 48.13*). The direction and magnitude of these forces must be known to solve the equations of motion during stance and can be measured directly by force plates. The characteristics of the ground reaction force during gait are discussed in the following section.

The example presented in Examining the Forces Box 48.1 assumes that only one muscle group is active. However, the EMG data described earlier in this chapter provide convincing evidence that there is co-contraction of the hamstrings and quadriceps during late swing and early stance and sometimes at

the transition from late stance to early swing as well. Ligaments also apply significant loads to the knee joint during gait [67,160]. Thus there is more than one structure applying force at the knee joint, producing a dynamically **indeterminate** system. As noted in Chapter 1 and elsewhere in this book, sophisticated mathematical solutions for indeterminate systems exist, and they are applied frequently in locomotion research to approximate the muscle and joint reaction forces [27,158].

Using inverse dynamics, many studies report the joint reaction forces in the body during the gait cycle [3,17,33, 44,67,94,158,165]. Peak joint reaction forces at the hip, knee, and ankle reported in the literature are presented in *Table 48.3*. These data reveal wide variation in the forces reported at each joint. Several factors influence these calculations, including the estimates of the body segment parameters of mass and moment of inertia, the accuracy of the displacement data and the procedures to determine accelerations, the use of two- or three-dimensional analysis, as well as the analytical approach used to complete the calculations [1,4,36,39,96,191]. Values reported here are intended to demonstrate that regardless of the precise magnitude, all of the joints of the lower extremity sustain large and repetitive loads during locomotion. Running and jumping produce even larger muscle loads and joint reaction forces [21,112,172].

To avoid the problem of indeterminacy, researchers often solve only the moment equations, calculating the **external moments** applied to the limb by external forces such as weight and ground reaction forces and inferring the **internal moments** applied by the muscles and soft tissue [85]. Authors report either the internal [181] or external moment [88,98], and the reader is urged to read the literature carefully to identify which moment is reported. The limitation of this approach is that it prevents calculations of the forces in specific muscles and at the joints, but joint moments provide insight into the primary roles of muscle groups during gait and support the roles already suggested by EMG.

Typical internal moments generated at the hip, knee, and ankle in the sagittal plane during normal locomotion are reported in *Fig. 48.14*. The internal moment at the hip joint at ground contact and contact response is an extension moment, consistent with the EMG activity of the gluteus maximus and hamstrings [54,82]. The moment changes direction in midstance at about the time the hip extensors cease their activity and the flexors become active. The moment at the hip in swing is minimal until late swing when the hip extensors resume activity.

The knee demonstrates a small and brief flexor moment at ground contact, consistent with hamstring activity, but then a

TABLE 48.3: Reported Peak Joint Reaction Forces during Normal Gait in Units of Body Weight

	Anderson et al. [3]	Komistek [94]	Duda et al. [44]	Seireg and Arvikar [158]	Hardt [67]	Simonsen et al. [165]
Hip	4	2.0–2.5	3	5.25	6	6
Knee	2.7	1.7–2.3	n.r.[a]	7	2.75	4.5
Ankle	6	1.25	n.r.	5	3.5	4

[a]Not reported.

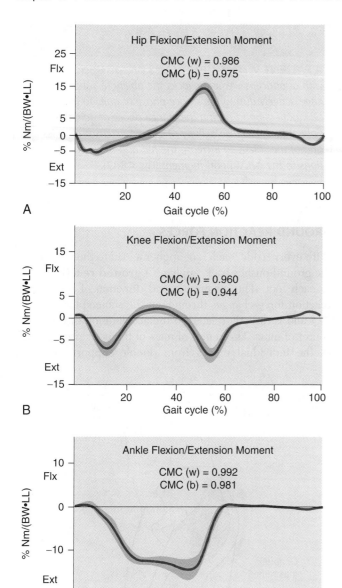

Figure 48.14: Internal moments at the hip, knee, and ankle in the sagittal plane. (Reprinted with permission from Kadaba MP, Ramakrishnan HK, Wootten ME, et al.: Repeatability of kinematic, kinetic, and EMG data in normal adult gait. J Orthop Res 1989; 7: 849–860.)

provide convincing evidence that these muscles contribute some of the propulsion moving the body forward [126, 142,144,153]. A very small dorsiflexion moment following toe off pulls the foot and toes away from the ground.

Moments in the transverse and frontal planes also are reported and appear to be important in the mechanics and pathomechanics of locomotion [46,73,107]. However, less consensus exists regarding the magnitude and even the pattern of these moments. Moments in the frontal and transverse planes are smaller than those in the sagittal plane, and smaller moments are more sensitive to measurement errors, including the location of the joint axes and the kinematics of the movements [20,72].

Clinical Relevance

KNEE ADDUCTION MOMENT: *The external frontal plane moment at the knee, known as the **adduction moment,** has been implicated in the development and progression of knee osteoarthritis (OA) as well as the pain and disability associated with knee OA* (Fig. 48.15) *[73].*

(continued)

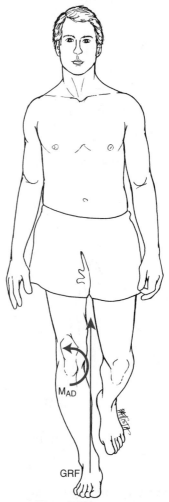

Figure 48.15: Adduction moment on the knee in gait. The ground reaction force (GRF) applies an external adduction moment (M_{AD}) on the knee during the stance phase of gait.

larger and more prolonged extensor moment that is consistent with quadriceps activity. In midstance, the knee exhibits a small flexor moment that is attributable to activity of the gastrocnemius. A small extension moment helps control knee flexion at the end of stance and in early swing, just as the flexion moment at the end of swing slows the rapid knee extension.

A small dorsiflexion moment at ground contact and contact response reflects the dorsiflexor activity controlling the descent of the foot onto the ground. It is followed by a steadily increasing and prolonged plantarflexion moment controlling advancement of the tibia through the rest of stance. Although there has been disagreement about whether the plantarflexors actually propel the body forward [135], recent studies

(Continued)

Treatments to reduce the adduction moment and reduce pain include lateral shoe wedges, knee braces that apply a valgus stress to the knee, and surgical osteotomy to realign the knee joint [6].

Winter describes a **support moment** for the stance phase of gait that is the sum of the internal sagittal plane moments in which all of the moments that tend to push the body away from the ground or support the body are positive (*Fig. 48.16*) [70,181]. The net support moment during stance is positive, indicating the overall role of the muscles to support the body and to prevent collapse during weight bearing. Data suggest that although the net support moment is consistent across walking trials, individuals without pathology demonstrate variability in the individual joint moments, indicating that individuals with normal locomotor systems may exhibit flexibility in the ways they provide support [182].

GROUND REACTION FORCES

With every stride, each foot applies a load to the ground and the ground pushes back, applying a **ground reaction force** to each foot. The magnitude and direction of this ground reaction force changes throughout the stance phase of each foot and is directly related to the acceleration of the body's center of mass. The center of mass of the body rises and falls as the individual moves from double support when the

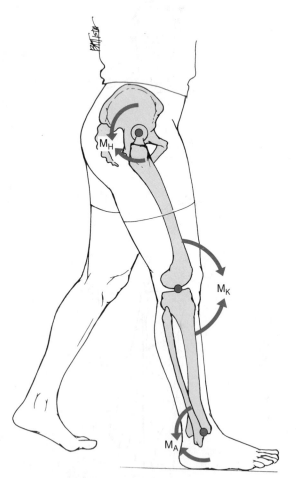

Figure 48.16: The support moment is the sum of the moments at the hip (M_H), knee (M_K), and ankle (M_A) needed to support the body weight during stance.

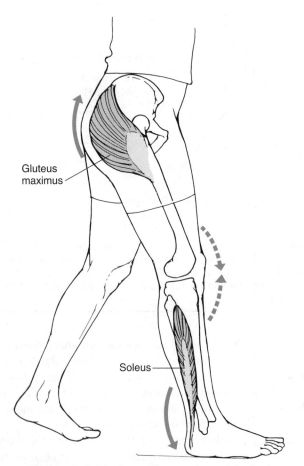

Gluteus maximus

Soleus

Figure 48.17: An individual may increase the activity in the soleus and the gluteus maximus to support the knee in extension by preventing forward movement of the tibia or the femur, respectively.

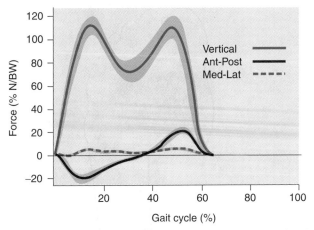

Force (% N/BW)

120
100
80
60
40
20
0
−20

Vertical
Ant-Post
Med-Lat

20   40   60   80   100

Gait cycle (%)

Figure 48.18: Ground reaction forces during gait. (Reprinted with permission from Meglan D, Todd F: Kinetics of human locomotion. In: Rose J, Gamble JG, eds. Human Walking. Philadelphia: Williams & Wilkins, 1994; 23–44.)

center of mass is low to single support when the center of mass is high [77,119,154]. Similarly, the center of mass moves from side to side as the individual passes from stance on the right to stance on the left [119]. The ground reaction force is measured directly by **force plates** imbedded in the walking surface.

The ground reaction force typically is described by a vertical force as well as anterior–posterior and medial–lateral shear forces. The vertical ground reaction force under one foot is characterized by a double-humped curve (*Fig. 48.18*). The two peaks are greater than 100% of body weight and occur when the body accelerates upward. The valley between the peaks is less than 100% of body weight and occurs during single limb support. *Examining the Forces Box 48.2* uses dynamic equilibrium to demonstrate how acceleration of the center of mass of the body alters the ground reaction force. The vertical ground reaction force also is characterized by a brief but high peak just following ground contact, which reflects the impact of loading [164].

Clinical Relevance

GROUND REACTION FORCES AND JOINT PAIN: *Vertical ground reaction forces contribute significantly to joint reaction forces, and large joint reaction forces contribute to pain in patients with joint pathology such as arthritis. Patients with arthritis walk more slowly [84], and their vertical ground reaction forces demonstrate smaller peaks and valleys as the result of smaller vertical accelerations [163,166]. A reduction in walking speed, producing a reduction in accelerations, may be an effective way to reduce joint loads and, consequently, joint pain. These changes may represent appropriate adaptations to protect a painful joint and to maintain overall function.*

The posterior and anterior shear components of the ground reaction force also demonstrate a consistent pattern in normal locomotion. The ground exerts a posterior force on

EXAMINING THE FORCES BOX 48.2

THE CONTRIBUTION OF ACCELERATION TO THE VERTICAL GROUND REACTION FORCE

Using the dynamic equilibrium condition, $\Sigma F_Y = ma_Y$, provides a direct demonstration of the role of the acceleration of the body's center of mass in generating the vertical ground reaction force (GRF).

$\Sigma F_Y = ma_Y$

$\Sigma F_Y - ma_Y = 0$

$-W - ma_Y + GRF = 0$

$GRF = W + ma_Y$

When the body is accelerating toward the ground, the acceleration, a_Y, is negative, and the GRF is less than body weight, W. When the body accelerates upward away from the ground, acceleration, a_Y, is positive, and the GRF is greater than body weight, W.

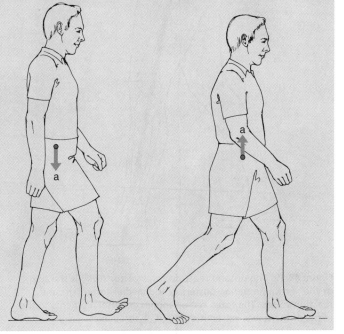

the foot during the initial portion of stance, decelerating the foot; consequently this period is known as the **deceleration phase.** In midstance, the ground applies an anterior shear force on the foot, contributing to the forward propulsion of the body. The second half of the stance phase is known as the **acceleration phase** of the gait cycle. Walking on ice demonstrates the importance of these posterior and anterior shear forces. Because there is little friction between the foot and the ice, the posterior and anterior shear forces between the ground and the foot are small when walking on ice, and forward progress is impaired. In the absence of any posterior and anterior shear forces, forward progress is impossible.

The medial and lateral shear forces during gait are smaller and more variable than the vertical forces or posterior–anterior shear forces. They reflect forces associated with the shift of the body from side to side between the supporting feet. Although plots of the ground reaction forces demonstrate rather stereotypical shapes, it is important to recognize that like kinematic variables, these forces exhibit normal intra- and intersubject variability [55,68].

The **ground reaction force vector** is the sum of the individual components of the ground reaction force. Whether described as a single force vector or as three individual components, the ground reaction force generates external moments on the joints of the body in all three planes (*Fig. 48.19*). Realistic computation of joint moments and

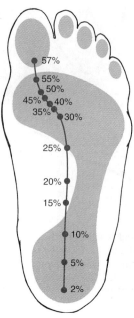

Figure 48.20: Progression of the center of pressure during locomotion. (Reprinted with permission from Sammarco GJ, Hockenbury RT: Biomechanics of the foot and ankle. In: Nordin M, Frankel VH, eds. Basic Biomechanics of the Musculoskeletal System. 3rd ed. Philadelphia: Lippincott Williams & Wilkins, 2001; 222–255.)

forces during gait must include the three components of the ground reaction force or the force vector.

The location of the ground reaction force with respect to the foot indicates the path of the **center of pressure** through the foot. In the normal foot, the center of pressure progresses in a relatively straight line from the posterior aspect of the plantar surface of the heel through the midfoot and onto the forefoot where it deviates medially onto the plantar surface of the great toe [64,66] (*Fig. 48.20*). Inability to roll over a painful toe or the interrupted forward progress of the body's center of mass because the knee suddenly hyperextends, are examples of gait deviations that produce changes in the pattern of the progression of the center of pressure.

Energetics of Gait: Power, Work, and Mechanical Energy

Normal locomotion appears to be a remarkably efficient movement. Individuals without impairments, walking at a self-selected cadence, require less oxygen consumption than when walking at lower or higher cadences [12,116]. Individuals with locomotor impairments expend more energy during ambulation than individuals without impairments [18,111,167]. The efficiency of locomotion depends on many factors, including the mechanics of the muscular control of gait described earlier in this chapter and the conservation of mechanical energy that results from the synergistic movement of the limb segments.

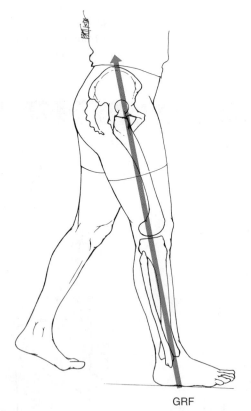

GRF

Figure 48.19: The ground reaction force vector (*GRF*) is the sum of the vertical, anterior–posterior, and medial–lateral ground reaction forces. The force vector applies external moments to the joints of the lower extremities about all three axes.

JOINT POWER

Mechanical power is the product of force and linear velocity or, in rotational motions such as the joint movements in locomotion, the product of joint moment and angular velocity:

$$P = \mathbf{M} \cdot \omega \qquad \text{(Equation 48.4)}$$

where P is power in watts, **M** is a joint moment, and ω is the angular velocity of the limb segment. Power is a useful indication of the muscles' role in controlling motion; it is negative when the body absorbs energy during eccentric muscle activity and is positive when the body generates energy during concentric muscle activity. Power also can be described as work (**W**) per unit time (t) (i.e., W/t), where work is the product of force and displacement, or in angular terms, the product of moment (**M**) and angular displacement ($\boldsymbol{\theta}$):

$$W = \mathbf{M} \cdot \theta \qquad \text{(Equation 48.5)}$$

Angular velocity, ω, is equal to angular displacement over time ($\omega = \theta/t$) and therefore:

$$P = \mathbf{M} \cdot \theta/\mathbf{t} \qquad \text{(Equation 48.6)}$$

and

$$P = W/t \qquad \text{(Equation 48.7)}$$

Thus concentric muscle activity generates power, or does work, and eccentric activity absorbs power, and work is done on the segment [187]. A pogo stick (Pogo™) provides a useful example of positive and negative power, work done on or by the pogo stick (*Fig. 48.21*). In landing, the weight of the child does work on the pogo stick, and energy is absorbed by its spring, but in takeoff, the spring releases its energy and performs work on the child, pushing the child and pogo stick off the ground.

Analysis of joint powers provides increasing understanding of the role of muscles in propelling and controlling movement during locomotion [144,151]. The joint powers at the hip, knee, and ankle during gait derived from two-dimensional analysis are pictured in *Fig. 48.22*. These demonstrate that positive power generation, when muscles are generating power and doing positive work, occurs at the hip at loading response as the hip extends and again at the end of stance as it flexes. Both of these periods are characterized by concentric muscle contractions. In contrast, the knee has only a brief period of power generation, producing only a small amount of power. Like the hip, the ankle generates considerable positive power at the end of stance when the plantarflexors contract concentrically. These data suggest that the hip flexors and extensors and the plantarflexors contribute important energy to the lower extremity during normal locomotion. It is worth noting that the power generated by the plantarflexors is considerably larger than that of any other muscle groups. The plantarflexor muscles, particularly the gastrocnemius muscles, appear to play an essential role in forward propulsion [60,142].

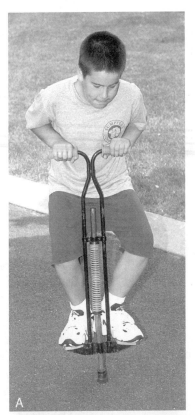

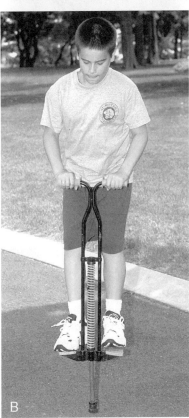

Figure 48.21: Energy storage and release. **A.** Weight bearing on the Pogo stick™ compresses its spring and work is done on the stick. **B.** As weight is removed, the spring is released, and the Pogo stick™ does work on the body, lifting it into the air.

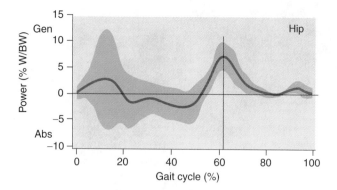

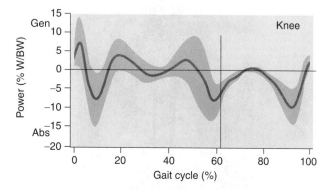

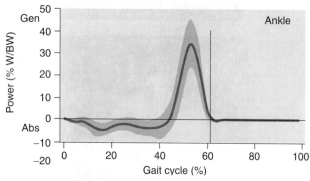

Figure 48.22: Joint powers at the hip, knee, and ankle from two-dimensional analysis. (Reprinted with permission from Meglan D, Todd F: Kinetics of human locomotion. In: Rose J, Gamble JG, eds. Human Walking. Philadelphia: Williams & Wilkins, 1994; 23–44.)

Clinical Relevance

JOINT POWERS IN INDIVIDUALS WITH GAIT

DYSFUNCTIONS: *Joint powers during free-speed walking are altered in elders and in individuals with weaker lower extremity muscles [41,114]. The decrease in plantarflexion power and concomitant increase in hip flexor power generation noted in elders and in individuals with weakness may help to explain the decrease in velocity and step length reported in these individuals, as well as their mechanisms of compensation [41,113,114]. As an individual is unable to generate power through plantarflexion for forward progression, active hip flexion appears to provide the forward propulsion needed to swing the limb forward. These patients*

may benefit from exercise to improve plantarflexion force production.

The use of joint kinetics in conjunction with EMG is also useful in evaluating the complex gait deviations in individuals with central nervous system disorders such as cerebral palsy. These analyses provide more insight into the mechanics of the gait abnormalities than can be provided solely by clinical observation and lead to more informed treatment decisions [132,148].

MECHANICAL ENERGY

The cyclic movement inherent in locomotion and the ability of the muscles to store energy contribute to the inherent efficiency of normal gait. The cyclic nature of gait has led to its description as an **inverted pendulum** in which the body swings repeatedly over the stance limb [128]. The **mechanical energy** of a pendulum changes form from **potential** to **kinetic energy,** thereby maintaining its swing with little additional energy input. The image of gait as the movement of an inverted pendulum has spurred investigators to study the mechanical energy of gait as a means of assessing its efficiency. Potential (PE) and kinetic (KE) energy are related to the distance of a body's center of mass from the earth and to the body's linear and angular velocity, as indicated by the following relationships:

$$PE = mgh \qquad \text{(Equation 48.8)}$$

where m is the mass of the body, g is the acceleration due to gravity, and h is the distance from the body's center of mass to the earth; and

$$KE = \tfrac{1}{2} mv^2 + \tfrac{1}{2} I\omega^2 \qquad \text{(Equation 48.9)}$$

where m is the body's mass, v is its linear velocity, I is its moment of inertia, and ω is its angular velocity. In an ideal system, conservation of energy dictates a complete transformation between potential and kinetic energy, so that an ideal roller coaster continues in motion indefinitely (*Fig. 48.23*). When the cars are at their peak height, potential energy is maximized and kinetic energy is minimized. At its lowest point, the roller coaster's potential energy is minimum and its kinetic energy is maximum. Since the work done on a body equals the change in total energy, an ideal system requires no work to continue moving, since the change in the body's total energy is zero. Studies of the mechanical energy of the limb segments during gait suggest that an exchange of kinetic and potential energy can account for most of the energy change in the distal leg at the beginning and end of swing [146,186]. This energy exchange improves when walking normally at free speed and is greater at steady-state walking than at the initiation of gait [109,117,177]. Assessment of the energy transfer during locomotion demonstrates the efficiency of gait and suggests that minimizing the expenditure of mechanical energy may actually be a dominant characteristic of normal gait [141].

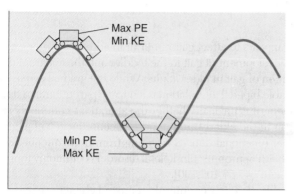

Figure 48.23: In an ideal roller coaster, potential and kinetic energy are transformed from one form to the other with no loss of energy. Potential energy (PE = mgh) is maximum when the roller coaster is farthest from the ground, at the same time the kinetic energy (KE = 1/2 mv²) is at its minimum. As the roller coaster descends the track it gains speed, increasing its kinetic energy while it is losing potential energy as it moves closer to the ground.

The ability of the muscles to absorb and generate energy contributes to the overall efficiency of gait and explains how many of the movements can proceed without muscle contraction [156]. Energy flows between adjacent limb segments during locomotion in much the same way that energy flows between the vaulter and the pole during a pole vault or among children playing "crack the whip." Like the pole used by the vaulter, much of the energy released by the muscles in gait is elastic energy stored within the passive elastic components of the muscle [156]. (See Chapter 4 for details about the passive elements of muscle.) Examination of the energy flow between limb segments reveals that the energy generated by the plantarflexors at push off is transferred passively to the leg and thigh, facilitating the initiation of swing. Similarly, the hamstrings absorb energy at the end of swing, and that energy is transferred to the trunk at ground contact, assisting in the trunk's forward progression. The transfer of energy from segment to segment depends on the normal sequencing of the angular changes described earlier in this chapter.

Thus normal, efficient gait consists of complex motions of several limb segments whose movement and control are interdependent. Alterations at a single joint are likely to produce changes in movement patterns throughout the body and diminish the efficiency of the movement.

Clinical Relevance

ENERGY TRANSFER AMONG LIMB SEGMENTS IN ABNORMAL GAIT: *Energy transfer among limb segments depends on the power generated and absorbed at joints and requires precise coordination among the moving segments. Since power is a function of the velocity of a limb segment, a limb segment that has a low angular velocity also has low power generation or absorption and, consequently, has less ability to transfer energy from one segment*

to another. A patient with arthritis producing a stiff knee is unable to transfer energy from the plantarflexors to the thigh; a patient with Parkinson's disease, which is characterized by generalized rigidity, has difficulty transferring energy through the lower extremity and into the trunk because the joints lack the freedom of movement to allow the sequential movement patterns of the joints of the lower extremity. A study of patients with multiple sclerosis demonstrates an inverse relationship between the metabolic cost of walking and the patients' ability to rapidly flex and extend the knee. This finding is consistent with a diminished capacity to transfer energy through the knee joint [130]. Thus treatments directed toward reducing joint stiffness or rigidity may lead to improved gait efficiency in these individuals.

FACTORS THAT INFLUENCE PARAMETERS OF GAIT

Several factors influence gait performance and must be considered by clinicians evaluating and treating a person with a locomotor dysfunction. Factors considered here are gender, speed, and age.

Gender

Although most observers would report differences between the gait patterns of males and females, few studies provide direct comparisons. Women walk with higher cadences than men and shorter strides [15,88,119]. Yet when the distance characteristics of the gait cycle are normalized by height, females demonstrate a similar or slightly larger stride length [47,88].

A study directly comparing 99 males and females of similar ages reports statistically different joint kinematics, although these differences are on the order of 2–4°, and the clinical significance of these differences is negligible [88]. The same study also reports that females exhibit a statistically greater extension moment at the knee at initial contact and a greater flexion moment in preswing with increases in power absorption or generation at the hip, knee, and ankle. A similar study found no gender differences in flexion or adduction moments at the knee during stance [90]. These studies suggest that while slight differences exist in some kinetic variables of gait, none of these differences are enough to explain the higher incidence of knee osteoarthritis in women.

Walking Speed

Gait speed affects several parameters of gait performance. As noted in the discussion of the temporal and distance characteristics of gait, cadence, step length, and stride length increase with increased walking speed and decrease with decreased speed [7,119]. Increased speed appears to increase the variability of some temporal and spatial gait parameters such as step width [159]. Angular excursions generally increase with walking speed, but these changes vary with the joint and the direction of motion [34,170,173]. Increases in joint excursions at the proximal joints are related to the increase in stride length associated with increased speeds [34].

Increased walking speeds also lead to increased ground reaction forces [7,28] and changes in the pattern of muscle activity. The relationship between walking speed and muscle activity is somewhat complex and depends on the muscle [71,178]. In general, peak muscular activity increases with walking speed [173,178]. The duration of muscle activity may increase at both very fast and very slow walking speeds [118,173]. In general, muscle activity during free-speed walking is more reproducible than that at speeds slower or faster than free speed [26,93]. With increased peak muscle activity, it is not surprising that joint moments and joint reaction forces also increase with walking speed [13,103,191]. Similarly increased mechanical work and power at all of the lower extremity joints accompany increased walking speed [80,103]. However, the relative contribution of the hip flexors and extensors to propulsion increases with walking speed [142,143].

Clinical Relevance

WALKING SPEED IN INDIVIDUALS WITH GAIT IMPAIRMENTS: *Many abnormal gait patterns found in individuals with impairments are characterized by decreased walking velocities. Patients with dysfunctions associated with low back pain, stroke, hemiparesis, and anterior cruciate ligament tears all frequently exhibit altered gait patterns that include decreased step length, smaller joint excursions, and decreased walking speed. Because decreased walking speed is associated with decreased step length and joint excursion, are the gait deviations exhibited by these patients merely the consequence of their walking speed? If a goal of treatment is to improve the gait pattern, the clinician must attempt to discern what characteristics of the gait pattern are attributable to the gait speed alone, and what characteristics are the result of the patient's impairments.*

Age

Age appears to affect gait rather dramatically, as witnessed by the development of gait in the toddler and the apparent deterioration of gait in older adults. While the gradual acquisition of stable bipedal ambulation is a normal part of human development, it is unclear whether the alterations commonly seen in gait in the elderly are the normal consequence of aging or reflect functional deficits resulting from impairments associated with neuromusculoskeletal disorders commonly found in elders [37,47,56,102,190].

Table 48.4 lists commonly reported changes in gait with aging. The ages of the elders studied range from approximately 60 years to over 100 years, and studies vary in the magnitude of changes reported. Despite the overwhelming data demonstrating changes in gait with increasing age, the nature of the relationship between age and locomotor function remains unclear. One of the most consistent findings with age is a decrease in free-walking speed [50,69,86,102,105,121], but many of the other changes reported with aging also are consistent with the changes reported earlier in this chapter for walking speed alone [48]. Specifically, decreased walking speed produces reductions in step length, joint excursions, and ground reaction forces [50,69,87,185]. Consequently, many of the changes that occur with aging appear to be secondary changes associated with walking speed. However, even when controlling for speed, elders demonstrate a significant increase in variability in gait characteristics as well as an increased energy cost of walking [19,108,133].

The decrease in walking velocity reported with age appears to depend on an individual's level of fitness and other factors besides age itself. Coexisting joint impairments; strength of the quadriceps, plantarflexors, and hip flexors; hip and knee passive ranges of motion; and maximal oxygen uptake all help explain the diminished walking velocity seen with age [22,37,47,56,81]. Treatment of gait dysfunctions in elders requires consideration of the contributions made to the dysfunction by discrete impairments in the neuromusculoskeletal and cardiorespiratory systems.

TABLE 48.4: Commonly Reported Changes in Gait in Older Adults

	Change with Increased Age
Speed	Decreased [50,69,86,102,105,121]
Cadence	Increased [50,80]
Step/stride length	Decreased [48,50,69,80,81,121,185]
Double support time	Increased [48,80,185]
Joint angular excursions	Decreased [80,87,121] Unchanged [50]
Muscle activity	Increased [50]
Joint powers	Decreased generation in hip extension and plantarflexion and increased generation in hip flexion [80,81,87,185]
Gait variability	Increased [19,133]
Energy cost of gait	Increased [108]

Clinical Relevance

EVALUATION AND TREATMENT OF GAIT DYSFUNCTION IN ELDERS: *Data describing the gait of elderly individuals reveal that many of the changes thought to be characteristic of aging can be explained by a reduction in walking speed. Consequently, a clinician must alter the standards of "normal" used to judge the adequacy of gait. The gait patterns of elders walking at reduced speeds are not comparable to the patterns of subjects walking at faster speeds, regardless of age. Similarly, treatment may be most successful when directed toward those factors that contribute to diminished speed, including strength of the quadriceps, plantarflexors, and hip flexors and extensors.*

SUMMARY

This chapter reviews the kinematic and kinetic variables of normal gait. The kinematic variables presented in this chapter include the more global parameters of time and distance as well as the discrete displacement patterns of joints. Although all of these variables are subject to intra- and intersubject variability, representative values from the literature are presented to provide the reader with a frame of reference for normal locomotion.

Joint excursions are largest in the sagittal plane and exhibit stereotypical patterns and sequences. In normal locomotion, the hip, knee, and ankle rarely move together toward or away from the ground. Activity of the major muscle groups of the lower extremity is reviewed. Their activity is typically brief, characterized by initial eccentric activity followed by concentric activity. In most cases, joint movement continues after muscle activity has ceased.

The kinetic variables described in this chapter include ground and joint reaction forces, muscle forces, and joint moments, as well as joint power and mechanical energy. The principle of dynamic equilibrium is used to explain the derivation of muscle and joint reaction forces, joint moments, and joint power. Like the kinematic variables, the kinetic variables exhibit intra- and intersubject variability that reflects the normal variability of individuals and populations, but kinetic parameters also are quite sensitive to differences in measurement procedures. The kinetic variables reveal that locomotion generates large muscle and joint forces. Kinetic analysis also demonstrates the remarkable efficiency of normal locomotion in which energy is stored and released, reducing the amount of work the muscles must perform to achieve the movement. Impairments in the neuromusculoskeletal system decrease the efficiency of gait.

Finally this chapter discusses factors that influence walking patterns, including gender, walking speed, and age. The discussion reveals a complex interdependence between walking speed and age effects on gait, and the clinician is cautioned to keep these factors in mind when judging the walking performance of an individual.

References

1. Alkjaer T, Simonsen EB, Dyhre-Poulsen P: Comparison of inverse dynamics calculated by two- and three-dimensional models during walking. Gait Posture 2001; 13: 73–77.
2. Anderson FC, Pandy MG: Individual muscle contributions to support in normal walking. Gait Posture 2003; 17: 159–169.
3. Anderson FC, Pandy MG: Static and dynamic optimization solutions for gait are practically equivalent. J Biomech 2001; 34: 153–161.
4. Andrews JG: Methods for investigating the sensitivity of joint resultants to body segment parameter variations. J Biomech 1996; 29: 651–654.
5. Andriacchi TP, Alexander EJ: Studies of human locomotion: past, present and future. J Biomech 2000; 33: 1217–1224.
6. Andriacchi T, Mundermann A: The role of ambulatory mechanics in the initiation and progression of knee osteoarthritis. Curr Opinion Rheum 2006; 18: 514–518.
7. Andriacchi TP, Ogle JA, Galante JO: Walking speed as a basis for normal and abnormal gait measurements. J Biomech 1977; 10: 261–268.
8. Annaswamy TM, Giddings CJ, Della Croce U, Kerrigan DC: Rectus femoris: its role in normal gait. Arch Phys Med Rehabil 1999; 80: 930–934.
9. Apkarian J, Naumann S, Cairns B: A three dimensional kinematic and dynamic model of the lower limb. J Biomech 1989; 22: 143–155.
10. Arnold AS, Anderson FC, Pandy MG, et al.: Muscular contributions to hip and knee extension during the single limb stance phase of normal gait: a framework for investigating the causes of crouch gait. J Biomech 2005; 38: 2181–2189.
11. Assaiante C, Woollacott M, Amblard B: Development of postural adjustment during gait initiation: kinematic and EMG analysis. J Mot Behav 2000; 32: 211–226.
12. Bastien GJ, Willems PA, Schepens B, et al.: Effect of load and speed on the energetic cost of human walking. Eur J Appl Physiol 2005; 94: 76–83.
13. Bergmann G, Deuretzbacher G, Heller M, et al.: Hip contact forces and gait patterns from routine activities. J Biomech 2001; 34: 859–871.
14. Bianchi L, Angelini D, Orani GP, Lacquaniti F: Kinematic coordination in human gait: relation to mechanical energy cost. Am Physiol Soc 1998; 79: 2155–2170.
15. Blanc Y, Balmer C, Landis T, Vingerhoets F: Temporal parameters and patterns of the foot roll over during walking: normative data for healthy adults. Gait Posture 1999; 10: 97–108.
16. Borghese NA: Kinematic determinants of human locomotion. J Physiol (Lond) 1996; 494: 863–879.
17. Bresler B, Frankel SP: The forces and moments in the leg during level walking. Trans ASME 1950; 27: 27–36.
18. Brown M, Hislop HJ, Waters RL, Porell D: Walking efficiency before and after total hip replacement. Phys Ther 1980; 60: 1259–1263.
19. Buzzi UH, Stergiou N, Kurz MJ, et al.: Nonlinear dynamics indicates aging affects variability during gait. Clin Biomech 2003; 18: 435–443.
20. Castagno P, Richards J, Miller F, Lennon N: Comparison of 3-dimensional lower extremity kinematics during walking gait using two different marker sets. Gait Posture 1995; 3: 87–87.
21. Cavanagh PR: The biomechanics of lower extremity action in distance running. Foot Ankle 1987; 7: 197–217.

22. Chang RW, Dunlop D, Gibbs J, Hughes S: The determinants of walking velocity in the elderly. Arthritis Rheum 1995; 38: 343–350.

23. Chao EY, Laughman RK, Schneider E, Stauffer RN: Normative data of knee joint motion and ground reaction forces in adult level walking. J Biomech 1983; 16: 219–233.

24. Chen WL, O'Connor JJ, Radin EL: A comparison of the gaits of Chinese and Caucasian women with particular reference to their heelstrike transients. Clin Biomech 2003; 18: 207–213.

25. Cheng CK, Chen HH, Chen CS, et al.: Segmental inertial properties of Chinese adults determined from magnetic resonance imaging. Clin Biomech 2000; 15: 559–566.

26. Chung SH, Giuliani CA: Within- and between-session consistency of electromyographic temporal patterns of walking in non-disabled older adults. Gait Posture 1997; 6: 110–118.

27. Collins JJ: The redundant nature of locomotor optimization laws. J Biomech 1995; 28: 251–267.

28. Cook TM, Farrell KP, Carey IA, et al.: Effects of restricted knee flexion and walking speed on the vertical ground reaction force during gait. J Orthop Sports Phys Ther 1997; 25: 236–244.

29. Cornwall MW, McPoil TG: Comparison of 2-dimensional and 3-dimensional rearfoot motion during walking. Clin Biomech 1995; 10: 36–40.

30. Craik RL, Dutterer L: Spatial and temporal characteristics of foot fall patterns. In: Craik RL, Oatis CA, eds. Gait Analysis: Theory and Application. St. Louis: Mosby-Year Book, 1995; 143–158.

31. Craik RL, Oatis CA: Gait Analysis: Theory and Application. St. Louis: Mosby, 1995.

32. Cromwell RL, Aadland TK, Nelson AT, et al.: Sagittal plane analysis of head, neck, and trunk kinematics and electromyographic activity during locomotion. J Orthop Sports Phys Ther 2001; 31: 255–262.

33. Cromwell RL, Schultz AB, Beck R, Warwick D: Loads on the lumbar trunk during level walking. J Orthop Res 1989; 7: 371–377.

34. Crosbie J, Vachalathiti R, Smith R: Age, gender and speed effects on spinal kinematics during walking. Gait Posture 1997; 5: 13–20.

35. Crosbie J, Vachalathiti R, Smith R: Patterns of spinal motion during walking. Gait Posture 1997; 5: 6–12.

36. Crowninshield RD, Brand RA: A physiologically based criterion of muscle force prediction in locomotion. J Biomech 1981; 14: 793–801.

37. Cunningham DA, Rechnitzer PA, Pearce ME, Donner AP: Determinants of self-selected walking pace across ages 19 to 66. J Gerontol 1982; 37: 560–564.

38. Das P, McCollum G: Invariant structure in locomotion. Neuroscience 1988; 25: 1023–1034.

39. Davy DT, Audu ML: A dynamic optimization technique for predicting muscle forces in the swing phase of gait. J Biomech 1987; 20: 187–201.

40. Dempster WT: Space requirements of the seated operator. In: Krogman WM, Fischer O, eds. Human Mechanics; Four Monographs Abridged AMRL-TDR-63-123. Wright-Patterson Air Force Base, OH: Behavioral Sciences Laboratory, 6570th Aerospace Medical Research Laboratories, Aerospace Medical Division, Air Force Systems Command, 1963; 215–340.

41. Devita P, Hortobagyi T: Age causes a redistribution of joint torques and powers during gait. J Appl Physiol 2000; 88: 1804–1811.

42. Dingwell JB, Cusumano JP: Nonlinear time series analysis of normal and pathological human walking. Am Inst Phys 2000; 10: 848–863.

43. Drillis R: Objective recording and biomechanics of pathological gait. Ann NY Acad Sci 1958; 74: 86–109.

44. Duda GN: Internal forces and moments in the femur during walking. J Biomech 1997; 30: 933–941.

45. Dujardin FH, Roussignol X, Mejjad O, et al.: Interindividual variations of the hip joint motion in normal gait. Gait Posture 1997; 5: 246–250.

46. Eng JJ, Winter D, Patla AE: Intralimb dynamics simplify reactive control strategies during locomotion. J Biomech 1997; 30: 581–588.

47. Escalante A, Lichtenstein MJ, Hazuda HP: Walking velocity in aged persons: its association with lower extremity joint range of motion. Arthritis Care Res 2001; 45: 287–294.

48. Ferrandez AM, Paihous J, Durup M: Slowness in elderly gait. Exp Aging Res 1990; 16: 79–89.

49. Finley FR, Cody KA: Locomotion characteristics of urban pedestrians. Arch Phys Med Rehabil 1970; 51: 423–426.

50. Finley FR, Cody KA, Finizie RV: Locomotion patterns in elderly women. Arch Phys Med Rehabil 1969; 140–146.

51. Frigo C, Carabalona R, Dalla Mura M, et al.: The upper body segmental movements during walking by young females. Clin Biomech 2003; 18: 419–425.

52. Fukunaga T, Kubo K, Kawakami Y, et al.: In vivo behaviour of human muscle tendon during walking. Proc R Soc Lond B Biol Sci 2001; 268: 229–233.

53. Gabell A, Nayak USL: The effect of age on variability in gait. J Gerontol 1984; 39: 662–666.

54. Ganley KJ, Powers CM: Determination of lower extremity anthropometric parameters using dual energy X-ray absorptiometry: the influence on net joint moments during gait. Clin Biomech 2004; 19: 50–56.

55. Giakas G, Baltsopoulos V: Time and frequency domain analysis of ground reaction forces during walking: an investigation of variability and symmetry. Gait Posture 1997; 5: 189–197.

56. Gibbs J, Hughes S, Dunlop D, et al.: Predictors of change in walking velocity in older adults. J Am Geriatr Soc 1996; 44: 126–132.

57. Goble DJ, Marino GW, Potvin JR: The influence of horizontal velocity on interlimb symmetry in normal walking. Human Movement Science 2003; 22: 271-283.

58. Goldberg SR, Anderson FC, Pandy MG, et al.: Muscles that influence knee flexion velocity in double support: Implications for stiff-knee gait. J Biomech 2004; 37: 1189–1196.

59. Goodwin CS: The use of the voluntary muscle test in leprosy neuritis. Leprosy Rev 1968; 39: 209–216.

60. Gottschall JS, Kram R: Energy cost and muscular activity required for propulsion during walking. J Appl Physiol 2003; 94: 1766–1772.

61. Gottschall JS, Kram R: Energy cost and muscular activity required for leg swing during walking. J Appl Physiol 2005; 99: 23–30.

62. Grieve DW, Gear RJ: The relationships between length of stride, step frequency, time of swing and speed of walking for children and adults. Ergonomics 1966; 5: 379–399.

63. Growney E, Meglan D, Johnson M, et al.: Repeated measures of adult normal walking using a video tracking system. Gait Posture 1997; 6: 147–162.

64. Grundy M, Blackburn, Tosh PA, et al.: An investigation of the centres of pressure under the foot while walking. J Bone Joint Surg 1975; 57B: 98–103.

65. Hageman PA, Blanke DJ: Comparison of gait of young women and elderly women. Phys Ther 1986; 66: 1382–1386.

66. Han TR, Paik NJ, Im MS: Quantification of the path of center of pressure (COP) using an F-scan in-shoe transducer. Gait Posture 1999; 10: 248–254.

67. Hardt DE: Determining muscle forces in the leg during normal human walking—an application and evaluation of optimization methods. J Biomech Eng 1978; 100: 72–78.

68. Herzog W, Nigg BM, Read LJ, Olsson E: Asymmetries in ground reaction force patterns in normal human gait. Med Sci Sports Exerc 1989; 21: 110–114.

69. Himann JE, Cunningham DA, Rechnitzer PA, Paterson DH: Age-related changes in speed of walking. Med Sci Sports Exerc 1988; 20: 161–166.

70. Hof AL: On the interpretation of the support moment. Gait Posture 2000; 12: 196–199.

71. Hof AL, Elzinga H, Grimmius W, et al.: Speed dependence of averaged EMG profiles in walking. Gait Posture 2002; 16: 78–86.

72. Holden JP, Stanhope S: The effect of variation in knee center location estimates on net knee joint moments. Gait Posture 1998; 7: 1–6.

73. Hunt MA, Birmingham TB, Giffin JR, Jenkyn TR: Associations among knee adduction moment, frontal plane ground reaction force, and lever arm during walking in patients with knee osteoarthritis. J Biomech 2006; 39: 2213–2220.

74. Hunt AE, Smith RM: Inter-segment foot motion and ground reaction forces over the stance phase of walking. Clin Biomech 2001; 16: 592–600.

75. Hunt AE, Smith RM: Interpretation of ankle joint moments during the stance phase of walking: a comparison of two orthogonal axes systems. J Appl Biomech 2002; 17: 173–180.

76. Hunt AE, Smith RM, Torode M: Extrinsic muscle activity, foot motion and ankle joint moments during the stance phase of walking. Foot Ankle Int 2001; 22: 31–41.

77. Iida H, Yamamuro T: Kinetic analysis of the center of gravity of the human body in normal and pathological gait. J Biomech 1987; 20: 987–995.

78. Isacson J, Gransberg L, Knutsson E: Three-dimensional electrogoniometric gait recording. J Biomech 1986; 19: 627–635.

79. Johnston RC, Smidt GL: Measurement of hip joint motion during walking: evaluation of an electrogoniometric method. J Bone Joint Surg 1969; 51A: 1083.

80. Judge J, Davis RB, Ounpuu S: Age-associated reduction in step length: testing the importance of hip and ankle kinetics. Gait Posture 1995; 3: 81–81.

81. Judge JO: Step length reductions in advanced age: the role of ankle and hip kinetics. J Gerontol A Biol Sci Med Sci 1996; 51: M303–M312.

82. Kadaba MP, Ramakrishnan HK, Wootten ME, et al.: Repeatability of kinematic, kinetic, and electromyographic data in normal adult gait. J Orthop Res 1989; 7: 849–860.

83. Katoh Y, Chao YS, Laughman RK, et al.: Biomechanical analysis of foot function during gait and clinical applications. Clin Orthop 1983; 177: 23–33.

84. Kaufman K, Hughes C, Morrey BF, et al.: Gait characteristics of patients with knee osteoarthritis. J Biomech 2001; 34: 907–915.

85. Kepple TM, Siegel KL, Stanhope SJ: Relative contributions of the lower extremity joint moments to forward progression and support during gait. Gait Posture 1997; 6: 1–8.

86. Kernozek TW, LaMott EE: Comparisons of plantar pressures between the elderly and young adults. Gait Posture 1995; 3: 143–148.

87. Kerrigan DC: Biomechanical gait alterations independent of speed in the healthy elderly: evidence for specific limiting impairments. Arch Phys Med Rehabil 1998; 79: 317–322.

88. Kerrigan DC: Gender differences in joint biomechanics during walking: normative study in young adults. Am J Phys Med Rehabil 1998; 77: 2–7.

89. Kerrigan DC, Riley PO, Lelas JL, et al.: Quantification of pelvic rotation as a determinant of gait. Arch Phys Med Rehabil 2001; 82: 217–220.

90. Kerrigan DC, Riley PA, Nieto TJ, et al.: Knee joint torques: a comparison between women and men during barefoot walking. Arch Phys Med Rehabil 2000; 81: 1162–1165.

91. Kitaoka HB, Crevoisier XM, Hansen D, et al.: Foot and ankle kinematics and ground reaction forces during ambulation. Foot Ankle Int 2006; 27: 808–813.

92. Kleissen RFM, Litjens MCA, Baten CTM, et al.: Consistency of surface EMG patterns obtained during gait from three laboratories using standardised measurement technique. Gait Posture 1997; 6: 200–209.

93. Knutson LM, Soderberg GL: EMG: use and interpretation in gait. In: Craik RL, Oatis CA, eds. Gait Analysis: Theory and Application. St. Louis: Mosby, 1995; 307–325.

94. Komistek RD, Stiehl JB, Dennis DA, et al.: Mathematical model of the lower extremity joint reaction forces using Kane's method of dynamics. J Biomech 1998; 31: 185–189.

95. Komura T, Nagano A: Evaluation of the influence of muscle deactivation on other muscles and joints during gait motion. J Biomech 2004; 37: 425–436.

96. Koopman B, Grootenboer HJ, de Jongh HJ: An inverse dynamics model for the analysis, reconstruction and prediction of bipedal walking. J Biomech 1995; 28: 1369–1376.

97. Krebs DE, Wong D, Jevsevar D, et al.: Trunk kinematics during locomotor activities. Phys Ther 1992; 72: 505–514.

98. Kuruvilla A, Costa JL, Wright RB, et al.: Characterization of gait parameters in patients with Charcot-Marie-Tooth disease. Neurol India 2000; 48: 49–55.

99. Kuster M, Sakurai S, Wood GA: Kinematic and kinetic comparison of downhill and level walking. Clin Biomech 1995; 10: 79–84.

100. Lafortune MA, Cavanagh PR, Sommer HJ, Kalenak A: Three-dimensional kinematics of the human knee during walking. J Biomech 1992; 25: 347–357.

101. Larsson L-E, Odenrick P, Sandlund B, et al.: The phases of the stride and their interaction in human gait. Scand J Rehabil Med 1980; 12: 107–112.

102. Leiper CI, Craik RL: Relationships between physical activity and temporal-distance characteristics of walking in elderly women. Phys Ther 1991; 71: 791–803.

103. Lelas JL, Merriman GJ, Riley PO, et al.: Predicting peak kinematic and kinetic parameters from gait speed. Gait Posture 2003; 17: 106–112.

104. Lemke MR, Wendorff T, Mieth B, et al.: Spatiotemporal gait patterns during over ground locomotion in major depression compared with healthy controls. J Psychiatr Res 2000; 34: 277–283.

105. Lundgren-Lindquist B, Aniansson A, Rundgren A: Functional studies in 79-year olds: III. Walking performance and climbing capacity. Scand J Rehabil Med 1983; 15: 125–131.

106. Macellari V, Giacomozzi C, Saggini R: Spatial-temporal parameters of gait: reference data and a statistical method for normality assessment. Gait Posture 1999; 10: 171–181.

107. MacKinnon CD, Winter DA: Control of whole body balance in the frontal plane during human walking. J Biomech 1993; 26: 633–644.

108. Malatesta D, Simar D, Dauvilliers Y, et al.: Energy cost of walking and gait instability in healthy 65- and 80-yr-olds. J Appl Physiol 2003; 95: 2248–2256.

109. Mansour JM, Lesh MD, Nowak MD, Simon SR: A three dimensional multi-segmental analysis of the energetics of normal and pathological human gait. J Biomech 1982; 15: 51–59.

110. Mansour JM, Pereira JM: Quantitative functional anatomy of the lower limb with application to human gait. J Biomech 1987; 20: 1: 51–58.

111. Martin PE, Morgan DW: Biomechanical considerations for economical walking and running. Med Sci Sports Exerc 1992; 24: 467–474.

112. McClay I, Manal K: Three-dimensional kinetic analysis of running: significance of secondary planes of motion. Med Sci Sports Exerc 1999; 31: 1629–1637.

113. McGibbon CA, Krebs DE: Discriminating age and disability effects in locomotion: neuromuscular adaptations in musculoskeletal pathology. J Appl Physiol 2004; 96: 149–160.

114. McGibbon CA, Puniello MS, Krebs D: Mechanical energy transfer during gait in relation to strength impairment and pathology in elderly women. Clin Biomech 2001; 16: 324–333.

115. McPoil T, Cornwall MW: Relationship between neutral subtalar joint position and pattern of rearfoot motion during walking. Foot Ankle 1994; 15: 141–145.

116. Mian OS, Thom JM, Ardigo LP, et al.: Metabolic cost, mechanical work, and efficiency during walking in young and older men. Acta Physiol 2006; 186: 127–139.

117. Miller CA, Verstraete MC: A mechanical energy analysis of gait initiation. Gait Posture 1999; 9: 158–166.

118. Miyashita M, Matsui H, Miura M: The relation between electrical activity in muscle and speed of walking and running. Med Sport 1971; 6: 192–196.

119. Murray MP: Gait as a total pattern of movement. Am J Phys Med 1967; 46: 290–333.

120. Murray MP, Drought AB, Kory RC: Walking patterns of normal men. J Bone J Surg 1964; 46: 335.

121. Murray MP, Kory RC, Clarkson BH: Walking patterns in healthy old men. J Gerontol 1969; 24: 169.

122. Murray MP, Kory RC, Sepic SB: Walking patterns of normal women. Arch Phys Med 1979; 51: 637.

123. Murray MP, Sepic SB, Barnard EJ: Patterns of sagittal rotation of the upper limbs in walking. Phys Ther 1967; 47: 272–284.

124. Nawoczenski DA, Baumhauer JF, Umberger BR: Relationship between clinical measurements and motion of the first metatarsophalangeal joint during gait. J Bone Joint Surg Am 1999; 81: 370–376.

125. Nene A, Mayagoitia R, Veltink P: Assessment of rectus femoris function during initial swing phase. Gait Posture 1999; 9: 1–9.

126. Neptune RR, Kautz SA, Zajac FE: Contributions of the individual ankle plantarflexors to support, forward progression and swing initiation during walking. J Biomech 2001; 34: 1387–1398.

127. Neptune RR, Zajac FE, Kautz SA: Muscle force redistributes segmental power for body progression during walking. Gait Posture 2004; 19: 194–205.

128. Neptune RR, Zajac FE, Kautz SA: Muscle mechanical work requirements during normal walking: the energetic cost of raising the body's center-of-mass is significant. J Biomech 2004; 37: 817–825.

129. Nester C: The relationship between transverse plane leg rotation and transverse plane motion at the knee and hip during normal walking. Gait Posture 2000; 12: 251–256.

130. Olgiatti R, Burgunder JM, Mumenthaler M: Increased energy cost of walking in multiple sclerosis: effect of spasticity, ataxia, and weakness. Arch Phys Med Rehabil 1988; 69: 846–849.

131. Ostrosky KM, VanSwearingen JM, Burdett RG, Gee Z: A comparison of gait characteristics in young and old subjects. Phys Ther 1994; 74: 637–646.

132. Ounpuu S, Thompson JD, Davis RB III, DeLuca PA: An examination of the knee function during gait in children with myelomeningocele. J Pediatr Orthop 2000; 20: 629–633.

133. Owings TM, Grabiner MD: Variability of step kinematics in young and older adults. Gait Posture 2004; 20: 26–29.

134. Patla AE: Adaptability of Human Gait—Implications for the Control of Locomotion. New York: Elsevier/North-Holland, 1991.

135. Perry J: Ankle foot complex. In: Gait Analysis: Normal and Pathological Function. Thorofare, NJ: Slack, 1992; 51–87.

136. Perry J: Hip. In: Gait Analysis, Normal and Pathological Function. Thorofare, NJ: Slack Incorporated, 1992; 119.

137. Perry SD, Lafortune MA: Influences of inversion/eversion of the foot upon impact loading during locomotion. Clin Biomech 1995; 10: 253–257.

138. Pierrynowski MR, Smith SB: Rear foot inversion/eversion during gait relative to the subtalar joint neutral position. Foot Ankle Int 1996; 17: 406–412.

139. Rao S, Saltzman C, Yack HJ: Segmental foot mobility in individuals with and without diabetes and neuropathy. Clin Biomech 2007; 22: 464–471.

140. Reinschmidt C, van den Bogert AJ, Lundberg A, et al.: Tibiofemoral and tibiocalcaneal motion during walking: external vs. skeletal markers. Gait Posture 1997; 6: 98–109.

141. Ren L, Jones RK, Howard D: Predictive modeling of human walking over a complete gait cycle. J Biomech 2007; 40: 1567–1574.

142. Requiao LF, Nadeau S, Milot MH, et al.: Quantification of level of effort at the plantarflexors and hip extensors and flexor muscles in healthy subjects walking at different cadences. J Electromyogr Kinesiol 2005; 15: 393–405.

143. Riley PO, Croce UD, Kerrigan DC: Propulsive adaptation to changing gait speed. J Biomech 2001; 34: 197–202.

144. Riley PO, Dellacroce U, Kerrigan DC: Effect of age on lower extremity joint moment characteristics to gait speed. Gait Posture 2001; 14: 264–270.

145. Rivest LP: A correction for axis misalignment in the joint angle curves representing knee movement in gait analysis. J Biomech 2005; 38: 1604–1611.

146. Robertson DGE, Winter DA: Mechanical energy generation, absorption, and transfer amongst segments during walking. J Biomech 1980; 13: 845–854.

147. Rose J, Gamble JG: Human Walking. Baltimore: Williams & Wilkins, 1994.

148. Rose SA, DeLuca PA, Davis RB III, Ounpuu S: Kinematic and kinetic evaluation of the ankle after lengthening of the

gastrocnemius fascia in children with cerebral palsy. J Pediatr Orthop 1993; 13: 727–732.

149. Rowe PJ, Myles CM, Walker C, Nutton R: Knee joint kinematics in gait and other functional activities measured using flexible electrogoniometry: how much knee motion is sufficient for normal daily life? Gait Posture 2000; 12: 143–155.

150. Sadeghi H: Local or global asymmetry in gait of people without impairments. Gait Posture 2003; 17: 197–204.

151. Sadeghi H, Allard P, Duhaime M: Contributions of lower-limb muscle power in gait of people without impairments. Phys Ther 2000; 80: 1188–1196.

152. Sadeghi H, Allard P, Prince F, Labelle H: Symmetry and limb dominance in able-bodied gait: a review. Gait Posture 2000; 12: 34–45.

153. Sadeghi H, Sadeghi S, Prince F, et al.: Functional roles of ankle and hip sagittal muscle moments in able-bodied gait. Clin Biomech 2001; 16: 688–695.

154. Saini M, Kerrigan DC, Thirunarayan MA, Duff-Raffaele M: The vertical displacement of the center of mass during walking: a comparison of four measurement methods. J Biomech Eng 1998; 120: 133–139.

155. Sarfaty O, Ladin Z: A video-based system for the estimation of the inertial properties of body segments. J Biomech 1993; 26: 1011–1016.

156. Sasaki K, Neptune RR: Muscle mechanical work and elastic energy utilization during walking and running near the preferred gait transition speed. Gait Posture 2006; 23: 383–390.

157. Saunders SW, Schache A, Rath D, et al.: Changes in three dimensional lumbo-pelvic kinematics and trunk muscle activity with speed and mode of locomotion. Clin Biomech 2005; 20: 784–793.

158. Seireg A, Arvikar RJ: The prediction of muscular load sharing and joint forces in the lower extremities during walking. J Biomech 1975; 8: 89–102.

159. Sekiya N, Nagasaki H, Ito H, Furuna T: Optimal walking in terms of variability in step length. J Orthop Sports Phys Ther 1997; 26: 266–272.

160. Shelburne KB, Pandy MG, Anderson FC, et al.: Pattern of anterior cruciate ligament force in normal walking. J Biomech 2004; 37: 797–805.

161. Shiavi R: Electromyographic patterns in adult locomotion: a comprehensive review. J Rehabil Res Dev 1985; 22: 85–98.

162. Siegel KL, Kepple TM, Stanhope SJ: A case study of gait compensations for hip muscle weakness in idiopathic inflammatory myopathy. Clin Biomech 2007; 22: 319–326.

163. Simkin A: The dynamic vertical force distribution during level walking under normal and rheumatic feet. Rheumatol Rehabil 1981; 20: 88–97.

164. Simon SR, Paul IL, Mansour J, et al.: Peak dynamic force in human gait. J Biomech 1981; 14: 817–822.

165. Simonsen EB, Dyhre-Poulsen P, Voigt M, et al.: Bone-on-bone forces during loaded and unloaded walking. Acta Anat (Basel) 1995; 152: 133–142.

166. Smidt GL, Wadsworth JB: Floor reaction forces during gait: comparison of patients with hip disease and normal subjects. Phys Ther 1973; 53: 1056.

167. Song KM: The effect of limb-length discrepancy on gait. J Bone Joint Surg Am 1997; 79: 1690–1698.

168. Stauffer RN, Chao EYS, Brewster RC: Force and motion analysis of the normal, diseased and prosthetic ankle joint. Clin Orthop 1977; 127: 189–196.

169. Stolze H, Kuhtz-Buschbeck JP, Mondwurf C, et al.: Retest reliability of spatiotemporal gait parameters in children and adults. Gait Posture 1998; 7: 125–130.

170. Taylor NF, Goldie PA, Evans OM: Angular movements of the pelvis and lumbar spine during self-selected and slow walking speeds. Gait Posture 1999; 9: 88–94.

171. Terrier P, Schutz Y: Variability of gait patterns during unconstrained walking assessed by satellite positioning (GPS). Eur J Appl Physiol 2003; 90: 554–561.

172. van den Bogert AJ, Read L, Nigg BM: An analysis of hip joint loading during walking, running, and skiing. Med Sci Sports Exerc 1999; 31: 131–142.

173. van Hedel HJA, Tomatis L, Muller R: Modulation of leg muscle activity and gait kinematics by walking speed and body-weight unloading. Gait Posture 2006; 24: 35–45.

174. Vogt L, Banzer W: Measurement of lumbar spine kinematics in incline treadmill walking. Gait Posture 1999; 9: 18–23.

175. Wagenaar RC, van Emmerick REA: Resonant frequencies of arms and legs identify different walking patterns. J Biomech 2000; 33: 853–861.

176. Wall JC, Devlin J, Khirchof R, Lackey B: Measurement of step widths and step lengths: a comparison of measurements made directly from a grid with those made from a video recording. J Orthop Sports Phys Ther 2000; 30: 410–417.

177. Wang WJ, Crompton RH, Li Y, et al.: Energy transformation during erect and 'bent-hip, bent-knee' walking by humans with implications for the evolution of bipedalism. J Hum Evol 2003; 44: 563–579.

178. Warren GL, Maher RM, Higbie EJ: Temporal patterns of plantar pressures and lower-leg muscle activity during walking: effect of speed. Gait Posture 2004; 19: 91–100.

179. Whittle MW, Levine DF: Sagittal plane motion of the lumbar spine during normal gait. Gait Posture 1995; 3: 82.

180. Winter D: Biomechanics and Motor Control of Human Movement. New York: John Wiley & Sons, 1990.

181. Winter DA: Overall principle of lower limb support during stance phase of gait. J Biomech 1980; 13: 923–927.

182. Winter DA: Kinematic and kinetic patterns in human gait: variability and compensating effects. Hum Move Sci 1984; 3: 51–76.

183. Winter DA: Biomechanics of normal and pathological gait: implications for understanding human locomotor control. J Mot Behav 1989; 21: 337–355.

184. Winter DA: The Biomechanics and Motor Control of Human Gait: Normal, Elderly and Pathological. Waterloo: University of Waterloo Press, 1991.

185. Winter DA, Patla AE, Frank JS, Walt SE: Biomechanical walking patterns in the fit and healthy elderly. Phys Ther 1990; 70: 340–347.

186. Winter DA, Quanbury AO, Reimer GD: Analysis of instantaneous energy of normal gait. J Biomech 1976; 9: 253–257.

187. Winter DA, Robertson DGE: Joint torque and energy patterns in normal gait. Biol Cybern 1978; 29: 137–142.

188. Winter DA, Yack HJ: EMG profiles during normal human walking: stride-to-stride and inter-subject variability. Electroencephalogr Clin Neurophysiol 1987; 67: 402–411.

189. Woodburn J, Turner DE, Helliwell PS, Barker S: A preliminary study determining the feasibility of electromagnetic tracking for kinematics at the ankle joint complex. Rheumatology (Oxford) 1999; 38: 1260–1268.

190. Woolley SM, Sigg J, Commager J: Comparison of change in level walking activities in three groups of elderly individuals. Gait Posture 1995; 3: 81.

191. Wu G, Ladin Z: Limitations of quasi-static estimation of human joint loading during locomotion. Med Biol Eng Comput 1996; 34: 472–476.

Index

Note: Page numbers followed by f, t, or b indicate figures, tables, or boxed text, respectively.

for low back pain, 613–616, 614f–616f
  for beginners, 617
  for osteoarthritis, 80
  for quadriceps femoris, 769, 774
  sit-ups, 613
  stretching, for rectus femoris, 769, 770f
  for vastus medialis, 774
Expiration, muscles of, 553, 553f
Extension pattern (synergy), in
    locomotion, 898
Extensive properties, 22
Extensor carpi radialis brevis, 304, 304f
  actions of, 305, 306f, 312, 312f
  attachments of, 305b
  innervation of, 305b
  moment arms of, 306f
  palpation of, 305b
  tennis elbow and, 324b
  tightness of, 305, 306b
  weakness of, 305
Extensor carpi radialis longus, 304, 304f
  actions of, 305, 306f, 312, 312f
  attachments of, 305b
  innervation of, 305b
  moment arms of, 306f
  palpation of, 305b
  tightness of, 305, 306b
  weakness of, 305
Extensor carpi ulnaris, 304f, 310
  actions of, 311–312, 312b, 312f
  attachments of, 311b
  innervation of, 311b
  palpation of, 311b
  tightness of, 312
  weakness of, 312
Extensor digiti minimi, 304f, 310
  actions of, 310
  attachments of, 311b
  innervation of, 311b
  palpation of, 311b
  tightness of, 310
  weakness of, 310
Extensor digiti quinti, 310
Extensor digitorum, 304f, 306–307, 307f
  actions of, 308–309
  attachments of, 307b
  innervation of, 307b
  moment arms of, 309
  palpation of, 307b
  tightness of, 309–310, 309f, 310f
  weakness of, 309
Extensor digitorum brevis, 859, 860b
Extensor digitorum communis, 306–310
Extensor digitorum longus, 842
  actions of, 842–843
  attachments of, 843b
  innervation of, 843b
  palpation of, 843b
  tightness of, 843
  weakness of, 843
Extensor hallucis longus, 842, 842b

Extensor hood mechanism, 346, 347f
Extensor indicis, 317f, 322
  actions of, 323
  attachments of, 323b
  innervation of, 323b
  palpation of, 323b
  tightness of, 323
  weakness of, 323
Extensor indicis proprius, 317f,
    322–323
Extensor lag, 744
Extensor pollicis brevis, 317f, 320
  actions of, 320, 320b–321b, 321f
  attachments of, 320b
  innervation of, 320b
  palpation of, 320b
  tightness of, 320
  weakness of, 320
Extensor pollicis longus, 317f, 321
  actions of, 321–322, 322f
  attachments of, 321b
  innervation of, 321b
  palpation of, 321b
  tightness of, 322
  weakness of, 322
Extensor retinaculum, at wrist, 343, 343f
External anal sphincter, 660
External fixation, Ilizarov, 43, 43f
External force, 12
External moments, 16
  flexion
    in knee, 797
    in thoracic spine, 556, 557b
  in locomotion, 904
  in standing, 884, 884f
External oblique, 597, 597b, 598f,
    602t, 606t
External urethral sphincter, 658–660
Extracellular matrix, of connective tissue,
    85–87, 86f
Extraocular muscles, 406–410, 407f
  weakness of, 409–410
Extrinsic defecation reflex, 670
Eyes
  extrinsic muscles of, 406–410, 407f
    weakness of, 409–410
  facial muscles affecting, 395–397, 395b,
    395f–397f, 396b

F

Facet joints
  lumbar, 571–572, 571f, 572f
    in low back pain, 572b
  thoracic, 526
Facial creases, 392b
Facial expression, muscles of, 392
  in nose, 397–399, 397b–399b, 397f, 398f
  in scalp and ears, 393–395, 393b,
    393f, 394f
  surrounding eyes, 395–397, 395b,
    395f–397f, 396b

Facial nerve
  distribution of, 391–392, 392f
  muscles innervated by, 392–406
  paralysis of, 394f, 400b, 400f
  psychological challenges in, 402b
Failure, in tension test, 27–29
Failure strength, static load resistance
    and, 515
Falls, lumbar spine in, 608
Fatigue, 31
Fatigue fracture, 31
Fatigue limit, 31
Feet. See Foot
Femoral anteversion, excessive, 697–698,
    697f, 698f
Femoral arcuate ligament, 689
Femur
  alignment of, 694–698, 694f–698f
  angle of inclination of, 690
  distal, 739–741, 739f, 740f
    lateral condyle of, 739f, 740–741,
      740f, 742–743, 742f, 773
    medial condyle of, 739–740, 739f,
      740f, 742–743
    motions of, 741–743, 742f
  head of, 689–690, 690f, 691f.
      See also Hip
    alignment of, 694–698, 694f–698f
    avascular necrosis of, 692, 734
    blood supply of, 691–692
    ligament of, 693, 693f
  motions of
    abduction, 742–743, 743f
    posterior rolling, 742–743, 743f, 743t
    rotation, 743, 743f, 743t
    tibiofemoral, 741–743, 743f, 743t
    translation, 742–743, 743f
  neck of, 689–690, 691f
    alignment of, 694–698, 694f–698f
    fractures of, 692
    retroversion of, 698
  palpation of, landmarks for,
    690–691, 744
  patellar contact with, 761, 761f
  proximal tibia and, 740, 740f. See also
      Tibiofemoral joint
  shaft of, 739–741, 739f, 740f
  structure of, 38f
Fibers. See Muscle fibers
Fibroblasts, 85
Fibrocartilage, 69. See also Cartilage
Fibrocartilaginous amphiarthrosis, 647
Fibrous capsule, of knee, 749, 749f
Fibrous layer, of joint capsule,
    104–105
Fibula, 808f, 810
  distal, fractures of, 810b
  proximal, 744–745
  tibia and, 815–816, 816b, 816f.
      See also Tibiofibular joint
Filum terminale, 625